DISCARD

ENCYCLOPEDIA OF
STRESS

SECOND EDITION

Volume 2 F–N

EDITORIAL BOARD

ENCYCLOPEDIA OF
STRESS

SECOND EDITION

Volume 2 F–N

EDITOR-IN-CHIEF
GEORGE FINK
Professorial Research Fellow (formerly Director)
Mental Health Research Institute of Victoria
Parkville, Melbourne, Victoria
Australia
Formerly Director, MRC Brain Metabolism Unit
Edinburgh, Scotland, UK.

ELSEVIER

AMSTERDAM • BOSTON • HEIDELBERG • LONDON • NEW YORK • OXFORD
PARIS • SAN DIEGO • SAN FRANCISCO • SINGAPORE • SYDNEY • TOKYO
Academic Press is an imprint of Elsevier

ACADEMIC
PRESS

Academic Press is an imprint of Elsevier
525 B Street, Suite 1900, San Diego, CA 92101-4495, USA
Linacre House, Jordan Hill, Oxford, OX2 8DP, UK

First edition 2000

British Library Cataloguing in Publication Data
A catalogue record for this book is available from the British Library

Library of Congress Catalog Number: 2007926917

ISBN: 978-0-12-088503-9

For information on all Elsevier publications
visit our website at books.elsevier.com

PRINTED AND BOUND IN UK
07 08 09 10 11 10 9 8 7 6 5 4 3 2 1

For Ann Elizabeth

CONTENTS

B

VOLUME 2

F

I

J

K

L

M

N

[†]Deceased.

VOLUME 3

O

P

T

U

V

W

VOLUME 4

CONTENTS BY SUBJECT AREA

DRUGS (TREATMENT)

GENERAL CONCEPTS AND MODELS

GENETICS AND GENOMICS

HUMAN COGNITION, EMOTION AND BEHAVIOR

HUMAN HEALTH AND PHYSICAL ILLNESS

HUMAN MENTAL HEALTH AND PSYCHOPATHOLOGY

IMMUNOLOGY, INFECTION AND INFLAMMATION

LABORATORY STUDIES AND TESTS

THERAPIES

Meditation and Stress
Problem-Solving Skills Training
Psychosomatic Medicine
Reenactment Techniques
Relaxation Techniques
Stress Management and Cardiovascular Disease
Stress Management, CAM Approach
Trauma Group Therapy

PHYSIOLOGICAL, PHARMACOLOGICAL AND BIOCHEMICAL ASPECTS

Acute Stress Response: Experimental
Acute Trauma Response
Adenylyl Cyclases and Stress Response
Adrenal Cortex
Adrenaline
Adrenal Medulla
Adrenocorticotropic Hormone (ACTH)
Adrenocortical Function, factors controlling development thereof
Aging and Stress, Biology of
Aging and Adrenocortical Factors
Alcohol and Stress: Social and Psychological Aspects
Aldosterone and Mineralocorticoid Receptors
Ambulatory Blood Pressure Monitoring
Amenorrhea
Amygdala
Anatomy of the HPA Axis
Androgen Action
Angiotensin
Angiotensin receptors
Annexin
Anti-CRF
Antidepressant Actions on Glucocorticoid Receptors
Apoptosis
Arterial Baroreflex
Autonomic Nervous System
Autotolerance
Avoidance
Beta-Endorphin
Blood–Brain Barrier, Stress and
Blood Pressure
Brain and Brain Regions
Brain Natriuretic Peptide (BNP)
Brain Trauma
Calbindin
Calcium-Dependent Neurotoxicity
Calcium, Role of
Cardiovascular System and Stress
Catecholamines
Central Stress Neurocircuits
Cerebral Metabolism, Brain Imaging

Chaperone Proteins and Chaperonopathies
Cholesterol and Lipoproteins
Comparative Anatomy and Physiology
Congenital Adrenal Hyperplasia (CAH)
Corticosteroid-Binding Globulin (Transcortin)
Corticosteroid Receptors
Corticosteroids and Stress
Corticotropin Releasing Factor (CRF)
Corticotropin Releasing Factor-Binding Protein
Corticotropin Releasing Factor Receptors
Critical Thermal Limits
Dopamine, Central
Drosophila Studies
Electrodermal Activity
Endocrine Systems
Estrogen
Ethanol and Endogenous Opioids
Excitatory Amino Acids
Excitotoxins
Familial Patterns of Stress
Febrile Response
Feedback Systems
Fibrinogen and Clotting Factors
Feeding Circuitry (and Neurochemistry)
Fetal Stress
Food Intake and Stress, Human
Food Intake and Stress, Non-Human
Food Shift Effect
GABA (Gamma Aminobutyric Acid)
Gastrointestinal Effects
Gender and Stress
Ghrelin and Stress Protection
Glia or Neuroglia
Glucocorticoid Negative Feedback
Glucocorticoid Effects on Memory: the Positive and Negative
Glucocorticoids – Adverse Effects on the Nervous System
Glucocorticoids, Effects of Stress on
Glucocorticoids, Overview
Glucocorticoids, Role in Stress
Glucose Transport
Glycobiology of Stress
Gonadotropin Secretion, Effects of Stress on
Heart Rate
Heat Resistance
Heat Shock Genes, Human
Heat Shock Proteins: HSP60 Family Genes
Heat Shock Response, Overview
Hippocampal Neurons
Hippocampus, Corticosteroid Effects on
Hippocampus, Overview
Homeostasis
11β-Hydroxysteroid Dehydrogenases
Hypothalamic-Pituitary-Adrenal Axis

PSYCHOLOGICAL THERAPY

PSYCHOSOCIAL AND SOCIOECONOMIC ASPECTS

PREFACE TO FIRST EDITION

"Stress" remains one of the most frequently used but ill-defined words in the English language. Stress is a phenomenon that has quite different meanings for the politician, social scientist, physician, nurse, psychotherapist, physiologist, molecular biologist, and perhaps you and me. This diversity of meanings was one impetus for creating the *Encyclopedia of Stress*, the aim being to derive a definition of stress from a variety of expert descriptions. The second impetus was the obvious need for an up-to-date compendium on one of the most important social, medical, and psychological phenomena of our age. We were fortunate in attracting stars for our Editorial Board and a set of most distinguished contributors for the 400 or so entries—indeed, the list of contributors is a Who's Who in stress research.

We anticipate that the diversity of our readers will equal the diversity of the topics covered. They will find that the coverage of the Encyclopedia extends well beyond the general adaptation theory of Hans (Janos) Selye and the fight-or-flight response of Walter Cannon. Nevertheless, the general principles annunciated by these two great pioneers in the field still underpin our understanding of the biology of the stress phenomenon. That is, stress is a real or perceived challenge, either endogenous or exogenous, that perturbs body equilibrium or "homeostasis." The stressor may range from overcrowding, traffic congestion, violence, bereavement, redundancy, or unemployment to physical, chemical, biological, or psychological insults. Whether the person can adapt to or cope with the stress will depend on the nature and severity of the stressor and the person's physical and mental state, which in turn depends on genetic, experiential, social, and environmental factors. These issues are discussed in depth in the Encyclopedia, as are the mechanisms of coping and the impact of stress on health and predisposition to diseases such as cancer, infection, rheumatoid arthritis, heart disease, high blood pressure, and mental disorder.

Aggression remains a hallmark of human behavior, even as we move into the third millennium, and so the Encyclopedia covers several topical areas that have only recently been analyzed systematically. These include war and specific wars, posttraumatic stress disorder (PTSD; formerly thought of vaguely as "shell shock"), rape, torture, marital discord and spousal abuse, and the Holocaust. In tackling these topics we accept that our entries may not include all the nuances that are necessary for a full understanding of what these phenomena are all about and described so graphically and sensitively in Tolstoy's *War and Peace* or Pat Barker's monumental *Regeneration* trilogy on the horrific psychological traumas of the First World War. Nevertheless, an important start has been made in that we now accept that PTSD is not just a lack of "bottle" (courage or "guts"), but rather a syndrome that needs to be and can be understood within the framework of medicine and psychology.

Biologically, the stress response reflects a set of integrated cascades in the nervous, endocrine, and immune defense systems. As in most areas of biology, molecular genetics has made a significant difference in the precision with which we now understand the physiopathological processes of the stress response. And so the adage formerly applied to diabetes mellitus may now apply equally to stress: "Understand stress and you will understand medicine."

In summary, we hope that this first *Encyclopedia of Stress* will indeed define the phenomenon and at the same time provide a valuable source of information on a phenomenon that affects us all. In setting out on this adventure we were aware that there is nothing new under the sun and that stress has been around since the first biological particles, bacteria, or even viruses competed for the same mechanisms of replication.

There is a tendency for each generation to imagine that stress and its untoward effects are uniquely harsh for them, but it is not this misconception that underlies this work. Rather, the stress of "stress" itself—the massive accumulation of knowledge—made it seem propitious to bring the information together in a systematic manner that allows ready access to all who need or wish to understand the phenomenon.

The idea of producing this Encyclopedia was conceived at an Academic Press reception in San Diego held in conjunction with the annual meeting of the Society for Neuroscience in 1996. I am deeply indebted to Erika Conner for enabling conversion of the idea to a concept and then a project and to Jennifer Wrenn, Christopher Morris, and Carolan Gladden, all of Academic Press, for their enthusiasm, encouragement, and herculean efforts that converted the concept into a reality. For giving generously of their intellect, expertise, sound advice, and unstinting work, I am greatly indebted to my friends and colleagues on the Editorial Board, who made the project such a satisfying experience. To all our contributors go our profound thanks for taking time out from wall-to-wall schedules to produce their entries, which together have made this Encyclopedia.

George Fink
August 1999

PREFACE TO THE SECOND EDITION

The popularity of the first edition of the Encylopedia of Stress, the several major stressful conflicts that have occurred since 1999, and the significant advances in our knowledge of stress prompted the production of this second edition. In addition to more than 140 new articles, most of the original 400 first edition articles have been updated for the second edition to reflect, for example, advances in our understanding of corticotropin releasing factor (CRF) and urocortin receptors, ideas about the role of central CRF in the overall control of the psychological/mental as well as neuroendocrine response to stress, and the novel discoveries of the complex neuropeptide regulation of hunger and satiety. The effects of maternal and perinatal stress on subsequent body development and function in the adult, the adverse effects of stress on brain (and particularly hippocampal memory function), the role of the amygdala in fear and aggression, and the role of stress in the etiology of obesity and the metabolic syndrome all feature prominently in this new edition. 9/11 and the many new conflicts since 1999 have engendered new articles on terrorism, suicide bombers and their effects, as well as a retrospective on previous human apocalypses such as Hiroshima. Coverage of the whole field of post traumatic stress disorder (PTSD) has been expanded, reflecting the greater recognition and understanding of PTSD, and possibly related disorders such as *combat fatigue* and *burnout*. Stress and depression and anxiety, already touched on in the first edition, now feature prominently. On the conceptual side, *allostasis* (modified from Hans Selye's *heterostasis*), or stability through centrally regulated change in physiological set points, receives greater emphasis than it did in the first edition.

Overall, our understanding of stress mechanisms in the human has benefited from two major quantum leaps in technology. First, the advances in molecular genetics and genomics and sequencing of the human genome (published after the first edition had appeared) have increased the rigor and precision of our understanding of the molecular neurobiology of stress. Thus, new to the second edition are a series of articles on the genetic factors that play a role in susceptibility to stress and in various components of the stress response. Secondly, functional brain imaging has enhanced our understanding of the neurobiology of stress in the human. Many of the articles in the second edition reflect the positive impact of these two advances.

Accessibility to the second edition of the Encyclopedia of Stress will be facilitated by virtue of the fact that it is published online as well as in hard copy. My profound thanks for their selfless work go to our team of distinguished authors and to my friends and colleagues on the Editorial Board. Production of the Encyclopedia would not have been possible without our colleagues at Elsevier, and in particular Bob Donaldson and Hilary Rowe whose dedication, commitment and excellent work I am pleased to acknowledge.

George Fink
November 2006

Note on Terminology of Corticotropin Releasing Factor/Hormone and the Catecholamines

The central nervous regulation of the anterior pituitary gland is mediated by substances, mainly peptides, which are synthesized in the hypothalamus and transported to the gland by the hypophysial portal vessels. Because these compounds are transported by the blood, the term "hormone" gained acceptance in the neuroendocrine literature. The major hypothalamic peptide involved in the stress response is the

41-amino acid corticotropin releasing factor (CRF). The Endocrine Society (USA), following convention, adopted the term corticotropin releasing hormone (CRH). However, this nomenclature has been challenged. Hauger et al. (*Pharmacol Rev* 55: 21–26, 2003), in liaison with the International Union of Pharmacology Committee on Receptor Nomenclature and Drug Classification, argued that the CRF's function extends well beyond the biology of a hormone, and that therefore it should be termed corticotropin releasing factor (CRF) rather than hormone. Since the terminology of CRF versus CRH has yet to be resolved, the two terms and abbreviations are here used interchangeably, depending on author preference.

Adrenaline and *noradrenaline* are catecholamines that play a pivotal role in the stress response. These terms are synonymous with *epinephrine* and *norepinephrine*, respectively. Both sets of terms are used interchangeably in the endocrine, neuroendocrine and stress literature, and this principle has been adopted for the Encyclopedia. Style has depended on author preference, but wherever possible within-article consistency has been ensured.

George Fink
November 2006

Hauger, R. L., Grigoriadis, D. E., Dallman, M. F., Plotsky, P. M., Vale, W. W., and Dautzenberg, F. M. (2003). International Union of Pharmacology. XXXVI. Current status of the nomenclature for receptors for corticotropin-releasing factor and their ligands. *Pharmacological Reviews* 55(1), 21–26.

GUIDE TO THE ENCYCLOPEDIA

The *Encyclopedia of Stress* is a complete source of information on the phenomenon of stress, contained within the covers of a single unified work. It consists of four volumes and includes 545 separate articles on the entire scope of this subject, including not only the physiological, biochemical, and genetic aspects of stress, but also the relationship of stress to human health and human cognition and emotion. Each article in this Encyclopedia provides a brief, but complete overview of the selected topic to inform a broad spectrum of readers, from research professionals to students to the interested general public. In order that you, the reader, will derive the greatest possible benefit from your use of the *Encyclopedia of Stress*, we have provided this Guide.

ORGANIZATION

The *Encyclopedia of Stress* is organized to provide maximum ease of use for its readers. All of the articles are arranged in a single alphabetical sequence by title. Articles whose titles begin with the letters A to E are in Volume 1, articles with titles from F to N are in Volume 2, and articles from M to Z are in Volume 3. Volume 4 includes a complete subject index for the entire work and an alphabetical list of the contributors to the Encyclopedia. So that information can be located more quickly, article titles generally begin with the specific noun or noun phrase indicating the topic, with any general descriptive terms following. For example, "Korean Conflict, Stress Effects of" is the article title rather than "Stress Effects of the Korean Conflict" and "Circadian Rhythms,

Genetics of" is the title rather than "Genetics of Circadian Rhythms."

TABLE OF CONTENTS

A complete table of contents for the *Encyclopedia of Stress* appears at the front of each volume. This list of article titles represents topics that have been carefully selected by the Editor-in-Chief, George Fink, and the Associate Editors. The Encyclopedia provides coverage of 17 specific subject areas within the overall field of stress. For example, the Encyclopedia includes 71 different articles dealing with human cognition and emotion. (See p. xxiii for a table of contents by subject area.) The list of subject areas covered is as follows:

Animal Studies and Models
Conflict, War, Terrorism
Disasters
Diurnal, Seasonal and Ultradian Rhythms
Drugs (Effects)
Drugs (Treatment)
General Concepts and Models
Genetics and Genomics
Human Cognition, Emotion and Behavior
Human Health and Physical Illness
Human Mental Health and Psychopathology
Immunology, Infection and Inflammation
Laboratory Studies and Tests
Therapies
Physiological, Pharmacological and Biochemical
    Aspects

Psychological Therapy
Psychosocial and Socioeconomic Aspects

ARTICLE FORMAT

Articles in the *Encyclopedia of Stress* are arranged in a standard format, as follows:

- Title of article
- Author's name and affiliation
- Outline
- Glossary
- Defining statement
- Body of the article
- Cross-references
- Further Reading

OUTLINE

Entries in the Encyclopedia begin with a topical outline. This outline highlights important subtopics that will be discussed within the article. For example, the article "Cushing's Syndrome, Medical Aspects" includes subtopics such as "Epidemiology," "Etiology," "Pathophysiology," "Clinical Picture," "Laboratory Findings," "Radiographic Findings" and "Treatment."

The outline is intended as an overview and thus it lists only the major headings of the article. In addition, second-level and third-level headings will be found within the article.

GLOSSARY

The Glossary section contains terms that are important to an understanding of the article and that might be unfamiliar to the reader. Each term is defined in the context of the article in which it is used. The Encyclopedia has approximately 2000 glossary entries. For example, the article "Cholesterol and Lipoproteins" includes this glossary term:

> *cholesterol* A fat-soluble particle in the body used to form cholic acid in the liver, steroid hormones in the gonads and adrenals, and for the formation of cell membranes.

CROSS-REFERENCES

Virtually all articles in the Encyclopedia have cross-references directing the reader to other articles. These cross-references appear at the conclusion of the article text. They indicate articles that can be consulted for further information on the same topic or for other information on a related topic. For example, the article "Economic Factors and Stress" contains references to the articles "Coping Skills," "Health and Socioeconomic Status," "Industrialized Societies," "Job Insecurity: The Health Effects of a Psychosocial Work Stressor," "Social Status and Stress".

FURTHER READING

The Further Reading section appears as the last element in an article. The reference sources listed there are the author's recommendations of the most appropriate materials for further reading on the given topic. The Further Reading entries are for the benefit of the reader and thus they do not represent a complete listing of all the materials consulted by the author in preparing the article.

FOREWORD

This is the second edition of the *Encyclopedia of Stress*, the three heavy volumes that first appeared in 2000 under the overall editorial guidance of George Fink. From its original coining in reference to rather unusual and unpleasant situations, the word *stress* is now quasi synonymous with *life*, i.e. modern life! This second edition of the *Encyclopedia of Stress* presents several hundreds of articles written by experts in that particular field, especially for this series, discussing, clarifying, explaining to the average-reader as well as to anyone more educated in one field or another, the extraordinary involvement of stress and our normal or abnormal reactions to it, both in our physical body and its accompanying mind. The table of contents is truly amazing, from the stress of being born to the stress of dying and so many circumstances in between, with clear presentations of the pertinent, current knowledge about them. This is truly an encyclopedia where, surely, you will find some explanation and answer to your own stresses (and those of others).

Roger Guillemin, MD, PhD
Nobel laureate in Physiology & Medicine

Familial Patterns of Stress

A Bifulco
University of London, London, UK

This article is a revision of the previous edition article by A Bifulco, volume 2, pp 103–107, © 2000, Elsevier Inc.

Measurement of Stressors
Stress and Disorder
Shared Stressors and Disorders in Families
Transmission of Stress Intergenerationally

Glossary

Childhood stressors	Adverse events or difficulties impacting on an individual in childhood; they typically involve specific experiences impinging on the child (e.g., parental loss; neglect, and physical, sexual, or psychological abuse), adverse family circumstances for the child (e.g., poverty, parental conflict, or parental psychiatric or criminal disorder), and child life events and difficulties. Childhood stressors can have an immediate impact or a longer-term impact in adult life.
Family environment	Experiences potentially common to the whole family unit. Thus, shared environment refers to experiences held in common, particularly within the household; nonshared environment refers to experiences that are different for various family members, specifically siblings, including the school and social arena.
Family studies	Studies that assess family members to look at the concordance of both experience and psychological disorders, as well as the intergenerational transmission of risk; they include parent to child comparisons, intrasibling and twin comparisons, and nontraditional family arrangements such as step-parent households, lone parents, and adoptive parents and siblings.
Intergenerational transmission	The passing of the risk of disorder and adversity from parent to child and within families across generations; several mechanisms are likely to be involved, including social (perpetuation of high rates of adversity/stressors), psychological (poor parenting and negative interpersonal style), and biological (genetic or constitutional) factors.
Psychological disorder	A disorder that results from the negative impact of stressors on psychological health (i.e., being stressed), such as major depression and anxiety disorders; these disorders have been studied in relation to familial stress in both adults and young people.
Sibling relationships	Relationships between monozygotic (identical) twins, dizygotic (fraternal) twins, full siblings, half-siblings, and adoptive siblings. Studies of these relationships are central to behavioral genetic studies of families and include designs to show cascade effects when comparing similarities in characteristics and behavior in siblings and studies examining similarities and differences in siblings brought up together and apart. Likely genetic contributions can be inferred from the known genetic similarity of different types of sibling pairs and the similarity of their measured characteristics.
Stress agency	The quality of bringing about stressful situations through poor coping with adversity and mismanagement of interpersonal interactions. People with high agency in producing stress are more likely to have externalizing disorders, such as delinquency, antisocial personality disorder, substance abuse, and criminal behavior, which impact negatively on close others and family members. Assessing agency or independence of life events

Stress carriers   Individuals who are both the recipients and bearers of high levels of stressors, which, although having no direct agency in their generation, can nevertheless transmit the stress to other family members. Mechanisms may be through passive and helpless coping styles, which perpetuate or increase difficulties. This is more common among those with the internalizing disorders such as depression and anxiety. For example, the choice of a partner with antisocial behavior may lead to a higher experience of stressful circumstances for both parents and children, even though specific difficulties are only indirectly brought about by the individual concerned.

Stressors   Adverse events or difficulties impacting on an individual.

Vulnerability factors   Characteristics that increase an individual's susceptibility to the impact of stressors; they interact with stressors to increase the risk of the onset of psychiatric disorder for particular individuals. Such factors can be psychological (e.g., low self-esteem and insecure attachment style), social (e.g., interpersonal conflict and lack of close confidants), or biological (e.g., irregular cortisol patterns). Vulnerability factors can be recent and ongoing or stem from early life experiences such as neglect or abuse in childhood.

Measurement of Stressors

The psychiatrist Adolf Meyer was the first modern practitioner in the 1950s to suggest that life events relate to psychopathology, developing a life chart system for recording the temporal relationships of life experiences and disorder. This method was developed further in the 1960s by Holmes and Rahe, with a questionnaire based on a summation of the quantity of environmental change in a given period in terms of a list of items representing both normative and non-normative changes such as moving one's residence or bereavement. The approach was then revolutionized in the 1970s both in psychiatry (by Paykel) and in social science (by Brown) by measuring the contextual threat or unpleasantness of events in more detail and by using more sophisticated assessment techniques to incorporate meaning into experience. This involved attending to the characteristics of events (such as whether they were undesirable or involved losses, entrances, or exits) by taking the context of the event into account when assessing its likely

unpleasantness, by examining the duration of the stressor (i.e., both chronic and acute), and finally by having the researcher assess the severity of the event according to benchmarked examples to circumvent the biases raised by self-report. Relevant context is crucial; for example, in the case of a pregnancy it is necessary to collect factual details of the experience including whether it was planned, the state of the marriage/partnership, the health of the individuals, and their financial and housing situation in order to assess its negative and potentially depressogenic characteristics. Although more attention was paid to life events because of their clear dating in relation to disorder, a role for chronic stressors or difficulties was also found. These involved problematic situations that continued over time and that frequently generated new events, for example, a financial difficulty involving debts that fluctuates in severity as new financial events occur. Severe events, matched to areas of ongoing marked difficulties, were found to be particularly pathogenic.

Studies in inner-London in the 1970s showed that severe life events (those that are highly threatening or unpleasant) were relatively common in the community with approximately one in three individuals experiencing at least one in a year. They were also found to be more common in working-class groups, in inner-city locations, and among single-parent families. Among events judged to be severe, three-quarters involved close relationships and these more often led to depression outcomes. The extension of this methodology to children was undertaken in the 1980s simultaneously by Goodyer and by Sandberg, following the Paykel and Brown traditions, respectively. A similar role for stressor and disorder was found in children but with chronic difficulties given a more prominent role. Parallel work looked at stressors simultaneously in parents and children and showed a large degree of familial patterning.

Stress and Disorder

Prior to the 1970s a relationship between the occurrence of life events and relapse of schizophrenia had been confirmed, and in the 1970s and 1980s the main development was the exploration in adults of the relationship of life events and the onset of affective disorder, particularly major depression. The relationship between severe life events and the onset of major depression was confirmed largely in samples of women and among mothers, in whom higher rates of depression are typically found.

A model was investigated prospectively, looking at the vulnerability characteristics of individuals who later succumbed to affective disorder when encountering stressors. In prospective community studies, it was possible to identify interpersonal and cognitive factors that placed an individual at higher risk of affective disorder when later experiencing a severe life event. For adults, vulnerability factors encompassed family conflict (negative interaction with a partner or child), lack of a close confidant outside the home, and low self-esteem. When negative family interactions, low self-esteem, and severe life events all occurred, the risk for the onset of major depression was raised more than fourfold (47% versus 10% in the community at large). When lifetime experience was examined, the presence of neglect or abuse in childhood was highly related both to disorder and adult vulnerability, with one-third of women with adverse childhoods becoming depressed in a 12-month study period. A similar model is emerging for children, whereby family conflict and low self-esteem increase a child's susceptibility to disorder on encountering severe stressors. Stress can also have negative biological impacts, for example on stress hormones. Thus, abnormal cortisol patterns are associated with stressors and with a range of psychological and physical illnesses. Children experiencing chronic neglect and abuse have been shown to have abnormal diurnal cortisol patterns associated with behavior problems and poor functioning.

Lifespan models of disorder have examined linkages in early life adversity with later life impacts on disorder. In particular, neglect or abuse in childhood has been linked with adverse social trajectories, including unplanned home-leaving, teenage pregnancy, lone parenthood, high rates of adult life events and difficulties, and lower social class. The same early life experiences have been linked with negative psychological impacts at different life stages, including low self-esteem, helplessness, poor coping, and insecure attachment styles. These provide causal links between early-life family adversity and later-life stressors, which often impact subsequent family formation.

Shared Stressors and Disorders in Families

Studies have consistently shown that both stressors and disorder congregate within families and that these provide simultaneous, as well as later, life risks for both parents and children. Not only do family conflicts and severe events increase the risk of disorder in both, but there is also evidence that disorder in parents provides additional risk for children, and vice versa. Although most studies have shown links between mothers' and children's disorder, associations have also been shown with the fathers' psychological disorder. Disorder in both parents increases the risk for

the children substantially. Contributory risk factors from mothers include a history of affective disorder, current depressed symptoms, vulnerability characteristics, and ongoing chronic stressors, all of which play a part in the children's disorder. Although chronic stressors predict children's disorder independently of mental illness in the parents, the accompanying maternal impairment and poor parenting are associated with higher negative outcomes. This is likely because common stressors (e.g., marital conflict) affect the mothers and children and, in addition, mothers who are depressed are emotionally unavailable as a protective influence to help the children to cope. Thus, without the buffering effect of maternal support, the children are additionally susceptible to stress and can become symptomatic. The role of types of family stressors, family structure, sibling stressors, parenting, and parental disorder in familial patterning of stressors is now examined.

Types of Family Stressors

The types of family stressors that have proved to be important in predicting disorder in children involve family conflict and parental loss and bereavement. Children in families with parental affective disorder experience more acute stressful events, particularly those of an interpersonal nature, than children with parents with other problems, such as medical illnesses. However, chronic stressors are equally high in both. The mothers' disorder itself also acts as stressor for the children, thereby increasing risk. Children's responses to stressors is another contributor to risk, with negative self-concept being not only more common in children with higher numbers of stressors but also increasing the risk of disorder, particularly depression. These negative cognitions are associated with criticism and noninvolvement by the mothers. Although little work has been done on the agency of the stressors, aspects of both stress agency and stress carrying are likely to be present in the parents and children, consistent with the disorders and associated vulnerability.

Family Arrangements

Nontraditional family structures following the loss of a biological parent have been examined in relation both to stress and parenting and to its differential effects on siblings raised together and raised apart explored. Siblings brought up apart in different family arrangements show the greatest difference in adjustment, although even siblings raised together show different responses to family conflict and stressors. Studies agree that the loss of parents affects children differentially, even when objective aspects of the loss are assessed. Poor parenting in terms of neglect and physical abuse are more common in certain family structures, such as when a biological and step-parent are present.

Sibling Stressors

Siblings' experiences have mainly been studied in the context of genetic studies to identify the sources of shared and nonshared environments to help explain the differences and similarities between siblings. These have used a variety of research strategies involving family studies, adoption studies, and twin studies to look at variations between siblings in personality, disorder, and experience of parenting. Interestingly, siblings have been shown to be largely different from one another in most assessments, and thus a large focus of such studies has been on assessing the role of the nonshared environment in explaining experience, personality, and psychopathology. The reasons for differences in siblings' environments include their relative ages, position in the family, gender, extra-familial experience such as school and social experience, and more random accidental or idiosyncratic experience. Although less work has been conducted on the degree to which stressors are shared by siblings, studies that do exist show a high degree of sharing of life events but less sharing of the negative impact of these events. Thus only approximately one-third of events held in common have a similar degree of negative impact for different family members. Twin studies have shown there to be a high degree of concordance for severe life events and a greater impact of such events in monozygotic than dizygotic twins.

In the late 1990s, an approach opposing the importance of family stressors emphasized the importance of children's experiences outside the family. Nonshared environmental influences in terms of school and social life were postulated as the critical environmental influences on child development and disorder, with familial influences being accounted for by genetic inheritance. Thus, sibling comparisons examining nonshared and usually nonfamily-based stressors, as well as positive experiences, have also been investigated.

Parenting

The quality of parenting has mainly been assessed around issues of the care and control of children. Poor parenting involves low levels of care and high control; at one extreme, this can involve the neglect and abuse of children. Parenting styles have also been categorized as authoritative, authoritarian, permissive, and disengaged, with the first of these being the most adaptive and related to positive child development. At the more extreme levels of poor parenting,

involving neglect and physical abuse, there is a high degree of shared experience among same-sex siblings. But where cold or critical parenting is involved, differential treatment by parents is much more common. with both favoritism and scapegoating of individual offspring occurring quite frequently. A process model of parenting shows the effects of the parents' own early development and personality, adult work history, marital relationship, and social network on parenting. This, in turn, impacts on child development and characteristics.

Parent Disorder

Psychiatric disorder in the parents can act as a magnet for familial stress, both in provoking the disorder and in perpetuating it. There is a strong relationship between concurrent disorder in parents (particularly mothers) and children. However, the chronicity and severity of the impairment by the disorder are more highly related to child's adjustment than to the actual parental diagnosis. Although the fathers' diagnoses exert weaker effects than mothers', the presence of disorder in both parents substantially increases the likelihood of disorder in the offspring. Because adults with depression have a higher likelihood of being partnered by people who have a psychiatric disorder, the likelihood of two parents being affected increases. Thus, 25% of husbands of women with depression have been shown to have disorders themselves, and as many as 41% of wives of men with a psychiatric diagnosis were similarly affected. This is argued to occur not only through assortative pairing, whereby individuals with a disorder appear to select partners with a similar impairment but also through the subsequent development of a disorder in the partner of an affected individual. This may be due to existing spousal difficulties or to the psychiatric disorder in both being caused by prior conditions in the family, such as poverty or conflict.

Transmission of Stress Intergenerationally

Because disorders and interpersonal difficulties run in families, three mechanisms of intergenerational transmission from parent to child have been investigated, with most studies suggesting that all three are likely to play a role.

Genetic Transmission

The genetic investigation of family influences on psychiatric disorder is engaged in the disentangling of genetic and environmental influences. A case has consistently been made for gene–environment correlations, with children appearing to inherit some biological qualities that later result in depression and some environments that shape and pull their experiences in ways that lead to depression and other disorders. Three types of gene–environment correlations have been identified, and the current challenge in the field lies in assessing the role of each of these in the intergenerational transmission of both disorders and susceptibility to a disorder.

1. Passive genotype–environment correlations occur when children passively inherit an environment from parents that is correlated with their genetic predisposition.
2. Reactive genotype–environment correlations occur when children actively evoke environments associated with their genetic endowment.
3. Active genotype–environment correlations occur when the children actively seek out environments correlated with their genetic endowment.

Some progress is being made in seeking molecular genetic modes of transmission for adversity and disorder. For example, genetic deficiencies in mono-amine oxidase A (MAOA) activity, responsible for metabolizing neurotransmitters such as norepinephrine (NE), serotonin (5-HT), and dopamine (DA), have been linked with aggression. The examination of violent offending using the Dunedin longitudinal study of children followed from birth showed a functional polymorphism in the gene encoding MAOA, which moderated the effects of childhood maltreatment on subsequent violent behavior in boys. An interaction between the level of maltreatment in childhood and low MAOA activity predicted a three-fold higher conduct disorder rate and a tenfold higher violent convictions rate. This is an example of genetic factors playing a moderating or protective role. Thus, the low activity of MAOA and maltreatment accounted for only 12% of one male cohort studied but for 44% of the cohort's violent convictions. Eighty-five percent of cohort males who had the low-activity MAOA genotype and who were also maltreated developed some form of antisocial behavior.

Direct Impact of Parental Disorder

Another likely mechanism of transmission of stressor and susceptibility to disorder from parents to children is through the direct effect of the parents' disorder. In addition to providing additional stress for the children, the parents' disorder also presents the children with a poor role model for coping and reduces the possibility of any buffering effect from parental support. Three generations of influence have been identified, with women raised in dysfunctional families likely to have impaired parenting skills from their parents (i.e., the grandparent generation), in turn increasing the risk of disorder in the children (i.e., the grandchild generation). However, evidence that individuals with disorders are more likely to be partnered with others with disorders means that this does not operate exclusively through the maternal line; disorder in both parents has been shown to provide the greatest risk for children.

The mother–child interaction is, however, particularly critical in intergenerational transmission, and this can trigger episodes either in the mothers or children, with evidence of influence in both directions. Depressed mothers have been shown to relate differentially to their children, with more negativity to dysfunctional children than to a normally functioning ones. In contrast, nondepressed mothers are less likely to acknowledge dysfunctionality in their children and therefore treat them more similarly. Thus, characteristics of both the parents and the children play a part.

Correlates of Parental Disorder

For children, as for their parents, psychiatric disorder is a consequence of adversity, but it also leads to the perpetuation of adversity. The most common family adversity associated with disorder is interpersonal, involving both marital conflict and conflict with children, although poverty and social isolation are also implicated. Susceptible individuals are thus capable of either being the agents of stress for close others or being the recipients and carriers of such stress and passing it on to others. Where both parents in a family have disorder, the accumulation of stressors for all family members is likely to be great. Thus negative family interaction can be a function both of parents' vulnerability characteristics (e.g., poor interpersonal relating, poor support, and low self-esteem) and of symptoms of psychological disorder (e.g., depression, anxiety, and antisocial behavior). Thus, intergenerational studies with mothers and young adult offspring interviewed independently show an important role for neglect/abuse in the offspring in disorder but with separate causal linkages from maternal depression and maternal vulnerability. It is of note that the perpetrators of physical abuse in children are rather more likely to be the fathers or surrogate fathers, despite the intergenerational impact observed for mothers. Thus, the mothers' role can be both a carrier and agent in stress, with both being conveyed to the offspring.

The reasons for familial stress patterning are therefore varied. The congregation of stressors within family groupings is due to both common and individual influences. Negative interpersonal functioning, poor parenting, poor coping, and family disadvantage are key factors. Biological factors involving the genetic transmission of risk and the physical impacts of stress are increasingly being discovered as contributing to final explanatory models.

Further Reading

Belsky, J. and Vondra, J. (1989). The determinants of parenting: a process model. In: Cicchetti, D. & Carlson, V. (eds.) *Child maltreatment – theory and research on the causes and consequences of child abuse and neglect*, pp. 153–203. Cambridge, UK: Cambridge University Press.

Bifulco, A. and Moran, P. M. (1998). *Wednesday's child: research into women's experience of neglect and abuse in childhood and adult depression*. London: Routledge.

Bifulco, A., Moran, P. M., Ball, C., et al. (2002). Childhood adversity, parental vulnerability and disorder: examining inter-generational transmission of risk. *Journal of Child Psychology and Psychiatry* **43**, 1075–1086.

Brown, G. W. and Harris, T. O. (1978). *Social origins of depression*. London: Tavistock.

Caspi, A. (2002). Role of genotype in the cycle of violence in maltreated children. *Science* **297**, 851–854.

Eley, T. C. and Stevenson, J. (2000). Specific life events and chronic experiences differentially associated with depression and anxiety in young twins. *Journal of Abnormal Child Psychology* **28**, 383–394.

Goodyer, I. (1990). *Life experiences, development and childhood psychopathology*. Chichester, UK: John Wiley.

Hammen, C. (1991). *Depression runs in families: the social context of risk and resilience in children of depressed mothers*. New York: Spring Verlag.

Harris, J. R. (1998). *The nurture assumption: Why children turn out the way they do*. New York: The Free Press.

Kendler, K. S., Kessler, R. C., Walters, E. E., et al. (1995). Stressful life events, genetic liability, and onset of an episode of major depression in women. *American Journal of Psychiatry* **152**, 833–842.

Plommin, R. (1994). *Genetics and experience: the interplay between nature and nurture*. Thousand Oaks, CA: Sage Publications.

Reiss, D., Plomin, R., Hetherington, E. M., et al. (1994). The separate worlds of teenage siblings: an introduction to the study of the nonshared environment and adolescent development. In: Hetherington, E. M. & Reiss, D. (eds.) *Separate social worlds of siblings: the impact of nonshared environment on development*, pp. 63–109. Hillsdale, NJ: Lawrence Erlbaum Associates.

Rutter, M. (1989). Intergenerational continuities and discontinuities in serious parenting difficulties. In: Cicchetti, D. & Carlson, V. (eds.) *Research on the consequences of child maltreatment*, pp. 317–348. New York: Cambridge University Press.

Family Therapy

B Jalali
West Los Angeles Veterans Administration Medical Center and UCLA School of Medicine, Los Angeles, CA, USA

Stress and the Family
Theoretical Models of Family Therapy
What Family Therapy Can Achieve
Indications for Family Therapy

Glossary

Differentiation of self	The degree of emotional separation between a person and his or her family of origin. More differentiated individuals have a better awareness of the influence of their emotions, behavior, and actions and are less dependent on approval of others for their decisions.
Double bind	Communication characteristics of a system that produces conflicting definitions of incongruous messages between members of a family, leading to stress and anxiety.
Enmeshment/ disengagement	Enmeshment is a type of family relationship in which the family members are fused and are unable to define their roles and boundaries. Subsystems are not well defined, and the hierarchy of executive functions is unclear. Disengagement refers to a lack of relatedness and binding between family members, who appear uninvolved and distant.
Homeostasis	Steady state of any living system that is regulated and maintained as it faces the external environment. If the system faces stress and breaks down, it attempts to repair itself so that a state of constancy and balance is maintained.
Identified patient	The person who bears the symptoms and is the reason for the family to seek treatment. However, from the family system

point of view, individual psychopathology is maintained and or amplified by the family, if not a consequence of family pathology.

Pseudo-mutuality A facade of harmony and pretending to share same behavior, feelings, and attitude in a family at the expense of lack of individuation in its members. Anything that threatens to deviate from the sameness of the structure and roles provokes a great deal of anxiety.

Rubber fence A specific state of relationship between the family system, its members, and the social environment. It protects the family from any intrusion or departure from its norm and incorporates items that fit and rejects those that appear noncomplimentary.

Scapegoat A person who is recruited by the family system to become the problem, instead of the family system attempting to resolve its conflicts.

Schism and skew Schism is a pattern of marital relationship in which the members of a couple fail to reach an agreement on role reciprocity and therefore undercut or coerce each other. Skew in a marital relationship means that one member of the couple has significant pathology, but the other goes along with it, and all conflicts, while present, are hidden.

Triangle When conflict or anxiety rises in a dyadic or a two-person relationship and a third person is included to diffuse the conflict. The pathological form of triangle is a rigid triangle wherein conflicts are never resolved in the dyad, and the third person is put in a position of either conflict of loyalty or alliance with one member against the other.

Stress and the Family

In a living system, nothing is static. Different psychological, biological, and social forces are continuously impinging on the system to synchronize and change. Stress on the family system disturbs its homeostatic equilibrium. In response, the system must mobilize its internal and external resources, become flexible enough to produce alternative modes of adaptation, be able to exchange roles and functions across its subsystems, reorganize to meet the demands of the stress, and redefine itself after adjustment to the stress.

The family system must be assessed as a whole, with a set of functions, relationships, and roles, which are continuously changing as the social structure surrounding the family system is changing. Therefore, in evaluating the effects of stress on the family system, one must be aware of the cultural, social, and historical makeup of the family, as it influences the experience of, meaning of, and response to stress.

The types of stress on the family are mainly the following:

1. The stress of transitions in the family's developmental stages (becoming a couple, birth of first child, children transitioning into adolescence, first child leaving home, last child leaving home, retirement and empty nest, sudden illness and death of a family member, chronic illness in a family member, threat of dissolution of the family such as separation and divorce, remarriage and blended family, illness or death of grandparents, etc.)
2. Outer stressors, such as loss of job, a move to a new location, changing schools, economic loss, catastrophic events such as flood and earthquake, and crime.

Regardless of the type of stress, the family system must first recognize the stress, then attempt to adjust and reorganize in order to cope with it. Adjustment and reorganization include changes in the structure, function, and roles of the system, which will be new and unfamiliar to the members and may bring anxiety and uncertainty with them.

If the family characteristics and functioning were problematic and conflictual to begin with, including poor communication skills, unclear boundary definition, poor parental skills, and marital conflicts, then the family structure may skew further in the face of stress and will have difficulty in reorganizing and readjusting. This may result in either poor adaptation or development of symptoms in vulnerable members (biologically or constitutionally), such as substance abuse, depression, suicide attempt, school or behavioral problems, eating disorder, infidelity, and threats of separation or divorce.

These families may mobilize pathological coping mechanisms, such as denial, blame, scapegoating, detouring of conflicts, and developing rigid triangulations, which may result in an increase of perceived stress in its members. Although denial can serve as a protective defense mechanism at first, if it persists it will impede the family's coping, because the family will resist change and continue to limp along as if no modifications were required. However, their established patterns will not be sufficient, and the stress may plunge the family into a state of crisis. The functioning of the family system will halt, and the system will be incapacitated, in a state of disequilibrium, and unable to function.

Lack of flexibility in gender roles and division of labor can cause rigidity and restrictions in the system, which will reduce resources necessary for coping. Families that are isolated from their social network and community also have restricted coping resources. The family system can recover from the state of crisis with the help of family therapy.

Family members can grow from the experience of stress and learn how to manage future stresses. Family therapy can help them to identify the stress, become more cohesive, communicate better among themselves and with the outer environment, recruit social and community resources, respect interpersonal boundaries, and avoid blame.

Theoretical Models of Family Therapy

Overview

Family therapy is a type of psychotherapy in which the unit of treatment is the family (whether nuclear or extended), and not the individual. It assumes that problems and symptoms emanate from unhealthy interactions in the family system and not solely from the psychological or subconscious problems of the individual. The theory uses circular rather than linear thinking; each individual is part of the larger group, with continuous interaction and feedback processes between the two.

In general, family therapy is based on family system theory. It examines family interactions, interpersonal relationships, and communications and aims to change unhealthy patterns. This theoretical model was introduced in late 1940s and early 1950s, emanating from the study of schizophrenic patients and the link between exaggerations of their symptoms and their family interactions. Family system theory assumes that the family system is in a constant state of change and balance, and it attempts to achieve homeostasis and adaptation to change by mobilizing alternative interactions. When the system can not adapt successfully due to stress, rigidity of patterns, and/or psychological features, problems and symptoms ensue in different members. Consequently, adaptation is inappropriate, and a state of dysfunctional homeostasis settles in.

The early family therapists hypothesized that whenever the family system's homeostasis is threatened, symptomatic behavior in one member may become a way to preserve the family's equilibrium. Therefore, the concepts of scapegoating and the identified patient were introduced.

Early family therapists also hypothesized that many of the preceding phenomena occur through a feedback process and nonverbal communications, through sequence of interactions. At first they attempted to examine the communication of schizophrenic patients and their families, and concluded that there are series of contradictory messages transmitted to the patient. The concept of double bind was introduced, which was considered the essential ingredient in the child–parent interaction, specifically the mother (the concept of the schizophrenogenic mother), in which a family member receives two contradictory messages that he or she can not obey or disobey. Later the concept of double bind was extended from a two-person system to a three-person system, as attention was drawn to fathers as well as mothers. Interactions in the marital relationship were found to be dysfunctional and pathological, and the concepts of schism and skew were introduced. They highlighted patterns of hostility, undercutting, domination, passivity, and distortion.

Other family therapists studied communication patterns and family roles in schizophrenia and identified pseudomutuality as a feature of families with a schizophrenic member. These families appear cohesive on the surface but are in deep conflict underneath. They may also erect a boundary around the family that will extrude any input that will not fit their norm (a rubber fence) and will only allow input that will fit their norm.

These theories were later applied to other family systems with a member identified as carrying a psychiatric diagnosis, such as an eating disorder, depression, or substance abuse. Although all family therapists agree on the basic principle of how a dysfunctional family can lead to stressing a vulnerable member(s) so that symptoms develop and are maintained and amplified, the techniques that have been developed to treat families are quite different from each other. However, each strives to establish a less stressful state in the family.

The length of a course of family therapy is usually shorter than individual therapy, ranging from several sessions to several months. On the whole, the therapist attempts to change the dysfunctional structure and functioning of the system, rather than address changes in the individual member. When therapists attend to symptoms, they are treated as part of a complex system of interaction and feedback processes in which symptoms have become faulty resolutions for other family problems. The therapist strives for a change in rigid behavioral patterns, increased communication, healthier interactions, and improved problem solving among all members.

Examples of Theoretical Models

Major theoretical orientations of family therapy include psychoanalytic (Ackerman), systems (Bowen), structural (Minuchin), strategic (Haley, Madanes), experiential (Whitaker), communicational (Satir, Bateson, Watzlawick), object relations (Framo, Nagy), and a few others, such as constructivist and Milan's system of counter paradoxical family therapy.

Psychoanalytic family therapy Ackerman theorized that a healthy family is in a state of constant homeostatic balance, which is dynamic and changing as the family grows in its developmental stages and as new stresses occur to which the family needs to adapt. The dysfunctional family cannot adapt to the required changes, and therefore the various family functions become faulty and lead to problems and symptoms in its members and possibly to disintegration of the family. Therefore, change can occur through implementing improved problem solving, learning healthier communication, and diminishing the scapegoating of its members.

Family Systems Therapy

Bowen developed family systems therapy, theorizing that the basis of human relationships is not a two-person system but a three-person one. He stated that when conflicts and anxiety develop in a relationship, invariably a third person becomes involved who will side with one of the other two. In this threesome, two individuals are close, and the third one is on the outside. This is the basis for the concept of triangles in the family. The triangle may appear to diffuse the anxiety, but conflicts remain unresolved.

Triangles are constantly shifting and unstable and have a tendency to interlock with other triangular relationships. Individuals learn from their family of origin how to operate in triangles. When the adaptive level of functioning in a family is pathological, the individuals in that family are more likely to resolve anxiety with triangulation and are less differentiated. The concept of triangles and triangulating was later applied to larger systems such as organizations and small groups.

Bowen stated that each family is part of an undifferentiated ego mass, and each member strives to differentiate from it, to develop one's own sense of self, and to detriangulate oneself. He also stated that patterns of relationships and handling stress are a part of a process that is transmitted across generations. When getting caught in triangulated relationships with their family becomes too intense and stressful, members may try to distance themselves emotionally or physically, or they may try to cut themselves off from the family. However, similar patterns will be re-created and repeated in other relationships that the individual develops.

This model also introduced the concept of family projection process, which means that the emotional processes are transmitted, for example, to a child, who as a result may develop difficulties in differentiation of self.

The family system theory of Bowen states that historical patterns are factors in symptom production as well as change; therefore, the main tool of treatment is using a genogram or diagram of the family's three generations in detail, demonstrating sets of relationships, conflict areas, and triangular relationships, and then exploring methods of unlocking and changing them. Bowen encouraged families to resolve issues with their families of origin and attempt to achieve separation and differentiation from them.

The goal of treatment is understanding the three-generation system of involvement in the symptoms. The main therapeutic technique is helping and teaching the family to differentiate and detriangulate themselves from their family of origin ego mass, which will lead to healthier relationships on the whole.

Structural family therapy Structural family therapy (Minuchin) presents a clear model of what is considered a normal family system. This is a system with a clear hierarchy of power, clear boundaries between members and the family subsystems (subsystem of parents and children), no cross-generational coalition, and clear cross-generational boundaries.

Minuchin presented a model of pathological family enmeshment in which boundaries are blurred, the hierarchy of power is unclear, cross-generational alliances and coalitions are present, and executive functions of the family are hampered. He stated that a dysfunctional family cannot adapt to developmental and extrafamilial stresses and it therefore recruits a vulnerable member who becomes symptomatic.

Minuchin applied his methods to severe problems of childhood and later to eating disorders. Structural family therapy's major contribution to the field was in the treatment of psychosomatic illnesses such as asthma and illnesses in which an emotional component was detrimental to control and compliance, such as diabetes. Research with diabetic and asthmatic patients done by structural family therapists clearly showed that family stress levels correlated with induction of an asthmatic attack or a rise in blood glucose level of the patient, and when the stress subsided, the asthma subsided and the blood glucose level returned to normal. Conflicts in the family correlated with exacerbation of medical symptoms, which was supported by laboratory data. Minuchin demonstrated that family therapy and reducing the family's conflicts and stress can indeed reduce the number of emergency visits for both the asthmatic and the diabetic family member.

Structural family therapy was also applied to patients with eating disorders, ranging from bulimia to anorexia, and to patterns of lack of conflict resolution and rigidity that were dysfunctional and therefore maintained and amplified the preceding symptoms. Once these patterns were addressed and changed, the eating disorder improved. Techniques used in this theoretical framework include joining, establishing clear subsystems, expanding the alternative ways of problem solving, strengthening the boundaries between generations, relabeling symptoms, creating intensity leading to change, increasing flexibility, modifying dysfunctional interactions, clarifying the hierarchy of power, and restructuring.

Strategic family therapy Strategic family therapy and the problem-oriented approach (Haley) also adhere to a systemic model of family interaction, stating that symptoms maintain homeostasis. Strategic family therapy studies the sequence of interactions among family members that leads to symptoms and then attempts to change this sequence to a better-functioning one and a healthier hierarchy. The symptom is also a solution, although an unsatisfactory one. It is both supported and opposed by other members' behavior. Therefore, the therapist has to identify the sequence of interactions that both reinforces and exacerbates it.

In this model, a historical perspective of the family is not studied, nor is the larger context or where the meaning of the symptom is embedded. The focus is on the presenting problem or symptom and not on the family. However, in order for the problem to improve, the organizational sequence that maintains the problem must change. Change is accomplished by prescribing strategies, positive reframing, changing dyadic relationships that are involved with the symptom, reversal of roles, and use of paradoxical assignments and interventions. Symptoms are changed through changes in hierarchy, coalitions, and communication. This model clearly adheres to a briefer period of therapy.

Experiential family therapy The experiential model (Whitaker) focuses on process and growth in therapy. The family is challenged by being offered a variety of alternative ways of interacting, including absurd ones, as a method to unstick the family. Change is induced by creating new experiences, personal growth, and marking boundaries between generations. Individual and family creativity and growth are promoted. The problems or symptoms are viewed as systems problems. In this model, an attempt is made to join the system in the beginning, but later in treatment the therapist distances and becomes an outside consultant to the system, encouraging the family to take the initiative in making changes.

Counter paradoxical family therapy The counter paradox model of the Milan group suggests that in a dysfunctional family, the members' response to each other is often paradoxical and illogical. This model attempts to counter the paradox by the use of a team of therapists, circular questioning (to gather more information), positive connotations, remaining neutral, increasing the time interval between the sessions, prescribing family rituals, and systemic prescriptions.

What Family Therapy Can Achieve

Family therapy can achieve the following:

- Help the family to understand the patterns of their interactions and relationships as a whole, instead of focusing on one member as the scapegoat.
- Identify conflicts and defects within the family structure and help members to develop new methods of resolving problems.
- Identify internal and external resources and strengths.
- Provide support, education, and guidance in handling inner and outer stresses.

The main rule of thumb in conducting family therapy is that all members who are identified as key members must participate; otherwise, it will not be effective.

Indications for Family Therapy

Indications that family therapy is needed include the following:

- Substance abuse in one or more family member
- Chronic psychosomatic disorder or other chronic medical illness in one member
- Physical or emotional abuse in the family
- Marital conflict
- Poor parental skills
- Eating disorder in one member
- Diagnosis of major psychiatric disorder in one member such as schizophrenia or bipolar disorder
- Depression in the family
- Any behavioral problems or psychological symptoms in a child or adolescent
- A dysfunctional adult offspring in the family
- A traumatic event experienced by the family

See Also the Following Articles

Depression and Manic-Depressive Illness; Eating Disorders and Stress; Familial Patterns of Stress; Schizophrenia.

Further Reading

Bateson, G. (1977). *The steps to an ecology of mind.* New York: Ballatine Books.

Boscolo, L., Cecchin, G., Hoffman, L. and Penn, P. (eds.) (1987). *Milan systemic family therapy: conversations in theory and practice.* New York: Basic Books.

Broderick, C. B. (1993). *Understanding family process: basics of family system theory.* California: Sage Publishers.

Bumberry, W. (1998). *Reshaping family relationships: the symbolic therapy of Carl Whitaker.* New York: Brunner Mazel.

Framo, J. L. (1992). *Family-of-origin therapy. An intergenerational approach.* New York: Brunner Mazel.

Gurman, A. S. (1981). *Handbook of family therapy.* New York: Brunner Mazel.

Haley, J. and Richeport-Haley, M. (2003). *The art of strategic therapy.* New York: Brunner-Routedge.

Hoffman, L. (1981). *Foundations of family therapy.* New York: Basic Books Publishers.

Lidz, T., Fleck, S. and Cornelison, A. R. (1965). *Schizophrenia and the family.* New York: International Press.

Kerr, M. I. and Bowen, M. (1988). *Family evaluation.* New York: W.W. Norton Press.

McGoldrick, M., Gerson, R. and Shellenberger, S. (1999). *Genograms: assessment and interventions.* New York: W.W. Norton.

McGoldrick, M., Giordano, J. and Garcia-Preto, N. (eds.) (2006). *Ethnicity and family therapy.* New York: Guilford Press.

Minuchin, S., Rosman, B. L. and Baker, L. (1978). *Psychosomatic families.* Cambridge, MA: Harvard University Press.

Minuchin, S., Wai-Yung and Simaon, G. M. (1996). *Mastering family therapy: journey of growth and transformation.* New York: John Wiley and Sons.

Minuchin, S., et al. (2006). *Assessing families and couples: from symptoms to system.* New York: Allyn and Bacon.

Nichols, M. P. (1984). *Family therapy: concepts and methods.* New York: Gardner Press.

Wynn, E., Ryckoff, J. M., Day, J. and Hirsch, S. I. (1958). Pseudomutuality in the family treatment of schizophrenia. Psychiatry. **21**: 205–220.

Zeig, J. L. and Haley, J. (2001). *Changing directives: the strategic therapy of Jay Haley.* Phoenix, AZ: Milton Erickson Foundations Press.

Fatigue and Stress

A Appels
University of Maastricht, Maastricht, Netherlands
W J Kop
Uniformed Services University of the Health Sciences, Bethesda, MD, USA

This article is a revision of the previous edition article by A Appels, volume 2, pp 108–110, © 2000, Elsevier Inc.

Psychiatric Approach
Organizational and Occupational Health Approach
Psychophysiological Approach
Psychosomatic Approach
Conclusion

Glossary

Burnout	A state characterized by emotional exhaustion that may occur after exposure to prolonged stress.
Hypothalamic-pituitary-adrenal (HPA) axis	Part of the neurohormonal stress system. Both increased and decreased activity of the HPA axis can be observed, depending on the nature of the disorder.
Neurasthenia	A state characterized by fatigue, impaired cognitive functioning, and increased emotional sensitivity.
Vital exhaustion	A state characterized by unusual fatigue and loss of energy, increased irritability, and feelings of demoralization; often precedes cardiac events. In the original conceptualization of the exhaustion construct, the term vital was included to reflect the far-reaching consequences of this condition on daily life function (similar to vital depression).

Fatigue is a common symptom that can substantially interfere with daily functioning and quality of life. A large literature indicates that episodes of extreme fatigue are precipitated and maintained by emotional distress. A substantial number of individuals (5–20% of the general population) suffer from persistent fatigue that interferes with routine daily life activities, and fatigue is one of the most common presenting complaints in primary care. Prevalence estimates of fatigue depend on the measurement instruments, cut-off points for presence versus absence, and the persistence of the complaint. Patients generally regard fatigue as important because it is disabling, whereas physicians often do not place a strong emphasis on fatigue because it is diagnostically nonspecific for most if not all diseases.

Several theories have been developed to conceptualize and investigate fatigue. These theories describe fatigue as a pollution of the *milieu interieur*, as an energy problem, as a breakdown in nervous system functioning, or as an evaluative motivational assessment of an individual's psychophysiological condition in relation to exogenous demands, resulting in a decision to either continue or discontinue an activity. These theories have strengths and limitations, and reflect the way in which scientists organize and operationalize their approaches to investigating a coherent set of symptoms. There are overlaps and distinctions between the approaches to the origins and treatment of fatigue, depending on the investigator's fields of interest and scientific background. In the following sections we provide a selective review of these approaches.

Psychiatric Approach

Since the late 1800s, much debate has arisen addressing the question of whether fatigue states should be distinguished from depressive mood disorders. There is little doubt that depressed individuals often feel tired and that fatigue is one of the diagnostic symptoms for depression. However, not all individuals who feel depleted of energy suffer from mood disturbances, lack of self-esteem, or guilt feelings. Therefore, psychiatric constructs have been developed to describe a condition that is mainly characterized by profound fatigability. In 1869, George M. Beard introduced the concept neurasthenia to describe an organically based disorder characterized by fatigability of the body and mind, largely resulting from environmental factors. Neurasthenia was primarily treated by rest and reportedly common among well-educated and professional individuals. Other concepts that have been developed to describe fatigue states include effort syndrome, neurocirculatory asthenia, or postinfectious fatigue syndrome.

More recently, the chronic fatigue syndrome (CFS), myalgic encephalomyelitis (ME), and also posttraumatic stress disorder (PTSD) have been introduced as conditions in which fatigue and distress play a primary role. CFS is an operationally defined syndrome characterized by a minimum of 6 months of severe physical and mental fatigue and fatigability made worse by minor exertion. Because of the similarities among the prior neurasthenia construct, CFS, and ME, it has been questioned whether these more recent

concepts are mainly "old wine in new bottles." PTSD describes the sequels of exposure to severe psychological distress, such as occur during major disasters, war, and other life-threatening events. Increased fatigue and fatigability belong to the major characteristics of PTSD. Detailed research has revealed that some symptoms are relatively specific for PTSD and CFS, justifying their heuristic value. There is, nonetheless, substantial overlap among the symptoms that constitute these postulated syndromes, which may suggest that stress is a common factor.

Psychiatric classifications and diagnoses were originally based on the presumed pathophsyiological origins of a complaint. In contrast, contemporary diagnostic classifications, such as the *Diagnostic and Statistical Manual of Mental Disorders* (4th edn.; DSM-IV), are predominantly based on the description and classification of symptomatology. DSM-IV includes PTSD, but does not include any of the other fatigue-related constructs or syndromes. DSM-IV lists decreased energy, tiredness, and fatigue among the symptoms of depressive mood disorders or dysthymia. Thus, the most commonly used classification system for mental disorders does not make a distinction between depression and other fatigue states.

Organizational and Occupational Health Approach

In occupational medicine and occupational psychology, fatigue is mainly approached as the result of an imbalance between demand and supply or as a breakdown in adaptation to stress. During the last decades, much attention has been given to burnout as the end point of long-lasting work-related stress. Burnout is a negative state of physical, emotional, and mental exhaustion that is the result of a gradual process of disillusionment. The concept of burnout was first used by Freudenberger in the mid-1970s to describe a common psychological characteristic observed in health-care professionals. Freudenberger observed that many of the volunteers with whom he was working experienced a gradual emotional depletion and a loss of motivation and commitment. Burnout has three main components: emotional exhaustion, depersonalization, and reduced personal accomplishment.

There has been substantial debate about the optimal definition of the burnout construct. However, this debate has not prevented fruitful empirical research, including Maslach's successful development of a reliable scale to measure burnout. This scale assesses the three dimensions of burnout (emotional exhaustion, depersonalization, and reduced personal accomplishment) and has become the gold standard for the assessment of burnout. Empirical research has shown that the emotional exhaustion component is related to depression, whereas the relationships between depersonalization and personal accomplishment with depression are less strong.

The burnout literature is more concerned with situational antecedents than with individual differences as the determinants of burnout, probably because of the occupational health origins of this construct. The extension of the burnout concept to nonoccupational domains (e.g., feelings of emotional exhaustion caused by marital conflicts) has been controversial, especially because the concepts of depersonalization and reduced personal accomplishment are less applicable outside the realm of occupational settings. Therefore, the contributions of research on burnout to fatigue lie primarily in the identification of social and occupational determinants.

Psychophysiological Approach

Psychophysiological approaches address behaviors, emotions, and cognitions that correspond with physiological reactions to normal and abnormal, internal or external stimuli. For example, psychophysiologists and other behavioral scientists investigate the influence of fatigue on inflammation, as well as how the mental state is influenced by inflammation. The stress system receives much attention in these types of psychophysiological research designs.

The autonomic nervous system and neurohormonal processes play a crucial role in the human stress response. The autonomic nervous system involves two branches: the sympathetic nervous system (involved in the acute stress response) and the parasympathetic nervous system (which is commonly more active in periods of rest and, in general, counterbalances the sympathetic nervous system). The neurohormonal stress response is complex and involves the sympathetic-adreno-medullary (SAM) system and the HPA system. The stimulation of the SAM system is characterized by increased secretion of the cathecholamines epinephrine and norepinephrine, as well as increased heart rate and blood pressure, sweating, palpitations and other vegetative symptoms (i.e., related to autonomic nervous system activation). Most of the autonomic nervous system and neurohormonal responses in response to stress exposure are normal, enabling the organism to adapt to environmental changes.

The HPA axis response displays important divergent concomitants of increased versus decreased activity. Increased HPA axis activity is observed in response to acute stress; increased HPA axis activity characterized by increased secretion of cortisol is also well documented among individuals with melancholic depression, panic disorder, central obesity, and Cushing's syndrome. These elevated cortisol levels may coincide with the suppression of inflammation. In contrast, decreased HPA axis activity has been observed in chronic stress, persistent fatigue, atypical depression (i.e., hyperphagia and hypersomnia), and nicotine withdrawal. These conditions are associated with a decreased production of cortisol and purportedly with the activation of immune-mediated inflammation.

During inflammation, the body produces cytokines, which play a pivotal signaling role in immune system activation. Some of these cytokines reach the brain or elicit the release of cytokines in the brain, resulting in what has been labeled sickness behavior, characterized by locomotor retardation, general malaise, anorexia, and inhibition of sexual behavior. Sickness behavior is part of the defensive response to infection or inflammation. Evidence consistently demonstrates that fatigue and inflammation are interrelated. Thus, there is probably a bidirectional or circular association between inflammation and fatigue, which is mediated in part by the central and autonomic nervous systems. The psychophysiological approach makes a unique contribution to the study of fatigue by investigating which symptomatic and physiological reactions belong to normal health-protecting behaviors and which reactions are markers of a breakdown in adaptation to environmental challenges.

Psychosomatic Approach

In psychosomatic medicine, fatigue is approached in several ways, depending on the nature of the coinciding medical disorder. For example, among patients with cancer, fatigue is considered as a (still poorly understood) consequence of the disease and its treatment. Programs are mainly directed at coping with the fatigue. In patients with multiple sclerosis, fatigue is particularly disabling symptom, distinct from depressed mood or physical weakness.

In coronary artery disease, fatigue and exhaustion are of particular interest because it is well established that exhaustion (i.e., feelings of unusual fatigue, loss of energy, and increased irritability and demoralization) is an important precursor of myocardial infarction and sudden cardiac death. Exhaustion and depression also predict recurrent cardiac events among high-risk populations, and more research is needed to further document the divergent validity of these two partially overlapping constructs.

Based on the predictive value of exhaustion and depression for future adverse cardiovascular outcomes, two different intervention approaches have been investigated recently. Many scientists interpret the premonitory symptoms of extreme fatigue as manifestations of a clinical or subsyndromal depression; consequently, Beck's cognitive therapy has been used to treat coronary disease patients with depressive symptomatology. Other investigators have approached the same symptoms as manifestations of a sustained state of exhaustion resulting from long-term exposure to uncontrollable emotional distress. This perspective emphasizes the similarity between exhaustion and the psychological consequences of decreased HPA activity following chronic stress. Interventions targeting exhaustion use group therapy, including relaxation and reducing stressors that can lead to exhaustion. The effects of both types of interventions on the risk of new coronary events have been tested in well-designed, randomized, controlled intervention trials. Neither of the two strategies succeeded in demonstrating that a reduction of depression or exhaustion reduced the risk of a new coronary event. However, the interventions were successful in subsamples (determined *a posteriori*). It is reasonable to assume that future trials will profit from the lessons learned in these pivotal studies. Such trials may demonstrate that a behavioral treatment of fatigue and depressive symptomatology will not only improve quality of life but also reduce the risk of recurrent cardiac events.

Conclusion

Fatigue is a ubiquitous phenomenon. Less than 10% of patients presenting with fatigue in primary care present with a disease that plays a direct causal role in this symptom. The law of parsimony has accompanied fatigue research and will accompany future work. It has been debated whether concepts such as neurasthenia, burnout, and vital exhaustion are needed and whether the procrustean bed of DSM-IV does more harm than good in stress research. Each of the aforementioned approaches has contributed to our obtaining more insight into the origins of fatigue, its biological and physiological correlates, and the possibilities and limitations of helping individuals who suffer from unusual fatigue. The domain of fatigue research has unique epistemological problems, which require further scientific attention. More research is needed on the distinction between fatigue as a health-protecting factor and fatigue as a marker of overtaxing of the body. The precipitating and maintaining factors of chronic fatigue conditions are complicated because some of the original etiological factors may have become undetectable (e.g., the long-term consequences of viral infections). It will be difficult to answer the question of whether chronic fatigue can be best approached as a form of psychological adaptation to prolonged and uncontrollable environmental challenges or whether fatigue is a manifestation of depression and/or a dysfunctional neurohormonal system. Future multidisciplinary research will continue to add to our understanding of the role of stress and other psychological factors in the origins, mental and somatic consequences, and treatment of fatigue, particularly in conditions in which fatigue is a known predictor of adverse medical prognosis.

See Also the Following Articles

Burnout; Chronic Fatigue Syndrome; Depression Models; Sleep Loss, Jet Lag, and Shift Work; Sleep, Sleep Disorders, and Stress; Workplace Stress; Night Shift-work; Posttraumatic Stress Disorder – Clinical; Posttraumatic Stress Disorder – Neurobiological basis for.

Further Reading

American Psychiatric Association (1994). *Diagnostic and statistical manual of mental disorders* (4th edn.). Washington DC: American Psychiatric Association.

Appels, A. (1990). Mental precursors of myocardial infarction. *British Journal of Psychiatry* **156**, 465–471.

Appels, A. (1997). Depression and coronary heart disease: observations and questions. *Journal of Psychosomatic Research* **43**(5), 443–452.

Appels, A., Bar, F., van der Pol, G., et al. (2005). Effects of treating exhaustion in angioplasty patients on new coronary events: results of the Randomized Exhaustion Intervention Trial (EXIT). *Psychosomatic Medicine* **67**(2), 217–223.

Berkman, L. F., Blumenthal, J., Burg, M., et al. (2003). Effects of treating depression and low perceived social support on clinical events after myocardial infarction: the Enhancing Recovery in Coronary Heart Disease Patients (ENRICHD) Randomized Trial. *Journal of the American Medical Association* **289**(23), 3106–3116.

Chrousos, G. P. (1995). The hypothalamic-pituitary-adrenal axis and immune-mediated inflammation. *New England Journal of Medicine* **332**(20), 1351–1362.

Kop, W. J. (1999). Chronic and acute psychological risk factors for clinical manifestations of coronary artery disease. *Psychosomatic Medicine* **61**(4), 476–487.

Kop, W. J. (2003). The integration of cardiovascular behavioral medicine and psychoneuroimmunology: new developments based on converging research fields. *Brain, Behavior & Immunity* **17**(4), 233–237.

Krupp, L. B. (2003). Fatigue in multiple sclerosis: definition, pathophysiology and treatment. *CNS Drugs* **17**(4), 225–234.

Maslach, C. and Jackson, S. E. (1986). *Maslach burnout inventory*. Palo Alto, CA: Consulting Psychologists Press.

Sharpe, M. and Wilks, D. (2002). Fatigue. *British Medical Journal* **325**(7362), 480–483.

Siegrist, J. (1991). Contributions of sociology to the prediction of heart disease and their implications for public health. *European Journal of Public Health* **1**(1), 10–29.

Skapinakis, P., Lewis, G. and Mavreas, V. (2003). Unexplained fatigue syndromes in a multinational primary care sample: specificity of definition and prevalence and distinctiveness from depression and generalized anxiety. *American Journal of Psychiatry* **160**(4), 785–787.

Wagner, L. I. and Cella, D. (2004). Fatigue and cancer: causes, prevalence and treatment approaches. *British Journal of Cancer* **91**(5), 822–828.

Wessely, S. (1990). Old wine in new bottles: neurasthenia and "ME." *Psychology and Medicine* **20**(1), 35–53.

Fear

A Öhman
Karolinska Institutet, Stockholm, Sweden

This article is a revision of the previous edition article by A Öhman, volume 2, pp 111–115, © 2000, Elsevier Inc.

Components of Fear

Measures of Fear

Fear Stimuli

Fear Learning

Pathological Fear: Phobias

The Neurophysiology of Fear

Glossary

Agoraphobia	An intense fear and avoidance of situations in which one would be helplessly exposed in case of a panic attack.
Amygdala	A collection of interconnected nuclei in the anterior medial temporal lobe, which is the hub of the brain network controlling the activation of fear responses.
Autonomic nervous system	A part of the peripheral nervous system concerned with the metabolic housekeeping of organisms. In general, the activation of its sympathetic branch results in the expenditure of energy and the activation of the parasympathetic branch results in the restoration of energy.
Fear	The emotional state associated with attempts to cope with threatening events.
Social phobia	An intense fear and avoidance of being socially evaluated or scrutinized.
Specific phobia	An intense fear and avoidance of specific objects or situations.

Fear is an activated, aversive emotional state that serves to motivate attempts to cope with events that provide threats to the survival or well-being of organisms. The coping attempts are typically centered on defensive behaviors such as immobility (freezing), escape, and attack.

Components of Fear

A fear response comprises several partially independent components, such as subjective feelings (accessible through verbal reports), peripheral physiological responses, and overt behavior. In humans, the phenomenological quality of fear is best described as an aversive urge to get out of the situation. This is a familiar feeling for every human being and a frequent target for artistic representation.

Fear is closely associated with the activation of the autonomic nervous system. Depending on situational constraints, the direction of this activation may differ. If the threat is not imminent and appears stationary, the typical response is one of freezing or immobility. This is associated with enhanced attentiveness toward the environment and the potential threat stimulus and with a vagally mediated deceleration of the heart. If the threat is imminent or approaching, there is a pervasive mobilization of the sympathetic branch of the autonomic nervous system, including heart rate acceleration and increases in blood pressure and circulating catecholamines (primarily epinephrine) from the adrenal medulla. These responses lay a metabolic foundation for taxing overt reactions of flight or fight.

In terms of behavior, there is an important distinction between expressive and instrumental overt acts. Expressive behavior includes automatic tendencies to withdraw from the threat and a typical facial expression of fear. The latter is composed of elevated eyebrows, wide open eyes, and a mouth that is either slightly opened or shut with depressed mouth corners. Instrumental behavior primarily concerns escape from and avoidance of the fear stimulus.

Measures of Fear

Measures of fear can be readily derived from the various components of fear. The intensity of the subjective component of fear can be directly assessed through ratings that may be anchored, for example, at a zero level of no fear at all, with a maximal level of fear corresponding to the most intense fear ever experienced by the subject.

Many fear indices have been derived from effectors innervated by the autonomic nervous system. Some of these measures, such as heart rate deceleration and skin conductance responses, are primarily related to the increased attentiveness associated with the initial stages of fear. Other measures, such as increases in heart rate or blood pressure, reflect the sympathetic mobilization that supports active coping attempts. Endocrine indices are available from the adrenal medulla and the adrenal cortical hormones. Measures among the former, such as circulating epinephrine, are often assumed to index successful coping, whereas measures from the latter, such as cortisol, are regarded as related to failing coping attempts.

Many behavioral measures have been used to assess fear. Typically they focus on avoidance behavior. For example, in a standard behavioral avoidance test to assess specific human fears, subjects are encouraged to approach their feared object as close as they dare, and the minimal achieved distance (touching included) is taken as inversely related to avoidance. In animals, the strength of escape behavior or the duration of freezing responses can be measured, depending on the experimental situation. In rodents, who typically freeze when fearful, the effect of a fear stimulus can be assessed by its interfering effect on a regular background behavior, such as operant lever pressing for food rewards on a variable interval schedule.

On the premise that defensive reflexes are primed by an induced fear state, the modulation of such reflexes by fear stimuli can provide accurate information about fear both in animals and humans. Typically, the startle reflex is studied using whole-body startle in rodents and the eyeblink component of startle in humans. The typical result is an enhancement of the startle reflex to a standard startle probe stimulus (e.g., a white noise with abrupt onset) when it is presented against a background of a fear stimulus compared to when the probe is presented alone.

It is important to realize that different measures of fear are not necessarily highly intercorrelated, even when assessing the effects of a common fear stimulus. This is because the fear response is better conceptualized as a loosely coupled ensemble of partially independent response components, sensitive to various modulating parameters, than as a unitary internal state mechanically elicited by the appropriate fear stimulus.

Fear Stimuli

There are innumerable events and situations that are feared by humans. Loosely speaking, they have in common that they provide a threat to the integrity of the individual, either in a physical or in a psychological sense. Many of the stimuli that are feared by humans are feared by other mammals as well. They include, for instance, loud noises, predators, and dominating conspecifics.

Classification of Fear Stimuli

In general, behaviors can be classified as communicative or noncommunicative depending on whether they elicit an active response from the environment. Communicative behavior is directed toward other living creatures, whereas noncommunicative behavior is directed toward the physical environment. Communicative behavior can be further subdivided into behavior directed toward members of another species, such as in predator–prey relationships, and members of the own species in what is commonly regarded as social behavior. Applied to fear, this classification system distinguishes among fear of physical stimuli, fear of animals, and social fears.

Physical stimuli Humans and other animals fear many types of physical stimuli, particularly those that may inflict tissue damage, thus inducing pain. A primary stimulus dimension is that of intensity. Highly intense stimuli of any modality may induce pain, and certainly they elicit fear and associated attempts to escape in most animals. Complex events that incorporate high-intensity stimulation, such as lightning and thunder, often evoke intense fright. But there are other complex events or situations whose fear-eliciting power is less directly dependent on simple stimulus dimensions. The effectiveness of such situations can be understood only in relation to the recurrent threat they have provided throughout evolution. Examples that come to mind include heights, small enclosures, wide-open spaces, and darkness or light (for species primarily active in daylight or at night, respectively).

Animal stimuli Species typically share ecological niches, and thus the presence of other animals has been a shaping force in evolution. Species compete for similar food supplies, and in predation, one species provides the food supply for another. In this latter case, avoiding capture as prey is a prerequisite for reproduction; therefore, potential prey species fear their predators. There is also a widespread fear of potentially poisonous animals, such as snakes, spiders, and insects, and these fears may be better represented as fear of (and disgust for) contamination rather than as fear of the animal itself.

Social stimuli No animal is more dangerous to humans than other humans; the most dangerous predators are humans who are ready to use violence to exploit the resources of other humans. Conflicts with fellow humans, however, are not restricted to fights about tangible resources. Typically they deal with something more abstract, but also more pervasive – power. Like other primates, human groups are structured in terms of dominance, that is, some members dominate others. Fear is part of the submissiveness shown by the dominated group members when confronting a dominant conspecific. This fear is not automatically connected to escape or (least of all) to attack, but it is shown in a readiness to emit signals of submissiveness and in refraining from competition. In humans (and other primates), it denotes a fear of being negatively evaluated, of losing face in front of the group, rather than of physical harm.

Moderating Factors

Several general dimensions modify the fear elicited by these types of fear stimuli. One of them is closeness. In general, the closer the fear stimulus, the stronger the fear response. This may, in fact, provide an explanation for the effect of stimulus intensity on fear – an intense stimulus is likely to be very close. Prey animals (e.g., gazelles) show a minimal reactive distance before they overtly take notice of a predator (e.g., a lion). If the predator is far away or appears to be resting, it is monitored only by increased attention. If it gets closer or appears to be hunting, the attention enhancement is accompanied by defenses such as immobility. When the predator gets dangerously close, finally, there is active defense such as flight.

A second moderating factor is movement of the stimulus and the direction of the movement. Approaching objects, in general, elicit more fear than stationary objects or objects moving away. For example, more fear is generated by a fearsome authority figure who is heading in our direction than by one who is heading in another direction.

A third class of moderating factors involves predictability and/or controllability of the fear stimulus. An abruptly occurring stimulus is, by definition, not predicted and elicits immediate fear. Fear stimuli that are predictable may also be behaviorally controlled, for example, through avoidance. Less predictable or controllable stimuli elicit more fear. However, it is only reasonable to talk about increasing fear as long as the uncontrollability does not completely undermine the coping attempts. When the situation is too uncontrollable to support active attempts to cope, fear is replaced by anxiety, and when the organism eventually gives up and becomes helpless, anxiety is replaced by depression (see **Anxiety**).

Fear Learning

Events such as obstructed breathing, physical constraints, and rapidly approaching large objects can be regarded as innate fear stimuli and may be called natural fear triggers. However, even though evolution has equipped us with defenses for a number of events that have threatened our survival in the long past of our species, modern humans, for good reason, fear many stimuli that simply were not around during our evolution. Thus, these stimuli must have acquired their fear-eliciting power through learning. They may be called learned fear triggers.

Pavlovian conditioning is the central mechanism for associative fear learning. Through Pavlovian conditioning, a natural fear trigger may transfer its potential to a new, previously neutral stimulus, thus turning it into a learned trigger. The procedure for achieving this is simply to present the two stimuli together, so that the to-be-learned trigger serves as a signal for the natural trigger. This is direct Pavlovian conditioning, but the procedure also works in a social arrangement in which one individual sees another individual express intense fear of the to-be-learned trigger. In this way, fear may transfer to new stimuli and circumstances, and, particularly for a species that has access to language, with its associative structure, this means that fear may come to be elicited from large classes of new stimuli only remotely associated with the original natural trigger.

An interesting possibility is that fear is more easily transferred to some stimuli that by themselves do not elicit fear, even though throughout evolution they have occurred in threat-related contexts. However, because of this long historic association with threats to survival, they may be evolutionarily prepared to enter easily into association with fear after only minimal aversive experience. For example, even though rhesus monkeys do not show an innate fear of snakes, they easily learn such fear after seeing conspecifics in fearful interactions with snake-related stimuli. Similar easy fear learning to neutral stimuli such as flowers is not obvious.

Pathological Fear: Phobias

Fear may sometimes be excessive to the extent that it interferes with normal adaptive functioning. Intense, involuntary, and rationally unfounded fear of a specific object or situation that provokes maladaptive avoidance is called a phobia. Phobias are classified into three categories depending on the feared object or situation.

Specific Phobias

Specific phobias concern circumscribed objects or situations, such as knives, other sharp objects, and dental treatments. One subgroup of specific phobias involves nature fears, such as fears of water or thunderstorms. Another important category centers on fear of animals; snakes, spiders, dogs, cats, and birds are typical examples. A third category involves fear of blood, taking injections, and mutilated bodies. Contrary to other anxiety disorders, which often incorporate a fear of fainting, this type of phobia is the only one actually associated with fainting as a result of a pronounced vasovagal response to exposure to the phobic situation.

Social phobias Some people tremble at the mere thought of meeting new people or having to formally address a group. In general, they fear social situations that involve being scrutinized or evaluated by others and the associated risk of being socially humiliated. Social phobia is more debilitating than specific phobia because social situations are central to human adjustment. For example, consistently avoiding such situations or enduring them only with intense dread may be detrimental both to academic and vocational careers.

Agoraphobia Agoraphobia (from the Greek *agora*, which means marketplace) denotes an intense fear of being out among people in crowded places such as in supermarkets or on public transportation vehicles. However, the fear is less concerned with this particular situation than with an intense fright of being overwhelmed by fear or anxiety in a situation in which no help or assistance is available; the common denominator is that the person would be left helpless without any escape route back to safety in the event of a sudden fear attack. Safety typically is defined as being at home, and thus many agoraphobics become captives in their homes, only able to leave if accompanied by a trusted companion.

Preparedness and Phobias

It is reasonable to assume that phobias derive primarily from learned fear triggers. Even though phobias are fairly common in the population, the overwhelming majority does not show a phobia-level fear of, say, snakes, knives, blood, underground trains, or airplanes. Thus, the assumption that phobics somehow have associated fear to the phobic situation is readily invoked. If this were the case, we would expect a correlation between common ecological traumas and phobias. However, there is an obvious discrepancy between the distribution of phobic situations and the distribution of traumas in our environment. For example, many people have aversive experiences with broken electrical equipment, but there are few bread-toaster phobics needing clinical assistance. On the other hand, clinicians encounter many spider and bird phobics, even in environments completely lacking poisonous spiders or threatening birds. This discrepancy between traumas and phobias can be accounted for by the preparedness hypothesis because phobic objects and situations appear more obviously related to threats in an evolutionary than in a contemporary perspective. In fact, most phobic situations (animals, heights, enclosures, dominant conspecifics, lack of escape routes, etc.) have provided recurrent threats to humans and our predecessors throughout evolution. As a result, humans may have become biologically predisposed easily to associate such situations with fear even after only minimal trauma. Nonprepared situations, such as cars, on the other hand, may not come to elicit fear even after having been paired with excessive traumas.

The Neurophysiology of Fear

Research during the last 2 decades has delineated a neural network in the brain that controls fear responses and fear learning. This network is centered on the amygdala, a small set of nuclei in the anterior temporal lobe that has long been identified as a limbic structure associated with emotion.

A primary role for the amygdala appears to be the evaluation of input to the brain in terms of its potential threat. This purpose is achieved by the lateral nucleus, which receives fully processed sensory information from the cortex as well as only preliminarily processed information from subcortical structures such as the thalamus. These two routes to the amygdala have been described as the high and the low routes, respectively. Because the low route depends on monosynaptic linkage between the thalamus and the amygdala, the incompletely processed information conveyed by this route reaches the amygdala faster than the polysynaptically wired information conveyed by the high route. As a consequence, the amygdala can start recruiting defense responses even before the veridicality of the threat stimulus is confirmed by the full cortical analysis.

The high route, therefore, is not necessary for eliciting fear, but the low route may be necessary both for fear elicitation and fear learning. Fear may be elicited and learned in animals even after the ablation of the relevant sensory cortices, and in humans, fear responses can be elicited and learned via stimuli that are prevented from conscious recognition through backward masking. Thus, fear responses are recruited after a quick and nonconscious analysis of the stimulus, which explains the automatic, nonvoluntary character of intense fear, such as in phobias.

After threat evaluation in the lateral and basolateral nuclei of the amygdala, the information is conveyed to the central nucleus, which controls various efferent aspects of the fear response. Neural pathways to the lateral hypothalamus activate sympathetically controlled responses, such as heart-rate acceleration and skin conductance responses, and parasympathetically dominated responses, such heart-rate decelerations, are influenced through the vagal motor nucleus and the nucleus ambiguus of the brain stem, which also can be controlled from the amygdala. Through connections between the central nucleus and the paraventricular nucleus in the hypothalamus, corticotropin releasing hormone can be released, which, via adrenocorticotropic hormone from the anterior pituitary, activates corticosteroid stress hormones from the adrenal cortex. Paths to the tegmentum, including the locus coeruleus, activate the dopaminergic, noradrenergic, and cholinergic arousal systems of the forebrain, resulting in electroencephalogram (EEG) activation and increased vigilance. Overt motor responses associated with fear such as freezing, fight, and flight are activated by connections between the central nucleus of the amygdala and the dorsal and ventral periaqueductal gray of the brain stem. The facial expressions of fear are activated through the facial motor nucleus and the seventh cranial nerve, the nervus facialis. The modulation of the startle reflex, finally, is accomplished through neurons connecting the central nucleus of the amygdala with the central nexus for the startle reflex, the nucleus reticularis pontis caudalis in the brain stem. This circuit accounts both for peculiarities of fear activation such as its independence of conscious recognition of the fear stimulus and the complex efferent organization of the fear response. Furthermore, its sensitization through various procedures may contribute to the understanding of pathological fear and anxiety.

See Also the Following Articles

Anxiety; Fear and the Amygdala.

Further Reading

Davis, M. and Whalen, P. J. (2001). The amygdala: vigilance and emotion. *Molecular Psychiatry* 6, 13–34.
Lang, P. J., Bradley, M. M. and Cuthbert, B. N. (1997). Motivated attention: affect, activation, and action. In: Lang, P. J., Simons, R. F. & Balaban, M. T. (eds.) *Attention and orienting: sensory and motivational processes*, pp. 97–135. Mahwah, NJ: Lawrence Erlbaum.
LeDoux, J. E. (1996). *The emotional brain*. New York: Simon & Schuster.
Öhman, A. and Mineka, S. (2001). Fears, phobias, and preparedness: toward and evolved module of fear and fear learning. *Psychological Review* 108, 483–522.
Rosen, J. B. and Schulkin, J. (1998). From normal fear to pathological anxiety. *Psychological Review* 105, 325–350.

Fear and the Amygdala

R Norbury
Warneford Hospital and University of Oxford, Oxford, UK
G M Goodwin
University of Oxford, Oxford, UK

Amygdala Anatomy
Afferent and Efferent Connections
The Amygdala and Fear Conditioning in Animals
The Amygdala and Fear in Humans

Glossary

Amygdala	A complex brain structure with numerous subnuclei located deep within the temporal lobe of the brain.
Backward masking paradigm	A paradigm in which an initial emotional face (e.g., fear) is presented for a very short duration (17–33 ms) and then immediately replaced by a neutral face presented for a longer duration (~200 ms). In this situation, the initial image is subliminal; subjects report that they have seen only the neutral expression.

Excitatory postsynaptic potential (EPSP)	A depolarization of the postsynaptic membrane.
Fear	An unpleasant, powerful emotion caused by anticipation or awareness of potential or actual danger.
Fear conditioning	A form of emotional learning in which an emotionally neutral or conditioned stimulus acquires the ability to elicit behavioral and physiological responses associated with fear after being associated with an aversive unconditioned stimulus.
Long-term potentiation (LTP)	The long-lasting strengthening of the connection between two neurons.
Neuroimaging	A number of powerful noninvasive techniques, including positron emission tomography (PET) and functional magnetic resonance imaging (fMRI), that allow the examination of regional patterns of brain activation in the living human brain with considerable spatial resolution, but limited temporal resolution, in the order of seconds as determined by vascular responses associated with neural activity.
Startle response	An innate reflex observed in nearly all animals, including humans, that manifests as an involuntary motor response to any unexpected noise, touch, or sight. In studies of emotion, it has been used to measure the aversiveness of emotive stimuli.

Amygdala Anatomy

The amygdala is an almond-shaped structure located deep within the temporal lobe of higher animals. It was first identified by Burdach in the early nineteenth century, who described a group of cells, or nuclei, now referred to as the basolateral complex. Subsequently, however, the amygdala was shown to be both more complex and more extended, comprising more than twelve subnuclei. In rats, current nomenclature divides the amygdala nuclei into three main groups: (1) the basolateral complex, which includes the lateral nucleus, the basal nucleus, and accessory basal nucleus; (2) the cortical nucleus, which includes the cortical nuclei and the lateral olfactory tract; and (3) the centromedial nucleus, comprising the medial and central nuclei.

Afferent and Efferent Connections

The amygdala receives input from all sensory systems: olfactory, somatosensory, gustatory, visceral, auditory, and visual. Olfactory inputs arise at the olfactory bulb and project to the lateral olfactory tract. Somatosensory inputs pass via the parietal insular cortex in the parietal lobe and via thalamic nuclei to the lateral, basal, and central nuclei. Primary gustatory and visceral sensory areas project to the basal nucleus and central nucleus. In contrast, auditory and visual information, thought to be important in fear conditioning, arise from association areas rather than from the primary sensory cortex.

The amygdala has widespread efferent connections to cortical, hypothalamic, and brain-stem regions. The basolateral complex projects to the medial temporal lobe memory system (e.g., the hippocampus and perirhinal cortex), and the basal nucleus has a major projection to prefrontal cortex, nucleus accumbens, and the thalamus. Thus, the anatomy of the amygdala is consistent with its role in fear processing. The amygdaloid complex receives inputs from all sensory modalities and activates brain regions important to measurable neurobehavioral correlates of fear. How it works offers an insight into the nature of emotion in humans and animals.

The Amygdala and Fear Conditioning in Animals

Much of the scientific interest in the amygdala stems from its established role in fear conditioning, research that has been carried out mostly in rats. Classical Pavlovian fear conditioning is a type of emotional learning in which an emotionally neutral conditioned stimulus (CS), often a tone, is presented in conjunction with an aversive unconditioned stimulus (US), typically a small electric shock to the foot of the animal. After one or more pairings, the emotionally neutral stimulus (CS) is able to elicit a constellation of species-specific conditioned responses (CRs) that are characteristic of fear, such as freezing or escape behavior, autonomic responses (elevated heart rate and blood pressure), potentiated acoustic startle to aversive acoustic stimuli, and increased neuroendocrine responses (release of stress hormones). Fear conditioning therefore allows new or learned threats to activate ways of responding to threat that have been long established in evolution.

Numerous studies have demonstrated that lesions to the amygdala impair the acquisition and expression of conditioned fear in rats. The basolateral complex of the amygdala is a substrate for sensory convergence from both the cortical and subcortical areas, and it is considered a putative locus for CS–US association during fear conditioning. Thus, its cells encode this emotional learning. By contrast, the central nucleus of the amygdala projects to brain regions implicated in the generation of fear responses, such as the hypothalamus; it may therefore act as a common output pathway for the generation of fear-conditioned responses. Consistent with this hypothesis, lesions to either the basolateral or central nucleus of the amygdala impair the both the acquisition and expression of conditioned fear.

The amygdala pathways involved in fear conditioning have also been studied using electrophysiological studies (see **Figure 1**). During fear conditioning, the convergence of CS and US inputs to the basolateral complex results in sustained enhancement, or long-term potentiation, of EPSPs evoked by the CS (**Figure 1**). Thus, the amygdala is able to both integrate and associate sensory information and influence the motor and physiological responses associated with fear conditioning.

The Amygdala and Fear in Humans

Evidence from Lesion Studies

Damage to the amygdala, or areas of the temporal lobe that include the amygdala, also produces deficits in fear processing in humans. In a recent study, a patient with Urbach–Wiethe disease (S.M.), a rare congenital lipoid storage disease that results in the bilateral degeneration of the amygdala, underwent fear conditioning with either visual or auditory CSs and a loud noise as the US. Compared to normal control subjects, S.M. showed no evidence of fear conditioning (as measured by galvanic skin response). Notably, S.M.'s recall of events associated with fear conditioning was intact. These data support the hypothesis that the amygdaloid complex plays a key role in the acquisition of Pavlovian fear conditioning, whereas the hippocampus is important in acquiring declarative knowledge of the conditioning

contingencies. In a further study with the same patient, it was demonstrated that bilateral amygdala damage impaired the recognition of fearful facial expressions. Other patients with Urbach–Wiethe disease have also been shown to be impaired in recognizing fearful facial expressions. S.M., however, had no difficulty in recognizing people by their faces or in learning the identity of new faces. These results suggest that the human amygdala is directly involved in the processing of emotion but not in recognizing aspects of facial appearance. There is also evidence to suggest that the impairment of the perception of expressive signs of fear in patients with amygdala damage extends beyond facial expressions; bilateral amygdala damage has also been associated with impairment in the recognition of vocalic expressions of threat.

The effect of amygdala damage on the startle response has also been studied in humans. A recent study compared the startle response in a 32-year-old male with a localized legion in the right amygdala with that of eight age-matched controls. The control subjects displayed the well-documented effect of aversive stimuli potentiating startle magnitude. In the patient with the right-amygdala lesion, no startle potentiation was observed in response to aversive versus neutral stimuli. Together, studies of patients with amygdala damage suggest that this structure plays a key role in the perception and production of negative emotions, particularly fear.

Evidence from Neuroimaging Studies

During the early 1990s, researchers began to explore the role of the amygdala in fear processing using neuroimaging (e.g., positron emission tomography, PET; and functional magnetic resonance imaging, fMRI) and continue to do so today. So far, amygdala activity has been assessed predominantly using two

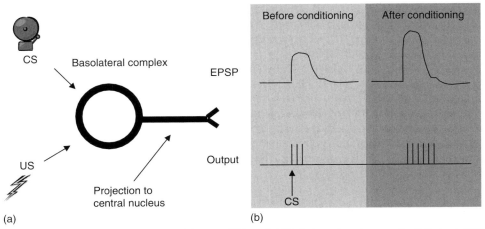

Figure 1 During fear conditioning convergence of inputs (CS and US) induce long-term potentiation of EPSPs evoked by the CS. a, Schematic; b, graphs. CS, conditioned stimulus; EPSPs, excitatory postsynaptic potentials; US, unconditioned stimulus.

basic paradigms: fear conditioning and presentation of emotional facial expressions.

Functional MRI experiments have demonstrated increased amygdala activity during both the early acquisition and early extinction of fear conditioning to a visual stimulus. Indeed, it has been suggested that the amygdala's role is limited to early conditioning or early extinction, when response contingencies change. That is, the amygdala is particularly important for forming new associations as relationships – emotional learning and unlearning.

The amygdala may also be responsible for generating coordinated reflexive behavioral responses to highly aversive stimuli. The animal literature shows that the amygdala, specifically the central nucleus, generates conditioned autonomic, behavioral, and endocrine responses in acute stress paradigms. CSs, which may be interpreted as changing the animal's emotional set, increase the response in startle paradigms, for example. Clearly, this kind of response may be quite primitive, but lesioning experiments demonstrated definite mediation by the amygdala. It is usually assumed the amygdala may be involved in the selection of more purposive motor-behavioral responses in response to more subtle aversive conditions.

The second major neuroimaging protocol for assaying amygdala activity is the presentation of faces expressing different emotions. It is difficult to overemphasize the importance of facial expressions in social communication. Facial expressions act at a number of levels to signal important information; expressions of disgust enable the avoidance of the ingestion of harmful substances, and fearful facial expressions rapidly communicate the presence of imminent threat. More subtly, cues from the faces

of others are continuously informing us of our social impact and acceptability, and we, in turn, communicate our feelings and intentions through our own facial gestures and expressions.

It is no surprise, therefore, that facial expressions have provided a useful experimental tool to measure fear-related amygdala activity. Many studies have demonstrated that the amygdala is preferentially activated during the presentation of fearful facial expressions. Moreover, even when subjects are unaware of seeing a fearful face, by the use of a masking protocol or when attention is directed away from the fearful face, the amygdala is still activated. Such findings suggest that the extraction of potentially threatening information within the amygdala may not be sufficient for conscious face perception but it may well be necessary. The amygdala may act to direct attention toward emotionally salient events that are ambiguous or require further processing. Indeed, anatomical studies in rats suggest that sensory information travels to the amygdala via two distinct pathways: a short, rapid thalamic route, and a longer cortical pathway. It is proposed that the short thalamic pathway rapidly prepares the animal for a potentially aversive encounter independent of conscious processing, which occurs later via the slower cortical route. A similar two-way route to the amygdala has yet to be anatomically defined in humans; however, evidence from a number of well-designed fMRI experiments point to the existence of these two pathways (**Figure 2**). First, as already described, the amygdala responds to fearful faces even when presented outside conscious awareness. Second, in an extension of the masking paradigm, Whalen and colleagues presented degraded versions of fearful and happy expressions

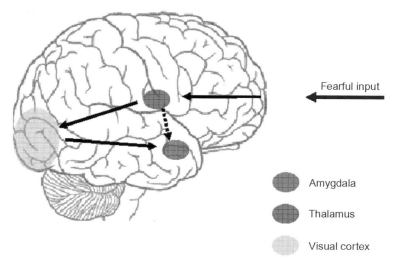

Fearful input

Amygdala

Thalamus

Visual cortex

Figure 2 Two-pathway hypothesis for amygdala activation to fear. The short, rapid thalamic route is shown by the dashed arrow; the longer cortical pathway is shown by bold arrows. (For clarity, subcortical structures are shown overlaid on brain surface.)

by displaying only the eye whites immediately masked by a complete image of a neutral expression. Fearful faces are typically associated with the enlarged exposure of the sclera, and it was observed that the crude information provided by the wide eyes of fearful expressions was sufficient to stimulate the amygdala. Analogously, Vuilleumier and coworkers used fMRI to compare amygdala and cortical responses to rapidly presented (200 ms) fearful and neutral faces that had been filtered to extract either low-spatial-frequency information (giving a blurry image) or high-spatial-frequency information (giving a finely detailed, sharp image) (**Figure 3**). As detected by fMRI, the finely detailed images elicited a greater response in a region of the cortex called the fusiform face area, a brain region widely implicated in the conscious recognition of faces and facial expressions. The amygdala was relatively unresponsive to these images even if they were fearful in nature. Low-spatial-frequency fearful faces, however, produced a robust response in the amygdala. Although these findings could imply the existence of a two-pathway route to the amygdala in humans, with dissociation between neural responses in amygdala and fusiform gyrus across different spatial frequency ranges for face stimuli, they do not prove it. However, they suggest that the amygdala does not require very complex configural stimuli, such as presented by the complete image of a face, in order to respond to emotion. It is obviously possible that crude fragmentary information related to emotionally salient signals could be rapidly communicated via a subcortical route. Extreme facial expressions of emotion may be well adapted to attract immediate attention via this mechanism.

Given the involvement of the amygdala in fear processing, there is increased interest in the role of this structure in anxiety disorders, such as post-traumatic stress disorder (PTSD), and obsessive-compulsive disorder (OCD), and in depression. For example, patients with PTSD show increased blood flow in the right amygdala (as measured by PET) in response to the presentation of images designed to activate traumatic memories, compared to neutral images. Using fMRI, it has also been demonstrated that individuals with OCD have significantly increased activity bilaterally in the amygdala in response to ideographically tailored stimuli designed to provoke their symptoms.

Functional MRI can also be used to investigate how pharmacological treatment for anxiety and depression modulates amygdala activity. A number of studies have demonstrated that the increased amygdala response to negative facial expressions seen in depression is reduced following effective treatment with serotonergic antidepressants. Although these results suggest an important role for the amygdala in the recovery from depression, it remains unclear if this normalization of amygdala response to fearful faces with time is a direct action of the drug or, rather, a reflection of the current symptom state (the scans of patients when depressed and when they had recovered were compared). Work from our laboratory, in healthy volunteers, demonstrated that the short-term administration (7 days) of either serotonergic (e.g., citalopram) or norepinepherine (e.g., reboxetine) antidepressants reduces the amygdala response to the masked expressions of fear compared to placebo controls. Significantly, these effects on the amygdala were observed in the absence of changes in mood. These

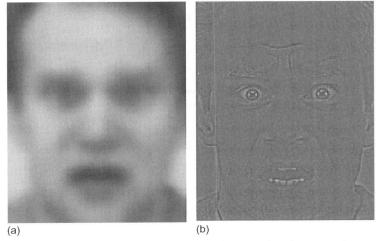

(a)　　　　(b)

Figure 3 Processing of images by the amygdala and cortical regions. a, Low-frequency image; b, finely detailed image. The rapid subcortical pathway may allow low-frequency inputs to reach the amygdala rapidly, whereas finely detailed images are further processed in cortical regions (e.g., fusiform gyrus).

results suggest that antidepressants have rapid, direct effects on the amygdala. Moreover, if similar effects are seen in clinical populations, drug modulation of amygdala activity in response to negative stimuli may be a key component in patients' recovery from depression and anxiety.

See Also the Following Articles

Anxiety; Fear; Posttraumatic Stress Disorder, Delayed; Posttraumatic Stress Disorder – Clinical; Posttraumatic Stress Disorder – Neurobiological basis for.

Further Reading

Harmer, C. J., Mackay, C. E., Reid, C. B., et al. (2006). Antidepressant drug treatment modifies the neural processing of nonconscious threat cues. *Biological Psychiatry* **59**, 816–820.

Ledoux, J. (2003). The emotional brain, fear, and the amygdala. *Cellular and Molecular Neurobiology* **23**, 727–738.

Phelps, E. A. and LeDoux, J. E. (2005). Contributions of the amygdala to emotion processing: from animal models to human behaviour. *Neuron* **48**, 175–187.

Sah, P., Faber, S. L., de Armentia, L., et al. (2003). The amygdaloid complex: anatomy and physiology. *Physiological Reviews* **83**, 803–834.

Vuilleumier, P., Armony, J. L., Driver, J., et al. (2003). Distinct spatial frequency sensitivities for processing faces and emotional expressions. *Nature Neuroscience* **6**, 624–631.

Whalen, P. J., Kagen, J., Cook, R. G., et al. (2004). Human amygdala responsivity to masked fearful eye whites. *Science* **306**(5704), 2061.

Febrile Response

S Gatti McArthur
F. Hoffmann-LaRoche, Basel, Switzerland
T Bartfai
The Scripps Research Institute, CA, USA

This article is a revision of the previous edition article by S Gatti McArthur and T Bartfai, volume 2, pp 116–123, © 2000, Elsevier Inc.

Introduction
Thermal Control in Endotherms
Endogenous Pyrogens and Fever Induction
Stress and Fever Induction

Glossary

Anterior hypothalamus/ preoptic area	Hypothalamic area representing the major center of control of the temperature set point of the body.
Basal metabolic rate	The minimal (or steady state) energy use, keeping the body temperature constant under conditions of no net work carried out.
Cytokines and interleukins	Small proteins with regulatory functions produced and secreted mostly by immunocompetent cells.
Endogenous pyrogens	Proinflammatory cytokines or endogenous compounds that function as humoral mediators of fever induction.
Hypothalamic-pituitary-adrenocortical axis	The central and peripheral system sustaining the physiological response to stressors.
Intraperitoneal and intracerebroventricular injections	Usual ways to administer exogenous pyrogens, i.e., lipopolysaccharide or endogenous pyrogens to study their peripheral and central proinflammatory effects.
Lipopolysaccharide	A fraction of the *Escherichia coli* bacterial wall used in different experimental models of gram-negative bacterial infection.
Thermoneutral zone	A range of ambient temperatures compatible with a control of the core body temperature achievable solely by cardiovascular changes in the peripheral compartment of the body.

Introduction

Fever is a transient change of the hypothalamic temperature (HT) set point causing the rise of the core body temperature (BT) of about 2–4°C in humans. This physiological response to inflammatory stimuli is always associated with peripheral and central events: massive hepatic production of acute-phase proteins, sleep induction, and anorexia, defined globally as the acute-phase response. Fever is triggered by the peripheral and central production of interleukin-1β (IL-1β), tumor necrosis factor α (TNF-α), and interleukin-6 (IL-6) and is caused by the local production of prostaglandins (PGE_2) in the anterior hypothalamus/preoptic area (AH/POA). The rise of the BT during febrile response is achieved by reducing heat loss (vasoconstriction) and by increasing simultaneously the heat production (facultative thermogenesis) via the activation of the sympathetic system. The sudden heat production associated with acute stress, usually described as hyperthermia, is also triggered by the activation of the sympathetic system. It is a common observation that subchronic, chronic, or exhaustive stresses are associated either with fever-like episodes or with an impairment of the whole inflammatory response. Experimental data demonstrate the endogenous production of IL-1β in rat hypothalamus during unescapable stress, pointing to the tight molecular control exerted by glucocorticoids (GCs) and corticotropin-releasing factor (CRF) on the production and effects of pyrogenic cytokines.

Thermal Control in Endotherms

Heat production is a sign of metabolic activity. Heat storage/heat exchange mechanisms are strikingly different in living organisms, resulting from the evolution of specialized systems (e.g., enzymes, organs, and cell types) required to survive and acclimate in different environmental conditions. **Figure 1** shows a summary of the mechanisms controlling thermal balance in endotherms. The core BT is the result of both heat production and heat exchange with the environment under the control of different pools of thermal sensors present in skin, viscera, main cardiovascular districts, spinal cord, and brain. The whole body can be divided in three main compartments (core, periphery, and skin), which regulate the exchange of heat mainly by modifying blood flow in the different districts. Cardiovascular, respiratory, and perspirative effects are always accompanied by behavioral changes in order to obtain an effective increase or drop of the BT. The main metabolic exothermic reactions contributing to heat production are listed in **Figure 1b**. The brown fat tissue (BAT), which is very rich in mitochondria, can produce heat by uncoupling the electron transport/proton gradient in the inner mitochondrial membrane thanks to the presence of uncoupling protein-1 (UCP-1) (nonshivering thermogenesis). Other gene products of the same family, UCP-2 and UCP-3, are expressed in white fat tissue/liver and in the muscular tissue, respectively. The contribution of UCP-2 to thermogenesis during fever is under debate.

Transient (or prolonged) temperature changes, observed during fever, have a deep metabolic impact, being associated with kinetic changes in all enzymatic reactions, in membrane conductance, and change

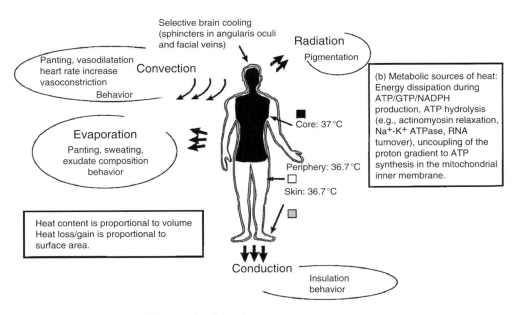

ATP, adenosine triphosphate; GTP, guanosine triphosphate;
NADPH, nicotinamide adenine dinucleotide phosphate; RNA, ribonucleic acid.

Figure 1 Schematic view of the mechanisms of heat production and heat exchange in endotherms. (a) Conduction, convection, radiation, evaporation, and metabolic heat production contribute in an additive manner to the definition of the temperature in the different districts of the body: skin, periphery, and core. The mechanism of selective brain cooling controls the facial venous flow in order to locally control the brain temperature by circulatory means. (b) The main exothermic metabolic reactions.

of permeability of ionic channels. Furthermore, to actively increase the BT of a human by 1°C within 1 h requires the net heat storage of about 3.48 J kg^{-1} with an energy cost for a human of 70 kg (in thermoneutral conditions) of about 243.6 J. GCs do support the metabolic heat requirements of the febrile response by enhancing several thermogenic reactions. Endogenous pyrogens (EPs) are also responsible for the metabolic changes observed during the acute-phase response. In particular leptin, a protein controlling white fat tissue metabolism and energy expenditure, exerts a necessary role in sustaining facultative thermogenesis during fever. Considering the energy required to mount a febrile response, it becomes understandable why starvation, cachexia, extreme ambient temperature, or other causes of metabolic distress would reduce the magnitude of the febrile response if not abolish it completely.

Temperature Set Point

Figure 2 shows effector systems activated in endotherms to keep the core BT constant while the ambient temperature changes progressively. During cold exposure, shivering is controlled by the activation of the motor system, whereas changes in superficial microcirculation and nonshivering thermogenesis are signs of the activation of the sympathetic system. The energetic requirement of the cold-induced thermal response is reduced progressively as the ambient temperature reaches the thermoneutral zone. Within this narrow range of temperatures, energy requirements to keep the BT constant (in absence of stress and motor activity) are met by the basal metabolic rate (BMR). The response to a warm environment is conversely characterized by vasodilatation, panting, and sweating. Shivering frequency and BMR are inversely correlated on a logarithmic scale with the body mass. Furthermore, the BMR is constantly adapted in different individuals in response to climatic conditions, diet, and motor activity under the control of the thyroid hormones. The BT in the different compartments and the range of temperatures triggering the effector systems in order to increase alternatively heat storage or heat loss are defined by the integration of thermoafferent signals and their comparison with a temperature set point defined in the AH/POA. Among the signals integrated in AH/POA, it is important to point at the local HT, reported by several studies as the stimulus able to overcome peripheral inputs. The local HT cannot fluctuate freely more than 0.1–0.2°C in a narrow range of temperatures that is defining the set point. Whatever change of the local temperature outside the limits of this range would trigger the effector response to a warm or cold environment (**Figure 2**). During fever the hypothalamic set point is shifted upward with a

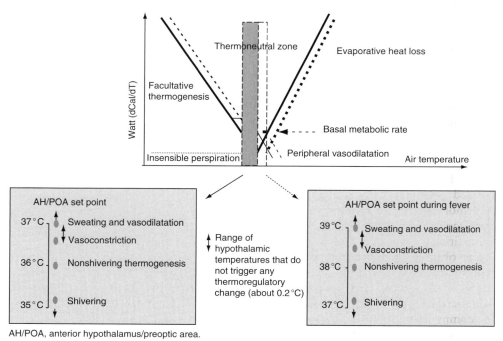

Figure 2 Thermal control in endotherms: the sympathetic and parasympathetic systems are alternatively activated by changes of the ambient temperature exceeding the thermoneutral zone in order to keep the core BT constant. The thermoneutral range is defined by the HT set point. The whole system is transiently shifted upward during fever.

reset of the range of HTs triggering the different effector responses. Because the body would need increased heat storage and heat production to reach the new temperature in the different districts, fever, in its initial phase, would cause a thermal response mimicking the normal reaction to a cold environment.

Thermosensitive Neurons

There are no known molecular markers for the neurons involved in the central control of the temperature set point. The only information available about the neuronal populations involved is that they share the common feature of being thermosensitive. Neuronal thermosensitivity (TS) can be characterized by measuring the neuronal firing rate in a paraphysiologic range of temperatures and calculating the thermal coefficient for each cell. The range of thermal sensitivity of AH/POA neurons may vary quite extensively and it is generally linear within a narrow range of temperatures. Two distinct populations of TS neurons have been characterized in the hypothalamus: cold-sensitive and warm-sensitive neurons. Cold-sensitive neurons are less studied, mostly because they represent less than 10% of the TS neurons in AH/POA. Warm sensitivity has been studied quite extensively using hypothalamic slices. These studies demonstrate that TS is an intrinsic cellular property. Warm-sensitive neurons are present in several brain regions: in AH/POA, in lower centers in the brain stem, and in the spinal cord. The presence of TS neurons in different brain regions may suggest temperature differences in the cerebral versus peripheral compartment. However, it has been demonstrated that thermal curves are similar both in time course and in absolute values in the cerebral cortex and the peritoneum under basal conditions, during fever, and pharmacological hypothermia.

Fever and Thermosensitivity

Fever depresses the TS of neurons whose firing rates had been increased previously by local AH/POA warming. Furthermore, local injections in the AH/POA of EPs or prostaglandin E2 (PGE$_2$) cause a reduction of the tonic firing of warm-sensitive neurons similar to the one observed when lowering locally the HT. The plasticity of warm-sensitive neurons and their responsivity to bath-applied IL-1 or IL-6 has yet to be characterized properly, and moreover, the molecular components of neuronal activity changes in AH/POA during fever have yet to be determined. Few studies reporting intracellular recordings from warm-sensitive neurons are opening up a key path of research in this respect.

Endogenous Pyrogens and Fever Induction

IL-1β was among the first cytokines described, and its biological properties as EP, the leukocytic pyrogen, were described long before the purification of the protein. In general, the concept of a humoral mediator of a fever response is older than the discovery of pro-inflammatory cytokines and was initially related to the observation that bacterial debris lipopolysaccharide (LPS) could cause fever with almost a 2-h delay from the time of the injection. The LPS effect was also characterized by priming and tolerance, further suggesting the presence of endogenous mediators. The progressive discovery of several pyrogenic cytokines present in the plasma only during an inflammatory reaction, and the study of their synergism and production in hypothalamus during a febrile response, further clarified the definition of EP. All EPs cause fever when administered by the intracerebroventricular (ICV) route and in the periphery and they are released into the circulatory system during the fever response to exogenous pyrogens. The magnitude and time course of the fever response could be related to the plasma and hypothalamic levels of the EP only in the case of IL-6. IL-1β or TNF-α seems to trigger the febrile response more than sustaining it because several endogenous antagonistic systems (such as IL-1 receptor antagonist (IL-1ra), in the case of IL-1α and IL-1β) are buffering or suppressing *in vivo* the initial EPs effects both peripherally and centrally (**Figure 3a**). The list of known EPs would then contain interferons (IFN-α, -β, and -γ), IL-1α/β, TNF-α/β, and IL-6. IL-1β is the most potent: a 30-ng kg^{-1} intravenous injection is sufficient to cause fever in humans. IL-6 and chemokines (IL-8, macrophage inflammatory protein-1) would trigger the fever response only when injected centrally into the AH/POA or ICV. The generation of mice carrying null mutations for the different EPs or their receptors has been extremely important in demonstrating the presence of a hierarchy of EP in the generation of the fever response, with IL-6 acting probably downstream of IL-1β and TNFα.

The most relevant results of the studies can be summarized as follows:

- Studies on IL-1 type 1 receptor (IL-1RI) knockout (KO) mice and IL-1R accessory protein (IL-1Rap) KO mice have demonstrated that IL-1RI mediates the fever response induced by an intraperitoneal (IP) injection of IL-1α and IL-1β. The fever response to LPS is rather normal in these animals, suggesting that TNF and other EPs can bypass the IL-1 system in the generation of the febrile response.

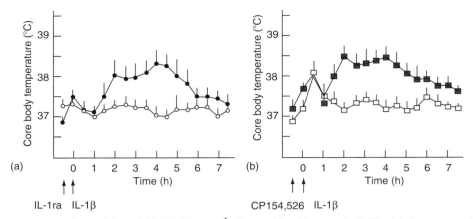

Figure 3 (a) Fever response in rats injected IP with 5 μg kg^{-1} of recombinant human IL-1β.The febrile response is blocked by the injection of recombinant human IL-1ra (2.5 mg kg^{-1}). (b) Fever response in rats injected IP with human recombinant IL-1β (5 μg kg^{-1}). The effect is blocked by the previous injection of the nonpeptidic CRF receptor antagonist CP154,526 (0.16 mg kg^{-1}, IP). Data are means $\pm$ standard error means. Data were recorded using a telemetry system and averaged every 30 min. Open circles, IL-1ra plus IL-1β (n = 5), closed circles, IL-1β (n = 3), open squares, CP154 526 plus IL-1β (n = 4), and closed squares, IL-1β (n = 8).

- IL-1β KO mice show hyperresponsive fever mostly in terms of magnitude of the effects in response to IL-1α and IL-1β IP injection.
- IL-6 KO mice are unable to mount a febrile response on injection of IL-1β or LPS in the periphery. Only the parallel co-injection of IL-6 IP seems to restore a sort of fever response to LPS IP injection. Very interesting genetic studies on different autoimmune familiar disorders like Mediterranean fever are pointing future research towards proteins such as pyrin and cryopyrins which are possibly upstream EP production.

Exogenous Pyrogens

The most used experimental model of fever response in the presence of an endogenous stimulus is represented by LPS injection in the periphery. This model mimics a response to gram-negative bacterial infections. Fever is also present during gram-positive bacterial infections because macrophages can produce somnogenic and pyrogenic muramyl peptides during the digestion of staphylococci fractions. Furthermore, agents such as turpentine are broadly used as an experimental model of aseptic inflammation, which is almost uniquely mediated by IL-1β. However, the broadest spectrum of exogenous pyrogens is offered by viral proteins 2 or by the etiological agents of parasitic infections such as schistosomiasis or malaria. In case of viral infections, interferons (IFNs) are the principal responsible of the observed febrile response with IL-1β contributing as EP. EP and Toll-like proteins responsive to exogenous pyrogens are probably present in all vertebrates. Equally ancient from the

phylogenetic point of view is the complement cascade of proteins which interact with EPs and EP production mainly via anaphylatoxins.

Expression of Endogenous Pyrogens and their Receptors in the Hypothalamus

IL-1α/β, TNF-α, and IL-6 gene expression can be induced in AH/POA on peripheral immune challenge (with LPS or IL-1β for instance). The peripheral administration of LPS induces IL-1β production in meninges, choroid plexus macrophages, some perivascular cells, and microglial cells shortly after IP injection (1–8 h). Constitutive expression of IL-1β and IL-6/IL-6R in neuronal cell types has been reported by some authors, but the matter is still controversial. Receptors for the different EPs, particularly IL-1RI, are expressed constitutively in AH/POA. Their expression is modulated by GCs and EP, particularly IL-1β. At the same time, pharmacological doses of corticosterone block the LPS-induced fever response and IL-1α/β and TNF-α mRNAs expression in the hypothalamus, suggesting a causal role for the hypothalamic production of cytokines in fever induction. The control by GC and EPs on the expression of EPs/EP receptors is mostly transcriptional. The promoter regions of EP genes contain an unusually high number of GC receptor response elements. In the case of IL-1β and TNF-α, posttranscriptional control of GC at the mRNA and proteic level has been demonstrated to be extremely important in controlling the cellular production of these EPs in immunocompetent cells and the activation/secretion of the mature form of these cytokines.

Humoral Versus Neuronal Mediators of Fever Induction

How does the brain sense EPs? This key question has several answers. In fact, circulating pro-inflammatory cytokines can reach the brain via the interaction with saturable carriers in the plexus chorioideus. However, this mechanism would account for the entrance of a limited amount of protein, eventually able to trigger local cytokine production AH/POA. Several pathologic conditions cause damage to the blood–brain barrier. In this case the amount of circulating EPs reaching the hypothalamus could be higher. There is also a specialized circumventricular organ, the organum vasculosum lamina terminalis (OVLT), located along the margin of the ventricular system that has fenestrated capillaries and, therefore, direct contact with the circulatory system. The role of the OVLT has been demonstrated in the case of peptides such as angiotensin II and cholecystokinin and is probably also essential for the transduction of the plasmatic levels of EPs into central effects. A third mechanism of immune signaling, essential in the case of peritoneal immune challenge, is the peripheral stimulation of sensory nerves, particularly the afferent part of the vagus nerve. IL-1Rs are present in vagal paraganglia, chemosensory bodies, all along the course of the vagal nerve in the cervical region, and in thoracic and abdominal cavities. Subdiafragmatic vagotomy is able to block the central production of IL-1β in response to the IP injection of IL-1β or LPS. The immediate c-fos mRNA induction has been used to trace the neuronal pathway activated in response to the peripheral loading of LPS, and several studies would point to the presence of a selective activation of neurons in the hypothalamus (paraventricular nucleus, ventromedial POA), brain stem (A1 and A2 region), nucleus of the solitary tract, and ventrolateral medulla. In some cases the activated pathways represent antipyretic responses that are initiated during fever, such as the activation of neurons that contain α-melanocyte-stimulating hormone (α-MSH) and arginine-vasopressin.

Role of Prostaglandins in Fever

The role of prostaglandins (PG) of the E series in fever induction was first described by Milton and colleagues in 1970. PGs of the F class can also cause fever. Their effect is, however, mediated by the release of CRF. Both PG series are thus EPs. The fever response triggered by pro-inflammatory cytokines is always mediated by the local production in AH/POA of PGs. In fact, the pyrogenic effect of peripheral LPS and EPs can be blocked by cyclo-oxygenase inhibitors injected locally into AH/POA. A dense distribution of PGE$_2$-binding sites is present in the anterior wall of the third ventricle surrounding the OVLT in the rat brain. Moreover, a study on mice carrying a null mutation for the different PG receptors demonstrated that receptor EP3 selectively mediates the PGE$_2$-induced fever response in the presence of IL-1β or LPS. It is important to note that PG synthesis inhibitors are excellent antipyretic agents but have few or no effects on stress. So the picture is not complete. A missing link for fast hypothalamic events triggered by EPs could be the C2-ceramide pathway.

Stress and Fever Induction

Stress-induced fever can be measured using several experimental protocols of stress in rodents, e.g., unescapable stress or restriction. In some cases, it should be noted, however, that the stress response would modify the circadian rhythms of BT and that the results obtained should be normalized considering possible shifts of the circadian rhythm of the BT of the animals. The development of a fever response to certain kinds of stress is also confirmed by the increased expression in the hypothalamus and hippocampus of EPs; particularly IL-1β mRNA and protein. The effects of IL-1β on all the levels of the hypothalamus-pituitary-adrenocortical (HPA) axis are significant and very well characterized by several studies. IL-1β can activate CRF synthesis and release and adrenocorticotropic hormone (ACTH) secretion acting locally at the hypothalamic and pituitary level, respectively. Hence, IL-1β is one of the few known agents able to induce CRF release, although the direct effect of IL-1β on the production/release of GC is still controversial. In contrast, the GC effect on cytokine production is dual and depends on the circulating levels of GC. In fact, physiological levels of GC would support the metabolic requirement of the acute-phase reaction, leading also to increased GC production as the HPA is activated. As a result, the increased GC release during inflammation buffers the pro-inflammatory cytokine effects by restricting their expression. A special note should, however, be taken while discussing the effect of GC on IL-6. In rodents, IL-6 mRNA expression is higher in the hypothalamus after chronic treatment with high doses of corticosterone, and mice overexpressing IL-6 in astrocytes exhibit higher plasmatic levels of corticosterone, reduced ACTH response, and adrenal hyperplasia. This may suggest a direct effect of IL-6 at the level of the adrenal glands. Furthermore, both IL-6 and GC are responsible for the production of different sets of hepatic proteins carrying GC-responsive elements and nuclear factor–IL-6 response elements in the promoter region of their genes, and they are both probably involved in controlling the duration and the magnitude of the acute-phase response. Increased plasmatic cytokine levels during stress have been explained considering the possible bacterial translocation from the gastrointestinal tract to the mesenteric lymph nodes.

The presence of this phenomenon is, however, seldom considered when planning an experimental protocol, and the impact of bacterial translocation on central and peripheral IL-1 production has not yet been characterized clearly. When examining the activation of the HPA axis during fever response, it is important to keep in mind that a central role is played by CRF and vasopressin. Central injection of CRF causes fever in rats and it also activates thermogenesis in the BAT. Furthermore, neutralizing antibodies to CRF or synthetic CRF antagonists block the pyrogenic response associated with IL-1β or TNF injection (**Figure 3b**). CRF plays a necessary but indirect role in the development of the fever response. Vasopressin is an endogenous antipyretic hormone. New synthetic selective antagonists will possibly allow in the future a better understanding of which receptor is mediating fever and HPA-axis effects.

Finally, the role of the sympathetic system in the development of stress or the cytokine-induced thermal response has to be redefined on the basis of the demonstrated presence of the constitutive production of IL-1β and IL-6 in the sympathetic ganglia and in adrenal medulla. *In vivo* during an inflammatory reaction and fever induction, the presence of EP and EP receptors at different levels can ensure a tight control on the activation of the sympathetic system in terms of magnitude and duration of the effect based on the presence of a local or systemic inflammatory reaction.

See Also the Following Articles

Homeostasis; Hyperthermia; Hypothermia; Prostaglandins.

Further Reading

Chai, Z., Alheim, K., Lundkvist, J., et al. (1996). Subchronic glucocorticoid pretreatment reversibly attenuates IL-1 beta induced fever in rats; IL-6 mRNA is elevated while IL-1 alpha and IL-1 beta mRNAs are suppressed, in the CNS. *Cytokine* **8**, 227–237.

Dinarello, C. (1998). Interleukin-1, interleukin-1 receptors and interleukin-1 receptor antagonist. *International Review of Immunology* **16**, 457–499.

Elmquist, J., Scammell, T. and Saper, C. (1997). Mechanisms of CNS response to systemic immune challenge: The febrile response. *Trends in Neurosciences* **20**, 565–570.

Kluger, M. (1991). Fever: role of pyrogens and cryogens. *Physiological Reviews* **71**, 93–127.

Lundkvist, J., Chai, Z., Teheranian, R., et al. (1996). A non peptidic corticotropin releasing factor receptor antagonist attenuates fever and exhibits anxiolytic-like activity. *European Journal of Pharmacology* **308**, 195–200.

Nguyen, K. T., Deak, T., Owens, S. M., et al. (1998). Exposure to acute stress induces brain interleukin-1beta protein in the rat. *Journal of Neuroscience* **18**, 2239–2246.

Rolfe, D. and Brown, G. (1997). Cellular energy utilisation and molecular origin of standard metabolic rate in mammals. *Physiological Reviews* **77**, 731–758.

Sanchez-Alavez, M., Tabarean, I. V., Behens, M. M., et al. (2006). Ceramide mediates the rapid phase of febrile response to IL-1beta. *Proceedings of the National Academy of Sciences USA* **103**, 2904–2908.

Schobitz, B., Reul, J. and Holsboer, F. (1994). The role of the hypothalamic-pituitary-adrenocortical system during inflammatory conditions. *Critical Reviews in Neurobiology* **8**, 263–291.

Schonbaum, E. and Lomax, P. (eds.) (1990). *International encyclopedia of pharmacology and therapeutics, sect. 131, Thermoregulation: physiology and biochemistry.* New York: Pergamon Press.

Kluger, M. J., Kozak, W., Leon, L. R., et al. (1998). Fever and antipyresis. In: Sharma, H. S. & Westman, J. (eds.) *Brain function in hot environment. Progress in brain research* (vol. 115), pp. 465–475. Amsterdam: Elsevier Science.

Sundgren-Andersson, A., Gatti, S. and Bartfai, T. (1998). Neurobiological mechanisms of fever. *Neuroscientist* **4**, 113–121.

Sundgren-Andersson, A. K., Ostlund, P. and Bartfai, T. (1998). Simultaneous measurement of brain and core temperature in the rat during fever, hyperthermia, hypothermia and sleep. *Neuroimmunomodulation* **5**, 241–247.

Ting, J. P., Kastner, D. L. and Hoffman, H. M. (2006). CATERPILLERS, pyrin and hereditary immunological disorders. *Nature Reviews Immunology* **6**, 183–195.

Ushikubi, F., Segi, E., Sugimoto, Y., et al. (1998). Impaired febrile response in mice lacking the prostaglandin E receptor subtype EP3. *Nature* **392**, 281–284.

Feedback   *See:* Glucocorticoid Negative Feedback; Feedback Systems.

Feedback Systems

G Fink
Mental Health Research Institute, Parkville, Victoria, Australia

This article is a revision of the previous edition article by G Fink, volume 2, pp 124–137, © 2000, Elsevier Inc.

Introduction

Overview

Interaction between Negative Feedback and Circadian Rhythm in the HPA System

Corticosteroid Feedback on the Hypothalamus and Pituitary Gland: Phase Differences

Glucocorticoid Feedback Effects on Stress Neurohormone Biosynthesis

Role of Atrial Natriuretic Peptide in Glucocorticoid Inhibition

Role of Hippocampus and Amygdala in Glucocorticoid Negative Feedback

Glucocorticoid Negative Feedback at the Pituitary Level

Possible Role of 11β-Hydroxysteroid Dehydrogenase

Functional Importance of Glucocorticoid Negative Feedback

Clinical Manifestations of Disordered Glucocorticoid Feedback Regulation of the HPA System

Allostasis and Allostatic Load

Conclusion

Glossary

Allostasis — Maintaining stability (or homeostasis) through change; term introduced by Sterling and Eyer in 1988 to describe cardiovascular adjustments to resting and active states.

Homeostasis — The maintenance of equilibrium, or constant conditions, in a biological system by means of automatic mechanisms (generally feedback systems) that counteract influences (stressors) that tend toward disequilibrium (term introduced by Walter Cannon in 1932).

Hypercortisolemia — Excessively high concentrations of adrenal corticosteroids in plasma.

Hypophysial portal vessels — A group of small venules that connect a primary plexus of capillaries in the median eminence of the hypothalamus (base of the brain) with a secondary plexus of sinusoids in the pituitary gland. Blood flowing in these vessels, which run down the pituitary stalk, transports hypothalamic-pituitary regulatory neurohormones, released at nerve terminals in the median eminence of the hypothalamus, to the anterior pituitary gland, where they stimulate or inhibit the release of anterior pituitary hormones.

Limbic system — An extensive brain region that includes the cingulate and parahippocampal cortex, hippocampus, amygdala, hypothalamus, septal nuclei, and other structures. The precise interaction of the several components of the system is poorly understood, but since the proposal by Papez, the limbic system has been implicated in emotion. The connections between the limbic system and the neocortex, hypothalamus, and the olfactory bulb via the olfactory tract suggest that it serves as an important analyzer-integrator of signals, which it conveys from the neocortex to the hypothalamus. The input of olfactory information to the limbic system has led to its alternative name, the rhinencephalon (olfactory brain), and possibly reflects the strong emotive and signaling effects of smell in many animals. The structure and relative size of the limbic system have remained remarkably constant through evolution; in humans it is overshadowed by the massive development of the neocortex.

Neurohormones — Chemical neurotransmitters released from nerve terminals into the hypophysial portal vessels or the systemic circulation at neurohemal junctions and conveyed to their target cells by the blood stream. This contrasts with classical neurotransmitters that reach receptors on target cells by crossing synaptic clefts or neuromuscular junctions.

Suprachiasmatic nuclei — Two small hypothalamic nuclei located immediately above (dorsal to) the optic chiasm that are responsible for regulating most circadian rhythms of the body.

Introduction

Feedback control systems are fundamental for the normal physiological functioning of the body. There are two types of feedback, negative and positive, of which the former is the more common. Removal of the main pituitary target glands, the adrenals, gonads, and thyroid, the most reproducible and reproduced experiment in classical endocrinology, demonstrates that the secretion of pituitary adrenocorticotropin (ACTH), gonadotropins, and thyrotropin is controlled by negative feedback exerted by the adrenal corticosteroids, gonadal steroids, and thyroid hormones, respectively. Interruption of the negative feedback loop caused, for example, by surgical or pharmacological adrenalectomy, gonadectomy, or thyroidectomy, or an enzymatic defect in steroid or thyroid hormone biosynthesis, results in massive hypersecretion of pituitary ACTH, gonadotropin, or thyrotropin.

Crucial for homeostasis, negative feedback control mechanisms are composed of a system in which the output moderates the strength of the controller to a predetermined set point level (**Figures 1** and **2**). The set point–stimulator complex contains a comparator (error detector), which compares the strength of the feedback signal with a preset level. An increase in the strength of the feedback signal above the preset level reduces the output of the stimulator, whereas a decrease in the strength of the feedback signal below the preset level results in an increase in output of the feedback signal and corrects the error. Negative feedback control operates widely throughout the body at the molecular (e.g., end product inhibition of enzyme activity), cellular, and whole system/body levels. The mechanisms by which the set point is determined vary between systems: in the case of the hypothalamic-pituitary-adrenocortical (HPA) feedback system, the set point is regulated by the central nervous system. GABAergic and glutamatergic neural projections from the limbic system and other brain regions to the paraventricular nuclei (PVN) of the hypothalamus may play a key role in HPA set point regulation.

Positive feedback, whereby the output of a system increases the output of the stimulator (gain in the system) (**Figure 2b**), is far less common than negative feedback, possibly because taken to its logical conclusion, a positive feedback system, uncontrolled, will eventually self-destruct. Some systems loosely termed positive feedback are, in fact, servomechanisms. A servomechanism is a closed loop control system, which increases significantly the power of a small signal. Positive feedback is exemplified by (1) estrogen stimulation of gonadotropin secretion, which results in ovulation, and (2) the release of oxytocin induced during parturition by pressure of the fetal head on the uterine cervix. The latter triggers volleys of impulses that, by way of a multisynaptic pathway to the hypothalamus, stimulate oxytocin release. Oxytocin stimulates further contraction of the uterus, which results in a further increase in pressure on uterine cervix. This vicious cycle is broken only when the fetus is expelled. Servomechanisms are illustrated by the way that, just before ovulation in humans as well as in other spontaneously ovulating mammals, elevated plasma estrogen concentrations increase the responsiveness of the anterior pituitary gland to gonadotropin-releasing hormone (GnRH) by 20- to 50-fold. This estrogen effect, reinforced by the priming effect of GnRH, whereby a small pulse of GnRH further potentiates pituitary responsiveness to itself, ensures the occurrence of a massive ovulatory gonadotropin

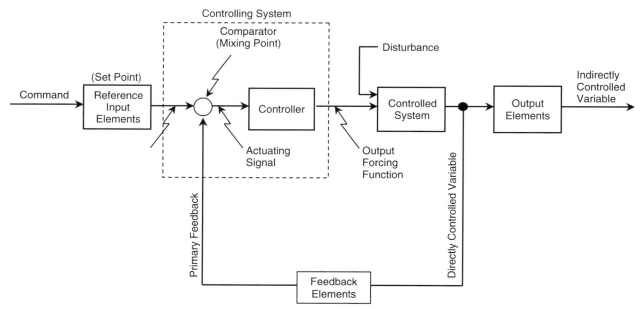

Figure 1 A generalized feedback control system. Modified from Milhorn, H. T. J. (1966). *The application of control theory to physiological systems,* with permission from Saunders, Philadelphia, PA.

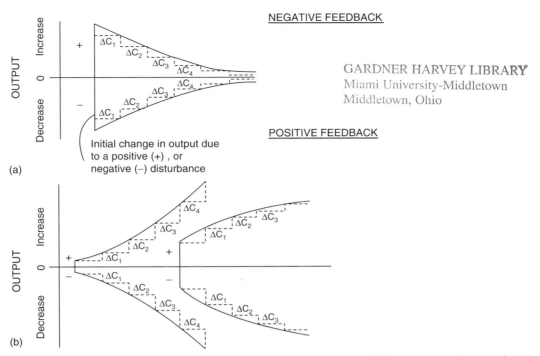

Figure 2 (a) Negative feedback minimizes the disturbance to a regulator, resulting in a system in which the output tends to remain constant. In this case, the ratios of the decrements of the controlled variable C (C_2/C_1, C_3/C_2) are less than unity. (b) In positive feedback (left-hand curves) an initial disturbance results in a continuous increase in output (vicious cycle). The increments of the controlled variable (C_2/C_1, C_3/C_2) are greater than unity. When the response does not result in a vicious cycle, the ratios of C_2/C_1, C_3/C_2, and so on are less than unity (see right-hand curves in B). From Milhorn, H. T. J. (1966). *The application of control theory to physiological systems,* with permission from Saunders, Philadelphia, PA.

surge in response to a small surge or increased pulse frequency of GnRH.

This article focuses on the principles of negative feedback control in the HPA system with emphasis on neurohormone and hormone release. While the discussion concentrates on negative feedback maintenance of homeostasis, the same mechanisms are involved in allostasis that is brought about by a change in set point so as to enable the organism to deal with the physiological challenge or stress.

Overview

In the normal state, with the negative feedback loop intact, the set point in the brain-pituitary module maintains the secretion of ACTH within a relatively narrow bandwidth. Within this bandwidth, the basal secretion of ACTH is pulsatile. Plasma ACTH concentrations also show a circadian rhythm, with a peak in the morning and a trough approaching a nadir around midnight. In nocturnal animals, such as rodents, the phase of this rhythm is reversed so that plasma ACTH concentrations reach a peak just before the onset of darkness. The circadian rhythm of ACTH results in a circadian rhythm in the plasma concentrations of adrenal corticosteroids: cortisol in

humans and corticosterone in rodents. A key feature in both diurnal and nocturnal animals is that corticosteroid plasma concentrations reach a peak just before the animal is due to wake from sleep; the levels are lowest just before or during sleep.

Glucocorticoids (cortisol in the human; corticosterone in rodents) secreted by the adrenal cortex exert their inhibitory action both on the brain and on the pituitary gland (**Figures 3** and **4**). The PVN of the hypothalamus contain the final common pathway neurons that mediate the neural control of pituitary ACTH synthesis and release (see **Secretagogue**). The PVN receive stimulatory and inhibitory neural inputs and an important projection from the suprachiasmatic nuclei (SCN), the key circadian oscillator in brain. PVN drive is mediated by stress neurohormones, corticotropin releasing factor-41 (CRF-41) and arginine vasopressin (AVP), which are released into hypophysial portal vessel blood. ACTH is released into the systemic circulation and stimulates adrenal corticosteroid synthesis and release. In keeping with revised standard nomenclature, CRF-41 will be abbreviated to CRH (corticotropin-releasing hormone).

The release of ACTH is pulsatile in humans and is cleared rapidly from the blood by both metabolic degradation and distribution into several body

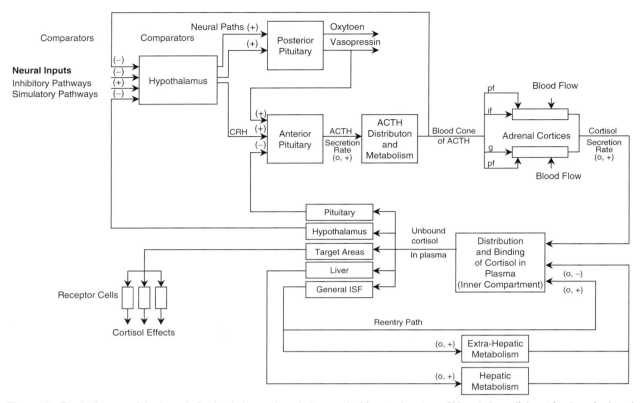

Figure 3 Block diagram of the hypothalamic-pituitary-adrenal glucocorticoid control system. Abbreviations: if, input forcing of adrenal by ACTH; pf, parametric forcing of adrenal (hypertrophic effect) caused by ACTH over a longer time period. The parametric effect of changes in adrenal blood flow is also indicated. The designators 0, + and 0, − indicate that signals in pathways are restricted in values (e.g., there are no negative masses or frequencies, and removal processes or inhibitors are negative in effects). From Yates, F. E. and Maran, J. W. (1975). In: Knobil, E. & Sawyer, W. H. (eds.) *Handbook of physiology* (pp. 367–404). Washington, D.C.: American Physiological Society, with permission.

compartments. The glucocorticoids are bound rapidly by albumin and a specific corticosteroid-binding protein, transcortin, and are metabolized by several organs, especially the liver and kidney (**Figure 3**). Only unbound (free) glucocorticoids inhibit ACTH release, and therefore the degree of glucocorticoid binding and metabolism, as well as the magnitude of adrenal secretion (**Figure 3**), determines the strength of the negative feedback signal. The HPA feedback system might also be influenced by a CRH-binding protein in plasma (first discovered by Orth and Mount in 1987). The physiological role of the CRH-binding (glyco) protein, which is synthesized in the liver, awaits to be determined – in humans, CRH-binding protein concentrations in plasma increase during the third trimester of pregnancy (see **Corticotropin Releasing Factor-Binding Protein**).

Interaction between Negative Feedback and Circadian Rhythm in the HPA System

The circadian rhythm of ACTH and (the consequent) glucocorticoid secretion, which has a peak at the end and a nadir at the beginning of the sleep phase, is driven by a neural mechanism mediated mainly by the stress neurohormones. The twofold increase in the ACTH signal between the nadir and the peak of the circadian rhythm in the rat results in a ninefold increase in corticosterone due to an increase in the responsiveness of the adrenal cortex.

In the unstressed state, the HPA system operates in an approximately linear domain with all the loop variables (**Figure 3**) showing circadian periodicity. Ultradian rhythms in plasma cortisol concentration, independent of ACTH concentration, occur in humans and rhesus monkeys, in which they are highly synchronized between animals with a predominant periodicity of 85–90 min.

The circadian rhythm of ACTH secretion is driven by the SCN. In addition to the diurnal rhythm of corticosterone, the SCN are involved in other key rhythms in the body, such as the sleep–wake cycle, motor activity, thermoregulation, pineal N-acetyl transferase activity, and the regular occurrence of ovulation. If any one of these functions is abnormal, then there is a high probability that the others will

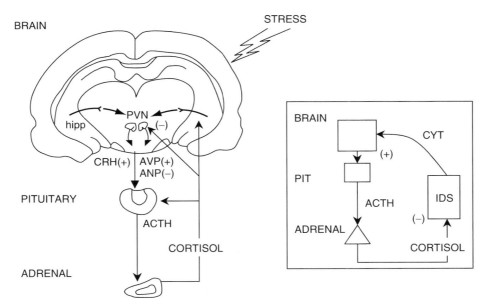

Figure 4 Schematic diagram of the elements involved in glucocorticoid negative feedback. The paraventricular nuclei (PVN) contain the main stress (final common pathway neurons) secreting both CRH and AVP. The negative feedback action of cortisol (corticosterone in rodents) is exerted mainly on the PVN and the pituitary corticotropes. However, long-term effects mediated through the hippocampus (Hipp) and amygdala (not shown) cannot be excluded. There are several possible indirect connections between the hippocampus and PVN. Neural control of ACTH secretion may also be mediated by a corticotropin inhibitory peptide, atrial natriuretic peptide (ANP). The inset shows the important inhibitory action of cortisol on the immune defense system (IDS). The IDS produces cytokines (CYT), which act on the brain to stimulate ACTH secretion. Cytokine secretion is inhibited by the negative feedback effect of glucocorticoids.

also be abnormal. The corticosterone rhythm is especially sensitive in that even partial lesions of the SCN, which have no effect on any of the other circadian functions, do disrupt the adrenal rhythm.

The SCN receive afferent projections from (1) the retina (direct as well as indirect after a relay in the ventral lateral geniculate nucleus), (2) the 5-hydroxy-tryptamine (5-HT) raphe neurons, and (3) the hippocampus by way of the medial corticohypothalamic tract. Each of these inputs to the SCN is likely to affect the periodicity of the pacemaker: the retinal input affects the time of the light–dark cycle; the hippocampal input may be related to the sleep–wake cycle; the raphe input may be related to paradoxical sleep. The raphe input also plays a major role in determining the amplitude of diurnal ACTH oscillations.

Although the central action of glucocorticoids is mainly on the PVN, the 5-HT neurons of the dorsal raphe nuclei, which project to the SCN, have high concentrations of glucocorticoid receptors. The SCN have direct projections to the PVN and may also affect PVN function by way of their projections to the subparaventricular zone. While circadian rhythmicity of the HPA is modulated by glucocorticoids and other factors, the intrinsic rhythmicity of the SCN circadian pacemaker is primarily under genetic control (see **Circadian Rhythms, Genetics of**).

Corticosteroid Feedback on the Hypothalamus and Pituitary Gland: Phase Differences

The seminal modeling studies of Eugene Yates and associates suggested that corticosteroid negative feedback on ACTH release occurs in three phases: a fast and immediate rate-sensitive phase of about 30 min, followed by a level-sensitive phase that occurs 2–3 h after the start of corticosteroid administration, followed by a long-term chronic phase. Fink and associates investigated the effect of corticosteroids on the release of stress neurohormones into hypophysial portal blood (see **Neuroendocrine Systems**) in the intermediate and chronic phase. They found that adrenalectomy induced a three- to fourfold increase in the release of both CRH and AVP into hypophysial portal blood. Administration of the synthetic glucocorticoid dexamethasone 2.5 h before portal blood collection significantly reduced the release of AVP, but not CRH (**Figure 5**), and also blocked the ACTH response to CRH (**Figure 6**). These findings suggest that intermediate-delayed (2–3 h) glucocorticoid feedback is mediated by the blockade of pituitary responsiveness to CRH and a reduction in AVP output into hypophysial portal blood. That is, in this situation AVP is the regulatory or signaling neurohormone,

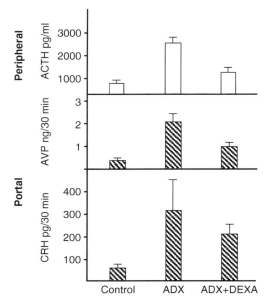

Figure 5 The delayed negative feedback action of glucocorticoid in adult female Wistar rats anesthetized with sodium pentobarbitone. ACTH was measured in plasma taken immediately before sectioning of the pituitary stalk for the collection of hypophysial portal vessel blood. Adrenalectomy (ADX) resulted in a fourfold increase in ACTH concentration and a similar increase in the output of AVP and CRH release relative to that in intact, untreated animals (control). The administration of dexamethasone (DEXA) significantly reduced the levels of ACTH and AVP, but not CRH. Modified from Fink, G., Robinson, I. C. A. F. and Tannahill, L. A. (1988). Effects of adrenalectomy and glucocorticoids on the peptides, CRF-41, AVP and oxytocin in rat hypophysial portal blood. *Journal of Physiology* **401,** 329–345, with permission of the authors and Cambridge University Press.

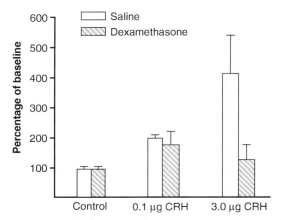

Figure 6 Mean (±SEM, *n* = 5) percentage increase over the basal concentration of ACTH after the injection of saline, 0.1 μg CRH, or 3 μg CRH. Female Wistar rats that had been adrenalectomized 3 weeks earlier were treated with either saline or dexamethasone 3 h before injection of CRH. Note that dexamethasone blocked the ACTH response to 3.0 μg of CRH. From Fink, G., Robinson, I. C. A. F. and Tannahill, L. A. (1988). Effects of adrenalectomy and glucocorticoids on the peptides, CRF-41, AVP and oxytocin in rat hypophysial portal blood. *Journal of Physiology* **401,** 329–345, with permission of the authors and Cambridge University Press.

Glucocorticoid Feedback Effects on Stress Neurohormone Biosynthesis

Glucocorticoids have potent inhibitory effects on CRH biosynthesis as well as release. Thus, adrenalectomy is followed by a significant increase in CRH mRNA levels in the parvocellular PVN, and this increase can be reduced by either corticosterone or dexamethasone. As assessed by CRH-intron *in situ* hybridization, the stimulation of CRH gene transcription can be detected as early as 15 to 30 min after the injection of the glucocorticoid synthesis inhibitor metyrapone. This increase in CRH gene transcription in the PVN was associated with a coincident increase in c-fos mRNA in the PVN. An increase in the levels of CRH mRNA in the PVN after metyrapone injection was delayed by about 60 min, possibly a function of the high resting levels of CRH mRNA and the time taken to assemble mRNA from the CRH primary transcript.

The effects of corticosterone and dexamethasone are dose dependent and can be demonstrated by systemic administration of the steroid, as well as by implantation of steroid pellets into the brain. This effect of glucocorticoids is cell specific in that the glucocorticoid-induced decrease in CRH mRNA was localized to the dorsomedial parvocellular neurons of the PVN, the major source of CRH fiber projections to the median eminence. In contrast, glucocorticoid increased the levels of CRH mRNA in parvocellular

whereas CRH is the permissive neurohormone. In contrast, studies on the long-term effects of corticosterone administered by a subcutaneous pellet suggested that long-term negative glucocorticoid feedback is due to a decreased release of CRH, as well as AVP, into portal blood. That is, both stress neurohormones are sensitive to the long-term effects of corticosteroids.

These findings agree broadly with those of Plotsky and associates, which showed that pharmacological adrenalectomy with metyrapone and aminoglutethimide (which block glucocorticoid biosynthesis) resulted in a significant increase in the release of both CRH and AVP into hypophysial portal blood. The intravenous infusion of corticosterone inhibited nitroprusside-evoked CRH release into portal blood, but had no effect on AVP release.

Data in the rat are complemented by those obtained in the sheep. Thus, the concentrations of CRH and AVP in hypophysial portal blood collected from conscious sheep were (1) similar to those in the rat, (2) increased by volume depletion, fear-associated audiovisual stimuli, and insulin-induced hypoglycemia, and (3) inhibited by dexamethasone.

neurons that project to the brain stem and the spinal cord. The implantation of dexamethasone micropellets in cerebral cortex, dorsal hippocampus, ventral subiculum, lateral septum, or amygdala had no effect on CRH mRNA levels in the PVN.

The molecular mechanism by which glucocorticoids regulate CRH gene expression remains unclear. Recent data show that the repressor isoform of cAMP response element modulator (CREM) is involved in CRH gene regulation, and that, *in vivo*, stress-induced glucocorticoids do not limit CRH gene transcription, in spite of the fact that the CRH promoter has a glucocorticoid receptor response element. The inhibitory effect of glucocorticoids on CRH gene transcription may be mediated, at least in part, by GABAergic, glutamatergic, and monoaminergic projections to the PVN from the forebrain and hindbrain limbic system.

The concentration of AVP mRNA in the dorsomedial parvocellular neurons of the PVN paralleled those of CRH mRNA, that is, levels increased after adrenalectomy and decreased after treatment with glucocorticoids. Corticosterone treatment also produced a modest reduction in the levels of enkephalin mRNA in all four regions of the PVN, but glucocorticoid manipulation had no significant effect on the PVN concentrations of the mRNAs for angiotensin, cholecystokinin, preprotachykinin, and tyrosine hydroxylase. There is, therefore, a close correlation between the synthesis and the release of CRH and AVP. Whether this means that synthesis and release are mechanistically coupled is not established.

Data on the release and synthesis of stress neurohormones suggest that even though corticosteroid receptors are present in high concentration in parts of the brain remote from the hypothalamus, including the hippocampus, amygdala, and the monoaminergic nuclei of the hindbrain, central inhibition of CRH and AVP synthesis and release may be due in large part to corticosteroid action mainly at the level of the PVN. Although a role for mineralocorticoid receptors cannot be excluded, glucocorticoid receptors predominate.

Role of Atrial Natriuretic Peptide in Glucocorticoid Inhibition

Fink and associates showed that atrial natriuretic peptide (ANP) is released into hypophysial portal blood and, by immunoneutralization, that ANP is possibly an inhibitor of ACTH release. This suggests that the glucocorticoid inhibition of ACTH release may be mediated in part by ANP. A consensus sequence for the glucocorticoid response element is present in the second intron of the ANP gene, and ANP gene expression in and ANP release from cardiac cells are increased significantly by glucocorticoids.

A pathophysiological role for ANP is suggested by multiple trauma and septic shock in humans, where, paradoxically, plasma ACTH concentrations are decreased but plasma cortisol concentrations are increased. These results raise the possibility that under conditions of extreme stress, increased levels of ANP inhibit ACTH release while cortisol secretion is stimulated by a direct action of endothelin-l on the adrenal gland. ANP inhibition of ACTH release might also explain the dissociation between plasma ACTH and CRH in patients who have undergone cardiac surgery or sustained myocardial infarction. Dissociation between plasma concentrations of ACTH and CRH under extreme, and especially cardiopulmonary, stress is relevant to allostatic override of the normal glucocorticoid negative feedback system.

On the basis of all the present *in vivo* and *in vitro* data, Engler and colleagues conclude that studies with ANP have so far provided the most compelling evidence that a neuropeptide may inhibit ACTH release.

Role of Hippocampus and Amygdala in Glucocorticoid Negative Feedback

It has long been assumed that the hippocampus and the amygdala, major components of the forebrain limbic system, play a key role in the stress response. The forebrain limbic system, together with the thalamus and neocortex and brain stem structures, form an analyzer-integrator system involved in neuroendocrine control. The hypothalamus can be considered an intermediate relay station in the reciprocal circuits between the limbic forebrain and brain stem structures, receiving inputs from both. The forebrain limbic system is thought to be involved in stressors that require analysis by higher brain structures (processive stressors), whereas direct brain stem projections to the PVN subserve stressors that pose an immediate physiological threat (systemic stressors).

Projections to the PVN from the hippocampus are mainly multisynaptic, involving (1) the hippocampal fimbria-fornix system involving the lateral septum, bed nucleus of the stria terminalis (BNST), and anterior hypothalamus, which all project to the parvocellular PVN, and (2) the medial corticohypothalamic tract from the anteroventral subiculum to the ventromedial, arcuate, and suprachiasmatic nuclei of the hypothalamus. The PVN also receive direct projections from the amygdala as well as projections that relay in the BNST.

Many, but not all, studies in which HPA activity was assessed by the assay of corticosterone and, less frequently, ACTH suggest that the hippocampus inhibits HPA activity. Hippocampal inhibition of the

HPA appears to be due mainly to corticosteroid negative feedback inhibition, although there is also evidence that the hippocampus may exert an inhibitory tone on the HPA independently of corticosteroid feedback. However, the hippocampus is neither the only site nor necessarily the major site of corticosteroid negative feedback, since removal of its input to the hypothalamus reduces, but does not abolish, the efficacy of corticosteroid inhibition. Thus, for example, (1) although electrical stimulation of the PVN resulted in a two- to threefold increase in CRH release into hypophysial portal blood, stimulation of the hippocampus had no effect on the release of CRH, AVP, or oxytocin; (2) transection of the fornix, the major hippocampal-hypothalamic connection, had no significant effect on either basal or stress (nitroprusside-induced hypotension) evoked CRH release into hypophysial portal blood; and (3) implantation of dexamethasone pellets in hippocampus had no effect on CRH synthesis in the PVN. Nevertheless, fornix section did elevate AVP concentrations in portal blood and blocked corticosterone reduction of elevated CRH, but not AVP, levels in portal blood during hypotensive stress.

Further evidence that the hippocampus normally moderates the synthesis of stress neurohormones is suggested by the finding that lateral fimbria-fornix lesions increased CRH mRNA and AVP mRNA in medial parvocellular PVN, and also plasma ACTH concentrations.

Feldman and Weidenfeld showed that, in freely moving male rats, photic and acoustic stimuli depleted the CRH content of the median eminence with a concomitant increase in plasma ACTH and corticosterone levels. This photic/acoustic activation of the HPA was inhibited by the systemic administration of dexamethasone. HPA inhibition by dexamethasone was in turn inhibited by hippocampal implants of glucocorticoid and, to a lesser extent, mineralocorticoid receptor antagonists. These results suggest that in conscious animals the hippocampus does play a role in corticosteroid feedback inhibition of stress-induced ACTH release.

Herman and associates have underscored the role of the BNST as a nucleus that integrates or processes hippocampal and amygdaloid modulation of the HPA. This hypothesis is based, first, on the anatomical connections of the BNST in that the nucleus receives rich projections from the amygdala and hippocampus and projects to the parvocellular PVN. Second, lesion of the anterior BNST resulted in a 30% decrease in CRH mRNA levels in the PVN, whereas lesion of the posterior BNST resulted in a 13% increase in the level of CRH mRNA in the PVN. On the basis of these data, Herman and colleagues

inferred that the anterior BNST integrates excitatory inputs mainly from the amygdala, whereas the posterior BNST integrates inhibitory inputs mainly from the hippocampus.

In summary, the hippocampus plays an important role in moderating the HPA both by mediating corticosteroid negative feedback and by exerting an endogenous inhibitory tone on the HPA. Corticosteroid negative feedback is also exerted directly on the PVN and the pituitary gland. The hippocampus is a heterogeneous structure; thus, for example, Dunn and Orr found that electrical stimulation of the CA1 region increased corticosterone levels, whereas stimulation of the CA3, dentate, and subiculum decreased plasma corticosterone concentrations. This heterogeneity will need to be considered in the design of further studies on the role of the hippocampus in negative feedback control of the HPA.

Glucocorticoid Negative Feedback at the Pituitary Level

As well as exerting a central effect, corticosteroids inhibit ACTH synthesis and release by an action at the level of the anterior pituitary gland. As in brain, the inhibitory action of corticosteroids on pituitary corticotropes is mediated by glucocorticoid (type II) receptors.

Studies on dispersed pituitary cells with inhibitors of mRNA and protein synthesis have shown that both the rapid and delayed glucocorticoid inhibition of ACTH release depends upon mRNA and protein synthesis. Glucocorticoids also exert potent inhibitory effects on the expression of the ACTH precursor proopiomelanocortin (POMC) in the anterior lobe of the pituitary gland. In male Sprague-Dawley rats, transcription assays showed that dexamethasone inhibited POMC gene transcription by 10-fold within 30 min of a single injection of the glucocorticoid. Inhibition of POMC transcription was paralleled by a dramatic fall in plasma ACTH concentrations. The same study showed that CRH stimulated POMC transcription by nearly twofold within 15 min, which coincided with a massive increase in ACTH release. The action of dexamethasone is cell specific in that the steroid had no effect on the transcription rate of POMC in primary cultures of neurointermediate lobe cells.

Studies in transgenic mice showed that no more than 769 base pairs of the rat POMC promoter are required for cell-specific expression and glucocorticoid inhibition of the POMC gene in the anterior pituitary gland. A good deal is known about the glucocorticoid response elements in the POMC promoter and the transcription factors involved in POMC expression, but the precise molecular mechanism of glucocorticoid inhibition of POMC transcription remains to be elucidated.

In addition to a direct action on POMC gene expression, which determines the amount of ACTH available for release, glucocorticoids inhibit ACTH release by a mechanism mediated by adenylate cyclase (see **Adenylyl Cyclases and Stress Response**).

Possible Role of 11β-Hydroxysteroid Dehydrogenase

Two types of 11β-hydroxysteroid dehydrogenase play a pivotal role in glucocorticoid synthesis and metabolism. This enzyme is involved in glucocorticoid negative feedback (see **11β-Hydroxysteroid Dehydrogenases**).

Functional Importance of Glucocorticoid Negative Feedback

Glucocorticoid feedback inhibition of ACTH release protects the organism against the deleterious effects of hypercortisolemia (excessive concentrations of cortisol in blood). Whether due to endocrine disorders, such as Cushing's syndrome, or other causes such as trauma or chronic stress, hypercortisolemia is associated with at least three major deleterious effects. First, it suppresses the immune-inflammatory defense system and so incapacitates the animal's ability to respond to infection by pathogenic microorganisms or to chemical or physical insult. Second, persistent hypercortisolemia has major adverse effects on intermediary metabolism, resulting eventually in all the features of Cushing's syndrome, that is, android obesity, diabetes mellitus, hyperlipidemia, hypertension, and osteoporosis. Third, hypercortisolemia and/or stress are associated with reduction in hippocampal volume (atrophy) in several neuropsychiatric disorders, such as depression and posttraumatic stress disorder, as well as in Cushing's syndrome. In all three disorders, the hippocampal atrophy is associated with explicit memory deficits.

Clinical Manifestations of Disordered Glucocorticoid Feedback Regulation of the HPA System

No attempt is made here to give a detailed account of the clinical effects of disruption of feedback control within the HPA system. Rather, this section considers two clinical examples that underscore the principles of negative feedback and illustrate the consequences of disruption of normal HPA feedback control.

The first example is of enzyme defect in the adrenal cortex that results in the absence or deficiency of the afferent glucocorticoid signal of the HPA negative feedback system, whereas the second is probably due to an alteration in the central set point of the negative feedback control system.

Congenital Adrenal Hyperplasia: Failure of Glucocorticoid Negative Feedback

There are several types of inherited enzymatic defects in cortisol synthesis known to result in congenital adrenal hyperplasia (CAH), also known as the adrenogenital syndrome. By far the most common form is due to a deficiency of $P450c_{21}$ (21-hydroxylase; see **Figure** 7), which leads to a deficiency in cortisol biosynthesis. Excessive androgen secretion results from a failure of glucocorticoid negative feedback and consequent, uncontrolled, high ACTH secretion. Excessive androgen levels may lead to virilization of females *in utero*. About two-thirds of patients also have mineralocorticoid deficiency, resulting in salt wasting. If not obvious during the neonatal period, androgen excess may appear in early infancy, resulting in sexual precocity in boys and clitoral enlargement and pubic hair growth in girls. Excess androgen accelerates linear growth and epiphyseal closure, leading ultimately to diminished adult height. In adult women with untreated CAH, reproductive function is impaired due to (1) the disturbance of normal menstrual cycles as a consequence of the high plasma progesterone and androgen concentrations and (2) labial fusion, which prevents successful coitus. The former can be corrected by glucocorticoid replacement therapy, whereas the latter can be treated surgically.

The $P450c_{21}$ deficiency is transmitted as a single gene autosomal recessive trait linked to the major histocompatibility complex locus on the short arm of chromosome 6. An allelic variable of classical 21-hydroxylase deficiency results in a late-onset type, which frequently presents with clinical features similar to those of polycystic ovarian disease.

Deficiency of $P450c_{11}$ (11β-hydroxylase) is a much less common cause of CAH. As in the case of $P450c_{21}$ deficiency, it is transmitted as an autosomal recessive disorder but is not linked to the HLA locus. As in the case of $P450c_{21}$ deficiency, a deficiency in $P450c_{11}$ results in impaired glucocorticoid feedback and a consequent hypersecretion of ACTH and adrenal androgens. The condition is treated with glucocorticoid replacement therapy.

Much more rare forms of CAH are produced by deficiencies of 17α-hydroxylase and 3β-hydroxysteroid dehydrogenase, which result in defective adrenal androgen, as well as glucocorticoid secretion.

Cholesterol

VI ↓ P-450_SCC

| Δ5-Pregnenalone | P-450_c17 → V | Δ6-17-OH-Pregnenolone | P-450_c17 → Lyase | Dehydroeplandrosterone | 17B-HSO → | Androstenediol |

IV ↓ 3β-HSD   IV ↓ 3β-HSD   IV ↓ 3β-HSD   IV ↓ 3β-HSD

| Progesterone | P-450_c17 → V | 17-OH-Progesterone | P-450_c17 → Lyase | Δ4-Androstenedlone | 17B-HSO → | Testosterone |

II ↓ P-450_c21   1+II ↓ P-450_c21   ↓ P-450_SCC   ↓ P-450_SCC

| Deoxycorticosterone (DOC) | | Deoxycortisol | | Estrone | 17B-HSO → | Estradiol |

III ↓ P-450_c11   III ↓ P-450_c11

| Corticosterone | | Cortisol |

↓ (18-OH) P-450_c11

| 18-OH-Corticosterone |

↓ (18-Oxidase) P-450_c11

| **Aldosterone** |

MINERALCORTICOIDS   GLUCOCORTICOIDS   GONADAL STEROIDS

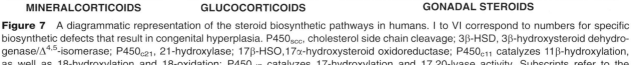

Figure 7 A diagrammatic representation of the steroid biosynthetic pathways in humans. I to VI correspond to numbers for specific biosynthetic defects that result in congenital hyperplasia. P450_scc, cholesterol side chain cleavage; 3β-HSD, 3β-hydroxysteroid dehydrogenase/$\Delta^{4,5}$-isomerase; P450_c21, 21-hydroxylase; 17β-HSO,17α-hydroxysteroid oxidoreductase; P450_c11 catalyzes 11β-hydroxylation, as well as 18-hydroxylation and 18-oxidation; P450_cl7 catalyzes 17-hydroxylation and 17,20-lyase activity. Subscripts refer to the steroidogenic enzymatic action of the several cytochrome P450 enzymes. From Grumbach, M. M. and Conte, F. A. (1998). Disorders of sexual differentiation. In: Wilson, J. D., Foster, D. W., Kronenberg, H. M. & Larsen, P. R. (eds.) *Williams textbook of endocrinology* (9th edn., pp.1303–1425). Philadelphia, PA: Saunders, with permission.

Hypercortisolemia in Major Depression: Possibly due to an Altered Set Point in Glucocorticoid Negative Feedback

Major depressive disorder is characterized by a significant increase in plasma cortisol concentrations (hypercortisolemia), which is most prominent at the nadir of the circadian rhythm around midnight. It was first thought that hypercortisolemia and resistance to the suppression of endogenous cortisol secretion by dexamethasone were specific features of major depression, which led to the hope that the dexamethasone suppression test could be used as a specific biological marker of depression. However, extensive studies have shown that hypercortisolemia and resistance to dexamethasone suppression are also associated with other types of psychoses, such as schizoaffective disorder and organic dementia, including Alzheimer's disease.

As shown by Goodwin and associates, hypercortisolemia in major depression is associated with a threefold increase in the mean plasma concentration of β-endorphin. In fact, resistance of β-endorphin to dexamethasone suppression appears to be a more robust marker of major depression than cortisol. Thus, in a study by Young and associates of 73 patients

with major depressive disorder, 39 (53%) showed β-endorphin nonsuppression to dexamethasone, while only 8 patients (11%) showed cortisol nonsuppression. These findings suggest that hypercortisolemia in major depression is due to a resistance of the brain-pituitary-ACTH module to glucocorticoid negative feedback, that is, an elevation of the set point for glucocorticoid feedback. The precise mechanism remains to be determined, but decreased responsiveness of the limbic system, PVN, and/or pituitary gland to glucocorticoid negative feedback is a likely explanation. Reduced responsiveness of the PVN could be caused by transynaptic changes triggered by changes in function of the limbic system and frontal cortex. Because the serotonergic raphe neurons determine the amplitude of the circadian excursions of plasma ACTH and corticosterone, it is also conceivable that hypercortisolemia reflects dysregulation of serotonergic function, which seems to occur in major depression.

Allostasis and Allostatic Load

Allostasis and allostatic load are mentioned here to clarify the link between homeostasis and allostasis.

The latter refers to maintenance of stability through change or adaptation and is illustrated by the increase in blood pressure on wakening or sex to cope with extra circulatory demands. In normal subjects, the increased blood pressure required to match increase in load does not necessarily reflect all but a transitory override of blood pressure control mechanisms involving baroreceptors (pressure receptors in the carotid sinus) and chemoreceptors (chemical sensors in the carotid body). Rather, there is a shift or adaptation in set point of the blood pressure control system so that it maintains mean arterial blood pressure within narrow limits around the new set point commensurate with the new load. Simply put, this is the same as altering the set point of a thermostat in a room to increase or decrease the mean ambient temperature – the set point has been changed, but the control mechanisms remain the same. The same principle may be applied to the control of plasma cortisol or adrenaline concentrations. The ability to alter the set point of one or more feedback control systems is termed regulation. In the case of the HPA and systemic blood pressure, set point regulation is located within the CNS. The elements that change the controlled variable (e.g., blood pressure, cortisol, adrenaline) toward the new set point are the control mechanisms.

Allostatic load was first introduced and defined by McEwen and Stellar (McEwen 2001) "as the cost of chronic exposure to fluctuating or heightened neural or neuroendocrine response resulting from repeated or chronic environmental challenge that an individual reacts to as being particularly stressful." That is, allostatic load reflects the hidden cost of chronic stresses to the body that act as a predisposing factor for the adverse effects of acute, stressful life events.

Conclusion

The HPA system, together with the sympathetic-medullary system, plays a pivotal role in the neuroendocrine response to stress. Homeostasis within the HPA is maintained by a precise negative feedback system by which the adrenal glucocorticoids (the afferent inhibitory signal), cortisol in humans or corticosterone in rodents, moderate ACTH synthesis and release (efferent output signal). Allostasis – that is, change in HPA activity to cope with increased stress load – is brought about by change in feedback set point. The major sites of negative feedback are the PVN, where glucocorticoids inhibit CRH and AVP synthesis and release, and the pituitary gland, where they block the ACTH response to CRH and inhibit POMC/ACTH synthesis. The limbic system of the brain, especially the hippocampus and amygdala, plays an important role in glucocorticoid negative feedback control.

Disruption of the HPA negative feedback system has serious deleterious effects, a point illustrated by the congenital adrenogenital syndrome and hypercortisolemia associated with serious mental illnesses. The adrenogenital syndrome, due to defective or absent cortisol secretion (loss of the afferent feedback signal) consequent on a congenital enzyme defect in the adrenal cortex, results in massive uncontrolled pituitary ACTH release. The latter induces excessive androgen production that in turn causes precocious puberty in males and masculinization of females. Hypercortisolemia, a prominent feature of major depressive disorder and other psychoses and organic dementias, is probably due to elevation of the set point of the HPA negative feedback system. Elucidation of the precise cause of this change in feedback set point may provide insight into the central disorder in depression. Hypercortisolemia may exert adverse effects by (1) inhibiting immune-inflammatory defense mechanisms, (2) disrupting intermediary metabolism, (3) inducing effects akin to Cushing's syndrome that lead to obesity, diabetes type II, and osteoporosis, and (4) compromising hippocampal structure, neurogenesis, and function that might lead to cognitive impairment.

See Also the Following Articles

11β-Hydroxysteroid Dehydrogenases; Adenylyl Cyclases and Stress Response; Allostasis and Allostatic Load; Circadian Rhythms, Genetics of; Corticotropin Releasing Factor-Binding Protein; Food Shift Effect; Glucocorticoid Negative Feedback; Glucocorticoids – Adverse Effects on the Nervous System; Major Depressive Disorder; Neuroendocrine Systems; Pituitary Regulation, Role of.

Further Reading

Bremner, J. D. and Vermetten, E. (2004). Neuroanatomical changes associated with pharmacotherapy in posttraumatic stress disorder. *Annals of the New York Academy of Science* **1032**, 154–157.

Christie, J. E., Whalley, L. J., Fink, G., et al. (1986). Raised plasma cortisol concentrations are a feature of drug-free psychotics and not specific for depression. *British Journal of Psychiatry* **148**, 58–65.

Christie, J. E., Whalley, L. J., Fink, G., et al. (1987). Characteristic plasma hormone changes in Alzheimer's disease. *British Journal of Psychiatry* **150**, 674–681.

Copolov, D. L., Rubin, R. T., Stuart, G. W., et al. (1989). Specificity of the salivary cortisol dexamethasone suppression test across psychiatric diagnoses. *Biological Psychiatry* **25**, 879–893.

Engler, D., Redei, E. and Kola, I. (1999). The corticotropin-release inhibitory factor hypothesis: A review of the evidence for the existence of inhibitory as well as stimulatory hypophysiotropic regulation of adrenocorticotropin secretion and biosynthesis. *Endocrine Review* 20, 460–500.

Feldman, S. and Weidenfeld, J. (1999). Glucocorticoid receptor antagonists in the hippocampus modify the negative feedback following neural stimuli. *Brain Research* 821, 33–37.

Fink, G. (1979). Feedback actions of target hormones on hypothalamus and pituitary with special reference to gonadal steroids. *Annual Review of Physiology* 41, 571–585.

Fink, G. (1988). The G. W. Harris Lecture: steroid control of brain and pituitary function. *Quarterly Journal of Experimental Physiology* 73, 257–293.

Fink, G. (1995). The self-priming effect of LHRH: a unique servomechanism and possible cellular model for memory. *Frontiers in Neuroendocrinology* 16, 183–190.

Fink, G. (1997). Mechanisms of negative and positive feedback of steroids in the hypothalamic-pituitary system. In: Bittar, E. E. & Bittar, N. (eds.) *Principles of medical biology* (vol. 10A), pp. 29–100. New York: JAI Press.

Fink, G., Robinson, I. C. A. F. and Tannahill, L. A. (1988). Effects of adrenalectomy and glucocorticoids on the peptides, CRF-41, AVP and oxytocin in rat hypophysial portal blood. *Journal of Physiology* 401, 329–345.

Fink, G., Dow, R. C., Casley, D., et al. (1992). Atrial natriuretic peptide is involved in the ACTH response to stress and glucocorticoid negative feedback in the rat. *Journal of Endocrinology* 135, 37–43.

Grumbach, M. M. and Conte, F. A. (1998). Disorders of sexual differentiation. In: Wilson, J. D., Foster, D. W., Kronenberg, H. M. & Larsen, P. R. (eds.) *Williams textbook of endocrinology* (9th edn., pp. 1303–1425). Philadelphia, PA: Saunders.

Herman, J. P. and Cullinan, W. E. (1997). Neurocircuitry of stress: central control of the hypothalamo-pituitary-adrenocortical axis. *Trends in Neurosciences* 20, 78–84.

Malberg, J. E. and Schechter, L. E. (2005). Increasing hippocampal neurogenesis; a novel mechanism for antidepressant drugs. *Current Pharmaceutical Design* 11, 145–155.

Malkoski, S. P. and Dorin, R. I. (1999). Composite glucocorticoid regulation at a functionally defined negative glucocorticoid response element of the human corticotropin-releasing hormone gene. *Molecular Endocrinology* 13, 1629–1644.

McEwen, B. S. (2002). Sex, stress and the hippocampus: allostasis, allostatic load and the aging process. *Neurobiology of Aging* 23, 921–939.

Milhorn, H. T. J. (1966). *The application of control theory to physiological systems.* Philadelphia, PA: Saunders.

Munck, A., Guyre, P. M. and Holbrook, N. J. (1984). Physiological functions of glucocorticoids in stress and their relation to pharmacological actions. *Endocrine Reviews* 5, 22–44.

Roth-Isigkeit, A., Dibbelt, L., Eichler, W., et al. (2001). Blood levels of atrial natriuretic peptide, endothelin, cortisol and ACTH in patients undergoing coronary artery bypass grafting surgery with cardiopulmonary bypass. *Journal of Endocrinology Investigation* 24, 777–785.

Sapolsky, R. M., Armanini, M. P., Sutton, S. W., et al. (1989). Elevation of hypophysial portal concentrations of adrenocorticotropin secretagogues after fornix transection. *Endocrinology* 125, 2881–2887.

Sawchenko, P. E. and Swanson, L. W. (1983). The organization of forebrain afferents to the paraventricular and supraoptic nuclei of the rat. *Journal Comparative Neurology* 218, 121–144.

Schulkin, J. (ed.) (2004). *Allostasis, homeostasis, and the costs of physiological adaptation*, pp. 1–372. Cambridge: Cambridge University Press.

Shepard, J. D., Liu, Y., Sassone-Corsi, P. and Aguilera, G. (2005). Role of glucocorticoids and cAMP-mediated repression in limiting corticotropin-releasing hormone transcription during stress. *Journal of Neuroscience* 25, 4073–4081.

Tannahill, L. A., Sheward, W. J., Robinson, I. C. A. F. and Fink, G. (1991). Corticotropin-releasing factor-41, vasopressin and oxytocin release into hypophysial portal blood in the rat; effects of electrical stimulation of the hypothalamus, amygdala and hippocampus. *Journal of Endocrinology* 129, 99–107.

Watts, A. G., Tanimura, S. and Sanchez-Watts, G. (2004). Corticotropin-releasing hormone and arginine vasopressin gene transcription in the hypothalamic paraventricular nucleus of unstressed rats: daily rhythms and their interactions with corticosterone. *Endocrinology* 145, 529–540.

Yates, F. E. and Maran, J. W. (1974). Stimulation and inhibition of adrenocorticotropin release. In: Knobil, E. & Sawyer, W.H. (eds.) *Handbook of physiology*, pp. 367–404. Washington, D.C.: American Physiological Society.

Young, D. A., Kotun, J., Haskett, R. F., et al. (1993). Dissociation between pituitary and adrenal supression to dexamethasone in depression. *Archives of General Psychiatry* 50, 395–403.

Feeding Circuitry (and Neurochemistry)

S E La Fleur, J J G Hillebrand and R A H Adan
Rudolf Magnus Institute of Neuroscience, University Medical Centre Utrecht, Utrecht, The Netherlands

Neural Circuitry Involved in Food Intake
Interactions with the Stress Circuitry
Effects of Stress on Food Intake
Effects of Feeding (or Fasting) on Stress Responses
Concluding Remarks

Glossary

Anorexigenic	Inhibiting food intake (e.g., POMC (α-MSH), CART, leptin).
Arcuate nucleus	A collection of neurons (nerve cells) in the hypothalamus.
Hypothalamus	Region of the brain linking the nervous system to the endocrine system by synthesizing and secreting neurohormones and neuropeptides. The hypothalamus is also the area of the brain that controls hunger and thirst, body temperature, and circadian cycles.
Orexigenic	Stimulating food intake (e.g., AgRP, NPY, ghrelin).

Neural Circuitry Involved in Food Intake

Food intake involves several aspects of different behaviors, such as hunting for food and decision making. The complexity of feeding behavior is reflected in the number of brain areas involved; several nuclei in the caudal brain stem, hypothalamus, and the corticolimbic area are part of the feeding circuitry. Despite the large number of brain areas involved in feeding behavior, the hypothalamus is regarded as the main center for regulation of homeostatic feeding in the brain. Within the hypothalamus, the arcuate nucleus is central to the regulation of food intake. The arcuate nucleus contains at least two distinct groups of neurons controlling food intake: neurons that contain the orexigenic neuropeptides agouti-related protein (AgRP) and neuropeptide Y (NPY) and neurons that contain the anorexigenic neuropeptides pro-opiomelanocortin (POMC) and cocaine- and amphetamine-regulated transcript (CART). These arcuate neurons contain different receptors of hormones that are secreted in the periphery by adipocytes, the pancreas, and the gut in response to nutrients passing or being stored. Leptin, for example, is secreted by adipocytes, reflecting the amount of fat stores in the body. When the body becomes fat, leptin will silence orexigenic neurons and trigger anorexigenic neurons in the arcuate nucleus to secrete α-melanocyte-stimulating hormone (α-MSH) (derived from POMC) and CART to decrease food intake. In contrast to leptin, the hormone ghrelin, which is released from the (empty) stomach and which has been associated with the anticipation of meals, activates NPY/AgRP neurons and inhibits POMC/CART neurons in the arcuate nucleus. The neurons of the arcuate nucleus project to several nuclei within the hypothalamus, such as the paraventricular (PVN) and the lateral hypothalamic (LHA) nuclei, which also receive and send information from and to the caudal brain stem and corticolimbic areas. In addition to the anorexigenic and orexigenic neuropeptides in the arcuate nucleus, within the PVN corticotropin-releasing hormone (CRH) and within the LHA melanin-concentrating hormone and orexin(s) are peptides also involved in food intake regulation. Within the brain stem, groups of catecholamine cell groups are localized that project to the hypothalamus and are important for the regulation of feeding behavior, for example, in response to a glucoprivation. In the brain stem, integration of signals from the periphery (such as cholecystokinin [CCK]) takes place, carrying information on gastrointestinal distention and presence of meals in the gastrointestinal tract and signals from the hypothalamus indicating long-term nutritional status. For instance, leptin and α-MSH affect meal size, probably by determining the sensitivity for CCK at the level of the brain stem, which is released when fat-containing foods reach the duodenum. Furthermore, within the corticolimbic area, the amygdala and nucleus accumbens are implicated in the evaluation of taste and rewarding aspects of food. Taken together, this complex neural circuitry holds many brain areas, in which neuropeptides and neurotransmitters convey information important for the regulation of feeding behavior.

The brain, however, does not function on its own. To maintain a stable body weight, food intake needs to be tuned to the needs of the peripheral body. This means that when fat stores are increasing or depleting, satiety or hunger factors (e.g., hormones) are produced by different organs to change feeding behavior. For example, leptin that is secreted from adipose tissue acts on its receptor in the arcuate nucleus to decrease food intake. In addition, glucocorticoids secreted by adrenals in response to fasting act as factors to adjust feeding behavior.

Interactions with the Stress Circuitry

During stress, several neuropeptides and hormones are affected that are part of the previously described neural circuitry involved in feeding behavior. CRH in the PVN plays an initiating role in hypothalamic-pituitary-adrenocortical (HPA) axis activity and is increased with acute stress and decreased with chronic stress (through feedback effects of released glucocorticoids). In addition, acute stress increases NPY mRNA in the arcuate nucleus. In the amygdala, which is also part of processing taste information, NPY mRNA will decrease whereas CRH mRNA will increase after a stressful event. Thus, during stress, depending on the anatomical site, anorexigenic (CRH) as well as orexigenic (NPY) signaling is increased. This might result in conflicting food intake signals. Interestingly, some eat more while others eat less following stressful experiences. The individual sensitivity and reactivity in these different neural circuits may underlie the response of food intake to a stressful situation. It has also been shown that NPY induces changes in the daily rhythm of circulating corticosterone (which shows a rhythm over the day–night cycle) when rats' food intake is restricted. Interestingly, AgRP, but not NPY, mRNA levels are reduced following a stressful event. Thus, although both orexigenic neuropeptides are colocalized in the arcuate nucleus and their expression appears similarly affected following fasting, their expression is differently regulated following a stressor. Also, α-MSH interacts with the stress circuitry; central administration of α-MSH stimulates grooming and the release of ACTH and corticosterone in rats, and this activation is further increased in stressed rats.

Another overlapping system for food intake and stress responsivity is the catecholaminergic pathway between the brain stem and the hypothalamus, which is involved in feeding behavior as well as in stress responsivity. Physiological evidence that these systems indeed interact is provided by data showing effects of stress on food intake and vice versa.

Effects of Stress on Food Intake

Human studies showed that the psychophysiological response to stress is related to greater food consumption. Stress is the main trigger for obese patients to start binge eating. Moreover, people that release more cortisol due to a stressor are consuming more calories and eat significantly more sweet foods across days. Stress eaters gain more weight and are at greater risk for cardiovascular disease and type II diabetes. In Cushing's disease as well as in patients treated with corticosteroids for longer periods, a typical visceral form of obesity is induced. Generally, adrenal insufficiency is accompanied by reduced food intake and body weight. Removal of the adrenal glands in rodents results in reduced food intake and body weight, which demonstrates that corticosteroids are essential for maintaining a normal body weight. More severe traumatic environmental stressors (e.g., the loss of a spouse) can have an opposite effect, decreasing food intake and fat stores. Stress is also thought to play a central role in anorexia nervosa. The neurodevelopmental model of anorexia nervosa proposes that chronic stress in predisposed individuals results in (maladaptive) hyperactivity of the HPA axis, resulting in a loss of nutritional homeostasis. Other models, however, state that the principles of anorexia nervosa are starvation and physical activity, and that the consequential activation of the HPA axis is rewarding for the patient.

In animal models, the influence of stress (ranging from physical stress to social stress) on food intake has been studied extensively. The typical response of rodents to a wide range of stressors is to decrease food intake. Only in Syrian hamsters has it been shown that social stress increases food intake and fat stores. Most experiments studying effects of stress on food intake in rats and mice have been done using normal lab chow, which is balanced, healthy, and high in carbohydrates. In daily society, however, humans have choices, and often have easy access to cheap foods with high fat and sugar content. Providing rats with a greater choice of food results in different food intake responses when animals are subjected to a chronic stressor. Rats were given access to normal lab chow, lard, and a bottle of 1 M sugar water and were repeatedly restrained for 5 days, 3 h/day. Rats increased their intake of the more palatable items, lard and sugar, and consumed more of those as compared to the nonstressed animals.

Effects of Feeding (or Fasting) on Stress Responses

Although stress alters food intake regulation, the absence of food (fasting or starvation) is itself a stressful event. For instance, stress hormones and CRH (anorexigenic) are chronically increased in anorexia nervosa patients, which may contribute to the difficulty these patients experience in trying to reverse their illness. Stress from absence of food is, however, different from stressors such as restraint stress. Glucocorticoid receptors (GRs) in the hypothalamus are downregulated following chronic, repeated restraint, thus decreasing negative feedback on CRH mRNA in the PVN. The decreased inhibition of CRH mRNA results in fewer anorexigenic effects of the PVN CRH during starvation. Furthermore, the ACTH response to stress is altered during fasting.

Not only does the absence of food change stress responsivity, but eating palatable (e.g., sugar- and fat-containing) food also changes the response to stress. Rats that voluntarily choose the percentage of lard in their diets (composing their own high-fat diet) have reduced HPA responses to restraint stress; however, when forced to eat a high-fat diet the response of the HPA axis to restraint is high or similar compared to rats that consume only chow. Some controversy exists regarding the stress responsivity when animals are eating a high-fat diet. Although the choice to eat fat seems important for the response to stress, rats that were force-fed a high-fat diet for a longer time did have decreased responses in activity and body temperature when socially stressed (social defeat).

Concluding Remarks

Stress clearly affects the neural circuitry regulating food intake at several levels. Some people react to stress by overeating, which contributes to the development of obesity, whereas others (e.g., anorexia nervosa patients) reduce their food intake. Differences in these coping strategies may originate in subtle differences between individuals in the neural circuitry underlying food intake and stress. A better insight into how the stress system interacts with the food intake circuitry, as well as into the mechanism underlying individual responsiveness to stress, is necessary to find new strategies to treat eating disorders such as obesity and anorexia nervosa. The type of diet also affects the stress response. Future research is needed to understand the mechanisms underlying how palatable food interacts with the neural circuitry of the stress response.

See Also the Following Articles

Food Intake and Stress, Human; Food Intake and Stress, Non-Human; Food Shift Effect; Oxidative Stress; Leptin, Adiponectin, Resistin, Ghrelin; Orexin.

Further Reading

Bergh, C. and Sodersten, P. (1996). Anorexia nervosa, self-starvation and the reward of stress. *Nature Medicine* **2**, 21–22.

Berthoud, H. R. (2004). Mind versus metabolism in the control of food intake and energy balance. *Physiology and Behavior* **81**, 781–793.

Buwalda, B., Blom, W. A., Koolhaas, J. M., et al. (2001). Behavioral and physiological responses to stress are affected by high-fat feeding in male rats. *Physiology and Behavior* **73**, 371–377.

Connan, H., Campbell, I. C., Katzman, M., et al. (2003). A neurodevelopmental model for anorexia nervosa. *Physiology and Behavior* **79**, 13–24.

Conrad, C. D. and McEwen, B. S. (2000). Acute stress increases neuropeptide Y mRNA within the arcuate nucleus and hilus of the dentate gyrus. *Molecular Brain Research* **79**, 102–109.

Dallman, M. F., Akana, S. F., Bhatnagar, S., et al. (2000). Bottomed out: metabolic significance of the circadian trough in glucocorticoid concentrations. *International Journal of Obesity and Related Metabolic Disorders* **24**(supplement 2), S40–S46.

Dallman, M. F., Pecoraro, N. C. and la Fleur, S. E. (2004). Chronic stress and comfort foods: self-medication and abdominal obesity. *Brain Behavior and Immunity* **19**, 275–280.

Donohoe, T. P. (1984). Stress-induced anorexia: implications for anorexia nervosa. *Life Science* **34**, 203–218.

Epel, E., Lapidus, R., McEwen, B., et al. (2001). Stress may add bite to appetite in women: a laboratory study of stress-induced cortisol and eating behavior. *Psychoneuroendocrinology* **26**, 37–49.

Foster, M. T., Solomon, M. B., Huhman, K. L. and Bartness, T. J. (2006). Social defeat increases food intake, body mass and adiposity in syrian hamsters. *American Journal of Physiology. Regulatory, Integrative and Comparative Physiology* **290**, R1284–R1293.

Hillebrand, J. J., De Wied, D. and Adan, R. A. (2002). Neuropeptides, food intake and body weight regulation: a hypothalamic focus. *Peptides* **23**, 2283–2306.

Inui, A. (2001). Eating behavior in anorexia nervosa – an excess of both orexigenic and anorexigenic signaling? *Molecular Psychiatry* **6**, 620–624.

Kas, M. J., Bruijnzeel, A. W., Haanstra, J. R., et al. (2005). Differential regulation of agouti-related protein and neuropeptide Y in hypothalamic neurons following a stressful event. *Journal of Molecular Endocrinology* **35**, 159–164.

la Fleur, S. E., Houshyar, H., Roy, M., et al. (2005). Choice of lard, but not total lard calories, damps adrenocorticotropin responses to restraint. *Endocrinology* **146**, 2193–2199.

Makino, S., Kaneda, T., Nishiyama, M., et al. (2001). Lack of decrease in hypothalamic and hippocampal glucocorticoid receptor mRNA during starvation. *Neuroendocrinology* **74**, 120–128.

Solomon, M. R. (2001). Eating as both coping and stressor in overweight control. *Journal of Advanced Nursing* **36**, 563–572.

Von Frijtag, J. C., Croiset, G., Gispen, W. H., et al. (1998). The role of central melanocortin receptors in the activation of the hypothalamus-pituitary-adrenal-axis and the induction of excessive grooming. *British Journal of Pharmacology* **123**, 1503–1508.

Fetal Stress

M Eleftheriades, P Pervanidou and G P Chrousos
Athens University Medical School, Athens, Greece

Fetal Programming and Fetal Origins of Adult Disease
Mediators of the Predictive Adaptive Response
Fetal Distress – Clinical Evaluation
Fetal Growth Restriction (FGR)
Preterm Birth

Glossary

Biophysical profile	A noninvasive test that identifies a compromised fetus. It integrates five parameters to determine the biophysical profile score: the nonstress test, ultrasound measurement of the amniotic fluid volume, observation of the presence or absence of fetal breathing movements, gross body movements, and fetal tone.
Cardiotocography (CTG)	A method of monitoring fetal heart rate using either an abdominal transducer or a probe on the fetal scalp; in addition, another transducer placed over the uterine fundus monitors uterine activity (contractions).
Cordocentesis	An invasive procedure that involves the aspiration of fetal blood from the umbilical cord under sonographic guidance for diagnostic (fetal-karyotyping) or therapeutic (blood/platelet-transfusion) purposes.
Doppler ultrasound	A noninvasive technique of blood-flow velocity measurement. The Doppler effect (named after Christian Andreas Doppler) is the apparent change in frequency and wavelength of a wave that is perceived by an observer moving relative to the source of the waves; the total Doppler effect may result from either the motion of the source or motion of the observer. For the velocity measurement of blood, ultrasound is transmitted into a vessel and the sound that is reflected from the blood is detected.
Preeclampsia	A pregnancy-specific multisystem disorder that is characterized by the development of hypertension of 140 mmHg or higher systolic or 90 mmHg or higher diastolic after 20 weeks of gestation in a woman with previously normal blood pressure and proteinuria of 0.3 g or more of protein in a 24-h urine collection (usually corresponds to 1+ or greater on a urine dipstick test).
Programming	The process whereby a stimulus or insult, when applied during a critical or sensitive period of development, results in a long-term or permanent effect on the structure or function of the organism.

Fetal Programming and Fetal Origins of Adult Disease

Experimental and clinical studies have highlighted the importance of the fetal environment in the subsequent growth and development of an individual. Indeed, a poor *in utero* environment elicited by maternal malnutrition or placental insufficiency may increase the susceptibility of the fetus to the later development of metabolic and cardiovascular disease. The fetal origins of adult disease hypothesis originated from the epidemiological research of Barker and colleagues, which demonstrated an association between low birth weight and cardiovascular disease, hypertension, insulin resistance, and dyslipidaemia later in life. In an attempt to explain this association, Hales and Barker proposed the thrifty phenotype hypothesis, according to which the fetus in a poor intrauterine environment maximizes the uptake and conservation of fuel resources by altering its metabolism. This alteration is adaptive in a deprived environment but maladaptive in an environment of plentiful resources.

The fetal programming response to environmental stressors, predictive adaptive response (PAR), however, is much broader that the one suggested by Barker and colleagues, extending well beyond energy use and conservation. PAR uses developmentally plastic processes to set a postnatal physiological and behavioral phenotype that the fetus predicts will offer an optimal chance for survival and reproduction during adulthood. The prediction of an adverse, deprived, risky, and hence stressful environment leads to adaptive changes in body size, body composition, organ size, neurohormonal activity, and many aspects of behavior. These predictive adjustments could be advantageous in a deprived environment but are maladaptive under abundant conditions.

Mediators of the Predictive Adaptive Response

The fetal adaptive response to stressors is mediated largely by the stress system. The hypothalamic-pituitary-adrenal (HPA) axis and the locus ceruleus–norepinephrine–sympathetic nervous system (LC-NE-SNS) and their mediators corticotropin releasing hormone (CRH), arginine vasopressin (AVP), norepinephrine (NE), epinephrine (E), and cortisol are responsible for both the concurrent adaptive response to the stressor and for causing the long-term organizational changes in the brain and periphery that constitute the PAR. Indeed, CRH and cortisol have been shown to have strong activating and organizational effects.

Fetal Distress – Clinical Evaluation

In perinatology practice, the term fetal distress has been employed as the condition in which the fetal heart rate (FHR) pattern detected by cardiotocography (CTG) is abnormal during antepartum surveillance. The generation of reactive FHR patterns constitutes a complex process involving appropriately for gestational age mature brain-stem centres, normally functioning sympathetic and parasympathetic system, intact electrical pathways to conduct the contractile stimulus, appropriately functioning cardiomyocytes' neurohormone receptors, and normal cardiac partitioning and development.

CTG tracing patterns indicative of fetal hypoxemia and/or acidemia are characterized by fixed FHR baselines, loss of FHR variability, absence of accelerations and are described as 'non-reassuring'. Documentation of spontaneous late decelerations is associated with a significant risk of fetal compromise. CTG patterns can be influenced by constitutional and environmental parameters, such as fetal congenital abnormalities, fetal maturation (depending mainly on gestational age) and movements. Moreover, maternal emotional or physical stress and the use of medication can also generate abnormal FHR patterns. Fetuses exhibit restricted central nervous system maturation and therefore cerebral activity before 28 weeks of gestation. Thus, CTG monitoring before this gestational age usually demonstrates reduced variability and benign spontaneous decelerations. Fetal sleep cycles are frequent and longer monitoring is required to record reactivity.

In addition FHR patterns are correlated to the nature of the hypoxic insult. Acute hypoxemia generates abrupt and profound declines in FHR baseline and variability and fetal activity. Chronic hypoxemia is associated with a more gradual deterioration in these parameters and therefore may remain undiagnosed by CTG monitoring for days to weeks.

Numerous studies have assessed CTG sensitivity, specificity, and predictive values. Most of them have documented relatively high specificity (>90%) but much lower sensitivity (averaging 50%). Positive and negative predictive values are less than 50% and more than 90%, respectively, suggesting that the non stress test (NTS) is better at excluding than diagnosing fetal compromise.

Despite extensive research, the association between a compromised fetus (invasively traceable by altered biochemical parameters) and a nonreassuring CTG pattern remains an unresolved issue. In addition, the correlation between an acute or chronic intrauterine adversity and the extent of fetal compromise caused by it, is not clearly defined regarding stressor's threshold level, intensity and duration required to impair fetal developmental, physiological and metabolic mechanisms. Furthermore, fetal capability to sustain a stressor is characterized by a wide range of adaptive mechanisms whose efficacy depends on gestational age and other only partially elucidated factors.

Fetal hypoxemia can be categorized, depending on the severity and duration of the *in utero* adversity, as acute or chronic. Acute hypoxemia as a stressor activates the fetal stress system. There is evidence from experimental studies that acute hypoxemia is associated with bradycardia and compensatory tachycardia, elevated blood pressure, reduced fetal breathing and reduced gross body movements, and increased cerebral blood flow, indicating cardiac redistribution. The fetal ovine HPA axis responds to acute hypoxemia with elevated arterial plasma concentrations of ACTH and cortisol. Furthermore, catecholamines and vasopressin concentrations are elevated in the hypoxic ovine fetus. In the sheep fetus during late gestation, episodes of acute stress induce endocrine responses that promote fetal adaptation and survival during the period of adversity.

Chronic hypoxemia is associated with the progressive return of fetal body movements, heart rate, and blood pressure to normal. However, cardiac output redistribution is maintained, as documented by increased cerebral blood flow. In fetal sheep, the partial compression of the umbilical cord for a period of three days causing a 30% reduction in umbilical blood flow can produce reversible mild fetal asphyxia, a transient increase in fetal plasma ACTH concentration, and a progressive and sustained increase in fetal plasma cortisol. Chronic hypoxemia is associated with increased NE concentrations. On the contrary epinephrine concentrations are restored to control levels during the course of hypoxemic period.

Hypoxia can activate a sequence of systemic, cellular, and metabolic responses, allowing tissue adaptation to the adverse effect of the lack of oxygen. Furthermore, hypoxia can induce altered gene expression with long-term detrimental outcome. The underlying molecular mechanisms that determine fetal development in response to hypoxia are not clearly defined, and it is suggested that placental gene upregulation is associated with the inflammatory response after the hypoxic exposure. Hypoxia may cause placental insufficiency or may induce preeclampsia through an inflammatory response, leading to FGR or even to *in utero* demise. Additionally pro-inflammatory molecules, such as cytokines, are considered responsible for the systemic maternal inflammatory response observed in pregnancies complicated with preeclampsia.

Current research suggests that exposure to inflammatory stressors during the critical developmental windows may induce altered gene expression of the neuroendocrine–immune axis. Evidence of HPA axis and autonomic nervous system (ANS) activation during inflammation supports the hypothesis that inflammatory stress during fetal development induces the programming of both the neuroendocrine and immune systems, influencing vulnerability to disease development later in life. Moreover, both clinical and experimental studies suggest that low-grade systemic inflammation is present in the metabolic syndrome participating in the development of atherosclerosis and cardiovascular disease.

Fetal Growth Restriction (FGR)

Genetically predetermined fetal growth potential influenced by environmental parameters determines fetal growth and birth weight. These parameters can be physiological (fetal and maternal health and placental function), behavioral (maternal emotional stress), social (socioeconomic status, life-style and malnutrition), and ecological (starvation/famine). The interaction between genome and environment in the regulation of fetal growth and development constitutes a complex process. Intrauterine adversities challenge the growing fetus, forcing it to reallocate its energy resources between the adaptation to the challenge and growth in order to ensure survival, reproduction enhancement and genome preservation. Thus, FGR is the evolutionary result of adaptation to a suboptimal intrauterine milieu.

FGR occurs in approximately 5% of all human pregnancies and is associated with a substantially increased risk of perinatal mortality and long-term morbidity. The definition of FGR excludes small for gestational age (SGA) fetuses that are constitutionally small. Based on growth curves, growth-restricted fetuses are considered to be those with estimated weights below the 10th percentile for gestational age, below the 5th percentile for gestational age, or two standard deviations (<3%) below the mean for gestational age. Approximately 80% of fetuses with estimated weights below the 10th percentile for gestational age are constitutionally small (normal small), 15% are starved small due to placental insufficiency,

and 5% are abnormal small. The lower the percentile that defines SGA, the higher the likelihood of FGR.

FGR is further categorized as symmetric or asymmetric. Symmetric FGR is characterized by proportional reduction in growth velocity of both the fetal head circumference (HC) and abdominal circumference (AC), indicating a constitutionally small fetus. Symmetric FGR can also be indicative of *in utero* adversities such as chromosomal abnormalities, genetic syndromes, congenital infections, use of medication or teratogenic agents. Asymmetric FGR is characterized by a disproportional reduction in growth velocity of the fetal HC to AC and is mainly associated with placental insufficiency. However, body proportionality does not always specify the causes of FGR. Snijders et al. performed fetal blood karyotyping on 458 fetuses between 17 and 39 weeks gestation who had been referred for evaluation of intrauterine growth restriction (IUGR) and they demonstrated that the relative shortening of the femur can be found in both chromosomally normal and abnormal fetuses. In the same study, fetuses with triploidy had been found to have severe, early-onset, asymmetric FGR, whereas fetuses with chromosomal abnormalities other than triploidy were symmetrically growth retarded at <30 weeks. Chromosomally abnormal IUGR fetuses diagnosed after 30 weeks are usually asymmetrically growth restricted. The authors suggested that the asymmetry results from superimposed starvation due to placental insufficiency.

Placental insufficiency and fetal abnormalities (chromosomal, structural and congenital infections) are responsible for the majority of FGR cases in singleton pregnancies. According to histopathological studies, placental insufficiency is associated with abnormal trophoblast invasion and villous development that impairs placental vascular function, restricting nutrient and oxygen transfer to the fetus. The severity of placental insufficiency can be manifested in both maternal and fetal vascular compartments, (uterine and umbilical arteries respectively). The discrepancy between fetal growth demands and environmental conditions, mainly defined by placental vascular dysfunction, determines the severity of the compromised growth velocity that may manifest as FGR or even as fetal demise.

Clinical studies have documented the correlation between increased blood flow impedance in the uterine arteries and the subsequent development of preeclampsia, and FGR. Abnormal Doppler waveform in the uterine arteries is associated with a 70% chance of developing preeclampsia and an approximately 30% chance of developing growth restriction. In FGR pregnancies increased Doppler indices in the umbilical arteries are associated with fetal hypoxemia and acidemia correlated to the severity of the impedance of the umbilical flow. Fetal cardiovascular adaptations to placental insufficiency result in the redistribution of cardiac output. As a consequence, there is an increase in the blood supply to the brain, myocardium, and the adrenal glands at the expense of the kidneys, gastrointestinal tract, and lower extremities. The aforementioned redistribution of cardiac output can be documented by the reduced impedance of the blood flow in the middle cerebral artery. Fetuses exhibiting blood flow redistribution are usually hypoxemic, while acidemia may still not be clinically apparent. Further deterioration of fetal circulatory status is manifested by cardiac decompensation due to the exhaustion of adaptive mechanisms to hypoxia, indicated by right heart failure and abnormal organ autoregulation.

Elegant studies investigating the metabolic status of growth-restricted fetuses by cordocentesis have documented fetal compromise by hypoxemia, hypercapnia, hyperlacticemia, and acidosis. Growth-restricted fetuses are deprived of glucose and amino acids and are hypertriglyceridemic. In addition, some of these fetuses are hypoinsulinemic and their degree of hypoinsulinemia is disproportional to the degree of hypoglycemia, suggesting pancreatic dysfunction. In growth-restricted fetuses, the plasma cortisol concentration is increased and inversely correlated to fetal hypoglycemia. There is evidence of a significant correlation between umbilical cord plasma CRH and both ACTH and cortisol concentrations, as well as a significant negative correlation between CRH and dehydroepiandrosterone sulfate (DHEAS) levels in the growth-restricted fetuses. The umbilical cord plasma CRH level is extremely elevated compared to that of normal fetuses.

Placental CRH synthesis and release, in contrast to hypothalamic CRH, appears to be stimulated by glucocorticoids. In pregnancies complicated by uteroplacental insufficiency, placental CRH production may be enhanced by increased fetal glucocorticoids. In turn, placental CRH may modulate fetal pituitary-adrenal steroidogenesis to favor increased cortisol secretion. Conditions of chronic stress may stimulate hypothalamic as well as placental CRH, modulating fetal pituitary-adrenal function and consequently fetal response to a compromised intrauterine environment.

In FGR fetuses there is delayed maturation of biophysical parameters is apparent in IUGR fetuses. Fetal behavioral responses to placental insufficiency can affect heart-rate control by delaying the physiological decline of the baseline heart rate and maturation of reactivity and by decreasing short- and long-term variability.

Diagnostic Approach to Fetal Growth Restriction

The best method to diagnose the growth-restricted fetus and determine its growth velocity is ultrasound evaluation. The diagnostic approach to the FGR fetus is based on a detailed biometric and anatomic assessment evaluating for growth, chromosomal and structural defects, and congenital infections. Compared to other fetal biometric parameters, the AC is regarded as the most accurate measurement with the highest sensitivity and negative predictive value for identifying FGR. However, assessment of the estimated fetal weight (EFW) requires additional measurement of the HC and femur length.

The assessment of fetal growth velocity by serial ultrasound evaluation of AC and EFW is superior to single estimates of AC and EFW in the prediction of FGR. Moreover, it is important to assess the amniotic fluid volume. Placental insufficiency and fetal hypoxemia cause fetal oliguria and consequently oligohydramnios. Decreased amniotic fluid volume is regarded as an early sign of IUGR and oligohydramnios is defined as the presence of a largest vertical pocket of amniotic fluid less than 2 cm or amniotic fluid index (AFI) less than 5 cm.

The next essential step in the diagnostic process of FGR is based on Doppler blood-flow studies. It is well established that Doppler ultrasound assessment of the uterine and umbilical arteries helps to distinguish growth restricted fetuses due to impaired placentation from constitutionally small fetuses. In FGR fetuses, abnormal blood flow in the umbilical artery usually precedes other cardiovascular adaptations. Abnormal Doppler findings indicative of uteroplacental insufficiency include increased impendance with absent or reversed end-diastolic flow in the umbilical artery.

The further evaluation of the fetal cardiovascular system involves the assessment of the middle cerebral artery and the ductus venosus. When redistribution occurs, ductus venosus blood flow is usually normal and biophysical abnormalities are generally not clinically apparent. Abnormal ductus venosus blood flow indicates a decompensation of the cardiovascular system, which is followed by abnormalities in biophysical parameters. The biophysical profile consists of fetal tone, breathing movements, gross body movements, amniotic fluid volume assessment, and CTG monitoring, and it reflects the fetal behavioral status. The deterioration of the fetal biophysical profile associated with Doppler evidence of right heart failure indicates intrauterine fetal jeopardy. Optimizing the time of delivery, in which iatrogenic intervention should be delayed to avoid the risks of premature birth without increasing the risks of exposure to an adverse intrauterine environment, remains a challenge for perinatologists.

Perinatal mortality and long-term morbidity, including neurodevelopmental delay, is considerably increased in FGR fetuses with evidence of abnormal ductus venosus blood flow. The delivery decision should not be based merely on the umbilical artery waveform alone but mainly on the combination of abnormal venous Doppler indices and abnormal biophysical profile parameters. Furthermore, if early delivery is required, the gestation- and birth weight-specific charts produced by a study by Draper et al. should be used to determine the likelihood of survival.

Preterm Birth

Stress experienced during pregnancy increases the risk of preterm labor. Preterm birth, i.e. delivery before 37 weeks of gestation, occurs in approximately 10% of all pregnancies constituting the leading cause of neonatal morbidity and mortality. It is noteworthy that the incidence of premature labor remains unaffected by improvements in social health care and socioeconomic level observed in Western countries during the last 50 years. A substantial body of evidence has emphasized the role of stress as a major risk factor for preterm delivery. Furthermore, a correlation has been documented between maternal stress, either physical or emotional and premature delivery and it is proposed that the earlier in pregnancy the adversity is experienced, the earlier parturition occurs.

It has been suggested that premature activation of placental CRH gene expression in response to stressors induces early fetal neuroendocrine maturation and premature labor. Indeed, maternal and placental endocrine dysfunction triggered by a variety of stressors and the consequent occurrence of fetal stress may generate the process leading to preterm delivery. Although the early expulsion of the stressed FGR fetus from an adverse intrauterine environment carries the evolutionary advantage of genome maintenance it has the cost of increased risk of perinatal morbidity and mortality as well as the development of dysmetabolic syndrome in adulthood.

Further Reading

Barker, D. J. (2002). Fetal programming of coronary heart disease. *Trends in Endocrinology and Metabolism* 13(9), 364–368.

Barker, D. J. P., Osmond, C., Forsen, T. J., et al. (2005). Trajectories of growth among children who have coronary events as adults. *New England Journal of Medicine* 353, 1802–1809.

Baschat, A. A. (2004). Pathophysiology of fetal growth restriction: implications for diagnosis and surveillance. *Obstetrical and Gynecological Survey* 59(8), 617–627.

Baschat, A. A., Gembruch, U. and Harman, C. R. (2001). The sequence of changes in Doppler and biophysical parameters as severe fetal growth restriction worsens. *Ultrasound in Obstetrics and Gynecology* 18(6), 571–577.

Challis, J. R. G., Sloboda, D., Matthews, S. G., et al. (2001). The fetal placental hypothalamic-pituitary-adrenal (HPA) axis, parturition and post natal health. *Molecular and Cellular Endocrinology* 185(1–2), 135–144.

Chrousos, G. P. and Gold, P. W. (1992). The concepts and stress and stress systems disorders. *Journal of the American Medical Association* 267, 1244–1252.

Devoe, L. D. and Jones, C. R. (2002). Nonstress test: evidence-based use in high-risk pregnancy. *Clinical Obstetrics and Gynecology* 45(4), 986–992.

Dole, N., Savitz, D. A., Hertz-Picciotto, I., et al. (2003). Maternal stress and preterm birth. *American Journal of Epidemiology* 157, 14–24.

Draper, E. S., Manktelow, B., Field, D. J., et al. (1999). Prediction of survival for preterm births by weight and gestational age: retrospective population based study. *British Medical Journal* 319(7217), 1093–1097.

Gluckman, P. D. and Hanson, M. A. (2006). The consequences of being born small – an adaptive perspective. *Hormone Research* 65(supplement 3), 5–14.

Gluckman, P. D., Hanson, M. A. and Spencer, H. G. (2005). Predictive adaptive responses and human evolution. *Trends in Ecology and Evolution* 20(10), 527–533.

Hales, C. N. and Barker, D. J. P. (2001). The thrifty phenotype hypothesis. *British Medical Bulletin* 60, 5–20.

Huang, S.-T. J., Vo, K. C. T., Lyell, D. J., et al. (2004). Developmental response to hypoxia. *FASEB Journal* 18(12), 1348–1365.

Kofman, O. (2002). The role of prenatal stress in the etiology of developmental behavioural disorders. *Neuroscience and Biobehavioral Reviews* 26(4), 457–470.

Laplante, D. P., Barr, R. G. and Brunet, A. (2004). Stress during pregnancy affects general intellectual and language functioning in human toddlers. *Pediatric Research* 56(3), 400–410.

Latini, G., De Mitri, B., Del Vecchio, A., et al. (2004). Foetal growth of kidneys, liver and spleen in intrauterine growth restriction: "programming" causing "metabolic syndrome" in adult age. *Acta Paediatrrica* 93(12), 1635–1639.

McMillen, I. C. and Robinson, J. S. (2000). Developmental origins of the metabolic syndrome: prediction, plasticity and programming. *Physiological Reviews* 85, 571–633.

Nicolaides, K. H., Bilardo, C. M., Soothill, P. W., et al. (1988). Absence of end diastolic frequencies in umbilical artery: a sign of fetal hypoxia and acidosis. *British Medical Journal* 297(6655), 1026–1027.

Ozanne, S. E. and Hales, C. N. (2002). Early programming of glucose-insulin metabolism,. *Trends in Endocrinology and Metabolism* 13(9), 368–373.

Phillips, D. (2002). Endocrine programming and fetal origins of adult disease. *Trends in Endocrinology and Metabolism* **13**(9), 363.

Seckl, J. R. (2001). Glucocorticoid programming of the fetus; adult phenotypes and molecular mechanisms. *Molecular and Cellular Endocrinology* **185**(1–2), 61–71.

Snijders, R. J. M., Sherrod, C., Gosden, C. M., et al. (1993). Fetal growth retardation: associated malformations and chromosome abnormalities. *American Journal of Obstetrics and Gynecology* **168**(2), 547–555.

Smith, J. F., Jr. and Onstad, J. H. (2005). Assessment of the fetus: intermittent auscultation, electronic fetal heart rate tracing, and fetal pulse oximetry. *Obstetrics and Gynecology Clinics of North America* **32**(2), 245–254.

Soothill, P. W., Nicolaides, K. H. and Campbell, S. (1987). Prenatal asphyxia, hyperlacticaemia, hypoglycaemia, and erythroblastosis in growth retarded fetuses. *British Medical Journal Clinical Research Edition* **294**(6579), 1051–1053.

Ward, A. M., Syddall, H. E., Wood, P. J., et al. (2004). Fetal programming of the hypothalamic-pituitary-adrenal (HPA) axis: low birth weight and central HPA regulation. *Journal of Clinical Endocrinology and Metabolism* **89**(3), 1227–1233.

Fever *See:* Febrile Response.

Fibrinogen and Clotting Factors

E Brunner
University College London, London, UK

This article is a revision of the previous edition article by E Brunner, volume 2, pp 138–142, © 2000, Elsevier Inc.

Molecular Biology
Physiology
Pathophysiology
Epidemiology

Glossary

Acute-phase reactant	A blood constituent (e.g., C-reactive protein, leukocytes, fibrinogen, or albumin) that shows a transient change in concentration in response to infection or inflammation.
Endothelium	The tissue lining the inside surface of blood vessels.
Fibrinolytic activity	A measure of the ability of blood to dissolve a thrombus.
Mendelian randomization	An approach to testing causal associations in epidemiology using the influence of a common genetic polymorphism on the risk factor being studied.
Monocyte/ macrophage	A type of phagocytic leukocyte.
Restriction site polymorphisms	The differences in the DNA base sequence of a gene identified by fragmentation of the gene with a DNA-cutting enzyme.
Thrombus	A blood clot; formed by platelet aggregation and the conversion of soluble fibrinogen to an insoluble mesh of polymerized fibrin.

Fibrinogen is a large protein synthesized by the liver that makes up some 5% of total plasma protein. Various stimuli, including injury, activate a sequence of clotting factors that cause soluble fibrinogen to be converted enzymatically to fibrin, an insoluble polymer matrix that is the structural component of blood clots. Raised fibrinogen levels indicate an increased risk of ischemic heart disease and stroke. It is uncertain whether fibrinogen is a risk factor that causes cardiovascular disease (CVD) or a marker of developing disease. Fibrinogen is an acute-phase reactant, and the circulating level increases in response to infection, chronic inflammation, smoking, and other environmental stressors.

Molecular Biology

Structure

Fibrinogen is a large soluble protein of approximately 340 kDa. It is made up of two tripeptide units, each

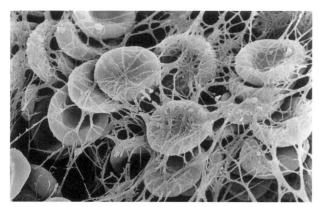

Figure 1 High-resolution electron micrograph of a fibrin polymer matrix. Red blood cells are trapped within the mesh. Courtesy of Dr. D. W. Gregory, University of Aberdeen/Wellcome Trust Medical Photographic Library.

consisting of Aα, Bβ, and γ peptides held together by covalent disulfide bonds. The three-dimensional structure has the form of a rod of dimensions 7×48 nm with a globular domain at each end and a third globular domain at the center of the rod, where the two units are joined together by further disulfide bonds. Free N-terminal residues project radially from the central domain. This negatively charged region prevents the aggregation of fibrinogen molecules by electrostatic repulsion. Fibrin is formed when the four N-terminal peptides are cleaved to release fibrinopeptides A and B. With the loss of the negatively charged peptides, staggered end-to-end polymerization takes place to produce fibrin fiber bundles (**Figure 1**). The clot is completed by the reinforcement of the fibers with covalent cross-links. More than 20 enzymes and protein cofactors are involved in clot formation and dissolution. Blood platelets interact with and possess receptors for fibrinogen. These nonnucleated bodies originate from bone marrow cells (megakaryocytes) and circulate at a concentration of some $150–500\,000$ mm^{-3}.

Biosynthesis and Genetics

Fibrinogen is synthesized primarily by hepatic parenchymal cells and to a lesser extent by megakaryocytes. The fibrinogen peptides are encoded on chromosome 4. A 50-kb span contains the genes for the Aα, Bβ, and γ chains separated by untranslated base sequences. These promoter sequences appear to coordinate the expression of the three genes. After translation and assembly, with the formation of the disulfide bonds, the molecule is glycosylated before release into the circulation from secretory vacuoles.

Serious congenital abnormalities of fibrinogen biosynthesis are uncommon. Absent or very low levels of fibrinogen have been identified, but congenital hyperfibrinogenemia has not. Major abnormalities are probably due to translation, transcription, or secretion defects rather than gross fibrinogen gene defects. Less dramatic abnormalities are associated with bleeding or thrombosis, or may be asymptomatic. Several restriction site polymorphisms exist on the α and β genes. Common genetic variants have been shown to account for some 15% of within-population differences in plasma fibrinogen levels and may explain susceptibility to CVD in some families. Genetic epidemiology uses this variation in association studies of unrelated individuals to test the causal link with coronary heart disease (CHD), applying the method of Mendelian randomization.

Physiology

The Clotting System

The clotting, or coagulation, system functions to maintain the integrity of blood vessels and is essential to homeostasis. Two mechanisms initiate formation of a thrombus: (1) injury of the vascular lining (endothelium) to expose anionic surfaces causes binding and activation of factor XII, the first step in the intrinsic pathway, and (2) exposure of the transmembrane protein factor III or tissue factor (TF) at the site of injury leads to the initiation of the extrinsic pathway (so called because it relies on a substance not usually present in the circulation).

The main reaction of the extrinsic pathway involves the binding of factor VII and calcium ions (Ca^{2+}) to the exposed tissue factor receptor to form the catalyst TF-VIIa-Ca^{2+}, which converts inactive factor X to active Xa. The cascade of four reactions in the intrinsic pathway also generates an increase in the local concentration of factor Xa. If each step in this pathway activates 100 enzyme molecules, the initial event will produce a signal amplified by 10^6. The two clotting pathways lead to the formation of the same prothrombinase complex (Va-Xa-Ca^{2+}-phospholipid), which catalyses the hydrolysis of prothrombin to thrombin. Thrombin has three major roles: it splits fibrinopeptides A and B from the Aα and Bβ chains of fibrinogen to form fibrin and promotes the aggregation of platelets at the site of injury. The clotting process is self-controlling by means of inhibitory mechanisms in which thrombin and protein C are central.

Blood Platelets

Low platelet counts are associated with capillary bleeding, and high counts are associated with intravascular thrombosis. Platelet aggregation is initiated in two ways. First, thrombin and receptors on damaged endothelial cells cause the exposure of a receptor for fibrinogen (integrin α_{IIb}/β_3 or glycoprotein GPIIb/IIIa) on the platelet membrane. Fibrinogen binds the activated platelet to other platelets or to collagen. Second, high shear conditions, such as those occurring in narrowed atheromatous vessels, activate a second receptor that binds von Willebrand factor (vWF). This glycoprotein is released by activated platelets to form links between platelets and to anchor the growing thrombus to the vessel wall. Aspirin inhibits the aggregation mechanism involving fibrinogen but not shear-induced aggregation involving vWF.

The Fibrinolytic System

The thrombus is broken down to restore normal blood flow by the proteolytic action of plasmin on the fibrin matrix when, for example, the wound has healed. This enzyme is converted from the inactive form by tissue plasminogen activator (t-PA), which is secreted by endothelial cells of the vessel wall. Fibrin degradation products are detectable in the blood of healthy individuals, indicating that thrombus formation and fibrinolysis proceed continually. Inhibitors of fibrinolysis include lipoprotein (a) and plasminogen activator inhibitor.

Blood Viscosity

The plasma level of fibrinogen is an important influence on the flow properties of blood. Plasma viscosity increases exponentially with fibrinogen concentration. Because blood contains cells, among which the erythrocyte (red blood cell) predominates at some 5 million mm^{-3}, it is a non-Newtonian fluid exhibiting an apparent viscosity depending on local flow conditions. Viscosity is lower when blood flow is turbulent and under high shear conditions; it is higher under the opposite conditions. The blood flow rate is inversely related to viscosity and directly proportional to the fourth power of the vessel diameter. A small change in diameter thus produces a large change in tissue perfusion.

Pathophysiology

Thrombus Formation

Thrombus formation is involved in several important causes of death and disability. Coronary thrombosis may precipitate sudden coronary death or heart attack, whereas cerebrovascular thrombosis leads to stroke. A small proportion of women possess an abnormally sensitive clotting system and an increased tendency to form venous thrombi in response to raised circulating estrogen levels with oral contraceptive use or in pregnancy. Clot-busting or thombolytic

drugs, such as recombinant t-PA, administered within hours of heart attack are effective in restoring blood supply to the damaged heart muscle and in reducing subsequent mortality.

Atheroma Formation

The clotting system is involved in the slow evolution of atheroma, the plaques that produce arterial narrowing. Fibrinogen and fibrin are found in atherosclerotic lesions. Histological studies show that small thrombi formed at the vessel wall can be incorporated into the evolving plaque. Platelets or platelet fragments are detectable in many plaques. Fibrinogen and its degradation products interact with platelets, endothelial and smooth muscle cells, and monocytes. These processes include the transfer of cholesterol from lipoproteins and platelets to monocytes to form giant foam cells and their incorporation into the growing plaque.

Acute-Phase Reaction

The acute response to infection or inflammation includes an increase in plasma fibrinogen concentration. This is, in part, stimulated by a rise in monocyte secretion of interleukin (IL)-6, one of a group of inflammatory mediators known as the cytokines. An IL-6-responsive element has been identified in the promoter region of the β-fibrinogen gene, and IL-6 thus appears to be a major regulator of fibrinogen synthesis. The size of the inflammatory response appears to be tuned by a vagally mediated anti-inflammatory pathway. Parasympathetic outflow via cholinergic neurons inhibits release of pro-inflammatory cytokines from liver, spleen, and other organs of the reticuloendothelial system. The connection between the nervous and immune systems has been demonstrated in animal models employing direct electrical stimulation of the efferent vagus nerve.

The higher fibrinogen levels seen in smokers may be due to chronic inflammation of the pulmonary epithelium and consequent raised IL-6 production. Long-term low-level inflammatory processes may also be involved in atheroma development as a result of chronic asymptomatic infections, such as gastric *Helicobacter pylori* infection.

Epidemiology

Cardiovascular Epidemiology

It is not clear whether hemostasis is causally involved in early development of coronary atherosclerosis, as opposed to the thrombotic processes that precede an acute CVD event. Internationally, levels of hemostatic factors reflect underlying rates of CHD. Fibrinogen levels measured around 1980 were high in Czechoslovakia and Finland and low in urban Gambia. Mean fibrinolytic activity was highest in Gambia, intermediate in Scotland, and lowest in Finland. Plasma fibrinogen measured in the United States and Japan in 1987 showed substantially higher levels in White American men than in Japanese men. The difference was evident in nonsmokers; among Japanese nonsmokers mean fibrinogen was 2.2 g l^{-1}, whereas among American nonsmokers it was 2.8 g l^{-1}. These ecological associations, which parallel rates of disease, could be the product of cause or consequence.

At the individual level, a high plasma fibrinogen concentration in adulthood has been shown to predict CVD in a meta-analysis of 31 large cohort studies. Other hemostatic factors, including factor VII, white blood cell count, plasma viscosity, and fibrinolytic activity, predict CHD, although the evidence is less extensive. Fibrinogen level may be a mediator of the relationship between smoking and CVD. Likewise, the alcohol–fibrinogen relationship is consistent with the protective effect of moderate alcohol consumption on heart attack risk, and the fibrinogen level is lower in those taking regular leisure time physical activity. Fibrinogen remains predictive of CVD after taking into account smoking, blood pressure, body mass index, and serum cholesterol level. However, from prospective observational studies this evidence does not constitute proof of causation. The alternative interpretation, that fibrinogen is not a causal factor but a marker of the disease process, remains plausible. One deficiency in the evidence is the lack of fibrinogen-lowering trials that might demonstrate reduction of coronary risk.

Mendelian Randomization

Evidence that fibrinogen, and by implication hemostasis, is not causal for CVD comes from genetic epidemiology. Employing the method of Mendelian randomization, the lifelong influence of a common genetic variant in the promoter region of the β-fibrinogen gene that raises the plasma fibrinogen level was found to be without effect on CHD risk. In the same large case-control study, as in many other observational studies, plasma fibrinogen levels were substantially higher in coronary cases. The conflicting findings for phenotype and genotype suggest that plasma fibrinogen is raised as a result of the presence of developing atherosclerotic plaques. If replicated, the conclusion that raised fibrinogen is a consequence, rather than a cause of disease, becomes more likely.

Infancy and Childhood

Poor intra-uterine and early postnatal development are important elements in the genesis of adult disease. In this context, poor early growth and poor childhood socioeconomic conditions are related to elevated fibrinogen levels in adulthood. In addition, height in adulthood (reflecting early environment and genetic endowment) is inversely related to fibrinogen level and to cardiorespiratory mortality risk. These findings are consistent with the long-term *in utero* and childhood influences on CVD risk. It remains unclear whether the association with hemostatic factors is a direct result of early life conditions or the indirect consequence of accelerated disease processes that raise fibrinogen levels secondary to damage of the arterial wall. If the latter explanation emerges as the correct understanding, the measurement of hemostatic factors will remain important as a marker of subclinical disease in studies of the early origins of CVD.

Social Position and Psychosocial Factors

Plasma fibrinogen level is related to several social and psychosocial factors in adulthood. This is consistent with a contribution of hemostasis to the high rates of coronary disease experienced by people in unfavorable socioeconomic circumstances or, alternatively, with plasma fibrinogen being a marker of socially patterned disease processes. Mean fibrinogen levels are strongly and inversely related to grade of employment in the British civil service (**Figure 2**) and to social class based on occupation in a stratified sample of the population of England and Wales. Among civil servants, approximately one-half of the inverse association with social position was accounted for by health-related behaviors and degree of obesity.

Low job control, a measure of an adverse psychosocial work environment, has been linked to higher fibrinogen levels in both sexes in several studies. This association has been found when the work environment was assessed either subjectively, using standard self-completion questionnaires, or externally, by personnel managers. Complementing the link with adverse psychological conditions, positive affect is associated with a small plasma fibrinogen response to behavioral stress tasks (color-word and mirror tracing) in the laboratory.

It is plausible that psychosocial factors exert effects on the hemostatic system and thereby influence disease risk. Acute effects include increased platelet stickiness in the fight-or-flight response via increased circulating catecholamines. In a study of astronauts, spaceflight evoked raised urinary IL-6 on the first day

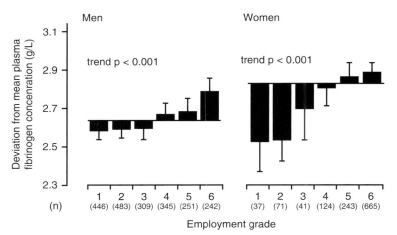

Figure 2 Plasma fibrinogen levels by employment grade (the Whitehall II study). Civil service employment grade classifications: 1, unified grades 1–6; 2, unified grade 7; 3, senior executive officer; 4, higher executive officer; 5, executive officer; 6, clerical/office support. Reproduced with permission from Brunner, E. J., Davey Smith, G., Marmot, M. G., et al. (1996), Childhood social circumstances and psychosocial and behavioural factors as determinants of plasma fibrinogen, *Lancet* **347**, 1008–1013. © The Lancet Ltd.

but not on other days before or after launch, which is consistent with a psychological explanation because infection does not appear to be implicated. Cytokine release in response to psychosocial stimuli, and thereby increased fibrinogen synthesis, is feasible in view of the observation that mRNA for IL-6 is expressed within the brain. Over decades, such small effects may add to the formation of arterial plaques to increase risks of heart disease and stroke.

Further Reading

Brunner, E. J., Davey Smith, G., Marmot, M. G., et al. (1996). Childhood social circumstances and psychosocial and behavioural factors as determinants of plasma fibrinogen. *Lancet* **347**, 1008–1013.

Danesh, J., Collins, R., Appleby, P., et al. (1998). Association of fibrinogen, C-reactive protein, albumin, or leukocyte count with coronary heart disease. *Journal of the American Medical Association* **279**, 1477–1481.

Dang, C. V., Bell, W. R., Baltimore, M. D., et al. (1989). The normal and morbid biology of fibrinogen. *American Journal of Medicine* **87**, 567–576.

Davey Smith, G., Harbord, R. and Ebrahim, S. (2004). Fibrinogen, C-reactive protein and coronary heart disease: does Mendelian randomization suggest the associations are non-causal? *Quarterly Journal of Medicine* **97**, 163–166.

Fibrinogen Studies Collaboration (2005). Plasma fibrinogen level and the risk of major cardiovascular diseases and nonvascular mortality: an individual participant meta-analysis. *Journal of the American Medical Association* **294**, 1799–1809.

Meade, T. W., Ruddock, V., Stirling, Y., et al. (1993). Fibrinolytic activity, clotting factors, and long-term incidence of ischaemic heart disease in the Northwick Park Heart Study. *Lancet* **342**, 1076–1079.

O'Brien, J. R. (1990). Shear-induced platelet aggregation. *Lancet* **335**, 711–713.

Rabbani, L. E. and Loscalzo, J. (1994). Recent observations on the role of hemostatic determinants in the development of the atherothrombotic plaque. *Atherosclerosis* **105**, 1–7.

Stein, T. P. and Schluter, M. D. (1994). Excretion of IL-6 by astronauts during spaceflight. *American Journal of Physiology* **266**, E448–E552.

Steptoe, A., Wardle, J. and Marmot, M. (2005). Positive affect and health-related neuroendocrine, cardiovascular, and inflammatory processes. *Proceedings of the National Academy of Sciences* **102**, 6508–6512.

Vaisanen, S., Rauramaa, R., Penttila, I., et al. (1997). Variation in plasma fibrinogen over one year: relationships with genetic polymorphisms and non-genetic factors. *Thrombosis and Haemostasis* **77**, 884–889.

Fibromyalgia

P B Wood
Louisiana State University Health Sciences Center,
Shreveport, LA, USA and McGill University, Montreal,
Quebec, Canada

Introduction
Background
Epidemiology
Etiology: The Role of Stress
Experimental Findings
Hypothetical Mechanisms of Abnormal Pain Processing
Future Directions

Glossary

Allodynia	Pain produced by normally nonpainful stimulation such as touch, gentle pressure, cold, or gentle joint movement.
Central sensitization	The development within the central nervous system of an exaggerated, pathological response to a stimulus that was originally innocuous, which depends on plasticity in function of N-methyl-D-aspartate (NMDA) glutamate receptors.
Hyperalgesia	Abnormally increased pain sensation.
N-*methyl-D-aspartate (NMDA)-receptors*	Class of glutamate receptors that act as ion channels characterized by their affinity for NMDA that are crucial for neural plasticity.
Nociception	The perception of pain.
Pain	An unpleasant sensory and emotional experience associated with actual or potential tissue damage, or described in terms of such damage.
Tender points	Discrete areas of hyperalgesia/allodynia where localized pressure will elicit pain.
Wind-up	A frequency-dependent increase in the nervous system response to repeat stimulation thought to be dependent on glutamate and NMDA receptors in the dorsal horn of the spinal cord; temporal summation to pain produced by repeat stimulation.

Introduction

Fibromyalgia is a disorder characterized by chronic widespread pain and tenderness to light palpation, sleep disturbance, and chronic fatigue. A diagnosis of fibromyalgia is made by the presence of diffuse tenderness to light palpation in nonarticular soft tissues in a characteristic distribution in the absence of specific laboratory or radiological abnormalities, along with a history that typically includes exposure to significant stressors. Fibromyalgia can occur as an isolated condition, sometimes termed primary fibromyalgia, or it may occur in the presence of other painful conditions such as rheumatoid arthritis, a condition known as secondary fibromyalgia. In addition to the core features of chronic widespread pain and fatigue, patients are typically afflicted by a variety of other symptoms involving multiple organ systems, which has led in turn to the development of a more comprehensive construct: the fibromyalgia syndrome.

Background

The current concept of fibromyalgia is primarily derived from the work of Gowers and Stockman, who, in 1904, proposed that chronic widespread pain likely resulted from fibrositis, or diffuse inflammation of fibrous connective tissues. Subsequent analysis of said tissues has failed to demonstrate such changes, and, in fact, no peripheral pathology has been elucidated to date, despite extensive investigations. Given the lack of inflammation, the name was subsequently changed to fibromyalgia, which literally translated means simply pain in the muscles and fibrous tissues. The diagnostic criteria for classification and research purposes were formalized by the American College of Rheumatology, based on findings of the Multicenter Criteria Committee in 1990, which rely on the presence of discrete areas of tenderness to light palpation occurring diffusely in a primarily axial distribution that have been present for a minimum of 3 months (see **Figure 1**).

In the original documentation of the disorder, patients with fibromyalgia were noted to experience, in addition to chronic widespread pain, symptoms in multiple systems including disturbed bowel function, genitourinary problems, and allergic phenomena such as sinus drainage and congestion. An increased incidence of affective- and anxiety-related symptoms is also well known. More recently, the Canadian Case Definitions has been published, which places an increased emphasis on a variety of neurological phenomena associated with the disorder, including nondermatomal parasthesias, headache, temporospatial dysmetria, and restless legs syndrome. In addition, patients frequently complain of cognitive dysfunction (commonly referred to as "fibro fog") characterized

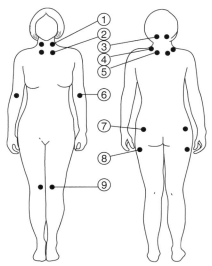

Figure 1 A diagnosis of fibromyalgia is based on (1) the presence of chronic widespread pain of at least 3 months duration in a distribution above and below the waistline, on the left and right sides of the body, and in a primarily axial distribution and (2) pain on palpation with a 4-kg force in 11 of 18 tenderpoints.

by impaired concentration and short-term memory consolidation, impaired speed of performance, inability to multitask, and frequent cognitive overload.

The combination of a lack of readily demonstrable pathology to which symptoms might be ascribed and the dependence on subjective patient report has fueled much of the controversy surrounding fibromyalgia and led to large segments of the medical community dismissing such patients as neurotic complainers aspiring to fashionable diagnoses. However, although the exact pathology underlying the disorder's cardinal feature, namely, chronic widespread pain, remains one of medicine's enduring mysteries, recent advances have shed increasing light on the nature of the disorder. As investigations into potential peripheral pathologies have remained largely fruitless, increasing attention has been focused on mechanisms within the central nervous system. Accordingly, fibromyalgia is increasingly conceptualized as an aberration of information processing in pain-related pathways and thus is considered a form of central sensitization.

Epidemiology

Fibromyalgia is a common condition with an estimated prevalence of 2% of the general population: 3.4% for women and 0.5% for men. Although all ages are affected, the prevalence increases with age, reaching greater than 7% in women aged 60 to 79 years. Fibromyalgia is the second most common diagnosis in rheumatology clinics. Given that the vast majority of fibromyalgia patients are female, many

researchers have suggested that gender-specific factors likely play a role in the development and/or maintenance of symptoms.

Etiology: The Role of Stress

Fibromyalgia has been characterized as a stress-related disorder due to the recognition of its frequent onset after acute or chronic stressors and apparent exacerbation of symptoms during periods of physical or emotional stress. Factors associated with the onset of fibromyalgia include severe infectious illness, physical trauma, and severe emotional distress. In addition, many of the comorbid conditions that affect fibromyalgia patients are likewise considered to be stress-related disorders, including irritable bowel syndrome, chronic fatigue syndrome, interstitial cystitis, and such neuropsychiatric disorders as depression and posttraumatic stress disorder. Patients with fibromyalgia also report a higher incidence of adverse early life events than unaffected individuals. While the experience of adverse early life events has been demonstrated to produce a variety of changes to the neuroendocrine function and to have an adverse impact on the brain limbic system in susceptible individuals, the specific contribution of these events to the etiology of the disorder is not clear, nor is there a strict correlation between the experience of adverse early life events and the development of chronic widespread pain.

While a number of phenomena associated with fibromyalgia have been attributed to the stress of chronic pain, basic science has demonstrated that the experience of chronic stress per se produces harmful sequelae such as disrupted immune and neuroendocrine function, alterations of neurotransmitter release, and damage to the very substance of the brain itself. These observations have in turn informed some of the more recent theoretical considerations concerning the etiopathogenesis of the disorder, which are explored later. In addition, a growing body of evidence supports a component of genetic heritability in the development of the disorder. Taking into account the contribution of both genetic as well as environmental factors, the development of fibromyalgia likely results from of a combination of genetic predisposition and subsequent exposure to critical environmental conditions that must reach a critical load in order to initiate the changes that result in the development of chronic widespread pain and tenderness. (One might therefore suggest that what fibromyalgia represents is a rather bizarre form of allostasis.) As such, individuals with high susceptibility would require little or no stress in order for symptoms to develop, while others might endure years of duress prior to symptom onset.

This suggestion raises the possibility of a prodromal period during which subtle changes are occurring within the susceptible nervous system during periods of prolonged stress.

Experimental Findings

An unfortunately intransigent misconception among many clinicians is the notion that the patient with fibromyalgia essentially has nothing wrong with him or her, a position that stems in large part from a frustrating lack of readily demonstrable pathology in the soft tissues or blood. On the contrary, research has demonstrated a variety of abnormalities are in fact associated with the disorder, which are detailed below.

Polymodal Sensitivity

Results from studies examining responses to experimental stimulation have shown that fibromyalgia patients display sensitivity to pressure, heat, cold, and electrical and chemical stimulation. Experiments examining pain regulatory systems have shown that fibromyalgia patients also display a dysregulation of diffuse noxious inhibitory control, an exaggerated wind-up response, and an absence of exercise-induced analgesic response. Together, these results point to dysregulation of the nociceptive system at the central level.

Sleep Disturbances

The first objective findings associated with the disorder were reported in 1975 by Moldofsky and colleagues, who reported the presence of anomalous alpha wave activity (typically associated with arousal states) on sleep electroencephalogram (EEG) in fibromyalgia patients during non-rapid eye movement sleep. In fact, by consistently disrupting stage IV sleep in young, healthy subjects, Moldofsky was able to reproduce a significant increase in muscle tenderness similar to that experienced by fibromyalgia patients but that was resolved when the subjects were able to resume their normal sleep patterns. Since that time a variety of other EEG sleep abnormalities has also been reported in subgroups of fibromyalgia patients. While chronic sleep disruption has been documented to disrupt normal brain function and produce a variety of deleterious neuroendocrine and metabolic consequences, the specific mechanism whereby increased tenderness might result remains to be determined, as does the exact relationship of sleep disruption to the disorder, whether as a contributing factor or rather an additional manifestation of an underlying pathology.

Neuroendocrine Disruption

Patients with fibromyalgia have been demonstrated to have a disruption of normal neuroendocrine function, characterized by mild hypocortisolemia, hyperreactivity of pituitary adrenocorticotropin hormone release in response to challenge, and glucocorticoid feedback resistance. A progressive reduction of serum growth hormone levels has also been documented – at baseline in a minority of patients, while most demonstrate reduced secretion in response to exercise or pharmacological challenge. Other abnormalities include reduced melatonin secretion, reduced responsivity of thyrotropin and thyroid hormones to thyrotropin-releasing hormone, and a mild elevation of prolactin levels with disinhibition of prolactin release in response to challenge and hyposecretion of adrenal androgens. These changes might be attributed to the effects of chronic stress, which, after being perceived and processed by the central nervous system, activates hypothalamic corticotropin-releasing hormone neurons. Thus, the multiple neuroendocrine changes evident in fibromyalgia have been proposed to stem from chronic overactivity of corticotropin-releasing hormone releasing neurons, resulting in a disruption of normal function of the pituitary-adrenal axis and an increased stimulation of hypothalamic somatostatin secretion, which, in turn, inhibits the secretion of a multiplicity of other hormones.

Sympathetic Hyperactivity

Functional analysis of the autonomic system in patients with fibromyalgia has demonstrated disturbed activity characterized by hyperactivity of the sympathetic nervous system at baseline with reduced sympathoadrenal reactivity in response to a variety of stressors including orthostatic challenge and mental stress. Fibromyalgia patients demonstrate lower heart rate variability, an index of sympathetic/parasympathetic balance, indicating sustained sympathetic hyperactivity, especially at night. In addition, plasma levels of neuropeptide Y, which is colocalized with norepinephrine in the sympathetic nervous system, have been reported to be low in patients with fibromyalgia. Incongruent with this finding, there have been inconsistent reports of low, normal, and high circulating levels of epinephrine and norepinephrine. Administration of interleukin-6, a cytokine capable of stimulating the release of hypothalamic corticotropin-releasing hormone, which in turn stimulates the sympathetic nervous system, resulted in a dramatic increase in circulating norepinephrine levels and a significantly greater increase in heart rate over baseline in fibromyalgia patients as compared to healthy controls.

Cerebrospinal Fluid Abnormalities

Perhaps the most reproducible laboratory finding in patients with fibromyalgia is an elevation in cerebrospinal fluid levels of substance P, a putative nociceptive neurotransmitter. While this finding is intriguing, a review of the literature reveals that an elevation in substance P levels is not specific to this disorder, nor has any correlation between these levels and clinical pathology been determined. In addition, metabolites for the monoamine neurotransmitters serotonin, norepinephrine, and dopamine – all of which play a role in natural analgesia – have been shown to be lower, while reports of changes in cerebrospinal fluid concentrations of endogenous opioids (i.e., endorphins and enkephalins) have been contradictory. The mean concentration of nerve growth factor, a substance known to participate in structural and functional plasticity of nociceptive pathways within the dorsal root ganglia and spinal cord, has been reported to be elevated in fibromyalgia patients. In addition, evidence for increased excitatory amino acid release within cerebrospinal fluid has also been reported, with a correlation between levels for metabolites of glutamate and nitric oxide and clinical indices of pain.

Brain Imaging Studies

Evidence of abnormal brain involvement in fibromyalgia has been provided via functional neuroimaging. The first findings reported a decreased blood flow within the thalamus and elements of the basal ganglia and mid-brain (i.e., pontine nucleus) in patients with fibromyalgia. Differential activation in response to painful stimulation has also been demonstrated. Brain centers showing hyperactivation in response to noxious stimulation include such pain-related brain centers as the primary and secondary somatosensory cortex, anterior cingulate cortex, and insular cortex, while relative hypoactivation at subjectively equal pain levels appears to occur within the thalamus and basal ganglia. In addition, patients exhibit neural activation in brain regions associated with pain perception in response to nonpainful stimuli, in such areas as the prefrontal, supplemental motor, insular, and cingulate cortices. Some of the brain abnormalities seem to be amenable to pharmacological intervention, as a few studies have reported changes on neuroimaging in response to effective therapeutic intervention, although replication of such findings is needed. Patients with fibromyalgia also have evidence of hippocampal disruption indicated by reduced brain metabolite ratios and reduced gray matter concentration. Finally, positron emission tomography using radiolabeled DOPA, a precursor to dopamine synthesis, has demonstrated a diffuse reduction in monoaminergic (i.e., dopamine, norepinephrine, and epinephrine) metabolism specifically in brain areas in which dopamine plays a critical role in natural analgesia, including the anterior cingulate cortex, insula, and thalamus.

In summary, the abnormalities associated with fibromyalgia show evidence of enhanced nociception associated with increased cortical excitability (as evidenced by abnormal arousal patterns on sleep EEG and increased activation in response to stimulation), subtle changes in brain chemistry, and a dysregulation of both arms of the stress response, i.e., the HPA axis and the sympathetic nervous system. As a review of these findings might suggest, one problem facing both patients and clinicians is that the type of abnormalities reviewed herein are generally detected by assays not typically available to primary care or even tertiary referral clinics. Given the lack of more readily demonstrable pathology, the difficulty that the medical culture has had coming to terms with fibromyalgia and related conditions seems to stem from the pervasive philosophical tradition of Cartesian dualism, in which human phenomena are categorized as belonging to one of two domains, i.e., psyche or soma – the mind or the body. Thus, if an individual presents to a clinician with somatic complaints for which no pathological change is evident in the organ from which the symptoms seem to originate, and if stress appears to play a contributory role, then the patient is liable to be dismissed as somatizing or expressing psychic distress by way of physical symptoms. This unfortunate attitude on the part of uninformed clinicians represents what essentially amounts to a medical form of being politically correct in suggesting that a patient's problems are all in his or her head – a phrase that tacitly avoids the pejorative and clinically irrelevant label "crazy".

Hypothetical Mechanisms of Abnormal Pain Processing

While the preceding findings are intriguing, the fact is that the exact mechanism of enhanced nociception in fibromyalgia remains a matter of debate and continuing inquiry. Accordingly, the following represents a synopsis of some hypothetical considerations regarding the potential pathologies that might contribute to the phenomenon of enhanced nociception.

There exists a school of thought that considers the pain of fibromyalgia to represent a primarily psychic phenomenon. Accordingly, those who ascribe to this perspective consider the enhanced nociception displayed by fibromyalgia patients to represent a form of secondary hyperalgesia, attributed to such processes as hypervigilance or increased attention to somatosensory stimulation suggesting a perceptual style of amplification. This conclusion is derived in part from the consistent observation of increased activation of the anterior cingulate cortex, which plays a role in both the attentional and affective, or emotional, dimensions of pain perception. Enhanced activation of the anterior cingulate cortex in response to stimulation has also been demonstrated in another stress-related disorder characterized by enhanced somatosensory perception: irritable bowel syndrome.

On the other hand, the hyperalgesia and other forms of polymodal sensitivity that characterize the disorder have been conceptualized as a form of central sensitization in which elements of the central nervous system have become pathologically sensitive to stimulation, thereby making stimuli that were previously innocuous (light touch, for example) excruciating. The phenomenon of central sensitization has been demonstrated to depend on the plasticity in function of N-methyl-D-aspartate (NMDA) subtype glutamate receptors, which play a fundamental role in the flow of information within the brain and spinal cord. In support of this notion, it has been demonstrated that a large subgroup of patients respond to very small doses of the anesthetic ketamine, which at sufficient doses antagonizes NMDA receptors, with dramatic reductions in the painful symptoms. It is then intriguing that NMDA receptors play a critical role in pain perception, specifically within the hippocampus and anterior cingulate cortex, wherein a variety of stress-related factors such as corticotropin-releasing hormone, cortisol, norepinephrine, substance P, and histamine contribute to neuronal excitability specifically by enhancing NMDA receptor activity. Thus, the pain of fibromyalgia (and perhaps other related disorders) might stem from stress-related changes within brain centers involved in overlapping mechanisms of nociception (i.e., attentional and affective dimensions), in which stress-related factors reduce the threshold for excitation. As such, these changes provide a credible organic basis for what might otherwise be appreciated as psychic phenomena.

A relative increase in the amount of information flowing out of the body and toward the brain might also result in enhanced pain perception. One naturally expects this in scenarios involving tissue damage, whether related to mechanical causes (as in an injury or a degenerative condition such as arthritis) or a chemical or thermal exposure. Likewise, inflammatory processes result in the release of various chemicals within affected tissues that sensitize peripheral pain receptors (nociceptors), thereby amplifying the flow of information from the area of inflammation.

The adaptive value of such an increased amount of painful information originating from injured tissue is clear: the organism protects the area and allows it to heal. On the other hand, no such peripheral pathology has been described in fibromyalgia; therefore, an area of intense focus regarding the potential source of increased information flowing toward the brain has been potential pathological changes within the dorsal root ganglion and dorsal horn of the spinal column, which collectively represent the interface between the peripheral and central nervous systems. Both of these regions contain high densities of NMDA receptors, which are thought to contribute substantially the phenomenon of wind-up, and both have been demonstrated to undergo pathological transformation under certain conditions, thereby resulting in hyperalgesia and allodynia in the affected area. Intriguingly, recent investigations using rat models have demonstrated that stress exposure results in increased metabolic activity within the dorsal horn. However, the relevance of these findings to fibromyalgia remains unknown.

Somatosensory information processing represents a two-way flow of information within the spinal cord: information concerning the status of the body is transferred from the peripheral nervous system to the central nervous system and ascends the spinal cord toward the brain, while a variety of filtering mechanisms descend from the brain to modulate the amount of information transferred specifically within the dorsal horn. The vast majority of neurons that carry descending inhibition run along tracks within the dorsal spinal column (i.e., the part furthest toward the back). Research has demonstrated that interruption of the dorsal descending systems leads to hyperactivity of pain-related neurons within the spinal cord characterized by an increase in background activity, lowering in stimulation threshold, and increase in response magnitude to noxious stimuli. Collectively, the findings suggest that if such an interruption were to occur in humans, such impairment would likely result in spontaneous deep pain, tenderness to palpation, and hyperalgesia of deep tissues – all of which characterize patients with fibromyalgia. Accordingly, some researchers are focused on determining the potential contribution of restrictive lesions, specifically within the cervical spinal cord, to the experience of chronic widespread pain. Likewise, an increase in descending facilitation involving medullary brain centers might also contribute to the amplification of sensory information.

The apparent dysregulation of the sympathetic nervous system detailed previously has led to the hypothesis that fibromyalgia might represent a sympathetically maintained pain syndrome. In support of this notion, proponents of the hypothesis observe that, like other so-called sympathetically maintained pain conditions (e.g., complex regional pain syndrome, or reflex sympathetic dystrophy), the pain associated with fibromyalgia may be characterized by its frequent posttraumatic onset and by the presence of chronic stimuli-independent pain accompanied by allodynia, paresthesias, and distal vasomotor changes. Limited reports suggest that fibromyalgia pain may be aggravated by peripheral administration of epinephrine. Historically speaking, it has been generally considered that sympathetically maintained pain is alleviated by maneuvers intended to block sympathetic activity, and there are (again, limited) reports reflecting that fibromyalgia patients respond to these as well. More recently, however, the contribution of sympathetic activity to those conditions traditionally considered to represent sympathetically maintained pain conditions has become a matter of some contention, while the specific mechanism whereby sympathetic activation might contribute to the development of chronic widespread pain remains to be elucidated.

The most recent hypotheses concerning the nature of pain in fibromyalgia have to do with a disruption of natural analgesia within the limbic system involving the neurotransmitter dopamine. Stressful experience has been robustly demonstrated to disrupt the normal function of dopamine neurons, which in turn plays an important role in natural analgesia in such brain centers as the thalamus, basal ganglia, nucleus accumbens, insular cortex, and anterior cingulate cortex. Recent insights regarding the pharmacology of ketamine have demonstrated that the drug activates dopamine D2 receptors, which may then explain its efficacy in relieving symptoms of fibromyalgia when given at very low doses. Intriguingly, many of the brain centers that have been shown to be involved in fibromyalgia using functional neuroimaging are among the same brain centers in which dopamine plays a role in analgesia. Dopamine acts within the thalamus and insular cortex to recruit mechanisms of descending inhibition, while in the anterior cingulate cortex dopamine opposes the activity of NMDA receptors specifically involved in nociception. In addition, the reactivity of dopamine neurons is controlled by excitatory output from the hippocampus, which in turn is exquisitely sensitive to the effects of stress-related factors. A stress-related increase in neuronal excitability within the hippocampus would be predicted to suppress the reactivity of dopamine neurons, thereby producing a relative increase in painful sensations. Other neurotransmitters whose dysfunction has been proposed to contribute to the development of chronic widespread pain include serotonin and norepinephrine. In general,

medications that act chiefly to boost serotonergic activity have met with disappointing results, while those with mixed activity for serotonin and norepinephrine are somewhat more promising.

Future Directions

Among the current concepts driving investigations into the nature of fibromyalgia is the growing awareness that patients with fibromyalgia likely represent a homogenous population in which chronic widespread pain is the common denominator. This idea resonates with the conceptualization of two other categories of central nervous system disorders: epilepsy, which has as its common denominator stereotyped and uncontrollable movement stemming from pathology within a variety of brain centers, and depression, in which patients experience dysphoria stemming from the disturbance of a variety of neurohormonal factors. Thus, efforts to subclassify fibromyalgia patients along both organic and psychological lines are currently under way.

In order to effectively target the symptoms of a disorder for therapy, there must first be an understanding of the underlying pathology. In light of recent advances in our insights into the disorder, we indeed seem to be standing at the threshold of understanding. While the status of fibromyalgia as a bona fide disorder is a matter of continuing debate among the uninformed, the fact that major pharmaceutical companies have begun to develop large-scale trials to investigate the potential efficacy of existing drugs at relieving the various symptoms associated with the disorder is evidence of its increasing acceptance within the medical community as a whole. In general, there seems to be grounds for an increased sense of optimism regarding relief for patients, both from their symptoms and from the stigma previously associated with the diagnosis.

See Also the Following Articles

Chronic Fatigue Syndrome; Dopamine, Central; Hippocampus, Overview; Hypothalamic-Pituitary-Adrenal; Musculoskeletal Problems and Stress; Pain; Posttraumatic Stress Disorder, Neurobiology of.

Further Reading

Bennett, R. M. (ed.) (2002). *The clinical neurobiology of fibromyalgia and myofascial pain: therapeutic implications.* Binghamton, NY: Haworth Press, Inc.
Clauw, D. J. (1995). Fibromyalgia: more than just a musculoskeletal disease. *American Family Physician* 52, 843–851, 853–854.
Clauw, D. J. and Crofford, L. J. (2003). Chronic widespread pain and fibromyalgia: what we know, and what

we need to know. *Best Practice and Research: Clinical Rheumatology* **17**, 685–701.

Gracely, R. H., Petzke, F., Wolf, J. M., et al. (2002). Functional magnetic resonance imaging evidence of augmented pain processing in fibromyalgia. *Arthritis and Rheumatism* **46**, 1333–1343.

Jain, A. K., Heffez, D. S., Carruthers, B. M., et al. (2003). The fibromyalgia syndrome: a clinical case definition for practitioners. *Journal of Musculoskeletal Pain* **11**, 3–108.

Neeck, G. and Crofford, L. J. (2000). Neuroendocrine perturbations in fibromyalgia and chronic fatigue syndrome. *Rheumatic Diseases Clinics of North America* **26**, 989–1002.

Staud, R. (2002). Evidence of involvement of central neural mechanisms in generating fibromyalgia pain. *Current Rheumatology Reports* **4**, 299–305.

Wolfe, F., Smythe, H. A., Yunus, M. B., et al. (1990). The American College of Rheumatology 1990 Criteria for the Classification of Fibromyalgia. Report of the Multicenter Criteria Committee. *Arthritis and Rheumatism* **33**, 160–172.

Wood, P. B. (2004). Fibromyalgia: a central role for the hippocampus – a theoretical construct. *Journal of Musculoskeletal Pain* **12**, 19–26.

Wood, P. B. (2004). Stress and dopamine: implications for the pathophysiology of chronic widespread pain. *Medical Hypotheses* **62**, 420–424.

Yunus, M. B. (1992). Towards a model of pathophysiology of fibromyalgia: aberrant central pain mechanisms with peripheral modulation. *Journal of Rheumatology* **19**, 846–850.

Fight-or-Flight Response

R McCarty
Vanderbilt University, Nashville, TN, USA

This article is reproduced from the previous edition, volume 2, pp 143–145, © 2000, Elsevier Inc.

Emotional Stimulation and Epinephrine Secretion

The James–Lange Theory of Emotions

The Cannon–Bard Theory of Emotions

Contemporary Research on the Fight-or-Flight Response

Glossary

Cannon–Bard theory	A theory based on the work of the American physiologist W. B. Cannon and his student P. Bard. Their work indicated that portions of the brain stem and hypothalamus were essential for the expression of emotions and the peripheral physiological manifestations of the emotions.
Fight-or-flight response	A concept developed by W. B. Cannon that linked emotional expression to physiological changes in the periphery. Cannon emphasized the emergency function of the adrenal medulla in such situations. He reasoned that the increased discharge of epinephrine from the adrenal medulla stimulated increases in blood glucose and blood flow to skeletal muscles and a corresponding decrease in blood flow to the viscera.
James–Lange theory	A theory based on the independent work of the American psychologist W. James and the Danish physiologist K. Lange. The theory proposed that emotions resulted from afferent feedback from the periphery to the brain.

Emotional Stimulation and Epinephrine Secretion

Walter Cannon and his students and coworkers conducted an initial series of experiments from 1910 to 1911 that examined the link between emotional experiences and the secretion of epinephrine from the adrenal medulla. Employing an intestinal strip bioassay for the semiquantitative study of epinephrine secretion, he and his students determined that epinephrine secretion increased dramatically when a quiescent animal was exposed to a stressful or threatening stimulus. In addition, Cannon's laboratory used increases in glucose in the urine (glycosuria) as an indirect measure of epinephrine secretion with similar results. The connection between epinephrine secretion and increases in blood glucose led Cannon to write the following entry in his journal on January 20, 1911: "Got idea that adrenals in excitement serve to affect muscular power and mobilize sugar for muscular use – thus in wild state readiness for fight or run!" In time, "fight or run" was transformed into the more familiar fight or flight.

The initial description of the fight-or-flight response encompassed only the peripheral manifestations of the response, including a redirection of blood flow and

Table 1 Sympathetic-Adrenal Medullary Components of Fight-or-Flight Response

	Physiological effects	Physiological consequences
Heart	Increased rate	Increased rate of blood flow
	Dilation of coronary vessels	Increased availability of O_2 and energy to cardiac muscle cells
Circulation	Dilation of vessels serving skeletal muscle	Increased availability of O_2 and energy to skeletal muscle cells
	Vasconstriction of vessels serving digestive and related organs	Allows for shunting of blood to skeletal muscle cells
	Contraction of spleen	Increase in delivery of O_2 to metabolically active tissues
Respiration	Dilation of bronchi	Increased availability of O_2 in blood
	Increased respiratory rate	Increased availability of O_2 in blood
Liver	Increased conversion of glycogen to glucose	Increased availability of glucose for skeletal muscle cells and brain tissue

increased delivery of O_2 and glucose to the skeletal muscles as an organism prepared to confront a threatening or stressful situation (**Table 1**).

It was not until the 1920s that Cannon began a series of studies on the central control of sympathetic-adrenal medullary activity. This work focused initially on studies of sham rage in decorticate cats. The findings pointed clearly to the posterior hypothalamus and basocaudal subthalamus as brain structures important for the elevated adrenal medullary discharge of epinephrine during sham rage. This line of research has continued to the present as investigators have used ever more refined anatomical techniques to define the central neural circuitry underlying emotional expression.

The James–Lange Theory of Emotions

At the turn of the twentieth century, the prevailing physiological theory of emotions was based on the independent efforts of the American psychologist William James and the Danish physiologist K. Lange. The James–Lange formulation was as follows:

1. An emotionally charged event occurs and stimulates sensory receptors.
2. Afferent nerve impulses reach the cerebral cortex and the event is perceived.
3. Efferent nerve impulses are directed to the skeletal muscles and the viscera and alter their levels of activity in preparation for the event.

4. Afferent nerve impulses from the periphery go once again to the cerebral cortex and the emotionally charged aspect of the event is perceived.

James emphasized the importance of visceral afferent signals and emotion, whereas Lange drew attention to the relationship between vascular afferent signals and emotion. This was the prevailing theory when Cannon and coworkers began to examine the neural basis for visceral and behavioral control during stressful experiences.

The Cannon–Bard Theory of Emotions

Cannon recognized that a critical test of the James–Lange theory would involve an examination of emotional expression in a subject with no visceral afferent feedback. In such an experiment, the critical link between visceral changes and the feedback required to stimulate the cerebral manifestations of the emotion would be broken. At least three prevailing lines of evidence pointed to the inaccuracy of the James–Lange theory: Sherrington had reported in 1900 that dogs exhibited intense emotions following complete destruction of the sympathetic and spinal sensory roots; later, Cannon and colleagues noted that cats remained emotionally responsive following surgical destruction of the sympathetic nervous system; and, finally, clinical case studies demonstrated that spinally transected patients retained their emotional responses despite being completely paralyzed below the neck.

Cannon was joined in this research effort by several of his students, most notably Philip Bard. Their efforts, beginning in the 1920s, changed the focus of research on emotions to include the central nervous system as the primary site for receiving sensory information, directing peripheral visceral and vascular changes, and generating the psychological manifestations of the experience.

Contemporary Research on the Fight-or-Flight Response

The study of the neural bases of emotions remains an active and exciting area of research to the present. Researchers continue to examine the neural circuits involved in the classic fight-or-flight responses of laboratory animals. Studies suggest that central command neurons within hypothalamic and brain stem nuclei project via sympathetic outflow systems to both the heart and the adrenal medulla. These collections of central command neurons may direct multiple sympathetically controlled neural and endocrine responses that subserve the fight-or-flight response. The midbrain peraqueductal gray region has also been implicated in the physiological and behavioral changes attending the fight-or-flight response. In addition, research on the amygdala has revealed the importance of this brain region for memories of emotionally charged events. Finally, with the advent of imaging techniques (e.g., functional magnetic resonance imaging, fMRI) for studying regional brain activation in human subjects, it is now possible to determine which brain areas are activated during emotionally stimulating events in humans.

Cannon introduced the fight-or-flight concept to physiology and conducted some of the seminal studies in this area. It is impressive to note that his original research linking physiology with emotions is still frequently referenced more than 80 years later and that the fight-or-flight response continues to serve as a stimulating topic of inquiry for researchers in a variety of fields, including physiology, neuroanatomy, and psychology.

See Also the Following Articles

Emotions: Structure and Adaptive Functions; Evolutionary Origins and Functions of the Stress Response; Fear.

Further Reading

Bandler, R. and Shipley, M. T. (1994). Columnar organization in the midbrain periaqueductal gray: modules for emotional expression? *Trends in Neuroscience* **17**, 379–389.

Benison, S., Barger, A. C. and Wolfe, E. L. (1987). *Walter B. Cannon: the life and times of a young scientist.* Cambridge, MA: Belknap Press of Harvard University Press.

Brooks, C. M., Koizumi, K. and Pinkston, J. O. (1975). *The life and contributions of Walter Bradford Cannon 1871–1945: his influence on the development of physiology in the twentieth century.* Brooklyn, NY: State University of New York Downstate Medical Center.

Cannon, W. B. (1915). *Bodily changes in pain, hunger, fear and rage: an account of recent researches into the function of emotional excitement.* New York: Appleton.

Cannon, W. B. (1927). The James-Lange theory of emotions: a critical examination and an alternation. *American Journal of Psychology* **39**, 106–124.

Davis, M. (1992). The role of the amygdala in fear and anxiety. *Annual Review of Neuroscience* **15**, 353–375.

LeDoux, J. E. (1995). Emotion: clues from the brain. *Annual Review of Psychology* **46**, 209–235.

Firefighters, Stress in

T L Guidotti
George Washington University, Washington, DC, USA

This article is a revision of the previous edition article by T L Guidotti, volume 2, pp 146–148, © 2000, Elsevier Inc.

Firefighting as an Occupation
Physical Stress
Psychological Stress

Glossary

17-Ketosteroids	The metabolites of endogenous steroid hormones produced under sustained stress.
Aerial ladder	A very high extension ladder on a hook and ladder truck, used for rescue and to reach the fire with water from above.
Catecholamines	Endogenous hormones produced acutely under stress.
Ischemia	A condition of insufficient blood supply; in the heart, coronary artery ischemia may lead to angina (chest pain), arrhythmia (irregular heartbeat), or a heart attack.
Knockdown measures	Measures to suppress a fire, such as laying on water from a hose carried up a ladder.
Moonlighting	Holding a job or doing work in addition to one's regular employment, usually without the knowledge or approval of the principal employer; firefighters may have several days off between long shifts and often work other jobs to earn extra money.
Myocardial infarction	A heart attack, in which some of the heart muscle dies from lack of oxygen due to ischemia.
Personal protective equipment	The equipment used by firefighters during work to protect the individual workers from a hazard, as distinct from measures used to control the hazard itself; examples include self-contained breathing apparatus, gloves, helmet, and turnout gear (heavy coat and boots).

Firefighting as an Occupation

Firefighting is an intrinsically stressful occupation that attracts an unusual type of person. It is a commonplace saying that firefighters are unique people because they run into burning buildings when other people are fleeing them. The sad human toll of the World Trade Center attack, in which 121 firefighters died, trapped in the North Tower because their radios did not deliver warning messages due to lack of interoperability, demonstrates the risk that firefighters face in their work and their dependence on equipment and organization.

Firefighting, like most occupations involving emergency response, is characterized by prolonged periods of preparation for episodes of intensely stressful activity. Episodically, performance demands require exertion near the limits of human factors and cardiopulmonary conditioning. The risk of injuries is high in firefighting, as indicated by an increased hospitalization rate compared to other occupations for soft tissue injuries, burns, and overexertion. However, much of a firefighter's time is routine, spent in training and maintenance. The psychological stresses of firefighting include long periods of relative inactivity punctuated by highly stressful alarms and extremely stressful situations, such as rescues, as reflected in physiological and biochemical indicators. The literature on the health risks associated with firefighting is large and has been extensively reviewed with particular reference to human factors and ergonomics, chemical hazards, and work-related health outcomes.

The hazards associated with firefighting are changing in nature and magnitude. In the mid-twentieth century, the new composition of interior furnishings introduced new chemical hazards for firefighting, including combustion products from polyvinyl chloride (including phosgene, vinyl chloride) and acrylonitrile (including cyanide). In modern times, commercial and manufacturing facility fires may produce combustion products that are not well characterized and may not even be known. Although firefighting is generally becoming safer due to better and more available equipment and improved procedures, the terrible toll at the World Trade Center illustrates the growing potential for multiple fatalities and serious injuries when things go seriously wrong in ever-larger modern skyscrapers and large facilities.

Firefighters tend to take care of their own but on an informal basis. Firefighting is a close-in activity requiring teamwork under very threatening conditions, and firefighters tend to be very aware of the problems that their fellow firefighters might have in handling difficult situations. Individual firefighters who show early signs of illness are often selectively transferred out of active firefighting positions.

Physical Stress

Energy Requirements

Firefighting is a physically strenuous occupation that is sometimes performed under extreme environmental conditions. There are several components to the physiological demands of firefighting; these include the energy cost of performing firefighting activities, heat stress associated with heat from the fire, encumbrance by personal protection equipment, and psychological stress related to personal safety, protection of property, and protection of lives. The ergonomic demands of firefighting are extreme at peak activity because of high energy costs of activities such as climbing aerial ladders, the positive heat balance from endogenous and absorbed environmental heat, and encumbrance by bulky but necessary protective equipment. The use of personal protection equipment has imposed new physiological demands on firefighters despite the increased level of personal protection.

Physiological Stress

Firefighting is intrinsically stressful. Firefighters increase their urinary excretion of catecholamines (endogenous hormones produced acutely under stress) following workdays compared to days off. Paramedics, for whom job satisfaction was much less, had even higher levels of stress than firefighters. The urinary excretion of 17-ketosteroids (metabolites of endogenous steroid hormones produced under sustained stress) and catecholamines reflects perceived patterns of psychological stress and activity levels at the station.

Cardiovascular Stress

At the sound of an alarm, firefighters experience a degree of immediate anxiety because of the inherent unpredictability of the situation that they are about to encounter. Some investigators believe that the psychological stress experienced at this moment is as great and perhaps greater than any of the stresses that follow during the course of responding to an alarm. Studies of the cardiovascular response to the alarm itself show a marked and highly variable increase in heart rate during the response to a fire alarm, well before physical exertion begins at levels associated with maximal exertion or anxiety. Urinary catecholamine levels are particularly elevated among male firefighters during and after work in the alarm center, an assignment that is highly unpopular. There is also a gender-associated difference in the response, which is less pronounced in women. En route, hazardous traffic maneuvers and high noise levels from the sirens contribute to stress.

Fitness

Numerous studies have evaluated the fitness of firefighters and have shown fairly consistently that most firefighters are as fit or somewhat more fit than the general adult male population. They are not, however, fit to an athletically trained level. Recent studies of job performance requirements suggest that exercise programs for firefighters should be more comprehensive rather than emphasizing cardiovascular fitness and muscle strength, as is now the case.

An increasing number of female applicants are now competing for firefighting jobs. This has forced a re-evaluation of performance tests. As a group, women appeared to demonstrate lower scores on average than men in all performance items, but a subgroup of women performed nearly as well in some tasks. The overall difference in performance was attributed primarily to lower absolute lean body weight, which correlated most strongly and consistently with performance difference.

There is evidence that some firefighters may be stressed to the limit during the exertions of their work. Barnard et al. described an ischemic response in healthy young men, including firefighters, who engaged in sudden vigorous exercise without warm-up. They suggested a transient mismatch in oxygen supply and demand. Although this mechanism is probably not a cause of persistent or cumulative myocardial injury, it may play a role in unusual and emergent situations requiring sudden maximal exertion.

On this basis, it may be concluded that acute myocardial infarction occurring under these circumstances or shortly after maximal exertion in an emergency response may be directly associated with working as a firefighter. It could also be that such an event may happen at work to a firefighter with existing coronary artery disease, in which case it is reasonable to assume an association with firefighting activity. However, it is difficult to attribute myocardial infarction when off-service, hypertension, or chronic manifestations of coronary artery disease to firefighting at this time, given the available evidence.

Because of the high level of physical and psychological stress and the presence of chemical hazards known to injure the cardiovascular system, heart disease is a major occupational health concern in firefighting. Most studies of firefighters show no elevation in mortality from cardiovascular causes or, at most, a small excess risk. "The healthy worker effect expected in such a highly selected group may be offset by greater than expected mortality. A healthy worker effect is more readily visible when comparisons are made to similarly selected occupational groups such as police. Although the findings of individual studies may differ, the pattern that emerges after careful examination is that mortality from cardiovascular causes is not obviously increased in association with firefighting activity (either in terms of years of service or exposure opportunity).

Psychological Stress

There are many extraordinary sources of psychological stress in the life of a firefighter. The expectations for performance placed on firefighters are well beyond that of other civilian occupations, with the possible exception of police. Firefighters accept a level of personal risk beyond the range of normal human experience. Although this risk is controlled to the extent possible with fire equipment and personal protection, the reality of firefighting is that there is much that can go wrong at any fire and the course of a serious fire is often unpredictable. In addition to personal security, the firefighter must be concerned with the safety of others. A failed rescue or the death of a victim is so stressful that some firefighters who have experienced this cannot cope.

Studies of firefighters have shown high levels of job satisfaction and motivation compared to the general population, despite job-related anxiety and adjustment issues related to sleep deprivation, heavy workload or pace of work, constantly being on guard, unsatisfactory public interactions, rigid working conditions, personal risk, inconsistent instructions, and unforeseen situations. On the other hand, firefighters exert a great deal of control over their work in the selection of approaches to knocking down the fire and the use of protective equipment. They are continually faced with new challenges because every alarm presents a different story or situation.

However, firefighters who have experienced particularly threatening situations have demonstrated adverse emotional effects. Chief among these is loss of a life during a rescue attempt or the death or serious injury on the job of a fellow firefighter.

Firefighters have been intensively studied as a model population at risk for posttraumatic stress disorder. Posttraumatic stress disorder can significantly impair in their ability to maintain social and family relationships. Firefighters who do not show the full-blown posttraumatic stress disorder may still be affected by intrusive memories and anxiety. Incident debriefing sessions have been shown to be valuable and effective in assisting firefighters who would otherwise have difficulty coping and in reducing the short-term anxiety of those who would have been able to cope without assistance.

Firefighters are enmeshed in conflicting expectations and numerous technicalities related to the insurance industry, the legal profession, the fire service administration and politics, labor–management relations, and building codes and inspection. Firefighters may be highly trained in the technicalities of fire suppression, but may become so enmeshed unwillingly in the nontechnical aspects of the occupation that they may experience great frustration. When inevitable mistakes happen or their judgment is questioned, firefighters may feel psychologically threatened because of the pressure to accommodate all these expectations and still manage during an evolving emergency.

On the other hand, firefighters enjoy many positive aspects of their work and social status. Firefighters have a high social standing and are considered to belong to the most highly skilled blue-collar occupation. The work itself is interesting, although highly routine between alarms. There is a high degree of autonomy and a heavy emphasis on teamwork and mutual support. Between shifts many firefighters moonlight (have second jobs). Firefighters enjoy the high esteem of the community, the admiration of other citizens, the aspirations of children as role models, and widespread support as unequivocally positive defenders of the public good.

See Also the Following Articles

Heat Shock Response, Overview; 9/11, Religion and Stress; Temperature Effects; Workplace Stress; Night Shiftwork.

Further Reading

Barnard, R. J. (1975). Fire fighters – a fit population with ischemic heart disease. *Sports Medicine Bulletin* **10**, 7–9.

Barnard, R. J. and Duncan, H. W. (1975). Heart rate and ECG responses of fire fighters. *Journal of Occupational Medicine* **17**, 247–250.

Barnard, R. J., Gardner, G. W. and Diaco, N. V. (1976). "Ischemic" heart disease in firefighters with normal coronary arteries. *Journal of Occupational Medicine* **18**, 818–820.

Barnard, R. J., Gardner, G. W., Diaco, N. V., et al. (1978). Near-maximal ECG stress testing and coronary artery disease risk factor analysis in Los Angeles City fire fighters. *Journal of Occupational Medicine* **17**, 693–695.

Bos, J., Mol, E., Visser, B., et al. (2004). Risk of health complaints and disabilities among Dutch firefighters. *International Archives of Occupational and Environmental Health* **77**, 373–382.

Byrd, R. and Collins, M. (1980). Physiologic characteristics of fire fighters. *American Corrective Therapy Journal* **34**, 106–109.

Dutton, L. M., Smolensky, M. H., Leach, C. S., et al. (1978). Stress levels of ambulance paramedics and firefighters. *Journal of Occupational Medicine* **20**, 111–115.

Guidotti, T. L. (1992). Human factors in firefighting: ergonomic-, cardiopulmonary- and stress-related issues. *International Archives of Occupational and Environmental Health* **64**, 1–12.

Guidotti, T. L. (1993). Mortality of urban firefighters in Alberta, 1927–1987. *American Journal of Industrial Medicine* **23**, 921–940.

Guidotti, T. L. (1995). Occupational mortality among firefighters: assessing the association. *Journal of Occupational and Environmental Medicine* **37**, 1348–1356.

Guidotti, T. L. (1998). Emergency and security services. In: Stellman, J. M., McCann, M., Warshaw, L., Brabant, C. & Dufresne, C. (eds.) *The ILO encyclopaedia of occupational health* (4th edn. vol. 3), pp. 95.1–95.22. Geneva: International Labor Organization.

Guidotti, T. L. and Clough, V. (1992). Occupational health concerns of firefighting. *Annual Review of Public Health* **13**, 151–171.

Hytten, K. and Hasle, A. (1989). Fire fighters: a study of stress and coping. *Acta Psychiatrica Scandinavica* **80** (supplement 355), 50–55.

Kalimo, R., Lehtonen, A., Daleva, M., et al. (1980). Psychological and biochemical strain in firemen's work. *Scandinavian Journal of Work, Environment & Health* **6**, 179–187.

Kuorinka, I. and Korhonen, O. (1981). Firefighters' reaction to alarm, an ECG and heart rate study. *Journal of Occupational Medicine* **23**, 762–766.

Lee, D. J., Fleming, L. E., Gomez-Marin, O., et al. (2004). Risk of hospitalization among firefighters: the National Health Interview Survey, 1986–1994. *American Journal of Public Health* **94**(11), 1938–1939.

Markowitz, J. S., Gutterman, A. M., Link, B., et al. (1987). Psychological response of firefighters to a chemical fire. *Journal of Human Stress* **13**, 84–93.

Reischl, U. W. E., Bair, H. S. and Reischl, P. (1979). Firefighter noise exposure. *American Industrial Hygiene Association Journal* **40**, 482–489.

Rhea, M. R., Alvar, B. A. and Gray, R. (2004). Physical fitness and job performance of firefighters. *Journal of Strength and Conditioning Research* **18**, 348–352.

Romet, T. T. and Frim, J. (1987). Physiological responses to fire fighting activities. *European Journal of Applied Physiology* **56**, 633–638.

Rosenstock, L., Demers, P., Heyer, N. J., et al. (1990). Respiratory mortality among firefighters. *British Journal of Industrial Medicine* **47**, 462–465.

Selkirk, G. A. and McLellan, T. M. (2004). Physical work limits for Toronto firefighters in warm environments. *Journal of Occupational and Environmental Hygiene* **1**, 199–212.

Smith, D. (1988). *Firefighters: their lives in their own words*. New York: Doubleday.

Sothmann, M. S., Gebhardt, D. L., Baker, T. A., et al. (2004). Performance requrierments of phsyically strenuous occupations: validating minimum standards for muscular strength and endurance. *Ergonomics* **22**, 864–875.

von Hallmeyer, A., Lingbeil, M., Kohn-Seyer, G., et al. (1981). Physische und psychische Belastungskomponenten in der Tatigkeit des Feuerwehrmannes. *Zeitschrift für die Gesamte Hygiene und Ihre Grenzgebiete* **27**, 191–194.

Fish, Stress in

C B Schreck
Oregon State University, Corvallis, OR, USA

This article is a revision of the previous edition article by
C B Schreck, volume 2, pp 149–152, © 2000, Elsevier Inc.

Elements of the Stress Response
Factors Affecting the Stress Response

Glossary

Clearance dynamics	The temporal pattern of disappearance of a substance from the circulation, a body part, or the body.
Interrenal	The cells (tissue) located in the fish's head kidney responsible for secretion of corticosteroids; analogous to the adrenal gland of mammals.
Ontogenetic stage	Life history or life cycle stage.
Osmo-regulatory	Pertaining to water balance and related to hydromineral balance, which also includes electrolytes.
Stressor	The factor extrinsic to the fish that causes a stress response.

The physiological responses of fish to stressful situations are very similar to those of the other vertebrates, including humans. Perception of a threat is followed by a neuroendocrine cascade involving catecholamines and the corticosteroid cortisol. Together, these result in secondary stress responses that can be categorized as those concerned with provision of energy, hydromineral balance, the immune system, and pathways that affect behaviors. The psychogenically induced responses tend to be similar, irrespective of the stressful agent; specific stressors can also induce specific responses. While the inter- and intraspecific differences in characteristics of the stress response are ultimately determined by genetics, the animal's history and its extant environment determine the exact nature of the magnitude, duration, and consequences of the response to a particular stressor. Acutely stressful situations result in temporary impairment of necessary functions such as disease resistance, predator avoidance, and learning ability. In addition, prolonged or repeated exposure to stress can have negative effects on development, growth, and reproduction.

Elements of the Stress Response

The general physiological response of a fish to a stressful situation (stressor) is similar to that of the warm-blooded vertebrates. Upon perception of a stressor, the fish's central nervous system initiates a neuroendocrine cascade, resulting in release of catecholamines from chromaffin tissue and secretion of glucocorticosteroids from interrenal tissue (**Figure 1**). These affect other physiological systems (**Figure 2**). Of course, the nature of the stress response is quite polymorphic, and specific stressors also have specific consequences.

Stress Response Factors

Fish, including lamprey, produce catecholamines such as adrenaline. These hormones are important for the initial response to the stressor, assisting the fish in terms of energy and stamina. Compared to the steroid hormones, there is relatively little known about the function and dynamics of these peptides. They are secreted almost immediately following the onset of stress and have cardiovascular actions, increasing cardiac output and gill blood flow. Catecholamines have other metabolic actions such as elevating circulating levels of glucose and depleting liver glycogen; their effects can ultimately lead to elevated plasma lactate and altered free fatty acid concentrations. They also affect hydromineral balance, perhaps making the fish more leaky to water because of hypertensive actions, are diuretic, and influence drinking rate.

The jawed fish activate a hypothalamic-pituitary-interrenal axis (HPI) to secrete glucocorticosteroids when stressed. Some literature suggests that these hormones are important in agnathans, but the question is still open. Elasmobranchs produce 1α-hydroxycorticosterone while the other groups of fish produce cortisol. Cortisol is secreted from interrenal tissue located in the head kidney within minutes after the onset of a stressor upon stimulation by adrenocorticotropin. Upon perception of a stressor, a neural response triggers the synthesis of corticotropin-releasing hormone (CRH) in the hypothalamus of the brain. This peptide is transported neuronally to the pituitary gland to stimulate production and release into the circulation of corticotropin (CTH; ACTH in mammals). There appear to be other brain peptides that may also have a similar action. CTH stimulates the release of cortisol into the blood from the interregnal cells located in the head (anterior) kidney. There is only a small reservoir of stored cortisol, so

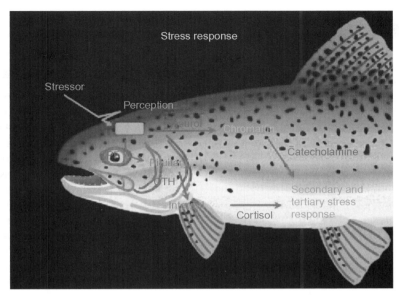

Figure 1 Schematic of the general stress response of teleostean fish leading from perception to the hormones that cause the secondary and tertiary stress responses.

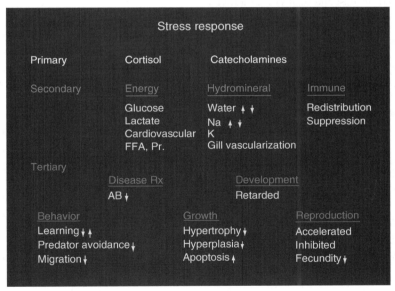

Figure 2 Primary, secondary, and tertiary stress response factors of teleostean fish.

new synthesis is also initiated. The rate of elevation of circulating cortisol varies greatly amongst the species of fish; increase can be seen in less than a minute in some species, while it appears to take hours in others. Cortisol also has a metabolic role during the stress response that serves to provide energy for fight-or-flight functions as well as for osmoregulation. It is essential for the active pumping of electrolytes such as sodium; it could thus help restore the water–ion imbalance consequent to stress by functioning as a mineralocorticoid (fish do not have a mineralocorticoid hormone like mammals). The glucocorticosteroids

might be beneficial to both resistance and recovery from stress. Cortisol is also immunosuppressive. The secondary stress responses are thus regulated via catecholamines and cortisol, acting via specific receptors for these hormones on tissues with target cells. The other elements of the HPI axis mentioned previously can also have direct effects independent of cortisol.

Responding to a stressor is an energetically costly process. That means that there is less energy available for other necessary life functions. The ability of fish to resist pathogens can be affected by stress. It appears that there can be enhancement of certain aspects of the immune response at some times after exposure to a stressor, but depression of immune system capability tends to be a more general and prolonged response. Cells of the fish's immune system also likely manufacture the stress-related hormones CRH and CTH. Behaviors such as general activity, swimming performance, schooling, thermoregulation, orientation taxis, avoidance, chemoreception, feeding, predation evasion, aggression territoriality, negative conditioning, and learning are all affected by stress, primarily negatively. CRH and several other brain neurotransmitters (e.g., serotonin and dopamine) affect stress-related behavioral responses.

Adult Pacific salmon, *Oncorhynchus* spp., die shortly after spawning. Mature fish of these species have activated HPI axes as encountered during stress and hence elevated circulating levels of cortisol; their ability to clear cortisol from the circulation also appears to be impaired. These fish die from something akin to Cushing's syndrome as described for mammals – i.e., depletion of energy reserves, deterioration of structural tissues, and infection with pathogens resulting from hypercortisolemia.

Nature of the Stress Response

The severity and duration of a stressful encounter influences the magnitude and duration of the physiological stress response. Fish are able to recover from acute, nonlethal stressors. The physiological stress response is initiated within fractions of seconds of when a stressor is first perceived. The physiological events happening soon thereafter (within an hour or so), representing the activation or getting started aspects (alarm phase of stress), are stereotypical (i.e., more predictable) than those of the later stages (resistance and compensation/recovery). Depending on species and environmental conditions, some physiological and behavioral components of the stress response recover quite rapidly following cessation of the stressor, perhaps in minutes to hours. Energy-regarding factors tend to require several hours to return to prestress levels, while those concerned with the immune system, disease resistance, and learning may take days to weeks to recover completely. Magnitudes and durations of response are extremely varied among species as stressor types and durations.

Sequential exposure to acutely stressful events can lead to cumulative physiological responses; it depends on the frequency and severity of the stressor. If the number of repeated exposure to stressors is substantial and frequent enough, fish can compensate and adapt to the experiences. Exposure to less-frequent repeated stressors may not lead to cumulative effects for physiological stress response factors but can have long-term negative effects on a fish's ability to grow, develop, or reproduce, presumably because there is less energy available for these functions.

Chronic exposure to a stressor can lead to exhaustion (death) or compensation if the stressor is not too severe. Severe but not acutely lethal stressors can result in eventual death via indirect mechanisms such as lowering resistance to pathogens. If fish have adapted to a chronically stressful situation, elements of the physiological stress response will likely not have the identical characteristics (e.g., circulating concentration, clearance dynamics, or rate of response) that they did in a resting state prior to the stressor. Also, the long-term fitness of a fish would be reduced under such circumstances.

When fish are exposed to more than one type of stressor simultaneously (e.g., crowding and temperature elevation), the closer a fish is to its tolerance limits to one stressor, the more severe will be the negative consequences of another concurrent stressor.

In general, the onset of stress in a fish can be determined, but science has not yet been able to establish how to determine when a fish has recovered from exposure to a stressor. In addition, we are not yet very capable of measuring the severity of a stressor. Higher order responses, such as resumption of feeding, appear to be better predictors of the absence of stress than clinical measurements regarding physiology.

Factors Affecting the Stress Response

The response to stressors is ultimately determined by the fish's genetic heritage. However, the stress response phenotype evident during any particular situation is strongly influenced by the fish's prior history, its extant environment, and its developmental stage.

Genetic Effects

There can be major interspecific differences in the nature of the stress response. While the basic elements are generally similar across groups, the magnitude and dynamics of the physiological responses to stressors can be quite different. Some species appear to respond quite slowly, at least in terms of the HPI axis, compared to others; there is a large variation in tolerance of stressors among different groups of fish. There are also genetic differences with reasonably high heritability between individuals within a species in the magnitude of the physiological response to stress. Similarly, there are genetically determined between-individual differences in tolerance of stressors, but it is unknown if these are related to the nature of the fish's physiological stress response.

The physiological stress response factors operate by activating and deactivating specific genes. The genes affected differ between organs. Functional genomics (which genes respond and what they do) of the fish stress response is a relatively new field of study. The liver, immune system, and brain have received the most attention to date, and are all very strongly affected by the stress response.

Environmental Effects

A fish's prior history and its present environment can affect how it responds to stressors. While the initial stages of the hormonal responses to stress are reasonably invariant in different environments, the persistence of the response and its secondary and tertiary (i.e., whole animal) consequences are very dependent on the nature of the extant environment. Temperature is important in affecting the rates of reactions. Other water quality variables can also be important as controlling or directing factors. Prior experiences with stressors can also harden the fish and hence lessen the apparent severity of subsequent, similar stressors. Nutritional history of the fish can also modify the magnitude and/or dynamics of certain physiological factors of the stress response, particularly with reference to factors concerned with energy.

Importantly, some environmental challenges, albeit lethal, might not necessarily invoke a general HPI stress response. It appears that stressors that are perceived by the central nervous system are those that elicit such a response.

Developmental Effects

Fish at different ontogenetic stages of their life cycle may respond to stressors differently. The basic elements of the physiological stress response, such as the hormones, are present at very early stages of development, and the system appears functional around hatching or soon thereafter. Transitional stages such as the onset of feeding by mouth, metamorphosis, or smoltification and reproduction appear very sensitive to stressors in regard to the increased magnitude of their physiological response and decreased tolerance limits (**Figure 3**).

Ecological Consequences

Exposure to acute stressors reduces the fish's capacity to resist other immediate threats (**Figure 3**). Longer-term or repeated exposure to relatively brief stressors depresses the capacity of fish during the time they

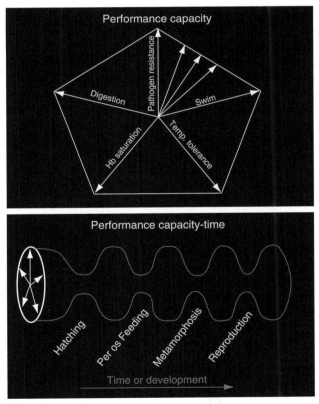

Figure 3 Top panel: Conceptualization of the performance capacity of a fish's necessary life functions that are determined genetically and limited by the environment and negatively affected by stress. The length of each arrow (vector) goes from zero in the center to some level of performance at the point (Hb = hemoglobin). Bottom panel: Cartoon representing the performance capacity of a fish as it changes through time, showing a smaller capacity to resist stress during transitional stages.

are adapting to carry on other necessary life functions. The fish will have less energy to channel into anabolic processes such as growth, development, and reproduction.

It is likely that longer-term stress can change a fish's developmental trajectory and thereby alter its life history strategy. For example, fish that are stressed during certain stages of reproductive maturation may change their spawning strategy. Depending on species of fish and the nature of the stressor, spawning could be accelerated, delayed, or totally inhibited. Stress experienced by females can lead to lower egg quality and subsequent progeny fitness.

While general disturbances and deteriorated water quality can cause a stress response, negative social interactions and low hierarchical status also result in a similar response. Fish of low social rank grow less well and tend to have reduced chances of survival. Submissive fish are stressed by aggressive displays, have activated HPI axes, and suffer its maladaptive consequences.

Temperature is one of the most important environmental controlling factors for fish because the fish are cold-blooded. The rates of biochemical reactions that drive physiological processes are directly dependent on the temperature of the water; in general, for each 10°C increase in temperature, the rates of biological reactions double or triple. Temperature is thus a key variable regarding how fish respond to a stressor, both physiologically and ecologically.

How fish interact with pathogens and parasites is also affected by stress. Stress can increase both the infection rate and pathogenicity of a microorganism.

See Also the Following Article

Animal Models (Nonprimate) for Human Stress.

Further Reading

Adams, M. S. (ed.) (1990). *Biological indicators of stress in fish*. Bethesda, MD: American Fisheries Symposium 8.

Ader, R., Felten, D. L. and Cohen, N. (eds.) (2001) *Psychoneuroimmunology* (vols. 1 and 2). San Diego, CA: Academic Press.

Balm, P. M. (1999). *Stress physiology in animals*. Sheffield, UK: Sheffield Academic Press.

Barton, B. A. and Iwama, G. K. (1991). Physiological changes in fish from stress in aquaculture with emphasis on the response and effects of corticosteroids. *Annual Review of Fish Diseases* 1, 3–26.

Fry, F. E. J. (1947). *Effects of the environment on animal activity*. University of Toronto Studies. Biol. Ser. No. 55. Publ. Ontario Fish. Res. Lab. No. 68. Toronto, Canada: Toronto University Press.

Iwama, G. K., Pickering, A. D., Sumpter, J. P. and Schreck, C. B. (eds.) (1997). *Fish stress and health in aquaculture*. Society for Experimental Biology, Seminar Series 62. Cambridge, UK: Cambridge University Press.

Pickering, A. D. (ed.) (1981). *Stress and fish*. London: Academic Press.

Schreck, C. B. (1996). Immunomodulation: endogenous factors. In: Iwama, G. & Nakanishi, T. (eds.) *The Fish Immune System*, pp. 311–337. Fish Physiology Series 15. San Diego, CA: Academic Press.

Wedemeyer, G. A., Barton, B. A. and McLeay, D. J. (1990). Stress and acclimation. In: Schreck, C. B. & Moyle, P. B. (eds.) *Methods for fish biology*, pp. 451–489. Bethesda, MD: American Fisheries Society.

Flashback *See:* Posttraumatic Stress Disorder – Clinical.

Floods, Stress Effects of

J O Brende
Mercer University School of Medicine, Macon, GA, USA

This article is a revision of the previous edition article
by J O Brende, volume 2, pp 153–157, © 2000, Elsevier Inc.

Introduction and Background
Postdisaster Coping
Postdisaster Effects on Children
Postdisaster Physical Symptoms
Postdisaster Effects on Emergency and Medical Personnel
Assessing Traumatic Exposure Severity and Symptoms

Introduction and Background

Flooding remains the most common catastrophe worldwide and accounts for an estimated 40% of all natural disasters and 26% of disaster-related deaths. Flash flooding kills more people in the United States than any other natural disaster, accounting for approximately 200 fatalities per year. Flash floods can occur within several seconds to several hours, with little warning and are deadly because they produce rapid rises in water levels and have devastating flow velocities. Several factors can contribute to flash flooding including rainfall intensity, rainfall duration, surface conditions, topography, and slope of the receiving basin. Urban areas are susceptible to flash floods because a high percentage of the surface area is composed of impervious streets, roofs, and parking lots where runoff occurs very rapidly. Mountainous areas also are susceptible to flash floods, as steep topography may funnel runoff into a narrow canyon. Floodwaters accelerated by steep stream slopes can cause the floodwave to move downstream too fast to allow escape, resulting in many deaths. One example of a deadly flash flood occurred after 37.5 cm of rain in 5 h from slow-moving thunderstorms killed 237 people in Rapid City, South Dakota, in 1972.

Floods can occur unexpectedly after excessive rainfall, tropical storms, hurricanes, or failing dams or levees. Deluges of heavy rains can quickly fill narrow ravines, mountain canyons, dry stream beds, or streets in a downriver community. Powerful torrents of water can roll bolders, tear out trees, destroy buildings and bridges, scour out new channels, trigger catastrophic mud slides, sweep away vehicles and houses, drown unsuspecting campers or residents, destroy property, kill or injure friends or family members, cause homelessness, spread disease, deplete financial resources, and cause emotional and psychological symptoms. Indeed, floods are major disasters and the Federal Emergency Management Agency (FEMA) has warned people to consider these facts:

- Most flood-related deaths are due to flash floods,
- 50% of all flash-flood fatalities are vehicle related. Individuals should not drive through floodwaters,
- 90% of those who die in hurricanes drown. People should heed the warnings and evacuate areas where flooding from storm surges has been predicted,
- Most homeowners' insurance policies do not cover floodwater damage. Flood insurance can be purchased through FEMA's National Flood Insurance Program.

Flooding can also take place from storm surges caused by major hurricanes and are unquestionably the most dangerous parts of hurricanes. Pounding waves create very hazardous flood currents and depths of water that can be greater than 60 m, depending upon the distance of water and the velocity of the wind. Nine out of 10 hurricane fatalities are caused by storm surges. Worst-case scenarios occur when storm surges occur concurrently with high tides. Stream flooding is also much worse inland during storm surges because of backwater effects. In September 1900, the hurricane and storm surge at Galveston, Texas, killed nearly 8000 people, making it the worst natural disaster in the nation's history.

Floods seem to have become more severe and commonplace in recent years. Within the boundaries of the United States, there have been many severe floods. One of the most significant of these was the Great Mississippi Flood of 1927. Rains began in the summer of 1926 and by May of 1927 the Mississippi River had flooded and was 97 km wide below Memphis, Tennessee, and flooded 109 km^2 in six states: Arkansas, Illinois, Kentucky, Louisiana, Mississippi, and Tennessee. There were 246 people killed in seven states and damages exceeded $650 million.

The floods of 1993 were also one of the greatest natural disasters ever to hit the United States. Major flooding primarily affected the Mississippi and Missouri rivers and extended into 150 major rivers and tributaries across nine states: North Dakota, South Dakota, Nebraska, Kansas, Minnesota, Iowa, Missouri, Wisconsin, and Illinois. Hundreds of levees failed and 600 river points were above flood stage at the same time. Fifty people were killed and damages approached $15 billion.

When tropical storm Alberto lingered over the Florida Panhandle on 3 July 3 1994, the ensuing rains continued until Georgia's flood of the century eventually devastated its central and southwest portions, killed 32 people, displaced 70 000 people, flooded 1214 km^2 of croplands, caused crop damage of $100 million, and a total monetary damage exceeding $500 million.

Two devastating floods inundated much of northern California in January 1995. Three different hurricanes struck the Caribbean and the United States Atlantic Coast in late summer and fall of 1996; Bertha struck in July, Fran in September, and then Hortense washed away southwestern Puerto Rico. From the early months of 1997, unprecedented floods affected eastern, mid-western, and northern United States, particularly devastating communities bordering the Red River which flooded the Minnesota and North Dakota border and continued into Canada in April 1997.

With the onset of El Niño, 1998 became an unusually severe year for flooding. The Pacific Coast was devastated by rain, rising rivers, ocean swells, and killer mud slides in January and February followed by significant flooding in the southeast and Midwest from February until June. Downpours, high ocean swells, and flooding rivers struck the West Coast and the Southeast Coast of the United States with a fury in early February 1998. Southern California was inflicted with the worst wind and rain storms in 5 years. Rain soaked hills and dikes began giving way, causing more flooding and destruction of homes and property.

While blizzards in the Upper Midwest paralyzed highways, roads, and air traffic, rain brought 30–50 cm of rainfall across the south during early March, 1998. The community of Elba, Alabama evacuated 2000 of its 4000 residents when a levee broke and killed two children from torrents of water roaring through the town without warning. Fierce thunderstorms swamped parts of seven states in the northeast. Flooding was so extensive that it required helicopter rescues. Vermont's Mad river, usually docile in summertime, lived up to its name when it jumped the banks to wash out roads and destroy homes, and drove campers in Vermont to higher ground.

On 24 August 1998, flash floods from tropical storm Charlie struck Del Rio, Texas on the Mexico–Texas border. Within the first few days, it was known that 15 people lost their lives although rescuers were continuing to look for missing persons during the following week. South Texas continued to be a target during mid-October as 37–45 cm of rain over a period of several days flooded the Guadalupe and Colorado Rivers, causing the deaths of 24 people.

The Gulf Coast was also stricken by flooding from hurricane Georges which first struck Puerto Rico on 21 September 1998, and devastated the Dominican Republic. It swept across the Caribbean, the eastern coast of Cuba, the Florida Keys, and continued northward through the Gulf of Mexico until its center crossed the coast at Gulfport and Biloxi, Mississippi, 8 days later. Storm surges and flooding caused extensive damage and drove 1.5 million Gulf Coast residents from their homes. In Mobile, Alabama, a 2.7 m storm surge from Mobile Bay sent chest-deep water into many neighborhoods so that more than 300 people had to be evacuated.

In 1998, the worst flooding to hit Central America began on 27 October when hurricane Mitch stalled over the isthmus of Central America. Its 180 mph winds, accompanied by 62 cm of rain over a 6-hour period, first devastated the Island of Guanaja near the coast of Honduras. In 2 days, torrential rain immobilized the Honduran Capital of Tegucigalpa, then moved inland where rainfall estimated to be 63–125 cm caused flooding and mud slides that wiped out complete villages in the mountains of Honduras and Nicaragua. On 30 October 1998, the rim of the Nicaraguan Volcano Casitas burst, releasing a deadly torrent of water and mud which destroyed the villages of Rolando Rodriguez and Posoltega as most of its residents and several thousand others in Nicaragua, were killed. Virtually all of Honduras, from the lowland marshes on the Atlantic coast to the mountains, hills, and plateaus of the interior, along with most of the highways, tens of bridges, and 70% of the national agriculture in Honduras, was destroyed. President, Carlos Flores Facusse, announced: "There are corpses everywhere from victims of landslides or floodwaters. The floods and landslides erased from the map many villages and households as well as whole neighborhoods of cities. We have before us a panorama of death, desolation, and ruin throughout the national territory." The number of dead in Honduras, Nicaragua, El Salvador, Guatemala, Costa Rica, Belize, and Mexico was estimated at 10 000 with 13 225 people missing, four million people homeless, and very little clean water, food, and medicine.

When hurricane Stan struck Central America on 5 October 2005 it brought several days of rain and caused major flooding which impacted 1000 Central American communities which were covered partially or completely by water and mud. Along the Southern Coast and western highlands of Guatemala flooding and landslides caused loss of life, injury, and displaced persons as well as damage to housing and infrastructure in 251 of 331 municipalities in 15 of the country's 22 departments. There were over 900 landslides and considerable damage to a high proportion of roads and bridges. In the highland and south-western departments of Solola and San Marcos, entire villages were swept away by landslides, with significant loss of life. One village was completely buried under tons of dirt and declared a Mayan mass grave site.

When category 3 hurricane Katrina struck the gulf states of Louisiana and Mississippi on 28 August 2005 there was flooding both from storm surges and heavy rains. The storm surge surpassed 6 m and caused major property destruction. The subsequent flooding of the City of New Orleans was unexpected and particularly devastating. Although hundreds of thousands of residents had left the danger zone prior to 29 August, there were yet thousands more who either refused to evacuate or were unable to leave. As Lake Pontchartrain rose to unprecedented heights, water began pouring into the city through broken levees. Over the next 2 days, the gradual rising water levels drowned the unfortunate who could not escape or forced them to their attics and rooftops.

On 4 September 2005, the Mayor of New Orleans speculated to reporters that the death toll might rise into the thousands after the clean-up was completed. By early November the number of confirmed fatalities in Louisiana reached a toll of 1056, a lower figure than previously estimated. Some fatalities were caused by self-destructive behaviors or violence, including one death at the Superdome evacuation site from a drug overdose and another from suicide. At least seven homicide victims were found in the city according to the medical examiner.

In early October 2005, heavy rain struck the eastern seaboard due to tropical storm Tammy and heavy rains and flooding which impacted five states and created enormous stress, according to the following time-table:

- Sunday, 9 October – Prolonged, heavy rain and flooding from North Carolina to New Hampshire. Hundreds of people evacuated, power lost, dams weakened and roads impassable. At least four people died, including two killed in New Hampshire when a car drove off a washed-out bridge into floodwaters. New Hampshire's Governor John Lynch declared a state of emergency and called in 500 National Guard for assistance.
- Monday, 10 October – At least 10 people dead and about six unaccounted for, including a couple whose house was washed away by a surge of water over Warren Lake dam in Alstead, New Hampshire.
- Tuesday, 11 October – Rescue crews and police dogs searched rivers and woods for people missing in New Hampshire after the weekend flooding. John Lynch said the floods are the worst the state had experienced in a quarter of a century.

- Thursday, 13 October – Steady rain fell around the saturated northeast, swamping roads, stalling airline passengers, and sending streams and rivers over their banks. Flood warnings covered parts of Connecticut, New York, and New Jersey.
- Friday, 14 October – Toilets backed up with sewage, military trucks plowed through headlight-high water to rescue people, and swans glided down the streets as rain fell for an eighth straight day around the waterlogged northeast. Overflowing lakes and streams forced hundreds of people from their homes, tens of thousands of sandbags were handed out in New Hampshire and flood warnings covered parts of New Jersey, New York, and Connecticut.
- Saturday, 15 October – The death toll from a week of driving rain and swelling floods across the Northeast rose to 11 after a 75-year-old Connecticut man was swept away by rushing water at a campground. Flooding also shut down major highways and forced hundreds to evacuate their homes. Massachusetts Governor Mitt Romney declared a state of emergency, following the lead of New Jersey. Flood warnings were in effect for New Jersey, New Hampshire, Connecticut, Massachusetts, Rhode Island, and southern New York.
- Sunday, 16 October – In Connecticut, the body of a woman who fell into the rapids of the Natchaug River in Chaplin was found.
- Tuesday–Saturday, 18–22 October – Taunton, Massachusetts. Population 50 000. Residents prepared for the worst after the 173-year-old, 3.6 m high Whitteton pond dam on the rain-swollen Mill river deteriorated, threatening a wall of water up to 1.8 m deep. Schools and businesses closed and thousands of residents were unable to return home as a weakened timber dam threatened to give way and spill a surge of water into downtown Taunton, Massachusetts. Over the next 4 days there was continuing heavy rain. About 2000 residents were evacuated and workers pumped millions of liters of water from the rain-swollen lake above the dam and begin shoring up the battered structure ahead of the new round of heavy rain that was forecast. Working in the rain, crews finished building a new rock dam and tore down the old wooden one that had buckled after a week of heavy downpours.

Postdisaster Coping

How do survivors cope with impending disasters related to rapidly rising water or flash floods? They have been observed to traverse through five psychological and emotional stress-related phases as follows.

Immediate Coping – Alarm and Outcry

In some cases victims become confused and overwhelmed by fear. However, most survivors respond to the danger with little or no expectation of personal risk, often with heroic efforts, clear thinking, and physical endurance. There are also those who refuse to believe the seriousness of the danger.

Early Adaptation – the Disbelief and Denial Response

Incredulity in the face of an extraordinary event should be perceived as normal, even potentially life-saving. But those who refuse to believe they will ever be overcome by life threatening circumstances can be at risk.

In some cases disbelief or denial can be a fatal response when individuals go too far and will not acknowledge they are in mortal danger. This attitude of omnipotence has been called the delusion of personal invulnerability. There are many examples throughout history. When the dikes broke, and 1835 people were drowned in The Netherlands in the early 1900s, many perished because they did not listen to those who warned of the danger. In somewhat similar circumstances, as the Rio Grande began to flood near Eagle Pass, Texas and Piedras Negras, Mexico in June 1954, warnings were issued for 36 h that a record crest was sweeping down the river. Nevertheless people refused to comprehend the danger and 130 persons were needlessly drowned.

Ideally, individuals will respond during this phase in a dramatic way to save lives. A very recent example occurred in Taunton, Massachusetts on 18 October 2005 when residents feared for the worst after the wooden Whittenton pond dam on the rain-swollen Mill River deteriorated and threatened to collapse (see earlier).

The fact that most survivors in the middle of a disaster are somewhat numb to the reality that they could be killed helps them contend with incredible circumstances as they organize themselves and other survivors in adaptive and innovative ways. Even after the disaster's force diminishes, survivors are likely to maintain an attitude of disbelief for a time until they begin to resume normal activities. In some cases, the demands on rescue workers and other helpers are exceedingly great during this time and the risk of developing significant physical and emotional symptoms is high. Reports from New Orleans' Methodist Hospital after hurricane Katrina had flooded New Orleans indicated that the medical staff worked unendingly in horrendous conditions and some succumbed to dehydration and exhaustion. Patients requiring ventilators were kept alive with hand-powered resuscitation bags. When the first floor of the hospital flooded the dead were stacked in a second floor operating room. Other hospitals reported even more dire conditions and in some cases the hospital staff were unable to evacuate the severely ill and they did not survive.

Mid-Phase Adaptation – Intrusions

The middle phase is marked by intrusive recollections alternating with periods of denial and numbing as survivors begin to remember and relive their experiences in the form of intrusive thoughts, emotions, and dreams several days or weeks later. Their intrusive symptoms may be intensified when survivors finally realize they may have lost lives, health, or property. This phase may be prolonged or delayed when the work of recovery, reconstruction, or self-preservation becomes all consuming and there may also be delayed resolution by the use of alcohol or drugs.

Survivors often contend with a variety of other stresses at this time including possible injuries, losses, role changes, displacement, cleaning up, repairing property damage, moving into temporary or even new housing, and preparing lengthy health, recovery assistance, and insurance claims. Thus, posttrauma symptoms are related not only to the disaster itself but other related difficulties, which has been called the dripping faucet syndrome. Taken individually, many small stresses seem minor but when taken collectively they can push a person to the edge and cause irritability, withdrawal from relationships, or loss of pleasure in activities.

Disaster workers subjected to prolonged or highly intensive exposure to the disaster tend to remain emotionally numb until the enormity of the disaster finally sinks in. Not until then do they develop sleep disturbances and nightmares but these are frequently resolved within 4–6 weeks.

Late Phase Adaptation – Anger and Physical Symptoms

After a period of time (from 1 to 3 months) survivors are more prone to experience negative and hostile reactions. There is a marked decrease in tolerance, an increase in complaining, a loss of humor, and mistrust of others. This becomes a problem for those trying to help victims of trauma and for the victims themselves, who keep others at a distance. Couples may become more easily aggressive and prone to violent outbursts. During this phase there is also a marked increase in physical complaints including headaches, nausea, diarrhea, vomiting, muscle aches, chest pain, restlessness, tremors, sweating, and general fatigue. These symptoms may also be associated with secondary victimization befalling those who are exploited by shysters, neglected by thoughtless people, and mistreated by dehumanizing agencies.

Resolution or Symptom Development

Finally, survivors either resolve their posttraumatic symptoms, develop recurring difficulties related to unresolved past stresses, or become victims of prolonged or worsening disorders associated with unresolved guilt, preexisting anxiety or depression, prior traumatization, drug or alcohol addiction, and organic syndromes. New symptoms may develop or prior difficulties may worsen including flashbacks, depression, obsessive–compulsive symptoms, panic attacks, nightmares, sleeplessness, interpersonal alienation, and emotional outbursts alternating with detachment. For some victims, these symptoms may extend indefinitely in the form of a chronic emotional or physical disorder requiring treatment.

Postdisaster Effects on Children

Children are vulnerable to all of the typical responses and symptoms following disasters and need special attention in order to prevent longstanding difficulties. Unfortunately, adults are not always aware of the full impact of traumatic stress on children nor do they always help them resolve their frightening dreams and memories. Most children, especially younger ones, become very fearful of being alone, overdependent, and sometimes clinging. They may also develop strong phobias, nightmares, night terrors, and regression to a previous level of function, including thumb sucking or bed wetting in younger children. Additional symptoms include clinging to parents, reluctance to go to bed, nightmares, fantasies that the disaster never happened, crying and screaming, withdrawal and immobility, refusal to attend school, school problems, inability to concentrate, and being poorly understood by parents and teachers.

Early intervention is particularly important for children. Parents need to recognize that withdrawal, fear, and overdependency will improve with time. Special care should be paid to helping the children resume normal daily routines within a safe and secure environment. Watching television programs about the flood can be helpful if parents are there to talk about what happened and reassure that being afraid is normal. Supervised trauma-related play can help children resolve their fears. They should be reassured with explanations like: "That hurricane is not a monster who took away children's toys and hurt people. The 'eye' will not seek children out or return again."

Postdisaster Physical Symptoms

Disaster survivors not uncommonly have physical complaints which often bring them to their doctor's offices. Following sudden disasters, many of the symptoms are associated with prolonged autonomic nervous system over-reactivity. Palpitations, tightness in the chest, shortness of breath, and feelings of dread may accompany intrusive memories. Headaches and gastrointestinal complaints are not uncommon. While survivors may have physical problems they often do not seek medical help. Researchers have found that only 40% of those reporting physical symptoms after a disaster consulted their doctors while 34% sought help from family members or friends. Most of them, 66%, sought medical help within 4 months while the remaining 33% waited until after 4 months to visit their physicians.

Survivors may also suffer from health problems indirectly linked to the disaster. For example, following the Iowa floods in the early summer of 1993, the national Centers for Disease Control (CDC) conducted a public health investigation. The CDC researchers discovered that survivors in seven Iowan counties had been hospitalized for flood-related illnesses or injuries, including carbon monoxide poisoning, hypothermia, electrocution, wound infections, and exacerbations of chronic illnesses.

Sometimes there are reports of unusual and long-term health problems. Investigators from the New York State Department of Health discovered some unusual health problems following a flood disaster in western New York in 1974. Within a population of 100 000 people exposed to flooding in three river valleys, scientists found a regional rise in spontaneous abortions as well as an increased incidence of leukemias and lymphomas of 4 years' duration, resulting in an excess of 30–35 malignancies. The reasons are not yet entirely clear.

After the flooding of New Orleans began on 29 August 2005, there was concern about a potential outbreak of serious health problems. Flood waters remained at high levels, over some roof tops, for a number of weeks and became toxic and a breeding area for bacteria. In addition to dehydration and food poisoning, New Orleans flood survivors were also at risk to contact hepatitis A, cholera, and typhoid fever, because of contaminated food and drinking water. Survivors also faced longer-term health risks due to prolonged exposure to the petrochemical tainted flood waters and mosquito-borne diseases such as yellow fever, malaria and West Nile Virus. *Escherichia coli* was detected in the water supply within a few days and at least five people died from bacterial infections caused by *Vibrio vulnificus* bacteria in the toxic waters. Other sources of contaminations included dead bodies lying in city streets and floating in still-flooded sections, causing an advanced state of decomposition of many corpses, some of which were left in the water or sun for days before being collected.

Medical assistance began in earnest within 3 days when an emergency triage center was set up at the regional airport at New Orleans. Helicopters and ambulances brought in the weak, elderly, sick, and injured and makeshift gurneys were used to transport persons from the flight line to a temporary hospital set up in the terminal. The captain in charge described the site as organized chaos but the emergency medical staff assembled from around the country kept pace and were able to handle anything from bruises to critical cases requiring ventilators. They triaged the seriously ill and injured to medical centers in the surrounding states and within 72 h had triaged up to 5000 people.

The potential health problems from flooding affected the residents of the city who had been evacuated. They were unable to return to their homes because of the length of time necessary for the Army Corps of Engineers to drain the flood waters. They managed to accomplish the task within 1 month but parts of the city re-flooded when hurricane Rita struck on 24 September. Many buildings that had withstood the initial storm and the direct force of the flooding were damaged beyond repair by the deleterious effect of long immersion and the rapid propagation of mold.

Hundreds of thousands of New Orleans residents that were displaced by the flooding lost their homes completely and the subsequent emotional effects will not be known for some time.

Postdisaster Effects on Emergency and Medical Personnel

Emergency medical technicians, law enforcement personnel, military medics or corpsmen, fire fighters, emergency room workers, physicians, intensive care nurses, and other crisis workers are exposed routinely to persons who are severely injured, killed, deathly ill, or have expired unexpectedly. These helpers usually adapt to their stress by becoming emotionally numb and detached from their feelings. As a result they can develop a pattern of maintaining emotional distance from people while preferring to throw themselves into their work. This accumulated exposure to traumatic events eventually causes posttraumatic symptoms: emotional detachment, sleep disturbance, irritability, marital problems, alcohol abuse, physiological symptoms, and an addiction to repetitive

stress. Helpers (health professionals, mental health workers, ministers, and even business executives) can feel used up. They eventually find it difficult, if not impossible, to meet the emotional and communication needs of their wives and children. They even ignore their own personal needs for rest and recreation as they often turn to work for gratification rather than their families. Eventually this leads to burnout.

Helpers may find it emotionally stressful and experience intense feelings in response to listening to victims' stories about disasters, assault, sexual abuse, and violent trauma. Those with little experience may even feel confused and even ashamed while empathically taking on the victim's emotional distress. The listener's experience may lead to symptoms of depression, bad dreams, irritability, excessive drinking, and other distressing difficulties caused by a process called vicarious traumatization (VT).

Assessing Traumatic Exposure Severity and Symptoms

The severity of symptoms, should they persist, often are frequently directly correlated with the enormity of the traumatic experience/loss or accumulation of prior unresolved traumatic experiences. Survivors may have experienced a seemingly unending series of stressors. For example, they may have suffered damage or destruction to their homes or personal belongings. They may have witnessed violence, injury, deaths of other victims, and they may have lost loved ones and pets.

When survivors fail to talk openly about the event(s); if they have been separated from family members; if they lack emotional support from friends or family members, the emotional aftermath is more severe. They are at risk to experience many or all of the following symptoms: flashbacks, sleep disorder, anxiety attacks, recurring nightmares or dreams, problems with concentration and memory, intrusive recollections, irritability, emotional outbursts alternating with periods of emotional numbing, misusing drugs or alcohol, and interpersonal conflicts. Clearly, individuals who are experiencing these symptoms should seek the help of an experienced trauma therapist. A successful resolution is possible when survivors find relief from their symptoms and discover new or broadened meaning in their lives.

See Also the Following Articles

Acute Stress Response: Experimental; Anxiety; Adrenaline; Hurricane Katrina Disaster, Stress Effects of; Other Natural Disasters, Illness Epidemics Related to Contamination.

Further Reading

Brende, J. O. (1998). Coping with floods, assessment, intervention, and recovery processes for survivors and helpers. *Journal of Contemporary Psychotherapy* **28**, 107–140.

Brende, J. O. (1995). *Coping with floods and other disasters: a workbook for physicians, helpers, and survivors.* Columbus, GA: Trauma Recovery Publications.

Clayer, J. R., Bookless-Pratz, C. and Harris, R. L. (1985). Some health consequences of a natural disaster. *Medical Journal of Australia* **143**, 182–184.

Figley, C. R. (ed.) (1985). *Trauma and its wake, volume 2: traumatic stress: theory, research, and intervention.* New York: Brunner/Mazel.

Forster, P. (1992). Nature and treatment of acute stress reactions. In: Austin, L. S. (ed.) *Responding to disaster, a guide for mental health professionals*, pp. 2–51. Washington DC: PA Press.

Kalayjian, A. S. (1995). *Disaster and mass trauma: Global perspectives on post disaster mental health management.* Long Branch, NJ: Vista Publishing.

McCann, I. L. and Pearlman, L. A. (1990). Vicarious traumatization: a contextual model for understanding the effects of trauma on helpers. *Journal of Traumatic Stress* **3**, 131–149.

Murphy, S. A. (1986). Perceptions of stress, coping, and recovery one and three years after a natural disaster. *Issues in Mental Health Nursing* **8**, 63–77.

Olson, L. (1993). After the flood: the dripping faucet syndrome. *Iowa Medicine* **83**, 324–327.

Pearlman, L. A. and Saakvitne, K. S. (1995). *Trauma and the therapist.* New York: WW Norton.

Robinson, D. (1959). *The face of disaster.* New York: Doubleday.

Tierney, K. J. (1986). The social and community contexts of disaster. In: Gist, R. & Lubin, B. (eds.) *Psychosocial aspects of disaster*, pp. 11–39. New York: Wiley.

Food Intake and Stress, Human

K Smith and G M Goodwin
Oxford University, Oxford, UK

This article is reproduced from the previous edition, volume 2, pp 158–161, © 2000, Elsevier Inc.

Effect of Stress on Food Intake

Effect of Food Composition and Intake on the Ability to Cope with Stress

Glossary

Dietary restraint	The tendency to control food intake consciously in order to prevent weight gain or promote weight loss.
Dieting	A behavior designed to bring about weight loss that demands a relatively severe degree of food restriction.
5-Hydroxy-tryptamine (serotonin)	A neurotransmitter, present in the brain, that is involved in controlling many different behaviors, including food intake, mood, motor output, learning, sleep, circadian pattern, aggression, and sexual behavior.
Macronutrients	Components of food, including carbohydrate, fat, and protein.
Satiety	The feeling of fullness that increases as food is ingested and that increases the drive to stop eating.
Tryptophan	An amino acid that forms one of the essential components of protein.

Effect of Stress on Food Intake

Under a variety of stressful conditions, food intake is altered in both animals and humans. However, different stressors seem to have different effects, with some resulting in an increase and some in a decrease in food intake. In human studies, some subjects appear to be nonresponders to stress, whereas of the responders, some markedly reduce their intake (stress fasters) while others increase their intake (stress eaters). Stress-induced eating is of particular interest because of the role it may play in contributing to obesity. Much overeating behavior is reported to be stress related, and some obese subjects report a decrease in anxiety after eating.

In everyday life there are a number of specific stressors that have an impact on food intake, particularly in women. Since the 1960s, Western society has placed increasing demands on the population, particularly women, to be slim and to aspire to an ideal of thinness. There has been an associated increase in body image dissatisfaction, particularly among young women. This has also coincided with a dramatic increase in the prevalence of dieting and of eating disorders such as anorexia and bulimia nervosa. The prevalence of eating disorders seems to be in direct proportion to the prevalence of dieting behavior in a given community, and longitudinal studies of young adults suggest that the risk of developing an eating disorder is significantly higher among dieters than non-dieters. Indeed, most of those suffering from an eating disorder report that their eating problem started as normal dieting that then got out of control.

Low self-esteem is an additional factor associated with dieting, body image dissatisfaction, and altera-tions in eating pattern, although it is difficult to know whether this is a cause or an effect. Subjectively, low mood and low self-esteem are often reported to be contributing factors to unwelcome weight gain. Experimentally induced stress or dysphoria in volun-teers causes an increased food intake in some indivi-duals. This effect occurs particularly in those subjects who are dieting or are restrained eaters, but not in those who are not restricting their food intake. Inter-estingly, subjects who binge eat often report that this occurs in response to stress or dysphoria and, at least initially, binges seem to relieve anxiety.

Dieting and dietary restraint are intimately bound up with mood and self-esteem. Subjects who restrict their food intake to lose weight record ratings of happiness that are directly related to weight loss or weight gain. In contrast, subjects who are not restricting intake report that weight change has little impact on ratings of happiness. Feedback to subjects about weight change will therefore alter mood, which in turn can affect food intake and weight. In a study where subjects were weighed regularly but the results were fed back to them as consistently heavier than their true weight, restrained eaters reported more mood changes than nonrestrained eaters in response to the feedback, including anxiety, depression, and low self-esteem. Interestingly, these restrained eaters, who experienced lowered mood, then ate more in a subsequent test meal.

Thus, there is growing evidence that stress can alter food intake. However, there is debate about how this effect is mediated. Stressful events can alter a number of different biological variables, which in turn could affect food intake. It has been hypothesized that stress-induced increases in food intake are mediated by endogenous opiates. Stress increases the release of β-endorphin, a naturally occurring opiate that increases food intake, but also reduces the perception of pain and the anxiety associated with stress.

An alternative is that these effects are mediated by the neurotransmitter 5-hydroxytryptamine (5-HT). 5-HT has attracted great interest because its function seems to be altered in disorders such as depression, which are known to be closely associated with the occurrence of stressful life events, and in eating dis-orders such as bulimia nervosa. In addition, altering 5-HT function (e.g., by using medication) has a pro-found effect on eating behavior. In human and animal studies, interventions that increase 5-HT function re-duce food intake; conversely, reducing 5-HT function increases food intake.

Could levels of 5-HT be altered by stress? Stress increases the level of a naturally occurring hormone, cortisol. When this occurs, 5-HT function is reduced. Reduced 5-HT function would be expected to lead to increased food intake, and experimental work sug-gests that this increase would occur particularly in carbohydrate intake, rather than protein. Interesting-ly, this alteration in the balance of macronutrients could itself affect 5-HT function. This is discussed in more detail in the next section.

Effect of Food Composition and Intake on the Ability to Cope with Stress

Research on the biological and psychological effects of varying food intake has focused on two main areas. First, there has been interest in the behavioral effects of dieting. Second, there has been interest in the effects of dieting on biological parameters, some of which may affect the ability to cope with stress. Research in the latter area has focused on the effects of dieting on the neurotransmitter 5-HT. 5-HT is biologically unusual in that the rate of its synthesis is entirely dependent on the supply of its essential amino acid precursor, tryptophan, in food. Furthermore, the availability of tryptophan to the brain depends on the balance of macronutrients (carbohydrate, protein, and fat).

Dieting is a very common behavior in Western cul-tures. Approximately 25% of men and 40% of women in the United Sates report that they are currently trying to lose weight. Dieting seems to be particularly com-mon among adolescent girls, but the rates are higher at all ages in women compared with men.

Behavioral Effects of Dieting

The first direct evidence on the behavioral effects of food restriction came from a study of World War II conscientious objectors who were placed on a 24-week semistarvation diet. The main findings were an increase in lethargy, tiredness, depression, and irri-tability and a lowering of energy. In contrast, other studies using less extreme dietary restriction have found less dramatic changes in mood.

Several studies have shown that dieters perform less well on cognitive tasks. Dieting impairs sustained attention and short-term recall and results in slower reaction times. Nondieters with high levels of restraint over eating showed intermediate cognitive performance between dieters and low restraint nondieters. Impairments in cognitive functioning, such as impaired vigilance, have also been noted among subjects with bulimia nervosa and anorexia nervosa, probably due to restricted eating.

Dieting itself affects eating behavior. In a series of well-replicated studies, Polivy and Herman showed that dieters failed to compensate for a modest calorie loading by decreasing their caloric intake at the next meal. They actually ate more after the preload than after no preload; they counterregulated rather than showing the normal compensatory regulation seen in the controls. It has been widely argued that counterregulation is a result of the preload causing disinhibition and abandoning of dietary restraint in the dieter. This cognitive explanation is supported by the finding that dieters also counterregulate when they perceive the preload as high in calories, regardless of the actual calorie content.

Severe dietary restriction in normal controls can result in binge eating. The World War II study of conscientious objectors described earlier also investigated the effects of refeeding. The men returned to their normal weights after the study but exhibited a persistent tendency to binge eat. This type of behavior had not occurred prior to the study. Healthy volunteer studies during short-term calorie-controlled diets show that subjects have increased preoccupation with thoughts of food, urges to eat more frequently, and feelings of being out of control with their eating. Rates of postwar binge eating in World War II combat veterans and prisoners of war show that binge eating is significantly more prevalent in veterans who lost large amounts of weight during their captivity.

Thus, dietary restriction and normal dieting have significant effects on behaviors such as food intake, mood, and cognitive functioning. There has been debate, however, about how these effects are mediated. One possibility is that dieting alters 5-HT function, discussed next.

Dieting and 5-HT

The rate of synthesis of 5-HT in the brain is critically dependent on the amount of its precursor, tryptophan, which is able to enter the brain. Tryptophan is available solely from the diet, and its availability in the brain can be critically affected by alterations in food intake, particularly in the balance of macronutrients. Tryptophan competes for entry to the brain across the blood–brain barrier with other amino acids (components of protein). Any change in food intake that alters this ratio of tryptophan to other amino acids will directly affect the amount of 5-HT synthesized.

Studies of the effects of a standard 3 week, 1000 kcal diet have shown that the diet results in a lowering of tryptophan in the plasma (blood). The key question is whether this affects 5-HT function itself. Studies using a variety of challenge tests for different aspects of 5-HT function show that it does, although the effect is significant only in women. It seems that female dieters can compensate to some extent for the reduction in 5-HT synthesis induced by dieting, but it is likely that dieting results in a reduction in 5-HT function. Because this effect is gender specific, women may be biologically more vulnerable to the effects of dieting on 5-HT function.

What might be the consequences of this lowered 5-HT function after dieting? First, decreased 5-HT function will reduce satiety and increase the drive to eat. This may be one of the reasons why it is often reported that dieting is difficult to sustain. Some subjects who are dieting report craving carbohydrate or even bingeing on high-carbohydrate, low-protein foods. Wurtman and colleagues have proposed that this craving may be explained by the fact that these foods increase 5-HT function indirectly. This occurs because a carbohydrate-rich meal causes secretion of the hormone insulin, increasing the ratio of tryptophan to other amino acids and an increase in the entry of tryptophan to the brain. The end result is an increase in the synthesis of 5-HT, which to some extent may correct the deficit induced by dieting.

It is also possible that the reduction in 5-HT function might affect mood. Experimental work using an artificial mixture of amino acids to temporarily lower 5-HT synthesis has shown that this can induce symptoms of depression, but only in women who have a strong previous history of depression. Animal and human work suggests that a key role of 5-HT is to promote resilience in the face of stressful circumstances. Failure of this system, thus reducing a person's ability to deal effectively with a stressful life event, may be one of the key factors contributing to the onset of depression. If dieting impairs 5-HT function directly, it may contribute to the onset of depression after a stressful life event. However, this may occur only in those people who have a vulnerability to depression because of their heredity or past history. Further research on the effects of dieting, particularly in people at risk of depression or eating problems, will need to performed before this hypothesis can be confirmed.

See Also the Following Articles

Eating Disorders and Stress; Self-Esteem, Stress and Emotion.

Further Reading

Cowen, P. J., Clifford, E. M., Williams, C., Walsh, A. E. S. and Fairburn, C. G. (1995). Why is dieting so difficult? *Nature* **376**, 557.

Deakin, J. F. W. and Graeff, F. G. (1991). 5-HT and mechanisms of defence. *Journal of Psychopharmacology* **5**, 305–315.

Hsu, L. (1997). Can dieting cause an eating disorder? *Psychological Medicine* **27**, 509–513.

Polivy, J. and Herman, C. (1993). Etiology of binge eating: psychological mechanisms. In: Fairburn, C. & Wilson, G. (eds.) *Binge eating: nature, assessment and treatment* (pp. 173–205). New York: Guilford Press.

Smith, K. A., Fairburn, C. G. and Cowen, P. J. (1997). Relapse of depression after rapid depletion of tryptophan. *Lancet* **349**, 915–919.

Wurtman, R. J. and Wurtman, J. J. (1995). Brain serotonin, carbohydrate-craving, obesity and depression. *Obesity Research* **3**(Supplement 4), 477s–480s.

Food Intake and Stress, Non-Human

Belinda A Henry and Iain J Clarke
Monash University, Melbourne, Australia

This article is a revision of the previous edition article by I J Clarke, volume 2, pp 162–166, © 2000, Elsevier Inc.

Introduction

Nonhormonal Responses to Nutritional Stress

Hormonal Responses to Nutritional Stress

Nutritional Stress and the Hypothalamic-Pituitary-Adrenal Axis

Neuronal Systems Underlying Endocrine Perturbations Induced by Nutritional Stress

Possible Hormonal Signals Involved in Mediating Nutritional Stress

Glossary

Basal metabolic rate	The rate of oxygen consumption, or calculated equivalent heat production, of an awake individual lying at rest who has had no food for at least 12 h.
Gluconeo-genesis	The formation of glucose from noncarbohydrate sources such as lactate or fatty acids.
Nutritional stress	A physiological, environmental, or metabolic stress that is imposed on an organism to disrupt metabolic homeostasis, thus causing a neural and/or endocrine response.
Orexigenic factor	A factor that acts to increase appetite and stimulate food intake.
Satiety factor	A factor that acts on the appetite-regulating regions of the brain to indicate satiety or to reduce food intake.

Introduction

Nutritional stress is, in some cases, an environmental stress and, in all cases, a metabolic stress. In particular cases, such as pregnancy and lactation, it could be construed that the nutritional demands of these states impose a physiological stress demanding increased food intake. In nonhuman species, nutritional stress occurs with a reduction in the availability of food or increased metabolic demand, but obesity is also associated with increased levels of stress hormones. In humans, a nutritional stress may be voluntarily imposed or due to psychogenic factors that have poorly defined etiology. The degree of impact varies among species depending on the type of metabolism of the organism (monogastric versus ruminant, for example) and also on the amount of body reserves of the organism.

Nutritional stress causes an alteration in the metabolic status of the animal and leads to altered concentrations of circulating metabolic substrates and metabolic hormones such as insulin and leptin. It is clear that blood-borne substances signal the metabolic status of the animal to the brain and that this leads to the alteration of hormonal output. These are responses of the organism to the stressor, but it is unlikely that a single factor that fulfils this signaling role. The neuroendocrine response to such a stress is probably the result of integrated effects of a composite of blood-borne substances. The gut may also signal directly to the brain by a neural route and through the altered secretion of ghrelin to regulate brain function and hormonal status.

Nonhormonal Responses to Nutritional Stress

Stress due to undernutrition produces a catabolic state, typified by changes in the levels of various substances in the bloodstream. Changes in metabolic factors, however, can be influenced by other physiological stimuli, so variations in the concentrations of singular components do not often reflect metabolic state. For example, fat is metabolized during a fast to produce nonesterified fatty acids (NEFA) that are used to synthesize carbohydrates via gluconeogenesis. Accordingly, plasma NEFA levels are elevated during a fast. On the other hand, prolonged undernutrition decreases body fat, leading to reduced NEFA levels, and obese subjects have increased NEFA levels, due

to increased body fat. Thus, plasma NEFA concentrations are increased in both fasting and obese states. Other changes indicative of a catabolic state include reduced plasma insulin and leptin levels and increased plasma urea concentrations (due to the breakdown of muscle tissue in an effort to mobilize amino acids for the production of carbohydrates via gluconeogenesis). Chronic undernutrition (and a reduction in gluconeogenic substrates such as NEFA and amino acids) is typically associated with a reduction in plasma glucose concentrations. Plasma levels of these metabolic factors are a reflection of nutritional state (undernutrition versus obesity) and also the extent of catabolic stress (fasting versus prolonged undernutrition).

Hormonal Responses to Nutritional Stress

Endocrine changes occur during food deprivation or food restriction and the effects of fasting are summarized in **Table 1**.

Table 1 Endocrine changes occur during food deprivation or food restriction[a]

Hormone	Change	Comments
Small monogastric animals (e.g., laboratory rat)		
Catecholamines	↑	Reflects the output of adrenalin from the adrenal medulla; catecholamines are lipolytic, mobilizing fat stores in response to reduced energy substrate
Insulin	↓	Insulin facilitates the uptake of sugar from the bloodstream
Growth hormone	↓	Response is opposite to that seen in large animals and also opposite to the response seen in humans
Gonadotropins (LH and FSH)	↓	Fasting for a period of 1–2 days can prevent the preovulatory LH surge in rats
Gonadal steroids (estrogen, testosterone, progesterone)	↓	
Prolactin	↓	With extended period of undernutrition
ACTH	↑	
Cortisol	↑	
TSH	↓	
T_3	↓	Through reduced conversion of T_4 to T_3
Nonhuman primates		
Insulin	↓	
Catecholamines	Not known	
Growth hormone	↑	
Gonadotropins (LH and FSH)	↓	LH is decreased, but there is a slower response in terms of FSH
Prolactin	Not known	
ACTH	Not known	
Cortisol	↑	
TSH	Not changed in the short term	
T_3	↓	
Ruminants		
Catecholamines	Not known	
Growth hormone	↑	
Gonadotropins (LH and FSH)	↓	LH is decreased, but there is a slower response in terms of FSH
Prolactin	Not changed	
Adrenocorticotropin	Not known	
Cortisol	↑	Morning levels only

[a]ACTH, adrenocorticotropic hormone; FSH, follicle stimulating hormone; LH, luteinizing hormone; T_3, triiodothyronine; T_4, thyroxine; TSH, thyroid stimulating hormone.

Nutritional Stress and the Hypothalamic-Pituitary-Adrenal Axis

General Considerations

The hypothalamic-pituitary-adrenal (HPA) axis is commonly activated by nutritional stress, which results in the increased secretion of glucocorticoids from the adrenal cortex. Most information to date has been derived from the laboratory rodent. The degree of activation of the HPA axis is dependent on a variety of factors, including:

- The species studied (monogastric small mammals such as rodents versus larger ruminant mammals such as sheep).
- The degree of intensity of undernutrition.
- The duration of undernutrition.
- The nutritional state of the animal prior to onset of catabolic state.
- The time of day; there is a diurnal pattern of glucocorticoid secretion.

Plasma glucocorticoids are elevated in states of undernutrition and in obese subjects, so both conditions might be regarded as stressors. The degree of change in body condition is an important factor. With undernutrition, the rapidity of change may also be a determinant of the stress response because animals can adapt over time to reduced energy stores. In obesity, the impact on the stress axis (glucocorticoid levels) depends on the obesity phenotype (where fat is distributed in the body).

There are species differences in the stress response to changing nutritional status and effects on plasma glucocorticoid levels are summarized in **Table 2**. It is important to note that the major glucocorticoid in rodents is corticosterone, whereas larger species including humans produce cortisol. Small monogastric mammals such as rodents exhibit robust activation of the HPA axis in response to fasting, but the same is not true for ruminants, in which digestion of nutrients is slower. Ruminants have a dynamic digestive system, with four stomach compartments (rumen, reticulum, omasum, and abomasum), which enables them to digest their primary dietary component, cellulose. Ruminant digestion takes a considerable time, so there is a delayed response to fasting. Furthermore, ruminants stringently maintain blood glucose levels by the mobilization of NEFA from fat stores. Small animals have higher basal metabolic rates, which impacts fuel utility. Small animals (rodents) also have very low fat stores (approximately 10%) in comparison to larger species, including both sheep and humans (approximately 20%).

The Effect of Fasting versus Food Restriction on Hypothalamic-Pituitary-Adrenal Axis Activity

The effect of nutritional stress on the HPA axis is dependent on the duration and the intensity of undernutrition. Fasting is often used in the laboratory as a nutritional stressor, and in rodents plasma corticosterone levels are elevated within 24 h. In sheep, the response takes longer and cortisol secretion is increased 48–72 h after the commencement of fasting. In rodents, chronic food restriction (animals fed a 50% maintenance diet) for 4 weeks increases plasma levels of corticosterone, but basal cortisol levels are minimally changed in sheep made lean by long-term food restriction. There is a perturbation of the diurnal pattern of cortisol secretion in fasting sheep, with higher morning levels.

Pregnancy and Lactation

Pregnancy and lactation can be considered physiological conditions that induce nutritional stress by virtue of the high energy demands consigned to the mother. In small mammals, it has been calculated that the energy demands of lactation are four times greater than those of nonpregnant females. The high metabolic demands of lactation are met by profoundly increased food intake, driven by changes in appetite-regulating systems in the brain. Unlike other typical nutritional stressors, however, lactation is associated with hyporesponsivity of the HPA axis; neuroendocrine responses to stress are blunted in lactating animals. adrenocorticotropic hormone (ACTH) and

Table 2 Species differences in glucocorticoid responses to nutritional stressors

	Laboratory rodent	Sheep	Nonhuman primate	Human
Fasting	↑ Corticosterone within 24–48 h	↑ Cortisol within 48–72 h	↑ Cortisol within 24 h	↑ Cortisol within 24 h
Food restriction	↑ Corticosterone	No change	Unknown	↑ Cortisol
Obesity	↑ Corticosterone in genetic models of obesity such as the fatty Zucker rat and the *ob/ob* mouse	No change in basal cortisol concentrations ↑ Cortisol response to stress	Unknown	↑ Cortisol (particularly in abdominal obesity)

cortisol levels are maintained during pregnancy, whereas corticotropin releasing hormone (CRH) levels are elevated due to peripheral synthesis and secretion by the placenta. This increase in CRH production is counteracted by increased circulating levels of CRH-binding protein (which sequesters CRH), thus preventing inappropriate secretion of ACTH. This phenomenon, however, occurs only in mammals that produce placental CRH.

Nutritional Stress and Negative Feedback Mechanisms of the Hypothalamic-Pituitary-Adrenal Axis

The HPA axis is tightly regulated by glucocorticoid (and mineralocorticoid) feedback to the hypothalamus and the anterior pituitary gland to regulate the secretion of hypophysiotropic hormones (CRH and arginine vasopressin, AVP) from the hypothalamus and ACTH from the pituitary corticotrophs. It has been hypothesized that abdominal obesity in humans and other species leads to dysfunction of the negative feedback actions of glucocorticoids, causing upregulation of the HPA axis and increased plasma levels of cortisol. In rodents, it has been hypothesized that decreased negative feedback actions within the brain actually precedes the obese state; animals susceptible to diet-induced obesity have decreased levels of glucocorticoid receptor mRNA within the hippocampus compared to diet-resistant animals.

Some work suggests that the sensitivity of the HPA axis to the negative feedback effects of glucocorticoids depends on carbohydrate ingestion. Adrenalectomized rodents suffer various abnormalities within the HPA axis, including increased expression of CRH mRNA in the paraventricular nucleus of the hypothalamus and decreased expression of CRH mRNA in the central nucleus of the amygdala. Interestingly, these perturbations in the adrenalectomized animal can be ameliorated by the ingestion of sucrose. Similarly, feeding animals a diet high in fat content also impacts on the HPA axis. For example, feeding rats a diet containing 20% fat (control diet, 4% fat) increases both basal and stress-induced secretion of ACTH and corticosterone. In contrast, feeding rats a diet very high (60%) in fat can decrease hormonal responses to stress. Thus, in animals, as in humans, the macronutrient dietary content impacts the reactivity of the HPA axis.

Nonadrenal Production of Glucocorticoids in Obesity

Peripheral tissues, other than the adrenal cortex, are able to produce glucocorticoids. This occurs by conversion of inert 11-keto steroids (11-dehydrocorticosterone in rodents and cortisone in humans) to active 11-hydroxy steroids (corticosterone in rodents and cortisol in humans). This process is regulated by the 11β-hydroxysteroid dehydrogenase (11β-HSD) enzymes; 11β-HSD-1 catalyzes the synthesis of active 11-hydroxy steroids, and 11β-HSD-2 catalyzes the synthesis of the inactive 11-keto steroids. The 11β-HSD-1 enzyme is predominantly expressed in white adipose tissue, the liver, and the central nervous system (particularly the paraventricular nucleus of the hypothalamus and the hippocampus). In genetic models of obesity such as the *ob/ob* mice (a naturally occurring mutation in the gene that encodes leptin) and the fatty Zucker rat (a mutation in the gene that encodes the leptin receptor), the expression of 11β-HSD-1 mRNA and 11β-HSD-1 enzymatic activity is increased within adipose tissue, whereas expression is reduced in the liver. Furthermore, overexpressing 11β-HSD-1 mRNA within the adipose tissue of transgenic mice specifically increases local concentrations of corticosterone. Such animals have an obese phenotype, but this is not associated with increased plasma levels of corticosterone.

The Role of the Hypothalamic-Pituitary-Adrenal Axis in the Predisposition to Obesity

In rodents, genetic obesity (the *ob/ob* mouse and the fatty Zucker rat) causes elevated concentrations of corticosterone. Adrenalectomy attenuates (or completely reverses) the obese phenotype in these animals. Furthermore, in nonmutated rodents, adrenalectomy reduces food intake, and corticosterone replacement restores normal feeding behavior. The stimulatory effect of glucocorticoids on food intake, however, cannot be displayed in an adrenal-intact rodent.

In rodents, mild pain induced by tail pinch initially increases food intake, but this effect is abolished by repeated experience; chronic exposure to tail pinch reduces food intake and body weight. Similarly, in rats repeated restraint stress reduces food intake and body weight, and this effect can be mimicked by chronic treatment with corticosterone. This decrease, however, is in comparison to rats fed *ad libitum*. In contrast, animals pair-fed to a similar (and lower) plane of nutrition tend to have lower body weights and reduced fat deposition compared to animals exposed to either repeated restraint stress or glucocorticoid treatment.

Neuronal Systems Underlying Endocrine Perturbations Induced by Nutritional Stress

There are numerous neuropeptides and neurotransmitters that are involved in both the regulation of appetite and neuroendocrine functions. Within the hypothalamus, this involves a number of interconnected nuclei. The arcuate nucleus is essential to the regulation of food intake and body weight and produces a number of neuropeptides, including the appetite stimulators neuropeptide Y (NPY) and agouti-related protein (AGRP) as well as the appetite inhibitors α-melanocyte stimulating hormone (α-MSH: derived from the proopiomelanocortin, POMC, gene) and urocortin 2. Other regions of the hypothalamus involved in regulating food intake and neuroendocrine function include the paraventricular nucleus, which produces the appetite inhibitors CRH, urocortin 1, urocortin 2 and urocortin 3; the lateral hypothalamic area, which contains the appetite stimulators melanin-concentrating hormone (MCH) and the orexin; and the ventromedial hypothalamic nucleus. Various appetite-regulating peptides impact on the HPA axis and these are summarized in **Table 3**.

In addition to the hypothalamus, several nuclei in the brain stem also regulate feeding behavior and the HPA axis. Brain stem nuclei can regulate HPA function by ascending projections to the forebrain or via descending spinal projections to the adrenal gland. For example, noradrenergic input from the locus ceruleus to the paraventricular nucleus of the hypothalamus is involved in the regulation of HPA function as well as food intake. In sheep and rats, various studies document the effects of nutritional stress on the expression of genes that encode appetite-regulating peptides. For example, in sheep made lean by chronic food restriction, the expression of genes encoding NPY, AGRP, and MCH is increased, indicative of increased hunger drive; these animals, however, have normal basal cortisol secretion. On the other hand, in fasted rodents, the expression of the same genes (NPY, AGRP, and MCH) is increased and there is activation of the HPA axis. Species differences in neuronal circuitry regulating the HPA axis may be relevant to the way that alteration in body weight affects the stress axis.

Possible Hormonal Signals Involved in Mediating Nutritional Stress

Various hormonal signals relay information about nutritional state to the appetite-regulating and neuroendocrine centers of the brain. Three hormones that play an important role are leptin, ghrelin, and insulin.

Leptin

Leptin is primarily produced by white fat tissue, and its plasma levels reflect the level of adiposity. In rodents, there is a tight negative correlation between the plasma levels of leptin and corticosterone. In rodents and sheep, the fasting-induced activation of the HPA axis is ameliorated by leptin treatment. Leptin also attenuates the ACTH and corticosterone responses to a physical stressor (hind-limb restraint) in rats. This suggests that leptin may in fact influence the neuroendocrine stress axis under conditions not associated with either nutritional or metabolic perturbations. The mechanisms by which leptin exerts such an effect are most likely to be centrally mediated. *In vitro* studies show that leptin can influence CRH secretion from isolated rat hypothalami but not ACTH secretion from cultured rat pituitary cells. A subpopulation of CRH-containing cells in the hypothalamus expresses the leptin receptor, allowing for direct action at this level of the HPA axis. Leptin receptors are also found in many cell types in the brain that provide afferents to the paraventricular nucleus, so there is likely to be relayed effects as well. Such cell types include those that produce NPY, MCH, and POMC.

Ghrelin

Ghrelin is primarily secreted from the stomach and has been shown to potently stimulate the secretion of

Table 3 The effect of hypothalamic appetite-regulating peptides on the HPA axis[a]

	Neuropeptide	Effect on food intake	Effect on HPA axis activity
Arcuate nucleus	NPY	↑	↑
	AGRP	↑	↑
	α-MSH	↓	↑ Basal ACTH and corticosterone ↓ IL-1-induced HPA axis activity
	CART	↓	↑
	Urocortin 2	↓	No effect
Paraventricular nucleus	CRH	↓	↑
	Urocortin 1	↓	↑
	Urocortin 2	↓	No effect
	Urocortin 3	↓	No effect
Lateral hypothalamic area	MCH	↑	↑
	Orexins	↑	↑
	Urocortin 1	↓	↑

[a]ACTH, adrenocorticotropic hormone; AGRP, agouti-related protein; CART, cocaine and amphetamine regulated transcript; CRH, corticotropin releasing hormone; HPA, hypothalamic-pituitary-adrenal; IL, interleukin; MCH, melanin-concentrating hormone; MSH, melanocyte stimulating hormone; NPY, neuropeptide Y.

growth hormone. In some species, ghrelin also acts within the brain to stimulate food intake. Studies in sheep show that a preprandial rise in ghrelin levels stimulates a postprandial rise in growth hormone levels. Plasma levels of ghrelin fall postprandially and are increased by fasting or reduction in body weight; levels are lower in obese individuals. In addition to the stimulation of growth hormone, ghrelin activates the HPA axis, although not in all species. Ghrelin mRNA levels are increased after both physical (tail pinch) and nutritional (fasting) stress. Thus, ghrelin may be an additional factor involved in the regulation of the HPA axis under stressful stimuli. Ghrelin acts via the growth hormone secretagogue receptor, which is present in both the central nervous system and the pituitary gland. In rodents, the *in vivo* action of ghrelin on the HPA axis is exerted centrally, via cells such as those that produce NPY and AGRP in the arcuate nucleus. The orexin system in the lateral hypothalamus has also been linked to ghrelin-induced corticosterone secretion.

Insulin

The role of insulin in the regulation of food intake and neuroendocrine function is sometimes confused with the confounding effects of insulin-induced hypoglycemia. The latter increases food intake due to glucose deprivation, whereas in other circumstances insulin acts to decrease food intake. In rodents, diabetes causes increased basal concentrations of ACTH and corticosterone but reduced responsiveness to stress. Streptozotocin-induced diabetes impacts various neuronal systems, which in turn may influence the HPA axis. For example, streptozotocin-induced diabetes increases the concentration of norepinephrine within the paraventricular nucleus of the hypothalamus, and this parallels increasing levels of corticosterone. This effect is dependent on insulin concentrations because insulin replacement restores levels of norepinephrine within the paraventricular nucleus and the peripheral concentrations of corticosterone. Interestingly leptin treatment, in the absence of insulin

replacement, also corrects these streptozotocin-induced perturbations. In addition to effects on catecholaminergic systems, diabetes-associated changes in HPA axis function may be mediated via hypothalamic peptides such as NPY. In the rat, the arcuate nucleus contains insulin receptors and insulin decreases NPY mRNA expression in this region.

Further Reading

Bronson, F. H. (1985). Mammalian reproduction: an ecological perspective. *Biology of Reproduction* **32**, 1–26.

Cameron, J. L. (1996). Regulation of the reproductive hormone secretion in primates by short-term changes in nutrition. *Reviews of Reproduction* **1**, 117–126.

Dallman, M. F., Pecoraro, N., Akana, S. F., et al. (2003). Chronic stress and obesity: a new view of "comfort food." *Proceedings of the National Academy of Sciences USA* **100**, 11695–11701.

Friedman, J. M. and Halaas, J. L. (1998). Leptin and the regulation of body weight in mammals. *Nature* **395**, 763–770.

Henry, B. A. (2003). Links between appetite regulating systems and the neuroendocrine hypothalamus: lessons from the sheep. *Journal of Neuroendocrinology* **15**, 697–709.

Horvath, T. L. and Diano, S. (2004). The floating blueprint of hypothalamic feeding circuits. *Nature Reviews Neuroscience* **5**, 662–667.

Krysiak, R., Obuchowicz, E. and Herman, Z. S. (1999). Interactions between the neuropeptide Y system and the hypothalamic-pituitary-adrenal axis. *European Journal of Endocrinology* **140**, 130–136.

Seckl, J. R. and Walker, B. R. (2004). 11β-hydroxysteroid dehydrogenase type 1 as a modulator of glucocorticoid action: from metabolism to memory. *Trends in Endocrinology and Metabolism* **15**, 418–424.

Smith, M. S. and Grove, K. L. (2002). Integration of the regulation of reproduction function and energy balance: lactation as a model. *Frontiers in Neuroendocrinology* **23**, 225–256.

van der Lely, A. J., Tschop, M., Heiman, M. L., et al. (2004). Biological, physiological, pathophysiological and pharmacological aspects of ghrelin. *Endocrine Reviews* **25**, 426–457.

Food Shift Effect

F K Stephan
Florida State University, Tallahassee, FL, USA

This article is reproduced from the previous edition, volume 2, pp 167–169, © 2000, Elsevier Inc.

Endogenous Circadian Clocks
Physiological Correlates of Entrainment by Meals
Shift Work and Jet Lag
Conclusion

Glossary

Circadian rhythm	A cycle with a period of approximately 24 h.
Entrainment	A zeitgeber forcing its period and phase on a rhythm.
Phase	A point in the circadian cycle.
Zeitgeber	A periodic external cue that entrains circadian clocks.

Endogenous Circadian Clocks

In 1972, the neural substrate responsible for the generation and entrainment of circadian rhythms by light was identified. Lesions of this small structure, the suprachiasmatic nucleus (SCN) of the hypothalamus, appeared to abolish circadian rhythms in behavior and physiology. However, despite such lesions, rats were still able to anticipate one meal per day by increased activity, a rise in core temperature and serum corticosterone, and other physiological changes that occurred approximately 2–4 h prior to meal access. There is now compelling evidence that these functions are mediated by an endogenous circadian clock: (1) meal anticipation occurs only if the interval between meals is in the circadian range (~22–30 h), (2) anticipatory activity persists for several days when rats are food-deprived or the activity free runs (in some rats) if meals are presented outside the circadian range, and (3) phase shifts of meal-time result in transients, that is, gradual daily adjustments until the activity reentrains to the new meal time (see **Figure 1**). Despite many efforts, this feeding-entrained oscillator (FEO) has not yet been localized. Nevertheless, most mammals, as well as some inframammalian species, are now known to have the capacity to anticipate daily meals, and it would be surprising if humans lacked such a circadian clock. It is well known that hunger sensations arise around the customary meal time. What has been difficult to explain from a purely homeostatic view is that the omission of a meal does not produce monotonically increasing feelings of hunger; instead, hunger subsides until the next customary meal time. However, this makes sense if hunger sensations are based in part on an internal timing signal and not entirely on an energy-deficit signal.

Physiological Correlates of Entrainment by Meals

Before addressing the potentially adverse effects of changes in meal time or meal omission, a brief summary of the main effects of feeding one meal per day on the rat's digestive physiology is in order. As mentioned earlier, serum corticosterone levels rise prior to expected meals. Corticosterone is both a metabolic and a stress hormone, and the brain has receptors for this steroid. Perhaps most surprising is the observation that disaccharidases (enzymes for digesting sugars) in the duodenum also increase before the meal is available. In addition, several aspects of liver function, cell division in the gastrointestinal tract, and intestinal motility become entrained to periodic meals. The increase in core temperature also may facilitate digestion. The general inference to be drawn from these observations is that the digestive physiology is not simply reactive to ingested nutrients but is capable of anticipating and preparing for meals, most likely under the influence of the circadian FEO. If the expected meal is displaced in time, these efforts are for naught and for several days these preparatory responses are out of synchrony with actual food consumption.

Shift Work and Jet Lag

Gastrointestinal malaise is a common complaint of shift workers and travelers across time zones. Along with impaired performance and other complaints, this has been attributed to the desynchronization of SCN-controlled rhythms (e.g., the sleep–wake cycle) from behavior. The discovery of a separate circadian clock raises the possibility that some of these symptoms are caused by forcing the FEO to phase shift to a new time. Unfortunately, the scientific literature regarding the role of meal timing and meal

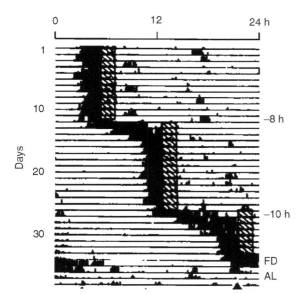

Figure 1 Anticipatory wheel running from a rat with a lesion of the suprachiasmatic nucleus (arrhythmic when fed *ad libitum*). Food is available for 2 h day^{-1}, indicated by the vertical cross-hatched bars. Most wheel running occurs approximately 3 h before meal time. When the meal time is delayed by 8 or 10 h, anticipatory activity takes 3 or 4 days to reentrain to the phase-shifted meal. The activity persists during food deprivation (FD), but is not observed during *ad libitum* (AL) feeding.

composition in producing jet-lag symptoms in humans is extremely sparse. Only very recently has an attempt been made to assess the consequences of limiting food intake to a single meal. A carbohydrate-rich meal in the morning for 3 consecutive days led to a phase advance of 1 h of the body temperature rhythm, whereas evening meals had no effect. A similar effect has been noted in mice in that the nocturnal activity rhythm is also phase advanced if they are limited to one meal per day. In rats, the FEO is easily phase shifted by a glucose meal, but seems less responsive to a fat meal. A number of other studies indicate that there are interactions between light-entrainable and food-entrainable circadian systems; the period and phase of one has an effect on the other. Thus, there is a possibility that particular meal schedules might facilitate adjustment to temporal shifts in daily routines, but this has not yet been specifically investigated. In an interesting study, patients in a vegetative state (which reduces or eliminates the effects of activity or other external factors) received intraduodenal infusions of a liquid diet continuously, only during the day or only during the night. No consistent temperature rhythms were observed with continuous infusions, whereas day infusions resulted in a peak temperature at 8 p.m. and night infusions resulted in a peak at 4 a.m. Because these peaks

occurred at different times relative to meal onset and end, they were probably not entirely due to the thermogenic action of food but may reflect the entrainment of some physiological processes by a circadian oscillator. When humans live in temporal isolation for more than 3 weeks, approximately one-half of the subjects display internal desynchronization. The core body temperature rhythm continues to free run with a period of approximately 25 h, but the sleep–wake cycle assumes a much longer period, between 30 and 48 h. When subjects were asked to eat only two meals per day (breakfast and lunch), the interval between meals was proportional to the wake time. Before internal desynchronization, the average interval between meals was approximately 7.4 h; after internal desynchronization (when the sleep–wake cycle had assumed a period of 35.4 h), the interval increased to 10.4 h. It should be noted that subjects were entirely unaware that their sleep–wake cycle had become abnormally long. It has long been suspected that internal desynchronization is evidence for two separate circadian clocks, but alternative explanations have also been offered. In particular, none of the studies establishes the existence of a separate feeding-entrained circadian clock in humans. Nevertheless, these studies at least suggest a circadian timing component to human hunger. However, in blind humans who have difficulties adhering to a 24-h schedule, regular meals and social routines have not been very effective in forcing entrainment of the sleep–wake cycle.

In other human studies regarding the effect of light or exercise on circadian rhythms, mealtime is either not reported or small meals are given at frequent intervals so that the effects of substantial meals on physiological measures cannot be assessed. Furthermore, temperature data (and other data) are often reported as group means or in other ways that make it impossible to determine even whether temperature or serum cortisol levels in humans rise in anticipation of meals. However, the evidence is quite compelling that such rhythms persist in constant conditions, that is, that they are controlled by one or more endogenous circadian oscillators.

A nearly universal observation is that circadian rhythms adjust more readily to phase delays (e.g., westward flights) than to phase advances (e.g., eastward flights). This asymmetry is even more pronounced in rats with SCN lesions that are entrained to one meal per day. As mentioned earlier, rats can anticipate meals at intervals as long as 30 h, but have difficulty anticipating meals presented at intervals shorter than 22 h, indicating that the FEO slows down more readily than it accelerates. When meals are shifted to a later time, anticipatory activity shifts by 2–4 h day^{-1} until it reaches the new phase position (see **Figure 1**). Conversely, after phase advances of 6 h or more, many rats display delays in anticipatory activity, again of about 3 h day^{-1}, i.e., the oscillator delays by 16–18 h over 5–6 days to catch up with the phase-advanced meal time. It is interesting that some humans also show delaying transients after rotating to an earlier shift (e.g., from the night to afternoon shift).

Conclusion

During the past decades, it has become increasingly clear that the regulation of energy balance is largely proactive rather than reactive. Circadian clocks, such as the FEO, entrain to predictable external events and ready the system for the arrival of nutrients. Phase shifts of mealtime temporarily disrupt these functions and probably account, at least partially, for the symptoms of jet lag or shift-worker malaise. The release of adrenal corticosteroids before meals could be a warning signal to the brain to replenish energy reserves. If food is consumed, serum levels decline, but if the meal is not available, serum levels might remain elevated for many hours. This, as well as other wasted physiological changes that occur in anticipation of meals, is undoubtedly not beneficial. There is no direct evidence as yet (because it has not been studied) that serious harm results from phase shifts of meals; however, it is conceivable that prolonged erratic eating habits contribute to the stress experienced by hectic modern lifestyles.

See Also the Following Articles

Circadian Rhythms, Genetics of; Sleep Loss, Jet Lag, and Shift Work.

Further Reading

Aschoff, J. (1998). Human perception of short and long time intervals: its correlation with body temperature and the duration of wake time. *Journal of Biological Rhythms* **13**, 437–442.

Czeisler, C. A. and Megan, E. J. (1990). Human circadian physiology: interaction of the behavioral rest-activity cycle with the output of the endogenous circadian pacemaker. In: Thorpy, M. J. (ed.) *Handbook of sleep disorders*, pp. 117–137. New York: Marcel Dekker.

Krauchi, K., Werth, E., Cajochen, C., et al. (1998). Are carbohydrate-rich meals a zeitgeber in humans? *Society for Research on Biological Rhythms* Abstract 96.

Mills, J. N., Minors, D. S. and Waterhouse, J. M. (1978). Adaptation to abrupt time shifts of the oscillator(s) controlling human circadian rhythms. *Journal of Physiology* **285**, 455–470.

Mistlberger, R. E. (1994). Circadian food-anticipatory activity: formal models and physiological mechanisms. *Neuroscience and Biobehavioral Reviews* **18**, 171–195.

Stephan, F. K. (1992). Resetting of a feeding-entrainable circadian clock in the rat. *Physiology & Behavior* **52**, 985–995.

Stephan, F. K. (1997). Calories affect zeitgeber properties of the feeding entrained circadian oscillator. *Physiology & Behavior* **62**, 995–1002.

Van Cauter, E., Sturis, J., Byrne, M., et al. (1994). Demonstration of rapid light-induced advances and delays of the human circadian clock using hormonal phase markers. *American Journal of Psychiatry* **266**, E953–E963.

Freud, Sigmund

D J Lynn
Thomas Jefferson University, Philadelphia, PA, USA

Introduction
Background and Personal Life
Freud the Theoretician and Proponent
Freud the Clinician
Freud the Organizer and Movement Leader
Freud and Stress
Freud in Perspective

Introduction

Sigmund Freud (1856–1939) is best known as the originator of psychoanalysis, which is at once a method of treatment for emotional disorders, a system of ideas concerning human emotional life (both healthy and disordered), and an intellectual movement. His historical significance stems from his activities in several frequently interlocking roles – theoretician, proponent, clinician, organizer, and leader. Although practitioners of psychoanalysis have divided themselves into diverging groups adhering to different doctrines, many psychoanalysts continue to rely on Freud's theoretical conclusions and technical recommendations, and his writings are still cited in current American textbooks of psychiatry. In addition, some writers in the humanities, literary critics and historians in particular, have relied extensively on Freud's theories. Indeed, Freud's ideas, or corruptions of them, have become commonplace in Western popular culture.

Background and Personal Life

Sigmund Freud was the oldest of eight children born to a Jewish family in what was then Freiberg, in the Austro-Hungarian Empire, and is now Pribor, in the Czech Republic. His father, Jakob Freud, was a wool merchant; during hard times he moved the family to Vienna when Sigmund was 4 years old. A strong student in gymnasium and then at the University of Vienna, Freud had adolescent ambitions of becoming a leader in progressive politics but put them aside to take up the natural sciences. The geographical and social context was the Austro-Hungarian Empire, which was undergoing very rapid industrialization and modernization. Much has been written on the question of how much influence Freud's Jewish ancestry had upon his experiences, attitudes, and beliefs.

Freud's first scientific mentor was Ernst Wilhelm von Brücke, and his early laboratory studies involved comparative neuroanatomy. He earned his medical degree in 1881, but he remained a laboratory researcher for a time. He did not engage in clinical work until 1882, after he had met Martha Bernays, his future wife, and had decided that his earnings in research would never support married life. His work in neuroanatomy reached its peak in his microscopic studies of the medulla in the laboratory of Theodor Meynert. His papers on axon tracts and on his method for using gold solutions for staining them were published in both German and English in 1884, but disappointment followed when his staining method could not be replicated. Freud chose the clinical specialty of neurology – not psychiatry, which in the late nineteenth century was largely concerned with treating and studying psychotic patients in mental hospitals. As a neurologist in office practice, Freud encountered patients with symptoms that were then classified into such syndromic categories as neurasthenia and hysteria. Freud's neurological studies included important work on aphasia and paralyses in children.

From October 1885 to February 1886, Freud studied in Paris with Jean-Martin Charcot, the premier French neurologist of the era. Charcot was then immersed in the study of hysteria, using hypnosis to explore patients histories and concluding that the paralyses and seizures that he saw in his patients, and demonstrated so dramatically in his clinical presentations, had their roots in ideas. Freud's interest in these clinical problems had been stimulated by the descriptions given by his friend and senior colleague, Josef Breuer, of Breuer's treatment of the woman known in later publications as Anna O.

Freud married Martha Bernays in 1886. The couple had three sons and three daughters. In 1923, he was first given a diagnosis of oral carcinoma. This neoplasm, related to his constant cigar smoking, required several surgical procedures and produced intermittent pain over the ensuing years. Freud lived and worked in Vienna until the Nazi Anschluss in March of 1938 placed him and his family in great peril. Through the intercession of Ernest Jones and Freud's patients Princess Marie Bonaparte and William Bullitt, and diplomatic pressure by the United States, Freud was allowed to leave Austria with his wife and children in June. A condition imposed by the Germans was that Freud state that he had been treated with due respect. In response, Freud is reported to have declared "I can heartily recommend the Gestapo to anyone" – a fine example of his celebrated sense of humor. Freud spent the last year of his life in London, seeing some patients and continuing to write, despite his advanced age, until July 1939. Pain and debilitation caused by his spreading oral carcinoma then became overwhelming. On September 23, 1939, he died in what would today be called an assisted suicide.

Freud the Theoretician and Proponent

Freud generated theoretical proposals and conclusions that spanned a breathtaking range of subjects, including the technique of clinical psychoanalysis, the etiology of mental disturbances, human psychological functioning in health and disease, the pattern of development of the human personality, and the basic forces motivating human life.

Concerning the technique of clinical psychoanalysis, Freud prescribed an approach based upon anonymity, neutrality, and confidentiality and requiring from the patient free associations, meaning the vocalization of an uncensored flow of thoughts. Freud emphasized the importance of interpretations expressed by the analyst and giving meaning to dreams, feelings, and symptoms experienced by the patient. Invariably, patients encountered difficulties in reporting, or even experiencing, uncensored thoughts. Freud reported that these difficulties, termed resistances, could themselves be understood and thus could serve to promote the exploratory process. The transference, the set of emotions experienced by the patient toward the analyst, initially seen as an obstacle to exploration, came to be seen as a crucial source of information for understanding the patient's development and reconstructing childhood relationships. The countertransference, defined as the psychoanalyst's attitudes and feelings toward the patient, subsequently received attention; Freud eventually prescribed that the analyst should undergo psychoanalysis in order to minimize its impact on the treatment.

Early in his psychoanalytic work, in 1896, Freud published his conclusion that the etiology of hysteria – the intermittent paralyses and other unexplained symptoms studied by Charcot and others – was invariably a delayed response by the patient to childhood experiences of seduction (sexual abuse or rape in today's terms) of the child by a trusted adult, typically the patient's father. Freud retracted this view within a few years and emphasized instead the significance of frustrated childhood wishes for sexual gratification by an adult.

Freud's initial psychoanalytic view of the functioning of the human mind involved what has been called a topographical model. In this conception, ideas, feelings, and wishes are processed in three different mental sectors. In the conscious sector, items that are not overly threatening could be remembered, considered, and acted upon. A preconscious sector would contain items that are not currently in awareness but that could be readily retrieved. An unconscious sector would contain extremely important memories, wishes, and feelings that would be too threatening to be recognized in consciousness. A postulated mental component known as the censor would perform the function of allowing, or preventing (through repression), items from reaching consciousness. Despite the functioning of the censor, unconscious ideation would be expressed in several interesting ways, through symptoms and symptomatic behavior, for example, or in dreams or parapraxes (slips of the tongue). In this view, an important function of psychoanalysis would be to strengthen the personality and resolve symptoms by interpreting these expressions and thereby making the unconscious conscious.

In later writings, Freud proposed a different model of mental functioning, although he never fully abandoned the topographic model. This tripartite model postulated three psychic structures. The id was described as a biologically rooted source of primitive urges. The superego, a rather rigid accumulation of prohibitions and rules imposed by parental and societal authorities, was thought to be formed in the resolution of the Oedipus complex, an emotional situation culminating in the fourth or fifth year of life, in which the boy experiences wishes to possess his mother (emotionally and sexually) and conflicting fears of paternal retaliation and general disapproval. The ego was described as the component of the mind that can think, perceive, adapt, learn, compromise, and create; this component faces the task of reconciling demands from the other components and from the external world and enabling the person to conduct a life. In this view of mental functioning, important features of emotional life, including symptoms, choices, capabilities, and limitations, were seen as arising from conflicts between the psychic components. The task of psychoanalysis in this view would be to strengthen the ego through the development of insight into these intrapsychic conflicts.

A persistent feature of Freud's theoretical views throughout his psychoanalytic writing was the notion that no mental life would occur without energy that would have biological drives or instincts as its ultimate sources. Initially, libido or eros, a sexual drive, manifesting itself in different transformations, was seen as the sole underlying source. Later, an aggressive or destructive drive, a death instinct, was postulated in addition. This latter drive remained controversial, neither universally accepted by Freud's followers nor consistently invoked by Freud himself.

Freud had superb talents as a writer. In general, his psychoanalytic contributions were in the form of essays that were not constrained by a conventional scientific format. At times he could deploy a formidable array of rhetorical devices to convince the reader that his points were valid or even inescapable. In 1930, the city of Frankfurt honored Freud's creativity and literary accomplishments with the Goethe Prize. All of his psychoanalytic writings, with the exception of *Thomas Woodrow Wilson: A Psychological Study*, co-authored by his patient, William C. Bullitt, have been translated into English in the *Standard Edition of the Complete Psychological Works of Sigmund Freud*.

Freud the Clinician

In his earliest years as a physician and neurologist, Freud had used the standard methods of the era: a limited array of drugs, electrical currents (Faradic and Galvanic treatments), minor surgery, and hypnosis. By 1896 he was concentrating on what he called psychoanalysis. In the beginning, his analytic treatments were brief and tended to culminate in a single interpretation, but by 1896 he had begun to see at least a few patients in treatments that would last for years.

His clinical work was important for several reasons. First, since he did not directly observe the psychoanalytic work of others, his own clinical work gave him his only opportunities to validate technical recommendations and to observe the clinical phenomena arising in psychoanalysis. Second, much of his analytic activity, especially after World War I, involved didactic psychoanalyses of trainees, and many of these trainees became productive, and useful, subordinates in the psychoanalytic movement. Third, even many of his patients who were not trainees and who never practiced psychoanalysis were prominent and wealthy people who retained a connection to Freud and his movement and proved to be helpful financially and in other ways.

Some of Freud's published discussions of individual cases, such as Schreber and Little Hans, do not refer to direct clinical psychoanalytic work conducted by Freud. His writings do contain extensive discussions of three of his own clinical cases. In the case of Dora, a young woman Freud treated in 1900, Freud reached a formulation involving an interpretation of her experience that was at variance with her own view. Freud concluded that the sexual advances from an older married man, which she had described as disturbing and unwanted, had been disturbing precisely because she had desired them, unconsciously. When Freud confronted her with this interpretation, she bolted in anger and terminated the treatment. He subsequently concluded that he had pressed this interpretation on her prematurely, but of course its validity, as well as its timing, is open to question.

Freud described the case of the Rat Man, a young army officer he treated in 1907, at length; in addition, his actual contemporaneous notes of the conduct of this analysis were discovered and published. Freud concluded that this patient suffered from an obsessional neurosis that Freud described as essentially cured by his interpretations. This case is usually seen as the most clinically successful of the ones that he described in his published works. Unfortunately, this man, later identified as Ernst Lanzer, died in 1914 at the onset of World War I, so that little longitudinal follow-up information is available.

The Wolf Man (later identified as Serge Pankejeff), a young Russian nobleman treated by Freud in 1909–1914 and later in 1919–1920, was Freud's best-studied case. Freud's published discussion focused on the Wolf Man's infantile neurosis, which Freud attempted to reconstruct. Central to Freud's formulation was his interpretation of the patient's wolf dream as symbolically referring to and describing a scene from this patient's infancy. This patient survived into the 1970s and was interviewed later in his life by two authors. Muriel Gardiner, a practicing psychoanalyst, described him as largely healed and contented. Karin Obholzer, a journalist, reported two

important findings. First, Pankejeff told her that he had received little or no clinical benefit from his psychoanalysis by Freud. Second, Pankejeff had never accepted Freud's interpretation of the wolf dream; he regarded Freud's reconstruction of a scene from his infancy as totally implausible.

Increasing quantities of information about many of Freud's psychoanalyses have gradually become available over the past half century in the form of Freud's letters, analysands' letters, memoirs and reports by analysands, and other sources. Recent revelations concerning his psychoanalytic treatments of some of his patients, such as Horace Frink, as described by Edmunds, or his daughter Anna, as described by Young-Bruehl, have sparked controversy. In a study of 43 of the cases he treated after 1907, Lynn and Vaillant found that in a majority of these cases, he deviated from the anonymity, neutrality, and confidentiality that he prescribed in his recommendations.

Freud the Organizer and Movement Leader

The development and maintenance of an organized group of psychoanalytic followers, forming a movement, always commanded Freud's attention, as shown especially in his correspondence with Ernest Jones and with Sandor Ferenczi. Freud was equally concerned with his followers' professional success, achievement of recognition, capacity to make intellectual contributions as members of his movement, and loyalty. Freud expressed his view of the optimal organization and functioning of the psychoanalytic movement in his essay On the History of the Psycho-Analytic Movement, first published in 1914. He envisioned a single leader with overwhelming authority. As the first leader, he wanted to find a successor who would be both capable and reliable. These considerations partly explain the pattern of his relations with a series of prominent male psychoanalysts. After apparently close collaboration, including personal friendship and mutual trust, there would be theoretical disagreement, a mutual sense of injury, competition for prominence, increasing estrangement, and repudiation. This series clearly included Carl Jung, Alfred Adler, Otto Rank, and (except for the overt repudiation), Sandor Ferenczi.

In 1912 Freud's most trusted followers, Sandor Ferenczi, Otto Rank, Karl Abraham, Ernest Jones, and Hans Sachs, formed a secret committee to oversee the movement, respond to criticisms, and assure Freud's continuing control. In his role of leader and organizer, Freud needed to reward loyalty and reliability rather than originality, creativity, or independent intellectual achievement. He generally saw new members as converts; he referred to critics as opponents or even enemies.

Freud and Stress

Freud viewed anxiety as a signal that could refer to a number of different dangers. He was especially concerned with anxiety arising from intrapsychic threats, such as the impending emergence of repressed wishes or conflicts. In many of these situations, even the anxiety itself would be unconscious; its existence could only be inferred or deduced by the psychoanalyst. Castration anxiety, anxieties concerning unconscious homosexual wishes, and anxieties concerning unconscious incestuous wishes were frequently invoked in the formulation and interpretation of patients' experiences and symptoms. Freud's work did not direct attention to the biological aspects of states of anxiety, nor to the role played by overwhelming external stressors. Even in his brief discussions of war neuroses, Freud emphasized intrapsychic conflict as the essential element that either made these neuroses possible or promoted them. Freud's influence was reflected in the official diagnostic terminology of American psychiatry codified in the *Diagnostic and Statistical Manual of Mental Disorders* (DSM-I) (1952) and retained in the DSM-II (1968). These listings explicitly described anxiety as an intrapsychic signal, included anxiety disorders as neuroses, and excluded any anxiety disorder specifically related to an external stressor (such as the current posttraumatic stress disorder).

Freud in Perspective

Sigmund Freud must be seen as one of the most influential intellectuals of the twentieth century. There is no indication that the influence of his system of ideas in such fields as literary criticism and historical analysis, or in the general popular culture, will recede.

Within the medical profession, Freud's ideas gained their greatest influence in American psychiatry in the middle of the twentieth century. As late as the 1970s, American psychiatry was divided into schools of thought, each of which had its own journals and took its own approach to the definition of problems to be studied, the terminology to be used, the clinical methods to be advocated, and the basic etiological assumptions to be adopted. An adherent of a particular school often felt no obligation to read or consider contributions from other schools. In this context, the extent of the influence that Freud's system of ideas had upon psychiatrists was very uneven. At one extreme, for some psychiatrists in some departments, Freud's conclusions were seen as scientifically established discoveries that served as the basis for any treatment or any academic discussion. In other departments, Freud's conclusions were either explicitly rejected or, more frequently, ignored. In recent years, American psychiatry has taken important steps toward a systematically scientific approach to clinical issues. In general, training programs no longer explicitly adopt locally accepted assumptions, and advocates of any treatment approach are expected to produce data supporting their claims.

In this current environment, Freud's conclusions will retain influence to the extent that they can be validated with reproducible results. (Advocates of psychoanalysis cannot, in this context, adequately deal with skeptics by simply maintaining that nobody has conclusively demonstrated that the method does not work.) Freud's own psychoanalytic publications have shortcomings that limit the extent to which they can be used as validation: a lack of raw observational data, an inadequate description of Freud's actual methods, and a commingling of postulates, hypotheses, observations, conclusions, and speculations without adequate designation. The psychoanalytic situation contains unavoidable difficulties for any clinical researcher in the collection and verification of data, in the generation of adequate numbers of cases, and in the standardization of technique between analysts. Efforts by latter-day psychoanalysts to validate conclusions through systematic outcome research have not produced any conclusive results, and it is unclear how, and by whom, such studies would be carried out in the future.

See Also the Following Articles

Child Sexual Abuse; Emotional Inhibition; Hysteria; Psychoanalysis; Psychotherapy.

Further Reading

Brabant, E., Falzeder, E. and Giampieri-Deutsch, P. (eds.) (1993). *The correspondence of Sigmund Freud and Sandor Ferenczi, vol. 1, 1908–1914.* Cambridge, MA: Belknap Press of Harvard University Press.

Brabant, E., Falzeder, E. and Giampieri-Deutsch, P. (eds.) (1996). *The correspondence of Sigmund Freud and Sandor Ferenczi, vol. 2, 1914–1919.* Cambridge, MA: Belknap Press of Harvard University Press.

Edmunds, L. (1988). His master's choice. *Johns Hopkins Magazine* 40, 40–49.

Ferris, P. (1997). *Dr. Freud, a life.* Washington, D.C.: Counterpoint.

Freud, S. (1957). *The standard edition of the complete psychological works of Sigmund Freud.* Strachey, J. (ed.). London: Hogarth Press.

Freud, S. and Bullitt, W. C. (1966). *Thomas Woodrow Wilson: a psychological study.* Boston, MA: Houghton Mifflin.

Gardiner, M. (1971). *The wolf-man by the wolf-man.* New York: Basic Books.

Gay, P. (1988). *Freud: a life for our time.* New York: Norton.

Gedo, J. (2002). The enduring scientific contributions of Sigmund Freud. *Perspectives in Biology and Medicine* **45**, 200–211.

Grosskurth, P. (1991). *The secret ring: Freud's inner circle and the politics of psychoanalysis.* Reading, MA: Addison-Wesley Publishing Co.

Jones, E. (1953–57). *The life and work of Sigmund Freud.* (vols. 1–3). New York: Basic Books.

Lynn, D. J. and Vaillant, G. E. (1998). Anonymity, neutrality, and confidentiality in the actual methods of Sigmund Freud: a review of 43 cases, 1907–1939. *American Journal of Psychiatry* **155**, 163–171.

Mahony, P. J. (1986). *Freud and the rat man.* New Haven, CT: Yale University Press.

Obholzer, K. (1982). *The wolf man – sixty years later.* Shaw, M. (trans.). New York: Continuum Publishing Co.

Paskauskas, R. A. (ed.) (1993). *The complete correspondence of Sigmund Freud and Ernest Jones 1908–1939.* Cambridge, MA: Belknap Press of Harvard University Press.

Roazen, P. (1976). *Freud and his followers.* New York: Knopf.

Shorter, E. (1997). *A history of psychiatry.* New York: John Wiley and Sons.

Westen, D. (1999). The scientific status of unconscious processes: is Freud really dead? *Journal of the American Psychoanalytic Association* **47**, 1061–1106.

Young-Bruehl, E. (1988). *Anna Freud: a biography.* New York: Summit Books.

GABA (Gamma Aminobutyric Acid)

J D C Lambert
University of Aarhus, Aarhus, Denmark

This article is reproduced from the previous edition, volume 2, pp 177–190, © 2000, Elsevier Inc.

Introduction to the Role of GABA as a Neurotransmitter
Neuronal Receptors for GABA
GABAergic Neurons and Their Role in Neuronal Activity

Glossary

Amino acid	A small organic molecule consisting of a backbone to which is attached an amino group (—NH$_2$) and an acidic group (—COOH). Twenty naturally occurring amino acids are incorporated into proteins under direct genetic control.
Benzo-diazepine	The generic name for a class of chemical substances that are in wide clinical use for their anxiolytic, sedative, and muscle-relaxant properties. These actions are produced by enhancing inhibitory transmission at synapses that use GABA as a transmitter.
Subunit	The receptors for many neurotransmitters are composed of a number of (usually five) distinct proteins encoded by separate genes. When the receptor is assembled from identical subunits encoded by a single gene, the assembly is termed homomeric; when subunits encoded by different genes are incorporated, the assembly is termed heteromeric.
Synapse	The very small contact area between two nerve cells where chemical transmission occurs. The chemical messenger (the neurotransmitter) is stored in vesicles in the presynaptic terminal. Nervous activity causes these vesicles to release the neurotransmitter into the synaptic cleft, following which it activates specific receptors on the postsynaptic membrane. These transduce the chemical message into an electrical signal, which can be either excitatory or inhibitory.

Gamma aminobutyric acid (GABA) is the principal inhibitory transmitter in the central nervous system (CNS). GABA acts on three distinct receptor complexes: GABA$_A$, GABA$_B$, and GABA$_C$ receptors. GABA$_A$ receptors are heteromeric structures assembled from 5 subunits selected from up to 16 different glycoprotein subunits. This heterogeneity confers discrete pharmacological and physiological properties on the assembled complex. The five subunits surround a central ion-selective channel, which conducts chloride ions into the neuron when GABA binds to the receptor. This inhibits the neuron by causing an increase in membrane potential and conductance. The GABA$_A$ receptor complex also contains a number of distinct modulatory sites that are the target for many neuroactive and therapeutic drugs, including benzodiazepines, barbiturates, steroids, alcohol, and a variety of general anesthetics. The activation of these modulatory sites generally enhances neuronal inhibition at GABA$_A$ synapses, which probably accounts for the anxiolytic, sedative, hypnotic, and anesthetic properties of these substances.

GABA$_B$ receptors are formed by a single protein molecule that is coupled with intracellular enzymes and effector systems. These can activate K$^+$-selective channels, which inhibits the neuron, or depress the activity of Ca^{2+}-selective channels, which decreases transmitter release from presynaptic terminals. GABA$_C$ receptors have many structural and functional similarities to GABA$_A$ receptors, but they exhibit sufficient pharmacological and mechanistic differences to merit classification as a separate receptor.

In view of its ubiquitous role in the integration of neuronal activity, it is hardly surprising that dysfunction of GABAergic transmission has been implicated in a wide variety of neurological and psychiatric disorders, including epilepsy, anxiety states, alco-holism, nociception, Huntington's chorea, and other movement disorders.

Introduction to the Role of GABA as a Neurotransmitter

GABA was already shown to be present in the CNS in 1950. Using the technique of microiontophoresis to apply pharmacologically active substances to single neurons in the CNS, it was subsequently shown that GABA caused a powerful inhibition of virtually every neuron to which it was applied. This, along with its simple structure and ubiquitous occurrence, meant that there was initially great skepticism as to whether GABA could fulfill the criteria required for a central inhibitory transmitter (see Box 1). These doubts were allayed by the use of two naturally occurring sub-stances that potently and selectively block the actions of exogenously applied GABA, as well as synaptic

---

Box 1
Classification of GABA Receptors

A single neurotransmitter usually activates a num-ber of distinct postsynaptic receptors. These are distinguished and identified on the basis of their responses to the actions of agonists and antagonists. Agonists are molecules that bear a chemical resem-blance to the natural transmitter and, on binding to the receptors, are able to operate the effector system and thereby mimic the response to the trans-mitter itself. As the name implies, antagonists pre-vent the agonist from evoking a response. There are two main classes of antagonist: competitive and noncompetitive. Competitive antagonists bind to the receptor site, but are unable to operate the effector system. However, they impede access of the agonist (including the natural transmitter) to the receptor site and thereby block the response. Bicu-culline is an example of a competitive antagonist at $GABA_A$ receptors, and CGP 55845A competiti-vely antagonizes responses at $GABA_B$ receptors. Noncompetitive antagonists do not interact with the receptor itself but block the action of the effector mechanism. Picrotoxin, for example, binds within the ionophore, which is gated by the $GABA_A$ receptor, and thereby inhibits the response to GABA.

On the basis of such pharmacological studies, three main families of postsynaptic receptors for GABA have been identified. These have simply been named alphabetically in the chronological order of their discovery: $GABA_A$, $GABA_B$, and $GABA_C$ receptors. The table shows the structural, pharmacological, and mechanistic features of these three receptors. $GABA_A$ and $GABA_C$ receptors are both pentameric structures surrounding a Cl^--selective ionophore. $GABA_C$ receptors have been accorded their own classification based primarily on their lack of sensi-tivity to bicuculline and lack of modulatory sites. $GABA_B$ receptors are coupled to intracellular enzymes and other mechanisms that mediate the response. Although $GABA_A$ and $GABA_B$ receptors obviously share the same natural transmitter, they otherwise have very little in common, either with respect to their molecular structure, pharmacology, or mechanism of action.

Specific properties of GABA receptors

	$GABA_A$	$GABA_B$	$GABA_C$
Receptor mechanism	Cl^--selective ionophore	G-protein-coupled metabotropic receptor	Cl^--selective ionophore
Receptor composition	Pentamer constructed from α_{1-6}, β_{1-4}, γ_{1-4}, δ_1, and ϵ_1	Dimer constructed from $GABA_BR1$ + $GABA_BR2$	Pentamer constructed from ρ_{1-2}
Single channel conductance	≈30 pS	—	≈8 pS
Mean channel open time	≈25 ms	—	≈150 ms
Receptor desensitization	Yes	No	No
Potency of GABA $(EC_{50})^a$	≈10 μM	≈10 μM	≈1 μM
Selective agonist	THIP,[b] P4S[c]	Baclofen	CACA[d]
Selective antagonist	Bicuculline	Saclofen, CGP 55845A	3-APA[e]

[a]Median effective concentration.
[b]4,5,6,7-Tetrahydroisoxazole[4,5-c]pyridin-3-ol.
[c]Piperdene-4-sulfonic acid.
[d]There are no potent selective agonists for $GABA_C$ receptors, but cis-4-amino crotonic acid is a partial agonist.
[e]3-Aminopropylphosphonic acid.

potentials evoked by the stimulation of inhibitory nerves. These substances are the alkaloids bicuculline and picrotoxin, which have played a pivotal role in past and present research on GABAergic inhibition. The ability of both alkaloids to cause sustained seizures and convulsions was known long before their actions on GABA receptors were resolved. However, this provided the first clue as to how manipulation of the GABAergic system could alter the state of excitability in the nervous system.

In 1980, a bicuculline-insensitive action of GABA was discovered that could be mimicked by the antispastic agent baclofen. A pharmacologically distinct receptor for GABA had been identified, and it was decided to name receptors alphabetically in chronological order of their discovery: bicuculline-sensitive receptors were termed $GABA_A$, and bicuculline-insensitive receptors were termed $GABA_B$.

Early studies of inhibition mediated by $GABA_A$ receptors at various sites in the CNS had disclosed discrete differences in the responses, which implied the existence of different isoforms of the receptor. Following its cloning in the late 1980s, it became apparent that the $GABA_A$ receptor is assembled from five subunits and that the identity of these determines the properties of the assembled complex. These studies also led to the identification of pharmacologically distinct $GABA_C$ receptors. The classification of the GABA receptors is given in Box 1.

Neuronal Receptors for GABA

$GABA_A$ Receptors

The $GABA_A$ receptor is a heterooligomeric complex that is probably assembled from five subunits. These are grouped around a central ion-conducting channel (ionophore), which is opened when two molecules of GABA (or another agonist) bind to the receptor. The subunits are encoded by at least 16 genes, which are grouped into five families: α_{1-6}, β_{1-4}, γ_{1-4}, δ_1, and ε_1. The degree of sequence homology of amino acids within each family is around 70%, whereas it is less than 30% between the families. Furthermore, the mature mRNAs for α_6, β_2, β_4, and γ_2 can be alternatively spliced to include or omit amino acid sequences, yielding long (L) or short (S) versions of these subunits, respectively. The subunits, which are composed of around 500 amino acids (molecular mass ranging from 48 to 64 kDa), have a similar topographical structure with the following features:

1. A large extracellular N-terminal domain containing the binding site (receptor) for GABA and a variety of modulatory ligands. This region also contains two to four glycosylation sites, which

could be important for the intracellular sorting and assembly of proteins.

2. Four hydrophobic transmembrane domains (TM1–4), which are linked by polypeptide chains. TM2 contains clusters of basic amino acids, which are believed to line the channel wall and determine its selectivity to anions.

3. A large intracellular loop connecting TM3 and TM4 that in some subunits contains sites that can be phosphorylated. Whether phosphorylation increases or decreases receptor function depends on the enzyme involved.

If there were no restrictions on how the subunits could assemble, an immense number of isoforms would exist. However, there are certain constraints on which combinations can form functional complexes. Thus, the presence of an α subunit is essential for producing a functional channel, and the $GABA_A$ receptor itself is probably located at the interface between two dissimilar subunits. The overall stoichiometry of the pentamer is likely to be two α, two β, and one γ subunits, which are arranged alternately (**Figure 1**). The α subunits need not be identical and the γ subunit can be replaced by a δ or an ϵ subunit. *In situ* hybridization and immunoprecipitation studies have shown that approximately 20 isoforms account for the vast majority of $GABA_A$ receptors, which are expressed in the CNS in a structure and cell-specific manner (**Table 1**). The most abundant combination is $\alpha_1 \beta_2 \gamma_2$, which accounts for almost half the receptors and is expressed in most brain regions. Different subunit combinations are often expressed within the same neuron.

This repertoire of 20 isoforms is sufficient to confer substantial functional and pharmacological diversity on the $GABA_A$ receptors. Examples of this diversity include the sensitivity to GABA, the kinetics of operation of the ionophore, and the actions of modulators. An interesting example of how these properties are exploited concerns the expression of $GABA_A$ receptors during development of the CNS.

$GABA_A$ receptors are expressed in the membrane some time before specialized synaptic contacts develop. The α subunit is selected from α_2, α_3, or α_5, which form receptors having a relatively high affinity for GABA and respond to ambient levels of GABA in the extracellular fluid. The intracellular Cl^- concentration is relatively high early in development: E_{Cl^-} is positive to the resting membrane potential and the activation of the $GABA_A$ receptors evokes an excitatory response (see Box 2). This depolarization activates voltage-dependent Ca^{2+} channels and the influx of Ca^{2+} activates a host of intracellular processes, which contribute to the neurotrophic response.

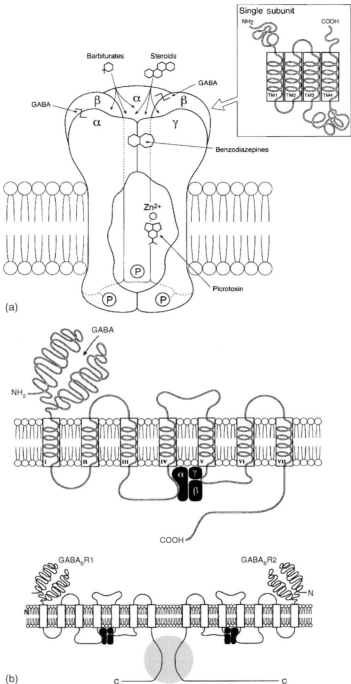

Figure 1 The molecular structure of GABA receptors. a, GABA$_A$ receptor complex; b, GABA$_B$ receptor. (a) The GABA$_A$ receptor complex is assembled from five individual subunits (with an overall stoichiometry of 2α, 2β, and 1γ) that surround a central chloride-selective channel (ionophore). The insert shows an individual subunit, which is composed of approximately 500 amino acids and has four transmembrane domains (TM1–4). Two GABA binding sites (receptors) are located between the α and β subunits. The GABA$_A$ receptor also contains a number of modulatory sites. The benzodiazepine receptor is located at the interface between α and γ subunits, whereas the receptors for steroids and barbiturates show little subunit specificity (indicated by the multiple arrowheads). Anesthetics, ethanol, and the convulsant picrotoxin exert their actions at sites associated with the channel. The areas marked by an encircled P on the inside of the channel denote sites that can be phosphorylated and that modify channel function. (b) The GABA$_B$ receptor has seven transmembrane domains (I–VII) with a large extracellular N-terminal region that forms the receptor for GABA. The complex is coupled to a G-protein complex on the inside of the membrane, which mediates the cellular effects following receptor activation. The lower diagram shows the functional GABA$_B$ receptor. This is a dimer formed by two receptors, GABA$_B$R1 and GABA$_B$R2, which associate at the C-terminal region. Adapted from (a) McKernan and Whiting (1996); (b) Kaupmann et al. (1998); Kuner et al. (1990).

Table 1 Distribution of the major GABAA receptor subtypes in the rat brain[a]

GABA$_A$ receptor subtype	Relative abundance (%)	Location and putative function
$\alpha_1 \beta_2 \gamma_2$	43	Most brain areas Interneurons in hippocampus and cortex Cerebral Purkinje cells
$\alpha_2 \beta_{2/3} \gamma_2$	18	Spinal cord motoneurons Hippocampal pyramidal cells
$\alpha_3 \beta_n \gamma_2/\gamma_3$	17	Cholinergic and monoaminergic neurons
$\alpha_2 \beta_n \gamma_1$	8	Bergmann glia Nuclei of the limbic system
$\alpha_5 \beta_3 \gamma_2/\gamma_3$	4	Predominantly hippocampal pyramidal cells
$\alpha_6 \beta \gamma_2$	2	Cerebellar granule cells
$\alpha_6 \beta \delta$	2	Cerebellar granule cells
$\alpha_4 \beta \delta$	3	Thalamus and hippocampus dentate gyrus
Other minor subtypes	3	Present throughout the brain

[a]Adapted from McKernan and Whiting (1996).

Synaptogenesis starts about 2 weeks after birth. The receptors cluster at the postsynaptic density and are exposed to a high concentration of GABA released from the presynaptic vesicles (see Box 3). These receptors predominantly contain the α_1 subunit, which has a relatively low affinity for GABA and is less susceptible to activation by extrasynaptic GABA. Meanwhile, an outwardly directed Cl$^-$ transporter reduces the intracellular Cl$^-$ concentration, and Cl$^-$ becomes negative with respect to the resting membrane potential. The activation of the synaptic GABA$_A$ receptors then produces the familiar inhibitory response.

Another example of the exploitation of receptor diversity is that α_1 subunits are expressed throughout the somatodendritic axis of hippocampal CA1 pyramidal neurons, whereas α_2 subunits are expressed on the initial segment of the axon (**Table 1**), where the output signal is generated (see Box 2).

Modulatory sites associated with GABA$_A$ receptors

The receptors for a number of therapeutically important drugs are associated with the GABA$_A$ receptor complex. Separate and distinct receptors have been identified for benzodiazepines, barbiturates, and steroids, whereas alcohol and some general anesthetics also act through the GABA$_A$ system (**Figure 1**). The binding of ligands to these receptors does not generally operate the GABA$_A$ ionophore directly. Rather, these act as modulatory sites that are allosterically coupled to GABA$_A$ receptors. The occupation of a modulatory receptor increases the affinity of the GABA$_A$ receptor and thereby increases the probability that the ionophore will open in response to GABA. Synaptic inhibition is prolonged, which depresses activity in neuronal networks. The therapeutic and behavioral effects of actions at modulatory sites are (in ascending order): anxiolytic → sedative → hypnotic → anesthetic.

Benzodiazepines The action of benzodiazepines shows subunit specificity. The minimum requirement for benzodiazepine sensitivity is an α subunit selected from α_1, α_2, α_3, or α_5, together with either a γ_2 or γ_3 subunit. The benzodiazepine receptor itself is probably located at the interface between the α and γ subunits. Benzodiazepines have no actions at receptors containing α_4, α_6, or γ_1 subunits, whereas the identity of the β subunit seems to have little influence on the effect of benzodiazepines.

The benzodiazepine receptor possesses the unique feature that the identity of the ligand determines whether it will interact positively or negatively with the GABA$_A$ receptor. Agonists at the benzodiazepine receptor (such as diazepam and flunitrazepam) increase the likelihood that the ionophore will open in response to GABA and have therapeutic profiles as anxiolytic, anticonvulsant, sedative, and hypnotic. On the other hand, inverse agonists such as the β-carbolines, β-CCM, and DMCM decrease the probability of channel opening, and their behavioral profile is correspondingly proconflict and proconvulsant. Benzodiazepine receptor antagonists block the actions of both agonists and inverse agonists.

In accordance with the intense efforts devoted to this therapeutically important locus, at least seven chemical classes of substances have been identified that interact with the benzodiazepine receptor. Investigations with representatives of these have shown further discrete subunit-dependent actions and have helped identify two main subtypes of benzodiazepine receptor. BZ$_1$ receptors have a high affinity for diazepam and β-CCM. They are characterized by containing an α_1 subunit and are widely expressed in the CNS (particularly the cerebellum). BZ$_2$ receptors have a high affinity for diazepam but a low affinity for β-CCM. BZ$_2$ receptors contain α_2, α_3, or α_5 subunits and are mainly expressed in a complementary pattern

Box 2
Why GABA Is an Inhibitory Transmitter

In order to understand why and how GABA acts as an inhibitory transmitter, it is necessary to consider the electrochemical basis of nenronal activity, which is illustrated in the accompanying diagrams.

(a) There is a potential difference across the membrane of the resting neuron, with the inside being approximately −70 mV with respect to the outside. This potential arises because of the asymmetrical distribution of the major monovalent ions (Na$^+$, K$^+$, and Cl$^-$) across the membrane. The diagram shows representative ionophores for these ions, along with their relative concentrations on both sides of the membrane. The resting membrane is relatively permeable to K$^+$ and Cl$^-$, but it is impermeable to Na$^+$ (indicated by the relative sizes of the channels through the ionophores). Each ionic species is under the influence of two gradients: a chemical gradient (**c**) favoring movement from high to low concentration and an electrical gradient (**e**) favoring movement toward the opposite polarity. The net driving force on a particular ion is given

by the sum (e.g., for Na$^+$) or difference (e.g., for K$^+$ and Cl$^-$) of these two gradients. In order to compare these gradients directly, the Nernst equation is used to convert the concentration gradient to an equivalent electrical gradient, the values of which are given on the arrows representing the chemical gradient and on horizontal lines in part (b). When the potential gradient exactly counterbalances the concentration gradient, equilibrium pertains and no net ionic movement occurs.

(b) A diagram of potential levels showing resting membrane potential (RMP), the equilibrium potentials for the ions (E_{Na^+}, E_{K^+}, E_{Cl^-}), and the threshold for action potential generation (E_{Thresh}). Zero potential is also shown for reference. A selective increase in membrane permeability to one of the ions causes it to move down its electrochemical gradient (ecg), and the membrane potential moves toward the equilibrium potential for that particular ion. Such a change in permeability can arise because the nerve cell membrane contains a multitude of

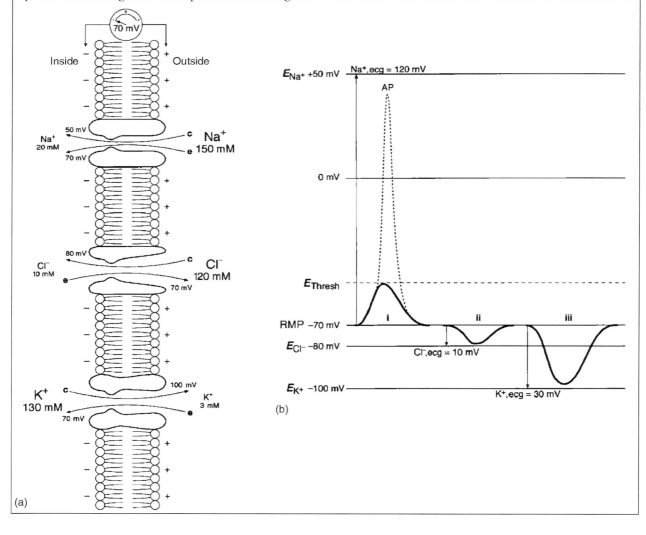

Box 2
Continued

different ion-selective channels that can be activated (gated) by changes in the transmembrane potential or by the binding of ligands and transmitters as to specific receptors (e.g., GABA). A selective increase in Na permeability (**i**) results in a depolarization and, if E_{Thresh} is reached, evokes a regenerative action potential (AP, stippled line). The AP is a positive-going potential of approximately 100 mV lasting for 1–3 ms and is the output signal of the neuron. Factors that move the membrane potential toward E_{Thresh} increase the likelihood of neuronal firing and are therefore termed excitatory. Conversely, increasing the membrane potential (hyperpolarization) makes it less likely that the neuron will fire an AP, and these influences are therefore inhibitory. GABA is an inhibitory transmitter because it acts on GABA$_A$ and GABA$_B$ receptors to cause a selective increase in permeability to Cl$^-$ ions (**ii**) and K$^+$ ions (**iii**). Because both E_{Cl-} and E_{K+} are more negative than the resting membrane potential, action at both receptors causes a hyperpolarization, which inhibits the neuron. This hyperpolarization is, however, not the only reason why the neuron is inhibited.

(c) It is also necessary to consider the spatial interactions between excitatory and inhibitory synapses. A typical nerve cell consists of a cell body (soma)

from which a more or less extensive dendritic tree arises. This acts as the receiving and integrating area for excitatory and inhibitory synaptic contacts. The axon also arises from the soma and conducts the APs to the terminals where it causes transmitter release. The initial segment of the axon (or axon hillock) has the highest density of voltage-gated Na$^+$ channels and therefore the lowest threshold for AP generation. As to whether this threshold is reached depends on the ongoing integration of synaptic activity on the somatic and dendritic membranes. (1) A representative excitatory synapse is selectively activated. These synapses use glutamate as a transmitter, which gates ionophores that are selectively permeable to Na$^+$. Positive current flows into the postsynaptic membrane at the synapse. Because the bilipid membrane has a high resistance, this current can flow relatively long distances within the neuron before exiting through the membrane and returning to the active synapse to complete the current loop. This spread of current allows the possibility of both spatial and temporal summation with activity at other synapses. For example, if a sufficient number of excitatory synapses are activated, the initial segment is depolarized to firing level and an AP arises. (2) Inhibitory GABA$_A$ synapses are

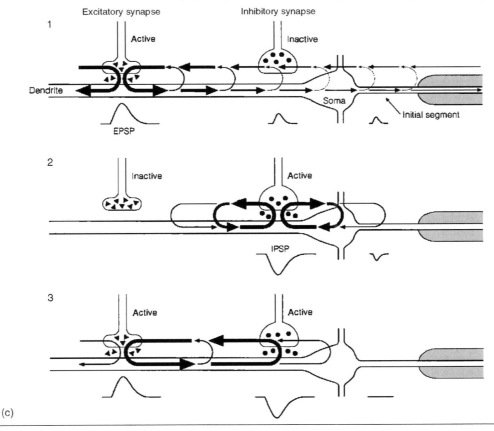

(c)

Box 2
Continued

usually located close to the soma, where they can exert a correspondingly greater influence on the initial segment. The selective activation of the inhibitory synapses causes Cl^- ions to move through the ionophore (which is equivalent to an outward movement of positive current, as shown by the direction of the arrowhead), which results in an IPSP. (3) When excitatory and inhibitory synapses are activated simultaneously, the $GABA_A$ ionophores provide a low-resistance pathway through which the excitatory current will pass. This means that much less depolarizing current reaches the initial segment and the output of the neuron is inhibited. Thus, $GABA_A$ synapses inhibit the neuron both by causing a hyperpolarization and by shunting excitatory synaptic activity.

---

to BZ_1 receptors (i.e., where the concentration of α_1 is low). Note that the aforementioned changes in receptor composition during development actually represented a shift from BZ_2 to BZ_1 receptors.

Barbiturates and steroids The $GABA_A$ receptor is also modulated by barbiturates and certain metabolites of gonadal and adrenal hormones (such as progesterone and deoxycorticosterone, respectively). When synthesized in the brain, these metabolites are termed neurosteroids (to distinguish them from neuroactive steroids, which may be synthesized elsewhere) and are therefore an endogenous ligand for a modulatory site associated with the $GABA_A$ receptor. Steroids were originally thought to interact with the barbiturate receptor until the separate identity of the two receptors was established.

The actions of barbiturates and steroids have much more in common with one another than they do with benzodiazepines. Barbiturates and steroids potentiate responses to GABA by prolonging the duration of channel open time, which contrasts to the increase in frequency of channel openings produced by benzodiazepine agonists. Furthermore, at concentrations greater than are required for the modulatory effect on $GABA_A$ receptors, both barbiturates and steroids can gate the ionophore directly by an action that does not involve the $GABA_A$ receptor itself. Such direct gating is never seen with benzodiazepines. Antagonists of the steroid receptor have been characterized (e.g., dehydroepiandrosterone), but so far no antagonists of the barbiturate receptor have been identified.

The actions of barbiturates and steroids do not show absolute subunit dependency, although their effects may be influenced more subtly by the actual composition of the receptor. The therapeutic and behavioral actions of barbiturates and steroids are generally much more pronounced than benzodiazepines. The former tend to cause heavy sedation and anesthesia, whereas benzodiazepines generally have milder effects. The lack of subunit specificity means barbiturates and steroids are likely to enhance $GABA_A$ergic actions more globally and indiscriminately. For example, the $GABA_A$ receptors expressed in the thalamus do not contain γ subunits (**Table 1**) and are not, therefore, responsive to benzodiazepines. The responses are, however, enhanced by barbiturates and steroids.

Other agents that modulate activity of the $GABA_A$ receptor In addition to the barbiturate anesthetics, a wide range of other anesthetics appear to potentiate responses mediated by $GABA_A$ receptors. These include the inhalation anesthetics halothane, isoflurane, and diethylether and the intravenous anesthetics propofol and etomidate. Augmentation of $GABA_A$ergic transmission is likely to make a marked contribution to the anesthetic action of these substances.

$GABA_A$ergic transmission is also modulated by ethanol. Interestingly, the effect of ethanol seems to be mediated by phosphorylation of the γ_{2L} subunit.

Side effects of agents that act at the $GABA_A$ receptor Familiar problems are associated with long-term therapeutic treatments with many agents that act at the $GABA_A$ modulatory sites. Prolonged use of benzodiazepines, barbiturates, and ethanol all cause tolerance, which is followed by dependence and addiction. There are also manifestly unpleasant symptoms on withdrawal of treatment. The increasing knowledge of the structure and function of the $GABA_A$ receptor subtypes has intensified efforts to develop drugs that act at specific subunits (or combinations thereof). These would have a narrower clinical profile with fewer side effects and could be used for conditions such as anxiety, epilepsy, and insomnia.

GABA_B Receptors

The $GABA_B$ receptor is formed by a single protein containing seven hydrophobic transmembrane domains and a large N-terminal extracellular domain that forms the receptor for GABA (**Figure 1**). This structure is characteristic of metabotropic receptors, which are not coupled directly to an ionophore but exert their

Box 3
Synaptic Transmission at a GABA_A Synapse

GABA fulfills the following criteria required for a neurotransmitter: it is present in the nerve terminal, it is released upon nerve stimulation, it activates specific receptors on the postsynaptic membrane, a specific uptake mechanism is available to remove it from the extracellular fluid, and its direct application to neurons mimics the effect of nerve stimulation. These aspects are illustrated in the accompanying diagram, which depicts the sequential steps (a–j) in synaptic transmission at a GABA_Aergic synapse.

The GABA_A synapse contains pre- and postsynaptic specializations at the area called the active zone. Four active zones are illustrated, each represented by a single presynaptic vesicle opposed by a single receptor complex in the postsynaptic membrane. The synaptic cleft is approximately 100 nm wide. (a.) Vesicles filled with GABA are docked at the presynaptic specialization in close proximity to a

voltage-sensitive Ca^{2+}-selective channel. (b.) On arrival of an action potential at the nerve terminal, the Ca^{2+}-selective channel opens transiently. (c.) Ca^{2+} ions pass into the terminal and bind to four Ca^{2+} sensors associated with the vesicle. This causes excytotosis of the vesicle and GABA is expelled into the synaptic cleft, where it quickly reaches a peak concentration of approximately 500 μM. The empty vesicle leaves the membrane and is recycled. (d.) The binding of two molecules of GABA to each receptor complex causes the subunits to tilt slightly. This opens the ionophores and allows Cl^- ions to flow across the postsynaptic membrane. (e.) Recordings from single-receptor complexes using the patch–clamp technique have shown that the ionophore flickers between open and shut states in the presence of GABA. Current flowing through the whole ensemble of 20–30 ionophores clustered together at the active zone creates a smooth, but transient, potential

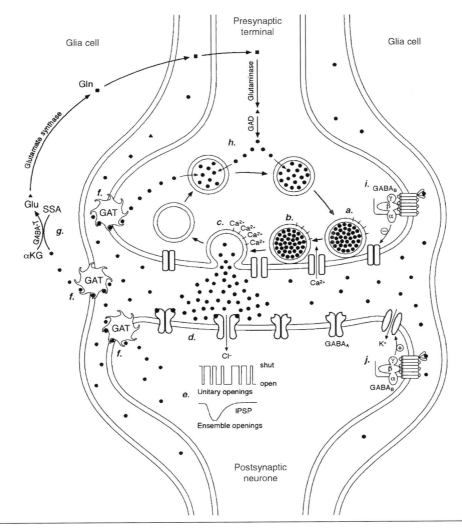

Box 3
Continued

change across the postsynaptic membrane. This is termed the inhibitory postsynaptic potential (IPSP), and lasts approximately 50 ms. The reasons why the IPSP depresses neuronal activity are given in Box 2. Although 90% of the GABA released from the vesicle has diffused away from the active zone within 0.5 ms, some molecules still remain bound to the receptor complexes. However, these ionophores close of their own accord. This process is known as desensitization, and it is thought to protect the $GABA_A$ receptors from overactivation. (*f.*) Synaptically released GABA is ultimately removed from the extracellular fluid by uptake transporters (GAT) located on both neurons and the supportive glia cells. (*g.*) The enzyme GABA-transaminase (GABA-T) catalyzes the conversion of GABA and α-ketoglutarate (KG; derived from glucose metabolism) to succinic semialdehyde (SSA) and glutamate (Glu). Glutamate, which cannot cross the extracellular space because it is neuroactive, is then converted to glutamine (Gln) by the enzyme glutamate synthase. Glutamine diffuses across the membranes and into the presynaptic terminal, where it is reconverted to glutamate by glutaminase, which in turn is converted to GABA by glutamic acid decarboxylase (GAD). (*h.*) Specific transporters fill the recycling vesicles with GABA, where it is stored at a concentration of approximately 100 mM. These dock with the presynaptic membrane at the active zone, thereby completing the cycle. (*i.*) $GABA_B$ autoreceptors located on the presynaptic terminal are activated by GABA present in the extracellular space. These are negatively coupled to the Ca^{2+} channels by G-proteins. The depression of Ca^{2+} entry through these channels decreases vesicle release in response to subsequent activation. (*j.*) Postsynaptic $GABA_B$ receptors are positively couples by G-proteins to K^+-selective channels. This mediates a slow IPSP, thereby inhibiting the postsynaptic neuron.

---

actions via second messengers that alter the activity of intracellular enzymes and other mechanisms.

Two splice variants of the $GABA_B$ receptor, $GABA_BR1a$ and $GABA_BR1b$, were originally cloned and tested for their ability to mimic the effects of native $GABA_B$ receptors. Although they showed a similar sensitivity to antagonists, their affinity for GABA was approximately 100 times less than the native receptors. Moreover, when expressed in mammalian cells, they showed poor translocation to the membrane and coupled only weakly to the effector mechanisms. The reasons for these anomalies have recently been resolved with the cloning and characterization of a second $GABA_B$ receptor, $GABA_BR2$. This has 35% sequence homology with the $GABA_BR1$ receptor and has a similar structure. The two receptors associate together at the C-terminus. This is expressed in the cell membrane as a functional dimer, where it displays the characteristics of the native $GABA_B$ receptor. The binding of GABA to this dimer causes the activation of GTP-binding proteins (G-proteins) on the inside of the membrane. Depending on the identity of the G-protein, this stimulates or inhibits effector enzymes (e.g., adenyl cyclase and phospholipase C) and proteins (e.g., ionophores), which mediate the cellular response. The binding of a single molecule of GABA to the $GABA_B$ receptor activates many molecules of G-protein, thereby amplifying the response greatly. However, due to the number of intermediate steps involved, G-protein-mediated transduction is characterized by a relatively long latency (around 40 ms), followed by a time course of action lasting a second or more.

$GABA_B$ receptors mediate two location-specific effects. On postsynaptic dendritic membranes, the G-proteins are positively coupled to a K^+ selective ionophore. Because E_{K^+} is negative to the resting membrane potential (see Box 2), the activation of these channels gives rise to a relatively large inhibitory postsynaptic potential (IPSP), which lasts for 1–2 s. $GABA_B$ receptors are also located on presynaptic terminals where they are negatively coupled to the voltage-dependent Ca^{2+} channels. The reduction of Ca^{2+} flux through these channels reduces the probability that a vesicle will be released in response to an action potential (AP) and thereby decreases synaptic transmission. These $GABA_B$ receptors are located on the presynaptic terminals of a variety of neurons that use a range of transmitters. In the special case in which they are located on the terminals of GABAergic neurons themselves, they are termed autoreceptors. During repetitive activity, these autoreceptors serve to decrease the synaptic release of GABA, which will promote the expression of postsynaptic excitatory responses from other sources.

Although pre- and postsynaptic $GABA_B$ receptors apparently show differences in their sensitivity to agonists and antagonists, it is presently unresolved as to whether these represent pharmacologically distinct receptors. Furthermore, it is not certain to what extent $GABA_B$ receptors are located within the postsynaptic density (see Box 1). They are certainly expressed at extrasynaptic sites, where they respond to ambient levels of GABA in the extracellular fluid (which partly arises as spillover from nearby GABA$_A$ synapses). This notion that GABA$_B$ receptors play more of a neuromodulatory role rather than a direct-transmitter role is supported by the fact that relatively strong stimulation of GABAergic neurons is required to activate pre- and postsynaptic GABA$_B$ receptors.

GABA$_B$ receptors show high concentrations in certain regions of the CNS, including the cerebellum, thalamus, and spinal cord. Although this pattern is distinct from that of GABA$_A$ receptors, there are many regions where the two receptors overlap. It is likely that the majority of single neurons express both GABA$_A$ and GABA$_B$ receptors.

Effects mediated by GABA$_B$ receptors have been implicated in the neuronal processes associated with memory (long-term potentiation), slow-wave sleep, muscle relaxation, and antinociception. The GABA$_B$ agonist, baclofen, has long been in clinical use as an antispastic agent and also shows promise in the treatment of chronic pain and withdrawal symptoms from cocaine. GABA$_B$ receptor antagonists do not presently have clinical applications, but have been shown to be effective in animal models of absence epilepsy and cognitive impairment.

GABA$_C$ Receptors

GABA$_C$ receptors are formed from homo- or heteromeric assemblies of ρ_1 or ρ_2 subunits and are structurally and functionally similar to GABA$_A$ receptors. Although ρ subunits are probably the ancestral form of the GABA$_A$ subunits, they do not apparently assemble together with other subgroups. GABA$_C$ receptors are characterized by their lack of sensitivity to bicuculline and high sensitivity to GABA (Box 3). The GABA$_C$-operated ionophores have a substantially lower conductance than the GABA$_A$ ionophores (probably because its diameter is slightly smaller), and they do not desensitize in the maintained presence of GABA. Finally, GABA$_C$ receptors lack the modulatory sites associated with the GABA$_A$ receptor. Functional GABA$_C$ receptors have so far been demonstrated only in the retina. However, ρ subunits occur at many other sites in the CNS (e.g., the cerebellum), and mRNA for ρ_2 is present throughout the brain.

GABAergic Neurons and Their Role in Neuronal Activity

Because the only known function of GABA is to act as an inhibitory neurotransmitter, GABAergic neurons may be identified by histochemical demonstration of the synthesizing enzyme, glutamic acid decarboxylase (GAD). The majority of GABAergic neurons are interspersed between the principal neurons of a given anatomical structure; then they are termed interneurons. However, they can also have long axons that project to other regions in the CNS. Although sharing the same transmitter, GABAergic neurons otherwise exhibit a wide range of morphological, histochemical, and functional characteristics. For example, at least a dozen distinct types of GABAergic neurons can be identified in the cerebral cortex.

Some of these have very narrow axonal fields confined to a cortical column, whereas others have extremely extensive axonal arborizations that can extend over large distances. GABAergic neurons themselves are under the control of other synaptic influences: they are excited by glutamatergic synaptic inputs and inhibited by other GABAergic neurons. The nature and degree of synaptic inhibition they produce on the neurons with which they form synaptic contacts depends on

1. Their intrinsic membrane properties and firing patterns. Many GABAergic neurons are able to fire APs at relatively high frequencies with little accommodation. This maximizes GABA release at the terminals (which in turn may be under the feedback control exerted by autoreceptors).
2. The number and location of the synaptic contacts on the postsynaptic membrane. Such contacts do not occur randomly but are placed in a strict topographical order on the postsynaptic membrane.
3. The identity of the postsynaptic receptors (e.g., GABA$_A$ or GABA$_B$ receptors and their possible subtypes).

By controlling the excitability of the postsynaptic neuron, GABAergic neurons participate in the regulation of network activity. Expressed in its simplest form, GABAergic inhibition curtails the activity of principal neurons in response to an excitatory synaptic input (feed-forward inhibition) and after an output signal has been generated (feedback inhibition) (**Figure 2**). These inhibitory influences act as a brake on the principal neuron, which could otherwise enter an unstable oscillatory state in which relatively modest excitation can result in an explosive response. Indeed, pharmacological blockade of GABAergic inhibition is often used in experimental situations to evoke activity that is reminiscent of epileptic discharges. It is becoming increasingly evident that GABAergic inhibition cannot be regarded simply as a counterweight to intrinsic and synaptic excitatory processes. GABAergic synapses participate in the spatiotemporal integration of activity in neuronal networks and thereby play a major role in the processing of information. GABAergic neurons are

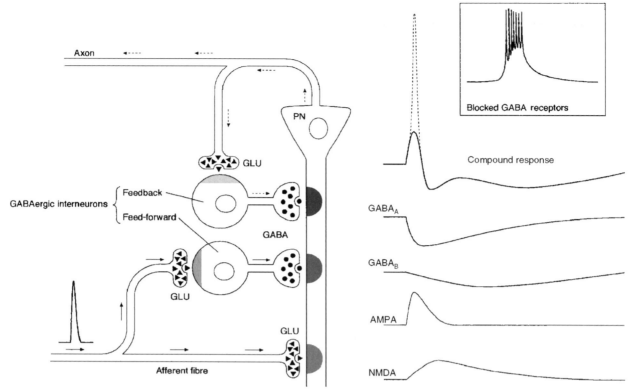

Figure 2 The role of GABA receptors in determining network excitability. The diagram shows how GABAergic inhibition controls the activity of principal neurons (PN). Only single synapses of each type are shown for clarity. Stimulation of the afferent input pathway (bottom left) evokes an action potential, which spreads in the nerve fiber (arrows). This ultimately results in a compound synaptic response in the PN (shown on the right), the components of which arise as follows. The initial response is a rapid depolarization by an excitatory postsynaptic potential (EPSP), which is mediated by two different types of excitatory receptors for glutamate (AMPA and NMDA). If sufficient excitatory synapses are activated, the threshold for the generation of an action potential (stippled line) may be reached. Meanwhile, collateral fibers also activate GABAergic interneurons. These release GABA on to the principal neuron after a short delay (feed-forward inhibition). The GABA activates both GABA$_A$ and GABA$_B$ receptors, which activate Cl$^-$- and K$^+$-selective ionophores, respectively. Both actions hyperpolarize the neuron, thereby ensuring that the membrane potential returns toward the resting level and prevents the overexcitation of the PN. If the PN fires an action potential (AP), this is transmitted down its axon (stippled arrows). Axon collaterals excite GABAergic interneurons, which feed back on to the PN and inhibit it (feedback inhibition). The insert shows the response to a single afferent stimulation following pharmacological blockade of the GABA receptors. The synaptic excitation is no longer curtailed and also recruits voltage-dependent ionic conductances in the membrane. This gives rise to a large depolarization surmounted by a number of action potentials, which is reminiscent of epileptic activity.

particularly prevalent in the cerebral cortex, where they serve to synchronize the firing of cortical pyramidal neurons into columnary activity.

See Also the Following Articles

Anxiolytics; Hippocampal Neurons.

Further Reading

Biggio, G., Sanna, E. and Costa, E. (eds.) (1995). *GABA$_A$ receptors and anxiety: from neurobiology to treatment.* New York: Rover.

Costa, E. (1998). From GABA$_A$ receptor diversity emerges a unified vision of GABAergic inhibition. *Annual Review of Pharmacology and Toxicology* 38, 321–350.

Johnston, G. A. R. (1996). GABA$_C$ receptors: relatively simple transmitter-gated ion channels. *Trends in Pharmacological Science* 17, 319–323.

Kaupmann, et al. (1998). *Proceedings of the National Academy of Sciences* 95, 14991–14966.

Kuner, et al. (1990). *Science* 283, 74–77.

McKernan, R. M. and Whiting, P. J. (1996). Which GABA$_A$-receptor subtypes really occur in the brain? *Trends in Neuroscience* 19, 139–143.

Miller, R. J. (1998). Presynaptic receptors. *Annual Review of Pharmacology and Toxicology* 38, 201–227.

Sieghan, VIT. (1995). Structure and pharmacology of gamma-aminobutyric acid$_A$ receptor subtypes. *Pharmacological Reviews* 47, 181–234.

Smith, G. B. and Olsen, R. W. (1995). Functional domains of GABA$_A$ receptors. *Trends in Pharmacological Science* 16, 162–168.

Gastrointestinal Effects

R Murison and A M Milde
University of Bergen, Bergen, Norway

This article is a revision of the previous edition
article by R Murison, volume 2, pp 191–195,
© 2000, Elsevier Inc.

Brain–Gut Interactions
Gastrointestinal Disorders and the Influence of Stress
Conclusion

Glossary

Amygdala	A walnut-shaped brain structure that plays a key role in fear.
Atropine	An anticholinergic drug.
Bombesin	A peptide important in various activities both in brain and other organs.
Brain-derived neurotrophic factor (BDNF)	A protein important for maintaining function in various brain areas.
Cholecysto-kinin (CCK)	A hormone produced by the mucosa of the upper intestine that stimulates contraction of the gallbladder.
Cholinergic	Liberating, activated by, or resembling the physiologic action of acetylcholine.
Functional dyspepsia	A nonorganic disorder typified by stomach discomfort and pains that can not be explained by organic changes.
Gastrin	A polypeptide hormone secreted by the pyloric mucosa that stimulates the pancreas to release pancreatic fluid and the stomach to release gastric acid.
Helicobacter pylori	A family of gram-negative bacteria whose members are spiral shaped, showing corkscrewlike motility; they are found in the vast majority of patients with peptic ulcer.
Hippocampus	A ridge that extends over the floor of the descending horn of each lateral ventricle of the brain.
Histamine	An amine derivative of histidine that is widely distributed in human tissues.
Hypophysec-tomy	Surgical removal of the pituitary gland.
Inflammatory bowel disease (IBD)	A group of organic disorders of the bowel, including ulcerative colitis and Crohn's disease.
Interferon	A protein that is produced by intact animal cells when they are infected with viruses; it acts to inhibit viral reproduction and to induce resistance in host cells.
Interleukins	Any of a class of proteins that are secreted mostly by macrophages and T lymphocytes and induce growth and differentiation of lymphocytes and hematopoietic stem cells.
Irritable bowel syndrome (IBS)	A functional (nonorganic) disorder characterized by discomfort and pain in the bowel.
Ischemia	Localized anemia as a result of obstruction of the blood supply or to vasoconstriction.
Neuro-peptide Y	A polypeptide released by axons at the synapse; it may act as a neurotransmitter and have a direct effect on synapse function or as a neuromodulator, having a long-term effect on postsynaptic neurons.
Neuroticism	A neurotic condition, character, or trait.
Nonsteroidal anti-inflamma-tory drugs (NSAIDs)	Drugs that are widely used for the treatment of inflammatory disorders (such as rheumatoid arthritis) and other painful conditions.
Nonulcer dyspepsia (NUD)	Functional dyspepsia.
Oxytocin	A polypeptide hormone secreted by the neurohypophysis that stimulates contraction of the uterine muscles.
Peptic ulcer	An ulcer involving the mucosa, submucosa, and muscular layers of the stomach or duodenum, due in part at least to the action of gastric acid–pepsin juice.
Rapid eye movement (REM) sleep	The part of the sleep cycle during which the eyes move rapidly, accompanied by a loss of muscle tone and a low-amplitude encephalogram recording.
Sacral nerves	Any of five pairs of spinal nerves in the sacral region that innervate the muscles and skin of the lower back, lower extremities, and perineum and branch to the hypogastric and pelvic plexuses.
Serotonin	A compound derived from tryptophan that functions as a local vasoconstrictor, plays a role in neurotransmission, and has pharmacological properties.
Sigmoid colon	The S-shaped portion of the colon between the descending colon and the rectum.
Somatostatin	A peptide secreted by the hypothalamus that acts primarily to inhibit the release of growth hormone from the anterior pituitary.
Vagotomy	An operative procedure involving cutting of the vagus nerve, previously used in treatment for ulcers.

Vagus nerve   The tenth cranial nerve, forming an important part of the parasympathetic system and carrying information in both directions between the brain and the periphery.

The functions of the gut encompass ingestion, digestion, absorption, and transport of ingested materials through the gastrointestinal (GI) tract. Digestive processes rely on the presence of acid and enzymes to break down the nutrients into individual molecules that can be absorbed across the intestinal lining for passage into the bloodstream. At the same time, the mechanical and chemical means to digest food particles also represent potential threats (aggressive factors) to the integrity of the gut mucosa. If the stomach lining secretes more hydrochloric acid than needed, it has the potential of irritating the duodenal and gastric lining, thus enhancing their sensitivity. Other aggressive factors include nonbeneficial bacteria (in particular *Helicobacter pylori* in humans) and our tendency to self-treatment with NSAIDs. Such a self-digesting potential is prevented by protective factors: (1) the secretion of protective mucus from various mucus glands throughout the GI tract, (2) the secretion of bicarbonate in saliva to remove hydrogen ions, and (3) a high rate of cell regeneration. Endogenous prostaglandins are important for the proper function of these protective factors, as is also an adequate mucosal blood flow. Various stressors are able to modulate all of these functions. Because many effects appear to be stressor-specific and indeed species-specific, several generalizations must be made in what follows.

Brain–Gut Interactions

For stress to impact the GI system, pathways must be in place to permit a bidirectional communication between the central nervous system (CNS) and the gut. Such mechanisms include both nerve pathways and the endocrine system. Among the former are parasympathetic vagal connections terminating in the enteric nervous system, which comprises two plexuses, or networks of neurons, embedded in the wall of the GI tract; the outermost collection of neurons, called the myenteric (or Auerbach's) plexus; and the innermost group of neurons, called the submucosal (or Meissner's) plexus. Included in the latter are the sympathetic innervations via the spinal cord. Among the hormonal influences are epinephrine, adrenocorticotropic hormone (ACTH), cortisol, and thyrotropin-releasing hormone (TRH). In addition, several immune-system substances (as interferon and interleukins) are now known to impinge on the GI tract.

Secretions

Gastric acid secretion is regulated by an interplay of several neural (cholinergic), hormonal (gastrin), and paracrine (histamine and somatostatin) mechanisms, where histamine is a potent inducer of acid secretion. TRH acts in the brain to stimulate gastric acid, pepsin, and serotonin secretion. TRH is also involved in mechanisms regulating mucosal blood flow, contractility, emptying, and activation of the parasympathetic outflow to the stomach, which may produce gastric ulcerations. Both vagotomy and atropine block this effect. It would appear that the main sites of TRH action in the brain for these effects lie in the dorsal vagal complex, nucleus tractus solitarius, nucleus ambiguous, and the dorsal motor nucleus of the vagus, which receive direct input from the amygdala and indirect input from the ventral hippocampus. Other centrally acting peptides shown to increase gastric secretion include CCK, gastrin, and oxytocin, whereas somatostatin inhibits the secretion of gastrin and histamine and appears to have a direct inhibitory effect on parietal cells.

Centrally acting corticotropin-releasing hormone (CRH), on the other hand, stimulates sympathetic activity while inhibiting parasympathetic activity. Injected into the paraventricular nucleus, CRH reduces acid secretion while increasing bicarbonate secretion. These central effects of CRH are independent of the hypothalamic–adrenocortical axis and vagal activity, but are prevented by adrenalectomy and noradrenergic blocking agents, suggesting that they are mediated by sympathetic outflow. CRH also inhibits the development of stress-induced gastric ulcerations. Apart from somatostatin, other peptides and proteins shown to inhibit gastric acid secretion include bombesin, neuropeptide Y, interleukin-1, platelet activating factor, and the opioid peptides.

Paradoxically, therefore, the immediate effect of central neuroendocrine stress-related peptides appears to be an inhibition of gastric acid secretion. Although the renowned Stewart Wolf and Harold Wolff studies from 1947 on the fistulated patient Tom suggested gastric hypersecretion in response to anxiety, resentment, and hostility, they also noted a transitory hyposecretion during situations associated with overwhelming despair and dejection. Results from animal studies indicate that acute stress is associated with a hyposecretion of acid followed by a hypersecretion (a rebound effect).

Mucus production is also inhibited by stress. The underlying mechanism for this effect appears to be related to the capacity of adrenal steroids to block the prostaglandin synthesis necessary for mucus production within the mucous epithelial cells, as well as modulating both gastric vasodilatation necessary for adequate circulation and hydrogen ion (H^+) release from the parietal cells. Of the other protective factors, CRH and stress promote bicarbonate secretion but reduce blood flow, leaving the mucosa at risk for focal ischemia. Conversely, Filaretova et al. suggest that corticosteroids may act to maintain gastric blood flow during stress.

The overall picture therefore suggests an acute response to stress of closing down the upper GI system to allow redistribution of energy resources to the organs involved in fight-or-flight behavior. Both human and animal data, however, point to the possibility of local rebound processes in the wake of this acute response. Because the various response systems (e.g., acid secretion, mucus secretion, and blood vessel constriction) do not necessarily follow the exact same time course, a rebound-related increase in acid secretion without the simultaneous reinstatement of adequate blood supply and mucus secretion represents a potential danger to the mucosal integrity.

Gastrointestinal Motility

GI motility is controlled by the reflex receptive relaxation mediated by vagal inhibitory fibers and endocrine influences. Perceived emotional stressors such as fear generally result in acute decreases in gastric motility and gastric emptying, evoked dysrhythmic gastric myoelectrical activity, and increases in colonic activity. These effects are mimicked by CRH and blocked by its antagonists. Pathways for these effects are believed to include higher brain functions that provide descending information to the gut via vagal and sacral nerve pathways rather than via the hypothalamo-adrenocortical axis. Motility is under the influence of several transmitters, most attention being focused on serotonin. Selective serotonin reuptake inhibitors (SSRIs) have proven effective in treatment of motility disorders.

Stomach The majority of mammalian animal studies (rats, mice, dogs, and guinea pigs) indicate that acute stress of various types (shock, avoidance, noise, and handling) leads to a delay in gastric emptying associated with reduced contractile activity or a series of slow contractions outlasting the stress period. It is important to take into account the nutrient content and nature of the meal (acoustic stress delays emptying but only with nutritive meals bulk) and the time course of events (cold increases gastric motility in rats, but this is followed by a decrease). The effects of stress in rat stomach are mimicked by the central application of CRH, which can be blocked by both vagotomy and norepinephrine antagonist drugs.

Early human studies suggested both increases and decreases in gastric motility in response to anger and resentment. Later studies have more consistently shown reduced motility in response to a number of stressors (cold pain, painful transcutaneous stimulation, and noise).

Small intestine The stomach connects the esophagus to the small intestine, and the majority of food digestion takes place here. Stress may alter normal transit time, the gut contents taking longer to travel from the small to the large intestine, and more liquid may be extracted, forming the basis for constipation. This is a potent symptom of the constipated predominant IBS, a functional, nonorganic, pathological bowel disorder.

Large intestine The large intestine is divided into the cecum, colon, and rectum, the cecum making up the first 2 or 3 in. of the large intestine. The colon is subdivided into the ascending, transverse, descending, and sigmoid colon. The last portion of the large intestine is the rectum, which extends from the sigmoid colon to the anus (approximately 6 in.). The nerve supply to the large intestine contains both sympathetic and parasympathetic nerves; sympathetic stimulation inhibits activity and parasympathetic stimulation causes an increase in defecation reflexes. The colon contains the majority of microorganisms in the intestines; these microorganisms weigh more than 1 kg and consist of both friendly and unfriendly bacteria.

Animal studies are fairly consistent in showing increases of colonic motility and colonic transport in response to acute stress or central CRH. The effects of CRH are abolished by noradrenergic blockers but not by adrenalectomy or hypophysectomy. Exposure of rats to psychological stress (as in water-avoidance stress) induces abnormal colonic motility (increased fecal pellet output), enhanced colorectal sensitivity (induced distention), and increased colonic permeability (e.g., urine secretion of 51-chromium ethylenediaminetetraacetic acid).

Gastrointestinal Disorders and the Influence of Stress

Background

The majority of studies have focused on the immediate effects of acute stress on GI function. Clearly, chronic effects of acute stress or effects of chronic stress on GI structure and function will have consequences for illness and disease states.

For decades there has been a clear dissociation in the literature between the functional and organic GI disorders. The former include functional dyspepsia (FD), (NUD), IBS, and constipation. Organic disorders include peptic ulcer, IBD, cancers, and acute stress ulcer. Traditionally, stress (psychosomatic factors) has been implicated in a number of GI disorders, including gastric and duodenal (peptic) ulcer, gastroesophageal reflux (GERD), and IBS. Apart from the obvious acute effects of stress on the gut, the clinical and epidemiological data support the notion that stress is associated with symptom worsening. A number of reports from war veterans and civilian woman indicate high rates of GI symptoms associated with posttraumatic stress disorder (PTSD). However, the relationship between PTSD and the GI system has not received the same research interest as, for example, PTSD's relationship to the cardiovascular system. It is important, as ever, that we be cautious in attributing a disease state to self-reports of prior stress. The presence of abnormal psychological or psychiatric profiles among a patient group does not mean that there is a psychological etiology to the disorder; the psychological changes are at least as likely to be a consequence of the disease (as is suggested for inflammatory bowel disorder). Equally, an absence of psychological/psychiatric abnormalities in a patient group is not sufficient to discard the role of stress in either the onset of the disease process or vulnerability to developing disease symptoms during the life span.

Functional Gastrointestinal Disorders

Patients diagnosed with functional GI disorders (FGID) are frequently reported to have been earlier exposed to severe and/or chronic psychosocial stress and to suffer from emotional disturbances. In recent years, an interest has emerged for studying pain circuits, brain activation, and metabolism (using functional magnetic resonance imaging and positron emission tomography) and neuroendocrine responses to various stressors. There is a consensus that psychological stress plays an important role in patients with IBS in precipitating and/or worsening the symptoms. This has been supported by animal studies of, for example, the long-term consequences of neonatal stress and maternal separation. Induced learned helplessness and chronic mild stress influence subsymptoms such as sleep abnormalities (in REM sleep in particular), production of BDNF, and γ-aminobutyric acid (GABA) receptor activity, which are central to symptoms of depression or anxiety.

Functional dyspepsia   FD is a chronic, upper-centered abdominal pain or discomfort characterized by the absence of organic changes that could explain the patient's predominant symptoms, which include nausea, early satiety, vomiting, abdominal distention,

bloating, and weight loss. Nonetheless, some patients may exhibit prepyloric erosive changes of the gastric mucosa that may be confused with acid-induced changes related to gastroesophogeal reflux disease (GERD). The role of *Helicobacter pylori* in FD is still under discussion. Although it is not believed to be a cause, testing for and treatment of the infection is regular medical procedure. There is considerable symptom overlap among FD, IBS, peptic ulcer, and GERD. Therefore, a more extended medical examination is often required (e.g., upper intestinal endoscopy). The pathophysiological mechanisms commonly proposed for FD include lowered vagal tone, impaired duodeno-jejunal motility, delayed gastric emptying, impaired gastric meal accommodation, and increased visceral sensitivity in both the stomach and duodenum. The role of stress in the etiology of FD remains unclear and clinical studies show a lack of consistency. Both stress responders and nonstress responders show delayed gastric emptying and increased rates of gastric motility. In addition, psychological profiles and personality traits of FD patients show similar inconsistency although there is some reason to believe that these patients are more prone to seek medical assistance due to general health worries, which may be connected to negative life experiences in early life.

A majority of FD patients presenting to a physician have some psychological or psychiatric abnormality, usually anxiety, mood disorder or neuroticism, or combinations of these, and they also report more adverse life events such as physical and sexual abuse, more relatives with illnesses, and failure to thrive. Personality factors such as trait anger reactivity and neuroticism, coping styles, life stressors, and degree of emotional support are shown to have predictive value in distinguishing among the FGID subgroups. Females with depression, state anxiety, and trait anger temperament are shown to have more FD-like symptoms.

Irritable bowel syndrome   Acute studies show that stress increases colonic activity. From the point of view of theories that explain IBS, we are more concerned with accounting for individual differences that can be traced back to earlier stress episodes (i.e., proactive effects). An interesting series of animal studies by Stam has adopted just this approach. A single short series of uncontrollable foot shocks failed to change basal colonic activity in rats but increased colonic activity in response to the presentation of an aversive novel stimulus (shock prod), despite there being no difference in the behavioral response. Such sensitization of the colonic response to a mild (and controllable) stressor after earlier experience with a more severe (and uncontrollable) stressor provides an attractive model for IBS. Indeed, patients with IBS do report that stressful life events exacerbate their symptoms, and early life stress may be an important contributory factor in the etiology of the disorder. Patients are characterized by higher levels of anxiety, and it is noteworthy that the levels and numbers of shock used by Stam are of the same order of magnitude as those known to induce heightened anxiety in rats. There appears to be an emotional component involved, and there is a gender difference, in that women are affected more than men across all age groups. In addition, there are ethnic differences, in that whites and Jews seem to be more affected than other ethnic groups.

The data are highly suggestive of a link between sexual abuse and later development of IBS symptoms. Twice as many IBS patients report a history of sexual abuse than the normal population, suggesting a sensitization effect of earlier stress on motility function and visceral sensitivity. Closer analysis, however, has led to the conclusion that sexual abuse is more likely to be associated with health-care use in general rather than to any specific GI disorder. In connection with this, IBS patients exhibit visceral hypersensitivity, although their peripheral pain thresholds are normal or even elevated compared to healthy individuals.

Recent studies with brain imaging techniques have revealed that normal subjects respond to rectal distention with the activation of the arcuate nucleus but that IBS patients do not. On the other hand, IBS patients respond to the same stimulus (or anticipation of it) with the activation of the prefrontal cortex. IBS nonpatients do not differ from normals in terms of psychosocial features, but IBS patients do. This may indicate that stress is not a major factor in the etiology of the disorder but rather in general illness behavior.

Organic Gastrointestinal Disorders

Peptic ulcer From being one of the classic psychosomatic diseases, peptic ulcers (stomach or duodenal lining eroded by stomach acid) have to a large extent been removed from the realm of stress-related disorders. The impetus for this radical change was the discovery that the overwhelming majority of patients harbored *H. pylori* and that the elimination of this particular bacterium was almost 100% successful in curing the disorder. A number of issues remain unresolved, however. The incidence of *H. pylori* in the population (50–80% in the older population) is considerably higher than the incidence of peptic ulcer (2–10% lifetime prevalence). The association between the disease and the infection is weaker for gastric peptic ulcer than for duodenal ulcer, as is the efficacy of the eradication treatment. *H. pylori* alone is therefore not sufficient to cause the disease. Other

putative factors include smoking, heavy drinking, and use of NSAIDs. There is considerable evidence from prospective studies that stress is also involved in both the onset and development of the disease. Several studies of groups exposed to chronic stress (e.g., prisoners-of-war and air traffic controllers) also provide evidence for the role of stress. Given the presence of *H. pylori*, it has been suggested that stress acts through the neuroimmune system to modify the rate of colonization of the bacteria. In the absence of the bacteria, it is suggested that peptic ulcer may develop from acute stress ulcerations. The role of *H. pylori* should not be underestimated in also having a potential role in slowing the healing process.

Inflammatory bowel disease IBD is a collective term that refers to both ulcerative colitis (UC) and Crohn's disease (CD). UC involves the inflammation of the mucosal lining of the large intestine, whereas CD may cause the inflammation of the lining and wall throughout the GI tract. The cause of IBD is not known, but there are several theories that combine genetics, immunology, and bacterial and neonatal factors. There is general agreement that UC and CD are not related to stress in any etiological manner; instead, the psychological symptoms associated with these disorders are the result of the poor quality of life in these patients, and stress may induce or exacerbate symptoms of the already existent disease state. Treatment programs focus on assessing possible stressors that may influence healing. Studies show that patients with active symptoms are more likely to report stressful experiences than patients with a more quiescent disease state. Some individuals are especially prone to symptom flare-ups and rehospitalization. Flare-ups of inflammation are reported to be elevated when the affected patients experience unpredictable or uncontrollable stress. The susceptibility to reactivate intestinal inflammation appears to be related to CD4 lymphocyte activity.

There are a number of animal models developed for studying the underlying interactions between stress and UC. Experimentally induced colitis in rats has been shown to be aggravated and sustained by stress. Animal studies also show that neonatal maternal separation sensitizes adult rats to chemically induced colitislike symptoms in addition to altering the intestinal microflora and disrupting the permeability of the intestine.

Stress Ulcer

All species studied develop gastric mucosal abnormalities in response to severe or chronic stress (see **Ulceration, Gastric**). In humans, the acute gastric ulcer is generally observed after severe physical trauma such as burns, surgery, sepsis, or injury to the CNS (Cushing's ulcer). The pathological background for these changes is most likely an exacerbation of superficial gastric erosions, caused by a combination of (1) restricted blood supply leading to local ischemia, (2) gastric acid, and (3) changes in gastric motility. There is no evidence that adrenocortical secretions play an aggressive role in this process; instead, the mediating mechanisms appear to be CRH-related sympathetic activation and vagally mediated gastric acid secretion.

Conclusion

Both animal and human studies provide clear evidence that stressors can and do impinge on the GI tract, most clearly at the gastric and intestinal levels. Although historically, many disorders were regarded as multifactorial, with stress as one of many contributory factors, the empirical evidence has been lacking due to methodological difficulties. There is no doubt that stress results from these disorders and that stress may exacerbate symptoms. In the case of the functional disorders, current medical attitudes have been influenced by the patients' visceral hypersensitivity. In the case of ulcer disease, the *Helicobacter* revolution has largely excluded a role for psychological stress factors. The basic physiological and psychobiological data together with comparative studies, however, clearly support the older notion that stress has an important contributory role in the etiology and maintenance of these multifactorial disease states.

See Also the Following Article

Ulceration, Gastric.

Further Reading

Bennett, E. J., Piesse, C., Palmer, K., et al. (1998). Functional gastrointestinal disorders: psychological, social, and somatic features. *Gut* **42**, 414–420.

Collins, S. M. (2001). Stress and the gastrointestinal tract IV. Modulation of intestinal inflammation by stress: basic mechanisms and clinical relevance. *American Journal of Physiology* **280**, G315–318.

Drossman, D. A. (1998). Presidential address: gastrointestinal illness and the biopsychosocial model. *Psychosomatic Medicine* **60**, 258–267.

Goebell, H., Holtmann, G. and Talley, N. J. (eds.) (1998). *Functional dyspepsia and irritable bowel syndrome: concepts and controversies*. Dordrecht: Kluwer Academic Publishers.

Hernandez, D. E. and Glavin, G. B. (eds.) (1990). *Special issue on neurobiology of stress ulcers. Annals of the New York Academy of Sciences* **597**.

Levenstein, S. and Kaplan, G. A. (1998). Socioeconomic status and ulcer: a prospective study of contributory risk factors. *Journal of Clinical Gastroenterology* **26**, 14–17.

Mayer, E. A., Naliboff, B. and Munakata, J. (2000). The evolving neurobiology of gut feelings. *Progress in Brain Research* **122**, 195–206.

Medalie, J. H., Stange, K. C., Zyzanski, S. J., et al. (1992). The importance of biopsychosocial factors in the development of duodenal ulcer in a cohort of middle-aged men. *American Journal of Epidemiology* **136**, 1280–1287.

Milde, A. M., Enger, O. and Murison, R. (2004). The effects of postnatal maternal separation on stress responsivity and experimentally induced colitis in adult rats. *Physiology & Behavior* **81**, 71–84.

Samuelson, L. C. and Hinkle, K. L. (2003). Insights into the regulation of gastric acid secretion through analysis of genetically engineered mice. *Annual Review of Physiology* **65**, 383–400.

Sapolsky, R. M. (2004). *Why zebras don't get ulcers* (3rd edn.). New York: Henry Holt and Company.

Sartor, R. B. and Sandborn, W. J. (2004). *Kirsner's inflammatory bowel diseases*. Edinburgh: Saunders.

Söderholm, J. D., Yates, D. A., Gareau, M. G., et al. (2002). Neonatal maternal separation predisposes adult rats to colonic barrier dysfunction in response to mild stress. *American Journal of Physiology* **283**, G1257–1263.

Stam, R., Ekkelenkamp, K., Frankhuijzen, A. C., et al. (2002). Long-lasting changes in central nervous system responsivity to colonic distention after stress in rats. *Gastroenterology* **123**, 1216–1225.

Thompson, W. G. (1996). *The ulcer story*. New York: Plenum Press.

Gender and Stress

R J Handa and W C J Chung
Colorado State University, Fort Collins, CO, USA

This article is a revision of the previous edition article by R J Handa and R F McGivern, volume 2, pp 196–204, © 2000, Elsevier Inc.

Evidence Supporting Gender Differences in Stress
    Responses
Basic Mechanisms of Sexual Differentiation of Neural
    Function
Clinical Implications for Gender Differences in Stress
    Responses

Glossary

5α-Dihydro-testosterone (DHT)	Androgen responsible for the masculinization of the genitalia during development. It is metabolized from testosterone by the enzymatic actions of 5α-reductase.
α-Fetoprotein	A protein produced by the liver. α-Fetoprotein can bind circulating estrogen and sequester it from the brain.
Activational actions of sex steroids	The actions of estrogens and androgens that occur transiently, in direct response to the presence of hormone. Activational effects can occur at any time during life.
Aromatase	An enzyme belonging to the P450 family of enzymes. Aromatase is primarily responsible for the metabolism of testosterone to estrogen.
Critical period of sexual differentiation	The period of time when the central nervous system is most sensitive to the organizing actions of sex steroids. The timing and length of the critical period can vary depending on the species, parameter, and hormone examined.
Estrogen	The main class of sex steroid hormones found in females. Estrogen is produced predominantly in the ovary; however, it can be produced *de novo* in other tissues and even in brain tissue in both women and men.
Organizational actions of sex steroids	The actions of estrogen and androgen that result in permanent changes in the structure or function of the brain. Organizational effects result from exposure during development or during a period of high sensitivity to the hormone in question.
Testosterone	The main class of sex steroid hormone found in males. Testosterone is produced predominantly by the testis; however, circulating testosterone is also found in females. Testosterone is metabolized to estrogenic as well as androgenic products.

Evidence Supporting Gender Differences in Stress Responses

Gender Differences in Adrenal Function

The early work of Hans Selye described adrenal gland function and its role in homeostasis. This work also provided the first compelling evidence for potential sex differences in stress responses. In supporting the observations of Selye, many studies showed that the adrenal gland is larger in females than in males, even when corrected for sex differences in body weight. Correspondingly, the rate of hormone secretion by the adrenal gland differs between males and females. Moreover, some studies in rodents reported that females show a greater diurnal fluctuation in corticosterone or cortisol, the main steroid hormone secreted by the adrenal cortex (corticosterone in the mouse and rat, cortisol in the hamster and human; **Figure 1**). Similarly, the adrenal response in secreting these glucocorticoid hormones following stressful, or perceived stressful, situations such as exposure to noxious fumes, exposure to a novel environment, immobilization, or a brief electric shock (see **Glucocorticoid Negative Feedback, Glucocorticoids, Effects of Stress on, Glucocorticoids – Adverse Effects on the Nervous System, Hippocampus, Overview**) resulted in peak elevations in adrenal glucocorticoid hormone levels that were 1.5–2 times greater in females than in males.

In adult animal models, sex differences in adrenal function appear to be relatively confined to glucocorticoids because gender differences in other adrenal cortex-derived steroid hormones, such as progesterone and androgen, have not been reported in the literature. Androgen and progesterone are secreted predominantly by the gonads at relatively high levels. Therefore, gonad-derived steroids may mask any sex differences in adrenal-derived steroids, which may underlie the absence of these types of studies in the literature.

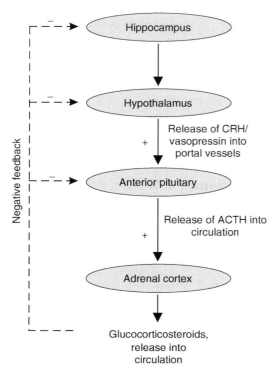

Figure 1 Schematic representation of the hypothalamic-pituitary-adrenal (HPA) axis. The positive feedback portion of the HPA starts at the level of the paraventricular nucleus of the hypothalamus. Neurons residing in this nucleus release corticotropin releasing hormone (CRH) and vasopressin into the hypophysial portal vessels to the anterior pituitary to stimulate the synthesis and release of ACTH. This in turn stimulates both synthesis and release of adrenal glucocorticoids into the general circulation to elicit an appropriate stress response. The presence of increased levels of glucocorticosteroids in turn induces an inhibitory effect (i.e., negative feedback) on the HPA axis, which is thought to be mainly mediated through glucocorticoid-responsive neurons in the hippocampus.

Sex Differences in Neuroendocrine Function

Pituitary hormone secretion The sex difference in adrenal function is in part due to sex differences in the neuroendocrine axis that regulates adrenal hormone secretion. This axis has been termed the hypothalamic-pituitary-adrenal (HPA) axis because of the interaction of each of these tissues in regulating one another's secretory activity (**Figure 1**). Similar to sex differences in the adrenal glucocorticoid release, adrenocorticotropic hormone (ACTH) is also released in a sexually dimorphic fashion. ACTH is a hormone secreted by the anterior pituitary gland into the general circulation, which in turn stimulates adrenal synthesis and secretion of glucocorticoids. Animal studies also demonstrated that the increases in circulating ACTH levels following physical or psychological stressors are greater and more prolonged in females than in males. An enhanced ACTH response in female

rodents seems to depend on the hypothalamic peptide called corticotropin releasing hormone (CRH), suggesting that the sex difference in ACTH response may, in part, be the result of a sex difference in anterior pituitary responsiveness to CRH.

Hypothalamic function The secretion of ACTH from the anterior pituitary is controlled by hormones that are synthesized in neurons residing in the paraventricular nucleus of the hypothalamus (PVN). These hormones are released into the hypophysial portal vasculature via the median eminence (**Figure 1**). The most important releasing factors for ACTH appear to be CRH and vasopressin. Both CRH and vasopressin are potent ACTH secretagogues, and vasopressin potentiates the ACTH-releasing activity of CRH several-fold. Animal studies have shown that the PVN in females contains more CRH neurons than in males. Moreover, females exhibited a more pronounced diurnal variation in hypothalamic CRH immunoreactivity than males. These data are consistent with physiological data demonstrating a greater activation of the HPA axis in females.

Studies have demonstrated sex differences in the release of vasopressin following a stressor. Indeed, vasopressin was released in female rats following immobilization stress, whereas this was not the case in male rats. Although, vasopressin immunoreactivity in the PVN is not sexually dimorphic, the presence of a sex difference in the functional sensitivity of vasopressin cells in the PVN to stressors may help explain sex differences in neuroendocrine responses.

Negative feedback regulation The stimulatory limb of the HPA axis (CRH, vasopressin, and ACTH) is kept in check by continuous feedback inhibition by circulating glucocorticoid hormones. Thus, it has been hypothesized that the intensity of this negative feedback action may be an underlying factor in the sexually dimorphic secretion of adrenal glucocorticoid hormones. The negative feedback glucocorticoids is mediated by two receptor types – mineralocorticoid receptor (MR) and glucocorticoid receptor (GR) – that reside in target neurons in the hypothalamus, hippocampus, and anterior pituitary gland, as well as other brain areas. Both receptors appear to be involved in differing aspects of the negative feedback regulation. Because of their high affinity for glucocorticoids, MRs are thought to regulate basal hormone secretion, whereas GRs, which exhibit a lower affinity for glucocorticoids, are thought to return stress-responsive elevations in glucocorticoids back to baseline. Assuming that the number of receptors accurately reflects the sensitivity of a tissue for a hormone, it is logical to conclude that sex differences in the HPA axis may result from a sex difference in the number of receptors in a given cell. A greater negative-feedback sensitivity would be indicated by more receptors and consequently result in lower basal and stress-activated hormone secretion. On the other hand, lower levels of receptors would indicate weaker negative feedback and thus result in higher basal and stress-responsive hormone secretion. This hypothesis has been supported by sex differences in the concentration and function of MRs and GRs. Overall, females tend to have lower levels of MRs and GRs in many brain regions, including the hypothalamus and hippocampus, which is consistent with the pattern found in other tissues, such as the thymus and liver. Given similar levels of hormone, GR- or MR-mediated functions (e.g., autoregulation of the receptors) was reported to be less sensitive to glucocorticosteroid modulation in females than in males.

Sex Differences in Behavioral Responses to Stress

Sex differences in behavioral responses to stress have been well-documented in humans and animals. Laboratory animals have provided much of what we know regarding gender differences in response to stress. When placed in a given stressful situation, animals undergo a series of well-described behaviors that have been interpreted to indicate the degree of fear or anxiety that is being experienced. Freezing, defecation, and vocalization are a few good examples of these behaviors. Females appear to be less sensitive to stress-associated novel or aversive environments. For example, when placed into a novel environment or an elevated plus maze, female animals show less freezing and defecation than males. Females also enter a compartment in which they have been previously shocked more readily. In these behavioral paradigms, females also show more activity and exploration, behaviors that have been interpreted as signifying a lesser expression of fear and anxiety. However, when exposed to a variety of chronic stress paradigms, females are found to habituate significantly less than males.

In a well-studied animal model of chronic stress known as learned helplessness, animals are subjected to a repeated inescapable stressor, such as an intermittent tail shock. Subsequently, when allowed to escape, male rats are impaired in their escape performance, whereas female rats do not show this deficit to the same extent. However, when stressed repeatedly over a long period of time, it appears that males adapt more readily (eventually do not show reduced activity), whereas females fail to adapt over the same time period. It appears that this sex difference in adaptability may be dependent on levels of glucocorticoids because the reduction of the poststress glucocorticoid

levels in females to levels attained in males allows the adaptation to repeated restraint. However, these effects are not always observed across studies. One reason may be related findings from studies showing that both strain and stress exposure during early development are important determinants in the expression of stress-related sex differences in behavior in adulthood.

Basic Mechanisms of Sexual Differentiation of Neural Function

Sexual differentiation of the brain occurs as a result of the presence of gonadal steroid hormones acting during either development or adulthood (**Figure 2**). The actions of gonadal steroid hormones on the brain have been classified as being either organizational or activational. Organizational actions are permanent changes in brain structure or function that occur during development. Generally, these permanent effects of gonadal steroid hormones are greatest during a defined critical window of opportunity, usually during gestation or early postnatal life. The removal of gonadal steroid hormones after this critical period does not alter the organization or function of the brain appreciably. In contrast, the activational effects of gonadal steroid hormones are those that occur transiently, in direct response to the presence of a gonadal steroid hormone. Indeed, the removal of gonadal steroid hormones from the circulation, through castration or ovariectomy, results in a loss of effect. The activational effects of gonadal steroid hormones can occur throughout life, but are generally thought to have a maximal influence on gender differences during adulthood.

The literature regarding sexual differentiation of the brain suggests that the mammalian brain is an undifferentiated or perhaps neutral state and that, in response to normal circulating levels of testosterone (from the fetal male gonad), it develops toward the male direction. In contrast, if testosterone is low or absent, the brain develops toward the default mode, which is female (see **Figure 2**).

Although testosterone or its androgenic metabolite DHT may play a role in the masculinization of the brain, through their intracellular androgen receptor, in rodent models the functional gonadal steroid hormone for the organizational sexual differentiation of the brain is considered to be estrogen (**Figure 2**). This steroid hormone is produced intracellularly as a metabolite of testosterone due to the actions of the enzyme aromatase. The defeminizing effects of estrogen on the developing brain are mediated by estrogen receptors (ERs), although the exact role of each of the two forms of ERs, ERα and ERβ, is not known.

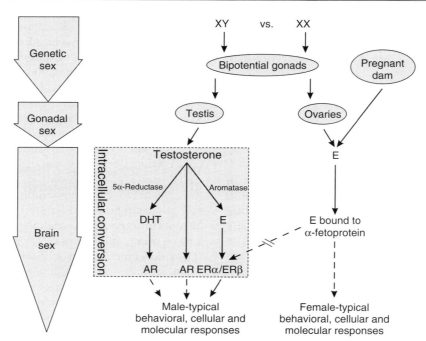

Figure 2 Schematic representation of the gonadal steroid hormones involved in the sexual differentiation of the vertebrate brain during development. According to this scheme, α-fetoprotein sequesters circulating estrogen, thereby preventing the defeminization (or masculinization) of the male or female brain. Therefore, the brain is thought to be initially programmed to develop in the female direction. However, α-fetoprotein is bypassed in the male brain because circulating testosterone is converted intraneuronally into estrogen by the enzyme aromatase, thus enabling estrogen to defemininize (or masculinize) the male brain, which is mediated through estrogen receptors. AR, androgen receptor; DHT, 5α-dihydrotestosterone; E, estrogen; ER, estrogen receptor.

Circulating estrogen from the mother or the developing ovary of the female is bound to a liver-derived protein called α-fetoprotein, which is present in high levels during perinatal development. Consequently, circulating estrogens are sequestered and cannot defeminize (or masculinize) the developing male or female brain. In contrast, defeminization (or masculinization) by estrogen can occur in the male brain because the estrogen-sequestering abilities of α-fetoprotein are circumvented due to its intracellular origin through the aromatization of testosterone. In rodents, the high levels of α-fetoprotein decrease during the second and third weeks of life, which coincides with increasing levels of unbound estrogens in the circulating, thus allowing the organizational and activational effects of estrogens to occur at puberty and in adulthood.

Organizational Effects of Gonadal Steroid Hormones on Stress Responses

Gonadal steroid hormones may act during early development to permanently organize adult responses to stress. This is best illustrated by examining the effects of perinatal hormone removal and replacement on the development of the adult pattern of behavior in response to stress. An example is the earlier described sex difference in the performance of the elevated plus maze and open-field test, in which female rats showed more activity and were less anxious than male rats. Indeed, the activity of an adult male rat that was castrated postnatally (a procedure that removes circulating levels of testosterone and its associated metabolites, such as estrogen) is similar to that of a female rat. The castration of male rats up to 21 days after birth prevents the development of the sex difference in activity. In contrast, neither the castration of adult males nor estrogen or testosterone replacement affects the sex difference in the level of activity. Similarly, the treatment of female rats with testosterone or estrogen up through 4 weeks after birth, but not in adulthood, results in a more malelike activity pattern. These studies indicate a critical period of sensitivity for the organizing actions of gonadal steroid hormones; moreover, they also show that sex differences in the activity level do not arise until after puberty.

Few studies have examined the occurrence of similar organizational effects of sex steroids on neuroendocrine responses to stress. The neonatal gonadectomy of male rats produces a more female-like hormonal response to stress in adulthood, but much of this may be due to the absence of hormones in adulthood because adult gonadectomy has a similar effect. On balance, it appears that the predominant effects of gonadal steroid hormones on neuroendocrine stress responses are activational in nature, with organizational influences contributing a much more modest amount to the overall sex difference.

Activational Effects of Gonadal Steroid Hormones on Stress Responses

The activational effects of gonadal steroid hormones on stress responses can be demonstrated easily by the gonadectomy of males and females in adulthood. The castration of male rats results in an increase in stress-responsive ACTH and corticosterone secretion. Similarly, the ovariectomy of female rats results in a decrease in stress-responsive HPA axis activity. These are gonadal steroid hormone-specific effects because they were reversed by the replacement of gonadal steroid hormones to gonadectomized animals. Moreover, androgen and estrogen have opposing actions in regulating stress-responsive hormone secretion. The treatment of gonadectomized male and female rats with estrogen augments subsequent ACTH and corticosterone responses to stress, whereas treatment with testosterone, or the nonaromatizable androgen, DHT, effectively inhibits HPA axis responses to stress. These studies provide a good mechanistic understanding as to why the stress-responsive hormone secretion is greatest in female rats during proestrus, when estrogen levels are highest.

Testosterone and estrogen can limit or augment the ACTH and corticosterone response to stress at several sites. These include the adrenal gland, anterior pituitary, hypothalamus, and higher brain centers such as the hippocampus. Receptors for androgen and estrogen exist in all these tissues, and the effects of estrogen and androgen on cellular parameters relevant to HPA activation have been demonstrated in all tissues.

At the level of the adrenal gland, estrogen has been shown to increase the adrenal secretory response to ACTH administration. Similarly, some studies showed that in the presence of estrogen the anterior pituitary gland responds to CRH with a greater secretion of ACTH than in the absence of estrogen. Increases in CRH immunoreactivity and mRNA have also been demonstrated in the hypothalamus in response to estrogen treatment. Whether these are direct actions on CRH neurons or mediated transsynaptically is currently in question. However, studies have demonstrated that the promoter sequence of the human CRH gene contains sequences (estrogen response elements) that respond to occupied estrogen receptors by increasing gene transcription, suggesting a direct action on the CRH gene. More recently, studies in rodents and humans showed the presence of ERs in some populations of CRH neurons of the PVN.

Similarly, androgen also appears to act at several sites. Castration increases adrenal enzyme activity and the synthesis of corticosterone by the adrenal gland *in vitro*, suggesting that testosterone acts to inhibit adrenal activity. Although testosterone does not appear to alter the anterior pituitary ACTH response to CRH administration, it does decrease CRH immunoreactivity in the hypothalamus of castrated rats. A direct action of testosterone on CRH synthesis or secretion does not seem to be the case because CRH neurons do not contain androgen receptors; thus upstream sites containing androgen receptors and projecting to CRH cells in the hypothalamus have been implicated, including the medial preoptic area, septum, and bed nucleus of the stria terminalis.

Sex differences in circulating estrogen and testosterone are also responsible for the sex differences in brain GR and MR levels or function. These effects underlie the reported sex differences in the negative feedback modulation of the HPA axis. Estrogen decreases GR and MR levels and their respective mRNAs in some brain areas and interferes with the ability of GR to autoregulate gene expression following changes in circulating glucocorticoids. These effects of estrogen could arise secondarily as a result of estrogen-induced increases in corticosteroid-binding globulin (CBG). In response to estrogen exposure, increased levels of CBG can sequester circulating glucocorticoid hormones from the brain, resulting in a decrease in negative feedback. However, estrogen has also been reported to increase GR in some tissues, such as the pituitary gland, and decrease the efficacy of corticosteroid receptor agonists that are not bound by CBG. Thus, it is likely that the actions of estrogen on the negative feedback are not solely mediated by an increase in CBG.

At the molecular level, interactions between ERs and GRs have been demonstrated with each modulating the functional response of the other. Testosterone also appears to interact with glucocorticoids in the regulation of GRs, but not MRs; however, a clear role for androgen receptors in altering negative feedback mechanisms has yet to be demonstrated.

Clinical Implications for Gender Differences in Stress Responses

Hans Selye's work in the 1940s also introduced the concept that stress accelerates the onset of disease through pathophysiological changes in endocrine and autonomic regulatory systems. Stress alone does not cause disease, but it is hypothesized to increase an individual's susceptibility to disease. In the past quarter century, this concept has been supported by results from numerous clinical and epidemiological studies related to cardiovascular disease, affective disorders, gastrointestinal disorders, diabetes, and physiological disorders associated with normal aging.

The mechanisms linking stress to disease states in humans are not fully understood, but hormonal changes, induced by the stress response, are recognized as a major influence. Glucocorticoids have a primary role but one that is modulated by gonadal steroid hormones. Androgen receptors, ERs, and GRs are found in many tissues that are stress-responsive. Some of these include the heart muscle, blood vessels, and immune tissues such as the spleen, thymus, and bone marrow. Gonadal steroid hormone receptors are also found in brain regions that mediate emotional and autonomic responses to stress, such as the hippocampus, hypothalamus, and amygdala. Thus gender differences in stress-related disease susceptibility appear to involve an interaction between glucocorticoid and gonadal hormones.

The role of stress in psychological and physiological disorders is complex. Animal studies have demonstrated that adult stress responsiveness is influenced developmentally by both genetics and the early environment. This bidirectional influence of both factors makes it difficult to predict the stress-related susceptibility to disease in individuals. However, physiological gender differences are still evident in humans regardless of early environment.

Many of these differences parallel sex differences in animals. For instance, the unstressed basal heart rate in women is greater than in men. Women also exhibit a larger exercise-induced increase in heart rate. However, in response to anger and psychological stress, men exhibit greater emotional and cardiovascular lability with respect to both heart rate and blood pressure. This lability, resulting in larger increases in systolic pressure, is thought to contribute significantly to the greater risk in men for cardiovascular morbidity. Protection from heart disease in women is also related to estrogen, which provides protection against arteriosclerosis until menopause. The anti-atherosclerotic effects of estrogen also appear to involve the presence of ERs in cardiovascular tissue.

Physical or psychologically stressful stimuli also produce a greater stimulation of the HPA axis in women than in men, similar to the stress effects observed in other mammals. Administering CRH to women induces a greater release of ACTH and a prolonged elevation of cortisol than administering it to men, indicating that these gender differences probably involve processes directly under the regulation of the central nervous system. However, unlike animals, gender differences in the human HPA axis responsiveness to psychological stressors appear to be much more dependent on the type of psychological stress and the environmental circumstances in which it occurs. Studies suggest that psychological factors associated with social stress, such as taking care of an elderly parent, have more impact on HPA reactivity in women than in men, perhaps placing women's health at greater risk under such circumstances.

A primary factor underlying gender differences in the HPA response to stress appears to be higher estrogen levels in women. During the normal menstrual cycle, HPA activity is enhanced during the follicular phase, when estrogen levels peak, and is reduced during the luteal phase, when progesterone levels are elevated. The removal of the ovaries prior to menopause reduces the HPA sensitivity to CRH stimulation. The effect of estrogen on HPA reactivity is not gender-specific because normal men who were administered a short-term regimen of estrogen also exhibited increased HPA activity. One possible explanation for such effects of estrogen is provided by observations that estrogen therapy increases circulating levels of CBG in women. Although not yet shown to be the case, such increases in CBG, and the resulting decreases in free cortisol, could play a role in the elevated HPA activity in response to stress reported in women (due to a decrease in cortisol bioavailability). Similarly, it remains to be determined whether men and women are equally sensitive to the influence of estrogen on the HPA and whether organizational influences of gonadal steroids confer a differential sensitivity to the later hormonal modulation of HPA activity.

The incidence of autoimmune disease is also sexually dimorphic, and the severity and onset are exacerbated by life stress. The overall incidence in women is approximately 2.5-fold greater then in men. In contrast to the protective role estrogen plays in cardiovascular disease, it appears to be a major contributory factor to the gender difference observed in autoimmune diseases such as multiple sclerosis, rheumatoid arthritis, and lupus. Estrogen can regulate immune responses through ERs present on thymocytes, macrophages, and endothelial cells, all of which also express GRs. The interaction between estrogen and glucocorticoids on immunomodulation is a rapidly expanding area of research interest and one that is likely to underlie the gender difference in autoimmune disease susceptibility.

Numerous clinical studies have reported a greater incidence of depression in women. The reasons underlying this gender difference are controversial, but both hormonal status and stress may be involved. Women have been reported to be more susceptible to depression during periods of fluctuations in estrogen and progesterone levels. However, although such changes have often been cited as causes of mood disorders in women, the literature does not provide strong support for a direct causal relationship between gonadal hormone status and depression or anxiety disorders. An additional mediating factor may be life stress. The onset of clinical depression is well known to be exacerbated by life stress, and data suggest that a link to a gender bias in mood disorders involves an increased susceptibility in some women to the combined effects of stress and hormonal status. Thus, fluctuations in estrogen and progesterone during the menstrual cycle have been proposed to confer a susceptibility to depression in women that can be exacerbated by life stress.

A gender difference is also observed in the incidence of posttraumatic stress disorder (PTSD), which is a stress-induced pathological condition that is clinically distinct from depression or other affective disorders. Long-term physiological changes are observed in PTSD patients that involve increased adrenergic tone and alterations in HPA function. Following exposure to prolonged psychological trauma, women exhibit PTSD symptoms twice as frequently as men, even when the type of trauma is equivalent. The organizational effects of hormones may also play a role in gender differences in the incidence of PTSD. This stems from findings showing that experiencing psychologically traumatizing events prior to puberty greatly increases the susceptibility to PTSD in adulthood in females compared to males. This increased susceptibility appears to relate specifically to experiencing childhood psychological trauma because accidents or injury during this period do not increase the risk for PTSD in either gender when later psychological trauma is experienced.

In summary, current research studying the interrelationships among gender, stress, and pathophysiology strongly implicate a role for gonadal hormones in predicting gender differences related to disease or psychopathology. However, a definitive understanding of the role of gender in the elicitation of stress-induced pathophysiology awaits a better understanding of the complex relationship among the environment, steroid hormones, and other stress-induced biochemical factors.

See Also the Following Articles

Adrenal Cortex; Androgen Action; Autoimmunity; Depression Models; Estrogen; Glucocorticoid Negative Feedback; Glucocorticoids, Effects of Stress on; Glucocorticoids – Adverse Effects on the Nervous System; Hippocampus, Overview; Learned Helplessness; Menopause and Stress; Selye, Hans.

Further Reading

Beatty, W. W. (1979). Gonadal hormones and sex differences in nonreproductive behaviors in rodents: organizational and activational influences. *Hormones and Behavior* **12**, 112–163.
Breslau, N., Glenn, C., Andreski, P., et al. (1997). Sex differences in posttraumatic stress disorder. *Archives of General Psychiatry* **54**, 1044–1048.
Chrousos, G. P., Torpy, D. J. and Gold, P. W. (1998). Interactions between the hypothalamic-pituitary-adrenal axis and the female reproductive system: clinical implications. *Annals of Internal Medicine* **129**, 229.
Gorski, R. A. (1985). The 13th J. A. F. Stevenson memorial lecture: sexual differentiation of the brain: possible mechanisms and implications. *Canadian Journal of Physiology and Pharmacology* **63**, 577–594.
Handa, R. J., Burgess, L. H., Kerr, J. E., et al. (1994). Gonadal steroid hormone receptors and sex differences in the hypothalamo-pituitary-adrenal axis. *Hormones and Behavior* **28**, 464–476.
Handa, R. J., Price, R. H., Jr. and Wilson, M. E. (1998). Steroid hormone receptors and the assessment of feedback sensitivity. In: VandeKar, L. (ed.) *Methods in neuroendocrinology: the cellular and molecular neuropharmacology series*, pp. 49–68. Boca Raton, FL: CRC Press.
Seeman, M. V. (1997). Psychopathology in women and men: focus on female hormones. *American Journal of Psychiatry* **154**, 1641–1647.
Turner, B. B. (1997). Influence of gonadal steroids on brain corticosteroid receptors: a minireview. *Neurochemical Research* **22**, 1375–1385.
Vogele, C., Jarvis, A. and Cheeseman, K. (1997). Anger suppression, reactivity and hypertension risk: gender makes a difference. *Annals of Behavioral Medicine* **19**, 61–69.
Wilder, R. L. (1995). Neuroendocrine-immune system interactions and autoimmunity. *Annual Review of Immunology* **13**, 307–338.

Gender-Specific Stress *See:* Gender and Stress.

Gene–Environment Interactions in Early Development

I S P Davis and R Plomin
Institute of Psychiatry, King's College London, London, UK

Quantitative Genetics

Molecular Genetics

Behavioral Genomics and GE Interplay

Future QTL Research on GE Interplay

Glossary

DNA pooling	A molecular genetic technique that combines DNA from individuals in order to estimate allele frequencies for the group of individuals.
Family chaos	A measure of the family environment derived from the Confusion, Hubbub, and Order Scale.
Genotype–environment correlation (rGE)	Genetic influence on exposure to environments.
Genotype–environment interaction (GxE)	Genetic sensitivity to environments.
Microarray	A technology that allows the genotyping of hundreds of thousands of polymorphisms simultaneously.
Quantitative genetics	The statistical study of the genetic and environmental origins of individual differences in complex traits, using information about the relatedness of individuals; in contrast to molecular genetics, which attempts to identify specific genes.
Quantitative trait locus (QTL)	A genetic polymorphism that plays a role in the etiology of a trait influenced by many such loci.
Single nucleotide polymorphism (SNP)	A genetic polymorphism involving the substitution of a single letter (nucleotide base pair) of the four-letter genetic alphabet.

The interplay between nature and nurture has long been characterized as adversarial; the truth is much more complex, and more interesting. Although there are many ways of thinking about the issue, this article considers genotype–environment (GE) interaction and correlation from a quantitative genetic perspective, where GE interaction refers to genetic sensitivity to environments and GE correlation refers to genetic influence on exposure to environments. Diathesis-stress theories predict that individuals' sensitivity to stressful events and access to social support networks depends on their genotype. Although evidence for such interactions is – as yet – inconclusive, a more convincing case can be made for genetic influence on environmental measures: gene–environment correlations. The ability to detect gene–environment interplay has traditionally relied on the use of specific environmental measures in genetically sensitive designs such as twin or adoption studies. This ability is greatly enhanced by incorporating genotyping for specific genes: new methods for doing this are likely to see future stress research making use of genetic measures as a matter of course.

Quantitative Genetics

Over the past two decades, there has been an increasing tendency to include measures of the environment in quantitative genetic research; without measures of the environment, quantitative genetic designs such as twin and adoption studies cannot contribute much to our understanding of GE interaction and correlation. This section begins with quantitative genetic research on GE interaction and correlation that incorporates measures of the environment and then turns to molecular genetic research that incorporates information from DNA. The effects of stressful environments on learning ability and disability are used as an example of how molecular genetics can contribute to our understanding of gene–environment interplay.

GE Interaction

The great advantage of research with animal models is the ability to manipulate both genes and environment experimentally so that main effects and interaction are assessed directly. That is, genetically different animals such as selected low and high lines or inbred strains can be studied in different environments. Animal models are powerful, but they have been hard-pushed to find GE interaction, especially for learning. The classic example in psychology textbooks is Cooper and Zubek's study of maze-bright and maze-dull rats reared in enriched or deprived environments. However, although it is highly cited, its conclusions are doubtful: Henderson studied GE interaction systematically using inbred strains of mice and found few such effects.

Adoption designs are similar to animal designs, except that they are only quasi-experimental in their separation of genes and environment (**Figure 1**). Parents usually share both genes and environment with their offspring, but adoption separates nature and nurture by creating a distinction between genetic parents whose children are adopted away and environmental parents who adopt these children. Using the phenotype of biological parents as an indicator of genetic risk and the phenotype of adoptive parents as an indicator of environmental risk, we can find genetic effects without environmental effects (**Figure 1a**) and environmental effects without genetic effects (**Figure 1b**). Studies usually reveal both genetic and environmental effects (**Figure 1c**). The adoption design can also identify GE interaction (**Figure 1d**), in which genetic effects depend on environmental effects or vice versa. However, as with animal studies, it has been difficult to find GE interaction, especially for cognitive abilities. Twin studies are much more limited in terms of finding GE interaction because they are essentially constrained to detecting differences in heritability as a function of the environment.

For example, in the Twins Early Development Study (TEDS) of a large twin sample assessed at 2, 3, 4, and 7 years, GE interaction was looked for,

but not much evidence for it was found using quantitative genetic methods. Despite this, one promising example of GE interaction is that heritability of verbal ability is significantly higher (about 0.60) in high chaos families and lower (about 0.30) in low chaos families. However, the twin design lacks power to detect even this limited type of GE interaction: about 1000 pairs of each type of twin are needed to detect a heritability difference of 60% versus 40%. As discussed later, the lack of quantitative genetic evidence for GE interaction does not preclude the likelihood that molecular genetic research will find interactions between specific genes and specific environmental stressors.

GE Correlation

In spite of the current interest in GE interaction, it is likely that GE correlation, the nature of nurture, will eventually be seen as more important. Animal models are powerful for investigating GE interaction, but laboratory research has rarely considered GE correlation because it requires a menu of environments from which individuals can choose. The first step in addressing GE correlation is to investigate the extent to which there is genetic influence on environmental measures. This can be done by treating environmental measures as dependent measures in quantitative genetic analyses. Dozens of such twin and adoption

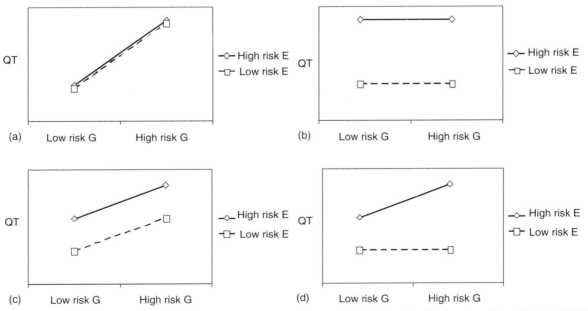

Figure 1 G, E, and GxE in an adoption study. G refers to low or high genetic risk, as indexed by the phenotype (quantitative trait [QT]) of the biological parents. E refers to the environment of the adoptive home. a, A main effect of G, but no effect of E on the phenotype. b, A main effect of E, but no effect of G. Very often, there is a main effect of both G and E, as illustrated in c. d, A main effect of both G and E, and a GxE interaction of the diathesis stress type, in which environmental risk (stress) has a disproportionately large effect on individuals at genetic risk (diathesis).

studies consistently find genetic influence on environmental measures: nearly all measures of family environment show genetic influence. Most studies that have addressed this question find genetic influence on environmental measures outside the family as well, such as peer groups, life events, and social support, which are of particular relevance to stress.

How can environmental stressors show genetic influence when environments do not have DNA? The answer is that our measures of stress are not independent of us – genetic influence on our behavior is reflected in our experiences. If genetics affects both environmental measures and behavioral measures, then the correlation between environmental measures and behavioral outcomes may be genetically mediated. Life events such as illness and injury have been shown to have a heritability of around 40%, implying that they do not happen capriciously to individuals: they happen, or are perceived to happen, more often to the genetically predisposed. As expected, those life events that the individual is involved in or has control over show more substantial heritability than those that happen to others. Recent research suggests that minor, chronic, daily stressors may be more important in determining outcomes than major life events. New studies are expected to show that these also show genetic influence. In a similar way, social support networks show heritability: studies have demonstrated that although the extensiveness of the network is not heritable, the quality of the relationships is.

The method underlying all these studies is to use multivariate genetic analysis to analyze genetic and environmental sources of covariance between environmental stressors and behavioral outcomes. Studies of this sort consistently show some genetic mediation of the association. In this sense, quantitative genetic research provides much more evidence for GE correlation than for GE interaction. GE correlation suggests an important model of environments that goes beyond the usual passive view in which the environment (and, by extension, stress) is what happens to us. Instead, environments are active: we select, modify, construct and, afterward, reconstruct our experiences partially based on our genetic propensities. From a molecular genetic point of view, GE correlation means that we ought to be able to find specific genes associated with environmental measures.

In summary, quantitative genetic research does not find much evidence for GE interaction, but it finds considerable evidence for GE correlation. This section has not gone into great detail because quantitative genetic results on GE interaction and correlation are not very relevant for future research in this area, which will use specific genes as well as specific environments. The rest of this article considers molecular genetic approaches.

Molecular Genetics

So far, evidence of the existence of interplay between genes and the environment has been considered. Research on GE interaction and correlation will be much more powerful when we are able to include specific genes as well as specific environments, that is, when the G in GE refers to genes in molecular genetic analyses rather than genotypes in quantitative genetic analyses. There have been several replicated linkages and associations, but most people would agree that progress has been slower than expected in terms of finding genes for complex behavioral traits. The problem is that we are looking for needles in a haystack, but we have only had the power to detect very large needles. Very rarely, the effects of a single gene can account for all the variance in a trait. This is the case with phenylketonuria (PKU), in which a mutation in both copies of a single gene results in the inability to metabolize the amino acid phenylalanine. This causes a buildup of toxic products that damage the developing brain. The environmental intervention of a low phenylalanine diet has the effect of preventing mental impairment in children with PKU but has no effect on other children: a dramatic example of a GE interaction.

Despite the slow progress in identifying quantitative trait loci (QTLs) associated with common disorders and complex traits, some evidence has been found for GE interaction using candidate QTLs that affect genetic sensitivity to environments. For example, there are reports that the influence of maltreatment in early life on the development of adult antisocial problems is moderated by a functional polymorphism in the promoter region of the *MAOA* (monoamine oxidase A) gene. Likewise, the influence of stressful life events on depression may be moderated by a functional polymorphism in the promoter region of the *5-HTT* (5-hydroxytryptophan [serotonin] transporter) gene. These examples of GE interaction emerged despite the absence of a main effect for these two genes.

For the vast majority of complex traits, the largest QTL effect is unlikely to account for more than 1% of the variance. Very large samples are needed to attain power to detect such small effects, and even larger samples are needed to detect GE interaction. Rather than just examining a few candidate genes, the trend in molecular genetic research is toward systematic genome-wide scans that require hundreds of thousands of DNA markers. The costs for such genome-wide association scans on very large samples are substantial.

One new method that goes some way to solving this problem is genotyping of pooled DNA on microarrays, a method called SNP-MaP (single nucleotide polymorphism microarrays and pooling).

The first application of SNP-MaP involved mild mental impairment (MMI), which can be seen as the low end of general cognitive ability (g). g was assessed in 10 000 children at 7 years, and two independent SNP-MaP studies using a microarray that assessed 10 000 SNPs (the 10K GeneChip) compared high and low g groups. Five SNPs were identified that remained significantly associated with g when individually genotyped for 5000 children. On average, each SNP in the set accounts for just 0.2% of the variance in g. However, as the effects of the SNPs are uncorrelated and additive, it is possible to combine their effects to create a composite SNP set using an additive model in which each SNP is scored 0, 1, or 2, depending on the number of high-g-associated alleles. The SNP set accounts for nearly 1% of the variance of g scores at 7 years. As shown in **Figure 2**, SNP set scores are normally distributed and almost linearly related to g. The difference between those scoring low on the SNP set and those scoring high is about one-third of a standard deviation, or 5 IQ points.

Repeating the analysis using the newly available 500K microarray should find many more SNPs accounting for much more of the variance. It will then be possible to use SNP set scores as genetic risk indicators in research into environmental stressors and to select genotypically for extreme SNP set groups to use in paradigms such as neuroimaging that cannot study large samples.

Behavioral Genomics and GE Interplay

Once genes or QTL sets associated with behavioral dimensions or disorders are found, the next phase of research will investigate the pathways between genes and behavior via the brain, which will represent a paradigm shift in research on GE interplay. The term functional genomics, which has been used to describe this direction for research, usually refers to bottom-up research that begins with understanding the gene product in a cell and works up toward the brain and behavior. However, other levels of analysis can also be useful in understanding pathways between genes and behavior: behavioral genomics refers to a complementary approach that begins with behavior of the individual and works down toward the brain. For example, we can investigate how genetic effects unfold during development or ask multivariate questions about heterogeneity and comorbidity. As the present concern is GE interaction and correlation, the focus will be on behavioral genomic analyses of GE interplay.

To return to the earlier example, the 5-SNP set associated with g at 7 years was used in behavioral genomic analyses of GE interaction and correlation. The environmental measures employed in these analyses included distal environmental measures such as parental occupation or education and proximal measures such as family chaos and discipline in early

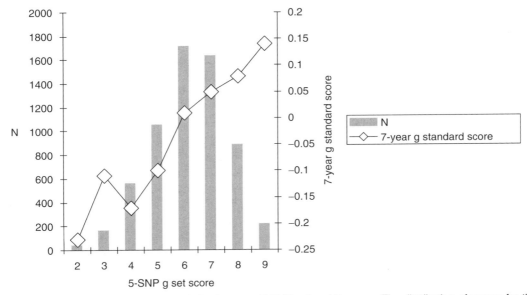

Figure 2 Distribution of 5-SNP g set and association between 5-SNP set and 7-year g. The distribution of scores for the SNP set (derived on the basis of higher scores for high-g-associated alleles) is normal (gray bars). The line represents the means of the 5-SNP set score plotted against means of the g composite score at 7 years.

childhood in those homes. Although GE interaction can be examined in several different ways, the extent to which environmental stressors moderate the SNP set association with g was investigated. Using family chaos as an example, the top panel (a) of **Figure 3** shows a main effect for family chaos (higher g scores

for children in families with less chaos) but no statistically significant interaction using linear and nonlinear continuous analyses.

The other three environmental variables shown in **Figure 3** yielded significant but modest GE interaction. For harsh parental discipline (**Figure 3b**),

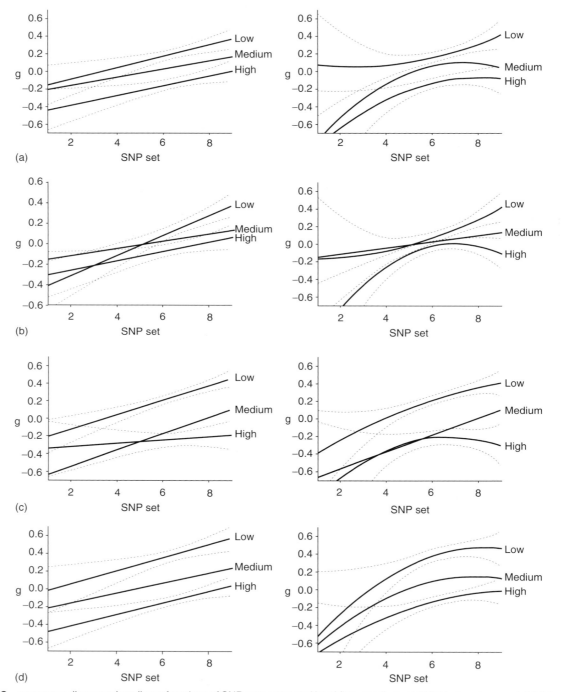

Figure 3 g scores as linear and nonlinear functions of SNP set scores and level (low, medium, and high) of environmental risk for chaos (a), harsh parental discipline (b), father's occupational class (c), and mother's highest qualification (d). Ninety-five percent confidence intervals (dotted lines) are shown for low and high levels of environmental risk.

environmental effects are greater at both the high and the low SNP set scores. For high SNP set scores, children with good environments (low harsh discipline) have higher than expected g scores, whereas children with low SNP set scores and harsh parental discipline have lower than expected g scores. In other words, this GE interaction suggests that children with a genetic propensity toward high g profit disproportionately from a good environment, and children with a genetic propensity toward low g suffer disproportionately from a bad environment. A similar sort of GE interaction was found for father occupation (**Figure 3c**): environmental effects were greater at both the high and the low genetic extremes.

We also found a significant GE interaction for the fourth environmental measure, maternal education (**Figure 3d**). However, this GE interaction represents a different sort of interaction, one that is compatible with recent findings from quantitative genetics suggesting that genetic effects on g are weaker for families with lower socioeconomic status. The result for maternal education is compatible with this finding: the association between SNP set and g is weakest for families with the least-educated mothers.

What about GE correlation? As noted earlier, GE correlation refers to the correlation between genes and environment. In contrast to GE interaction, which concerns environmental moderation of the association between the SNP set and g, GE correlation focuses on the extent to which the environment mediates the association between the SNP set and g. Such mediation requires that the environmental measure correlate with the SNP set and also correlate with g. Because the environmental measures were chosen for their correlation with g, the simplest GE correlation analysis was conducted, which was merely to correlate the environmental measures with SNP set scores, rather than conducting more formal mediation analyses. Both proximal measures of the family environment (harsh parental discipline and family chaos) were correlated significantly with the SNP set for g, suggesting GE correlation. It is interesting that the distal measures of family environment (father's occupation and mother's education) showed no GE correlation. Of the three types of GE correlation (passive, evocative, and active), finding GE correlation for distal environmental variables would be most easily characterized as passive GE correlation: the children's family environments would be correlated with their genetic propensities because their parents share the same genes. In contrast, these analyses suggest that GE correlation is stronger for proximal environments, implying evocative (reactive) GE correlation: children evoke reactions based on their genetic propensities.

In summary, there is evidence for both GE interaction and GE correlation in early development. One final caveat is that GE interactions may result from GE correlations under certain circumstances; true GE interaction should remain significant after controlling for GE correlation.

Future QTL Research on GE Interplay

In addition to using QTLs identified on the basis of their main effect in order to investigate GE interaction and correlation, future research on GE interplay will profit from identifying QTLs that contribute to GE interaction and correlation regardless of their main effect. In the previous example, SNPs were identified based on their association with g (regardless of environment) by comparing SNP allele frequencies for low versus high g groups. **Figure 4** shows a simple two-by-two interaction design in which cases are selected based on low versus high environmental stress as well as on low versus high g. Using DNA pooled separately for the four groups, QTL associations representing the main effect of the QTL on g regardless of environment stressors can be detected by comparing groups 1 and 2 versus groups 3 and 4. The important advantage of this design is that GE correlation and GE interaction can also be detected independent of their contribution to the main effect. GE correlation can be assessed as the main effect of the environment, comparing groups 1 and 3 versus groups 2 and 4, thus identifying QTLs that are associated with low versus high environmental stress. Finally, GE interaction can be detected by comparing the diagonals (groups 1 and 4 versus groups 2 and 3).

The future of research on genotype-environment interaction and correlation looks bright, especially as the G in GE increasingly comes to represent genes in molecular genetic analyses rather than genotypes in quantitative genetic analyses.

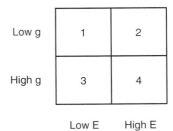

Figure 4 Identifying QTLs on the basis of GE interaction and correlation. Using four, rather than two, DNA pools will facilitate these studies. For example, comparing SNP allele frequencies for pools 1 and 2 versus pools 3 and 4 tests for a main effect for g. Comparing pools 1 and 3 versus 2 and 4 reveals GE correlation, a QTL association with E. Comparing pools 1 and 4 versus 2 and 3 assesses GE interaction, a QTL association for g that depends on E.

See Also the Following Articles

Animal Models (Nonprimate) for Human Stress; Antisocial Disorders; Depression and Manic-Depressive Illness; Dopamine, Central; Economic Factors and Stress; Education Levels and Stress; Environmental Factors; Familial Patterns of Stress; Genetic Factors and Stress; Genetic Predispositions to Stressful Conditions; Learning and Memory, Effects of Stress on; Life Events Scale; Major Depressive Disorder; Serotonin; Social Status and Stress; Social Support.

Further Reading

Asbury, K., Wachs, T. and Plomin, R. (2005). Environmental moderators of genetic influence on verbal and nonverbal abilities in early childhood. *Intelligence* 33, 643–661.

Butcher, L. M., Meaburn, E., Liu, L., et al. (2004). Genotyping pooled DNA on microarrays: A systematic genome screen of thousands of SNPs in large samples to detect QTLs for complex traits. *Behavior Genetics* 34, 549–555.

Butcher, L. M., Meaburn, E., Knight, J., et al. (2005). SNPs, microarrays, and pooled DNA: identification of four loci associated with mild mental impairment in a sample of 6000 children. *Human Molecular Genetics* 14, 1315–1325.

Caspi, A., McClay, J., Moffitt, T. E., et al. (2002). Role of genotype in the cycle of violence in maltreated children. *Science* 297, 851–854.

Caspi, A., Sugden, K., Moffitt, T. E., et al. (2003). Influence of life stress on depression: Moderation by a polymorphism in the 5-HTT gene. *Science* 301, 386–389.

Cooper, R. M. and Zubek, J. P. (1958). Effects of enriched and restricted early environments on the learning ability of bright and dull rats. *Canadian Journal of Psychology* 12, 159–164.

Harlaar, N., Butcher, L., Meaburn, E., et al. (2005). A behavioural genomic analysis of DNA markers associated with general cognitive ability in 7-year-olds. *Journal of Child Psychology & Psychiatry* 46, 1097–1107.

Henderson, N. D. (1972). Relative effects of early rearing environment on discrimination learning in housemice. *Journal of Comparative and Psychological Psychology* 72, 505–511.

Meaburn, E., Butcher, L. M., Liu, L., et al. (2005). Genotyping DNA pools on microarrays: tackling the QTL problem of large samples and large numbers of SNPs. *BMC Genomics* 6, 52.

Plomin, R. (1977). Genotype–environment interaction and correlation in the analysis of human behavior. *Behavior Genetics* 7, 83.

Plomin, R. (1994). *Genetics and experience: the interplay between nature and nurture.* Thousand Oaks, CA: Sage Publications Inc.

Plomin, R. and Crabbe, J. C. (2000). DNA. *Psychological Bulletin* 126, 806–828.

Plomin, R., DeFries, J. C., McClearn, G. E., et al. (2001). *Behavioral genetics* (4th edn.). New York: Worth Publishers.

Rowe, D. (2003). Assessing genotype–environment interactions and correlations in the postgenomic era. In: Plomin, R., DeFries, J. C., Craig, I. W. & McGuffin, P. (eds.) *Behavioral genetics in the postgenomic era,* pp. 71–86. Washington, D.C.: American Psychological Association.

General Adaption Syndrome (GAS) *See:* Alarm Phase and General Adaptation Syndrome; Selye, Hans.

Genetic Factors and Stress

C A Koch and C A Stratakis
National Institute of Child Health and Human Development, Bethesda, MD, USA

This article is reproduced from the previous edition, volume 2, pp 205–211, © 2000, Elsevier Inc.

Genes Regulating the Stress System
Stress Effects in Prokaryotes and Eukaryotes
Summary

Glossary

Allele	Alternative forms of a gene at a given locus.
Apoptosis	Programmed cell death inducible by DNA damage that exceeds the capacity of repair mechanisms.
Chaperone	Any protein that binds to an unfolded or partially folded target protein, thus preventing misfolding, aggregation, and degradation of the target protein and facilitating its proper folding.

DNA polymerase	The enzyme responsible for replication of DNA, which is accomplished by using each complementary strand of the DNA double helix as a template for the synthesis of a new strand.
Epistasis	The situation in which expression of one gene obscures the phenotypic effects of another gene.
Fitness	A measure of fertility and therefore of the contribution to the gene pool of the succeeding generation; for a given genotype, the number of offspring surviving to reproductive age is relative to the number of wild-type genotypes.
Genotype	The genetic constitution of an individual or the alleles at specific genetic loci.
Heavy chain-binding protein (bip)	A protein discovered by its interaction with the heavy chain of IgG antibodies in the endoplasmatic reticulum, keeping proteins unfolded and preventing misfolding.
Homology	Similarities between newly derived sequences and previously determined sequences.
Intron	A segment of a gene that is initially transcribed into RNA but is then removed from the primary transcript by splicing together the exon sequences on either side of it; intronic sequences are not found in mature mRNA.
Phenotype	The observed result of the interaction of the genotype with environmental factors.
Pleiotropy	The diverse effects of a single gene or gene pair on several organ systems and functions.
RNA primer	A short RNA sequence that is paired with one strand of DNA and provides a free 3' OH end at which a DNA polymerase starts the synthesis of a deoxyribonucleotide chain.

Stress is the response of the cell or the organism to challengers of homeostasis (a dynamic state of balance between the stress response and the stressors). Homeostasis is essential for the preservation of life. In humans and other higher organisms, components of the stress system include various neurotransmitters and hormones, which in most species constitute the effectors of the hypothalamic-pituitary-adrenal (HPA) axis. Thus, the cholinergic and catecholaminergic systems, corticotropin releasing hormone (CRH), arginine vasopressin, adrenocorticotropic hormone (ACTH), and the glucocorticosteroids are all essential parts of the stress system in higher organisms.

At the cellular level, the major players are different but still analogous to the effectors of the HPA axis: the DNA repair system, the heat shock proteins (hsp), and the products of many housekeeping genes that aim at maintaining homeostasis. In order to find genes that have a role in the regulation of the stress system in humans, it is essential to look at the effects of stress at all levels of development. This article reviews the effects of stress on various systems and notes the role of genetics in each one of them.

Genes Regulating the Stress System

Genetic loading can be described as follows. An individual with large innate susceptibility needs only a minor degree of internal or external stressors to reach the threshold for symptom expression and vice versa. The prevalence of psychosomatic symptoms among members of the same family suggests the existence of a genetic predisposition. When the fingerprints of 155 adult patients with psychosomatic abdominal pain since childhood were examined for congenital markers, digital arches were found in 64% of patients, compared to 10% of controls without abdominal pain. Genetic factors play an important role in the pathogenesis of psychiatric illnesses. The location of potential genes of interest for manic-depressive/bipolar disorder, a state of profound stress, has been summarized by Wahlstrom.

Role of the Corticotropin Releasing Hormone Gene and Other Components of the Hypthalamic-Pituitary-Adrenal Axis

CRH plays a key role in the regulation of the stress response with the CRH receptor type-1 (CRH-R1) as mediator. CRH-R1 is highly expressed in the anterior pituitary, neocortex, hippocampus, amygdala, and cerebellum. The activation of this receptor stimulates adenylate cyclase. CRH-R1-deficient mice show an impaired stress response as indicated by the absence of increased ACTH and corticosterone levels following stress.

Although acute and long-standing internal or external conflicts/stressors predispose to depression, a state associated with stress and elevated glucocorticosteroid levels, the CRH gene on human chromosomal region 8q13 is not linked to manic-depressive/bipolar disorder. Other components of the HPA axis have also been tested for linkage. On chromosome 5, the glucocorticoid receptor gene and the genes for β_2- and α_1-adrenergic receptors were excluded as candidates for manic-depressive disorder based on parametric lod score analyses. Mutation analysis in the gene for the adrenocorticotropin receptor located on chromosome 18p11.2 was negative. In addition, parametric methods of analysis excluded the area of the proopiomelanocortin gene on chromosome 2 for linkage to bipolar disorder.

Role of the Tyrosine Hydroxylase Gene

Another component of the stress system is the catecholaminergic system. Tyrosine hydroxylase (TH) catalyzes the rate-limiting step in catecholamine synthesis. The TH gene is regulated by an array of biochemical mechanisms in response to environmental factors. In animals, a long-term increase of TH activity can be elicited by electrical stimulation and environmental stress or drugs such as reserpine. In humans, the involvement of the TH locus in manic-depressive disorder is supported by association studies. However, the precise genes with a causative role in bipolar disorder are not yet known. It is possible that a particular variant of the tetrarepeat located in the first intron of the TH gene plays a role. Studying mechanisms of regulation of TH gene expression in rats showed the existence of stressor specificity and stressor-specific pathways. In rats exposed to cold or insulin stress, adrenal denervation (splanchnecotomy) prevented a rise in adrenal medullary TH mRNA levels, whereas immobilization-induced stress led to an increase in TH mRNA levels, suggesting that genetic changes in TH may indeed affect the stress response.

Role of Dopamine Receptors

The main effects of dopamine on the central nervous system include locomotion and behavior. Forebrain dopamine systems are involved in mediating the behavioral effects of chronic mild stress. At present, five subtypes of dopamine receptors are known and are classified as D1-like and D2-like, according to their similarity to the first and second cloned receptor. D1-like receptors are encoded by intronless genes and D2-like receptor genes are divided by intron sequences, suggesting that dopamine receptors have evolved from two main ancestral genes.

D1 receptors are predominant in the basal ganglia such as the nucleus accumbens and are involved in a prolactin stimulatory pathway in response to high environmental temperature stress. D1 receptor-deficient mice fail to thrive after weaning, with selective impairment of motivated behavior, including drinking and eating. These mice also demonstrated that the D1 receptor is important in drug addiction and reward mechanisms. The role of dopamine D1 receptor actions in reducing the function of the prefrontal cortex (a higher cognitive center) has been shown in various studies, including the infusion of a dopamine D1 receptor agonist in the prefrontal cortex, which induced cognitive deficits similar to those seen in stress. Increased catecholamine receptor stimulation in the prefrontal cortex leads to stress-induced working memory deficits, which can be ameliorated by agents that prevent catecholamine release or that block dopamine receptors.

Mice lacking D2 receptors have an impaired reproductive function. Alterations of the D3 receptor function may play a role in behavioral disorders associated with hyperactivity, such as attention deficit hyperactivity disorder, a disease of prefrontal cortex dysfunction.

Stress Effects in Prokaryotes and Eukaryotes

Effects of Stress on Life History Traits in *Drosophila*

In natural populations, there may be significant genetic variation for stress resistance and life history traits. Different genotypes may respond differently to environmental stress, and the variation in these norms of reaction may be of great importance to the maintenance of genetic variation in metabolic traits. Each physiological response may be mediated by different genes in different individuals. Similarity between parents and progeny may be altered if the genes that contribute to variation in a trait in one environment do not contribute in another environment. Responses of life history traits to selection may depend on environmental conditions in different ways. Heritabilities for morphological traits are more constant than for life history traits.

Interestingly, selection for stress resistance can alter many traits. In selected lines of *D. melanogaster* undergoing stress, including starvation, heat, radiation, and ethanol and acetic acid exposure, a decrease in metabolic rate, early fecundity, and early behavioral activity, as well as an increase in male longevity, occurred. In *D. simulans,* desiccation resistance was associated with resistance to starvation and toxic ethanol. In *D. serrata,* selection for desiccation resistance also resulted in an increased resistance to starvation. When *D. melanogaster* and *D. simulans* were selected for increased cold intolerance, cross-generational effects were detected in all lines with marked effects of selection on early fecundity. Selected lines in both species showed reduced fecundities specifically associated with the selection response.

However, not all responses to stressful conditions are associated with correlated changes in life history traits. For instance, selection for increased knockdown resistance to heat in *D. melanogaster* led to lines that were two- to fivefold more resistant to this stress. This selection response did not alter life history traits and was associated with allelic changes in two heat shock genes, suggesting that such genes may have specific effects on stress resistance and do not necessarily have life history costs.

These findings show that responses to stress can have many secondary effects unrelated to stress. Organisms under permanent stressful conditions may be expected to show life history changes that reduce their fitness under more favorable conditions. Many trait values seen in natural populations may reflect the effects of infrequent stressful conditions. The overall fitness of an individual that is unable to survive an infrequent stress will be zero, regardless of performance under normal conditions. The complexity of pleiotropic effects and epistatic interactions contribute to the likelihood that genotype and environment interactions play an important role in the maintenance of genetic variation.

Effects of Stress on Phenotype

In animals, most populations experience at least sporadically stressful conditions and change drastically in size when studied over long intervals. Environmental changes such as sudden climate changes can have many indirect effects, including competitive interactions and susceptibility to diseases. Animals developed many mechanisms for coping with sudden environmental shifts. For example, rapid changes at the cellular level involving the synthesis of enzymes and heat shock proteins occur in response to most stresses. Extreme conditions can influence the expression of phenotypic variability and the extent to which this variability is determined genetically. For instance, in *D. melanogaster* stress can produce abnormal morphological characteristics when the flies are exposed to stresses early in their development. However, the experimentally induced extreme conditions used to generate these mutant phenotypes probably do not exist under field conditions, and the resulting morphological peculiarities such as ultrabithorax in *Drosophila* would probably not survive in nature.

Effects of Cellular Stress on Genotype

Genetic variants may result from the ability of cells to repair damaged DNA or from the limited accuracy of the cellular machinery for DNA replication. By means of the fluctuation test, Luria and Delbrück attempted to clarify whether bacterial mutants arise spontaneously or specifically in response to a particular kind of stress. They concluded that genetic variants do originate randomly and without selective pressure. However, the possibility that, in addition to spontaneous mutants, genetic variants might have been induced by selective pressure was not excluded in that experiment; it was investigated and confirmed by Cairns in 1988. The degree of variation between parents and progeny differs enormously with different forms of life, depending on the stability of the living conditions.

Under nonstress conditions, variants predominantly result from replication errors. Eukaryotic organisms possess four (yeast, and probably other lower eukaryotes) or five (higher eukaryotes) different DNA polymerases. Cells do not need to assure a high accuracy of RNA primer synthesis because mistakes occurring during primer synthesis do not contribute to the mutation rate. Cells possess a battery of enzyme systems for DNA repair to avoid the loss of integrity of DNA genomes. The DNA repair system evolved to restore the original status of the damaged genome structure and to improve the ability of the cell to survive. However, some of the DNA repair processes are error-prone and are therefore important sources of genetic variants. In response to DNA breaks, recombination–repair mechanisms may construct a genome in an order that is different from the original. A cell will, naturally, rather survive as a variant than be killed as the original. Repairing DNA under the condition of prolonged stress may induce more genetic variants than absolutely necessary, as shown in starving bacterial cells that developed induced replication-independent mutants of selective advantage in the face of inhibited proliferation and threatened survival of the population. During severe stress, multiple mutations occur at high rates in cells that survived the hypermutable state with extensive DNA damage.

Effects of Stress on Heat Shock Gene Regulation and in Human Disease

Heat shock proteins: history Heat shock proteins were first described in 1962 when the chromosomes of the giant salivary gland of *D. busckii* were exposed to an elevated temperature that resulted in areas of swelling on the chromosome known as puffs. These puffs indicated transcriptionally active genes that were found to belong to the hsp family. The hsp are called molecular chaperones because they bind to unfolded proteins and thereby prevent the aggregation and misfolding of these proteins during cell stress.

Over the following years, stress protein research attracted the attention of basic and clinical investigators in many disciplines. Among other topics, studies on stress proteins include gene expression and the complex signal transduction pathways that control the regulation of stress genes; other studies focus on the role of stress proteins as molecular chaperones that regulate various aspects of protein folding and transport and on the role of stress proteins in human disease.

Heat shock proteins: function   Via the heat shock response as a homeostatic mechanism, cells are able to survive exposure to extreme environmental stress. Thermally induced stress proteins can also protect cells against other stresses that themselves induce stress protein synthesis. Such cross-protection is known as cross-tolerance.

The elevated synthesis of a few proteins following exposure to heat or other stressful stimuli, including ischemia; anoxia; hypoxia; cytokines; and certain drugs such as vasopressin, isoproterenol, and calcium channel blockers, occurs in all organisms ranging from prokaryotic bacteria such as *Escherichia coli* to mammals, including humans. After the genes encoding these stress proteins had been cloned, other genes encoding related stress proteins were identified based on their homology. Subsequently, many stress proteins were found to be encoded by multigene families encoding proteins with similar but distinct features. Major eukaryotic stress proteins are usually referred to as hsp with a number that reflects the molecular mass in kilodaltons, for example, hsp70 (**Table 1**).

Based on their molecular mass, the hsp are subdivided into two groups: large and small hsp. Small hsp possess a domain of homology to αA,B-crystallin proteins from the vertebrate eye and are less conserved than large hsp. Small hsp caught the attention of researchers because these proteins are able to induce protection against various toxic chemicals and interfere with inflammatory mediators. Cell death usually occurs by two distinct processes: necrosis and apoptosis. Small hsp protect cells against stress-induced necrosis and can also prevent differentiating cells from apoptosis. Therefore, small hsp participate in essential physiological processes in unstressed cells. There are at least 4 major small hsp in *Drosophila*, 3 in mammalian cells and yeast, and more than 20 in plants. Although small hsp in plants are represented by at least two multigene families, the small hsp27 in humans is encoded by a single gene located on chromosome 7.

There seems to be a link between small hsp expression and tumorigenicity. Several cancer cell lines, including breast cancer, were found to show changes in the expression of mammalian hsp25/27. Small hsp expression is also considered a prognostic parameter of some human tumors. For instance, in patients with breast cancer or osteosarcoma the expression of hsp27 is associated with a poor outcome.

Many of these stress proteins are also expressed in normal, unstressed cells, indicating that the function of hsp is likely to be required in normal cells but more so in stressed cells. Because this function has been conserved in evolution, it seems to be very important in all cells ranging from bacteria to humans. A large body of evidence shows that the primary role of the majority of hsp is creating the proper folding of other proteins in order to enable these proteins to fulfill their appropriate functions. Stressed cells produce aberrant proteins that are folded improperly and sometimes too abnormal to be refolded properly. For such situations, some stress-inducible proteins, such as the hsp ubiquitin, are involved in protein degradation.

Among the first genes that are transcribed from the embryonic genome are genes encoding stress proteins such as hsp90, emphasizing the importance of the complex regulatory processes of the stress proteins in normal and stressed cells.

Table 1   Eukaryotic stress proteins

Family	Member	Functional role	Comment
Ubiquitin	Ubiquitin	Protein degradation	In the nucleus found conjugated to histone H2A
Hsp27	Hsp27, Hsp26, etc.	Actin-binding proteins, protein folding	In different organisms very variable in size (12–40 kDa) and number
Hsp47	Hsp47	Protein folding of collagen and possibly other proteins	Homology to protease inhibitors
Hsp56	Hsp56 (=FKBP59)	Protein folding, in the steroid receptor complex associated with hsp90 and hsp70	Peptidyl prolyl isomerase activity, target of immunosuppressive drugs
Hsp60	Hsp60	Protein folding and mycobacterial unfolding, organelle translocation	Major antigen of many bacteria and parasites that infect humans
Hsp70	Hsp70, Hsc70, Hsx70, Grp78 (=Bip)	Protein folding and unfolding, assembly of multiprotein complexes	Hsx70 only in primates
Hsp90	Hsp90, Grp94	Maintenance of proteins such as steroid receptors in an inactive form until appropriate	*Drosophila* and yeast proteins known as hsp83
Hsp100	Hp104, Hsp100	Protein turnover	ATPase activity, role in tolerance to extreme temperature

The specific transcription factor heat shock factor 1 (HSF1) induces stress protein genes after exposure to heat or other stresses and exists in an inactive (monomeric) form in unstressed cells. The regulation of these stress protein genes in response to nonstressful stimuli or in normal cells remains to be elucidated.

Stress proteins seem to be essential for the survival of cells and organisms. Thus far in mammals there is no knockout mouse lacking specific hsp genes. In *Drosophila* and in yeast, the inactivation of the hsp90 gene turned out to be lethal. However, it is possible that the inactivation of an individual stress protein gene is not lethal in all cases if genetic and functional redundancy are present. If, however, the function of a specific family of stress proteins is completely eliminated, survival is unlikely.

Heat shock proteins and chaperones show specific expression patterns during development and cell differentiation as well as during aging. hsp genes do not act as developmental genes to direct development along one pathway or another. Rather, as important partners in differentiation, cell division, and apoptosis, hsp act at the cellular level to regulate development.

The maintenance of homeostasis in mammals is achieved by many mechanisms, including the release of cytokines in response to stressful challenges. It is well known that, via interleukin-6, tumor necrosis factor α and interleukin-1 activate the HPA axis, including the CRH neuron. Cytokines are redundant and functionally pleiotropic. By activating specific transcription factors that bind and transactivate hsp genes, cytokines are also capable of inducing stress proteins/hsp, such as hsp90, hsp70, and hsp27 (**Table 2**).

Mild stress, sufficient to induce hsp, could protect cells against a subsequent, more severe stress. Transgenic animals overexpressing hsp70 showed an enhanced resistance to cardiac ischemia. In the clinical setting, studies are underway to identify drugs that could induce the synthesis of stress proteins in a nonstressful manner and to find ways to deliver stress protein genes to damaged organs *in vivo* using gene therapy procedures.

On the other hand, the enhanced expression of stress proteins may play a role in many different human diseases. Several studies report that the synthesis of stress proteins is induced by stress caused by disease; this appears to be stress protein- and disease-specific. For instance, hsp90 is specifically overexpressed in a subset of patients with systemic lupus erythematosus, whereas the expression of other stress proteins is unaffected. General or specific overexpression of stress proteins can evoke an autoimmune response that leads to the production of antibodies or T cells that recognize these proteins and possibly cause a damaging immune response. Such immune responses to individual stress proteins, especially to hsp60, have been described in rheumatoid arthritis, multiple sclerosis, and diabetes mellitus type 1.

hsp90 is one of the most abundant proteins in eukaryotic cells. It makes up 2% of total cellular protein even under nonstress conditions and is highly evolutionary conserved with homologs in bacteria, yeast, *Drosophila*, and humans. hsp90 is needed for cell survival, as demonstrated by mutation analysis in yeast. hsp90 is important for the function of steroid receptors and perhaps certain viral oncogenic kinases. The hsp gp96, hsp90, and hsp70 isolated from tumors were able to immunize and elicit protective immunity specifically against the tumors from which the hsp were isolated. The hsp isolated from normal tissues were found to elicit immunity to any cancers tested. hsp96 molecules are not immunogenic per se but act as carriers of antigenic peptides. The hsp90 family may be a novel target for anticancer drug development such as vaccines, especially because cancer cells are very sensitive to the pharmacological disruption of hsp90 function.

Exciting work in yeast is centered around conformational alterations in prionlike proteins, which are believed to cause neurodegenerative diseases in humans, including Creutzfeld–Jacob, mad cow disease, and possibly even Alzheimer's. The delineation of an evolutionary-conserved chaperone related to hsp70 whose expression changes in response to environmental stress has been found to control the inheritance of a yeast prionlike element (release factor Sup35) called PSI. Further studies of this complex non-Mendelian genetic system may elucidate how the cellular response to stress may cause disease.

Summary

Stress, a state of threatened homeostasis, leads to an individual stress response that is subserved by the

Table 2 Candidate genes

Transcription factors	Glucocorticoid receptor, mineralocorticoid receptor, androgen receptor, estrogen receptor, progesterone receptor, aryl hydrocarbon receptor, heat shock factor 1, mutated p53
Protein kinases	Tyrosine kinases (Src family, sevenless, weel, p185), serine/threonine kinase (Raf-1/v-Raf, casein, heme-regulated eIF-2α, CDK4/CDK6, MEK)
Other proteins	Cytoskeletal proteins (tubulin, actin, intermediate filaments), calmodulin, proteasomes, G-protein βγ subunit

stress system(s). Each physiological response may be mediated by different genes in different individuals, perhaps explaining why the same/similar internal and external stressors affect individuals in different ways. This is complicated by the complexity of pleiotropic effects and the interactions between genotype and environment that contribute to the maintenance of genetic variation. At the molecular and cellular level, stress evokes the synthesis of enzymes and overexpression of certain genes, many of which encode heat shock/stress proteins. These stress proteins are expressed not only in stressed cells but also in normal cells underlining their essential function. For instance, a functional ubiquitin pathway that helps eliminate damaged proteins in the cytosol, nucleus, and endoplasmatic reticulum is an essential feature of the stress response in eukaryotes as well as of unstressed cells. All cells have multiple ubiquitin genes, each of which encodes a fusion between ubiquitin and another protein. In line with Aristotle's *in medias res* (everything in moderation), it appears that individuals and, at the molecular and cellular level, cells exposed to too much stress or to no stress at all have a shorter longevity than cells and individuals that are coping with mild stress sufficient to induce protective factors such as hsp against subsequent more severe stresses.

See Also the Following Articles

Apoptosis; Chaperone Proteins and Chaperonopathies; Dopamine, Central; Drosophila Studies; Heat Shock Proteins: HSP60 Family Genes.

Further Reading

Accili, D., Drago, J. and Fuchs, S. (1998). Dopamine receptors in human disease: lessons from targeted mouse mutants. In: Spiegel, A. M. (ed.) *Contemporary endocrinology: G proteins, receptors, and disease*, pp. Totowa, NJ: Humana Press.

Cairns, J., Overbaugh, J. and Miller, S. (1988). The origin of mutants. *Nature* 335, 142–145.

Clark, A. G. and Fucito, C. D. (1998). Stress tolerance and metabolic response to stress in *Drosophila melanogaster*. *Heredity* 81, 514–527.

Jenkins, N. L., Sgro, C. M. and Hoffmann, A. A. (1997). Environmental stress and the expression of genetic variation. *EXS* 83, 79–96.

Kvetañnský, R., Pacak, K., Fukuhara, K., et al. (1995). Sympathoadrenal system in stress: interaction with the hypothalamic-pituitary-adreno-cortical system. *Annals of the. New York Academy of Sciences* 771, 131–158.

Latchman, D. S. (ed.) (1999). *Handbook of experimental pharmacology: stress proteins*. Berlin: Springer.

Luria, S. and Delbrück, M. (1943). Mutations of bacteria from virus sensitivity to virus resistance. *Genetics* 28, 491–511.

Newnam, G. P., Wegrzyn, R. D., Lindquist, S. L., et al. (1999). Antagonistic interactions between yeast chaperones hsp104 and hsp70 in prion curing. *Molecular and Cellular Biology* 19, 1325–1333.

Stratakis, C. A., Sarlis, N. J., Berrettini, W. H., et al. (1997). Lack of linkage between the corticotropin-releasing hormone gene and bipolar affective disorder. *Molecular Psychiatry* 2, 483–485.

Thor, A., Benz, C., Moore, D., et al. (1991). Stress response protein (srp-27) determination in primary human breast carcinomas: clinical, histologic, and prognostic correlations. *Journal of the National Cancer Institute* 83, 170–178.

Timpl, P., Spanagel, R., Sillaber, I., et al. (1998). Impaired stress response and reduced anxiety in mice lacking a functional corticotropin-releasing hormone receptor 1. *Nature Genetics* 19, 162–166.

Uozaki, H., Oriuchi, H., Ishida, T., et al. (1997). Overexpression of resistance-related proteins (metallothioneins, glutathione-S-transferase, heat shock protein 27 and lung resistance-related protein) in osteosarcoma. *Cancer* 79, 2336–2344.

Wahlstrom, J. (ed.) (1998). *Genetics and psychiatric disorders*. New York: Elsevier Science.

Wintersberger, U. (1991). On the origins of genetic variants. *FEBS Letters* 285, 160–164.

Genetic Modifications of Stress Response   *See:* Genetic Factors and Stress; Genetic Predispositions to Stressful Conditions; Gene Environment Interactions in Early Development; Genetic Variation of HPA Axis Activity and Function in Farm Animals; Genetic Polymorphisms in Stress Response; Genetic Testing and Stress.

Genetic Polymorphisms in Stress Response

I W Craig
King's College London, London, UK

Genes and the Stress Responses
Polymorphisms of Genes in the Autonomic Stress
   Response Pathway
Polymorphisms of Genes in the Neuroendocrine Stress
   Response Pathway
Loci Whose Polymorphisms Interact with Stressful
   Influences in Mediating Behavioral Outcomes
Conclusion

Glossary

Allele	One of two or more possible forms of a gene. An individual may possess two identical or two different alleles, except for the genes on the X-chromosome in males (they possess only a single copy of this chromosome).
Body mass index (BMI)	A measure of body fat based on height and weight that applies to both adult men and women.
Case/control studies	Comparisons between groups of individuals with particular features or disorders and groups apparently normal for these aspects; often employed to search for differences in the genotype or allele frequencies between the two groups.
Genotype	The configuration of alleles at a genetic locus. If both alleles are identical the individual is homozygous; if the two alleles differ the individual is heterozygous.
Haplotype	The pattern of alleles at two or more polymorphic sites represented on one of the chromosome homologs.
Intragenic feature	A feature located within the conventional boundaries of a gene.
Kilobase (kb)	One thousand base pairs.
Linkage disequilibrium	The existence of combinations of alleles at two or more polymorphic sites within a region at frequencies greater than expected by random assortment.
Missense mutation	A base change in the coding region of the gene that results in the substitution of one amino acid in the encoded protein for another.
Polymorphism	The existence at gene locus of more than one allele with the rarest at appreciable frequency (usually assumed to be >1%) in the population.
Promoter	The section of DNA that precedes a gene and controls its activity.
Single nucleotide polymorphism (SNP)	A polymorphism at a single base position in DNA.
Stressor	Stimulus input that creates stress and initiates a response.

Genes and the Stress Responses

The genetic basis for the stress response is complex; nevertheless, the genes involved can be divided into two broad categories: those encoding the autonomic reaction to stressful situations and those involved in the neuroendocrine stress response. The typical rapid reactions to perceived stress are well recognized to be associated with the fight-or-flight response and are mostly mediated by the sympathetic nervous system with the release of norepinephrine from widely distributed synapses and epinephrine from the adrenal medulla. Implicit in this classic description of the rapid stress response is the recognition of the potential violent and aggressive outcomes that stress can engender. A more delayed response is mediated by the release of cortisol, the major glucocorticoid in humans. This is initiated by neural signals to the hypothalamus that releases corticotropin releasing hormone (CRH), which in turn results in the release of adrenocorticotropic hormone (ACTH) from the anterior pituitary, thereby stimulating cortisol production by the adrenal cortex. The production of cortisol assists in restoring homeostasis in response to stress; however, prolonged exposure can be potentially harmful.

Reactions to acute stress are also usually accompanied by perturbations of serotinergic activity, as indicated by altered levels of serotonin (5-HT) or its metabolites. Serotonin is a significant regulator of morphogenetic activities during early central nervous system development, including cell proliferation, migration, and differentiation.

Outcomes following exposure to stress may, therefore, be highly variable depending on a wide range of genetic factors controlling these various aspects. A simplified overview of some of the most important elements of stress response and relevant genes is shown in **Figure 1**. The significance of genetic variation in the better-characterized components of the stress response pathways is considered next. Several case/control studies have examined the association between genes involved in the stress response and somatic

The stress pathway and selected gene polymorphisms

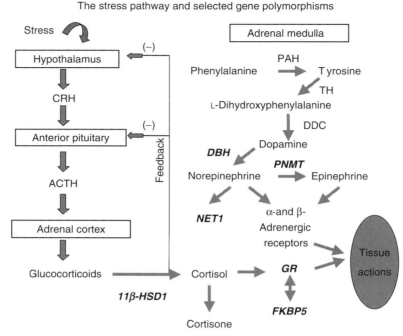

Figure 1 The stress pathway illustrating selected genes (in bold italics). 11β-HSD1, 11-β-hydroxysteroid dehydrogenase enzymes; ACTH, Adrenocorticotropic hormone; GR, glucocorticoid receptor; CRH, corticotropin releasing hormone; DBH, dopamine β-hydroxylase; DDC, DOPA decarboxylase; FKBP5, glucocorticoid receptor co-chaperone; NET1, norepinephrine transporter; PAH, phenylalanine hydroxylase; PNMT, phenylethanolamine *N*-methyl transferase; TH = tyrosine hydroxylase. α- and β-Adrenergic receptors include ADRA1A, ADRA1B, ADRA1D, ADRA2A, ADRA2B, ADRA2C, ADRB1, ADRB2, and ADRB3.

or behavioral traits. Some of these are noted; however, it is important to recognize that there are potential confounding factors to such studies and only consistent replication and supporting molecular evidence can establish the formal verification of such links.

Polymorphisms of Genes in the Autonomic Stress Response Pathway

The rapid stress response to stressful stimuli is mediated by the release of norepinephrine in the brain. This leads to the activation of the sympathetic nervous system and the adrenal medulla with release of epinephrine in the blood. Hence, the genes regulating the biogenesis and degradation of both epinephrine and norepinephrine and those encoding their cognate receptors are key players in the primary stress response. The epinephrine and norepinephrine metabolic pathways share components with those for other neurotransmitters. The steps in the synthesis of epinephrine from amino acid precursors are illustrated in **Figure 1**. The last two critical steps are undertaken by the enzymes dopamine β-hydroxylase (DBH) and phenylethanolamine *N*-methyl transferase (PNMT).

Dopamine β-Hydroxylase

The dopamine β-hydroxylase gene *(DBH)* is located on chromosome 9. A SNP in the presumed controlling region of *DBH*, which results in the substitution of a C to T substitution 1021 bp before the transcription start, accounts for up to 50% of the variance in plasma levels of the enzyme. Other variants flanking, or within, the potential promoter region include a polymorphism that depends on the copy number of an intragenic dinucleotide repeat approximately 4 kb upstream of the transcription start and a 19-bp insertion/deletion located 118 bp upstream.

In addition several SNPs have been reported within the coding region. Of these, an arginine to cysteine substitution in exon 11 has been suggested to be the most likely functionally significant variant. Several studies have linked a variation in plasma levels and *DBH* genotypes to various physiological and behavioral disorders, including hypertension, psychosis, depression, migraine, attention deficit hyperactivity disorder, and alcoholism. These reported associations await replication and consolidation.

There are also reports of individuals with undetectable levels of norepinephrine and epinephrine, together with elevated levels of dopamine. Such individuals have low, or absent, circulating DBH enzyme caused by deleterious mutations affecting both copies of the *DBH* gene and manifest a range of symptoms, including orthostatic hypotension.

Although alterations to this key enzyme in the synthetic pathway for norepinephrine and epinephrine are likely to have significant consequences for the stress response, no specific behavioral or physiological features relating to the reactions to stressors *per se* have been reported.

Phenylethanolamine *N*-Methyl Transferase

The gene for PNMT, a key enzyme, is located on chromosome 17. Two SNPs that may affect the regulation of the gene have been identified in the promoter. When tested in case/control studies, significant association was observed between these and early-onset, but not late-onset, versions of Alzheimer's disease, and there are data suggesting a possible association between these SNPs and hypertension in African American groups. In addition, there is evidence suggesting that a variant of this gene may be associated with blood pressure regulation abnormalities in the stroke-prone, spontaneously hypersensitive rat strain.

Norepinephrine and Epinephrine Receptors

The adrenergic receptors for epinephrine and norepinephrine are divided into two major classes, alpha (subdivided into α1 and α2) and beta (subdivided into β1, β2, and β3). These receptors are targeted by a variety of drugs, including the so-called beta-blockers; hence genetic variation in them may be an important feature for pharmacotherapy. The activation of the β-adrenergic receptors stimulates adenylate cyclase.

α1-Adrenergic receptors   The α1-adrenergic receptors are G-coupled trans-membrane receptors that are capable of binding both epinephrine and norepinephrine and thereby mediate some aspects of the sympathetic nervous system. The genes encoding them include *ADRA1A* (formerly known as *ADRA1C*, on chromosome 8), *ADRA1B* (formerly known as *ADRA1*, on chromosome 5) and *ADRA1D* (formerly known as *ADRA1A*, on chromosome 20). Of these, *ADRA1B* is of particular interest because fine mapping with highly polymorphic markers localizes it to a region that also contains the dopamine receptor gene *DRD1A*. Because this chromosome region has been linked to variability in systolic blood pressure, genetic variation in either *ADRA1B* or *DRD1A*, or both, may play an important role in influencing interindividual differences in this feature; however, specific functional variants in these have yet been described.

α2-Adrenergic receptors   The release of norepinephrine is controlled by negative feedback from α2-adrenergic receptors, which are located on the presynaptic side of nerve terminals, including nerve muscle junctions. The targets of the released norepinephrine on heart muscle cells (myocytes) are β1-adrenergic receptors. The individual roles of the three highly homologous α2-adrenergic receptors (ADRA2A, ADRA2B, and ADRA2C, encoded by genes located in humans on 10, 2, and 4, respectively) have been studied by gene disruption in mice. Both ADRA2A and ADRA2C subtypes were found to be required for the normal presynaptic control of transmitter release from sympathetic nerves in the heart and from central noradrenergic neurons. In addition, a small deletion (base pairs 322–325) in the *ADRA2C* gene in humans has been shown to decrease function and may act in concert with the beta-receptor gene *ADRB1* as a risk factor for heart attack.

A polymorphism leading to the deletion of three glutamic acid residues from a repeating motif in the third intracellular loop of *ADRA2B* has been associated with variations in basal metabolic rate.

β-Adrenergic receptors   β1-Adrenergic receptors encoded by the gene *ADRB1* (also known as *ADRB1R*, located on chromosome 10) are present in heart, and their stimulation causes an increase in heart rate. Many beta-blockers act on these targets (and on β2 receptors to a lesser extent). One variant of the β1-adrenergic receptor gene, which changes an arginine at position 389 in the protein to glycine, has been shown to possess increased function in tissue culture. There is also a polymorphic variant of a small deletion (base pairs 322–325) in the gene for the α2C-adrenergic receptor, *ADRA2C*, that has decreased function. A marked increase in the risk of heart failure among black patients has been observed for those who are homozygous for this and the *ADRB1* variant. This suggests that genotyping of these two genes may be a useful approach for identifying people at risk for heart failure. Further support for an interaction between these two genes has been provided by recent studies indicating that ADRA2A and ADRB1 proteins form heterodimers when expressed in tissue culture cells. In Caucasian women, it has been observed that the arg389 allele of *ADRB1* was associated with greater body weight and BMI.

β2-Adrenergic receptor   Several polymorphic variants have been described, the most common and significant of which is a substitution causing a change from glycine to arginine at position 16. β2-Adrenergic receptor agonist drugs are widely employed in the treatment of asthma. It is therefore of interest that an excess of the glycine allele has been observed in nocturnal asthmatics. It appears that this substitution imparts enhanced agonist-promoted downregulation of the receptor.

A second polymorphism is centered on amino acid 27, where a glutamine to glutamic acid replacement is observed. An association with obesity has been reported, with an excess of the glutamine version in nonobese individuals. Possible links of this variant with asthma have also been noted.

A third variant involving a threonine to isoleucine replacement at amino acid 64 exists at lower frequencies. This has a profound functional consequence that results in a fivefold reduction in sensitivity to β2-receptor agonist-mediated vasodilatation. This suggests a mechanistic explanation of decreased survival in patients carrying this variant.

β3-Adrenergic receptor The β3-adrenergic receptor, ADRB3, is located mainly in adipose tissue and for this reason has been studied in relation to obesity. A mutation resulting in the substitution of arginine for tryptophan at amino acid position 64 has been observed at a frequency of approximately 10%. Many studies have examined the relationship of the polymorphism to obesity, BMI, and noninsulin-dependent diabetes mellitus, with some concluding that the locus may have a role in predisposing these phenotypes; but other studies have failed to replicate the observations.

Norepinephrine Transporter

The norepinephrine transporter protein 1 (NET1) is also known as the norepinephrine transporter (NAT1) or the solute carrier family 6, member 2 (SLC6A2). The gene responsible is localized on chromosome 16. Approximately 80% of the reuptake of norepinephrine is mediated at nerve terminal synapses by the norepinephrine transporter. SLC6A2 is a target for the tricyclic antidepressants, including imipramine and desipramine and also for amphetamines and cocaine.

Following a report of SNP in the restriction site for the enzyme *Taq*I, a number of detailed investigations have revealed a range of rare mutations associated with orthostatic intolerance and more than 20 polymorphisms, some of which resulted in missense substitutions; however, no association with behavioral disorders were observed in the case/control studies. An insertion/deletion polymorphism of 4 bp in one of several AAGG repeat motifs in the promoter region at a position overlapping a transcription factor binding site has been reported, and there is some evidence supporting an association between the presence of the insertion and restricting anorexia nervosa. Rare genetic variants encoding a transporter with reduced affinity for norepinephrine have also been described. Carriers have been observed to manifest clinical symptoms (orthostatic intolerance) and metabolic evidence for disordered uptake of norepinephrine.

In summary, studies on the genes implicated in autonomic norepinephrine and epinephrine pathways have demonstrated the potential for a great deal of interindividual diversity. The consequences of this have major impact on a wide variety of disorders, including several with direct or indirect links to stress. Other autonomic pathways are mediated through acetylcholine release and detection.

Polymorphisms of Genes in the Neuroendocrine Stress Response Pathway

Further sources of genetic diversity in individual reactions to stress are the genes implicated in the delayed response of the hypothalamus-pituitary-adrenal (HPA) axis, leading to the release of cortisol from the adrenal cortex initiated by neural signals to the hypothalamus. Other genes are involved in the subsequent mobilization of hypothalamic peptide hormones (including CRH), resulting in the secretion of ACTH from the anterior pituitary and the release of glucocorticoid hormones (cortisol) from the adrenal cortex. Glucocorticoids are produced by the adrenal cortex and restore homeostasis in response to stress; however, prolonged exposure resulting from chronic stressful occurrences is potentially harmful. Cortisol (the most prominent glucocorticoid in humans) or corticosterone (in rats) is largely bound to corticosteroid-binding globulin in the systemic system. It has a classic steroid hormone mode of action via binding to a cognate intracellular receptor (the glucocorticoid receptor) and subsequent migration to the nucleus, where the complex interacts with a specific gene transcription apparatus. The loss or profound diminishment of glucocorticoid secretion leads to a state of deranged metabolism and an inability to deal with stressors, which, if untreated, is fatal. Functional genetic polymorphisms in some important genes of this pathway are recognized.

The Glucocorticoid Receptor

Two specific corticoid receptors are recognized: the glucocorticoid receptor (GR) and the mineralocorticoid receptor (MR). Whereas the latter binds aldosterone and glucocorticoids with similar high affinity, GR is selective for the glucocorticoids. It appears that the main response to raised levels of steroids resulting from stress is mediated primarily by GRs. There have been several polymorphisms described for the *GR* gene, including one in the promoter region. Because there is strong linkage disequilibrium across the gene, there are relatively few different combination of allelic patterns, with four major haplotypes recognized. Knowledge of the haplotype may help determine the response to glucocorticoid treatments. Variants within the coding region include two polymorphisms at adjacent codons for the amino acids 22 and 23 in the protein. Whereas the base change at codon 22 does not change the amino acid (glutamic acid), the polymorphism at codon 23 results in a change from arginine to lysine. Individuals with a specific combination of alleles at the promoter site and the codon 22–23 sites have an associated relative resistance to glucocorticoids. A further polymorphism resulting in a change from asparagine to serine at codon 363 appears to be associated with hypersensitivity to glucocorticoids. A *Bcl*I restriction enzyme polymorphism has also been employed in case/control studies, and there is evidence for an association with hypersensitivity to glucocorticoids that may be related to lower BMI in older individuals.

A wide variety of membrane-bound GRs have been reported in a range of tissues including the liver, lymphocytes, adrenal gland, and pituitary. There is a paucity of information concerning any structural features distinguishing these various forms, and there are no data on how any genetic variation may affect them, other than through changes affecting the GR itself. Significantly, however, the GR function depends on interactions with several components of a large molecular complex. Five co-chaperones of GR are recognized as significant in regulating its activity, and they are encoded by the following genes:

- *BAG1* – BCL2-associated anthanogene 1
- *STUB1* – STIP 1 homologous and U box-containing protein 1
- *TEBP* – Thyroid transcription factor 1 (TITF1)
- *FKBP4* – FK-506 binding protein 4
- *FKBP5* – FK-506 binding protein 5

A recent analysis of SNPs in these genes found three within the *FKBP5* locus to be significantly associated with the increased recurrence of symptom episodes in depressed patients and a rapid response to prescribed antidepressant treatment. Evidence for this apparent association was strengthened by genotyping a range of additional SNPs within and flanking the gene. One marker in particular (rs1360780) seems to track the tightness of the control of glucocorticoid signaling and HPA axis reactivity mediated by the reported interaction of the GR and FKBP5.

11-β-Hydroxysteroid Dehydrogenase Enzymes

Glucocorticoids are metabolized by the 11β-hydroxysteroid dehydrogenase enzymes (11β-HSD1). There are at least two forms of 11β-HSD1: type I (HSD11B1) and type II (HSD11B2). Both catalyze the conversion of cortisol to cortisone; however, the type I enzyme also catalyses the reverse reaction. Both are therefore important in the stress response. The HSD11B2 enzyme inactivates 11-hydroxysteroids in the kidney, the circumventricular organ of the brain, and some other tissues, thus protecting the nonselective MR from occupation by glucocorticoids. A base change confers a restriction-fragment-length polymorphism (detected by the enzyme *Alu*I) in exon 3 of this gene. This variant and a polymorphic microsatellite marker of the *HSD11B2* gene having 12 alleles have been employed to compare salt-sensitive (SS) and salt-resistant (SR) individuals in otherwise nonhypertensive white males. Homozygosity for one of the microsatellite alleles was higher in SS subjects than in SR subjects and the cortisol-to-cortisone ratios were higher in homozygous subjects than in the corresponding control subjects. It is possible that the decreased HSD11B2 activity observed in SS subjects reflects its involvement in the SS blood pressure response in humans and that variants of the gene contribute to different blood pressure responses to salt in humans.

Loci Whose Polymorphisms Interact with Stressful Influences in Mediating Behavioral Outcomes

The Serotonin Transporter

One particularly interesting connection between the perception of stress response and the serotinergic system is through the serotonin transporter, which removes the neurotransmitter from the synaptic cleft. The serotonin transporter (SERT, 5-HTT) plays a pivotal role in brain 5-HT homeostasis. It is also the initial target for both antidepressant drugs and drugs of abuse, some of which are potent neurotoxins. In humans, the gene for the transporter (variously designated as *SERT*, *HTT* or *SLC6A4*) is characterized by functional variants in the promoter region conferring high or low activity in expression of the locus. Several studies have linked variations of the two predominant alleles with anxiety response. Caspi and colleagues were the first to show that it appears that individuals with the low activity are more vulnerable to stressful life events and more likely to become clinically depressed as a result. Glatz and colleagues, in 2003, suggested a possible connection between stress and the serotonin system. They were able to demonstrate that a potent glucocorticosteroid hormone, dexamethasone, stimulates the expression of *SERT* in tissue culture at physiological concentrations. The hormone interacts with the promoter in an allele-specific manner, and this interaction may help to explain the differential vulnerability of individuals who are more susceptible to stressful experiences.

Monoamine Oxidase Type A

A similar picture emerges for variation of another gene involved in the serotonin system, the gene for monoamine oxidase type A, *MAOA*. Although this enzyme also has a role in metabolizing other neurotransmitters, including dopamine, drugs inhibiting its activity have long been employed in the treatment of behavioral disorders (particularly depression) and are thought to work through altering 5-HT levels. There are two major variants in the promoter of this gene that confer either high or low activity. Because the gene is X-linked, males exhibit either one or the other phenotype without complications from the presence of a second allele. There is a consensus view emerging that males who have the low-activity form of the gene are more sensitive to the effects of maltreatment and presumptive stressful environment manifested by their increased risk of antisocial behaviour and aggression. The high-activity form of the gene appears to provide protection against this outcome.

Conclusion

The response of individuals to stress varies considerably and depends on a wide range of environmental experiences, together with cognitive and genetic factors. Considerable progress has been made in characterizing some of the genes in the pathways relevant both to the fight-or-flight response and to those involved in the release and detection of glucocorticoid hormones. Many of the most significant changes to such genes are rare mutations. There are in addition, however, several variants of genes that are widely distributed in the population, and, although their impact may not be directly observable as an altered stress response, they may have important consequences with respect to a range of complex disorders including hypertension and allergic reactions. Furthermore, recent studies have shown common variants in the key enzymes involved in 5-HT metabolism (MAOA and SERT) can interact with stressful life experience to predispose individuals to manifesting antisocial behaviour or depression. Variants in several other related genes have subsequently also demonstrated an interaction with stress in predicting behavioral outcomes.

Further Reading

Caspi, A., McClay, J., Moffitt, T. E., et al. (2002). Role of genotype in the cycle of violence in maltreated children. *Science* **297**, 851–854.

Caspi, A., Sugden, K., Moffitt, T. E., et al. (2003). Influence of life stress on depression: moderation by a polymorphism in the 5-HTT gene. *Science* **301**, 386–389.

Cubells, J. F. and Zabetian, C. P. (2004). Human genetics of plasma dopamine β-hydroxylase activity: applications to research in psychiatry and neurology. *Psychopharmacology* **174**, 463–476.

Dionne, I. J., Garant, M. J., Nolan, A. A., et al. (2002). Association between obesity and a polymorphism in the beta-1-adrenoceptor gene (gly389arg ADRB1) in Caucasian women. *International Journal of Obesity* **26**, 633–639.

Small, K. M., Wagoner, L. E., Levin, A. M., et al. (2002). Synergistic polymorphisms of beta-1- and alpha-2C-adrenergic receptors and the risk of congestive heart failure. *New England Journal of Medicine* **347**, 1135–1142.

Stober, G., Nothen, M. M., Porzgen, P., et al. (1996). Systematic search for variation in the human norepinephrine transporter gene: identification of five naturally occurring missense mutations and a study of association with major psychiatric disorders. *American Journal of Medical Genetics: Neuropsychiatric Genetics* **67**, 523–532.

van Rossum, E. F. C., Koper, J. W., van den Beld, A. W., et al. (2003). Identification of the *Bcl*I polymorphism in the glucocorticoid receptor gene: association with sensitivity to glucocorticoids *in vivo* and body mass index. *Clinical Endocrinology* **59**, 585–592.

van Rossum, E. F. C., Roks, P. H. M., de Jong, F. H., et al. (2004). Characterization of a promoter polymorphism in the glucocorticoid receptor gene and its relationship to three other polymorphisms. *Clinical Endocrinology* **61**, 573–581.

Wüst, S., van Rossum, E. F. C., Federenko, et al. (2004). Common polymorphisms in the glucocorticoid receptor gene are associated with adrenocortical responses to psychosocial stress. *Journal of Clinical Endocrinology and Metabolism* **89**, 565–573.

Relevant Websites

Online Mendelian inheritance in man and Entrez SNP database, http://www.ncbi.nlm.nih.gov.

Genetic Predispositions to Stressful Conditions

D Blackwood and H Knight
University of Edinburgh, Edinburgh, UK

This article is a revision of the previous edition article by D Blackwood, volume 2, pp 212–217, © 2000, Elsevier Inc.

How Genes and Stressful Events Can Interact
Measuring Life Events
Twin Studies of Exposure to Stress
Molecular Genetic Approaches

Glossary

Genes	It is estimated the human genome contains approximately 30,000 genes distributed on the 23 pairs of human chromosomes, and about one-third of genes are expressed in the brain. Each gene is the specific DNA code for a protein.
Genetic association studies	Studies designed to detect differences in the frequencies of DNA polymorphisms in a group of individuals with a particular phenotype contrasted with a group of control subjects from the same population.
Genetic polymorphism	The occurrence of two or more variants (alleles) of DNA sequence in a population. There are many types of sequence variation in the human genome, including single nucleotide polymorphisms (SNPs), microsatellites, deletions, and insertions that have proved valuable for locating genes in human disease using linkage and association strategies. A well-known example of genetic polymorphisms is those giving rise to the proteins of the ABO blood groups.
Genotype	The complete genetic composition of an organism.
Life events	Events usually measured by a trained interviewer using standardized interview schedules to obtain a record of events over a stated time. The inventory is likely to cover common and major events, including financial and marital problems, bereavement, ill health, employment change and infringements of the law. Some investigators separate the effects of different classes of life events, for example, an independent event such as a close friend being involved in an accident is contrasted with the subject him- or herself being in an accident, an event over which the subject may have some control or which directly threatened him or her.
Phenotype	The physical expression of the genotype.
twin studies	In genetic research, studies based on the fact that identical (monozygotic, or MZ) twins have exactly the same genes and nonidentical (dizygotic, or DZ) twins share on average 50% of their genes. Both types of twins share similar environments. In characteristics that are genetically determined, MZ twin pairs are more alike (concordant) than DZ pairs, whereas MZ and DZ concordance rates are similar in phenomena due solely to environmental influences.

It has often been taken for granted that anxiety and depression are the natural consequences of stressful events such as sudden bereavement, loss of a job, or marital disharmony and that stresses in childhood such as those related to poor parenting, physical or emotional abuse, or loss of a family member may have an impact on behavior well beyond childhood. However, many early studies of the effects of stressful situations on behavior have not taken into account the effects of genes. It is now abundantly clear that genetic factors play an important and sometimes major role in many human behaviors, personality dimensions, and the development of specific patterns of illness.

How Genes and Stressful Events Can Interact

Kendler and Eaves gave a detailed account of three models to explain how genes and the environment can interact to cause psychiatric illness. These models also help us understand how genetic influences and stressful events interact in everyday life not necessarily associated with psychiatric symptoms. They form a useful basis for discussing a number of recent empirical studies.

The first and simplest model hypothesizes that symptoms of anxiety and depression are the result of the addition of genetic and environmental contributions. This assumes that people, regardless of their genotype, will respond in the same way to an environmental stress, and the probability of being exposed to a stress is independent of genetic background. This model has been the basis of much research in social psychiatry and has, for example, highlighted the importance of early loss and poor social support as risk factors for the development of depression during adulthood in women. Such a direct causal link between environmental challenges and behavior is illustrated by the normal physiological and behavioral response to a life-threatening situation that is often termed the fight-or-flight response. However, the assumption that environmental stresses and genotype act independently does not explain the empirical observation that some individuals appear to be more sensitive than others to stressful life events.

A second model proposes that genes influence the individual's response to stressful events in the environment. The experience of life events differs widely between individuals and is related to personal characteristics including self-esteem, social support, mood, and personality traits. An example might be that individuals with high scores on neuroticism (a trait that is in part genetically determined) respond to loss or personal threat differently than those with low scores on neuroticism. Animal studies provide an example of how gender differences influence response to stress. Shors and colleagues have reported that the effect of acute stress on memory in rats differs between males and females; the degree of retrograde amnesia or enhanced memory depends on the sex of the animal. This suggests that the genetic differences between the sexes may underlie the expression of different stress response strategies.

Environmental control of the expression of genes is illustrated by animal studies showing that the stress of maternal separation during early development influences the growth of specific brain structures, leading to changes in adult behaviors. Different strains of animals respond differently to early stress, confirming a genetic background to the response. Under this model, however, genotype and environment are not correlated. The model accounts for the influence of genetic factors on the response of an individual to stressful events, but it does not include an effect of genes on the probability that a person will be exposed to stressful environmental situations.

A third, and in many ways the most interesting, model states that a person's genotype alters the probability that he or she will be exposed to a stressful environment. Genes and environment do not act independently, but are correlated. In effect, individuals throughout their lives select the level of environmental stress to which they are exposed. Specific stressful events such as road traffic accidents and injuries at work relate to a number of factors, including personality, drug and alcohol intake, and psychiatric illness. A common but indirect example is a person who is alcoholic and exposed to the consequences of heavy drinking. Since alcoholism is partly a heritable condition, as shown by family twin and adoption studies, one of the effects of the genes that increase risk of drinking behavior is also to increase exposure of the alcoholic to a range of stressful life events, including marital difficulties, assaults, road traffic accidents, and homelessness. Genes may also influence how a person recalls, perceives, and reports on their experiences of stressful life events.

Measuring Life Events

Over the past 30 years the concept of life events has been developed and refined as a means to study the effects of stressful conditions in the environment on human behavior and psychopathology. Scales such as the Social Readjustment Rating Scale of Holmes and Rahe were developed to be used as a measure of an individual's exposure to environmental stress and have become well-researched tools in social psychiatry. However, the reporting of life events may be influenced indirectly by genetic factors. One of the first studies to address the issue of how life event reporting is governed by social and other factors was carried out in New Zealand by Fergusson and Horwood, who obtained information on life events exposure including financial problems, marital problems, bereavement, ill health, and employment changes over a 6-year period for over 1000 women. The results made it clear that reporting stressful events was not random, and two major determinants of vulnerability to reporting life events were the level of social disadvantage of the woman and her level of trait neuroticism derived from the Eysenk Personality Inventory. Women of socially disadvantaged backgrounds and women with high neuroticism scores consistently reported high exposure to life events over the 6-year period.

Twin Studies of Exposure to Stress

Twin studies that include the comparison of monozygotic (identical) and dizygotic (nonidentical) twin pairs provide a powerful means to quantify the relative contributions to human behaviors of genetic and environmental factors. Rigorous statistical analysis including correlations between twin pairs permits calculation of variance due to genetic factors and shared and individual environments. If a twin experiences a life event that is entirely random and not influenced by his or her personal characteristics, we would not expect the co-twin to show increased likelihood of experiencing a similar event. The co-twin would have the same risk as the general population. If shared family environment was responsible for the life event, both MZ and DZ twins would share an equally increased exposure. If genetic factors contribute to the event, MZ twins will show greater concordance than DZ twins for that variable because they have more genes in common.

Kendler, in a study of more than 2000 twin pairs selected from the population in Virginia, found clear evidence that reported life events were influenced by both genetic and environmental factors. There was a significant familial resemblance for reported total life events: the correlations for MZ twins (0.43) and DZ twins (0.31) both differed significantly from zero ($p < 0.001$), and the correlation for monozygotic twins consistently exceeded that for dizygotic twins. These results support the view that personality characteristics increase the probability of experiencing stressful life events. The genetic effect was observed only when life events were divided into those that affected the individual directly (personal events), for example, if the individual was in a car accident, as opposed to events involving someone else (network events), for example, if a close relative was in a car accident. Personal events included marital difficulties, being robbed or assaulted, interpersonal difficulties, financial problems, illness or injury, and legal problems, and these were all significantly influenced by genetic factors that explained nearly 20% of the variance. Shared environment had little effect on personal events. In contrast, network events affecting other people were not influenced by genetic factors, and the similarities between twins were entirely attributable to shared family environment. It is understandable that personal events should be under some degree of genetic control, since these events are dependent on the person's behavior whereas net work events are not.

This twin study confirmed that the occurrence of stressful life events is more than just bad luck. A combination of familial and genetic influences may predispose the individual to create for themselves a high-risk environment leading to a complex relationship between life events and stress-related disorders. In a further analysis of the female twins from the Virginia Twin Registry, Kendler and Karkowski-Shuman demonstrated that the genetic liability for depression in these twins was associated with an increased risk for stressful life events that included assault, marital problems, job loss, serious illness, financial problems, and social difficulties with relatives and friends. In the same twin sample, the genetic liability to alcoholism was related to the risk of being robbed and having trouble with the police. One of the ways that genes contribute to psychiatric illness is probably by causing individuals to select themselves into high-risk environments. Silberg, in a study of juveniles from the Virginia Twin Registry, proposed a model whereby depression in girls is partly influenced by genes that mediate adverse life events, and the influence of genes on life events is not stable but increases during adolescence.

Lyons specifically examined how genes influenced exposure to combat trauma in a study of more than 4000 male twin pairs who had served in the Vietnam War. A range of data was collected, including volunteering for service in Vietnam, actual service, a composite index of combat experiences, and the award of combat decorations. Correlations within twin pairs for actually serving in Vietnam were 0.41 (MZ) and 0.24 (DZ), and those for combat experiences were 0.53 (MZ) and 0.3 (DZ). These figures generated an estimate of heritability of 35 to 47%. The family environment had no significant effect on any of the variables, and the results are unlikely to be due to biases from self report because being awarded a combat medal gave similar correlations. The differences between MZ and DZ twin pairs show that exposure to combat is partly heritable and is not influenced by the socioeconomic status of the family of origin. A number of factors could influence combat experience, including the personality trait of novelty seeking, which is known to be genetically determined. Individuals scoring high on novelty seeking will be more likely to volunteer for active service. Similarly, genetic traits that increase the likelihood of a person suffering physical and psychiatric illnesses will act to decrease the likelihood that the person will seek out and experience exposure to trauma in combat.

A twin study by Stein extended these observations to noncombat situations in a study of 400 Canadian civilian twin pairs rated for exposure to trauma and symptoms of posttraumatic stress disorder (PTSD). Seventy-five percent of these twins reported experience of trauma that could be divided into assaultive (robbery or sexual assault) and nonassaultive (road traffic accident or natural disaster). Analysis of heritabilities showed that genetic effects contributed to risk of exposure to assaultive but not nonassaultive trauma, and there was a correlation between genetic effects and PTSD symptoms. It was concluded that many of the same genes that influence exposure to assaultive trauma appear to influence susceptibility to PTSD symptoms in their wake.

Studies of twins have provided important evidence that genetic predisposition has an important role in stress-related activity and the experience of stressful life events ranging from engagement in wartime combat to exposure to assault in civilian life. It is also clear that genetic factors influence how people respond to stress, explaining why some people and not others develop symptoms of PTSD. How these genetic influences are mediated is not known, but a variety of mechanisms have been proposed.

Molecular Genetic Approaches

We can now be fairly sure that a person's complement of genes strongly influences personality traits, but it is highly unlikely that in due course a gene for neuroticism or any other personality dimension will be uncovered. It is more probable that these traits are determined by a number of genes, and the inheritance of different variants of these genes will lead to the particular traits in a manner that has long been familiar to animal breeders.

Complex phenotypes including human personality characteristics are often termed quantitative traits because a number of different genes are thought to act additively in a quantitative manner to produce the phenotype. The genes contributing to the additive effect are termed quantitative trait loci (QTL). The terms polygenic (caused by many additive or interacting genes) and multifactorial (caused by many genes interacting with environmental factors) have also been used to describe the same situation in which a complex phenotype is under a variety of genetic influences. The completion of the sequencing of the human genome, followed by the Hapmap project, which catalogued hundreds of thousands of normal DNA sequence variants (polymorphisms) present at high-density across the genome, have given researchers unrivalled tools for detecting genes contributing to inherited human diseases and complex behavioral traits. Linkage studies use many markers on each of the 23 pairs of chromosomes to identify the small DNA region that is inherited along with a particular disease or trait within a particular family. Another approach for identifying genes contributing to monogenetic disease or complex disorders is to study very large cohorts of subjects rated for a particular quantitative trait and compare the frequency of selected DNA polymorphisms between cases and a matched sample of controls recruited from the same population. Association studies are used to study candidate genes or small selected regions of a chromosome previously identified by family linkage analysis. Candidate genes coding for proteins in neurotransmitter pathways, including the serotonin (5-HT) and dopamine systems, have been the focus of particular attention because these neurotransmitters are known from animal and clinical studies to play an important role in regulating mood and a variety of behaviors relevant to traits of impulsiveness, sensation seeking, and addictive behavior. The neurotransmitter 5-HT is an important regulator of early brain development, and 5-HT neurons play known roles in integrating emotion, cognition, and motor function. Genes related to 5-HT are good candidates for a role in human personality, and the 5-HT transporter gene apparently influences a constellation of traits related to anxiety and depression. Individuals who carry a common small deletion in the promoter region of the 5-HT transporter gene are more susceptible to depression. A possible role for the transporter gene as a mediator of the effects of environmental stress on moods was described by Caspi in a study of a New Zealand birth cohort of individuals. At the age of 26, these individuals were assessed for symptoms of depression and anxiety, and self-reported life events occurring in the previous 5 years were recorded. To address the question of why stressful experience leads to depression in some people and not in others, the 5-HT transporter gene was studied and a crucial difference was observed between individuals who became depressed after experiencing stress and those who were tolerant of stress. Those who became depressed were more likely than nondepressed individuals to carry a small deletion on the promoter region of the gene. This raises the possibility that different variants of the 5-HT promoter gene could moderate how a person is going to react to adverse life experiences.

The neurotransmitter dopamine, like 5-HT, is distributed widely in the nervous system and has a range of functions, including the modulation of mood. It is of considerable interest that a receptor in the dopamine family (DRD4) may influence novelty-seeking behavior. In a study described by Noble, a person who inherits one variety of the DRD4 receptor appears to be more likely to rate highly when assessed for novelty seeking. The same trait was also more common in boys with one particular set of variants in the DRD2 gene. However, the combined DRD4 and DRD2 polymorphisms contributed more markedly to novelty-seeking behavior than when these two gene variants were individually considered. Substantially more needs to be done to unravel the complex relations between stress and symptoms in populations, and it is likely that many more candidate genes will be examined by these methods in large populations to try to detect gene–environment interactions.

Neurotransmitter function is just one of many possible areas of gene–environment interaction providing a link between chronic stress and ill health. An entirely different approach was reported by Epel and colleagues, who investigated the effects on cellular aging of chronic psychological stress experienced by a group of mothers looking after a chronically ill child. They found a significant association between perceived stress and shorter telomere length in peripheral blood mononuclear cells. Telomeres are regions at the ends of each chromosome. It has been noted that telomere length becomes progressively shorter in cells as they age. In this study, the women who reported the highest levels of emotional stress had, on average, shorter chromosome telomeres than the women who looked after children without disability. Thus, reduced telomere length due to increased oxidative stress in the cell, a determinant of longevity of cells, was associated with perceived psychological stress. It was striking that telomere shortening in women presumed to be under the most stress was shorter on average by an amount equivalent to 10 years of aging compared to low-stress women.

Another area of current interest is how genetic factors during prenatal development and childhood may exert an influence on the way the adult responds to stress several decades later. Welberg and Seckl have extensively reviewed the role of steroids and the hypothalamic-pituitary-adrenocortical (HPA) axis as a system involved in prenatal programming in the brain. In animal studies, prenatal stress leads to long-lasting effects on the HPA axis function in adult offspring, in general programming a persistently hyperactive system and producing clear alterations in the animals' behavior and response to stressful situations. Adult rats exposed to prenatal stress show an increase in behaviors reminiscent of human anxiety. Extrapolation from animal studies to human situations requires extreme caution. However, in a number of clinical studies poor maternal nutritional status in pregnancy and low birth weight were correlated with increased blood pressure, obesity, and glucose intolerance later in life. A possible link between such early life stress and altered behavior or psychopathology in the offspring once they reach adulthood remains an interesting conjecture, and steroids in the HPA axis are the focus of considerable research as possible mediators of such a link.

See Also the Following Articles

Gene Environment Interactions in Early Development; Genetic Factors and Stress; Life Events and Health.

Further Reading

Brown, G. V. and Harris, T. O. (1993). Aetiology of anxiety and depressive disorders in an inner-city population 1. Early adversity. *Psychological Medicine* 23(1), 143–154.

Epei, E. S., Blackburn, E. H., Lin, J., et al. (2004). Accelerated telomere shortening in response to life stress. *Proceeding of the National Academy of Sciences USA* 101(49), 17312–17315.

Gaspi, A., Sugden, K., Moffitt, T. E., et al. (2003). Influence of life stress on depression: moderation by a polymorphism in the 5-HTT gene. *Science* 301(5631), 386–389.

Kendler, K. S., Neale, M., Kessler, R., Heath, A. and Eaves, L. (1993). A twin study of recent life events and difficulties. *Archives of General Psychiatry* 50(10), 789–796.

Kendler, K. S. and Karkowski-Shuman, L. (1997). Stressful life events and genetic liability to major depression: genetic control of exposure to the environment? *Psychological Medicine* 27(3), 539–547.

Lvons, M. J., Goldberg, J., Eisen, S. A., et al. (1993). Do genes influence exposure to trauma? A twin study of combat. *American Journal of Medical Genetics* 48(4), 22–27.

Mormede, P., Courvoisier, H., Ramos, A., et al. (2002). Molecular genetic approaches to investigate individual variations in behavioral and neuroendocrine stress responses. *Psychoneuroendocrinology* 27(5), 563–583.

Noble, E. R., Ozkaragoz, T. Z. and Ritchie, T. L. (1998). D2 and D4 dopamine receptor polymorphisms and personality. *American Journal of Medical Genetics* 88(3), 257–267.

Seedat, S., Niehaus, D. J. and Stein, D. J. (2001). The role of genes and family in trauma exposures and posttraumatic stress disorder. *Mol Psychiatry* 6(4), 360–362.

Shors, T. J. (2004). Learning during stressful times. *Learning and Memory* 11(2), 137–144.

Silberg, J., Pickles, A., Rutter, M., et al. (1999). The influence of genetic factors and life stress on depression among adolescent girls. *Archives of General Psychiatry* 56(3), 225–232.

Stein, M. B., Jang, K. L., Taylor, S., Vernon, P. A. and Livesley, W. J. (2002). Genetic and environmental influences on trauma exposure and posttraumatic stress disorder symptoms, a twin study. *American Journal of Psychiatry* 159(10), 1675–1681.

Veenema, A. H., Meijer, O. C., de Kloet, E. R. and Koolhaas, J. M. (2003). Genetic selection for coping style predicts stressor susceptibility. *Journal of Neuroendocrinology* 15(3), 256–267.

Welberg, L. A. and Seckl, J. R. (2001). Prenatal stress, glucocorticoids and the programming of the brain. *Journal of Neuroendocrinology* 13(2), 113–128.

Genetic Testing and Stress

V Senior and M Cropley
University of Surrey, Guildford, UK

Overview of Genetic Testing
Stress and Uptake of Genetic Testing
Emotional Impact of Genetic Testing
Cognitive Appraisal of Genetic Testing

Glossary

Autosomal recessive condition	A genetic condition in which both copies of a gene need to be faulty in order for the specific condition to develop.
Carrier testing	A test to identify whether an individual has one copy of the faulty genes that contribute to an autosomal recessive condition.
Human genome project	An international collaboration to map the entire human genome.
Mutation	An inherited change in a sequence of DNA.
Predictive genetic testing	A test to identify whether an asymptomatic individual has a genetic mutation that predisposes him or her to developing a specific disease.

Overview of Genetic Testing

The knowledge generated by the Human Genome Project has already started to revolutionize our understanding of health and illness. It is now possible to identify people who have a genetic predisposition to an increasing number and variety of diseases. This knowledge offers great potential for disease prevention, developing more effective treatments, and, indeed, the hope of treating diseases that are currently incurable. This new understanding of the human genome also brings with it a whole host of ethical, social, and psychological dilemmas. Although genetic testing for certain conditions means that those at risk can reduce their chances of developing the disease, for other conditions genetic testing means that some people have to live with the knowledge that they are almost certain to develop an incurable disease. Genetic testing has implications for decisions about whether to have children and who to have them with, what to do if a fetus is known to have a genetic disease, and whether individuals will be discriminated against when seeking employment or insurance.

In this article, we focus on the role of stress in predictive genetic testing. This is because most of the well-conducted psychological evaluations conducted to date that assess stress using validated measures concerned predictive genetic testing. Also, in other forms of genetic testing, such as carrier testing, the psychological issues primarily concern decisions about pregnancy and childbirth. Carrier testing is concerned with identifying people who have a copy of a deleterious mutation for an autosomal recessive condition. These people do not develop the disease in question, but if they have children with someone who is also a carrier of the mutation, each child has a 25% chance of having the condition. Examples of these conditions are Tay–Sachs disease, sickle cell disease, and cystic fibrosis. Predictive genetic testing is concerned with identifying people who are at high risk of developing the disease themselves. All of the predictive genetic tests currently available raise different medical, psychological, and ethical issues.

One of the first genetic tests developed was for Huntington disease, an incurable neurodegenerative condition that typically develops in middle age or later life. People who carry the mutation definitely develop Huntington disease at some point, and those who do not carry the mutation definitely do not develop the disease. There is understandable concern that offering at-risk families genetic testing will constitute an enormous psychological burden for those who test positive. There are a number of exemplary longitudinal studies conducted worldwide to evaluate the consequences of genetic testing for these families. There are also an increasing number of psychological evaluations of genetic testing for a predisposition to cancer, particularly breast and ovarian cancer but also forms of colon cancer. In these cases, the psychological issues include the stress that may be associated with being found to be a carrier of a predisposing mutation and behavioral responses to genetic risk information. These behaviors include whether people adhere to recommendations about surveillance to detect possible cancers and also decisions about whether to have surgery to remove tissues likely to be affected prior to the development of any cancer (called prophylactic surgery). In the case of an inherited predisposition to cancer, being a carrier of a mutation increases the cancer risk considerably, typically making the likeliness of developing cancer 60–80%, but it does not make cancer inevitable. In addition, those found not to carry the genetic mutation still have at least the same risk as the general population of developing cancer, which means it is important that these people do not believe they are not at risk. For other diseases, genetic testing is still in its infancy. For example, it is possible to offer predictive genetic testing for the predisposition to coronary heart disease and Alzheimer's disease. In the case of coronary heart disease, predictive genetic testing can be offered for familial hyper-cholesterolemia, an inherited predisposition to raised cholesterol levels. Because the treatment for this condition, in the form of cholesterol-lowering statin medication, is very effective, the psychological issues raised pertain particularly to preventative behavior, that is, whether those identified adhere to medication regimens and engage in other risk-reducing behaviors such as eating a low-fat diet and not smoking. Like Huntington disease, Alzheimer's disease is not curable at present. However, genetic testing for Alzheimer's indicates whether an individual has an increased risk for the disease rather than providing the information that an individual definitely will or will not go on to develop it. In this case, it is necessary for those undergoing testing to understand quite complicated probabilities.

Genetic testing programs differ in how they are organized. In some cases, everyone within a particular population may be offered genetic testing. Such population-based screening programs are most common for detecting carriers of recessive genes and for the prenatal and neonatal screening of infants. More common among predictive genetic testing programs is some form of cascade screening. These programs start with an individual who either has the disease or is at known risk (called the proband) and, if a deleterious mutation is identified in this individual, genetic testing is then offered to other biological relatives.

All these factors have an impact on the emotional state, risk perceptions, and expectations of those offered genetic testing and receiving the results of genetic tests. An interactional model of stress is widely accepted within the stress community, whereby stress is conceptualized as a process involving an interaction of individuals and their environment. One such example is the transactional model of stress and coping proposed by Lazarus and Folkman in the 1980s. Using this framework, we address three main questions with respect to genetic testing: does stress influence the decision to have a genetic test, is receiving the results of genetic testing stressful, and does genetic testing influence secondary appraisal processes and coping strategies? Each of these issues is now considered in turn.

Stress and Uptake of Genetic Testing

It is widely recognized that feelings of stress about health lead people to be more likely to engage in risk-reducing behaviors such as stopping smoking, taking exercise, and adopting a healthy diet. The picture with regard to disease-detecting behaviors, of which having a genetic test is one example, is less clear cut. Disease-detecting behaviors are actions that can inform the individual whether they have or are likely to develop a particular disease but that, in themselves, do not change the disease or risk status of the individual. Similar to models of stress and behavioral performance in nonhealth domains, it has been proposed that a certain amount of perceived stress motivates the performance of disease-detection behaviors. However, high levels of perceived stress are thought to lead to a greater likelihood of fear-control strategies and the subsequent avoidance of the behavior.

Only a proportion of those offered genetic testing will decide to have the test. There are a wide variety of factors influencing this decision, including the disease being tested for and whether treatment is available, sociodemographic factors, and the expectations and motivations of the individual. Whether greater perceived stress facilitates or inhibits the uptake of the offer of genetic testing has not been widely investigated. What is known is that people who believe they can cope with the results of genetic testing are the ones who have a greater interest in and uptake of genetic testing. In addition, people's perceiving themselves as being at greater risk for having the gene and developing the disease is typically associated with a greater uptake of genetic testing. In one of the early reports of genetic testing for Huntington disease, the Canadian Collaborative Study of Predictive Testing group found that participants who declined genetic testing (along with those who received uninformative test results) were the most distressed over a period of 12 months. In 1997 Caryn Lerman and colleagues explicitly tested the influence of distress on requesting the results of genetic testing for hereditary breast and ovarian cancer susceptibility. After controlling for sociodemographic factors and objective risk, those with higher levels of cancer-specific distress were nearly three times more likely to request the results of genetic testing. No evidence of a curvilinear (inverted-U) relationship between distress and genetic testing was found, although this may be because, on the whole, participants did not have high levels of distress. Although there are inherent difficulties in investigating whether stress predicts the uptake of genetic testing given that people who decline the offer of genetic testing are less likely to want to take part in psychological evaluations, there is clearly a need to attempt to understand this relationship. As genetic testing becomes more ubiquitous, there is a need to find out whether those who are offered genetic testing and decline it constitute a particularly vulnerable group.

Emotional Impact of Genetic Testing

Given the justifiable concern that finding out one has a high risk of developing a serious genetic disease may prove to be a huge burden, it is unsurprising that the most widely investigated issue over the past 20 or so years has been the emotional impact of receiving genetic test results. The original studies continue to report the long-term emotional effects of testing, and more studies are needed as new genetic testing procedures for various diseases are implemented. As already discussed, having an uninformative genetic test result for Huntington disease (along with declining the genetic testing) was found to be more distressing than receiving a positive result. An uninformative genetic test result is one in which it is not possible to definitively state whether or not the individual is a carrier of a deleterious mutation. In this study, the higher distress of those receiving uninformative results was quite possibly due to the motivation for testing. Many people who seek predictive genetic testing do so hoping to resolve the uncertainty they have been living with, and uninformative results fail to help them achieve this goal. Most studies, however, report the impact of positive and negative genetic test results and these are considered next.

Negative Genetic Test Results

As might be expected, across different genetic tests, a consistent finding is that immediately after individuals learn they do not have the predisposing gene they experience psychological relief. Thus levels of anxiety, depression, distress, and illness-specific measures of distress typically drop to significantly lower levels than they were at the time when baseline assessments were made. Some studies find that these lower levels of psychological stress are maintained over the coming months and years, whereas other studies find that the level of stress slowly rises back to the baseline level. This latter finding may well be explained by the fact that the threat of disease is but one of the problems that individuals face. Despite the relief invoked by not being a carrier of the disease-causing gene, other problems remain unresolved and quickly start to impinge on the individuals' emotional state. In addition, these people come from families affected by serious diseases and still need to cope with this

situation and, possibly, the feelings of guilt that others are affected when they are not.

A consistent finding across studies is that distress prior to testing is the biggest predictor of distress after testing, regardless of the test result. A positive effect on the mean stress levels in individuals who receive a negative test result can hide the fact that some individuals have problems coping with testing negative for the gene. These people may have lived their lives and made important decisions (such as not having children) on the basis of their expectation of developing the disease in the future. Almqvist and colleagues recently reported that one person who tested negative for the gene for Huntington disease attempted suicide on the day he received the test result. Therefore, it is important that it not be assumed that all patients who receive negative genetic test results do not require additional support and counseling.

Positive Genetic Test Results

Some studies found that, immediately after receiving positive genetic results, people's levels of distress are no different than their baseline levels. Other studies found increased levels of distress in this group. An unexpected and important finding is that any increased distress is usually transitory. As early as 1 month and for at least 1 year after being given this bad news, the levels of distress are consistently no different to those reported for the baseline levels. In some studies, the levels of distress up to 1 year later are no different than the levels reported by those receiving negative test results. As with the finding for negative test results, a concentration on the mean scores can hide the fact that some individuals do experience great and long-term difficulties coming to terms with the information that they are at high risk of developing a serious disease. There is a need to ensure that these individuals, in particular, receive appropriate support in the months and years following the receipt of genetic test results. Because distress prior to testing predicts distress following testing, the process of identifying potentially vulnerable individuals can be put in place as soon as they come forward for testing.

Huntington disease was the first disease for which a predictive genetic test was developed, and these studies were also the first to report the results of long-term psychological evaluations. These are crucial because they show whether those who receive positive genetic tests start to experience greater distress when they approach the time when they can expect to develop symptoms. In 2003, Almqvist and colleagues reported that for those who carry the gene for Huntington disease the levels of distress, which were reduced soon after testing and up to 2 years later, had increased at the 5-year assessment. However, this increase was no higher than the baseline levels of distress. Although some participants did report distress levels in the clinical range, the mean scores were below the clinical cut-off at all the times measured. Therefore, there are reasons to be optimistic that, for the majority of people, genetic testing does not result in psychological harm.

Many authors have noted that there are a variety of explanations to account for the finding that positive test results do not, on the whole, lead to long-term emotional difficulties. Most of the people undergoing predictive genetic testing have lived most of their lives with the knowledge that their family members are affected by this disease and that they are at risk. Thus, many enter genetic testing programs with the hope of resolving uncertainty about their own risk status and that of their relatives. In many contexts, living with uncertainty can be more stressful than certainty. In addition, only a proportion of those who are at risk decide to have genetic tests, and, as stated previously, these are typically those who feel they can cope with the results. Finally, many of the genetic testing programs evaluated to date have at their core the provision of excellent information and counseling, and this will make no small contribution to the psychological well-being of recipients of genetic testing. There is a need to ensure that, when genetic testing is expanded to other clinical environments and other diseases for which people may have less awareness of their own risk, it is still accompanied by the provision of high-quality information and support.

Cognitive Appraisal of Genetic Testing

There are rapid developments in the understanding of the genetic basis of multifactorial diseases such as cancer, cardiovascular disease, and diabetes, in which both genetic and behavioral factors can contribute to developing the disease. In this context, whether genetic testing influences the cognitive appraisal of the disease becomes a key issue. If having a genetic test leads people to appraise the disease differently, this may have implications for whether they will engage in behaviors that can reduce their risk.

In the general public, studies suggest that there is a common perception that the genetic risk of disease is less controllable than other risk factors. From a stress and coping perspective, the appraisal of a health threat as uncontrollable could initiate different coping procedures than its appraisal as controllable. Specifically, genetic risk information could invoke fatalism and could demotivate the individual from engaging in risk-reducing behaviors. This hypothesis

was tested – and was not supported – in a UK trial of genetic and nongenetic diagnoses of familial hypercholesterolemia. In this study, genetic testing appeared to influence the cognitive appraisal of the disease by reinforcing a biological model of the disease, such that the more genes were endorsed as contributing to coronary heart disease, the more medication was endorsed as an effective means of reducing risk. Thus, there is some preliminary evidence that genetic risks are indeed appraised differently and may lead to greater engagement in biological rather than behavioral ways of reducing risk. As with the majority of the studies conducted to date, this research was conducted with participants already highly aware of their increased risk of disease.

Some studies have found that genetic test results do have an impact on behavior, such as an increased adherence to surveillance behaviors in those with an inherited predisposition to cancer. Indeed, some people who are found not to have a genetic predisposition to cancer find it difficult to accept that their risk is at the same level as the general population and still desire regular screening to detect cancer. To date there is little evidence to suggest that such populations feel falsely reassured that a negative genetic test means they have no risk of developing the disease. Some people who do have an inherited predisposition to cancer opt to have prophylactic surgery (e.g., a mastectomy before any cancer has developed). Although this is clearly a difficult decision, the option to undergo surgery is an understandable coping strategy for those who have seen family members affected by cancer. Other studies, however, have not found any behavioral effects of genetic testing.

Given the equivocal findings across the few studies to date that have investigated behavioral outcomes, there is a need for improving our understanding of the mechanisms that may explain these differences. A number of authors are beginning to conceptualize the impact of genetic testing from a stress and coping and from a self-regulatory perspective. These conceptualizations should pave the way for developing an evidence base of the mechanisms by which cognitive and emotional appraisal and self-regulatory processes impact on behavior following genetic testing. This developing evidence base will lead to a greater certainty about how best to implement genetic testing for multifactorial diseases. In particular, as genetic testing for common diseases such as cancer and coronary heart disease becomes more widespread, there is a need to investigate the impact of genetic testing on cognitive appraisal and behavior in populations that have less prior awareness of their risk. These populations may have very different emotional responses and cognitive appraisals of their risk status than the highly aware populations studied so far. Based on the evidence to date, however, there is cause for cautious optimism that if attention is paid to providing high-quality information and support to at-risk families the potential medical benefits of genetic testing can be realized without causing emotional or behavioral harm.

Further Reading

Almqvist, E. W., Brinkman, R. R., Wiggins, S., et al. (2003). Psychological consequences and predictors of adverse events in the first 5 years after predictive testing for Huntington disease. *Clinical Genetics* **64**, 300–309.

Bleiker, E. M. A., Hahn, D. E. E. and Aaronson, N. K. (2003). Psychosocial issues in cancer genetics: current status and future directions. *Acta Oncologica* **42**, 276–286.

Broadstock, M., Michie, S. and Marteau, T. (2000). Psychological consequences of predictive genetic testing: a systematic review. *European Journal of Human Genetics* **8**, 731–738.

Butow, P. N., Lobb, E. A., Meisser, B., et al. (2003). Psychological outcomes and risk perception after genetic testing and counselling in breast cancer: a systematic review. *Medical Journal of Australia* **178**, 77–81.

Gooding, H. C., Organista, K., Burack, J., et al. (2006). Genetic susceptibility testing from a stress and coping perspective. *Social Science & Medicine* **62**, 1880–1890.

Lerman, C., Croyle, R. T., Tercyak, K. P., et al. (2002). Genetic testing: psychological aspects and implications. *Journal of Consulting and Clinical Psychology* **70**, 784–797.

Lerman, C., Schwartz, M. D., Narod, S., et al. (1997). The influence of psychological distress on use of genetic testing for cancer risk. *Journal of Consulting and Clinical Psychology* **65**, 414–420.

Marteau, T. M. and Richards, M. (eds.) (1996). *The troubled helix: social and psychological implications of the new human genetics.* Cambridge, UK: Cambridge University Press.

Marteau, T. M. and Weinman, J. (2006). Self-regulation and the behavioural response to DNA risk information: a theoretical analysis and framework for future research. *Social Science & Medicine* **62**, 1360–1368.

Senior, V. and Marteau, T. M. (in press). Causal attributions for raised cholesterol and perceptions of effective risk-reduction: self-regulation strategies for an increased risk of coronary heart disease. *Psychology & Health.*

Genetic Variation of HPA Axis Activity and Function in Farm Animals

P Mormède

INRA – Université Victor Segalen Bordeaux 2, Bordeaux, France

Evidence for Genetic Variability

Sources of Genetic Variability

Functional Consequences of Genetic Variability

Perspectives

Glossary

Corticosteroid-binding globulin (CBG)	A glycoprotein specifically carrying glucocorticoid hormone in blood plasma.
Genotype	The specific genetic makeup (the specific genome) of an individual. It codes for the phenotype of that individual.
Heritability	The proportion of the observed variation in a particular phenotype and, in a particular study, that can be attributed to the contribution of genotype (inheritance).
Hypothalamic-pituitary-adrenal (HPA) axis	The neuroendocrine system responsible for glucocorticoid hormone secretion.
Phenotype	A specific manifestation of a trait that varies between individuals. The phenotype is determined to some extent by genotype, or by the identity of the alleles that an individual carries at one or more positions on the chromosomes. Quantitative phenotypes are determined by multiple genes and are influenced by environmental factors.
Quantitative trait locus (QTL)	A polymorphic site on a chromosome containing alleles that differentially influence the expression of a quantitative trait.
Single nucleotide polymorphisms (SNPs)	Stable mutations consisting of a change at a single base in a DNA molecule. They are the most common type of genetic variation.

Evidence for Genetic Variability

A wide range of variability has been observed in hypothalamic-pituitary-adrenal (HPA) axis function, both basal and in response to stress. The contribution of genetic factors is shown by the differences among genetically defined stocks. Most available data have been obtained from pigs. Wild boars have the highest levels of cortisol, followed by Chinese breeds, including the most-studied Meishan. The highly selected lean breeds Large White and Landrace have the lowest levels, and Piétrain and Duroc pigs show intermediate levels. Few data are available in other species.

If a trait is influenced by genetic factors, it should be possible to increase or decrease the value of this trait by genetic selection. Indeed, divergent lines have been obtained by genetic selection in poultry (response to adrenocorticotropin [ACTH] or social stress), Japanese quail (response to immobilization), turkey (cold stress), and trout (confinement stress).

Sources of Genetic Variability

This article will not deal with major gene effects on HPA axis activity as seen in endocrine diseases induced by corticosteroid receptor or enzymatic defects. Traits such as circulating cortisol levels are normally distributed in genetically heterogeneous populations, suggesting that several genes may influence the phenotype, each gene with a small effect, and with complex gene × gene and gene × environment interactions. Several sources of genetic variability have been identified in farm animals.

Adrenal Sensitivity to ACTH

In the 1980s, D. P. Hennessy (Victoria, Australia) demonstrated in pigs that the increase of plasma cortisol after ACTH injection was variable among individuals but stable across time for a given animal. Similar differences in cortisol secretion were shown in response to corticotropin-releasing hormone (CRH), physical exercise, or insulin-induced hypoglycemia, although the release of ACTH was not different among individuals. Furthermore, the metabolic clearance of cortisol bears no relationship with the response to ACTH. Altogether, these data demonstrate that the key index of individual differences in HPA axis activity is the adrenal sensitivity to ACTH that was shown to be heritable in pigs. Several experimental results confirm genetic influences on the sensitivity of adrenal glands to ACTH. For instance, Meishan pigs (high cortisol levels) have a higher response to ACTH than Large Whites (low cortisol). In poultry, divergent lines could be selected on this trait. In quails, selection for high corticosterone to immobilization increased the steroidogenic response of adrenocortical cells to ACTH, and in turkeys, selection for a high corticosterone response to cold stress also increased the sensitivity of the adrenal gland to ACTH. In trout, the divergent cortisol response to confinement stress mostly results from the selection of animals with divergent interrenal gland response to ACTH, together with a large difference in the expression level of genes involved in corticosteroid hormone synthesis. Taken together, these data show that the adrenal sensitivity to ACTH is an important mechanism by which genetic factors influence HPA axis response to stress.

Hormone Bioavailability

Quantitative trait locus (QTL) analysis is a strategy to search for gene polymorphisms influencing a quantitative trait. It is based on the linkage between phenotypic value and genetic polymorphisms in a segregating population, usually an F2 intercross or a backcross. A QTL analysis run on an F2 intercross between the Large White and Meishan breeds revealed the large influence of a locus located at the end of the q arm of chromosome 7 on basal and post-stress (novel environment exposure) levels of cortisol, explaining, respectively, 7.7% and 20.7% of the phenotypic variance, with the Meishan alleles increasing cortisol levels. Other loci on chromosome 1 and 17 were shown to influence poststress ACTH levels. The comparison of genetic maps from different species shows that the end of the long arm of chromosome 7 is homologous to the telomeric end of the long arm of human chromosome 14. In this region corticosteroid-binding globulin (CBG), a glycoprotein specifically carrying cortisol in blood plasma, has been mapped. CBG is an important factor influencing bioavailability of the hormone, as it has been shown in humans that differences in CBG levels are a major determinant of differences in plasma cortisol levels. Therefore, the *Cbg* gene is an interesting positional and functional candidate gene to explain QTL influences on plasma cortisol levels. Indeed, comparison of gene sequences in Large White and Meishan pigs revealed several polymorphisms influencing CBG levels and function.

Corticosteroid Hormone Receptors

Two receptors (mineralocorticoid receptor [MR] and glucocorticoid receptor [GR]) mediate the biological effects of corticosteroid hormones. They act as transcription factors to increase or decrease the expression of target genes. The efficiency of corticosteroid hormone receptors is a major site of genetic variation, but few data are available in farm animals.

Functional Consequences of Genetic Variability

Physiopathological consequences of genetic variations in HPA axis activity reflect the wide range of corticosteroid hormone functions. Most data are related to growth and carcass composition. Indeed, glucocorticoid hormones influence feeding behavior; they also exert catabolic effects in peripheral tissues and anabolic effects in the liver so that they reduce growth rate and promote the accumulation of fat at the expense of proteins. In pigs, breeds with a higher body fat content such as Duroc and Meishan also produce more cortisol that lean breeds such as Large White and Landrace. In a segregating population (F2) of Large White × Duroc pigs, the fat content of the carcass was positively correlated with urinary levels of cortisol measured in the bladder after slaughter. In other studies in pigs, the magnitude of the adrenal response to ACTH – the main mechanism of genetic variability in HPA axis activity – was shown to be negatively correlated with body weight and growth rate. In sheep and turkeys, selection for leanness is accompanied by a reduction of HPA axis reactivity. Conversely, selection for a reduced adrenal response to cold stress in turkeys also increased body weight and egg production in turkeys, and growth rate was also inversely related to cortisol levels in divergently selected lines of rainbow trout.

Glucocorticoid hormones are also potent modulators of the immune system, and data obtained in chickens illustrate the consequence of genetic variation in HPA axis activity/reactivity on resistance to parasites or infectious diseases.

Perspectives

Current research in molecular genetics aims at the identification of gene polymorphisms responsible for individual phenotypic variation. For instance, there are documented mutations in the *Cbg* gene modifying its functional properties and associated with variable carcass fat content and meat quality of pigs. A single nucleotide polymorphism in the CRH gene was found to influence rib-eye area and carcass weight in beef cattle. In the future, it should be possible to optimize the functioning of the HPA axis by genetic selection based on molecular polymorphisms. When considering growth rate and carcass fat content, a low level of cortisol production should be favorable in the context of modern breeding for meat production. However, the picture is much less clear when considering the influence of HPA axis on other phenotypes. For instance, a lower cortisol response to social stress in poultry can either increase or decrease resistance depending on the infectious agent, and recently it was shown that plasma cortisol levels measured at birth are the best predictor of the genetic merit for piglet survival, with highest levels increasing survival. Further research will be necessary to better define the optimal activity of the HPA axis and to refine the molecular tools for farm animal selection.

See also the Following Articles

Adrenal Cortex; Comparative Anatomy and Physiology; Corticosteroid Receptors; Corticosteroid-Binding Globulin (Transcortin); Hypothalamic-Pituitary-Adrenal; Obesity, Stress and; Genetic Polymorphisms in Stress Response.

Further Reading

DeRijk, R. and de Kloet, E. R. (2005). Corticosteroid receptor genetic polymorphisms and stress responsivity. *Endocrine* **28**, 263–270.

Desautes, C., Sarrieau, A., Caritez, J. C., et al. (1999). Behavior and pituitary-adrenal function in large white and Meishan pigs. *Domestic Animal Endocrinology* **16**, 193–205.

Gayrard, V., Alvinerie, M. and Toutain, P. L. (1996). Interspecies variations of corticosteroid-binding globulin parameters. *Domestic Animal Endocrinology* **13**, 35–45.

Geverink, N., Foury, A., Plastow, G. S., et al. (2006). Cortisol-binding globulin and meat quality in five European lines of pigs. *Journal of Animal Science* **84**, 804–811.

Kino, T. and Chrousos, G. P. (2004). Glucocorticoid and mineralocorticoid receptors and associated diseases. *Essays in Biochemistry* **40**, 137–155.

Mormède, P., Courvoisier, H., Ramos, A., et al. (2002). Molecular genetic approaches to investigate individual variations in behavioral and neuroendocrine stress responses. *Psychoneuroendocrinology* **27**, 563–583.

Ousova, O., Guyonnet-Duperat, V., Iannuccelli, N., et al. (2004). Corticosteroid binding globulin: a new target for cortisol-driven obesity. *Molecular Endocrinology* **18**, 1687–1696.

Plastow, G. S., Carrion, D., Gil, M., et al. (2005). Quality pork genes and meat production: a review. *Meat Science* **70**, 409–421.

Tempel, D. L. and Leibowitz, S. F. (1994). Adrenal steroid receptors: interactions with brain neuropeptide systems in relation to nutrient intake and metabolism. *Journal of Neuroendocrinology* **6**, 479–501.

Genetics of Stress *See:* Genetic Factors and Stress; Genetic Predispositions to Stressful Conditions; Gene Environment Interactions in Early Development; Genetic Variation of HPA Axis Activity and Function in Farm Animals; Genetic Polymorphisms in Stress Response; Genetic Testing and Stress.

Ghrelin and Stress Protection

**T Brzozowski, M Pawlik, D Drozdowicz,
Z Sliwowski, S J Konturek and W W Pawlik**
Jagiellonian University Medical College, Cracow, Poland
P C Konturek
University Erlangen-Nuremberg, Erlangen, Germany

Pathogenesis of Stress-Induced Gastric Ulcerations

Discovery, Receptors, and Physiological Functions of Ghrelin

Role of Ghrelin in Maintenance of Gastric Mucosal Integrity

Mechanism of Gastroprotection Induced by Ghrelin

Neural Aspects of Gastroprotective Activity of Ghrelin

Ghrelin Attenuates Inflammation and the Generation of Reactive Oxygen Metabolites

Glossary

D cells	Endocrine cells belonging to the amine precursor uptake and decarboxylation (APUD) system known to release the hormone, somatostatin.
Endocrine cells (EC)	Release the hormone motilin and the neurotransmitter serotonin.
Enterochro-matoffin-like cells (ECL)	Known to release histamine, a potent stimulant of gastric acid secretion in the stomach. They are the predominant endocrine cell-type of the oxyntic (acid-producing) mucosa of the stomach. Histamine acts as the positive paracrine stimulator of the release of hydrochloric acid from the parietal cell.
Gastric blood flow (GBF)	Defined as the flow of the blood through submucosal vessels in the gastric mucosa.
Gr cells	Ghrelin-producing cells identified in the gastric mucosa.
N^G-*nitro-L-arginine (L-NAME)*	A nonselective inhibitor of the enzyme nitric oxide synthase. It has been used experimentally to induce hypertension.
Neuropeptides	Small proteins (peptides) comprised of a chain of amino acids that are synthesized in, and secreted by, nerves and serve as neurotransmitters (when released at synapses) and neurohormones (when released into the bloodstream)
Nitric oxide (NO)	Intracellular gaseous mediator released from vascular endothelium, sensory nerves, and gastrointestinal epithelial cells. It contributes to the mechanism of gastrointestinal mucosal integrity by increasing gastrointestinal microcirculation and protective mucus and bicarbonate secretion.
Prostaglandins (PG)	Metabolites of enzyme cyclo-oxygenase activity, the derivatives of arachidonic acid that exhibit cytoprotective activity.
Prostanoids	A group of compounds derived from unsaturated 20-carbon fatty acids, primarily arachidonic acid, via the cyclo-oxygenase pathway. They are extremely potent mediators of a diverse group of physiological processes. These compounds play an essential role in the control of gastrointestinal circulation and gastrointestinal mucosal defense. A group of arachidonic acid metabolites which include mainly prostaglandins and thromboxanes.
Vascular endothelial growth factor (VEGF)	One of the important growth factors, responsible for angiogenesis and acceleration of ulcer healing and process of gastrointestinal mucosal repair.

Pathogenesis of Stress-Induced Gastric Ulcerations

Stress ulcerations are defined as acute gastric mucosal lesions occurring as complications in severely ill patients after burns, sepsis, major surgery, or trauma to the central nervous system. Critically ill patients are at increased risk of developing stress-related gastric mucosal lesions and gastrointestinal bleedings. Stress can induce acute gastric mucosal lesions by a complex of psychological factors, psychosis, or brain trauma, influencing individual vulnerability and specific brain pathways regulating autonomic functions. These stress-induced gastric microbleeding erosions are accompanied by a marked decrease in the gastric blood flow (GBF), a substantial decrease in the gastric mucosal prostaglandin (PG) content and nitric oxide (NO) release, inhibition of gastric mucus and bicarbonate secretion, and the increased formation of free oxygen radicals in the gastric mucosa leading to gastric ischemia and inflammation. Among various stress models used in animals, the most reproducible results can be obtained by water immersion and restraint stress (WRS), which appear to act synergistically in the production of gastric ulcerations. Numerous studies have demonstrated the usefulness of cold-restraint stress and proved it to be a clinically relevant experimental model for studying of pathomechanism of acute gastric damage and protection. It has been shown that gastric acid plays an important role in the development of stress-induced gastric ulcer and is the most common endogenous factor responsible for the destruction of epithelial cells. Gastric mucosal lesions induced by different time-dependent exposures to WRS trigger time-course dependent changes of the ultrastructure of gastric parietal cells secreting gastric acid. Many physiological agents such as PG, NO donors, calcitonin gene-releasing factor (CGRP), and gastrointestinal hormones such as cholecystokinin (CCK) and leptin have been reported to attenuate the gastric erosions induced by stress of different origin and durations. The mechanism of the recovery of gastric mucosa from stress injury is not fully understood and the underlying healing of stress-induced gastric lesions appears to be multifactorial. It has been proposed that mucosal integrity and mucosal repair after stress damage, involve the enhancement of GBF and increased cell proliferation mediated by expression and subsequent release of growth factors such as epidermal growth factor (EGF) and transforming growth factor (TGF)-α.

Discovery, Receptors, and Physiological Functions of Ghrelin

Ghrelin is a recently described 28-amino acid peptide that has been discovered in rat and human gastrointestinal tracts, particularly in gastric mucosa, as an endogenous ligand for growth hormone (GH) secretagogue receptor (GHSR). Ghrelin stimulates food intake and body weight gain exerting a modulating effect on energy expenditure acting through afferent nerves and directly on hypothalamic feeding centers. This peptide was also shown to enhance the gastric motility and gastric secretion. Recent studies revealed that ghrelin is produced by special neuroendocrine cells located mainly in oxyntic mucosa but not in enterochromatoffin-like cells (ECLs), endocrine cells (ECs) or D cells. Ghrelin has no relevant homology with any known gastrointestinal peptides but

potently stimulates the release of GH and acts as a natural ligand for the GHRS which is the endogenous counter of the family of synthetic, peptidyl and non-peptidyl GH secretagogues. Ghrelin stimulates food intake and body weight gain exerting a modulating effect on energy expenditure. Administration of ghrelin causes weight gain via appetite stimulation and reduced fat oxidation. The release of ghrelin may be influenced by the status of fasting and nutrient feeding because central and peripheral administration to rats results in an increase in their feeding behavior. Previous studies in humans revealed that gastrectomy produced a dramatic fall in the plasma ghrelin levels, whereas fasting and anorexia nervosa were accompanied by elevated plasma ghrelin concentrations supporting the notion that the gastrointestinal tract, primarily the stomach, is a major source of circulating ghrelin, which could be considered as a starvation-related hormone. Interestingly, obestatin, which is encoded by the same gene as ghrelin has recently been reported to counteract physiological effects of ghrelin.

A recent study revealed that endocrine Gr cells of the stomach are a major source of circulating ghrelin acting via activation of two receptor subtypes. Two GHS-R subtypes are generated by alternative splicing of a single gene: the full-length type 1a receptor (GHS-R1a); and a carboxyl-terminally truncated GHS-R type 1b (GHS-R1b). The GHS-R1a is the functionally active, signal-transducing form of the GHS-R, while the GHS-R1b is devoid of high-affinity ligand binding and signal transduction activity. Ghrelin molecules, produced by endocrine cells of gastric glands exist in two major molecular forms, ghrelin and des-n-octanoyl ghrelin (des-acyl ghrelin). The acylation by n-octanoic acid of the hydroxyl group of their third residue, which is either serine or threonine, is essential for binding of ghrelin to GHS-R1a. The anorexia associated with cancer chemotherapy in rodents is reported to be alleviated by exogenous ghrelin and similar effects have been described in humans. This may be due to a reduction in activity of ghrelin-producing cells, present predominantly in the oxyntic mucosa.

Role of Ghrelin in Maintenance of Gastric Mucosal Integrity

Little is known about the factors that might affect ghrelin release in the stomach and whether this peptide can contribute the mechanism of gastric mucosa integrity. The role of ghrelin in the mechanism of gastric mucosal defense and gastroprotection has been investigated by revealing that peripheral administration of ghrelin reduces the formation of lesions induced by ethanol and cold stress (**Figure 1**).

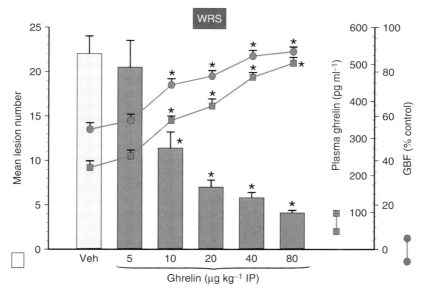

Figure 1 The mean number of water immersion and restraint stress (WRS)-induced gastric lesions, gastric blood flow (GBF), and plasma immunoreactivity of ghrelin in rats treated with vehicle (saline) or with various doses of ghrelin (5–80 μg kg^{-1} intraperitoneal). Please note a significant and dose-dependent reduction in the number of gastric lesions induced by WRS accompanied by a significant rise in the GBF and plasma ghrelin levels. Means $\pm$ standard error of means of 6–8 rats. Asterisk indicates a significant change as compared to the vehicle control values. Reproduced from *Regulatory Peptides* **120**, Exogenous and endogenous ghrelin in gastroprotection against stress-induced gastric damage. 39–51, 2004, with permission from Elsevier.

In agreement with the original hypothesis that prostanoids, NO, and sensory neuropeptides cooperate in the mechanism of maintenance of gastric integrity, it was proposed that NO and sensory neuropeptides may mediate these gastroprotective effects because the blockade of NO synthase (NOS) activity with N^{G}-nitro-L-arginine (L-NAME) and the functional ablation of sensory afferent nerves with capsaicin were both found to attenuate them. It is of interest that centrally applied ghrelin can influence gastric acid secretion, while attenuating lesions caused by stress and this effect is mediated by the vagal innervation and the expression of calcitonin gene related peptide (CGRP) messenger ribonucleic acid (mRNA), an important neuropeptide released from sensory nerve endings. Both these events are considered as important components of the brain-gastrointestinal tract axis involved in the gastroprotective effects of ghrelin especially against stress-induced gastric lesions.

In contrast, the *Helicobacter pylori* (*H. pylori*) infection of the human gastric mucosa which is now considered to play a role as the causal factor in the pathogenesis of gastritis and peptic ulcer was found to attenuate the mucosal expression and release of ghrelin and to reduce appetite. This was confirmed in *H. pylori*-infected gastric mucosa of Mongolian gerbils, which is now widely accepted as an appropriate model to study the mechanism of *H. pylori* infection under experimental conditions. It is of interest, that after successful cure of *H. pylori* in

healthy asymptomatic subjects the plasma ghrelin concentration increased, which in turn led to enhanced appetite and weight gain. This implies that increase in ghrelin in *H. pylori* cured gastric mucosa may contribute to the increasing obesity seen in Western populations, where the prevalence of *H. pylori* is low.

Mechanism of Gastroprotection Induced by Ghrelin

Recently, endogenous PGs have been implicated in the control of food intake and appetite but the possibility that these cytoprotective arachidonic acid metabolites could also play an important role in the gastroprotective effect of ghrelin has not been explored. Moreover, the question remains whether ghrelin contributes to gastroprotection against gastric lesions caused not only by artificial irritants such as ethanol, but also can protect against those caused by vascular disturbances resulting from stress or ischemia-reperfusion (I/R) that lead to severe microbleeding erosions and the fall in the microcirculation (**Figure 2**). Therefore it was important to confirm whether endogenous PGs as well as the expression of cyclo-oxygenase (COX)-1 and COX-2 are involved in the possible gastroprotective activity of ghrelin against stress-induced gastric erosions.

Our study supports the notion that ghrelin-induced protection and hyperemia involves co-activation of NO and sensory afferents and endogenous PG.

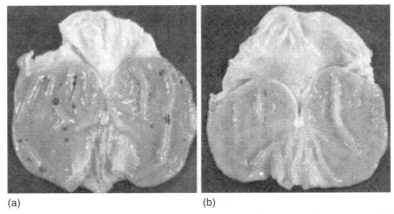

(a)   (b)

Figure 2 Representative photomicrograph showing gross appearance of gastric mucosa of rat pretreated 30 min before the exposure to 3.5 h of water immersion and restraint stress (WRS) with a, vehicle (1 ml of saline intraperitoneal (IP)) or b, ghrelin (20 µg kg^{-1} IP). Please note that many bleeding erosions are observed macroscopically in vehicle-pretreated gastric mucosa as compared to that treated with ghrelin indicating a protective activity of this hormone against the formation of WRS-induced gastric lesions.

Arachidonic acid metabolites were believed to act as the classic mediators of cytoprotection but recent studies revealed that in contrast to NO, endogenous PG do not appear to contribute to the observed gastroprotection by peptides such as leptin and CCK against ethanol-induced gastric lesions. Questions arose whether the suppression of COX by nonselective COX inhibitor, indometacin, or the highly selective COX-2 inhibitor, rofecoxib, could influence the gastroprotective and hyperemic activity of ghrelin. It has been documented that ghrelin-induced protection and hyperemia is accompanied by the enhancement in the mucosal PGE$_2$ generation. Both, indometacin and rofecoxib greatly attenuated the protective and hyperemic effects of ghrelin, indicating that endogenous PG possibly derived from COX-1 and COX-2 PG pathway may mediate these beneficial effects of this hormone on the stomach (**Figure 3**).

Ghrelin applied centrally exhibits comparable gastroprotective activity as when administered peripherally against the mucosal damage induced by corrosive substance such as ethanol and nontopical ulcerogen such as stress. This suggests that exogenous ghrelin could be considered as an important protective factor for the gastric mucosa. This notion is supported by observation that ghrelin attenuated the gastric lesions induced by ethanol in various concentrations and those provoked by stress while producing an increase in gastric mucosal blood flow and the plasma level of this hormone. The results of secretory studies revealed that ghrelin applied by the intracerebroventricular (ICV) and intraperitoneal (IP) routes in doses that were gastroprotective against stress and ethanol injury significantly raised gastric acid secretion suggesting that the protective effect of this peptide occurred despite an increase of the gastric secretory function,

thus representing genuine gastroprotective activity as previously proposed for the phenomenon of cytoprotection. The ghrelin-induced protection after its central administration was accompanied by a significant and dose-dependent rise in the plasma ghrelin concentrations by WRS suggesting that ghrelin-evoked gastric hyperemia could be an important mechanism of the protective effect of this peptide in rat stomachs (**Figure 1**).

It has been shown that ghrelin, primarily produced in the stomach, but also in the hypothalamus, is an orexigenic peptide and affects both feeding at the levels of hypothalamus (arcuate nuclei) and GH secretion partly due to an activation of gastric vagal afferents transmitting visceral sensory signals to the brain. The observation that ghrelin stimulates gastric acid secretion is in keeping with the original observation that an increase in gastric secretion was achieved after parenteral but not topical administration of ghrelin. The mechanism by which ghrelin increases gastric acid secretion after peripheral as well as central administration could be related to elevation of plasma gastrin concentration, since a considerable increase in this hormone level was notified following ghrelin application. Gastrin could contribute, at least in part, to the secretory as well as protective and hyperemic effects of ghrelin but its effect on histamine release should also be considered. The notion that the protective activity of ghrelin depends, at least in part, on gastrin release is at variance with some studies claiming that ghrelin release does not operate under gastrin; however, these studies failed to directly address the effect of ghrelin on gastrin release. It is not excluded that ghrelin, which is known for the release of GH, acts via GH release to protect gastric mucosa against stress damage as GH was shown to

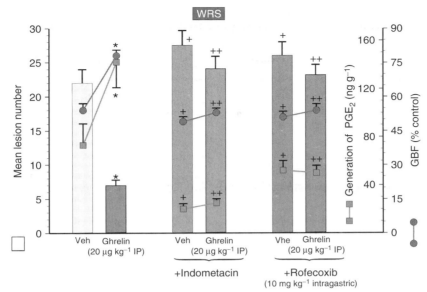

Figure 3 The mean number of gastric lesions induced by water immersion and restraint stress (WRS) and accompanying changes in gastric blood flow (GBF) in rats treated with vehicle (saline) and ghrelin (20 μg kg^{-1} intraperitoneal (IP)) with or without pretreatment with nonselective COX inhibitor, indometacin (5 mg kg^{-1} IP) or COX-2-selective inhibitor, rofecoxib (10 mg kg^{-1} intragastric). Mean ± standard error of mean of 6–8 rats. Asterisk indicates a significant decrease as compared to the value obtained in vehicle-control animals. Cross indicates a significant change as compared to the respective value obtained in animals without pretreatment with COX inhibitors. Double cross indicates a significant change as compared to the respective value obtained in ghrelin-treated animals without pretreatment with COX inhibitors. Reproduced from *Regulatory Peptides* **120**, Exogenous and endogenous ghrelin in gastroprotection against stress-induced gastric damage. 39–51, 2004, with permission from Elsevier.

enhance the healing of gastric ulcers, while increasing plasma gastrin level.

Neural Aspects of Gastroprotective Activity of Ghrelin

Ghrelin is an orexigenic peptide and affects both feeding at the levels of hypothalamus (arcuate nuclei) to stimulate neuropeptide Y (NPY) and Agouti-related peptide (AgPP)-related neurons and to release GH partly due to an activation of gastric vagal afferents transmitting visceral sensory signals to the brain. An experimental study in a stress model of gastric injury revealed that ghrelin mRNA was upregulated in the gastric mucosa exposed to WRS. This was followed by an increase in the plasma ghrelin level indicating that endogenous ghrelin might act as local integrity peptide to limit the extent of gastric damage provoked by WRS. This is similar to leptin, another gastric hormone involved in the control of food intake though acting in opposite direction than ghrelin. As expected, ghrelin-induced protection after its central administration was accompanied by a significant and dose-dependent rise in the plasma ghrelin concentrations and marked attenuation of the fall in the GBF caused by WRS suggesting that ghrelin-evoked gastric hyperemia could be an important

mechanism of the protective effect of this peptide in the rat stomach. This notion is based on the well-documented facts that an appropriate microcirculatory blood supply helps to orchestrate various lines of mucosal defense system in gastric mucosa. In addition, as mentioned before, ghrelin significantly increases the expression of mRNA for CGRP, which is known to increase the gastric mucosal blood flow. The mechanism by which ghrelin improves this gastric mucosal blood flow could be related to a direct effect of ghrelin on blood vessels due to a potent vasodilatatory activity of this peptide. It is assumed that the direct protective effect of ghrelin can not be ruled out; however, no study has been yet undertaken to demonstrate that ghrelin exerts direct effects on vasculature.

Since the mechanism of gastric mucosal defense include NO that could be released from vascular endothelium, sensory nerves, or gastric epithelial cells, the hypothesis was tested that ghrelin-induced gastroprotection involving NO could originate from the activation of afferent sensory neurons by this peptide. The deactivation of rat primary afferent nerves, using a neurotoxic dose of capsaicin about 2 weeks before the stress experiment, aggravated WRS-induced gastric damage as compared to rats without capsaicin denervation and significantly reduced the GBF when compared to that in animals with intact sensory nerves. Moreover, it has been demonstrated that such a capsaicin-induced deactivation of sensory nerves significantly attenuated the gastroprotective activity of central and peripheral ghrelin and completely abolished the ghrelin-induced rise in GBF. Moreover, the replacement therapy with exogenous CGRP, the major neuropeptide released from sensory afferent nerves, restored the protective and hyperemic activity of ghrelin against the WRS-induced gastric lesions (**Figure 4**). In addition, the expression of mRNA for CGRP, the major neuropeptide released from sensory afferent nerves, was enhanced in ghrelin-treated animals indicating that this major sensory nerve neuropeptide is essential for microcirculatory response and of crucial importance for the gastroprotective activity of ghrelin.

Involvement of sensory nerves in ghrelin-induced gastroprotection does not exclude the possibility that centrally applied ghrelin enhances the central parasympathetic outflow to the stomach and that also vagal efferent nerves are involved in gastroprotection afforded by centrally and peripherally administered ghrelin. It was proposed, for instance, that the inhibitory effects of ghrelin on gastric acid secretion require intact vagal pathways because vagotomy abolished the increase in gastric secretion induced by this peptide. Indeed, vagotomy significantly attenuated the ghrelin-afforded gastroprotection and the accompanying rise in the GBF after its central and peripheral administration indicating that vagal pathway plays an important role in the mediation of the protective and hyperemic effects of this peptide against lesions evoked by stress. These data could be interpreted that ghrelin induced protection against damage induced by stress might be due to the stimulation of vagal cholinergic pathways that are involved in the recruitment of CGRP from afferent sensory nerves. Thus, evidence was provided that these protective and hyperemic effects of ghrelin may affect vagal nerves, the principal component of brain-gastrointestinal tract axis and involve cooperation between endogenous NO and sensory nerves releasing neuropeptides such as CGRP.

The finding that centrally applied ghrelin raised NO in stress model, is consistent with the observations that protective effects of ghrelin against ethanol can be attenuated by the pretreatment with L-NAME suggesting an involvement of NOS-NO pathway in the gastroprotective effect of ghrelin applied ICV. This excessive gastric NO production by ghrelin may originate from the upregulation of constitutive NOS (cNOS) rather than inducible NOS (iNOS) in the gastric mucosa. It seems likely that NO contributes to gastroprotection afforded by central and peripheral

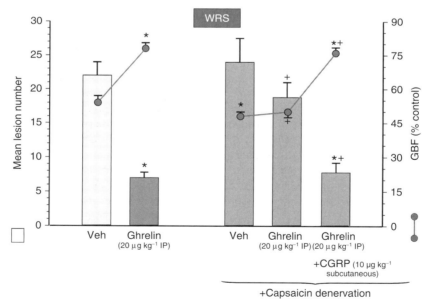

Figure 4 The mean number of WRS-induced gastric lesions and the alterations in the gastric blood flow (GBF) in rats with intact sensory afferent nerves and those with capsaicin denervation with or without pretreatment with vehicle (Veh; control) and ghrelin (20 μg kg^{-1} intraperitoneal). Please note that ghrelin-induced protection against WRS lesions and the accompanying increase in the GBF are almost completely abolished by functional ablation of afferent sensory neurons by capsaicin. These effects are further restored by the concomitant treatment of ghrelin with exogenous CGRP (10 μg kg^{-1} subcutaneous) in capsaicin-denervated animals. Mean ± standard error of mean of 6–8 rats. Asterisk indicates a significant change compared to the value in vehicle-treated rats. Cross indicates a significant change compared to the value obtained in rats without capsaicin denervation. Asterisk and cross indicate a significant decrease as compared to ghrelin-treated animals with capsaicin denervation of sensory afferents.

ghrelin as proposed earlier for CCK and leptin, both also implicated in control of appetite and gastroprotection.

Therefore, it is concluded that ghrelin, besides its recognized function in the control of appetite, energy homeostasis, fat, and carbohydrate metabolism and gastrointestinal motility, could be considered as an important gastroprotective factor, expressed locally in the gastric mucosa in response to mucosal injury. This notion is supported by recent observations that mRNA for ghrelin is upregulated in the gastric mucosa exposed to WRS. Furthermore, it has been demonstrated that beneficial effect of ghrelin involves an activation of the capsaicin-sensitive sensory nerves in the gastric mucosa that are responsible for the increased production of CGRP in gastric mucosa exposed to WRS. This notion is in keeping with the previous studies demonstrating the importance of the activation of capsaicin-sensitive sensory nerves in the protection of gastric mucosa against acute gastric injury. The contribution of CGRP to the ghrelin-induced gastroprotection is further supported by the observation that the functional ablation of sensory nerves by capsaicin attenuated significantly the protective activity of ghrelin and completely abolished the rise in GBF induced by this peptide. The addition of exogenous CGRP to ghrelin in rats with deactivated sensory nerves restored the protection and accompanying rise in the GBF with the extent similar to that observed in ghrelin-treated rats with intact sensory nerves. These results indicate that sensory nerves, and their neuropeptides such as CGRP, are essential for microcirculatory response and of crucial importance for the gastroprotective activity of ghrelin.

Previous studies revealed that CGRP released in response to acute gastric mucosal injury leads also to increased production of NO due to activation of constitutive endothelial NOS. The exposure of rats to WRS that produced gastric lesions was associated with a significant downregulation of cNOS mRNA expression as compared to vehicle-control rats. The treatment with ghrelin of such WRS exposed rats, dose-dependently increased the expression of cNOS which reached the level of this expression comparable to that observed in the vehicle-control gastric mucosa indicating that ghrelin is capable of preventing the decrease in expression of cNOS mRNA caused by the exposure of this mucosa to WRS. The implication of NO in gastroprotection induced by ghrelin was further determined by employing of an inhibitor of NOS, L-NAME injected IP without or with addition of L-arginine, the substrate of NOS. The gastroprotective and hyperemic effects induced by ghrelin were significantly attenuated by L-NAME, but reversed by addition to L-NAME of L-arginine. All these observations support the notion that NO plays a crucial role in the mechanism of gastric protection against WRS damage afforded by ghrelin.

Ghrelin Attenuates Inflammation and the Generation of Reactive Oxygen Metabolites

The beneficial effects of ghrelin on the protection of gastric mucosa against injury induced by WRS could be related to the suppression of free oxygen radicals and anti-inflammatory properties of this peptide. Recent studies indicate that ghrelin could be considered as an important mediator in the regulation of inflammation due to its anti-inflammatory activity. Pretreatment with ghrelin just before exposure to WRS and I/R caused a significant reduction in the mRNA expression of proinflammatory cytokine, TNF-α, confirming that anti-inflammatory effect of ghrelin contributes to the gastroprotection and hyperemia exhibited by this peptide. This mechanism seems to be of importance since the upregulation of TNF-α expression represent a central pathophysiological event in the mechanism of acute mucosal injury induced by stress. Further support for the potent anti-inflammatory effects of ghrelin is the fact that ghrelin inhibited the activation of NFκB, which is considered as a critical signaling molecule in inflammation. Previous studies revealed that transcription factor NFκB activation is involved in acute injury of stomach and other organs. In its inactive form, NFκB is sequestered in the cytoplasm and bound by members of I-κB family of inhibitor proteins. Phosphorylation of I-κB by an I-κB kinase complex leads to the translocation of NFκB-p65 into the nucleus. Activation of NFκB induces gene programs leading to transcription of factors that promote inflammation. Therefore, it is assumed that a potential mechanism whereby ghrelin could modulate inflammatory response is blocking of activation of NFκB. This notion was confirmed by observation that ghrelin inhibits an activation of NFκB in human endothelial cells *in vitro*.

Ghrelin not only prevents the acute gastric injury induced by WRS, but also accelerates the healing of these lesions. At 6 h after the end of standard 3.5-h WRS, a significant acceleration of healing of the WRS-induced lesions was observed in rats treated with ghrelin as compared to those treated with vehicle. The mechanism by which ghrelin could stimulate the healing of WRS-induced lesions is poorly understood. Previous studies demonstrated that the growth factors stimulating angiogenesis play a crucial role in the mechanism of healing process. The acceleration of healing of acute WRS-induced gastric erosions was accompanied by the increased expression of hypoxia-inducible factor-1α (HIF-1α). The increased expression of HIF-1α in the ulcerated mucosa leads to increased expression and activation of vascular endothelial growth factor (VEGF). For instance, the concomitant rise in the expression of HIF-1α and VEGF was observed at day 6 following the combination of ghrelin and I/R and this was accompanied by a marked decrease of the gastric mucosal lesions produced by I/R. At 24 h after the end of WRS and I/R, an increase in expression of HIF-1α, while resulting in downregulation of the VEGF expression was observed in ghrelin-treated animals. This early reduction of VEGF expression despite increased expression of HIF-1α at 24 h after I/R injury or following mucosal recovery from WRS lesions could be attributed to the increased generation of free oxygen radicals and increased lipid peroxidation which can inhibit the activation of VEGF. It is known that healing of WRS and I/R injury involves an activation of antioxidant enzymes resulting in the inhibition of free oxygen species generation and subsequent enhancement in VEGF mRNA expression. This could, at least in part, explain significant increase in the expression for

VEGF mRNA at 24 h following WRS damage and at day 6 after I/R-induced gastric injury.

In summary, the administration of exogenous ghrelin applied by the ICV or IP routes that is accompanied by a significant increment in its plasma levels, exhibits dose-dependent gastroprotection against the WRS-induced gastric lesions. Ghrelin is effective not only in gastroprotection against WRS damage but also accelerates the healing of these lesions. Existing evidence indicates that these protective and hyperemic actions of ghrelin may affect brain-gastrointestinal tract axis and involve cooperation between endogenous PG, NO, and sensory nerves releasing neuropeptides such as CGRP (**Figure 5**). Ghrelin exerts a potent anti-inflammatory activity and inhibits activation of NFκB, an important transcription factor, which seems to be an essential step in the formation of WRS injury. As CGRP and cNOS/NO system are activated in gastric mucosa of ghrelin-treated animals, it is assumed that these two factors could trigger the gastroprotective mechanisms and contribute to the maintenance of gastric mucosal integrity in experimental animals and possibly also in humans exposed to noxious agents and to adverse conditions such as stress.

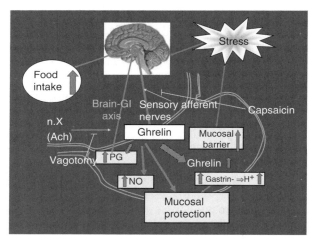

Figure 5 Scheme of the proposed mechanisms involved in gastroprotective action of ghrelin against the formation of mucosal damage induced by stress. Besides recognized involvement of ghrelin in the regulation of food intake and appetite behavior, this hormone exhibits gastroprotective and hyperemic activity. Ghrelin-induced protection may involve the activation of brain–gastrointestinal tract (GI) axis via vagal and sensory innervation and interactions of this hormone with potent gastroprotective factors including nitric oxide (NO), calcitonin gene releasing factor (CGRP) released from sensory afferent nerve endings and gastrin, known to exhibit gastroprotective and ulcer healing properties. The gastroprotective activity of ghrelin is impaired by suppression of sensory afferent and vagal efferent activities by capsaicin denervation and vagotomy, respectively, confirming the importance of neural aspects in the mechanism of gastroprotection induced by this hormone. n.X, vagal nerve; PG, prostaglandin.

Further Reading

Ariyasu, H., Takaya, K., Tagami, T., et al. (2001). Stomach is a major source of circulating ghrelin, and feeding state determines plasma ghrelin-like immunoreactivity levels in humans. *Journal of Clinical Endocrinology and Metabolism* **86**, 4753–4758.

Brzozowski, T., Konturek, P. C., Konturek, S. J., et al. (2000). Central leptin and cholecystokinin in gastroprotection against ethanol-induced damage. *Digestion* **62**, 126–142.

Brzozowski, T., Konturek, P. C., Konturek, S. J., et al. (2000). Expression of cyclooxygenase (COX)-1 and COX-2 in adaptive cytoprotection induced by mild stress. *Journal of Physiology* **94**, 83–91.

Brzozowski, T., Konturek, P. C., Konturek, S. J., et al. (2001). Classic NSAID and selective cyclooxygenase (COX)-1 and COX-2 inhibitors in healing of chronic gastric ulcers. *Microscopy Research and Technique* **53**, 343–353.

Brzozowski, T., Konturek, P. C., Konturek, S. J., et al. (2004). Exogenous and endogenous ghrelin in gastroprotection against stress-induced gastric damage. *Regulatory Peptides* **120**, 39–51.

Brzozowski, T., Konturek, S. J., Śliwowski, Z., et al. (1996). Role of capsaicin-sensitive sensory nerves in gastroprotection against acid-independent and acid-dependent ulcerogens. *Digestion* **57**, 424–432.

Date, Y., Kojima, M., Hosoda, H., et al. (2000). Ghrelin, a novel growth hormone-releasing acylated peptide, is synthesized in a distinct endocrine cell type in the gastrointestinal tracts of rats and humans. *Endocrinology* 14, 4255–4261.

Kojima, M., Hosoda, H., Date, Y., et al. (1999). Ghrelin is a growth-hormone-releasing acylated peptide from stomach. *Nature* 402, 656–660.

Konturek, P. C., Brzozowski, T., Pajdo, R., et al. (2004). Ghrelin – a new gastroprotective factor in the gastric mucosa. *Journal of Physiology and Pharmacology* 55, 325–336.

Konturek, P. K., Brzozowski, T., Konturek, S. J., et al. (1990). Role of epidermal growth factor, prostaglandin and sulfhydryls in stress-induced gastric lesions. *Gastroenterology* 99, 1607–1615.

Konturek, S. J., Brzozowski, T., Majka, J., et al. (1992). Adaptation of the gastric mucosa to stress. Role of prostaglandin and epidermal growth factor. *Scandinavian Journal of Gastroenterology* 27, 39–45.

Masuda, Y., Tanaka, T., Inomata, N., et al. (2000). Ghrelin stimulates gastric acid secretion and motility in rats. *Biochemical and Biophysical Research Communications* 267, 905–908.

Robert, A. (1979). Cytoprotection by prostaglandins. *Gastroenterology* 77, 761–767.

Sibilia, V., Rindi, G., Pagani, F., et al. (2003). Ghrelin protects against ethanol-induced gastric ulcers in rats: studies on the mechanisms of action. *Endocrinology* 144, 353–359.

Whittle, B. J. R., Lopez-Belmonte, J. and Moncada, S. (1990). Regulation of gastric mucosal integrity by endogenous nitric oxide: interactions with prostanoids and sensory neuropeptides in the rat. *British Journal of Pharmacology* 99, 607–611.

Glia or Neuroglia

G W Bennett and D E Ray
University of Nottingham Medical School, Nottingham, UK

This article is a revision of the previous edition article by G W Bennett, volume 2, pp 218–223, © 2000, Elsevier Inc.

Introduction
Anatomy and Structure
Physiology and Pharmacology
Neuron–Glial Cell Interactions

Glossary

GABA	Gamma-aminobutyric acid, the major inhibitory neurotransmitter in the brain.
CR3	Complement receptor 3, a marker for immune cells.
ED1	Product of the ectodermal dysplasia 1 gene, a marker of immune activation.

Introduction

In the past, neuroscientists concentrated almost exclusively on the electroactive components of the nervous system (neurons) because of their direct relationship to function, and neglected the nonelectroactive silent cells (glia), which outnumber them by at least 10 to 1 in much of the nervous system. Classically, glia were named for and relegated to the status of glue responsible for binding together the more important neurons, although Ramón y Cajal and others classified them and made useful proposals about their functions. This neglect has now been partly redressed, and their important roles in development, in maintaining function in the face of physiological stresses, and in the response to injury and infection are now recognized.

Subsequent studies confirmed that there are basically three types of glial cells, namely:

1. Macroglia:
2. Astrocytes: cells with many processes and possible function
3. Oligodendrocytes: cells with few processes that form the myelin of myelinated nerve fibers
4. Microglia:
5. Macrophages: cells in white matter specifically activated in injury and degeneration

In addition to these glial cells, the normal brain also contains pericytes and perivascular macrophages. Pericyte processes partially cover the basement membrane of brain blood vessels in a way similar to those of astrocytes. Pericytes, however, express smooth muscle actin and are contractile. Both pericytes and perivascular macrophages express immune markers and have sentinel phagocytic functions.

Astrocytes are the most abundant cells in the mammalian brain and consist of (1) those located in white matter (nerve fibers), which were termed fibrous astrocytes due to the large numbers of fibrils present in the cells, and (2) those located in grey matter (nerve cell bodies), which have fewer fibrils and were termed protoplasmic astrocytes. Despite the survival of this early attempt at classification, it is evident that many other intermediary forms exist.

Functions of Glial Cells

Macroglial cells, astrocytes, and oligodendrocytes all possess complex roles during development and, in the adult, involve complex interactions with neurons. Suggested supportive roles include metabolic supply of energy and other substrates (though the extent of this remains to be substantiated) and the ability to mop up released neurotransmitters (e.g., Glu and GABA) and ions (e.g., K^+ ions). Astrocytes are often closely associated with blood vessels. They regulate endothelial cell function and the permeability of blood vessels as well as producing many factors present in extracellular space, including growth factors and steroids that have multiple regulatory roles. Oligodendrocytes specialize in myelination in the central nervous system (CNS), a role confined to the Schwann cell in peripheral nerves. Such functions are critical to the function of the normal, healthy brain, but microglial cells become activated in pathological states and share many functions of the macrophages of the immune system. Such cells become cytotoxic during inflammatory responses and produce and respond to specialized proteins called cytokines, which mediate the complex interactions between microglia, astrocytes, and neurons, as well as infiltrating immune cells resulting from disruption of the normal blood–brain barrier during these pathological processes.

Specific biochemical markers of glial cells have contributed enormously to our understanding of the roles of these cells. Immunohistochemical studies in the 1970s identified a glial fibrillary acidic protein (GFAP) as an associated marker of fibrous astrocytes, though many GFAP-negative cells predominate in gray matter and various other markers for these have emerged.

In Vitro Studies of Glial Cells

In the 1980s glial cell culture techniques were developed in which the cell-specific markers enabled cell identity to be confirmed. Such *in vitro* methods have been coupled with imaging techniques to record changes in intracellular Ca^{2+} and other ions and patch clamp methods to study individual cells and those in more intact brain slice preparations.

Applications of these techniques have demonstrated that glial cells have complex signaling processes similar to neurons. Compared to neurons, glial cells generally have a more negative resting membrane potential due to a higher permeability to potassium. Glial cells therefore usually do not produce action potentials and remain passive (or silent) during intracellular recording, though more recent studies using patch clamping techniques have identified complex membrane properties. In addition, glial cells in culture, especially astrocytes, have been widely used to characterize membrane voltage-dependent channels (predominantly potassium channels and also low densities of sodium and calcium channels).

Many pharmacological and molecular studies indicate that glial cells possess a variety of transmitter, hormonal, and other receptors, though most glial cells appear to communicate with each other through specialized gap junctions rather than chemical synapses. This enables cytoplasmic exchange of many molecules, and such syncytial coupling may explain the lack of active membrane properties of glia cells *in situ*.

Anatomy and Structure

The staining techniques of Golgi (first described in 1885) provided the means for the earliest identification and morphology of neuroglial cells and neurons in the vertebrate nervous system.

Astrocytes

Astrocytes are the most abundant cells in the mammalian brain but are somewhat polymorphic. Those close to nerve fibers (white matter) are termed fibrous, since they are relatively hypertrophic with prominent intermediate filaments. The less prominent astrocytes associated with nerve cell bodies and synapses (gray matter) are termed protoplasmic, although intermediate forms exist, such as those associated with blood vessels.

All these share a common phenotype, with uniform expression marker proteins such as aldolase 3, but expression of others such as S-100 and GFAP may vary markedly. The most extreme instance of this phenotypic diversity within astrocytes is represented by the adult neuronal precursor cells in the subventricular zone, which have most of the characteristics of the astrocytes seen elsewhere yet retain the ability to dedifferentiate and form neurons by asymmetrical division.

Oligodendrocytes and Schwann Cells

Similarly, oligodendrocytes, which were found in early anatomical studies to produce the myelin sheath in the CNS, are analogous to the Schwann cells associated with peripheral neurons; they also exhibit structural diversity and heterogeneity, including possible distinct perivascular as opposed to perineuronal oligodendrocytes. Although various subtypes have been identified, the growth and development of oligodendrocytes and their specific interaction with the neuron have been less well studied than those of the astrocyte.

Schwann cells function to protect peripheral neurons and nerve fibers from the surrounding tissues, are separated by a basal lamina, and are broadly of two types. The major group is ensheathing Schwann cells that are associated with unmyelinated nerve axons in parts of the autonomic and sympathetic nerves and dorsal root ganglia, where they offer strength and protection. Better known are the cells that form myelin sheaths around larger, fast-conducting nerve fibers (myelinating Schwann cells). The myelin sheath occurs in blocks with intervening nodes of Ranvier that possess high concentrations of potassium ion channels. This segmental arrangement, as well as providing important neuronal insulation, allows conduction of ionic currents within the enclosed fiber and facilitates saltatory (jumping) conduction along the fiber, resulting in a marked increase in conduction velocity of impulses. Recent research has strengthened the long-held view that Schwann cells are also metabolically active in facilitating regeneration processes and thereby enable peripheral nerve fiber recovery from injury, a capacity absent in central neural processes that lack Schwann cells. This prompted studies that have shown that in some situations it is feasible to experimentally transfer populations of Schwann cells into the CNS and thereby activate brain axonal regeneration.

A special type of CNS glial cell is the ependymoglial (radial glia) cells, which line the ventricular spaces of brain. These are specially modified astrocytes of a characteristic bipolar structure with a ciliated apical pole protruding into the cerebrospinal fluid (CSF). In many vertebrate species, some of these cells include specialized sensory epithelia that develop mechanoperception (e.g., organ of corti and vestibular organs). They also include tanycytes, which have a specialized role in the transportation of molecules between local blood vessels and brain circumventricular organ regions of the ventricular system; they are of particular importance in regions of the hypothalamus for the distribution of neuropeptide hormones. Other radial glial cells have important roles in development and demonstrate transitory existence.

Microglia

Microglial cells in the brain may outnumber nerve cells, and in the adult become particularly important in pathological states. Those present in the normal (nonpathological) brain are termed resting or ramified (many branched appearance) microglia, while activated (or reactive) microglia cells may be nonphagocytic or become phagocytic microglia in fully activated pathology. Microglia derived from the systemic immune system invade during development and take up a quiescent resting morphology, their fine processes establishing nonoverlapping territories that cover the whole brain. A number of immune marker proteins such as CR3 can be used to identify resting microglia, and when activated they express a wide variety of markers characteristic of immune signaling and cytolytic functions such as ED1, interleukins, and nitric oxide synthase.

Physiology and Pharmacology

Ion Channels and Receptors

With their many processes surrounding synapses and cell bodies, astrocytes are well placed to dominate and regulate extracellular homeostasis, especially since they express a variety of ion channels, including potassium (K^+), sodium (Na^+), calcium (Ca^{2+}), and ligand-gated channels. The latter reflects the local pattern of neuronal neurotransmitter types, and all have largely been studied using primary astrocytes in culture and patch clamp techniques. Similarly, whole cell patch clamp methods have been applied to *in situ* preparations using hippocampal or other brain slices. These studies have identified many types of K^+ channels in astrocytes, indicating an important function of these cells in the regulation of extracellular levels of this ion, consistent with the notion that maintaining K^+ homeostasis is an important function of astrocytes.

Astrocytes, oligodendrocytes, and Schwann cells also possess voltage-gated Na^+ and Ca^{2+} ion channels, but at much lower densities than those in neurons. This causes some difficulties regarding understanding their precise function, since there are insufficient levels for action potentials to be generated. With respect to Schwann cells, some authors have suggested that the ion channels may be a local store of channels that can be passed to neighboring neural axons, since they share similar properties, but this remains to be directly demonstrated. Na^+ channels may also produce sufficient Na^+ exchange for the activation of astrocyte Na^+/K^+-ATPase activity. Like with many other cells, modulation of glial intracellular Ca^{2+} may be an important signaling mechanism, since Ca^{2+} influx is activated by various stimuli, although the roles of calcium in astrocytes and other glia remain to be clarified.

Such ionic changes may be regulated by ligand-gated channel receptors, including $GABA_A$, that also occur in the membranes of cultured astrocytes. Astrocytes also express high-affinity carrier systems for various neurotransmitter-like molecules, especially amino acids (e.g., Glu and GABA), and amino acid uptake into these cells may well contribute to the physiological regulation of these transmitter synapses as well as offer possible cytotoxic protection from such amino acids. Recent work suggests similar regulation of arginine, which is the precursor of nitric oxide, now considered a fundamental signaling molecule in neural tissues.

Astrocytes also contribute to extracellular ionic homeostasis by sequestering potentially neuronotoxic metals such as mercury and aluminum.

Metabotropic Receptors

Metabotropic (G-protein-coupled) receptors are also present in glial cell membranes, and there is good evidence for functional roles for glutamatergic (Glu), GABA$_B$, cholinergic (ACh), serotonergic (5-HT), adrenergic (NA), and various peptidergic (including angiotensin II, somatostatin, endothelium peptides, and substance P) receptors in cultured astrocytes, as shown by binding studies, the use of receptor-selective antibodies, and *in situ* hybridization methods. Similarly, biochemical analyses of second messenger systems, such as cyclic AMP, as well as cytosolic ionic changes, have demonstrated the pharmacological properties of such receptors. Similar receptors for hormones and growth factors are also present.

Gap Junctions

Gap junctions are predominant intercellular cytoplasmic communications between glial cells, though they also occur in other cells, including neurons. They consist of specialized membrane protein channels that enable the flow of inorganic and organic molecules between cells, usually consisting of six similar connexin molecules. Various types of connexin have been identified as products of a specific family of genes and have been associated with specific glial cells and neurons.

Intercellular communication via gap junctions provides a mechanism whereby the whole local population of astrocytes can make a coordinated contribution to maintaining ionic homeostasis in the face of physiological or pathological stress. The potential depolarizing effect of an accumulation of extracellular potassium during transiently high levels of neuronal activity can be minimized by its movement into and distribution between astrocytes within the active region until activity returns to normal. In addition, these astrocytic end feet that are in contact with capillaries show a high level of expression of aquaporins, which may play a role in bulk movement of water within the brain.

Neuron–Glial Cell Interactions

Metabolism

The physical location of astrocytes between metabolic supply via the vasculature and metabolic demand in the neuron, combined with their unique possession of an energy reserve in the form of glycogen granules, is a clear indication of their potential role in energy metabolism. Furthermore, since astrocytes express glutamine synthetase, which is lacking in neurons, there is important metabolic cycling of glutamate and glutamine between neurons and glia. In addition to the considerable physiological importance of this cycle, astrocytic glutamine synthetase also plays an important role in defending the brain against hyperammonemia. Perivascular astrocytes are also the first casualties in hepatic encephalopathy.

Although there is no analogous compartmentation of the enzymes involved in glycolysis, it has been proposed that astrocytic conversion of glucose to lactate is followed by transfer of this lactate to neurons (the lactate shuttle hypothesis) and that this is the major pathway for glycolysis. There is recent evidence that the glycolytic response seen within 10 s of neuronal activation is specifically localized within astrocytes. Circulating lactate (elevated during fatiguing muscle activity) can also effectively substitute for glucose as an energy supply in the brain.

While astrocytes have been the primary focus of research, oligodendrocytes also respond metabolically to increased demand (as after traumatic myelin damage) in a complex manner with changes appropriate to the activation of sphingoglycolipids for myelination.

Neurotransmitter Inactivation

Astrocytes are closely associated with neuronal synapses in the CNS and are equipped with the means to degrade most neurotransmitters. Work in the late 1960s showed that various transmitters flowing out of the synaptic cleft are taken up and inactivated by glial elements. However, the question remains regarding the physiological importance of such processes during normal transmitter function, and it is possible that such processes function as a protective process during excess transmitter release and/or during pathological states. However, it is well established that astrocytes participate in the glutamate-glutamine cycle, in which metabolized transmitters can be taken up by the astrocyte and returned to neurons as a precursor.

Response to Injury: Microglia and Inflammatory Disease and Neuroglia and Stress

Response to local injury Although the brain does not participate in the normal systemic response to inflammation, the local presence of abnormal material (e.g., plasma proteins, cell debris, bacteria) or cytokines in the brain extracellular space activates both sentinel microglia and astrocytes. These recruit circulating neutrophils and monocytes, which arrive by vascular transcytosis, and all begin the process of cell killing and removal of debris. In addition to producing pro-inflammatory cytokines, activated microglia themselves become phagocytic. This local inflammation is normally self-limiting, and results in a glial scar that persists long after the initial damage has resolved. During inflammation, the normally tight blood–brain barrier becomes open to small molecules, under the influence of locally secreted cytokines and vascular endothelial growth factor. Normal vascular integrity is restored as the inflammatory process dies down. The later phase of the inflammatory process is associated with debris removal and replacement of nonneuronal elements, after which recruited macrophages leave the brain. However, the persistence of hypertrophic astrocytic processes within the scar severely limits the degree of axonal regrowth that is possible, although surviving axons passing through lesions can be remyelinated. In contrast, peripheral nervous system Schwann cells activate in a manner analogous to that seen during early development and facilitate axonal regeneration. In the future it may be possible to overcome the inhibitory influence of astrocytes and oligodendrocytes on axonal regrowth by blocking astrocyte-derived signaling molecules.

Local autoimmune reactions are seen in some disease states, most notably multiple sclerosis. In multiple sclerosis, apparently random, but most commonly periventricular, oligodendrocytes are targeted with primary demyelination and secondary neurodegeneration. The process of focal vascular infiltration and cytolysis progresses slowly, either continuously or, more commonly, at irregular intervals (the relapsing remitting form). The acute inflammatory process never extends beyond these focal areas, although magnetic resonance studies do show minor abnormalities in otherwise normal white matter. The precipitating factors that direct the immune system to what is to become a new focal area of damage are unknown, but may be minor vascular lesions that would be asymptomatic in a person without autoantibodies. A similar condition (relapsing experimental allergic encephalitis) can be produced in experimental animals autoimmunized with myelin basic protein.

Response to systemic injury and stress Glial cells express a variety of hormonal and growth factor receptors, which seem to be critical during development as well as during stress-induced injury or disease. Evidence indicates that thyroid hormones, especially T_3, which are well known for their requirement in the maturation of neurons, also bind to stem cell astrocyte nuclei and regulate glial differentiation during development. A number of developmental neurotoxicants are known to act by targeting glial proliferation, and maternal stress can have marked and irreversible effects on brain maturation.

More significantly, it is now well documented that astrocytes and oligodendrocytes synthesize many steroid hormones during development, while adult cultured cells have been shown to express receptors for several steroids, including estrogen, progesterone, glucocorticoids, mineralocorticoids, and androgens. Moreover, recent developments indicate that many such steroids elicit rapid nongenomic effects on both neuron and glial cells via membrane-bound receptors in addition to the established intracellular and nuclear genomic receptors known to activate RNA and protein synthesis.

The term neurosteroid describes the neuroactive steroids that are synthesized and released from glial cells and act as local neuromodulators in the brain. Such local steroids may be modulated in turn by the rise of hormones in the circulation during stress. For example, neurosteroids such as dehydroepiandrosterone (DHEA) alter in stress and during depression and may inhibit or reverse the stress effects of corticosteroids and other stress- or drug-induced behaviors. Furthermore, recent evidence suggests that cortisol-induced loss of brain hippocampal neurons may be attenuated by DHEA; an interesting possibility is that glial steroids may function as part of a neuroprotective mechanism.

The adult brain participates in systemic inflammation or trauma by producing sickness behavior (fever, loss of appetite, social withdrawal, and inactivity). This is thought to be mediated via the few small open barrier brain areas (notably the area postrema) that lack a blood–brain barrier and have resident macrophages that can respond directly to circulating cytokines and then signal to activate resident microglia elsewhere in the brain.

There is also some evidence that residual semi-activated states in resident microglia from prior brain damage or the accumulation of minor damage seen in normal aging may render otherwise normal brain areas sensitive to systemic cytokines. This has been suggested as a mechanism whereby systemic infections may precipitate a sudden deterioration in chronic neurodegenerative conditions such as Alzheimer's disease.

A number of studies have reported generalized increases in blood–brain barrier permeability in animals subjected to stress. Of those studies showing increased leakage into the brain parenchyma, several have not proved reproducible, and others did not allow sufficient time for markers to be cleared from the normal brain vasculature. The better methodologies have shown no evidence for blood–brain barrier compromise with stress, other than in extreme hypertension. However, in the case of dural blood vessels on the brain surface, there is some evidence that stress can lead to increased permeability. This stress effect, in rats and mice, is mediated by trigeminal activation of resident dural mast cells, and the effect may be relevant to the genesis of migraine headaches.

See Also the Following Articles

Blood–Brain Barrier, Stress and; Inflammation; Infection; Macrophages.

Further Reading

Abbott, N. J. (2002). Astrocyte-endothelial interactions and blood-brain barrier permeability. *Journal of Anatomy* 200, 629–638.

Kettermann, H. and Ransom, B. R. (1995). *Neuroglia.* Oxford: Oxford University Press.

Kreutzberg, G. W. (1996). Microglia; a sensor for pathological events in the CNS. *Trends in Neurosciences* 19(8), 312–318.

Martin, P. (1997). *The sickening mind.* London: HarperCollins.

Merrill, J. E. and Benveniste, E. N. (1996). Cytokines in inflammatory brain lesions: helpful and harmful. *Trends in Neurosciences* 19(8), 331–338.

Perry, V. H. (2004). The influence of systemic inflammation on inflammation in the brain: implications for chronic neurodegenerative disease. *Brain, Behavior, and Immunity* 18, 407–413.

Verkhratsky, A. and Kettermann, H. (1996). Calcium signalling in glial cells. *Trends in Neurosciences* 19(8), 346–352.

Glucocorticoid Effects on Memory: the Positive and the Negative

O T Wolf
University of Bielefeld, Bielefeld, Germany

Introduction
Effects of Stress on Different Memory Systems
Clinical Implications
Summary and Conclusion

Glossary

Classical conditioning	A form of learning caused by the association (or pairing) of two stimuli.
Declarative memory	The conscious (explicit) long-term memory for events or facts, mediated by the medial temporal lobe.
Gluco-corticoids (GCs)	Steroid hormones secreted from the adrenal cortex in response to stress. Cortisol and corticosterone are naturally occurring GCs in humans and animals.
Meta-analysis	A statistical procedure used to pool the results of multiple studies investigating a particular effect. This approach leads to a quantitative summary of a specific field of interest.
Procedural memory	Different forms of nonconscious (implicit) long-term memories that express themselves through changes in performance. These forms of memories are largely independent of the medial temporal lobe memory system.
Working memory	A system for temporarily (short-term) storing and managing information. This system is dependent on regions of the prefrontal cortex.

Introduction

Everyone has experienced instances of stress influencing his or her memory. There are situations in which we are unable to retrieve prior well-learned information, an example of how stress might interfere with our memory. In contrast, we remember very well specific embarrassing, shameful, or frightening events from the past; this is an example of how stress can enhance our memory. Finally, there are situations of chronic stress or stress associated psychiatric disorders that are characterized by hypo- or hyperamnesia. This article provides a brief and selective overview of what is known about the role of GCs in mediating some of these effects. Advances in the field of psycho-neuroendocrinology within the past few years have contributed substantially to a more differentiated and balanced view of the effects of stress hormones on memory in animals and humans.

Interaction with a stressor leads to a cascade of neuroendocrine stress responses designed to facilitate adaptation to the changing demands. The hypothalamic-pituitary-adrenal (HPA) axis, together with the sympathetic nervous system (SNS), is one of the most important systems in this respect. The hypothalamus activates the HPA axis in response to input from several other brain regions. Corticotropin releasing hormone (CRH) and vasopressin reach the pituitary through the portal blood system, which leads to the secretion of adrenocorticotropic hormone (ACTH). In response to ACTH release from the pituitary, the adrenal secretes GCs. In most laboratory rodents (rats and mice) corticosterone dominates, whereas in humans cortisol is the main adrenal GC. GCs, as lipophilic steroid hormones, enter the brain relatively easily and exert multiple effects in regions throughout the brain. These effects are often mediated through the binding to the two receptors for the hormone: the mineralocorticoid receptor (MR) and the glucocorticoid receptor (GR). These two receptors differ in their affinity for cortisol (with the MR having a much higher affinity) and also in their localization in the brain. In addition, GCs can exert rapid nongenomic effects by influencing ion channels or neurotransmitter receptors at the membrane level. We emphasize that CRH, vasopressin, and ACTH can, on their own, influence cognition; the focus of this article, however, is on the effects of GCs on the memory of humans and animals.

To date, there is a substantial, almost overwhelming, literature on stress and memory. A PubMed search conducted with the two search terms stress and memory produced more than 3000 hits. Even a more focused search using glucocorticoids and memory as search terms still resulted in almost 400 hits. In order to provide a structured overview of this large and rapidly growing field, I use the concept of multiple memory systems in the brain to guide the reader through this jungle. Within each discussed memory domain, animal and human data are discussed. Acute stress effects are described, followed by chronic effects.

Effects of Stress on Different Memory Systems

There is a general agreement that there is not a single memory system in the brain but multiple interacting memory systems. Abundant literature exists on this topic, and it is not the goal of the current review to

provide an in-depth overview of different models and ideas; the important question of the comparability of different memory systems in different species is not addressed here either. I focus instead on declarative or explicit long-term memory because this domain has been, until now, investigated most intensely with respect to stress effects. In addition, I briefly outline the findings for procedural memory, working memory, and conditioning (or associative learning); these three memory systems have been sparsely investigated, at least in humans.

Declarative Memory

Acute effects Declarative memory is the explicit storage of facts and events, which can later be intentionally retrieved. It is a relational and flexible memory system. This type of memory is tested in the laboratory with word lists, paired associates, or short stories in humans. In animals, spatial maze tasks are used most often, the most famous one being the Morris water maze (MWM). Long-term memory can be further divided into different memory phases: acquisition (or initial learning), consolidation (or storage), and retrieval (or recall). For the successful completion of declarative tasks, an intact medial temporal lobe region (the hippocampus and surrounding cortical structures) is essential for the acquisition of the task. The role of the hippocampus in retrieval is under debate, and it might fulfill a time-limited role only. Especially in humans, it is the prefrontal cortex regions that are of great importance for (effortful) retrieval. The literature regarding the effects of stress on declarative memory is quite diverse and confusing, with groups reporting enhancing as well as impairing effects of GCs on this form of memory. However, it has become apparent that this is largely due to the fact that the different memory phases are modulated by GCs in an opposing fashion.

GCs enhance memory consolidation, and this aspect represents the adaptive and beneficial mode of GCs central nervous system action. **Figure 1a** depicts the chain of events underlying this phenomenon. This process has been conceptualized as the beneficial effects of stress within the learning context or intrinsic stress, emphasizing that a stressful episode is remembered better. This effect is mediated by the action of stress-released GCs on the hippocampal formation, and it is very well documented in animals. Studies by Roozendaal and McGaugh showed that adrenergic activation in the basolateral amygdala (BLA) appears to be a prerequisite for the modulating effects of GCs on other brain regions (e.g., the hippocampus). Lesions of the BLA, as well as β blockade, abolish the enhancing effects of posttraining GC administration.

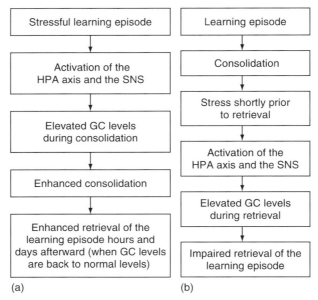

(a) (b)

Figure 1 Schematic diagram of the cascade of events underlying the effects of GCs. a, Positive effects on long-term memory consolidation; b, negative effects on long-term memory retrieval. GC, glucocorticoid; HPA, hypothalamic-pituitary adrenal; SNS, sympathetic nervous system.

Although the enhanced memory consolidation is adaptive and beneficial, this process appears to occur at the cost of impaired retrieval (see **Figure 1b**). Using a 24-h delay interval, deQuervain and colleagues were the first to show that stress or GC treatment shortly before retrieval testing impairs memory retrieval in rats in the MWM. Further studies revealed that, again, an intact BLA and adrenergic activation appear to be necessary for the occurrence of this negative GC effect. Roozendaal summarized these findings as indicating that stress puts the brain into a consolidation mode, which is accompanied by impaired retrieval. Such a retrieval reduction might facilitate consolidation by reducing interference.

In humans, the literature on the acute effects of cortisol on declarative memory is somewhat divergent. Few studies reported beneficial effects, some reported negative effects, and several others found no acute effects. We recently conducted a meta-analysis in order to provide a quantitative summary of the current state of the field. The results supported the model derived from animal studies showing that cortisol impairs memory retrieval. Similar observations have been made in humans who were exposed to a psychosocial laboratory stressor shortly before retrieval testing took place.

To date, the beneficial effects on consolidation could not be clearly established using a meta-analysis, which in part might reflect a power problem. At least some studies, using emotionally arousing learning material and a sufficiently long retention delay in order to assure that GCs can influence consolidation

and in addition are back to baseline at the retrieval testing, observed enhanced memory consolidation for emotionally arousing material.

Interestingly, the beneficial effects on consolidation as well as the impairing effects on retrieval in humans are more pronounced for emotionally arousing material. This observation fits nicely with the observation in animals that GCs can exert effects on memory only in the presence of adrenergic activity in the amygdala. This arousal could be the result of specifics of the learning material and/or specifics of the testing conditions.

In the meta-analysis, time of day appeared as a second modulatory factor. Studies that administered cortisol before initial acquisition observed impairing effects on memory when they were conducted in the morning, a time of high endogenous cortisol levels in humans. In contrast, studies in the evening were more likely to observe beneficial effects. This supports an inverted U-shaped function between cortisol levels and memory in humans with both too low and too high levels at the time of acquisition being associated with impairments, especially when retrieval is tested at times when cortisol levels are still elevated.

In sum, studies in animals and humans converge on the idea that GCs acutely enhance memory consolidation of emotional arousing material while impairing memory retrieval. In addition, within this framework, emotional arousal and a nonlinear dose–response relationship are important modulatory variables.

Cortisol also influences declarative memory consolidation during sleep. Here the relationships appear to be different than in the daytime. Low cortisol levels during the first half of the night are a prerequisite for a sleep-induced enhancement of declarative memory consolidation. Moreover, blocking the rise in cortisol levels, which typically occurs during the second part of the night, leads to enhanced emotional memory facilitation.

The interesting issue of individual differences in responsiveness to GCs has received little attention so far. Such differences might be able to account for some of the variance observed within as well as between studies. Individual differences could reflect genetic factors, differences in tissue GC sensitivity, or differences in lifetime cortisol exposure. Attempts to characterize subgroups with high versus low cortisol sensitivity could be one important venue for future research.

Chronic effects   The picture is different for more chronic effects as a result of prolonged stress or GC treatment – here negative effects prevail. Chronic stress in animals has repeatedly been shown to result in impaired spatial-memory performance. The neurobiological underpinnings of those effects are still under debate. Stress-induced dendritic atrophy (or dendritic remodeling) in the hippocampus is one possible mechanism for the negative effects of chronic stress on spatial memory in rodents. However, several additional mediators such as reduced neurogenesis and dysregulation of several catecholamines have to be considered. Recent studies demonstrated substantial plasticity in the adult rodent brain. For example, stress-induced dendritic atrophy appears to be reversible.

Interestingly, the negative effect of chronic stress on spatial memory might occur only in male rats and not in females. In fact, similarly, acute stress appears to impair spatial memory only in males. The area of sex differences in response to stress is an important and still relatively neglected field. However, authors who went through the extra effort of studying male and female animals have often observed quite striking sex differences in the effects of stress on a wide range of target systems. These observations in combination with evidence for sex differences in emotional memory lateralization and sex differences in the effects of adrenergic manipulations on emotional memory emphasize that caution should be used when generalizing findings obtained in one sex to predict responses in the opposite sex.

In humans, the effects of chronic long-term GC treatment cannot, of course, be studied experimentally due to ethical considerations. Studies that administered GCs for several (3–10) days observed declarative memory impairments. Moreover, studies of patients receiving GC therapy and studies of hypercortisolemic Morbus Cushing patients observed reduced declarative memory performance, which was associated with hippocampal atrophy. Some treatment studies in Cushing patients suggest that hippocampal atrophy in Cushing is reversible, which fits the observations in rodents previously mentioned.

Aging leads to alterations of HPA activity. Basal activity seems to increase and negative feedback is less efficient. Animal studies have suggested that enhanced HPA activity is associated with poorer memory. In older, otherwise healthy humans, several observational studies also reported associations between elevated or rising cortisol levels and declarative memory impairments. Whether these associations are specific for declarative memory or are, in fact, broader (also including working memory or attention) is currently under debate. Obviously all these human studies do not allow a clear cause and effect interpretation. Moreover, in most of these studies, the acute effects of cortisol cannot be differentiated from the chronic effects. In addition, the possible structural correlate of these hormone-performance associations remains to be firmly established. Hence, the possible association between rising cortisol levels and atrophy of the hippocampus is still not sufficiently understood, and the current empirical situation is somewhat mixed.

Finally, it has to be reiterated that other hormonal influences also might be important. With respect to aging, elevated cortisol levels could be part of the metabolic syndrome. Other aspects of this nonfavorable endocrine condition are impaired glucose tolerance and hypertension. These alterations have also been associated with memory impairment during aging, so future studies on this issue should consider taking a broader set of neuroendocrine measurements.

Procedural (Nondeclarative) Memory

This implicit and automatic form of (long-term) memory is not dependent on the medial temporal lobe. The brain areas involved depend on the specific content of the learning material. The neocortical areas, as well as the cerebellum and the basal ganglia, are involved in procedural memory. This is assessed in the laboratory with priming tasks (e.g., word-stem priming) or with skill-learning tasks (e.g., mirror tracing). In the few studies that used such tasks in the context of stress or GC research, a modulating effect of GCs was not observed, thus supporting the assumption that this memory form is not strongly influenced by GCs.

Working Memory

Working memory refers to the ability to store for the short term and manipulate material. This framework has replaced the older notion of short-term memory and emphasizes the active processing capacity of this system. Neuroanatomically, this function has been linked to the prefrontal cortex (PFC). There are a large number of GRs in the PFC, but, in contrast to the effects of GCs on the hippocampus, the effects on the PFC are less well characterized. Acute impairing effects on working memory have been reported in animals and in some studies in humans, but the results have been somewhat inconsistent.

Regarding the chronic effects of GCs on working memory, impaired performance has been reported in animals and humans. In animals, chronic stress was associated with dendritic atrophy in prefrontal regions, which was reversible. In humans, elevated basal GC levels have been associated in some studies with smaller PFC volumes. The PFC is, of course, not only involved in working memory but also in executive functions. These domains have not been well investigated in humans with respect to GC effects and additional research efforts are still needed.

Classical Conditioning (Associative Learning)

Classical conditioning is one of the most basic forms of learning, and it can be demonstrated in snails, fruit flies, rodents, and humans. The brain regions involved depend on the specific stimuli used and the timing of the conditioned stimulus (CS)–unconditioned stimulus (UCS) association. For example, the cerebellum is involved in simple eyelid conditioning, whereas the amygdala is critical for fear conditioning and the hippocampus is important for contextual conditioning and trace conditioning. In rodents, the effects of stress on conditioning has been studied repeatedly. For eyelid conditioning, Shors and coworkers observed that stress enhanced conditioning in male rats. This was true for delay as well as trace conditioning. Interestingly, they observed the opposite effect in female animals – stress impaired conditioning. These findings are the opposite of the effects of acute stress on spatial memory, in which stress enhanced memory in female rats while impairing it in males. Although the enhancing effects of stress or GCs have been observed for fear conditioning, the issue of sex differences has not been addressed systematically. With respect to chronic stress, enhanced fear conditioning in the presence of hippocampal dentritic atrophy has been detected. In humans, classical conditioning has not been studied intensively in the context of neuroendocrine stress research; however, the available studies also observed sex differences. Because this form of learning and memory is of relevance for several psychiatric disorders, more research appears to be necessary.

Clinical Implications

The basic-science studies discussed thus far are also of substantial clinical relevance. For example, patients with posttraumatic stress disorder (PTSD) have been reported to show reduced basal cortisol levels, which is probably due to an enhanced negative feedback of the system. Recent small-scale clinical studies suggested that cortisol treatment shortly after the trauma might help to prevent PTSD. Moreover, even patients with chronic PTSD appear to benefit from a low-dose cortisol treatment. For such patients, the impaired emotional memory retrieval, in combination with an enhanced and more elaborate (place and time) reconsolidation, might help to reduce the core symptoms of the disorder, illustrating that basic science studies in the field of stress neuroendocrinology can help us to understand and possibly treat major psychiatric disorders.

Summary and Conclusion

Research over the past decade has substantially helped us gain a better understanding of the effects of GCs on memory. It is obvious that a more differentiated picture of stress effects on memory has evolved and that oversimplifications such as "stress impairs memory" are no longer supported by the existing literature. Increases in GCs induced by acute stress enhance memory consolidation but impair memory retrieval. These impairing effects of stress-induced GC secretion might hinder us in performing well in an important exam or at an important job interview. In addition, GCs also appear to reduce the amount of items that can be stored in working memory, but this is less well documented than the effects on declarative long-term memory. Interestingly, there is now convincing evidence that adrenergic activation in the amygdale is a prerequisite for several acute effects of GCs on memory. This activation can be induced either through the cognitive task itself, through the test situation (e.g., novel unfamiliar environment), or through the test material (e.g., emotional slides).

Substantial sex differences have been observed in several animal studies, but evidence in humans is still sparse. The direction of the effect appears to be task-specific. More knowledge about sex differences should, in the long run, help us understand sex differences in stress-associated disorders. Future studies need to investigate whether these sex differences are related to differences in the neuroendocrine stress response or differences in the response of the brain to endocrine stress messengers.

Chronic stress or chronic GC treatment has mostly negative effects on the brain and on the body. These observations are relevant to psychiatric disorders as well as to the aging process. However, it is encouraging that recent research has repeatedly observed evidence for preserved plasticity and structural remodeling once the stress has ceased or GCs return to normal levels.

Especially rewarding for all basic-science research that has been done on stress is that already several clinical applications have been implemented or are on the horizon.

Acknowledgments

The author's work was supported by grants from the German Research Foundation (DFG WO 733/6-1 and WO 733/7-1).

Further Reading

Aerni, A., Traber, R., Hock, C., et al. (2004). Low-dose cortisol for symptoms of posttraumatic stress disorder. *American Journal of Psychiatry* 161, 1488–1490.

Buchanan, T. W. and Lovallo, W. R. (2001). Enhanced memory for emotional material following stress-level cortisol treatment in humans. *Psychoneuroendocrinology* 26, 307–317.

Cahill, L. (2003). Sex-related influences on the neurobiology of emotionally influenced memory. *Annals of the New York Academy of Sciences* 985, 163–173.

Conrad, C. D., Jackson, J. L., Wieczorek, L., et al. (2004). Acute stress impairs spatial memory in male but not female rats: influence of estrous cycle. *Pharmacology Biochemistry & Behavior* 78, 569–579.

Conrad, C. D., LeDoux, J. E., Magarinos, A. M., et al. (1999). Repeated restraint stress facilitates fear conditioning independently of causing hippocampal CA3 dendritic atrophy. *Behavioral Neuroscience* 113, 902–913.

Convit, A. (2005). Links between cognitive impairment in insulin resistance: an explanatory model. *Neurobiology of Aging* 26(supplement1), 31–35.

Croiset, G., Nijsen, M. J. and Kamphuis, P. J. (2000). Role of corticotropin-releasing factor, vasopressin and the autonomic nervous system in learning and memory. *European Journal of Pharmacology* 405, 225–234.

De Kloet, E. R., Joels, M. and Holsboer, F. (2005). Stress and the brain: from adaptation to disease. *Nature Reviews Neuroscience* 6, 463–475.

De Kloet, E. R., Oitzl, M. S. and Joels, M. (1999). Stress and cognition: are corticosteroids good or bad guys? *Trends in Neurosciences* 22, 422–426.

de Quervain, D. J., Roozendaal, B. and McGaugh, J. L. (1998). Stress and glucocorticoids impair retrieval of long-term spatial memory. *Nature* 394, 787–790.

Het, S., Ramlow, G. and Wolf, O. T. (2005). A meta-analytic review of the effects of acute cortisol administration on human memory. *Psychoneuroendocrinology* 30, 771–784.

Kuhlmann, S., Piel, M. and Wolf, O. T. (2005). Impaired memory retrieval after psychosocial stress in healthy young men. *Journal of Neuroscience* 25, 2977–2982.

LaBar, K. S. and Cabeza, R. (2006). Cognitive neuroscience of emotional memory. *Nature Reviews Neuroscience* 7, 54–64.

Luine, V. (2002). Sex differences in chronic stress effects on memory in rats. *Stress* 5, 205–216.

Lupien, S. J. and Lepage, M. (2001). Stress, memory, and the hippocampus: can't live with it, can't live without it. *Behavioural Brain Research* 127, 137–158.

Lupien, S. J., Schwartz, G., Ng, Y. K., et al. (2005). The Douglas Hospital Longitudinal Study of Normal and Pathological Aging: summary of findings. *Journal of Psychiatry & Neuroscience* 30, 328–334.

MacLullich, A. M., Deary, I. J., Starr, J. M., et al. (2005). Plasma cortisol levels, brain volumes and cognition in healthy elderly men. *Psychoneuroendocrinology* 30, 505–515.

McEwen, B. S. (2002). Sex, stress and the hippocampus: allostasis, allostatic load and the aging process. *Neurobiology of Aging* 23, 921–939.

Roozendaal, B. (2000). Glucocorticoids and the regulation of memory consolidation. *Psychoneuroendocrinology* 25, 213–238.

Roozendaal, B., Okuda, S., de Quervain, D. J., et al. (2006). Glucocorticoids interact with emotion-induced noradrenergic activation in influencing different memory functions. *Neuroscience* 138(3), 901–910.

Schelling, G., Roozendaal, B. and de Quervain, D. J. (2004). Can posttraumatic stress disorder be prevented with glucocorticoids? *Annals of the New York Academy of Sciences* 1032, 158–166.

Shors, T. J. (2004). Learning during stressful times. *Learning & Memory* 11, 137–144.

Squire, L. R. (1992). Memory and the hippocampus: a synthesis from findings with rats, monkeys, and humans. *Psychological Review* 99, 195–231.

Tulving, E. (2001). Episodic memory and common sense: how far apart? *Philosophical Transactions of the Royal Society of London B Biological Sciences* 356, 1505–1515.

Wagner, U., Degirmenci, M., Drosopoulos, S., et al. (2005). Effects of cortisol suppression on sleep-associated consolidation of neutral and emotional memory. *Biological Psychiatry* 58, 885–893.

Wolf, O. T. (2003). HPA axis and memory. *Best Practice & Research: Clinical Endocrinology & Metabolism* 17, 287–299.

Wolkowitz, O. M., Reus, V. I., Canick, J., et al. (1997). Glucocorticoid medication, memory and steroid psychosis in medical illness. *Annals of the New York Academy of Sciences* 823, 81–96.

Yehuda, R. (2002). Post-traumatic stress disorder. *New England Journal of Medicine* 346, 108–114.

Glucocorticoid Negative Feedback

M F Dallman
University of California, San Francisco, CA, USA

This article is reproduced from the previous edition, volume 2, pp 224–228, © 2000, Elsevier Inc.

Characteristics of Feedback in the Hypothalamic-Pituitary-Adrenocortical Axis

Site(s) of Negative Feedback in the Hypothalamic-Pituitary-Adrenocortical Axis

Glossary

Adrenocorticotropic hormone (ACTH)	A hormone made in corticotroph cells of the anterior pituitary; it stimulates the synthesis and secretion of corticosteroids from the adrenal cortex.
Arginine vasopressin (AVP)	A hormone that, when cosecreted with CRH, potentiates ACTH release.
Corticotropin releasing hormone (CRH)	A hormone synthesized in the hypothalamus; it stimulates ACTH synthesis and secretion from anterior pituitary corticotropic cells.
Dexamethasone	A potent synthetic glucocorticoid that does not bind to transcortin (corticosteroid-binding globulin, CBG).
Glucocorticoid receptor (GR)	Low-affinity intracellular corticosteroid receptor that prefers dexamethasone, cortisol, and corticosterone.
Limbic system	A system of neural structures (amygdala, bed nuclei of the stria terminalis, hippocampus, septal nuclei, and hypothalamic and midbrain cell groups) that subserve the emotional and other associative memory, determining overall responsiveness to stressors.
Mineralocorticoid receptor (MR)	High-affinity intracellular corticosteroid receptor that selectively binds aldosterone, corticosterone, and cortisol.
Paraventricular nucleus (PVN)	Hypothalamic site of neuronal synthesis of CRH and AVP, which are secreted from axonal endings in the median eminence to act on pituitary corticotrophs.
Stressors	Stimuli that challenge the physical or psychological stability of the organism and cause the activation of the hypothalamic-pituitary-adrenal axis.
Transcortin (CBG)	A high-affinity binder for cortisol and corticosterone made by the liver; it reversibly binds corticosteroids in the circulation; also called corticosteroid-binding globulin.

Negative feedback inhibition by adrenal glucocorticoids is the means by which the brain is informed that the pituitary ACTH-secreting cells and adrenocortical fasciculata cells have done its bidding. However, a great deal of flexibility is required for an effective feedback system to serve its appropriate function. Thus, there are various time domains and mechanisms by which the glucocorticoids act to inhibit further brain-induced stimulation of the hypothalamic-pituitary-adrenocortical (HPA) axis, the different sites at which the steroids act, and the state-dependent modifications of the brain response to the feedback action of the steroids. The net result of this seeming complexity is a spectacularly functional feedback system that maintains glucocorticoid levels at values appropriate for the physiology of the organism at most times.

Characteristics of Feedback in the Hypothalamic-Pituitary-Adrenocortical Axis

The wide variation in total circulating corticosteroid levels, from the low nanomolar range during the daily circadian trough to the micromolar range during stress, provides a problem for feedback regulation by corticosteroids; the solution is to use two receptors of differing affinities to regulate the brain activation of the adrenocortical system. In addition, there are three temporal domains for the inhibitory effects of corticosteroids and the brain also manages to modify the apparent efficacy of the negative feedback effects of corticosteroids under persistently stressful conditions, thus maintaining an HPA axis that is responsive under conditions in which circulating corticosteroid levels are higher than the usual set point.

Two Receptors Mediate the Feedback Effects of Glucocorticoids

Figure 1 indicates the problem that must be solved by a corticosteroid feedback system in order to control accurately the activity of the HPA axis under circadian and stressful conditions. During the trough of the basal rhythm, total cortisol levels range between 50 and 100 nM. Because at low values ~99% of this represents cortisol bound to CBG, the free cortisol levels that can diffuse from the vascular compartment into the interstitial fluid to bathe cells range between ~0.5 and 1.0 nM. By contrast, at the peak of the circadian rhythm and after stress, total cortisol ranges up to micromolar concentrations and free

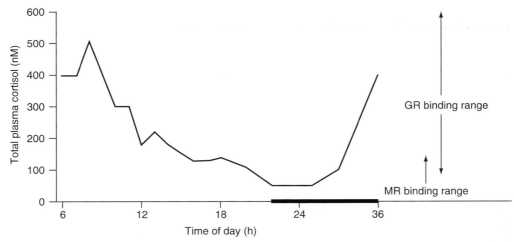

Figure 1 The two-receptor system that provides feedback information to the central HPA axis about adrenocortical performance. A hypothetical normal circadian rhythm in total plasma cortisol (CBG-bound and free) in humans. The dark bar on the abscissa represents the hours of darkness and sleep. The peak occurs just prior to awakening and the beginning of the daily activity cycle. The trough (MR occupancy) occurs early in the hours of sleep and inactivity before values rise again. Stressor-induced increases in cortisol can reach micromolar concentrations. Clearly, if GRs are occupied, MRs are as well. The estimated occupancy of MRs and GRs by free steroid at the various levels of total steroid is shown on the right.

cortisol levels approach 100–300 nM or even higher. Because receptors characteristically bind hormone over a 100-fold range, it is clear that a single receptor for cortisol cannot control the range of cortisol concentrations required during the normal physiological excursions of the HPA axis. The solution is the use of two receptors of differing affinities to inform the brain of adrenocortical activity.

1. The MR is a high-affinity receptor (K_d 0.5–1 nM) that has roughly equally high affinity for aldosterone, cortisol, and corticosterone. In cells that are selectively responsive to aldosterone, such as the principal cells of the renal nephron, there is an enzyme (11-β-hydroxysteroid dehydrogenase type II) that oxidizes the 11-hydroxyl groups of cortisol and corticosterone to the inactive 11-keto form. Aldosterone exists as an 11-18-hemiketal in solution and is not oxidized by this enzyme; therefore, it can exert its actions selectively in these target cells. Cells that do not contain the enzyme but do have MRs bind all three steroids; however, cortisol and corticosterone circulate in higher concentrations and gain entry to the brain much more easily than aldosterone; therefore, these steroids primarily occupy MRs in the brain. In the brain, MRs have a highly discrete distribution, primarily in neurons in entorhinal cortex, limbic structures, and motor output neurons. There is a very low density of MRs in the neurons of the hypothalamus.

2. The GR is a lower-affinity (K_d 10–30 nM) corticosteroid receptor that prefers dexamethasone ≫ cortisol, corticosterone > aldosterone. The GRs are distributed in every cell type in the organism. The distribution of GR in the brain is very widespread in both glial cells and neurons. CRH neurons in hypothalamus are well endowed with GRs, as are the neurons in the limbic system, the monoaminergic systems, and others.

Both occupied MRs and GRs dimerize in the cell nucleus to alter transcriptional rates of tissue-specific genes. In addition, MRs and GRs in the same cell can heterodimerize and act transcriptionally. Moreover, it is increasingly clear that the hormone receptor complexes can function in protein–protein interactions with other transcription factors to alter transcription rates. At this time, the specific effect of occupancy of MRs and GRs on transcription is impossible to predict. Nonetheless, occupancy of MRs and GRs by cortisol or corticosterone serves to inhibit activity in the HPA axis, generally by an action on brain.

Feedback regulation in the animal and its utility Using adrenalectomy and infusion of MR and GR agonists as well as treatment with specific antagonists in intact animals, it is clear that occupancy of the MRs is required to maintain ACTH secretion at low levels during the trough of the circadian rhythm. By contrast, at the circadian peak and during stress, the occupancy of both MR and GR restrains ACTH secretion, maintaining it within the normal limits observed in intact organisms. Because occupied GRs and MRs are powerful modulators of cell function, it is important to maintain their overall concentrations at tightly regulated levels. Many corticosteroid-sensitive end points change their levels and activity when there is slight deviance on either side of the normal daily mean value. In studies of the daily mean of plasma cortisol in humans, values range from 6 to 8 μg dl^{-1} when levels collected over 24 h are averaged. Similarly, in rats, the 24-h mean corticosterone concentration ranges between 4.5 and 7 μg dl^{-1}. Both species have relatively high circulating CBG levels. Above or below these ranges in unstressed humans and rats, untoward metabolic, behavioral, and immunological changes occur.

Temporally Discrete Effects of Corticosteroids on Hypothalamic-Pituitary-Adrenal Axis Function

Feedback inhibition of (CRH, AVP, and) ACTH secretion can be shown to exist in fast, intermediate, and slow time domains when corticosteroids are administered exogenously. Normally these segue smoothly from one to the other, but they can be distinguished mechanistically, and the degree of inhibition increases as the duration and amount of the corticosteroid exposure increases. In all time domains, the magnitude of the effect is strictly proportional to the dose of steroid, between the limits of threshold and saturating quantities.

1. The fast effects occur within milliseconds on neurons and must be exerted by an effect at the cell membrane. A membrane receptor has not yet been characterized. The iontophoresis of corticosteroids onto neurons or bathing tissue slices with corticosteroids shows effects within milliseconds to seconds on membrane function. Similarly, in animals the stimulation of pathways to CRH neurons does not evoke the normal response within minutes of a systemic injection of corticosteroids. At the pituitary corticotroph, CRH-stimulated ACTH secretion is inhibited within a few minutes of the application of corticosteroids; this inhibition is not altered by the inhibition of RNA or protein synthesis, showing that it is not mediated by the usual genomic effects of corticosteroids, although it may be mediated by interference with the generation of adenyl cyclase, the intracellular messenger for CRH. The magnitude of the fast inhibition of ACTH secretion by corticosteroids acting on the corticotroph is small (~25% of the maximal inhibition possible); thus, fast feedback leaves the organism responsive to further stressors and capable of secreting nearly normal amounts of ACTH.

2. Intermediate feedback has its onset at approximately 30 min after a pulse or continuous exposure to the steroid and lasts for a period of hours. The inhibition of protein synthesis with cyclohexamide blocks this feedback and, although it is powerful and can

completely inhibit CRH-induced ACTH secretion in the whole animal, ACTH secretion can usually be stimulated by further treatment with CRH or AVP. This temporal domain of corticosteroid feedback appears to dampen the excitability in the HPA axis without abolishing it (i.e., excitability is returned to prestress levels so that subsequent responsivity is not excessive). At the pituitary, AVP-stimulated ACTH secretion is less sensitive than CRH to corticosteroid inhibition.

3. Slow feedback is found in conditions in which the supraphysiological levels of exogenous corticosteroids have been provided for days or weeks. All components of the HPA axis are unresponsive to stimulation, both by intense stressors and, at the pituitary, by CRH and AVP. The CRH and AVP mRNA expression in the hypothalamus and proopiomelanocorticoid expression in the pituitary is markedly decreased. This condition is most frequently observed in humans with active Cushing disease or after prolonged treatment of disease with high levels of synthetic glucocorticoids; it takes months to recover from this inhibition when the high levels of steroid are removed.

Conditional Feedback in the Hypothalamic-Pituitary-Adrenal Axis

Up to this point, glucocorticoid feedback properties have been discussed with respect to the normal unstressed organism. Under conditions of persistent or chronic stress, the axis appears to change, and sensitivity to the feedback action of corticosteroids is slightly to markedly reduced. Thus, under chronic stress, mean daily plasma corticosteroid concentrations increase, frequently only because circadian trough levels are elevated but occasionally because there are major stressor-induced elevations throughout the circadian cycle. With chronic stress, the degree of the inhibition of stimulated ACTH secretion by exogenous (or endogenously secreted) glucocorticoids is decreased. In rats, chronic stress often stimulates increased expression of AVP in CRH-synthesizing neurons, thus providing a means for amplifying the corticotroph response to the CRH and AVP secreted. However, it also appears that neural sites upstream from the final hypothalamic CRH and AVP motor neurons of the HPA axis are less sensitive to corticosteroid feedback.

A decreased number of GRs has been reported, primarily in hippocampus, after many chronic stressors and after treatment with exogenous glucocorticoids, suggesting that one mechanism of reduced feedback sensitivity may reside in GR downregulation. This is not the only explanation for reduced feedback sensitivity during chronic stress, however, because there are several examples in which both MR and GR numbers are normal throughout brain but glucocorticoid feedback insensitivity is found.

Because the strength of inputs to the CRH and AVP cells stimulates dose-related output, it is likely that, although corticosteroid dose-related functions are occurring normally under chronic stress conditions, the level of input to the CRH and AVP cells increases. Thus, normal responsivity in the HPA axis is maintained, whereas the apparent feedback efficacy of glucocorticoids is reduced. It does appear that new stimuli presented to chronically stressed animals causes facilitated responses in the central neural pathways to the CRH and AVP neurons.

The result of the apparent decrease in glucocorticoid feedback under conditions of chronic stimulation of the HPA axis is that there is dampening of the response to the ongoing stimulus but full or even exaggerated responsiveness to a new and different stimulus. Both effects are useful – the degree of hyperglucocorticoidism is limited by ongoing glucocorticoid feedback, but the organism is still capable of responding to a new stimulus that may demand a momentary shot of the hormones for optimal response.

Site(s) of Negative Feedback in the Hypothalamic-Pituitary-Adrenocortical Axis

Feedback is primarily exerted in the brain under normal conditions, with only moderate increases in mean corticosteroid levels or low-magnitude acute stressors. Although the CRH and AVP neurons in the PVN are plentifully supplied with GRs, this site does not appear to be inhibited directly by the naturally occurring corticosteroids. Instead, the corticosteroids appear to inhibit the activity of neuronal pathways that eventually impinge on CRH and AVP neurons. At high sustained corticosteroid levels, there is also clearly negative feedback on anterior pituitary corticotrophs.

Feedback in the Brain

Microinfusions of low amounts of MR and GR antagonists into the cerebral ventricles or into specific brain sites augment the magnitude of ACTH responses to a variety of stressors, strongly suggesting that stress-induced glucocorticoid secretion decreases the stimulatory input to the PVN during both the fast- and intermediate-feedback time domains. Small crystalline implants of corticosterone placed chronically into prefrontal cortex, the preoptic area, and the dorsal hippocampus have been shown to reduce stress or adrenalectomy-induced ACTH secretion. However, it appears that steroids implanted into brain must bathe those neurons that are activated by the specific stressor used to excite the HPA axis. That is, there appear to be distributed sites at which steroids may inhibit HPA responses to stressors, not a single feedback site that globally inhibits PVN neuronal responses to stressors. Corticosteroids, acting through both MRs and GRs, have been shown to alter neuronal properties and activity in the hippocampus, and antagonists infused into both the amygdala and hippocampus have been shown to alter conditioned behaviors. However, it has not yet been directly demonstrated that implants in these sites alter the amount of ACTH secreted in response to a stressor. It may well be that corticosteroid receptors in these sites have little to do with modulating CRH and AVP secretion directly. In the brain, it appears that for feedback effects of steroid implants to be observed on ACTH secretion the steroid must act on sites that are also activated by stress; the feedback action is selective and specific.

Feedback at the Pituitary

Corticotrophs contain GRs but not MRs, and the direct inhibitory effects of corticosteroids are evident at the anterior pituitary. The concentrations of the naturally occurring steroids required to effect the inhibition of ACTH secretion are relatively high. This is probably because corticotrophs contain the high-affinity CBG corticosteroid binder apparently taken up from the circulation. The CBG in the corticotrophs sequesters the natural corticosteroids and high concentrations (10^{-8} M) are required to observe inhibition, although dexamethasone, which does not bind to CBG, is a more effective inhibitory agent. Moreover, corticotrophs tend to maintain sensitivity to AVP, although sensitivity to CRH decreases when corticosteroid levels are elevated. The relative insensitivity of the corticotroph to corticosteroid inhibition is useful because it allows the corticotroph to be the site of last resort, requiring the highest levels of signal, for the global inhibitory control of the HPA axis.

See Also the Following Articles

Adrenocorticotropic Hormone (ACTH); Corticotropin Releasing Factor (CRF); Feedback Systems; Glucocorticoids, Effects of Stress on; Hypothalamic-Pituitary-Adrenal.

Further Reading

Antoni, F. A. (1993). Vasopressinergic control of pituitary adrenocorticotropin comes of age. *Frontiers in Neuroendocrinology* 14, 76–122.
Bamberger, C. M., Schulte, H. M. and Chrousos, G. P. Molecular determinants of glucocorticoid receptor function and tissue sensitivity to glucocorticoids. *Endocrine Review* 17, 245–261.

Dallman, M. F., Akana, S. F., Cascio, C. S., Darlington, D. N., Jacobson, L. and Levin, N. (1987). Regulation of ACTH secretion: variations on a theme of B. In: Clark, J. H. (ed.) *Recent progress in hormone research*, pp. 113–173. Orlando, FL: Academic Press.

Dallman, M. F., Akana, S. F., Scribner, K. A., et al. (1992). Stress, feedback and facilitation in the hypothalamo-pituitary-adrenal axis. *Journal of Neuroendocrinology* 4, 517–526.

Dallman, M. F. and Bhatnagar, S. (1999). *Chronic stress and energy balance: role of the hypothalamo-pituitary-adrenal axis.* Washington, DC: American Physiological Society.

De Kloet, E. R. (1991). Brain corticosteroid receptor balance and homeostatic control. *Frontiers in Neuro-endocrinology* 12, 95–164.

Joels, M. (1997). Steroid hormones and excitability in the mammalian brain. *Frontiers in Neuroendocrinology* 18, 2–48.

Keller-Wood, M. E. and Dallman, M. F. (1984). Corticosteroid inhibition of ACTH secretion. *Endocrine Review* 5, 1–24.

Glucocorticoid Receptor Mutant Mice as Models for Stress-Induced Affective Disorders

P Gass
Central Institute of Mental Health (CIMA), University of Heidelberg, Heidelberg, Germany

Corticosteroids, Corticosteroid Receptors, and Depression
Animal Models of Depression
Mice with Targeted Mutations of GR
GR Mutant Mice Represent a Tool to Study Molecular Correlates of Depression-like Behavior

Glossary

Corticosteroids	Hormones synthesized in the adrenal glands, secreted in a circadian rhythm and in response to stress. The main endogenous glucocorticoids are corticosterone in rodents and cortisol in humans.
Corticosteroid receptors	Intracellular receptor molecules for corticosteroid hormones. On hormone binding they function as transcription factors in the nucleus of the cell to regulate the expression of target genes. There are two types: mineralocorticoid receptors and glucocorticoid receptors.
Depression	Psychiatric disorder characterized by core symptoms such as depressed mood, anhedonia, and loss of interests. The syndrome also includes changes in cognition, psychomotor alterations, and vegetative symptoms (changes in sleeping, eating, and sexual behaviors).
Hypothalamic-pituitary-adrenocortical (HPA) axis	The brain-controlled activation pathway for the secretion of corticosteroid hormones after stress through a hormonal signaling cascade, involving release of corticotropin-releasing hormone from the paraventricular nucleus of the hypothalamus in the brain and adrenocorticotropic hormone from the pituitary gland.
Learned helplessness	A psychobiological concept that predicts that stressors are particularly apt to induce depressive states when they are unpredictable and uncontrollable.
Stress	A physiological and psychological state caused by a real or perceived challenge to homeostasis, which is accompanied by a hormonal stress response.
Transgenic mice	Animals with a gene knockout (loss of function) or a transgene expressing an additional gene product (gain of function), designed by targeted mutagenesis. With modern techniques, genes can be overexpressed or shut down in a brain regional or temporal-specific way.

Corticosteroids, Corticosteroid Receptors, and Depression

Dysregulations and dysfunctions of corticosteroid receptors have been implicated in the pathogenesis of stress-related psychiatric disorders such as depression and posttraumatic stress disorder. It is still unclear, however, whether these corticosteroid receptor disturbances are a cause or a consequence of affective disorders. Clinical studies have demonstrated a hyperactivity of the hypothalamic-pituitary-adrenocortical (HPA) system with elevated plasma cortisol levels in many patients with major depression. In these patients, diminished corticosteroid receptor expression or function has been postulated as a causative factor for a deficient feedback of cortisol that may explain their increased HPA activity and stress sensitivity. An alternative hypothesis claims that the primary cause of the HPA dysregulation is an upregulation of hypothalamic corticotropin-releasing hormone (CRH) levels, which secondarily leads to corticosteroid receptor downregulation in the limbic system and the hypothalamus that perpetuates the disease state. According to the latter concept, the changes of the HPA system may result from a primary disturbance of monoaminergic systems and their widespread connections to higher brain centers, including cortex, limbic system, and hypothalamus.

Corticosteroids exert their effects via two types of receptors: high-affinity receptors for cortisol called mineralocorticoid receptors (MRs) because of their ability to bind also mineralocorticoids (e.g., aldosterone), and low-affinity receptors called glucocorticoid receptors (GRs), which mainly bind cortisol or corticosterone. MRs are predominantly found in the limbic system, in particular in the hippocampus, whereas GRs are ubiquitously expressed throughout the central nervous system. Functionally, MRs are thought to be involved in the physiological maintenance of the HPA system, while GRs are supposed to control the recovery from stress. Corticosteroid receptors are intracellular proteins and function as transcription factors. Their ligands are lipophilic and can easily cross the cytoplasmic membrane. Inside the cell, activation of the receptors provokes their translocation to the nucleus, where they bind to specific sequences on the DNA (glucocorticoid response elements [GREs]) and enhance or repress the transcription rate of their target genes. GRs can also up- or downregulate gene transcription by direct interaction with other transcription factors such as CREB or AP-1.

Activation of corticosteroid receptors in neurons can influence diverse cellular processes such as energy metabolism, signal transduction, and even structural plasticity. Functional consequences include the control of excitability in limbic brain regions, in particular in the hippocampus. The corticosteroid receptor-mediated effects at the cellular level have consequences for processes in which the hippocampal formation plays an essential role, e.g., in the neuroendocrine regulation of the HPA system and also in behavior. Thus, apart from emotional behavior, corticosteroids also influence perception as well as learning and memory.

According to current concepts, GR-mediated functions in particular are disturbed in patients with severe depressive episodes. However, since studies of the GR in the human brain are not feasible *in vivo*, such evidence is mostly derived from pharmacological challenge tests, such as the dexamethasone suppression test, which indirectly measures GR function in the pituitary and maybe in part also in the central nervous system. Thus, the analysis of direct effects of GR dysfunction and its potential role in emotional behavior is restricted to animal models. For this purpose, targeted mutagenesis in mice seems to be particularly promising.

Animal Models of Depression

Good animal models of human depression should fulfill the following criteria as best as possible: strong behavioral similarities (e.g., similar core symptoms), common etiology, similar pathophysiology, and common treatment. Such a model could then be used to elucidate molecular and biochemical mechanisms underlying the pathogenesis of depression. One of the core symptoms of severe depression in humans and mice is anhedonia, i.e., the lack of interest in pleasurable activities. In mice, anhedonia can be measured by a loss of preference for sweet solutions over tap water. Another core symptom is coping deficits in aversive but avoidable life situations. Confusion between a model and a test should be avoided. A model can be defined as an organism or a particular state of an organism that reproduces aspects of human pathology, providing a certain degree of predictive validity. A test is an end-point behavioral or physiological measure designed to assess the effect of a pharmacological or environmental manipulation. In this respect, models of depression are different from the tests used to monitor the effects of antidepressants. Behavioral despair paradigms such as the Porsolt forced swim test and the tail suspension test cannot be considered models of depression, even though their efficiency to screen for antidepressant-like activity is widely accepted. Nevertheless, increased despair behavior in these tests can be regarded as part of a depressive syndrome.

Two paradigms induce anhedonia in mice: the chronic mild stress model and the learned helplessness paradigm. In the chronic mild stress model, animals are subjected for several weeks to a series of mild stressors (intermittent food and water deprivation, overnight illumination, cage tilt, noise, etc.). This treatment induces a reduction of sucrose preference, decreased intracranial self-stimulation, altered sexual and aggressive behavior, loss of body weight, sleep disturbances, and overactivation of the HPA system. These symptoms are reversible upon administration of antidepressants. In the learned helplessness paradigm, animals are exposed to inescapable electric footshocks, which induce a number of deficits similar to those observed after chronic stress: failure in avoidance learning, lower preference for sucrose solution, decreased appetite, loss of body weight, and overactivation of the HPA system. Again, these effects are reversed by the administration of antidepressants. Thus, the behavioral and somatic deficits observed in these two models mimic the human depressive syndrome.

A major drawback of the previous models is the difficulty of knowing whether the pathological changes observed are due to the animals' depressive state or rather reflect the manipulation by which this state was induced, e.g., stress or pharmacological treatment. An alternative animal model of affective disorders would be an endogenous, genetic model, independent of external factors, which mimics essential aspects of the human disorder and responds to standard regimens of therapy. Mouse mutants with altered HPA system activity are candidate strains for a murine depression-like syndrome, because HPA system imbalances are a key biological marker for a major depression in humans. In particular, alterations of corticosteroid receptors appear promising in modeling affective disorders. Different strains of mutant mice have been or can be obtained with over- or underexpression of glucocorticoid receptors. Current techniques even allow a conditional gene disruption in specific brain regions, in the best case inducible at a selective time point.

Mice with Targeted Mutations of GR

Several mouse strains with altered GR expression or function have been generated (**Table 1**). The mice produced earlier (before 2000) did not exhibit a behavioral depression-like phenotype. Thus, mice with a GR point mutation (GR^{dim}) that prevents GR dimerization and binding to its cognate element GRE have not revealed any changes in emotional behavior. Surprisingly, a GR antisense model with reduced expression in the brain as well as a strain with a

Table 1 Mouse strains with targeted GR mutations

Mouse strain	Reference
Transgenic mice with reduced GR expression in the brain	Pepin et al. (1992)
Mice with destructed GR dimerization (GR^{dim})	Reichardt et al. (1998)
GR^{NesCre} mice with CNS-specific GR knockout	Tronche et al. (1999)
Transgenic mice with increased GR expression (YGR mice)	Reichardt et al. (2000)
Mice with forebrain-specific GR overexpression	Wei et al. (2004)
GR^{CamKIICre} mice with forebrain-specific GR knockout	Boyle et al. (2004)
GR$^{+/-}$ mice	Ridder et al. (2005)

brain-specific GR knockout (GR^{NesCre}) exhibited reduced depression-like behaviors. However, these paradoxical findings may be explained by the fact that a complete lack of GR prevents all stress- or corticosterone-induced effects usually mediated by GRs and results in a stress-resistant phenotype. With respect to human genetics and psychopathology, the genetic defects generated in these early mouse strains are very unlikely to occur in humans.

To mimic certain quantitative or functional alterations of GRs – as postulated for depressive patients – mice were generated that have either a 50% reduced or a twofold increased GR gene dosage (**Figures 1** and **2**). Moreover, in these mice the genetic context controlling the GR gene was preserved as much as possible to maintain the regulatory principles governing the normal gene. Such mice have been generated by homologous recombination (GR$^{+/-}$ mice) and by a transgenic approach (YGR mice). The latter strain contains two additional copies of the GR gene. This strain was generated by transfer of a yeast artificial chromosome of 290 kb in length, providing the transgenes with the natural chromosomal context of the mouse genome, resulting in expression of the GR transgenes in a copy number-dependent and position-independent manner. According to the molecular hypotheses of depression, one would expect that mice with reduced expression levels of GR (GR$^{+/-}$) have a predisposition to develop depression-like behavior. Current hypotheses would also predict that mice overexpressing GR (YGR) are more resistant to developing depression-like features than wild-type mice. To test these hypotheses, GR$^{+/-}$ and YGR mice were subjected to a standardized battery of tests for emotional behavior, including tests for depression-like signs such as despair and helplessness. Furthermore, the HPA system was analyzed under baseline conditions, after stress, and following a Dex/CRH challenge. Moreover, the content of brain-derived neurotrophic factor (BDNF) was determined in the hippocampus, since BDNF has been postulated to play a critical role in pathogenesis and therapy of affective disorders.

GR$^{+/-}$ Mice Exhibit a Depression-like Behavioral and Neuroendocrinological Phenotype

GR$^{+/-}$ mice did not exhibit phenotypical changes under basal conditions in a test battery for locomotor, exploratory, anxiety-related, and emotional behaviors. In this context, it is of interest that a selective loss of GR function in hepatocytes did not affect gluconeogenesis under basal conditions, but caused a gluconeogenesis deficit under challenge conditions by fasting the animals. Similarly, GR$^{+/-}$ mice exhibited a depression-like phenotype, i.e., increased

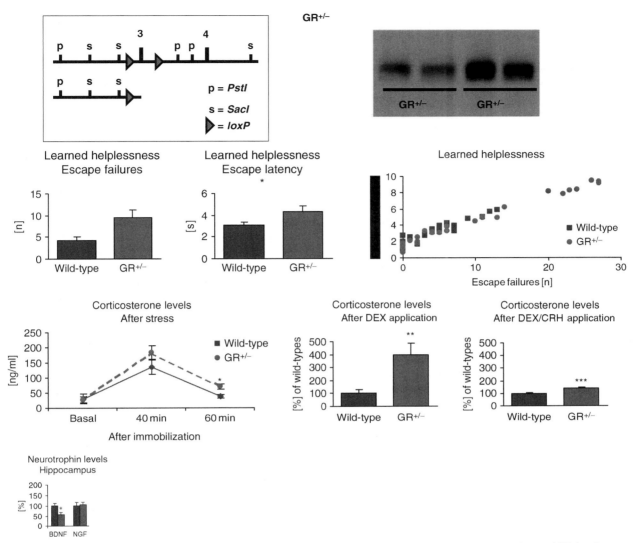

Figure 1 Genetic manipulation. The GR null allele was obtained by deleting the third exon (and a subsequent frame shift), leading to a truncated GR protein without functional domains. Heterozygous mice that underexpress GR exhibit normal baseline behaviors, but after stress exposure they demonstrate significantly increased learned helplessness. Similar to depressed patients, they show a disinhibition of the HPA system and a pathological Dex/CRH test. In agreement with the neurotrophin hypothesis of depression, they have reduced BDNF levels in the hippocampus. Thus, these mice represent a strain with a predisposition to develop depression-like features after stress.

helplessness, after being challenged by environmental stress (**Figure 1**). The learned helplessness model is a rodent depression model with good face and construct validity. It is based on the concept that depressed individuals show a loss of coping strategies in aversive environmental situations. $GR^{+/-}$ mice demonstrated significantly prolonged escape latencies and increased failures in the active avoidance task of the learned helplessness paradigm after two sessions of footshock exposure. The impaired coping behavior strongly indicated the development of depression-like behavior in $GR^{+/-}$ mice.

This altered behavioral reactivity to stress was accompanied by depression-like alterations of the HPA system. Similar to the behavioral level, changes of the HPA axis were not present under basal conditions in $GR^{+/-}$ mice, but a significant disinhibition occurred after stress. Furthermore, $GR^{+/-}$ mice exhibited a pathological Dex/CRH test, currently the most relevant biological marker in patients for both florid depression and the risk of developing a depressive episode. This test combines the suppressive effect of dexamethasone with the stimulatory potency of CRH. In 70–80% of severely depressed patients the CRH-elicited adrenocorticotropic hormone (ACTH) and cortisol response is blunted, and dexamethasone pretreatment does not elicit a suppressive effect and paradoxically induces enhanced cortisol levels

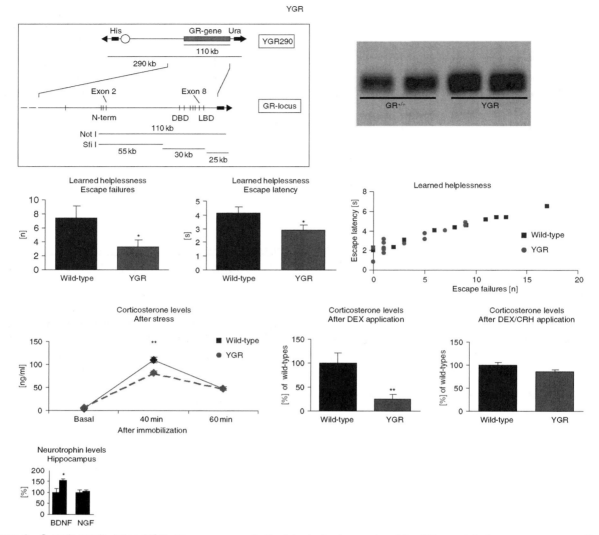

Figure 2 Genetic manipulation. YGR mice were generated by introducing two copies of the GR gene into the mouse genome with the help of the yeast artificial chromosome (YAC), which contains the entire GR locus of 110 kb with all regulatory sequences. Transgenic mice that overexpress GR in the brain are less sensitive to stress. Following immobilization, their HPA system returns to homeostasis faster than in wild-type. Behaviorally, they demonstrate better coping when exposed to stress than control littermates, even though baseline behavior is unaltered. Therefore, these mice represent a depression-resistant strain.

following a CRH challenge. In healthy individuals, in contrast, the Dex/CRH test creates the situation of a pharmacological (partial and transient) adrenalectomy in which hypothalamic CRH expression is increased due to a decrease in plasma cortisol. Similarly to depressed patients, GR[+/−] mice display a characteristic nonsuppression following dexamethasone treatment and the paradoxical increase of corticosterone levels after combined Dex/CRH application.

Normal Baseline Behavior and Neuroendocrinology of GR[+/−] Mice May Reflect Developmental Compensation

Using modern transgenic techniques, recently a mouse strain was generated with a forebrain-specific

complete GR knockout, induced by the calcium-calmodulin-dependent protein kinase II (CamKII) promoter. In contrast to GR[+/−] mice, these mice exhibited at 3 weeks of age a depression-like phenotype under basal (unstressed) conditions. This indicated that GR underexpression from early development on does not lead to an overt phenotype under baseline conditions with low levels of stress. This could be due to a mere gene dosage effect. Furthermore, a complete GR knockout in some brain areas with preserved GR levels in other regions may have resulted in a different phenotype than a more subtle and homogenous GR reduction throughout the brain. However, the depressive phenotype of forebrain-specific GR knockout mice also indicated that crucial brain regions responsible for the phenotype of GR$^{+/-}$ mice may be located in the forebrain. On the other hand, the lack of a phenotype under baseline conditions of GR$^{+/-}$ mice might also be caused by early ontogenetic compensatory or adaptive processes, possibly reflecting the condition of patients with a high genetic (familiar) risk for depression who are initially inconspicuous but develop depressive episodes following stressful life events.

Since depression is a multifactorial disease, the moderate dysregulation of a single system may not be sufficient to induce depression-like alterations in mice under basal conditions. Therefore, provoking or destabilizing factors, such as stress or early childhood environmental factors, may be needed in addition to the existing genetic predisposition to effectively elicit a behavioral and also a neuroendocrinological phenotype. This concept may explain why the depression-like phenotype of GR$^{+/-}$ mice manifests only after stress. The latter fact, however, can be regarded as a strength of the heterozygous model, because depression-vulnerable humans often develop a depressive episode only following external or internal stress factors.

YGR Mice Overexpressing GR Are Stress Resistant

A genetic approach to prove the specificity of the depression-like alterations of GR$^{+/-}$ mice seemed to be the behavioral and neuroendocrinological examination of mice overexpressing GR. In these mice one would expect the opposite phenotype of GR$^{+/-}$ mice. Indeed, YGR mice carrying four copies of the GR gene demonstrate a stress resistance on both the behavioral and the hormonal level. These animals exhibit less helplessness, lower corticosterone levels after stress, and oversuppression following dexamethasone treatment (**Figure 2**). This result was in good agreement with the predictions of the GR hypothesis of depression.

Recently it was also reported that mice overexpressing GR specifically in the forebrain displayed increased emotional lability in the Porsolt forced swim test, indicated by increased baseline immobility. Furthermore, these animals exhibited increased anxiety-like behavior in the elevated plus-maze and in the dark–light box. This was not observed in the YGR mice that express GR under control of its own regulatory sequences. These contradictory results could be explained by the late onset and forebrain restricted mutation induced by CamKII promotor used in the former study. Conflicting results also come from the human field. While enhanced glucocorticoid feedback has always been considered positive for better limiting the stress response, it is important to remember that overactive GR may transduce a stronger

glucocorticoid signal, i.e., it may produce effects of glucocorticoid excess. In a large elderly Dutch (Rotterdam) population cohort, two different polymorphisms in GR have been found, one that enhances sensitivity to dexamethasone and the other that confers resistance to dexamethasone. However, the group with increased sensitivity to dexamethasone (and lower basal cortisol) shows a glucocorticoid excess phenotype with greater incidence of dementia and reduced overall survival. Thus, our understanding of the animal models needs to examine additional possibilities of what reduced or increased glucocorticoid signaling entails beyond HPA feedback or learned helplessness models.

GR Mutant Mice Represent a Tool to Study Molecular Correlates of Depression-like Behavior

The results in GR$^{+/-}$ mice resemble the human situation in depressive disorders, in which individuals at risk are predisposed to develop depressive episodes after stress. In this respect, GR$^{+/-}$ mice differ from mice with a forebrain-specific complete GR knockout, which already demonstrate depression-like behavioral and neurochemical alterations under baseline conditions. However, the findings in both strains indicate that compromised GR function constitutes a crucial molecular risk factor in the pathophysiology of depression. This suggests that the mouse lines with altered GR expression are suitable tools for further physiological, biochemical, and pharmacological investigations of GR function with regard to depressive disorders. These analyses are also of clinical relevance, since in preliminary studies GR antagonists have been of value in the treatment of severe depressive episodes with psychotic features.

Recently, the so-called neurotrophin hypothesis of depression postulated that a downregulation of brain-derived neurotropic factor (BDNF) is crucial for the pathogenesis of depression in humans and rodents. A stress- or corticosterone-induced BDNF downregulation in the hippocampus can be partially blocked by adrenalectomy or can be reversed by antidepressant therapy. In accordance with this hypothesis, GR$^{+/-}$ mice – which have a predisposition to stress-induced depression-like behavior – show a significant downregulation of BDNF in the hippocampus, while YGR mice exhibit a significant BDNF upregulation. Indeed, this was the first experimental evidence that compromised GR function concurrently evokes a BDNF dysregulation and a predisposition to depressive behavior. Future experiments should investigate in these strains further mechanisms of neural plasticity thought to be involved in the molecular and cellular pathogenesis of depression, e.g., monoaminergic systems, arginine vasopressin, and neurogenesis. Using modern molecular techniques such as transcriptomics and proteomics, completely new or even unknown gene products that are involved in the pathogenesis of depression may be detected. Such gene products may represent new targets for antidepressive treatment and could help to develop therapeutic strategies that are faster and more efficient than those currently in use.

See Also the Following Articles

Corticosteroid Receptors; Corticosteroids and Stress; Depression Models; Glucocorticoid Negative Feedback; Glucocorticoids, Effects of Stress on; Glucocorticoids – Adverse Effects on the Nervous System; Glucocorticoids, Overview; Glucocorticoids, Role in Stress; Mineralocorticoid Receptor Polymorphisms.

Further Reading

Akil, H. (2005). Stressed and depressed. *Nature Medicine* **11**, 116–118.

Altar, C. A. (1999). Neurotrophins and depression. *Trends in Pharmacological Science* **20**, 59–61.

Beato, M., Herrlich, P. and Schütz, G. (1995). Steroid hormone receptors: many actors in search of a plot. *Cell* **83**, 851–857.

Belanoff, J. K., Rothschild, A. J., Cassidy, F., et al. (2002). An open label trial of C-1073 (mifepristone) for psychotic major depression. *Biological Psychiatry* **52**, 386–392.

Boyle, M. P., Brewer, J. A., Funatsu, M., et al. (2005). Acquired deficit of forebrain glucocorticoid receptor produces depression-like changes in adrenal axis regulation and behavior. *Proceedings of the National Academy of Sciences USA* **102**, 473–478.

Charney, D. S. (1998). Monoamine dysfunction and the pathophysiology and treatment of depression. *Journal of Clinical Psychiatry* **59**(Supplement 14), 11–14.

Cryan, J. F. and Mombereau, C. (2004). In search of a depressed mouse: utility of models for studying depression-related behavior in genetically modified mice. *Molecular Psychiatry* **9**, 326–357.

De Kloet, E. R., Vreugdenhil, E., Oitzl, M. S. and Joels, M. (1998). Brain corticosteroid receptor balance in health and disease. *Endocrine Reviews* **19**, 269–301.

Heuser, I., Yassouridis, A. and Holsboer, F. (1994). The combined dexamethasone/CRH test: a refined laboratory test for psychiatric disorders. *Journal of Psychiatric Research* **28**, 341–356.

Holsboer, F. (2000). The corticosteroid receptor hypothesis of depression. *Neuropsychopharmacology* **23**, 477–501.

Pepin, M. C., Pothier, F. and Barden, N. (1992). Impaired type II glucocorticoid-receptor function in mice bearing antisense RNA transgene. *Nature* **355**, 725–728.

Reichardt, H. M., Umland, T., Bauer, A., Kretz, O. and Schutz, G. (2000). Mice with an increased glucocorticoid receptor gene dosage show enhanced resistance to stress and endotoxic shock. *Molecular and Cellular Biology* **20**, 9009–9017.

Reichardt, H. M., Kaestner, K. H., Tuckermann, J., et al. (1998). DNA binding of the glucocorticoid receptor is not essential for survival. *Cell* **93**, 531–541.

Ridder, S., Chourbaji, S., Hellweg, R., et al. (2005). Mice with genetically altered glucocorticoid receptor expression show vulnerability for stress-induced depressive reactions. *Journal of Neuroscience* **25**, 6243–6250.

Seckl, J. and Meaney, M. J. (2004). Glucocorticoid programming. *Annals of the New York Academy of Sciences* **1032**, 63–84.

Tronche, F., Kellendonk, C., Kretz, O., et al. (1999). Disruption of the glucocorticoid receptor gene in the nervous system results in reduced anxiety. *Nature Genetics* **23**, 99–103.

Wei, Q., Lu, X. Y., Liu, L., et al. (2004). Glucocorticoid receptor overexpression in forebrain: a mouse model of increased emotional lability. *Proceedings of the National Academy of Sciences USA* **101**, 11851–11856.

Glucocorticoid Receptor Mutations and Polymorphisms

J W Koper
Erasmus MC, Rotterdam, The Netherlands

Glucocorticoid Receptor Mutations
Glucocorticoid Receptor Polymorphisms

Glossary

Mutation	Changes to the genetic material.
Polymorphism	The occurrence in the same habitat (DNA sequence) of two or more forms of a trait in such frequencies (usually >1%) that the rarer cannot be maintained by recurrent mutation alone.
SNP	A DNA sequence variation, occurring when a single nucleotide: A, T, C, or G – in the genome differs between members of the species.

Glucocorticoid Receptor Mutations

Some abnormalities in glucocorticoid (GC) response may be explained by mutations in the gene coding for the GC receptor (GR; NR3C1). Such mutations can occur either in the germline, causing systemic GC resistance or hypersensitivity, or they can occur somatically, resulting in localized changes in GC sensitivity, e.g., in tumors.

Germline Mutations, Glucocorticoid Resistance, and Glucocorticoid Hypersensitivity

Based on the results of experiments with knockout mice, it is clear that total absence of the GR is not compatible with life, and the germline mutations that have been identified in the GR gene have always been found to confer a relative GC resistance, which was compensated by increased activity of the hypothalamic-pituitary adrenal (HPA) axis. Typically, the symptoms of most patients could be explained by the concurrent overproduction of adrenal androgens (hirsutism, fertility problems in women, male precocious puberty in a boy) and mineralocorticoids (hypokalemia, hypertension).

Worldwide, nine different cases of GC resistance caused by mutations in the GR gene have been described (**Table 1**). Seven of these nine mutations are located in the ligand-binding domain and resulted in reduced ligand affinity. One mutation resulted in the (heterozygous) destruction of a splice site, and hence in a reduced amount of GR messenger ribonucleic acid (mRNA) and GR protein per cell. One mutation was located in the deoxyribonucleic acid (DNA)-binding domain and resulted in the ablation of transactivating capacity. The low number of cases of GR-gene mutations stands in strong contrast to the situation with respect to the androgen receptor, where in patients with the partial- or complete androgen insensitivity syndromes hundreds of different mutations have been identified. Several explanations for this are possible: (1) the GR is more essential to (prenatal) survival than the androgen receptor, resulting in the occurrence of relatively mild mutations only, (2) the symptoms of GC resistance are relatively mild, resulting in an underestimation of the number of cases.

Several cases of GC hypersensitivity (typically, the presence of the symptoms of Cushing's syndrome combined with low serum cortisol levels) have been described; however, none of these have been explained by the presence of mutations in the GR gene. Due to the extremely low number of cases there are no data available on the effects of this type of mutations on the stress response.

Somatic Mutations in Tumors and Tumor Cell Lines

GCs play an important role in the treatment of a number of hematological malignancies and lack of response to this treatment might be associated with mutations in the GR gene. However, in the current literature only very limited numbers of such mutations has been reported. Similarly, involvement of GR-gene mutations in adrenocorticotropic hormone

Table 1 Mutations in the glucocorticoid receptor gene associated with glucocorticoid resistance

Amino acid change[a]	Nucleotide change[a]
R477H	1562G > A
I559N	1808T > A
V571A	1844T > C
2013-2014del, IVSF+1-+2del	2013delGAGT
D641V	2054A > T
G679S	2168G > A
V729I	2317G > A
I747M	2373T > G
L773P	2450T > C

[a]Numbering is based upon Genbank Accession number NM_000176.

Table 2 Polymorphisms in the glucocorticoid receptor gene associated with changes in glucocorticoid sensitivity

Amino acid change	Nucleotide change	rs number
NA	5'-UTR, 3447 bp upsteam of NM_000176, C → T	rs10052957
ER22/23EK	GAG AGG → GAA AAG	rs6189 and rs6190
N363S	AAT → AGT	rs6195
NA	IVS-2,+646 C → G	NA "Bcl-I"
NA	3'-UTR exon 9β, A → G	rs6198

NA, not available.

(ACTH)-secreting pituitary adenomas has been shown in only a small number of studies.

Glucocorticoid Receptor Polymorphisms

The National Center for Biotechnology Information (NCBI) single nucleotide polymorphism database currently shows 461 SNPs in the human GR gene. Most of these are in noncoding sequences of the gene and have not (yet) been investigated with respect to functionality. Five SNPs in the GR gene have been investigated more extensively (**Table 2**). The main effects that have been observed for these polymorphisms are on body composition and metabolic profile (fat mass, fat distribution, lean mass, and serum lipids), but two polymorphisms have also been associated with changes in the response to psychosocial stress. Carriers of the N363S polymorphism showed an increased HPA-axis response when challenged with the Trier Social Stress Test, while carriers of the Bcl-I polymorphism showed a reduced response.

In general it can be said that the effects of these polymorphisms are relatively small. They can barely be measured in individuals, and their effects have been suggested to be due to lifelong exposure to small changes in GC sensitivity, rather than to changes in the acute HPA response.

Further Reading

Bray, P. J. and Cotton, R. G. H. (2003). Variations of the human glucocorticoid receptor gene (NR3C1): pathological and *in vitro* mutations and polymorphisms. *Human Mutation* **21**, 557–568.

Brufsky, A. M., Malchoff, D. M., Javier, E. C., et al. (1990). A glucocorticoid receptor mutation in a subject with primary cortisol resistance. *Transactions of the Association of American Physicians* **103**, 53–63.

Charmandari, E., Kino, T. and Chrousos, G. P. (2004). Familial/sporadic glucocorticoid resistance: clinical phenotype and molecular mechanisms. *Annals of the New York Academy of Sciences* **1024**, 168–181.

Charmandari, E., Raji, A., Kino, T., et al. (2005). A novel point mutation in the ligand-binding domain (LBD) of the human glucocorticoid receptor (hGR) causing generalized glucocorticoid resistance: the importance of the C terminus of hGR LBD in conferring transactivational activity. *Journal of Clinical Endocrinology and Metabolism* **90**, 3696–3705.

DeRijk, R. H., Schaaf, M. and de Kloet, E. R. (2002). Glucocorticoid receptor variants: clinical implications. *Journal of Steroid Biochemistry and Molecular Biology* **81**, 103–122.

DeRijk, R. H., Schaaf, M. J. M., Turner, G., et al. (2001). A human glucocorticoid receptor gene variant that increases the stability of the glucocorticoid receptor β-isoform mRNA is associated with rheumatoid arthritis. *Journal of Rheumatology* **28**, 2383–2388.

Detera-Wadleigh, S. D., Encio, I. J., Rollins, D. Y., et al. (1991). A TthIII1 polymorphism on the 5′ flanking region of the glucocorticoid receptor gene (GRL). *Nucleic Acids Research* **19**, 1960.

Huizenga, N. A., Koper, J. W., De Lange, P., et al. (1998). A polymorphism in the glucocorticoid receptor gene may be associated with and increased sensitivity to glucocorticoids *in vivo*. *Journal of Clinical Endocrinology and Metabolism* **83**, 144–151.

Hurley, D. M., Accili, D., Stratakis, C. A., et al. (1991). Point mutation causing a single amino acid substitution in the hormone binding domain of the glucocorticoid receptor in familial glucocorticoid resistance. *Journal of Clinical Investigation* **87**, 680–686.

Karl, M., Lamberts, S. W., Detera-Wadleigh, S. D., et al. (1993). Familial glucocorticoid resistance caused by a splice site deletion in the human glucocorticoid receptor gene. *Journal of Clinical Endocrinology and Metabolism* **76**, 683–689.

Karl, M., Lamberts, S. W., Koper, J. W., et al. (1996). Cushing's disease preceded by generalized glucocorticoid resistance: clinical consequences of a novel, dominant-negative glucocorticoid receptor mutation. *Proceedings of the Association of American Physicians* **108**, 296–307.

Malchoff, C. D. and Malchoff, D. M. (2005). Glucocorticoid resistance and hypersensitivity. *Endocrinology and Metabalolism Clinics of North America* **34**, 315–326.

Mendonca, B. B., Leite, M. V., de Castro, M., et al. (2002). Female pseudohermaphroditism caused by a novel homozygous missense mutation of the GR gene. *Journal of Clinical Endocrinology and Metabolism* **87**, 1805–1809.

Murray, J. C., Smith, R. F., Ardinger, H. A., et al. (1987). RFLP for the glucocorticoid receptor (GRL) located at 5q11–5q13. *Nucleic Acids Research* **15**, 6765.

Ruiz, M., Lind, U., Gafvels, M., et al. (2001). Characterization of two novel mutations in the glucocorticoid receptor gene in patients with primary cortisol resistance. *Clinical Endocrinology* **55**, 363–371.

Schaaf, M. J. and Cidlowski, J. A. (2002). Molecular mechanisms of glucocorticoid action and resistance. *Journal of Steroid Biochemistry and Molecular Biology* **83**, 37–48.

Seckl, J. R. (2004). Prenatal glucocorticoids and long-term programming. *European Journal of Endocrinology* **151**, U49–U62.

van Rossum, E. F. C. and Lamberts, S. W. J. (2004). Polymorphisms in the glucocorticoid receptor gene: associations with metabolic parameters and body composition. *Recent Progress in Hormone Research* **59**, 333–357.

van Rossum, E. F. C., Russcher, H. and Lamberts, S. W. J. (2005). Genetic polymorphisms and multifactorial diseases: facts and fallacies revealed by the glucocorticoid receptor gene. *Trends in Endocrinology and Metabolism* **16**, 445–450.

Vottero, A., Kino, T., Combe, H., et al. (2002). A novel, C-terminal dominant negative mutation of the GR causes familial glucocorticoid resistance through abnormal interactions with p160 steroid receptor coactivators. *Journal of Clinical Endocrinology and Metabolism* **87**, 2658–2667.

Wüst, S., van Rossum, E. F. C., Federenko, I. S., et al. (2004). Common polymorphisms in the glucocorticoid receptor gene are associated with adrenocortical responses to psychosocial stress. *Journal of Clinical Endocrinology and Metabolism* **89**, 565–573.

Glucocorticoid Receptors   *See:* Corticosteroid Receptors; Membrane Glucocorticoid Receptors.

Glucocorticoids – Adverse Effects on the Nervous System

R M Sapolsky
Stanford University, Stanford, CA, USA

This article is a revision of the previous edition article by R M Sapolsky, volume 2, pp 238–243, © 2000, Elsevier Inc.

Background
GCs and the Function and Structure of Hippocampal Neurons
GCs and the Birth of Hippocampal Neurons
GCs and the Death of Hippocampal Neurons
GCs and the Health of the Human Hippocampus

Glossary

Dendritic atrophy	The shrinking of the dendritic processes by which neurons receive excitatory or inhibitory inputs from neighboring neurons.
Gluco-corticoids	Steroid hormones released by the adrenal gland basally and in response to virtually all stressors.
Hippocampus	A region of the brain that plays a central role in learning and memory and in the regulation of the adrenocortical axis; it is atypically vulnerable to a number of neurological diseases and has an atypically high concentration of receptors for glucocorticoids.
Neuron death	The death of brain cells that can be due to disease or as part of normal development (i.e., programmed cell death).

It has long been appreciated that prolonged stress or exposure to glucocorticoids (GCs) can have adverse effects throughout the body. In recent decades, it has become clear that these adverse effects can extend to the nervous system, particularly the hippocampus, a brain region critical to learning and memory and with an abundance of corticosteroid receptors. These effects of GCs and stress include (1) reversible atrophy of dendritic processes, (2) inhibition of neurogenesis in the adult hippocampus, (3) compromising of the ability to neurons to survive a variety of insults, and (4) overt neurotoxicity. This article considers the emerging insights as to the cellular and molecular mechanisms underlying these events, as well as the possible clinical implications (including in the realm of normative aging, treatment with exogenous GCs,

Cushing's disease, posttraumatic stress disorder, and depression).

Since the time of Walter Cannon, there has been recognition of the critical role of the stress response in maintaining allostatic balance in the face of insult and injury. However, since the time of Hans Selye, there has been the complementary recognition that excessive activation of the stress response can be deleterious, increasing the likelihood of a disease occurring or exacerbating some preexisting disease. The pages of this encyclopedia are filled with ample documentation of the adverse effects of overactivation of the stress response on metabolism, cardiovascular function, reproductive physiology, and so on, and these realms represent the cornerstones of stress pathophysiology. Only more recently has it become clear that excessive activation of the stress response can have deleterious effects on the nervous system.

Background

An array of physiological and psychological stressors causes secretion of catecholamines by the sympathetic nervous system and of glucocorticoids (GCs) by the adrenal cortex. While such peripheral catecholamines do not pass the blood–brain barrier, the steroidal GCs do so readily and appear to be the culprits in damaging the nervous system.

The deleterious effects of GC excess within the nervous system are centered in (but not exclusive to) the hippocampus, the limbic structure that plays a central role in learning and memory. The first hints of such deleterious actions came at a time when it was not yet obvious why the hippocampus should be particularly sensitive to GCs and thus were mostly ignored. This changed in the late 1960s, with the classic work of Bruce McEwen and colleagues, who demonstrated the extremely high levels of receptors for GCs (i.e., corticosteroid receptors) in the hippocampus. Since then, vast numbers of studies have documented the extensive neurochemical and electrophysiological sensitivity of the hippocampus to GCs, and it is basically impossible to think of stress, GCs, and the nervous system without thinking first about the hippocampus.

In the mid-1980s, E. Ron de Kloet and colleagues made the critical observation that there are two types of corticosteroid receptors in the nervous system, with the hippocampus having ample amounts of both. These are the high-affinity, low-capacity mineralocorticoid receptor (MR), and the low-affinity, high-capacity glucocorticoid receptor (GR). The existence of these two receptors, and their possessing such different affinities, clarify a key feature of GC action in the hippocampus. Specifically, mild

elevations of GCs, or mild transient stressors, enhance hippocampal-dependent cognition, as well as the synaptic plasticity that mediates such cognition (such long term potentiation [LTP]); this makes sense, in that mild, transient stressors are what we think of as stimulation, something that very much enhances cognition. In contrast, major and/or prolonged stressors or GC exposure has opposite, disruptive effects on cognition. This U-shaped curve of GC effects on hippocampal function (a concept popularized by David Diamond) was explained by the two-receptor system in the hippocampus. Specifically, the high-affinity MRs are mostly occupied basally and are then fully occupied by mild elevation of GC concentrations. Such MRs mediate the salutary effects of GCs upon cognition (i.e., the permissive effects of GCs basally, and the enhancing effects of mild stressors). In contrast, GRs, which are minimally occupied basally and are not heavily occupied until there is a major stressor, mediate the disruptive effects.

GCs and the Function and Structure of Hippocampal Neurons

As just discussed, mild stressors, via MR occupancy, enhance hippocampal-dependent cognition and LTP, whereas major stressors, via GR occupancy, disrupt both. The mechanisms underlying these actions are well understood.

Major stressors and prolonged GC exposure can also cause structural changes in hippocampal neurons. Neurons are highly arborized cells, with information flowing in from neighboring neurons via a dense tree of processes called dendrites, and with information flowing out through a major cable called the axon. The extent of dendritic arborization – the length and complexity of processes – is now recognized to be highly dynamic, being remodeled by a variety of local, systemic, and even experiential influences. Work initiated by McEwen and colleagues has shown that in the rat, sustained exposure to stress or to excessive GC levels over the course of weeks can cause atrophy of dendrites in hippocampal neurons. Reflecting the dynamic nature of dendritic remodeling, the atrophy appears to gradually reverse when the stress or GC overexposure stops. Subsequent work from this group and others has shown that the same atrophy occurs in the nonhuman primate hippocampus as well.

It is the GR receptor that appears to mediate the deleterious GC effects on the dendrites. Moreover, GCs appear to cause the atrophy through the glutamate neurotransmitter system. As evidence, atrophy can be prevented by blocking NMDA glutamate receptors in the hippocampus or by the use of drugs that blunt glutamate release (such as the seizure suppresser phenytoin). Thus, the phenomena of GC-induced dendritic atrophy and of neuroendangerment appear to be linked mechanistically.

What are the consequences of this dendritic atrophy? There are at least three possibilities. First, part of the staggering complexity of the nervous system comes from the multiplicity of synaptic connections between neurons, and a typical neuron can form thousands of synapses with neighbors both near and far. The existence of such neuronal networks is obviously dependent upon an intact dendritic tree, and dendritic atrophy is likely to disrupt and simplify networks within the hippocampus. Stress or GC overexposure on the scale needed to cause dendritic atrophy will also disrupt cognition, and it seems plausible that the two are interrelated. Second, as will be reviewed shortly, GCs and stress can make hippocampal neurons less likely to survive coincident neurological insults. It has been suggested that the dendritic atrophy represents, in effect, a hibernation, of a neuron, an involution that protects it from a coincident insult. Third, in contrast, others have suggested that the atrophy represents a marker of the neuron being made more vulnerable, rather than less, to an insult. While it remains unclear whether the first two models are correct, most existing evidence supports the last.

GCs and the Birth of Hippocampal Neurons

For much of the twentieth century, a central dogma of neuroscience was that the adult mammalian brain did not make new neurons. The 1990s saw an overthrow of this view, with the recognition that a handful of generally ignored pioneering studies in the 1960s disproved this maxim, and the study of adult neurogenesis is now one of the most vibrant fields of neuroscience. Such neurogenesis occurs in only two regions of the brain (the hippocampus being one of them) and is stimulated by environmental enrichment, learning, voluntary exercise, and estrogen. An enormous amount of work has demonstrated that these are, indeed, neurons, that they can migrate some distance from their site of birth, and that they form functional synapses with preexisting neurons. Some of the current issues in the field include (1) whether such neurogenesis occurs in other brain regions as well (particularly the cortex); (2) how much neurogenesis occurs (with estimates ranging from rates that would completely replace certain hippocampal cell fields throughout the lifetime to rates that place the levels orders of magnitude lower); and (3) whether these new neurons are necessary for any

aspects of hippocampal function. These issues are quite contentious in this often fractious field.

One of the more consistent findings is that stress and GCs potently and rapidly (over the course of hours) inhibit adult hippocampal neurogenesis, a finding pioneered by Elizabeth Gould and colleagues. The mechanisms underlying this are unclear. As but one example, early reports suggested that neural progenitor cells in the adult hippocampus do not express MRs or GRs, and that the inhibitory effects of GCs had to be through neuron/progenitor interactions; more recent work, using more sensitive assays, suggests that progenitors do indeed possess GRs. Also unclear is how much the effects of GCs on neurogenesis contribute to any of the disruptive effects of GCs upon hippocampal function.

GCs and the Death of Hippocampal Neurons

GC Endangerment

A body of work initiated by Robert Sapolsky and colleagues in the 1980s demonstrated the ability of transient bursts of GC excess to endanger hippocampal neurons, compromising their ability to survive a coincident neurological insult. As such, the greater the GC levels at the time of an insult, the greater the extent of hippocampal damage. Such insults include epileptic seizures, hypoxia-ischemia, hypoglycemia and other metabolic insults, oxidative insults, the β-amyloid peptide (the fragment of the amyloid precursor protein that has been implicated in the neuron death of Alzheimer's disease), and gp120 (the coat protein of the AIDS virus that is thought to play a role in the neurodegeneration seen in AIDS-related dementia). This endangerment is of a considerable magnitude, with stress levels of GCs causing manyfold increases in insult-induced damage in some cases.

Features of this endangerment include the following: (1) it is mediated by GRs, rather than MRs; (2) while most dramatic in the hippocampus, the endangerment can also occur in the cortex and striatum; (3) it is a direct GC effect in the hippocampus (rather than secondary to some peripheral GC action), as the same phenomenon occurs in hippocampal cultures and tissue slices; and (4) it consists of GCs increasing the amount of insult-induced necrotic death, rather than an increase in the amount of apoptotic death (a form of programmed cell death).

In vitro models have made it possible to uncover some of the mechanisms underlying the endangerment. One realm concerns the disruptive effects of GCs upon neuronal energetics. GCs inhibit glucose transport in many peripheral tissues (as part of the strategy to divert energy to exercising muscle during a stressful crisis); this effect is due to a reduction in the number of glucose transporter molecules in the cell membrane. GCs cause a similar inhibition in the hippocampus, leaving neurons energetically vulnerable, thereby worsening insult-induced declines in energy substrates (such as ATP). Such insults cause neurons to release damaging amounts of the excitatory neurotransmitter glutamate. This, in turn, causes a wave of calcium influx in the postsynaptic neuron, which causes an array of calcium-dependent degenerative events; of most significance is the generation of oxygen radicals. It is quite costly for a neuron to contain the excesses of glutamate, calcium, and oxygen radicals, and the mild energetic vulnerability caused by GCs makes each of these steps spiral a bit more out of control, increasing the likelihood of the neuron succumbing.

In addition to these energetic features, GC endangerment probably also arises from the demonstrated abilities of the hormone to increase calcium currents in hippocampal neurons, to decrease the activity of calcium-extrusion mechanisms, to suppress the levels or efficacy of neurotrophins (neuronal growth factors), and to disrupt some of the defenses normally mobilized by neurons during neurological insults.

At present, these data are derived exclusively from rodent and tissue culture studies. Should subsequent work demonstrate GC endangerment in the primate hippocampus, they have a number of disturbing implications. Numerous individuals are administered high-dose GCs to control autoimmune or inflammatory disorders, and this might well exacerbate the damaging effects of some neurological crisis. Plus, GCs are often administered after strokes in order to decrease brain edema (swelling). Most studies show that GCs are less effective at reducing such edema than nonsteroid anti-inflammatory compounds; the present studies suggest that the use of GCs might even worsen the neurological outcome. Finally, stroke, seizure, and cardiac arrest all cause massive GC secretion; such endogenous GC release might add to damage. In effect, what we have learned to view as the typical extent of neurological damage caused by these insults might well reflect the damaging effects of the maladaptive hypersecretion of GCs at that time.

GC Neurotoxicity

Independent of a coincident neurological insult, GCs can directly influence the life and death of a hippocampal neuron. In an unexpected finding, Robert Sloviter and colleagues reported that GCs are required for the survival of dentate gyrus neurons. In the complete absence of the hormone, such neurons undergo apoptosis within days, and

very low levels of GCs, via MR occupancy, prevent this effect.

A separate literature showed that truly prolonged exposure to elevated GC levels could directly kill hippocampal neurons. Studies initiated by Phil Landfield and colleagues showed that the loss was centered in the CA3 region of the hippocampus and was highly relevant to hippocampal aging. That region of the hippocampus loses neurons with age, and these studies suggested that it is the cumulative extent of GC exposure over the lifetime that acts as a major determinant of the extent of neuron loss (as well as of hippocampal-dependent memory problems) in old age. As such, stress has the capacity to accelerate hippocampal aging, whereas behavioral or social manipulations that reduce cumulative GC exposure can delay such aging. The finding of GC- and of stress-induced neurotoxicity was replicated by other investigators, including in the nonhuman primate hippocampus.

The mechanisms underlying such neurotoxicity are not well understood. The assumption by most in the field, however, is that it is on a continuum with GC neuroendangerment – in effect, if a day of GC overexposure can compromise the ability of a neuron to survive a massive neurological insult, months of overexposure can compromise its ability to survive the minor metabolic challenges of everyday life, especially during aging. The difficult studies required to test this idea remain to be carried out.

Despite the replication of the finding of GC neurotoxicity, the phenomenon is more controversial than the other adverse GC effects that have been discussed. The disagreements have focused on a number of issues. The basic finding of neuron loss during hippocampal aging has been called into question by some researchers counting neurons with the technique of stereology. Some investigators suggest that overt neurotoxicity can be caused only by massive amounts of ever-shifting stressors (to avoid habituation of the system) or by pharmacological GC exposure, questioning the relevance of the phenomenon to normative aging. GC hypersecretion and hippocampal neuron loss in old age are quite variable among rodents. There appear to be strains in which neither occurs to any dramatic extent. Moreover, dramatic differences in the extent of successful aging can occur within strains. Michael Meaney and colleagues, for example, have shown that remarkably subtle differences in the quality of early maternal care can change the entire trajectory of hippocampal and adrenocortical aging in a rat, in some cases completely avoiding the neuron loss or GC hypersecretion; thus, neither component of that cascade model is an inevitable part of aging. Finally, to the extent that primates and humans hypersecrete GCs in old age, it is a nonlinear phenomenon, emerging only in extreme old age or when coincident with an insult (such as major depression or Alzheimer's disease).

GCs and the Health of the Human Hippocampus

Work in the past decade suggests that these findings regarding the deleterious effects of GCs and stress apply to the human hippocampus. These findings have been most striking in a number of realms.

Cushing's Syndrome

Cushing's syndrome can arise from any of a number of different types of tumors and results in vastly elevated levels of circulating GCs. Magnetic resonance imaging (MRI) studies by Monica Starkman and colleagues of Cushingoid patients have shown selective atrophy of the hippocampus. More strikingly, it is the same patients who have the most severe GC hypersecretion, the most severe hippocampal atrophy, and the most profound cognitive deficits. Post mortem studies to uncover whether this atrophy is due to neuronal loss, atrophy, or compression remain to be carried out. However, when the GC hypersecretion is corrected by removal of the tumor, the hippocampal gradually returns to normal size, in agreement with the model of reversible dendritic atrophy.

Exogenous GC Administration

Synthetic GCs are frequently administered in different realms of clinical medicine. Most cases involve transient exposure to fairly low concentrations, often through routes that do not result in much access of the steroids to the brain. However, there are hundreds of thousands of individuals on long-term, systemic high-dose GC treatment to control various autoimmune or inflammatory diseases. Difficult case-controlled work by Pamela Keenan and colleagues demonstrates that independent of the disease, treatment with such steroids increases hippocampal-dependent cognitive deficits. The mechanisms underlying this effect (e.g., whether it is due to dendritic atrophy, inhibition of neurogenesis, and so on) are unknown.

Clinical Depression

Major clinical depression is an archetypical example of a stress-related disease; as but three pieces of evidence, exogenous GC treatment increases the risk of depression, major stressors do as well, and about half of patients with major depression present with GC hypersecretion. Yvette Sheline and colleagues have observed that a history of prolonged depression is associated with selective hippocampal atrophy on MRI. In this observation, since replicated, the more prolonged the depression, the more atrophy. While the necessary post mortem cell counting has not been carried out, the atrophy appears to be permanent in that it is demonstrable in individuals long after the depressions have resolved; whether this is due to loss of neurons or inhibition of neurons that would otherwise have been born is not clear. Some researchers have suggested a scenario of reverse causality, in which individuals who (for other unrelated reasons) have a smaller than average hippocampus are more at risk for clinical depression. However, such volume loss is not demonstrable shortly after diagnosis, and more prolonged depressions are associated with more volume loss; both findings argue against reverse causality.

Posttraumatic Stress Disorder (PTSD)

Probably the most contentious studies concerning GC effects on the human hippocampus concern PTSD. A large numbers of studies, with the first coming from J. Douglas Bremner and colleagues, demonstrate volume loss in the hippocampi of individuals with PTSD. Furthermore, the more volume loss, the more severe the cognitive impairments, and there is little evidence that either tends to reverse over time. The controversial issues are threefold.

First, are GCs the cause of the volume loss? This question is central to the second issue as well, but the first version of this question focuses on whether GC levels are elevated in PTSD. While it might seem intuitive that this is the case, many (but not all) studies suggest lower than normal levels and that such hyposecretion may even precede and predispose toward succumbing to PTSD. The studies showing hyposecretion, pioneered by Rachel Yehuda and colleagues, also suggest an enhanced sensitivity to GCs in these patients. This would then shift the issue from whether excessive GC levels play a role in the volume loss to whether excessive sensitivity to GCs plays a role.

The second controversy concerns when the volume loss occurs. There are three possibilities: (1) volume loss occurs in response to the trauma itself; (2) volume loss occurs in response to the biology of the prolonged posttraumatic period (i.e., the period of the PTSD); and (3) a small hippocampus (arising for reasons unrelated to stress or GCs) precedes and predisposes toward PTSD. This issue is not resolved, and, at present, there are some striking findings supporting, as well as arguing against, each of these possibilities. One reasonable solution is that from the standpoint of hippocampal neurobiology, PTSD is a heterogeneous disorders, with all three occurring on occasion. Such heterogeneity is certainly seen in the clinical profile of the disorder.

The final issue is whether the volume loss is due to loss of neurons, blockage of birth of new neurons, atrophy of dendritic processes, loss of glia, and so on. As with the other realms of studies of the human hippocampus, resolving this issue requires difficult quantitative postmortem studies.

Obviously, many issues remain to be resolved and are likely to have some important consequences in neurology, psychiatry, and gerontology. Most broadly, the interrelated phenomena of GC neuroendangerment, inhibition of neurogenesis, dendritic atrophy, and neurotoxicity shift the realm of stress-related disease to the nervous system. For nearly 70 years, stress physiology has taught that cardiovascular function, metabolism, and immunity can be sensitive to the adverse effects of stress. This newer literature demonstrates that this vital and fragile portion of our bodies, the brain, can be sensitive to stress as well.

See Also the Following Articles

Alzheimer's Disease; Brain Trauma; Corticosteroid Receptors; Corticotropin Releasing Factor (CRF); Cushing's Syndrome, Medical Aspects; Cushing's Syndrome, Neuropsychiatric Aspects; Glucose Transport; Hippocampal Neurons; Hippocampus, Corticosteroid Effects on; Posttraumatic Stress Disorder, Neurobiology of.

Further Reading

Gould, E. and Gross, C. (2002). Neurogenesis in adult mammals: some progress and problems. *Journal of Neuroscience* **22**, 619–623.

McEwen, B. (2002). Sex, stress and hippocampus: allostasis, allostatic load and the aging process. *Neurobiology of Aging* **23**, 921.

Sapolsky, R. (1999). Stress, glucocorticoids and their adverse neurological effects: relevance to aging. *Experimental Gerontology* **34**, 721.

Sapolsky, R. (2000). Glucocorticoids and hippocampal atrophy in neuropsychiatric disorders. *Archives of General Psychiatry* **57**, 925.

Glucocorticoids, Effects of Stress on

J C Buckingham
Imperial College School of Medicine, London, UK

This article is reproduced from the previous edition, volume 2, pp 229–237, © 2000, Elsevier Inc.

Mechanisms Controlling Glucocorticoid Secretion in Stress
Glucocorticoid Secretion in Repeated or Sustained Stress
Age- and Gender-Related Changes in the Stress Response

Glossary

Hypothalamo–hypophysial portal vessels	A specialized portal blood system responsible for the transportation of neurohormones (termed releasing hormones) from the median eminence area of the hypothalamus to the anterior pituitary gland.
Paraventricular nuclei (PVNs)	Specialized areas of the hypothalamus lying on either side of the third ventricle; these nuclei include the cell bodies of neurons that project to the median eminence area of the hypothalamus, and they play a key role in initiating the pituitary-adrenal response to stress.

The glucocorticoids (cortisol and/or corticosterone, depending on the species) are steroid hormones produced by cells in the zona fasciculata of the adrenal cortex under the influence of the hypothalamic-pituitary complex (**Figure 1**). They exert diverse actions in the body and thereby play a key role in the regulation of crucial homeostatic mechanisms, such as those concerned with metabolic control and immune/inflammatory responses. The actions of the steroids are effected intracellularly, mainly via glucocorticoid receptors (GRs) but also via mineralocorticoid receptors (MRs). In normal circumstances, the rate of glucocorticoid secretion is maintained within narrow limits, varying according to a circadian rhythm that is coupled to the sleep–wake cycle; serum levels of the steroids are thus normally maximal at the end of the sleep phase and fall to a nadir some hours after waking. However, glucocorticoid secretion is increased markedly in conditions of physical and emotional stress; hence, the glucocorticoids are frequently termed stress hormones. The stress-induced changes in circulating glucocorticoids are superimposed on the existing circadian tone and vary in their rate of onset, magnitude, and duration according to the nature, duration, and intensity of the insult. Significant

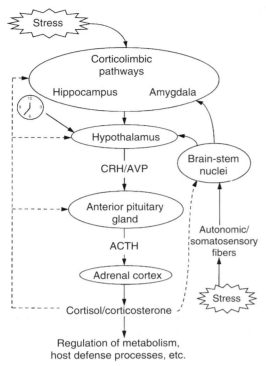

Figure 1 The hypothalamic-pituitary-adrenal axis. Dotted lines indicate inhibitory influences; intact lines indicate stimulatory influences; the clock indicates circadian influences. ACTH, adrenocorticotropic hormone; AVP, arginine vasopressin; CRH, corticotropin releasing hormone.

interspecies variations also occur; for example, humans are particularly sensitive to emotional trauma, whereas rats respond very readily to physical stimuli such as cold and pigs are relatively unresponsive to many stimuli (e.g., histamine and cold) but show a marked elevation in serum cortisol when deprived of food.

Mechanisms Controlling Glucocorticoid Secretion in Stress

The Hypothalamic-Pituitary-Adrenocortical Axis

The release of the glucocorticoids in stress is orchestrated mainly by the hypothalamus, which receives and integrates neural and humoral information from many sources and initiates the release of two neurohormones, termed corticotropin releasing hormone (CRH) and arginine vasopressin (AVP), into the hypothalamo-hypophysial portal vessels. These peptides are transported to the anterior pituitary gland via the portal vessels, where they act synergistically to cause the release of adrenocorticotropic hormone (ACTH), which, in turn, stimulates cortisol/corticosterone secretion. The hypothalamus thus provides a

vital link between the perception of physical and emotional stress and the regulation of key homeostatic mechanisms. The responsivity of the hypothalamic-pituitary-adrenocortical (HPA) axis to incoming stimuli is modulated by a servo system through which the sequential release of CRH/AVP and ACTH from the hypothalamus and anterior pituitary gland, respectively, is regulated negatively by the glucocorticoids themselves (**Figure 1**); the magnitude of the HPA response to stress thus depends on the preexisting glucocorticoid tone.

Adrenocorticotropic Hormone and Steroidogenesis

Cortisol and corticosterone are not stored to any great degree in the adrenal cortex but are synthesized on demand and promptly pass by diffusion across the cell membrane into the systemic circulation. The primary trigger for the synthesis of the steroids is ACTH, a polypeptide hormone produced by a specialized subgroup of cells in the anterior pituitary gland, the corticotrophs. ACTH acts via specific membrane-bound receptors, termed type 2 melanocortin (MC2) receptors, to activate the rate-limiting enzyme in the steroidogenic pathway; it thus causes the conversion of cholesterol to pregnenolone, from which cortisol and corticosterone are formed rapidly. In addition, ACTH acts on the vasculature to increase adrenal blood flow and thereby aid the passage of the newly synthesized steroids out of the cells and into the general systemic circulation. Increases in circulating glucocorticoids may be apparent within 10 min of the onset of the stress, although, in some instances (e.g., following an immune insult) the response may be delayed. Approximately 95% of cortisol/corticosterone in blood is protein bound, mainly to a specific high-affinity corticosteroid-binding globulin (CBG) but also to albumin, which has a lower affinity for the steroids. In principle, only the free steroid has ready access to the corticosteroid receptors (GRs and MRs), which are located intracellularly in the target cells. However, local mechanisms that release the steroid from its carrier protein(s) appear to exist in at least some target tissues; these include (1) interactions of the carrier protein with cell surface CBG receptors and (2) enzymatic cleavage of CBG (e.g., by serine proteases in inflamed tissues), a process that lowers the affinity of the binding protein for the steroids. The access of the steroids to their receptors is further regulated within the target cells by 11β-hydroxysteroid dehydrogenase (11β-HSD) enzymes, which control the interconversion of cortisol and corticosterone to their inactive counterparts, cortisone and 11-dehydrocorticosterone. The biochemical half-life of the steroids is approximately 90 min, but the biological effects may be sustained for very much longer. Metabolism is hepatic and the resulting metabolites are conjugated and excreted in the bile and the urine.

Synthesis and Secretion of Adrenocorticotropic Hormone

ACTH is synthesized in the corticotrophs by the post-translational cleavage of a large precursor molecule, proopiomelanocortin (POMC). POMC also gives rise to a number of other peptides that are coreleased with ACTH and are termed collectively ACTH-related or POMC peptides. These include an N-terminal peptide, N-POMC(1–76), of unknown function and β-lipotropin (β-LPH), which, in turn, may be partially degraded to β-endorphin (which is sometimes used as a marker of ACTH secretion) and γ-LPH. In some circumstances (e.g., adrenal insufficiency), more extensive N-terminal processing may occur, either within the pituitary gland or at the adrenal level, generating peptides that appear to augment the steroidogenic capacity of the adrenal cortex by potentiating the steroidogenic response to ACTH (γ-melanocyte-stimulating hormone) or enhancing adrenocortical mitogenesis (N-POMC(1–46)).

ACTH is released from the anterior pituitary gland into the bloodstream in an episodic manner under the direction of hypothalamic CRHs. The frequency of pulses is normally fairly constant over the 24-h period, and it is changes in the amplitude that give rise to the circadian profile of ACTH and, hence, glucocorticoid secretion. Increases in pulse amplitude also underpin the stress-induced excursions in pituitary-adrenocortical activity although, in some instances, changes in pulse frequency may also occur.

Hypothalamic Control of Adrenocorticotropic Hormone Secretion

The concept that the secretion of ACTH is driven by a neurohormone, termed corticotropin-releasing factor (CRF), that is released from the hypothalamus and transported to the pituitary gland via the hypothalamic-hypophysial portal vessels was first recognized in the late 1940s by Harris. However, some 35 years elapsed between Harris's pioneering work and the identification of the active principles. By the late 1970s it was becoming apparent that CRF activity of the hypothalamus could not be ascribed to a single factor, and the concept of a multifactorial CRF rapidly gained credence. Subsequent work identified a 41-amino-acid residue neuropeptide, termed CRH, as the principal component and also pointed to a key role for AVP.

Corticotropin releasing hormone The 41-amino-acid neuropeptide, CRH, was first identified in ovine hypothalami by Vale and colleagues; the human peptide was identified subsequently and shown to differ from the ovine peptide by seven amino acids but to be identical to the rat peptide. The CRH gene is well characterized in the rat, mouse, and human and is expressed at multiple sites within the central nervous system (e.g., the hypothalamus, amygdala, and brain stem) and also in the periphery. CRH destined for the anterior pituitary gland is synthesized in the cell bodies of parvocellular neurons, which originate in the paraventricular nucleus (PVN) of the hypothalamus and project to the external lamina of the median eminence. These neurons terminate in close apposition with the capillaries of the hypothalamo-hypophysial portal complex into which they release their secretory products for transportation to the anterior pituitary gland. The concentration of CRH in hypophysial portal blood is high (vs. peripheral blood) and alters in parallel with perturbations of pituitary-adrenal function (e.g., stress), as also does the expression of the peptide and its mRNA in the PVN–median eminence tract. The actions of CRH on the corticotrophs are effected by specific type 1 CRH receptors (CRH-R1s), and the blockade of these receptors with selective antagonists attenuates corticotropic responses to specific stressors and to exogenous CRH. The stress response is also impaired in mice in which genes encoding either CRH or CRH-R1 are ablated, although resting ACTH levels appear to be normal in mutant mice. CRH-R1s are coupled positively to adenylyl cyclase via a G_s-protein. The stimulation of the receptor therefore causes a rise in intracellular cAMP with subsequent activation of protein kinase A, which phosphorylates Ca^{2+} channels, thereby permitting Ca^{2+} influx and the release of ACTH by exocytosis. The activation of CRH-R1s in the pituitary gland also augments POMC gene expression and hence ACTH synthesis and, in the longer term, causes the proliferation of the corticotrophs.

Arginine vasopressin The ACTH-releasing activity of AVP was first recognized in the 1950s, and evidence that AVP may be an important component of a multifactorial corticotropin releasing complex emerged originally from studies performed in rats congenitally lacking AVP (Brattleboro strain) and was subsequently supported by work using specific antisera and antagonists to the peptide. AVP *per se* shows only weak ACTH-releasing activity, acting via the V1b subclass of AVP receptors, which use the phosphatidylinositol signal transduction system.

However, it also potentiates the corticotropic responses to CRH markedly and thus plays a key role in determining the magnitude of the stress response. Surprisingly, the biochemical basis of this important synergistic response is poorly defined, although it is apparent that the activation of the V1b receptor potentiates the accumulation of $3'5'$ cAMP induced by CRH, probably by a mechanism involving protein kinase C-dependent protein phosphorylation. AVP destined for the corticotrophs is derived primarily from a population of CRH-containing parvocellular neurons projecting from the PVN to the median eminence; thus, as for CRH, the concentration of AVP in the portal system is relatively high (vs. peripheral blood) and is increased further by stress. In addition, some AVP may be directed to the corticotrophs from magnocellular neurons of the neurohypophysial system (the primary source of AVP in peripheral blood) via the interconnecting short portal vessels. Within the parvocellular system, CRH and AVP are colocalized in the same secretory granules and may therefore be cosecreted. However, histological studies suggest that not all CRH-positive neurons express AVP in normal circumstances, thus permitting the ratio of AVP : CRH released to vary in a stimulus-specific manner; equally, not all corticotrophs express receptors for AVP, thereby permitting another level of control. Although AVP is generally considered to be the second CRH, this is not always the case. For example, in the sheep, AVP has precedence over CRH; similarly, in rodents and possibly in humans, AVP appears to be the dominant factor driving ACTH release in conditions of repeated or sustained stress.

Other hypothalamic factors Other hypothalamic factors may also contribute to the regulation of ACTH, including the pituitary adenylyl cyclase-activating peptide (PACAP), which exerts a stimulatory influence, and atrial natriuretic peptide (ANP) and substance P, both of which exert inhibitory influences.

Stress-Induced Activation of Corticotropin Releasing Hormone/Arginine vasopressin Neurons

The parvocellular CRH/AVP neurons in the hypothalamus are well positioned to monitor, integrate, and respond to emotional insults and physical changes in the internal or external environment that threaten homeostasis (i.e., stress). Significantly, they receive inputs from many ascending and descending nervous pathways; in addition, they are sensitive to a variety of substances that may be relayed by the bloodstream or the cerebrospinal fluid (e.g., glucose and steroids) and to local factors released from interneurons or glial cells (e.g., eicosanoids and cytokines). Major roles have been identified for (1) inputs from the brain-stem nuclei, particularly the nucleus tractus solitarius (NTS), that relay sensory information directly to the PVN and also to other parts of the brain and (2) pathways projecting to the PVN from the prefrontal cortex and the limbic system (hippocampus; amygdala; lateral septum; and the bed nucleus of the stria terminalis, BNST), but other pathways, such as those arising from raphe nuclei, are also likely to contribute. Although the precise complement of neural pathways, humoral substances, and local mediators that orchestrates the release of CRH/AVP in stress almost certainly depends on the nature of the stimulus and the status of the individual at the time of the stress, some classification according to the type of stress is now possible. For example, HPA responses to visceral homeostatic stressors that lack a cognitive component (e.g., acute hypotension) are initiated by afferent fibers that signal via the brain-stem nuclei and the noradrenergic pathways that project from the brain stem to the PVN; some homeostatic stressors also signal via humoral mechanisms; for example, the responses to hypoglycemia and hypertonicity involve intrahypothalamic glucose- and osmotic-sensitive neurons, respectively. Visceral stressors with a significant cognitive component (e.g., restraint, foot shock, or cold) use somatosensory afferents and central pathways involving both the brain-stem nuclei and the corticolimbic system to activate the PVN. The corticolimbic system also plays a fundamental role in effecting the HPA responses to emotional stressors; the importance of the hippocampus, which is critical to cognitive function, particularly learning and memory function, is well documented in this regard, as is the role of the amygdala, a key area in coordinating the behavioral, autonomic, and neuroendocrine responses to fear or anxiety.

Challenges to the host defense system, such as those provoked by infection, injury, or inflammation, pose a major threat to homeostasis and thus constitute a severe stress. Not surprisingly, in experimental animals and in humans the HPA axis responds to such insults with a marked increase in its activity. This response is driven by the army of mediators (e.g., interleukins, eicosanoids, histamine, and phospholipase A2) released from the activated immune/inflammatory cells. Some of these agents may target the HPA axis directly, acting mainly at the hypothalamic level to trigger CRH/AVP release but also on the anterior pituitary gland and adrenal cortex to augment or sustain the final adrenocortical response. Others may act locally at the site of the infection or inflammatory lesion to stimulate sensory fibers and thereby activate the central pathways that precipitate CRH/AVP release. In addition, many of the mediators provoke widespread pathological effects in the body (e.g., hypotension or hypoglycemia), which themselves stimulate the axis by the mechanisms outlined earlier. The HPA response to immune insults is thus a complex event potentially requiring the integration of a broad spectrum of stimuli, the complement of which reflects the nature and intensity of the insult. Much research has focused on the influence of the cytokines, interleukin (IL)-1β and IL-6, which are particularly important in initiating the HPA response to bacterial and viral infections. Three main mechanisms have been proposed to explain their actions.

1. The cytokines act directly on the PVN to trigger CRH release via a mechanism dependent on prostanoid generation. This mechanism has been refuted on the basis that the cytokines, which are large polypeptides (17–26 kDa), are unlikely to penetrate the blood–brain barrier and thereby gain access to their targets. However, the possibility that cytokines enter the brain via fenestrated regions of the barrier (e.g., organum vasculosum lamina terminalis, OVLT), areas in which the permeability is increased by local inflammation, or the recently described transporter system cannot be discounted.

2. The cytokines act at the level of the blood–brain barrier itself, exerting prostanoid-dependent actions on the endothelium that trigger CRH/AVP release by mechanisms that may include the activation of neural pathways and/or induction of *de novo* synthesis of cytokines in the hypothalamus and elsewhere in the brain that are required to drive the neuroendocrine response. This concept is supported by the presence of IL-1 receptors in the endothelial cells and by increased IL-1 mRNA expression in the hypothalamus and other brain areas of rodents subjected to endotoxin challenge.

3. Hypothalamic responses to peripheral cytokines involve the sequential activation of sensory fibers, brain-stem nuclei (notably the NTS), and the ventral noradrenergic pathways (and possibly others) to the PVN. This view concurs with claims that the expression of IL-1β mRNA in the hypothalamus and the hypersecretion of ACTH release induced by endotoxin are both dependent on the integrity of the vagus and that HPA responses to local inflammatory lesions induced by turpentine require C fibers. However, it is at odds with reports that cytokines activate the NTS, and hence connections between the NTS and the PVN, by mechanisms that are independent of the vagus but which may involve local prostanoid-dependent interactions with the blood–brain barrier.

Negative Feedback Control of the Hypothalamic-Pituitary-Adrenal Axis

Role of glucocorticoids Adrenocortical responses to incoming stimuli are effectively contained within appropriate limits by the glucocorticoids themselves, which exert powerful inhibitory influences on the secretion of ACTH and its hypothalamic-releasing hormones. Thus, elevations in circulating glucocorticoid levels brought about, for example, by the administration of exogenous steroids effectively suppress the HPA responses to stress and also the circadian rise in pituitary-adrenocortical activity. Conversely, the ACTH response to stress is exaggerated in subjects with adrenocortical insufficiency (e.g., Addison's disease) but corrected by glucocorticoid replacement therapy. The feedback actions of the steroids are highly complex because they are exerted at multiple sites within the axis, effected by multiple molecular mechanisms, and operate over three time domains: rapid or fast feedback, early delayed feedback, and late delayed feedback.

Phases of steroid feedback Rapid feedback develops within 2–3 min of an increase in glucocorticoid levels. It is of short duration (<10 min) and is followed by a silent period during which the stress response is intact, even though the circulating steroid levels may remain elevated. Rapid feedback is sensitive to the rate of change rather than the absolute concentration of steroid in the blood and may therefore provide an important means whereby the HPA response to stress is terminated; alternatively, it may serve to blunt the responses to a second stress incurred at a time when the steroid levels are still rising in response to the first stress. The early delayed phase of feedback develops approximately 0.5–2 h after an acute elevation in plasma steroid levels. It is normally maximal within 2–4 h and, depending on the intensity of the stimulus, may persist for up to 24 h. Both the circadian and the stress-induced excursions in ACTH secretion are suppressed with an intensity that is directly proportional to the concentration of steroid previously reached in the blood. Late delayed feedback, which has a latency of approximately 24 h, develops only after a very substantial rise in steroid levels and is frequently the consequence of repeated or continuous administration of high doses of corticosteroids. It may persist for days or weeks after the steroid treatment is withdrawn and is thus largely responsible for the potentially life-threatening suppression of the HPA axis associated with abrupt cessation of long-term treatment with high doses of steroids in, for example, rheumatoid arthritis.

Mechanisms of glucocorticoid feedback The rapid feedback actions of the glucocorticoids are exerted primarily at the hypothalamic level; weaker actions also occur at the pituitary level, but the contribution, if any, of extrahypothalamic sites in the central nervous system is ill defined. The underlying molecular mechanisms are poorly understood. Although there are some reports to the contrary, the majority of data suggests that these effects are nongenomic (and hence do not involve MRs or GRs) and that they may be mediated by receptors that are located close to or within cell membranes and which, when activated, inhibit exocytosis, possibly by blocking Ca^{2+}. In contrast, the early and late delayed phases of feedback inhibition are mediated by classic intracellular corticosteroid receptors located primarily in the anterior pituitary gland, the hypothalamus, and the hippocampus, but also elsewhere in the brain. Both the high-affinity MRs and the lower-affinity GRs are involved. Current evidence suggests that MRs (located predominantly in the hippocampus) may maintain the tonic inhibitory influence of steroids on HPA function in nonstress conditions because these receptors, which are not protected by 11β-HSD, are normally almost fully occupied by glucocorticoids, even at the nadir of the circadian rhythm. GRs, however (found in particular abundance in the anterior pituitary gland and hypothalamus) are occupied extensively only when the glucocorticoid level is raised by stress, disease, or the administration of exogenous steroids; thus, unlike MRs, these receptors serve to detect phasic changes in steroid levels and to adjust the activity of the HPA axis accordingly. Early delayed feedback requires the *de novo* generation of protein second messengers that serve to inhibit the release of ACTH and its hypothalamic-releasing factors; several proteins are likely to be involved, including lipocortin 1 (LC1, annexin 1), a Ca^{2+}- and phospholipids-binding protein strongly implicated in the anti-inflammatory and antiproliferative actions of the steroids. The genes encoding POMC in the pituitary gland and CRH/AVP in the parvocellular PVN neurons may also be repressed during the early delayed phase of feedback; however, the consequent downregulation of ACTH, CRH, and AVP synthesis emerges relatively slowly and, with existing techniques, is not normally discernible until some hours after the onset of inhibition of peptide release. Late delayed feedback is characterized by the inhibition of the synthesis and the release of CRH/AVP and ACTH in the hypothalamus and anterior pituitary gland, respectively. The inhibition of synthesis again reflects the inhibitory influence of the steroids on the genes encoding each of the three peptides, but the concomitant inhibition of peptide release cannot be explained fully in this way because peptide stores are rarely fully depleted.

Short loop and ultrashort loop feedback mechanisms In addition to the corticosteroids, other hormones of the HPA axis participate in the feedback regulation of ACTH secretion. Of particular importance are the POMC-derived peptides, ACTH and β-endorphin, both of which have been shown to exert powerful inhibitory actions on the secretion of CRH/AVP by the hypothalamus. Because neither peptide penetrates the blood–brain barrier readily, their short loop feedback actions are probably exerted at the level of the median eminence, which lies outside the blood–brain barrier. Ultrashort loop feedback actions have been attributed to both CRH and AVP, but the physiological significance of such responses is unclear.

Glucocorticoid Secretion in Repeated or Sustained Stress

The bulk of studies on stress and HPA function have focused on acute stresses, and relatively little is known of either the characteristics or the mechanisms controlling the HPA responses to repeated or sustained stress. Such conditions are, of course, inherent to our lifestyle and environment, and a deeper understanding of their influence on neuroendocrine function is thus highly desirable. However, for both ethical and practical reasons, it is difficult to develop appropriate animal models and, as described later, the available data suggest that the profile of the HPA responses observed may vary considerably according to the nature of the stress.

In some cases, HPA responses to repeated (successive or intermittent) or sustained (chronic) stressful stimuli are attenuated. For example, tolerance develops to stresses such as cold, handling, saline injection, or water deprivation (induced by the replacement of drinking water with physiological saline). Some degree of cross-tolerance may occur between stresses that invoke similar pathways/mechanisms to increase CRH/AVP release. Thus, for example, repeated handling reduces the subsequent adrenocortical response to a saline injection; however, rats tolerant to the C fiber-dependent stress of exposure to a cold environment respond to the novel stress immobilization with a normal or even exaggerated rise in serum corticosterone. In other situations, however, tolerance does not develop; thus, HPA responses to intermittent stresses of electric foot shock, insulin hypoglycemia, or IL-1β are maintained or even enhanced, as are those to the chronic stress of septicemia.

The sustained release of ACTH in repeated/chronic stress appears to be driven mainly by AVP. Thus, in rats subjected to repetitive foot shock, brain surgery, or injection of IL-1β or lipopolysaccharide (LPS), AVP is synthesized in and released from parvocellular neurons in the PVN in preference to CRH; in addition, the sensitivity of the pituitary gland to AVP is well maintained, whereas that to CRH is reduced. Similarly, the expression of AVP, but not CRH, in the parvocellular PVN is increased in rats with experimentally induced arthritis; moreover, although the arthritic rats respond to LPS with a rise ACTH secretion, they are relatively unresponsive to a novel neurogenic stress normally driven mainly by CRH. The switch to AVP as the principal driving force to the corticotrophs in repetitive/chronic stress may reflect the disruption of the negative feedback mechanism for the expression of MRs in the hippocampus, and GRs in the PVN are reduced in conditions of chronic stress; moreover, the capacity of dexamethasone to block the HPA response to IL-1β is impaired in rats pretreated 3 weeks with the cytokine. In the same vein, AVP and disrupted feedback have both been implicated in the etiology of the hypercortisolemia evident in depression, although others have advocated a role for CRH.

Age- and Gender-Related Changes in the Stress Response

Development

The functional development of the HPA axis begins in fetal life, and in the later stages of gestation the fetus secretes substantial quantities of cortisol/corticosterone. It also responds to stress with increases in adrenocortical activity, which are driven by the hypothalamic-pituitary axis and which are sensitive to the negative feedback actions of the glucocorticoids. Paradoxically, in the rat and several other species, HPA function regresses postnatally and a period ensues during which the ability of the axis to respond to stress is compromised. In the rat, this stress hyporesponsive phase (SHRP) normally persists from postnatal day 5 (P5) to P14, although depending on the stimulus a mature stress response may not emerge for up to 5–6 weeks. The refractoriness of the HPA axis to stress in the SHRP is not absolute and may be at least partially overridden in certain cases. For example, IL-1β, hypoglycemia, glutamate, and histamine all elicit modest rises in serum ACTH and corticosterone throughout this period. Exceptionally, the hypersecretion of ACTH provoked by LPS in the SHRP matches that observed in the adult, although the

associated rise in serum corticosterone does not; moreover, paradoxically, both the ACTH and the corticosterone responses to kainic acid are more robust at P12 than P18. These and many other data suggest that the processes involved in the maturation of the stress response are complex and stimulus-dependent. They are therefore likely to involve a variety of factors that act in concert at different levels of the axis during the developmental period. These include immaturity of the neural and humoral mechanisms effecting the release of CRH/AVP in stress, enhanced sensitivity of the axis to the regulatory actions of the glucocorticoids, and impairment of the synergy between CRH and AVP.

Perinatal Programming of the Stress Response

Glucocorticoids play a key role in developmental programming, and a growing body of evidence suggests that inappropriate exposure of the developing fetus/neonate to the steroids or to factors that influence the expression/function of their receptors may trigger a plethora of pathologies (e.g., growth retardation or impairment of central nervous system development) and predispose the individual in later life to conditions as diverse as hypertension, insulin resistance, cognitive and other behavioral disorders, and allergic/inflammatory disease. Because the SHRP coincides with an important phase of development, it seems likely that it may serve to protect the organism from the potentially harmful effects of overexposure to glucocorticoids.

Despite its tight control, the developing HPA axis exhibits a high degree of plasticity, and disturbances in its activity at critical stages of development precipitate abnormalities in glucocorticoid secretion that persist into adult life and may increase the susceptibility of the individual to disease. Perinatal manipulations that alter the expression of GRs (but not MRs) in the brain are particularly hazardous in this regard because, by disrupting the negative feedback mechanisms, they alter the responsivity of the HPA axis to stress throughout the lifetime of the individual. For example, exposure of neonatal rats to dexamethasone or LPS results in the adult in downregulation of GRs in the hippocampus and hypothalamus, decreased sensitivity of the HPA axis to the negative feedback actions of the glucocorticoids, and exaggerated HPA responses to stress. Similar long-term changes in GR expression occur in rats subjected to prolonged periods of maternal separation; the consequent impairment of the negative feedback system and changes in HPA function are associated with alterations in T-cell antibody responses and in the incidence of age-related neuropathies. In contrast, neonatal handling, which increases hippocampal GR expression by mechanisms involving serotonin, reduces the magnitude and duration of the stress response in the adult; maternal care may therefore help program events that regulate responses to stress in the adult and thus reduce vulnerability to disease.

Sexual Dimorphism in Hypothalamic-Pituitary-Adrenal Function

In adults, distinct sexually dimorphic patterns of glucocorticoid secretion emerge. Serum glucocorticoid concentrations are consistently higher in the female than in the male, with further increases occurring toward the middle of the menstrual/estrous cycle just prior to ovulation and in the late stages of pregnancy. These changes are due partly to the positive effects of estrogen on the expression of CBG. In addition, estrogen exerts significant effects at the hypothalamic level, increasing the synthesis and release of CRH, a phenomenon that may be implicated in the etiology of the relatively high incidence of emotional disorders (e.g., depression and anxiety) in the female that are characterized by enhanced CRH secretion. Further modulation may be brought about by progesterone, which, when present in large amounts (e.g., in the premenstrual phase or pregnancy), binds readily to but is only weakly active at MRs in the hippocampus.

Stress Responses in the Aging

In both sexes, serum glucocorticoid concentrations tend to increase in aging individuals, particularly in disease states; in addition, although sometimes delayed, the HPA responses to stress are frequently exaggerated and prolonged. This aging process has been attributed in part to the downregulation of the corticosteroid receptors (GRs and MRs) in the hippocampus and hypothalamus and to the consequent emergence of a resistance of the HPA axis to the negative feedback actions of the glucocorticoids. The consequences are potentially important because hyperglucocorticoidemia is considered to be an important contributory factor in a number of age-related diseases, including neurodegenerative conditions, cognitive dysfunction, osteoporosis, noninsulin-dependent diabetes mellitus, and the decline in immunocompetence.

See Also the Following Articles

Adrenal Cortex; Adrenocorticotropic Hormone (ACTH); Corticotropin Releasing Factor (CRF); Feedback Systems; Glucocorticoid Negative Feedback; Glucocorticoids, Role in Stress; Hypothalamic-Pituitary-Adrenal; Vasopressin.

Further Reading

Buckingham, J. C. (1996). Stress and the neuroendocrine immune axis: the pivotal role of glucocorticoids and lipocortin 1. *British Journal of Pharmacology* **118**, 1–19.

Buckingham, J. C., Gillies, G. E. and Cowell, A.-M. (1997). *Stress, stress hormones and the immune system*. Chichester, UK: John Wiley.

de Kloet, E. R., Vreugdenhil, E., Citzl, M. S., et al. (1988). Brain corticosteroid receptor balance in health and disease. *Endocrine Review* **19**, 269–301.

Ericsson, A., Arias, C. and Sawchenko, P. E. (1997). Evidence for an intramedullary prostaglandin-dependent mechanism in the activation of stress-related neuroendocrine circuitry by intravenous interleukin-1. *Journal of Neuroscience* **17**, 7166–7179.

Gillies, G. E., Linton, E. A. and Lowry, P. J. (1982). Corticotropin releasing activity of the new CRH is potentiated several times by vasopressin. *Nature* **299**, 355–357.

Harris, G. W. (1955). *Neural control of the pituitary*. London: Edward Arnold.

Kellerwood, M. E. and Dallman, M. F. (1984). Corticosteroid inhibition of ACTH secretion. *Endocrine Review* **5**, 1–25.

Li, H. Y. and Sawchenko, P. E. (1998). Hypothalamic effector neurons and extended circuitries activated in "neurogenic" stress: a comparison of footshock effects exerted accutely, chronically and in animals with controlled glucose levels. *Journal of Comparative Neurobiology* **393**, 244–266.

Lowry, P. J. (1984). Pro-opiocortin: the multiple hormone precursor. *Bioscience Reports* **4**, 467–482.

Muglia, L., Jacobson, L. and Majzoub, J. A. (1996). Production of corticotropin-releasing hormone deficient mice by targeted mutation of embryonic stem cells. *Annals of the New York Academy of Sciences* **780**, 49–59.

Rosenfeld, P., Surchecki, A. J. and Levins, S. (1992). *Neuroscience and Biobehavioral Reviews* **16**, 553–568.

Seckl, J. R. (1997). 11β-hydroxysteroid dehydrogenase in the brain: a novel regulator of glucocorticoid action? *Frontiers in Neuroendocrinology* **18**, 49–99.

Smith, G. W., Aubry, J. M., Dellu, F., et al. (1992). Corticotropin releasing factor receptor 1-deficient mice display increased anxiety, impaired stress response and observant neuroendocrine development. *Neuron* **20**, 1098–1102.

Tilders, F. J. and Solimidt, E. D. (1998). Interleukin 1β-induced plasticity of hypothalamic CRH neurons and long-term hyperresponsivity. *Annals of the New York Academy of Sciences* **840**, 65–73.

Vale, W., Spiess, J., Rivier, L., et al. (1981). Characterisation of a 41-residue ovine hypothalamic peptide that stimulates secretion of corticotropin and β-endorphin. *Science* **213**, 1394–1397.

Vamvakopoulos, N. C. and Chrousos, G. P. (1994). Hormonal regulation of human corticotropin releasing hormone gene expression: implications for the sexual dimorphism of the stress response and immune inflammatory reaction. *Endocrine Review* **15**, 409–420.

Glucocorticoids, Overview

B E Pearson Murphy
McGill University Health Center, Montreal, PQ, Canada

This article is a revision of the previous edition article by B E P Murphy, volume 2, pp 244–260, © 2000, Elsevier Inc.

Introduction
Evolution
Binding Proteins
Biosynthesis
Actions
Metabolism
Absorption
Regulation of Levels of Glucocorticoids
Measurement
Antiglucocorticoids
Uses of Glucocorticoids and their Inhibitors as
    Therapeutic Agents

Glossary

Gluco-corticoids	(From Greek γλυκος meaning sweet and Latin *cortex* meaning bark.) Steroids produced by the adrenal cortex which regulate carbohydrate metabolism; however their actions are by no means confined to carbohydrate metabolism.
Steroids	Chemicals containing the cyclopentanoperhydrophenanthrene nucleus (**Figure 1**).

Introduction

Chemistry

Structurally glucocorticoids (GCs) are all modifications of corticosterone (**Table 1**). Modifications which enhance activity include the addition of a 17α-hydroxy group (cortisol, **Figure 2**), a Δ1-double bond (prednisolone), a 9α-fluoro (fludrocortisol), a 16α- or 16β-methyl or a 16α-hydroxy group. The 11-keto analogs of these compounds are often included because, although they themselves are biologically inactive, they are readily converted to the active 11-hydroxylated forms. Cortisone, the 11-keto derivative of cortisol, was identified before cortisol, so that for many years cortisol was known as hydrocortisone (i.e., cortisone), with two additional hydrogens giving the 11-hydroxyl group. Oral cortisone and prednisone, the 11-keto analog of prednisolone, are widely used therapeutically since they are about 80% converted to the active forms as they pass through the liver after absorption in the gastrointestinal tract.

History

In the late 1930s and early 1940s many steroids were isolated from the adrenal cortex of animals and man. Glands from 20 000 cattle were collected to give 1000 kg of tissue from which 25 g of material was further processed to determine more than 30 different steroids, including the GCs and mineralocorticoids.

Evolution

Steroids are present throughout the whole of the biosphere of the Earth, and are thought to be ancient bioregulators, present throughout the plant and animal kingdoms, which evolved prior to the appearance of eukaryotes. They seem to be primordial biomolecules which are among the earliest chemical information transmitters and have had a crucial role in the evolution of life. Even bacteria, viruses, and blue–green algas contain steroids.

GCs are secreted in all vertebrates, but not in other life forms. In mammals and bony fish, the main GC is cortisol, except in some rodents where it is corticosterone. In birds, reptiles, amphibians, and cartilaginous fish, the main GC is corticosterone.

Binding Proteins

There are two types of binding proteins for steroids: one type which inactivates them, and the other which activates them.

Transport Proteins

Corticosteroid-binding globulin (CBG), present in blood, binds GCs noncovalently in such a way that their biological activity is suppressed; thus it is the

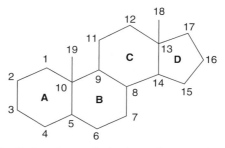

Figure 1 Cyclopentanoperhydrophenanthrene nucleus.

Table 1 Modifications of corticosterone to give other glucocorticoids, and their relative potencies in humans

Steroid	Modification of corticosterone	Anti-inflammatory potency	Salt-retaining potency	LHPA-axis suppression
Corticosterone	–	0.35	15	
Cortisol	17α-OH	1	1	1
Prednisolone	Δ^1-, 17α-OH	4	0.75	4
Methylprednisolone	6α-methyl-, Δ^1-, 17α-OH	6	0.5	4
Fludrocortisol	9α-fluoro-, 17α-OH	15	280	
Dexamethasone	16α-methyl-, Δ^1-, 9α-fluoro-, 17α-OH	26	<1	17
Betamethasone	16β-methyl-, Δ^1-, 9α-fluoro-, 17α-OH	25	<1	
Triamcinolone	16α-hydroxyl-, Δ^1-, 9α-fluoro-, 17α-OH	5	<1	4

LHPA, limbic-hypothalamic-pituitary-adrenal.

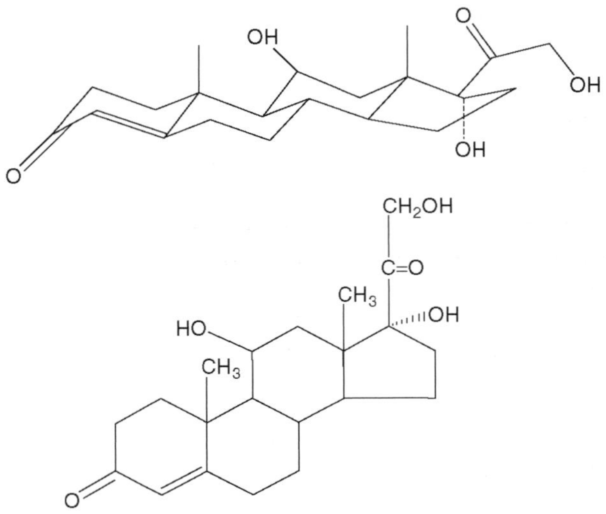

Figure 2 Structure of cortisol. Top: The three-dimensional structure. A dotted line denotes that the C17 OH is below the plane of the molecule, while a straight line, as for the C18- or C19-hydroxyl denotes that the CH_3 is above the plane. Asterisks indicate asymmetric carbon atoms. Bottom: Depicted in the customary fashion and showing numbering of the carbon atoms.

unbound or free hormone which is active. These proteins are found in virtually all vertebrates and their specificities for GCs vary; in some cases the binding is very highly specific and can be used to measure the steroid that is bound. They are saturable so that at high levels of GCs, proportionally less is bound. Such proteins are important in the transport of GCs since they prevent undue transfer of the steroid into tissues where it would be subject to enzymatic action and/or degradation. They thus provide a reservoir to damp down rapid changes. In conditions of severe stress, they are reduced. GCs are also bound reversibly and noncovalently to albumin, but this is a nonspecific and loose type of binding.

Glucocorticoid Receptors

Another kind of protein that binds GCs is the GC receptor (GR), which mediates the action of the steroid and is found in or on the target cells for the hormones. This binding is of high affinity and specificity and is saturable. In the nucleus, the hormone-receptor complex is activated and binds to deoxyribonucleic acid (DNA), leading to transcription.

The actions of GCs are mediated by two types of receptors: GRs and mineralocorticoid receptors (MRs). GRs bind GCs but not aldosterone, while MRs bind both GCs and aldosterone, the selectivity of the MRs being dependent upon the presence of 11β-dehydrogenase (particularly in the kidney) to inactivate the GCs. In the hippocampus where MRs are present in high concentrations, GCs serve to activate both.

Biosynthesis

The synthetic pathway appears to be much the same throughout the vertebrates: acetate → cholesterol → pregnenolone → corticosterone and/or cortisol (**Figure 3**). Each step is catalyzed by an enzyme. Some of these enzymes are known to occur also in plants and bacteria.

Steroidogenic tissues can take up low-density lipoprotein cholesterol from the plasma (about 80%), mobilize intracellular cholesteryl ester pools, or synthesize cholesterol *de novo* from acetate. GCs are synthesized from cholesterol by the P450 group of enzymes (oxidative enzymes that have a characteristic 450-nm absorbance maximum when reduced with carbon monoxide). The first step is achieved by P450$_{scc}$, the side-chain cleavage (SCC) enzyme, which cleaves the side chain from the C20 to give pregnenolone. This occurs in the inner mitochondrial membrane. 21-Hydroxylation occurs in the smooth endoplasmic reticulum while 11-hydroxylation occurs in the mitochondrion. In humans, the route to corticosterone and aldosterone production takes place in the adrenal zona glomerulosa while that to cortisol occurs in the zona fasciculata and the reticularis; the 11-hydroxylating enzymes involved differ slightly in the two regions, while the P450$_{C17}$-hydroxylase is

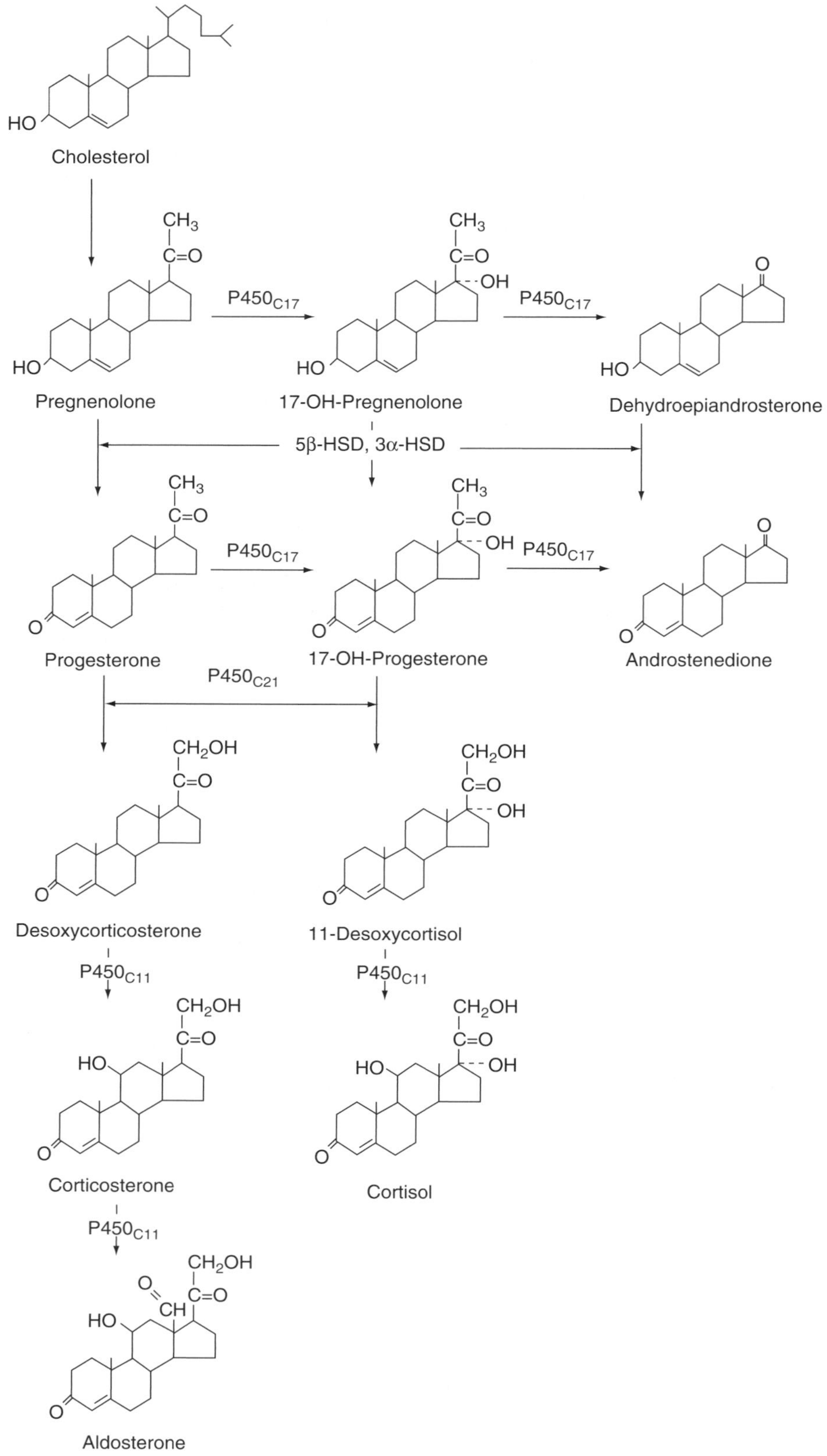

Figure 3 Biosynthesis of adrenal corticosteroids. 3α-HSD, 3α-hydroxysteroid dehydrogenase; 5β-HSD, 5β-hydroxysteroid dehydrogenase.

lacking in the zona glomerulosa. The $P450_{C17}$ enzyme also cleaves the C20–C21 from C17, giving rise to dehydroepiandrosterone (DHEA) and the adrenal androgen pathway. If the GC pathway is blocked, as in congenital adrenal hyperplasia, this route becomes prominent. DHEA is sulfated in the reticularis to give DHEA sulfate (DHAS), which is quantitatively, though not physiologically, the most important product of the adult adrenal cortex.

In fetal primates, the adrenal is relatively much larger than in the adult, and is made up mainly of a fetal zone which is lost at about the time of birth. This zone lacks 3β-hydroxysteroid dehydrogenase isomerase so that the major steroid produced by this zone is DHEA, mainly in the sulfated form. The function of this zone remains speculative.

Actions

GCs are necessary for life and affect every cell of the body. They are thought to enter the cell mainly by passive diffusion, and then bind to the GR. They also act nongenomically at membrane receptors.

Carbohydrate Metabolism

Adrenalectomized animals become hypoglycemic because they cannot maintain their hepatic glycogen stores. GCs activate glycogen synthase and inactivate the phosphorylase which mobilizes glycogen. Although glucagon and epinephrine are also gluconeogenic, they are ineffective in the absence of GCs which act permissively.

GCs enhance gluconeogenesis from protein, thereby raising blood glucose and repleting liver glycogen. This is accomplished by increasing release of glucogenic amino acids from peripheral tissues such as skeletal muscle. GCs also activate gluconeogenic enzymes, including glucose-6-phosphatase and phosphoenolpyruvate carboxykinase. Large amounts result in negative nitrogen balance, and if prolonged, depletion of body protein, observed clinically as thinning of the skin, muscle wasting, myopathy, osteoporosis, and in children, retarded growth.

Fat Metabolism

GCs, administered acutely, activate lipolysis in adipose tissue, so that plasma free fatty acid levels are reduced. However, when given chronically, increased availability of carbohydrate produces an antiketogenic effect, and clinically a redistribution of fat from the extremities to the face and trunk, especially in the supraclavicular and dorsocervical areas, the latter producing the characteristic buffalo hump seen in Cushing's syndrome.

Electrolyte and Water Metabolism

Although much less potent than the mineralocorticoids, GCs in high doses may produce sodium and water retention, hypokalemia, and hypertension. Conversely, in their absence, there is renal sodium wasting, with a concomitant loss of water, hemoconcentration, hyponatremia, and hypovolemia. Hypotension may occur, although this is usually avoided if sufficient mineralocorticoid is present. Vasopressin (VP) is increased and free water clearance is decreased in GC insufficiency, which may help to maintain normal blood pressure. GCs stimulate plasma atrial natriuretic peptide (ANP) production, and potentiate ANP action on the kidney.

Immunologic Function and Inflammation

GCs alter immune responses and inhibit inflammatory reactions. These actions can have both beneficial and deleterious results. While GCs are essential to maintain life in the face of stressors, excessive GCs may cause reactivation of latent infections such as tuberculosis. In contrast, they may benefit autoimmune diseases. A local inflammatory response involves the movement of cells and fluid to the site of inflammation. Histamine, a potent vasodilator, is released at the site, and prostaglandins are involved. Within 4 h after a rise in GCs in response to stress, peripheral lymphocyte and monocyte numbers fall, but granulocytes enter the circulation from lymphatic tissues and sites of inflammation. GCs inhibit synthesis of cytokines, proliferation of monocytes and their differentiation into macrophages; they also inhibit the phagocytic and cytotoxic functions of macrophages.

Effects on Bone and Connective Tissue

If GC excess is prolonged, osteopenia occurs because GCs inhibit osteoblast function – including downregulation of insulin-like growth factor I (IGF-I) which promotes osteoblast proliferation – thereby decreasing new bone formation. Osteoclast numbers and activity are increased. Intestinal calcium absorption is decreased and parathyroid hormone levels are secondarily increased; these effects can be reversed by giving vitamin D and calcium. Renal calcium reabsorption is decreased resulting in an increase in calcium excretion, and which may cause the formation of renal stones.

Since GCs also suppress synthesis of the extracellular matrix components collagen and hyaluronidate, clinically excessive GCs can impair wound healing and make connective tissue more friable, resulting in easy bruisability.

Oral administration of GCs may be associated with symptoms of gastric or duodenal ulcer; possibly this is only apparent, as ulcers caused by other factors, and which would heal if left alone, may become clinically troublesome if wound healing is impaired.

Neuropsychiatric Effects

GCs are released during learning and are necessary for establishment of an enduring memory. However excessive amounts impair spatial learning. Such processes involve the hippocampus.

Cortisol increases brain excitability, and emotional disturbances and even psychoses may occur in states either of deficiency or excess. In states of GC excess – either endogenous as in Cushing's syndrome or exogenous from therapeutic administration – altered behavior has been frequently noted.

Interestingly, in adrenal insufficiency, depression is also common, usually in association with apathy and lethargy; it improves with GC replacement.

The actions of GCs in the brain are mediated both genomically, whereby they enhance transcription, and nongenomically by direct effects on the excitability of neuronal networks, especially in the hippocampus, where GRs are present in the highest density. They can affect many neurotransmitter systems, including noradrenergic, serotonergic, cholinergic, dopamine, and GABAergic activity.

Development

Excessive concentrations of GCs, either endogenous or exogenous, inhibit skeletal growth in children. In the human fetus, the concentrations of circulating and tissue cortisol are kept low by the action of 11β-hydroxysteroid dehydrogenase type 2, which converts cortisol to inactive cortisone in almost all tissues until close to birth.

However GCs are important in stimulating differentiation of many cell types. In lung, they induce surfactant production, which is necessary for infant mammals to adapt to air-breathing at birth. GCs cause differentiation of the neural crest precursor cells of the adrenal medulla to differentiate into chromaffin cells which produce catecholamines.

Metabolism

Steps Involved

The GCs are metabolized primarily in the liver, and are excreted mainly through the kidneys in a series of steps catalyzed by enzymes (**Figure 4** and **Table 2**). These include:

1. Oxidation of the C11-hydroxyl to a ketone – the only reaction which is readily reversible

2. Reduction of the double bond at C4–5 to give 5α- and, mainly 5β-dihydro derivatives – these are almost entirely further reduced at the 3-ketone

3. Reduction of the 3-ketone to give 3α (mainly) and 3β-tetrahydro derivatives, which are in part further reduced at the C20-ketone

4. Reduction of the C20-ketone to give 20α- and (mainly) 20β-derivatives of any of the above compounds, but mainly of the tetrahydro derivatives to give the cortols (retaining the 11β-hydroxyl group) and cortolones (with the 11-ketone group)

5. Cleavage of the side chain of tetrahydrocortisol to give etiocholanolone

6. Oxidation of the 21-OH of the cortols to give the cortolic acids, and of the cortolones to give the cortolonic acids

7. Conjugation of the various metabolites with glucuronic acid (mainly at the 3β-hydroxyl) or sulfate (mainly 3α-hydroxyl), rendering the steroids more water-soluble

8. 6β-Hydroxylation of cortisol to give 6β-hydroxycortisol, also a much more water-soluble steroid

Factors Affecting Hepatic Metabolism

The following factors affect hepatic metabolism.

1. Thyroid hormones influence the rates of metabolism. In hyperthyroidism, metabolism of GCs is accelerated, while the opposite occurs in hypothyroidism. While these changes affect urinary excretion of metabolites, plasma corticoid levels are maintained, owing to the feedback mechanism which remains unaltered

2. In states of GC excess, hydroxylation to 6β-hydroxycortisol increases

3. In old age, corticoid metabolism decreases to some extent, while clearance of glucuronides is decreased; plasma levels usually rise slightly

4. In cirrhosis of the liver, 5-reduction is decreased

5. In obesity, greater amounts of metabolites are excreted, but the plasma levels remain essentially unchanged

6. Various drugs affect metabolism, e.g., rifampin accelerates metabolism, particularly to 6β-hydroxycortisol. Phenytoin, phenobarbital, and mitotane all divert metabolism toward 6β-hydroxycortisol

Extrahepatic Metabolism of Glucocorticoids

The kidney is another important site of metabolism, since its 11β-hydroxysteroid dehydrogenase (type 2) converts cortisol to cortisone, thereby limiting access of cortisol to the MR which binds both aldosterone

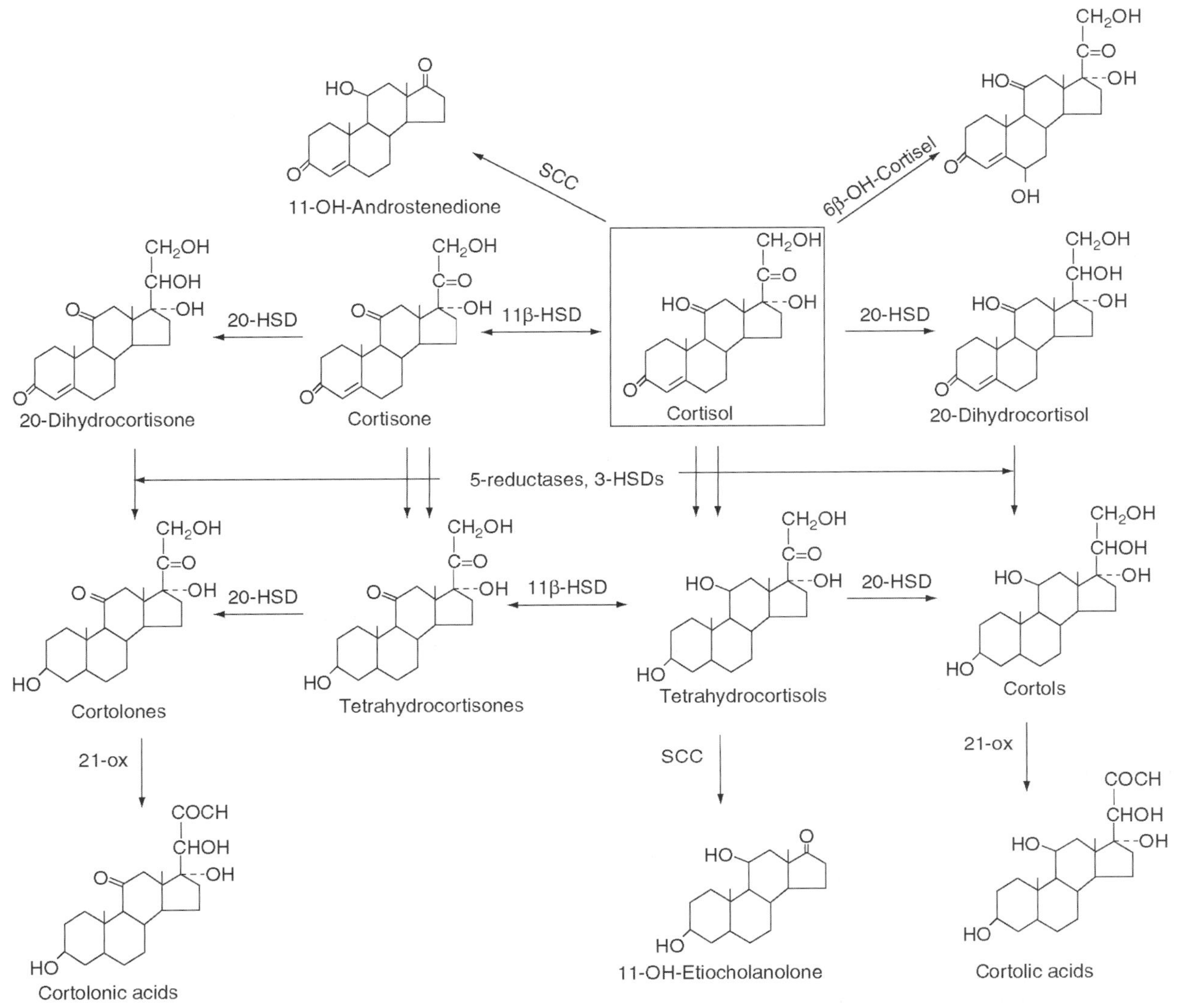

Figure 4 Metabolism of cortisol. HSD, hydroxysteroid dehydrogenase; ox, oxidase; SCC, side-chain cleavage.

Table 2 Cortisol and its metabolites in human urine[a]

Steroid	Approximate % of total
Tetrahydrocortisols (5β > 5α; 3α > 3β)	20
Tetrahydrocortisones (5β > 5α; 3α > 3β)	20
Cortolones	20
Cortols	10
Cortolic and cortolonic acids	10
11-OH-etiocholanolone	5
6β-OH-cortisol	1
11-OH-androstenedione	1
Cortisone, conjugated	1
Cortisol, conjugated	1
Cortisone, unconjugated	0.3
Cortisol, unconjugated	0.1

[a]With the possible exception of 6β-hydroxycortisol, all the metabolites occur mainly as conjugates, glucuronides exceeding sulfates.

and cortisol equally. Since aldosterone is present in much smaller amounts than cortisol, this permits aldosterone to exert its physiological action on the receptor. Genetic or pharmacologic alterations in the enzyme may cause mineralocorticoid problems.

Absorption

While steroids are generally administered via the oral route, they can be given effectively in many other ways including percutaneous, vaginal, rectal, nasal, and pulmonary, as well as intravenously, subcutaneously, and intramuscularly.

Intravenously administered steroids are diluted throughout the whole blood volume within a few minutes; subcutaneously injected steroids are absorbed within minutes to a few hours; intramuscularly injected steroids are more slowly absorbed, particularly if diluted in a medium which slows absorption, in which case absorption may be delayed for days to weeks. Absorption through skin (especially damaged skin) is rapid – usually detectable 30–100 min after application, and maximal by 16–24 h.

Regulation of Levels of Glucocorticoids

The Limbic-Hypothalamic-Pituitary-Adrenal Axis

Stimuli reaching the brain from extracerebral sites impact on the limbic system, where they are relayed to the hypothalamus, causing stimulation of corticotropin-releasing hormone (CRH) and VP. CRH and VP pass via the portal blood to the pituitary, causing pro-opio-melanocortin to be processed into adrenocorticotropic hormone (ACTH), endorphin, and other peptides, which enter the systemic circulation. ACTH stimulates the adrenal to produce cortisol and/or corticosterone which in turn feed back on GRs in the limbic system (principally the hippocampus and amygdala), hypothalamus, and pituitary to quench the stimulation, thus maintaining an ever-changing but essentially constant equilibrium (**Figure 5**).

Adrenocorticotropin ACTH acts by increasing synthesis of GCs, since adrenal storage of corticoids is minimal. ACTH stimulates the processing of cholesterol to Δ5-pregnenolone, the rate-limiting step in synthesis. It does this by binding to specific cell-surface receptors present on the adrenal cells, which activates adenylate cyclase thereby increasing cyclic adenosine monophosphate (cAMP), in turn activating cAMP-dependent protein kinase and phosphorylation of a number of proteins. If stimulation continues for more than a few minutes, increased synthesis of the various enzymes of the steroidogenic pathway are stimulated, as well as cell growth; if prolonged, the adrenal hypertrophies. Conversely, if ACTH levels fall for a prolonged period of weeks or months, the adrenal atrophies.

Other possible stimulators include direct effects of cytokines on the adrenal cortex and stimulation through neural connections.

Dexamethasone suppression test The dexamethasone-suppression test is often used to assess the suppressibility of the limbic-hypothalamic-pituitary-adrenal (LHPA) axis in humans; most commonly a 1 mg dose is given at bedtime, and blood samples are drawn once or more during the next day. The test is considered normal if the levels fall below 140 nmol l^{-1} (5 μg dl^{-1}, or preferably below 60 nmol l^{-1} (2.2 μg dl^{-1})).

Insulin tolerance test The insulin tolerance test is commonly used to evaluate the integrity of the LHPA axis. It measures the response to hypoglycemia induced by giving an injection of insulin, usually 1 μg,

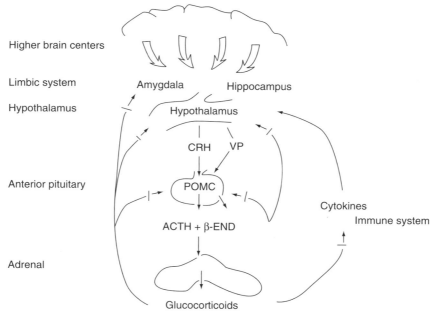

Figure 5 The limbic-hypothalamic-pituitary-adrenal (LHPA) axis. CRH, corticotropin-releasing hormone; VP, vasopressin; POMC, pro-opiomelanocortin; ACTH, adrenocorticotropic hormone; β-END, β-endorphin.

and following glucose and GC levels at 30, 60, and 90 min after injection. With normal CBG levels, the cortisol level should reach at least 500 nmol l^{-1} (18 µg dl^{-1}).

Plasma Levels of Glucocorticoids under Various Conditions

Plasma levels of GCs are generally in the range of 10–1000 nM. They vary diurnally, being highest shortly after awakening, and gradually falling during the period of activity (e.g., during the night in rodents, during the day in humans and monkeys). Plasma levels among species vary depending on the affinity and level of their CBG in plasma and of the GRs in the hippocampus, hypothalamus, and pituitary. GCs are also present in red blood cells in appreciable amounts.

In humans in the unstressed state, the plasma level of cortisol is 50–600 nmol l^{-1} during the day, being highest at 6–7 a.m. and lowest at midnight; corticosterone levels are about 10% of these and cortisone levels about 20%. Levels of cortisol in squirrel monkeys are higher at about 3000 nmol l^{-1} although their CBG levels are virtually undetectable. In rats, cortisol is absent, and corticosterone ranges at 50–200 nmol l^{-1}. Levels of corticosterone in fish (e.g., 15–200 nmol l^{-1} in trout) and reptiles are somewhat lower. In salmonids, and many animals, cortisol levels change seasonally, often in conjunction with CBG levels. In stressed animals, the levels of GCs rise within minutes to levels up to 10 or more times the resting levels.

Levels of Glucocorticoids in Other Tissues

GC levels in brain are as high or higher than those of plasma because brain is a fatty tissue and GCs are very fat soluble. GCs are found in all tissues but levels are usually lower than those in plasma and lymph. Levels are low in cerebrospinal fluid because the CBG level is low. They are very high in the adrenal cortex, the site of synthesis.

Cortisol–Cortisone Interconversion

Although in adult humans the level of cortisol greatly exceeds that of cortisone, the reverse is true in fetuses where oxidation by 11β-hydroxydehydrogenase (11β-HSD) greatly exceeds reduction. 11β-HSD consists of two enzymes: type 1 which predominates in adult liver and converts cortisone to cortisol; and type 2 which predominates in adult kidneys, allowing aldosterone to act in the presence of a 100-fold molar excess of circulating cortisol by converting cortisol

to cortisone. This type is also high in skin, salivary glands, and nonpregnant uterus.

In the fetus, type 2 predominates in all tissues except liver and intestine. It is particularly high in the placenta, converting maternal cortisol to cortisone, and corticosterone to 11-dehydrocorticosterone. This conversion, which inactivates cortisol and corticosterone, protects the fetus from excessive GCs which would interfere with growth. Type 2 11β-HSD is inhibited by licorice. The same enzyme converts prednisolone to prednisone but does not act on dexamethasone.

The human uterus, though oxidative in the nonpregnant state, becomes strongly reductive in late pregnancy, increasing the cortisol level eightfold so that the membranes are in contact with an environment high in cortisol. This increased cortisol concentration may play an anti-immune role in the uterine wall, the single maternal tissue, apart from maternal blood, in direct contact with fetal tissue.

A similar relationship between corticosterone and its 11-keto analog has also been demonstrated in rodents.

Conditions of Glucocorticoid Excess

Cushing's syndrome   In human Cushing's syndrome due to pituitary ACTH-secreting tumors (Cushing's disease), the morning cortisol levels are usually only minimally elevated, but the normal diurnal rhythm is lost so that the 24-h urinary cortisol, which reflects the integrated unbound cortisol level, is elevated. However the suppression of ACTH production by dexamethasone, although attenuated, is usually maintained.

In cases of ectopic ACTH-producing tumors, generally occurring in lung, cortisol levels are usually higher, and are frequently unsuppressed by dexamethasone.

Adrenal tumors cause varying levels of GCs, which are usually unresponsive to dexamethasone suppression, and are often associated with increases of adrenal androgens and/or mineralocorticoids.

Depression is common in Cushing's syndrome, and other behavioral disturbances may occur. In some cases the psychiatric features dominate over the physical features, leading to misdiagnosis. If the condition is successfully treated, either surgically or medically, the psychiatric manifestations usually subside.

Acute stress   When an acute stress (threat to homeostasis) is perceived by the brain, impulses to the hypothalamus stimulate the production of CRH and VP, which, through ACTH, stimulate the production of GCs. If the stimulus is prolonged, the axis usually adapts to it over several days, so that ACTH and GCs return to normal.

In rats, it has been shown that the response of GCs to stress in later life can be modified by neonatal handling, which appears to increase the efficiency of the stress response, and to protect the animal from potentially damaging effects of GCs.

Chronic stress   Should severe stress be continued for long periods, neurodegeneration or suppressed neurogenesis in the hippocampus occurs. Similar changes also occur after 3 weeks of treatment with a high dose of GCs.

Major depression   Increased levels of GCs in major depression (seen in 60–70%) are the best-documented biochemical abnormality in psychiatric disease. There is also a decrease in the diurnal variation and, in about 50%, a resistance to suppression of cortisol by dexamethasone. Major depression is twice as common in women as in men. Although CRH levels are increased, ACTH levels are not increased, so that there appears to be an alteration in adrenal responsiveness which is not understood. These changes are reversed on remission.

Conditions of Glucocorticoid Deficiency

Adrenal insufficiency (Addison's disease)   In adrenal insufficiency, first described by Addison in 1855, levels of GCs are low normal or low, and respond poorly or not at all to ACTH. Insufficiency may occur due to destruction of the adrenal cortex (primary), to deficient ACTH secretion (secondary), or to deficient hypothalamic secretion of ACTH secretagogues (tertiary).

Congenital adrenal hyperplasia (genetic defects in cortisol synthesis)   Inherited enzymatic defects of GCs synthesis may become manifest in fetal life, the most common being due to lack of the various enzymes involved. In order to maintain adequate GCs levels, ACTH levels are increased to overcome the block, and hypertrophy and hyperplasia of the adrenal cortex occur. Also, due to increased ACTH, synthetic steps which are not blocked produce increased quantities of their products, particularly of precursors of GCs and of adrenal androgens. While males are usually asymptomatic, the excess androgens usually cause ambiguous genitalia in female fetuses. When initially recognized, this syndrome of masculinization of female fetuses associated with enlarged adrenal glands was called the adrenogenital syndrome.

21-Hydroxylase deficiency is the most common defect accounting for 95% of all cases of congenital adrenal hyperplasia and is particularly prevalent among the Yupik Eskimos, where the incidence is 1 in 500 births and the heterozygote frequency is 1 in 11. Milder cases of 21-hydroxylase deficiency are masculinized while more severely affected infants have the salt-losing form, causing hyponatremia, hyperkalemia, acidosis, and dehydration, sometimes leading to vascular collapse. Very mild cases may not become manifest until puberty, when hirsutism becomes prominent. If suspected, this defect can be diagnosed prenatally and treated with small doses of dexamethasone, which crosses the placental barrier (unlike cortisol, which is converted to cortisone in the placenta).

Deficiency of the following enzymes may also occur but is rare: cholesterol desmolase, 3β-hydroxysteroid dehydrogenase/isomerase, 17-hydroxylase, and 11β-hydroxylase.

Measurement

Competitive Protein-Binding Assays

GCs are currently usually measured by competitive protein-binding (CPB, displacement analysis). In this type of assay, the steroid is measured according to its ability to displace a tracer form of itself from a protein which binds it with high affinity and specificity. Such proteins include endogenous plasma proteins (CBGs), endogenous GR proteins, enzymes, or most commonly, antibodies raised to GCs modified to make them antigenic. The sensitivity of such methods is very great (usually a few picograms) and depends on the affinity of the steroid for the protein (usually of the order of $10^9 \, M^{-1}$ or greater); thus for plasma only a few microliters of sample is required for the determination of cortisol or corticosterone concentrations. The specificity varies with the binding protein used, with the method of separating bound and free moieties, and with the steroid milieu in which the GCs are being measured. Since no protein is absolutely specific for any single ligand, each method must be carefully validated for the circumstances under which it is being used. The sample to be measured must be freed of any binding proteins that may interfere.

Assays Using Corticosteroid-Binding Globulin

Assays employing CBG were the first such assays to be used for GCs, and were introduced in 1963. Human CBG was the first to be used, but is less specific for cortisol than are dog or horse CBG. Each CBG has its own spectrum of specificity and can be chosen according to the milieu in which the GC is to be measured. These assays have the advantages that the binding properties of the CBG are essentially invariant, so that it is not necessary to determine the specificity or affinity of each batch of protein; also, no preparation beyond dilution is required.

Radioreceptorassays and Radioenzymaticassays

Receptor proteins can be used to measure their ligands, and enzymes can be used to measure their substrates in similar fashion, but are not usually used for GCs.

Radioimmunoassays

Immunoassays have the important advantage that a suitable protein can be raised to virtually any steroid, and since each antibody is slightly different, the most suitable one for the milieu in which the GC is to be measured can be chosen. A disadvantage is that each batch, even from the same animal, may vary with respect to affinity and specificity and must be characterized separately to ensure consistent results. Initially it was thought that the use of monoclonal antibodies might be advantageous but the sensitivity attained is usually less than with polyclonal antibodies.

Although radioactive isotopes have been the most common labels used (hence the term radioimmunoassay), other labels are now available (see below).

Fluorescence Immunoassays

Fluorescence immunoassays employ either a fluorophore label, or utilize enzyme-immunoassays in which substrates are converted to fluorescent endproducts.

Chemiluminescence Immunoassays

Chemiluminescence immunoassays use luminescent compounds which emit light during the course of a chemical reaction, usually enzymatic. Such assays have achieved the highest levels of sensitivity to date.

Determinations in Various Body Fluids

Plasma It is important to suit the method to the purpose. For example, a method which may be adequate for the measurement of cortisol in adult human blood may be, and usually is, entirely unsuitable for its measurement in neonatal or cord blood, which contain many steroids in high concentrations (e.g., progesterone and 17-hydroxyprogesterone) that are not present or are present in only minimal amounts in nonpregnant adult blood.

Urine Similarly, such a method is rarely, if ever, adequate to measure cortisol in urine, where there are very large amounts of competing steroids, so that extra steps such as extraction and chromatography must be performed first. Although the true mean value in human urine was established in 1980 to be about 60 nmol day^{-1}, published values continue to exceed these by a factor of 2–10 throughout the literature, so must be carefully scrutinized.

Saliva In saliva, which is convenient for the taking of samples, and more closely approximates free GCs, it must be taken into consideration that the level of cortisone (at least in humans) may exceed that of cortisol, so may interfere even with an antibody that ostensibly binds cortisone poorly. While saliva does not contain CBG, the salivary glands do contain 11β-hydroxysteroid hydroxylase type 2, which converts about half the cortisol reaching them to cortisone, so that salivary cortisol levels are about 50% of those of unbound plasma cortisol.

Indirect Methods

Prior to the development of CPB assays, GCs were measured by indirect methods. All of these are much less specific and less sensitive than CPB methods. They include fluorescence methods (steroids with an 11-hydroxyl group fluoresce under ultraviolet light in alkali or acid), the measurement of 17-hydroxycorticoids (Porter-Silber chromogens) as an approximation of GCs, the use of tetrazolium salts to measure compounds containing an α-ketol group, 17-ketogenic steroids minus 17-ketosteroids as an approximation of GCs, ultraviolet absorption after chromatography, and double isotope dilution derivative assay.

Antiglucocorticoids

Inhibitors of steroidogenesis

A selection of inhibitors of steroidogenesis is given in **Figure 6**.

Metyrapone mainly inhibits $P450_{C11}$, preventing 11-desoxycortisol from being hydroxylated at C11 to give cortisol, and 11-desoxycorticosterone from being converted to corticosterone, thereby lowering cortisol, corticosterone, and aldosterone and resulting in excessive amounts of the precursors due to stimulation of ACTH secretion.

Mitotane, which is related to the insecticide DDT (4,4′-(2,2,2-trichloroethane-1,1-diyl)bis(chlorobenzene)), is toxic to adrenal tissue, causing necrosis and hemorrhage. It also affects peripheral metabolism of cortisol, greatly increasing its conversion to 6β-hydroxycortisol

Aminoglutethimide affects GC synthesis in several ways: it inhibits $P450_{scc}$, thus decreasing the conversion of cholesterol to pregnenolone and the production of all the adrenal steroids. Although it may be useful in decreasing hypercortisolism, the blockade

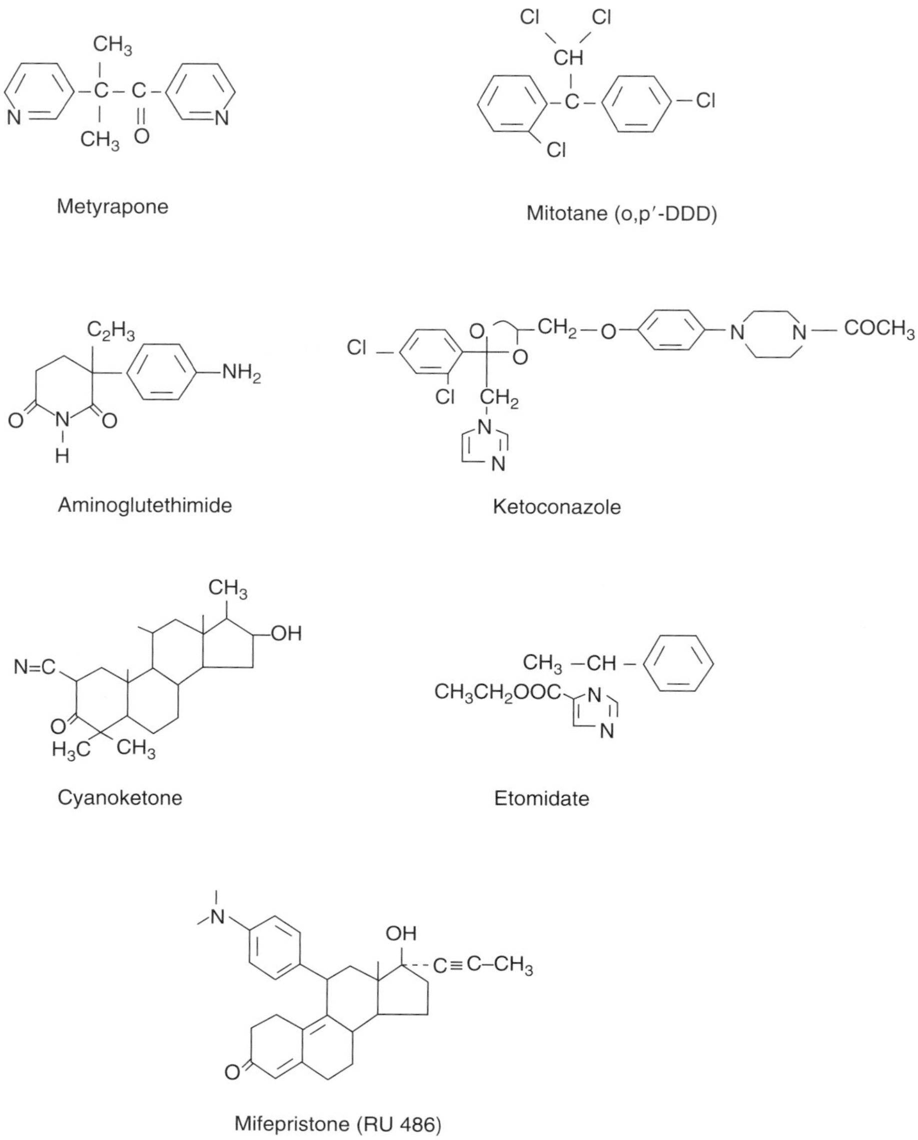

Metyrapone

Mitotane (o,p'-DDD)

Aminoglutethimide

Ketoconazole

Cyanoketone

Etomidate

Mifepristone (RU 486)

Figure 6 Structures of selected antiglucocorticoids.

is often overridden by increased secretion of ACTH in response to the lowered cortisol levels.

Cyanoketone inhibits 3β-hydroxysteroid dehydrogenase but it is not currently used clinically.

Ketoconazole is an antifungal agent which inhibits $P450_{scc}$ and $P450_{C11}$.

Etomidate is an anesthetic agent and its main effect is on $P450_{C11}$, although it also affects $P450_{scc}$.

Inhibitor of Glucocorticoid Receptor

Mifepristone (RU 486) inhibits GCs production by binding to the GR, and has been used successfully in some cases of Cushing's syndrome. As with agents that directly interfere with synthesis, the blockade

caused by this receptor inhibitor tends to be overcome by increased production of CRH and ACTH.

Uses of Glucocorticoids and their Inhibitors as Therapeutic Agents

Therapeutic Uses of Glucocorticoids

The first therapeutic use of GCs was that of cortisone by PS Hench and his coworkers in 1949 to treat rheumatoid arthritis. Since then, a great many disorders have been treated using a variety of GCs, including allergic diseases such as asthma and dermatitis, autoimmune diseases such as systemic lupus erythematosis and Graves' ophthalmopathy, and inflammatory disorders such as ulcerative colitis. They have also been used to decrease cerebral edema associated with intracerebral masses, to treat septic shock, and to suppress graft rejection after transplantation of organs.

When GCs are given therapeutically, a feeling of euphoria is commonly experienced, although prolonged use often results in depression, and less often mania, especially if higher doses are used. There is no typical presentation as a variety of mental symptoms is observed, including often irritability, insomnia, obsessive–compulsive behavior, and anxiety. Altered perception, sensory flooding, delusions and hallucinations, delirium, and even frank dementia may occur in about 5% of cases. The time required for mental symptoms to occur on treatment varies from almost immediate to several months, with a median onset of 11 days. These effects are usually largely reversible after reduction of dose or discontinuation of the steroid.

Cortisone itself is inactive but it is rapidly converted to cortisol in the liver. Although the natural GCs are very effective for many purposes, if given in large amounts they have many undesirable side effects, including bloating, hypertension, peptic ulcer, trunkal obesity, osteoporosis, and depression or mania.

Since GCs have so many different biological actions, much effort has been made to develop synthetic GCs that have a particular spectrum of effects deemed desirable but lack other effects deemed undesirable (**Table 1**). Examples are steroids which have strong anti-inflammatory effects but lack the mineralocorticoid effects. The modification of a double bond at C1–2 as in prednisolone (or its cortisone-like 11-keto analog prednisone) increases the GC activity while reducing the mineralocorticoid activity. Addition of a fluorine atom at C9 increases both GC (about 12-fold) and mineralocorticoid (about 25-fold) activity. Including both these modifications and adding a 16α-methyl group gives dexamethasone which has about 30-fold greater GC activity but relatively little mineralocorticoid activity. Since the steroids themselves are relatively insoluble in water, they are often formulated as organic esters such as acetates, which are somewhat more soluble, or as salts such as sodium succinates which are freely soluble.

Although extremely useful, GCs must be used with considerable caution, and preferably for only limited periods, because of their important side effects that can occur with all forms, and include bloating, osteoporosis, trunkal obesity, and other signs and symptoms of GC excess.

One of the most dangerous effects of large doses of GCs, whether natural or synthetic, is suppression of the LHPA axis. This can occur after only a few weeks of high-dose GC therapy and may require several months for recovery to occur. For this reason, therapy is never stopped abruptly but only very slowly so that the organism has time to adjust.

Uses of Antiglucocorticoids as Therapeutic Agents

Inhibitors of steroidogenesis are used to treat conditions of GC excess, including the various forms of Cushing's syndrome, and more recently, major depression. These agents may be effective for short periods, but their effects are often overcome after a few weeks or months by the normal feedback mechanism. In depressed patients, this may be long enough to induce a remission, in which case the levels remain normal after stopping the medication.

See Also the Following Articles

11β-Hydroxysteroid Dehydrogenases; Corticosteroid Receptors; Corticosteroid-Binding Globulin (Transcortin); Corticosteroids and Stress; Corticotropin Releasing Factor (CRF); Cushing's Syndrome, Medical Aspects; Cushing's Syndrome, Neuropsychiatric Aspects; Dexamethasone Suppression Test (DST); Glucocorticoid Negative Feedback; Glucocorticoids, Effects of Stress on; Glucocorticoids – Adverse Effects on the Nervous System; Hippocampus, Overview; Hypothalamic-Pituitary-Adrenal; Steroid Hydroxylases.

Further Reading

DeKloet, R. E., Vreugdenhil, E., Oitzl, M. S., et al. (1998). Brain corticosteroid receptor balance in health and disease. *Endocrine Reviews* 19, 269–301.

Dixon, P. F., Booth, M. and Butler, J. (1967). The corticosteroids. In: Gray, C. H. & Bacharach, A. L. (eds.) *Hormones in blood*, 2nd ed., vol. 2, London: Academic Press.

Ehrhart-Bornstein, M., Hinson, J. P., Bornstein, S. R., et al. (1998). Intraadrenal interactions in the regulation of adrenocortical steroidogenesis. *Endocrine Reviews* 19, 101–143.

Falkenstein, E., Tillmann, H.-C., Christ, M., et al. (2000). Multiple actions of steroid hormones – a focus on rapid nongenomic effects. *Pharmacological Reviews* 52, 513–555.

Fieser, L. F. and Fieser, M. (1959). *Steroids*. New York: Reinhold Publishing Corporation.

Meaney, M. J., Mitchell, J. B., Aitken, D. H., et al. (1991). The effects of neonatal handling on the development of the adrenocortical response to stress: implications for neuropathology and cognitive deficits in later life. *Psychoneuroendocrinology* 16, 85–103.

Murphy, B. E. P. (1967). Some studies of the protein-binding of steroids and their application to the routine micro and ultramicro measurement of various steroids in body fluids by competitive protein-binding radioassay. *Journal of Clinical Endocrinology and Metabolism* **27**, 973–990.

Murphy, B. E. P. and Branchaud, C. L. (1994). The fetal adrenal. In: Tulchinsky, D. & Little, B. (eds.) *Maternal-fetal endocrinology*, 2nd edn., pp. 275–295. Philadelphia: W. B. Saunders.

Murphy, B. E. P., Ghadirian, A. M. and Dhar, V. (1998). Neuroendocrine responses to inhibitors of steroid biosynthesis in patients with major depression resistant to antidepressant therapy. *Canadian Journal of Psychiatry* **43**, 279–286.

Sandor, T. and Mehdi, A. Z. (1979). Steroids and evolution. In: Barrington, E. J. W. (ed.) *Hormones and evolution*, vol. 1, pp. 1–72. New York: Academic Press.

Stewart, P. M. (2003). The adrenal cortex. In: Larsen, P. R., Kronenberg, H. M., Melmed, S., et al. (eds.) *Williams textbook of endocrinology* (10th edn., pp. 491–551). New York: W. B. Saunders.

Westphal, U. (1986). *Steroid-protein interactions II*. New York: Springer-Verlag.

Wild, D. (ed.) (2001). *The immunoassay handbook*, 2nd edn.). New York: Nature Publishing Group.

Wolkowitz, O. M. and Reus, V. I. (1999). Treatment of depression with antiglucocorticoid drugs. *Psychosomatic Medicine* **61**, 698–711.

Glucocorticoids, Role in Stress

J C Buckingham
Imperial College School of Medicine, London, UK

This article is reproduced from the previous edition, volume 2, pp 261–269, © 2000, Elsevier Inc.

Secretion in Stress, Delivery to Target Tissues, and Molecular Basis of Action

Functions of Glucocorticoids in Stress

Glossary

Cell-mediated immunity	The process by which thymus-derived lymphocytes (T cells) respond to specific antigens, undergo clonal expansion, and mount a cytotoxic response.
Humoral immunity	The process by which specific antigens activate bone marrow-derived lymphocytes (B cells), causing cell proliferation and the production and release of specific antibodies; also called antibody-mediated immunity.

Glucocorticoids are steroid hormones produced by the adrenal cortex. Their principal role is to restore homeostasis in conditions of stress. However, prolonged elevations in circulating corticosteroids, which may occur in conditions of chronic or repeated stress, are potentially harmful and may contribute to the pathogenesis of a wide range of disorders.

Secretion in Stress, Delivery to Target Tissues, and Molecular Basis of Action

Secretion of Glucocorticoids in Stress

The glucocorticoids (GCs), cortisol and/or corticosterone, depending on the species, are produced by cells in the zona fasciculata of the adrenal cortex. In normal circumstances, serum GC concentrations are maintained within narrow limits with pronounced excursions occurring only in accord with the well-documented circadian rhythm or in response to physical or emotional stress. Circadian and stress-induced increases in GC secretion are driven by neural and humoral factors that impinge on the hypothalamus to cause the release into the hypothalamo-hypophysial portal vessels of two neuropeptides, corticotropin releasing hormone (CRH) and arginine vasopressin (AVP); these peptides in turn act synergistically on the anterior pituitary gland to initiate the release of adrenocorticotropic hormone (ACTH), the primary trigger of steroidogenesis. The secretion of cortisol/corticosterone is regulated further by a complex servo mechanism through which the steroids themselves negatively regulate the release of ACTH and its hypothalamic-releasing hormones. The hypothalamic-pituitary-adrenocortical (HPA) responses to repeated or sustained stress are complex and depend on both the nature of the stress and the species. For example, in rats the adrenocortical response to cold stress is attenuated progressively with each exposure; that is, the axis becomes tolerant to the stimulus. In contrast, the HPA responses to repeated immune insults are well maintained and may become exaggerated, possibly because the feedback actions of the steroids are overcome.

Delivery of Glucocorticoids to Their Target Cells and Receptors

GCs in the systemic circulation are largely protein-bound (95%), mainly to a specific globulin, termed corticosteroid-binding globulin (CBG, or transcortin). but also to albumin. In principle, only the free steroid has ready access to the corticosteroid receptors, which are located intracellularly in the target cells. However, local mechanisms that release the steroid from its carrier protein(s) appear to exist in at least some target tissues: these include (1) interactions of the carrier protein with cell-surface CBG receptors and (2) enzymatic cleavage of CBG (e.g., by serine proteases in inflamed tissues), a process that lowers the affinity of the binding protein for the steroids. Access of the steroids to their receptors is regulated further within the target cells by 11β-hydroxysteroid dehydrogenase (11β-HSD) enzymes that control the interconversion of cortisol/corticosterone to their inactive counterparts, cortisone/11-dehydrocorticosterone.

Molecular Basis of Glucocorticoid Action

The actions of the GCs are exerted mainly via the classic pathway of steroid action – the free steroid enters the target cells and binds to an intracellular receptor that is subsequently translocated to the nucleus, where it initiates specific changes in DNA transcription and, hence, in protein synthesis. In many instances, the activated steroid–receptor complex induces or represses transcription by binding directly to specific response elements in the promoter region of the gene; in others, however, it may interfere with the activity of other transcription factors, such as activator protein (AP)-1 and nuclear transcription factor (NF)κB. In addition, the activated receptor may regulate posttranscriptional events, including mRNA transcript stability, RNA translation, and posttranslational processing of the protein.

In accord with the intracellular mode of action, the majority of biological responses to GCs are slow to emerge; some, however, are manifested more rapidly; for example, cortisol hyperpolarizes hippocampal neurons and coeliac ganglia within 1–2 min of contact. The mechanisms underlying these rapid action are unknown, but increasing evidence favors a membrane action of the steroids, possibly via a cell surface receptor.

Corticosteroid Receptors

Two distinct subtypes of intracellular corticosteroid receptors have been identified: the mineralocorticoid receptor (MR) and the glucocorticoid receptor (GR). The MR has a high and approximately equal affinity for aldosterone and the endogeneous GCs, corticosterone and cortisol ($K_d \sim 1$–2 nM). In contrast, the GR is of a lower affinity (K_d cortisol/corticosterone 10–20 nM), is glucocorticoid-selective, and does not bind aldosterone readily; a truncated form of this receptor, termed GR-β, which does not bind ligand but which has the capacity to bind DNA, also exists. MRs in the kidney are protected effectively from cortisol/corticosterone by type 2 11β-HSD (11β-HSD2), which acts primarily as a dehydrogenase and inactivates the steroids rapidly, thus permitting selective access of aldosterone to the receptors. MRs in the brain, however, are not always protected from GCs in this way and in many instances may be almost fully occupied at low physiological concentrations of cortisol/corticosterone. However, the delivery of GCs to GRs in organs such as the liver and white adipose tissues may be facilitated by type 1 11β-HSD (11β-HSD1), which acts primarily as a reductase and thereby regenerates the active steroids from their inactive 11-dehydro metabolites. Although the MR undoubtedly mediates several facets of glucocorticoid activity in nonstress conditions, particularly in the central nervous system (CNS), the responses to the raised levels of the steroids observed in, for example, stress are effected primarily via GRs. These receptors are widely distributed in the body; cell responsiveness depends not only on the presence of GRs, but also the receptor concentration, which is known to fluctuate during development, the cell cycle, following disturbances in endocrine status, and on the activation of 11β-HSD1 enzymes.

Functions of Glucocorticoids in Stress

General Considerations

The concept that corticosteroids play a key role in the body's responses to stress emerged from the work of Selye on the alarm reaction and the general adaptation syndrome. It is now evident that cortisol/corticosterone displays two modes of activity. The first is a permissive or proactive role in which the steroids (1) maintain the basal activity of the HPA axis and set its threshold for responding to stress and (2) normalize the body's response to stress by priming the body's defense mechanisms by, for example, facilitating the effects of catecholamines on lipid and carbohydrate metabolism; upregulating the expression of receptors for inflammatory mediators; and acting centrally to aid processes underlying selection attention, the integration of sensory information, and response selection. The second mode of cortisol/corticosterone action is suppressive or protective and enables the organism to cope with, adapt to, and recover from a stressful insult. Key to this mode are the powerful anti-inflammatory and immunosuppressive actions of the steroids that prevent the host defense mechanisms, which are activated by stress, from overshooting and damaging the organism. Other important protective actions include the ability of the steroids to redirect the metabolism to meet energy demands during stress, to exert important effects within the brain that promote memory processes, and to impair nonessential functions such as growth and reproductive function. The permissive actions of the steroids are evident at low physiological concentrations and are mediated at least partially, although probably not exclusively, by the high-affinity MRs. In contrast, the suppressive actions of the steroids emerge only when cortisol/corticosterone levels are raised by, for example, stress and are effected by the lower-affinity GRs.

The permissive and protective actions of GCs are complementary and enable the organism to mount an appropriate stress response and to maintain homeostasis. Dysregulation of either by genetic or environmental factors is potentially harmful and may predispose the individual to a variety of diseases that, depending on the site of the lesion, may include depression, disorders of the host defense system, osteoporosis, obesity, diabetes mellitus, hypertension, and other cardiovascular diseases. Long-term elevations in GC production that may occur in conditions of chronic stress are particularly hazardous and may have severe deleterious effects on the body. The effects of acute and sustained elevations in serum GCs are compared in **Table 1**.

Glucocorticoids and the Host Defense System

GCs exert multiple effects on the host defense system. In essence, they quench the early and late stages of the inflammatory response; that is, they suppress the initial vasodilation, the infiltration of leukocytes and pain, and the subsequent proliferative events associated with wound healing and tissue repair. They also oppose the changes in vascular permeability that occur in inflammation and thus reduce both edema formation and the increased permeability of the blood–brain barrier. In addition, GCs are powerful inhibitors of cell-mediated (i.e., T-cell-dependent) immune responses and may also modulate humoral (B-cell-dependent) responses. Chronic elevations in serum GCs thus induce immunosuppression and render the individual susceptible to infection.

The anti-inflammatory and immunosuppressive actions of the steroids are attributed to their powerful actions on the growth, differentiation, distribution,

Table 1 Response to acute and long-term elevations in serum glucocorticoids

System	Acute[a]	Long-term
Host defense	Protection from potentially harmful inflammatory mediators	Immunosuppression and vulnerability to infection Poor tissue repair/wound healing
Metabolism	Mobilization of energy stores ($\uparrow$ glycogen stores, $\uparrow$ gluconeogenesis, $\uparrow$ blood glucose, $\uparrow$ lipolysis, $\uparrow$ protein catabolism, $\downarrow$ peripheral glucose uptake/utilization)	Insulin-resistant steroid diabetes mellitus Centripetal obesity Protein depletion in muscle, connective, and other tissues Raised serum lipids and cholesterol
Musculoskeletal	Protein catabolism Altered Ca^{2+} homeostatsis	Impaired growth Muscle wasting Loss of connective tissue Osteoporosis and disturbed Ca^{2+} homeostasis
Central nervous system	Improved cognitive function	Mood changes (depression and psychotic episodes) Neurodegeneration
Cardiovascular	Salt and water retention Inhibition of the production of vasoactive inflammatory mediators	Hypertension and other cardiovascular disease
Reproductive	Inhibition of hypothalamic-pituitary-gonadal function	Menstrual irregularities Infertility (male and female)
Gastrointestinal tract	Reduced bicarbonate and mucus production	Increased susceptibility to ulcers

[a]$\uparrow$, increased; $\downarrow$, decreased.

function, and life span of monocytes, macrophages, polymorphonuclear cells, and lymphocytes. At the cellular level, GCs reduce the number of circulating lymphocytes, monocytes, and eosinophils by causing the cells to be marginated to the lymphoid tissues, mainly the bone marrow. In contrast, blood neutrophil levels rise as the steroids prevent the cells migrating to inflamed tissues by altering the expression of adhesion proteins on their surface and on the endothelium and thereby impairing the adherence and attachment processes. The profile of circulating white cells is also influenced by the fact that GCs also induce the apoptosis (programmed cell death) of thymocytes, mature T cells, and eosinophils, although not of neutrophils.

Several processes contribute to the suppression of cell-mediated immunity invoked by the steroids. These include (1) direction of the development of undifferentiated T helper (Th) cells away from the Th1 phenotype, which is critical to cell-mediated responses, and toward the Th2 phenotype, which facilitates B-lymphocyte-dependent responses; (2) inhibition of the synthesis of interleukin (IL)-1 and IL-2 by antigen-presenting cells and T cells, respectively, and hence the impairment of antigen presentation and T-cell proliferation; and (3) induction of T-cell apoptosis. Very high levels of GCs may also depress the synthesis of the immunokines required for immunoglobulin production and, with time, decrease serum immunoglobulins. However, lesser amounts of the steroids stimulate antibody production, probably because of their positive effect on the differentiation of Th2 cells. Other immune cell functions influenced by GCs include phagocytosis and antigen processing. GCs decrease Fc receptor expression on macrophages and thus prevent the recognition of particulate antigens that are antibody-bound or optimized for subsequent clearance. They also affect mast cell and basophil function in a number of rodent models, inhibiting IgE-dependent degranulation and hence the release of histamine and leukotriene C4.

The diverse effects of GCs on immune/inflammatory cell function are explained at a biochemical level by the striking ability of the steroids to inhibit the synthesis, release, and/or activity of the army of mediators normally produced when these cells are activated. Early studies focused on the powerful inhibitory action of the steroids on the phospholipase A2 (PLA2)-dependent generation of the pro-inflammatory eicosanoids (prostanoids, leukotrienes, and epoxides) and platelet-activating factor (PAF). Several lines of evidence indicate that GCs reduce the expression of the PLA2 subtype (group II) associated with the pathogenesis of inflammation and upregulate the synthesis of PLA2 inhibitory proteins, notably lipocortin 1 (also called annexin 1), which also influences other aspects of the inflammatory response. However, studies have shown that GCs also suppress prostanoid generation by repressing the expression of the inducible isoform of cyclooxygenase (COX II), which is normally expressed in abundance by activated monocytes, macrophages, fibroblasts, and endothelial cells.

GCs also exert profound inhibitory effects on the synthesis of many of the cytokines that are central to the manifestation of immune/inflammatory responses; these include IL-1, IL-2, IL-3, IL-6, IL-8, IL-12, granulocyte colony-stimulating factor (G-CSF), granulocyte–macrophage colony-stimulating factor (GM-CSF), interferon (IFN)-γ, tumor necrosis factor (TNF)-α, and monocyte chemotactic protein. Various mechanisms may contribute to these responses, including the downregulation of gene transcription and acceleration of mRNA degradation, together with effects at the translational and posttranslational levels. The biological actions of the cytokines may also be impaired; this may be explained in part by alterations in receptor expression and, for example, by the IL-2 receptor being downregulated by GCs. However, in many cases (e.g., IL-1, IL-6, and IFN-γ), the repression of cytokine expression is associated with the upregulation of the respective cytokine receptors (**Figure 1**); this phenomenon may help explain the permissive role of the steroids in priming the immune system for action as well as the ineffective responses mounted when GC levels are raised (e.g., by stress) or when adrenal function is impaired.

The release of many other inflammatory mediators may also be prevented by virtue of the powerful regulatory actions of the GCs on the enzymes responsible for their biosynthesis/degradation. For example, GCs suppress the inducible form of nitric oxide (NO) synthase and hence the generation of NO by macrophages. However, they promote the metabolism of nonlipid inflammatory mediators (e.g., bradykinin) by upregulating the enzymes responsible for their metabolism. Further important actions of the GCs include reductions in the serum complement components, in the release of mediators such as 5-hydroxytryptamine (5-HT), and in the production/activity of the proteolytic enzymes (e.g., elastase and collagenase) that are concerned with the late stages of inflammation.

Metabolic Actions of Glucocorticoids

GCs exert complex effects on carbohydrate, lipid, and protein metabolism; their principal actions are catabolic, and they thus mobilize energy stores and oppose the actions of insulin (**Figure 2**).

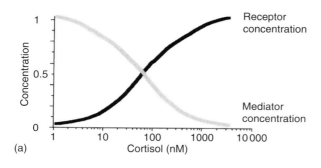

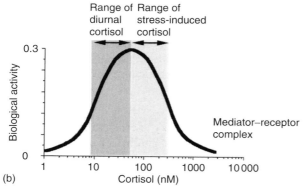

Figure 1 Mathematical model for the permissive and suppressive effects of glucocorticoids over a physiological concentration range. (a), Dose–response curves for a theoretical mediator and its specific receptors; (b), mathematical composite of mediator–receptor complex formation indicating biological activity and suggesting a mechanism by which low cortisol levels could be permissive and stress-induced cortisol surges suppressive in effect. From Munck, A. and Náraj-Fejes-Tóth, A. (1992), The ups and downs of glucocorticoid physiology: permissive and suppressive effects revisited, *Molecular and Cellular Endocrinology* **90**, C1–C4, copyright John Wiley & Sons Limited. Reproduced with permission.

Carbohydrate metabolism

The principal target is the liver, where GCs increase glycogen storage and gluconeogenesis. The effects of the steroids on glycogen storage reflect an increase in glycogen deposition due to the activation (dephosphorylation) of glycogen synthase and a concomitant decrease in glycogen breakdown due to inactivation of the glycogen-mobilizing enzyme glycogen phosphorylase. The increase in glucose synthesis is explained partly by the upregulation of key enzymes in the gluconeogenic pathway, such as phosphoenolpyruvate carboxykinase (PEPCK). In addition, the catabolic effects of the steroids on protein metabolism in peripheral tissues (e.g., muscle) and lipolysis in adipose tissue increase the availability of substrates (glucogenic amino acids and glycerol), while the fatty acids released with glycerol provide an important energy source for the process. The actions of GCs in the

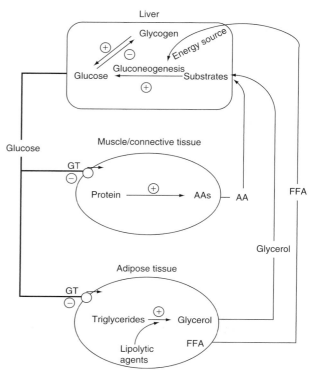

Figure 2 Schematic diagram illustrating the effects of glucocorticoids on carbohydrate, protein, and lipid metabolism. Note that the positive effects of the steroids on lipolysis involve interactions with other lipolytic agents (e.g., growth hormone and catecholamines). ⊕, stimulation; ⊖, inhibition; AA, amino acid; FFA, free fatty acid; GT, glucose transporter.

liver are effected by GR, and the delivery of the steroids to the receptors is facilitated by an abundance of 11β-HSD1, which serves mainly as a reductase.

Although much of the glucose formed in the liver in response to GCs is stored locally as glycogen, some is released into the circulation. Blood sugar levels are enhanced further by the actions of GCs in the peripheral tissues, which lead to the downregulation of the glucose transporters and, hence, to decreased glucose uptake and use.

Lipid metabolism GCs exert a permissive influence on lipid metabolism, producing an acute lipolytic action that appears to reflect an increased responsiveness to catecholamines, growth hormone (GH), and possibly other lipid-mobilizing agents. In the long term, however, GCs produce a striking redistribution of fat, with enhanced deposition in the trunk (centripetal obesity), dorsocervical and subcapsular regions (buffalo hump), and face (moon face), together with a loss of fat in the upper and lower limbs, giving rise to the 'lemon-on-sticks' appearance that is exacerbated by the changes in protein metabolism. Blood lipid and cholesterol levels are also raised. The underlying mechanisms are poorly defined; they may involve alterations in insulin secretion triggered by the changes in glucose homeostasis, and it is interesting to note that white adipose tissue is rich in GRs and 11 β-HSD1. Paradoxically, this pattern of fat redistribution is not seen in experimental animals.

Protein metabolism GCs have a powerfully catabolic effect on protein in muscle and other tissues with the consequent release of amino acids into the circulation, which are converted to glucose in the liver. Long-term elevations in serum GCs may cause severe muscle wasting.

Skeleton and Connective Tissue

Skeleton GCs exert direct and indirect effects on bone, and persistent elevations of serum GCs may lead to osteoporosis. The steroids decrease bone formation by inhibiting (1) the proliferation and differentiation of osteoclasts and (2) the production of type 1 collagen, osteocalcin, and other matrix components such as mucopolysaccharides and sulfate glucoaminoglycans while increasing the expression of collagen. In addition, they exert complex effects on the expression of growth factors and their receptors and reduce Ca^{2+} stores by decreasing intestinal Ca^{2+} absorption, increasing renal Ca^{2+} excretion, and raising serum parathyroid hormone (PTH) levels. GCs also promote bone resorption through mechanisms that are secondary to the rise in PTH and possibly also via direct actions on the bone.

Sustained elevations in serum GCs inhibit linear growth in children and experimental animals. The mechanisms responsible have yet to be defined but are likely to reflect the actions of the steroids on the bone, principally at the site of the epiphyses. Although there are reports to the contrary, the majority of data suggests that the serum levels of GH, insulin-like growth factor (IGF)-1, and IGF-binding proteins are normal in these subjects.

Connective tissue The actions of GCs on connective tissue lead to poor wound healing and tissue repair. The steroids decrease fibroblast proliferation and function; inhibit the production of the matrix proteins, collagen, and hyaluronidate; and augment the production of the matrix-degrading enzymes collagenase, elastase, and hyalurinidase. However, GCs augment the production of fibinonectin, a matrix glycoprotein.

Cardiovascular

Elevations in serum GCs raise blood pressure This may be at least partially explained by mineralocorticoid-like actions of the steroids, which cause increased salt and water retention, and by the anti-inflammatory actions of the steroids, which prevent the release of local vasodilator substances such as prostacyclin and bradykinin. However, other mechanisms also come into play. These include (1) the upregulation of vascular α_1-adrenoceptors and consequent increased sensitivity of the vessels to the vasoconstrictor actions of norepinephrine; (2) increased cardiac output, possibly as a result of increased β1-adrenoceptor expression in the myocardium; and (3) increased production of angiotensinogen and increased sensitivity of the blood vessels to the vasoconstrictor actions of angiotensin II. The endothelium is rich in GRs, and it is conceivable that the steroids also modulate the release/activity of other locally produced vasoactive substances. In addition, reports that GRs are abundant in the brain-stem nuclei raise the possibility that GCs may also act centrally to alter sympathetic outflow.

Mood and Behavior

GCs released in stress may exert significant effects on cognitive function, mood and behavior, and reception of sensory inputs. Subjects whose serum GCs are raised due to either Cushing's disease or exogenous steroids also show marked disturbances in sleep, with a reduction in time spent in the rapid eye movement phase.

Studies on laboratory animals have shown that GCs act in the neocortex and limbic system (hippocampus, septum, and amygdala) to modify learning and memory processes in a context-dependent manner. Thus, an acute rise in GCs may facilitate learning and memory processes but also eliminate learned behavior that is no longer of relevance. The complex actions of the steroids involve both MRs and GRs, with MRs effecting the appraisal of information and response selection and GRs promoting the processes underlying the consolidation of acquired information. The long-term effects of GCs on learning and memory are less well researched and the data available are conflicting, although, when given with neurotoxic agents, learned behavior is impaired by the steroids.

GC levels are raised in some patients with depression, but it remains to be determined whether this is cause or effect; indeed, the effects of GCs on mood appear variable. Thus, approximately one-half of patients with iatrogenic or endogenous Cushing's disease show psychological disturbances; depression is the most common but some subjects show euphoric or manic behavior and, in some cases, overt psychoses. Patients with adrenal insufficiency also frequently experience mood changes; paradoxically, the most common is also depression.

Increasing evidence suggests that sustained elevations in serum GCs, such as those that occur due to chronic stress, may contribute to the processes of neurodegeneration. The toxic actions of the steroids, which have been studied most widely in the hippocampus, are associated with altered glutaminergic transmission, a long-term enhancement of Ca^{2+} influx, and depletion of ATP stores, with a consequent impairment of essential energy-requiring processes such as glucose uptake. The vulnerability of the neurons may be enhanced further by a reduction in neurotrophic capacity because the elevations in serum GCs induced by chronic stress or the administration of exogenous steroids inhibit the expression of brain-derived neurotrophic factor mRNA and also tyrosine kinase, which is required for growth factor action.

Reproductive Function

GCs act at multiple sites within the hypothalamic-pituitary-gonadal axis to impair reproductive function; hence, chronic elevations in serum GCs lead to infertility and menstrual irregularities. An important site of action of the steroids is the hypothalamus. In addition, the steroids exert significant effects at the pituitary level to depress gonadotropin-releasing hormone (GnRH)-driven gonadotropin release and may also exert further regulatory actions within the gonads.

Development

GCs exert both positive and negative effects on cell growth. In addition, they fulfill complex organizational effects pre- and postnatally and thus play a key role in developmental programming. Not surprisingly, the HPA axis is tightly regulated during perinatal life and, in rodents, the stress response is attenuated during a critical phase postnatally. At this time, the developing HPA axis shows a high degree of plasticity, and a growing body of evidence suggests that disturbances in the GC milieu may (1) trigger a plethora of pathologies (e.g., growth retardation or impairment of CNS development) and (2) precipitate abnormalities in GC secretion that persist into adult life and may increase the susceptibility of the individual to conditions as diverse as hypertension, insulin resistance, cognitive and other behavioral disorders, and allergic/inflammatory disease. Perinatal manipulations that alter the expression of GRs (but not MRs) in the brain are particularly hazardous in this regard because, by disrupting the negative feedback mechanisms, they alter the responsivity of the HPA axis to stress throughout the lifetime of the individual. For example, the exposure of neonatal rats to stimuli that raise serum GCs, such as

an immune insult (the injection of bacterial lipopolysaccharide) or the administration of exogenous GCs, results in the adult in the downregulation of GRs in the hippocampus and hypothalamus, decreased sensitivity of the HPA axis to the negative feedback actions of the GCs, and exaggerated HPA responses to stress. Similar long-term changes in GR expression occur in rats subjected to prolonged periods of maternal separation; the consequent impairment of the negative feedback system and changes in HPA function are associated with alterations in T-cell antibody responses and in the incidence of age-related neuropathies. In contrast, neonatal handling, which increases hippocampal GR expression by mechanisms involving serotonin, reduces the magnitude and duration of the stress response in the adult; maternal care may therefore help to program events that regulate responses to stress in the adult and thus reduce vulnerability to disease.

Other Actions

GCs inhibit the production of mucus and bicarbonate in the stomach and small intestine by virtue of their ability to block prostaglandin production; sustained elevations in GCs thus increase susceptibility to gastric and duodenal ulcer formation. The steroids also promote Na^+ absorption in the colon by mechanisms that involve MRs and GRs while acting via GRs to augment Na^+ excretion by stimulating the synthesis of atrial natriuretic peptide (ANP) and augmenting the actions of ANP on the kidney, thereby opposing the Na^+-retaining influence exerted via MRs in the distal renal tubule. In addition, GCs may enhance free-water clearance by depressing the synthesis of vasopressin.

See Also the Following Articles

Adrenal Cortex; Adrenocorticotropic Hormone (ACTH); Cytokines; Glucocorticoids, Effects of Stress on; Glucocorticoids – Adverse Effects on the Nervous System.

Further Reading

Barnes, P. J. (1998). Anti-inflamatory actions of glucocorticoids: molecular mechanisms. *Clinical Science* **94**, 557–572.

Brann, D. W. and Manesh, V. B. (1991). Role of corticosteroids in female reproduction. *FASEB Journal* **5**, 2691–2698.

Buckingham, J. C., Gillies, G. E. and Cowell, A.-M. (1997). *Stress, stress hormones and the immune system.* Chichester, UK: John Wiley.

de Kloet, E. R., Vreugdenhil, E., Oitzl, M. S., et al. (1998). Brain corticosteroid receptor balance in health and disease. *Endocrine Review* **19**, 269–301.

Lukert, B. P. and Raiz, L. G. (1994). Glucocorticoid-induced osteoporosis. *Rheumatic Disease Clinics of North America.*

Munck, A., Guyre, P. M. and Holbrook, N. J. (1984). Physiological functions of glucocorticoids and their relation to pharmacological actions. *Endocrine Review* **51**, 25–44.

Munck, A. and Náraj-Fejes-Tóth, A. (1992). The ups and downs of glucocorticoid physiology: permissive and suppressive effects revisited. *Molecular and Cellular Endocrinology* **90**, C1–C4.

Nestler, J. E. and McClanahan, M. A. (1992). Diabetes and adrenal disease. *Baillière's Clinical Endocrinology and Metabolism* **6**, 829–851.

Pilkis, S. J. and Granner, D. K. (1992). Molecular physiology of the regulation of hepatic gluconeogenesis and glycolysis. *Annual Review of Physiology* **54**, 885–909.

Robinson, I., Gabrielsson, B., Klaus, G., et al. (1995). Glucocorticoids and growth problems. *Acta Paediatrica* **84**, 81–85.

Selye, H. (1952). *The story of the adaptation syndrome.* Montreal: Acta.

Tilders, F. J. and Schmidt, E. D. (1998). Interleukin 1 induced plasticity of hypothalamic CRH neurons and long-term stress hyperresponsiveness. *Annals of the New York Academy of Sciences* **840**, 65–73.

Vinson, G. P. and Anderson, D. C. (1996). *Adrenal glands, vascular system and hypertension.* Bristol, UK: Society for Endocrinology.

Glucose Transport

A L McCall
University of Virginia Health System, Charlottesville, VA, USA

This article is a revision of the previous edition article by A L McCall, volume 2, pp 270–275, © 2000, Elsevier Inc.

Introduction
Glucose Transport
Overview of Glucose Transport Regulation
Stress Hormones and Glucose Transport
GLUT1 as a Stress-Related Protein
Metabolic Stress and Glucose Transport
Overall Effects of Transport Regulation
Signaling Cascades and Glucose Transport
Summary

Glossary

ATP/ADP	Ratio of adenosine triphosphate to adenosine diphosphate, an index of cellular energy stores.
Dinitrophenol	A mitochondrial inhibitor associated with increased glucose transport *in vitro.*
GLUT	Glucose transport proteins enumerated in the order of their cloning, e.g., GLUT1, GLUT2.
Mitogen-activated protein kinase	A family of enzymes activated by hormones, cytokines, stress, and growth factors that result in a cascade of kinase activity and thereby influence cellular signaling.

Introduction

Glucose transport supplies fuel needed for energy metabolism by all mammalian cells. The supply of glucose is particularly important for cells, such as the neurons of the brain, that have a high metabolic rate supported by an obligate consumption of glucose as fuel. Transport is regulated by a variety of factors, including those associated with stress. The transport proteins that accomplish glucose transport are modulated in their expression, cellular distribution, synthesis, and half-lives by stress-related factors. Such factors include stress hormones, metabolic stress such as cellular energy demand or reduced supply of fuel or oxygen, and stress-related kinase signaling. The net effect of such regulation may be to ensure appropriate distribution of glucose fuel during stress to tissues that most require this particular fuel.

Glucose Transport

Simple diffusion of glucose across cellular phospholipid barriers is limited by its modest hydrophobicity. To overcome this, transfer of glucose across cell membranes uses a process known as facilitated diffusion, which is a carrier protein-mediated process. Two types of facilitated diffusion exist: energy dependent and energy independent. A few cells, such as the gut and kidney epithelium, are directly energy dependent and use a sodium-glucose cotransport. For most cells, however, energy-independent facilitated diffusion predominates. Facilitated diffusion via carrier proteins transports glucose down a concentration gradient in a saturable manner and is the major mechanism for glucose entry into mammalian cells. Such transport is accomplished by different isoforms of a superfamily of hydrophobic, integral membrane proteins often referred to as GLUTs or glucose transporters (see **Figure 1**). The cloning of the first member of this family, GLUT1, has facilitated much of the physiological investigation of glucose transport and these proteins. The homology of these transporters has led to additional members of this family of proteins being

identified. Their characterization physiologically in relation to stress signaling is as yet incomplete. **Table 1** lists the members of the GLUT family (excluding HMIT) of proteins and partially characterizes them. In brief, the GLUT family of transporters of hexoses and polyols now has 13 members, including 12 hexose transporters and one myoinositol transporter (HMIT). There are three classes within the transporter family: class I includes GLUT1–4, class II includes GLUTs 6, 8, 10, and 12, and class III includes 5, 7, 9, 11, and HMIT.

Overview of Glucose Transport Regulation

Glucose transport is a highly regulated process that varies considerably from one cell type to another. Some cells, such as red blood cells and brain neurons, have obligate consumption of glucose. For other cells, a facultative use of glucose exists, permitting other metabolic fuels, such as fatty acids, to supply the bulk of local energy requirements. Much evidence suggests that the regulation of glucose transport is also isoform specific. Regulation of transport occurs in response to altered energy requirements of tissues, so it is not surprising that one form of cellular stress, energy lack, is a potent regulator of glucose transport and transporter expression by different tissues. Regulation of GLUT proteins may occur by variation of the amounts of synthesis or degradation of the GLUT protein or mRNA. An increased transcription of GLUT mRNA or other regulatory effects on GLUTs

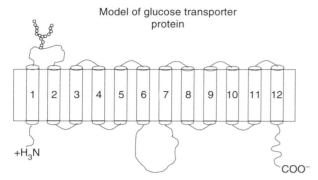

Model of glucose transporter protein

Figure 1 A model of glucose transporters. The diagram illustrates the putative 12 membrane-spanning domains of the glucose transporter's proposed structure, based on its cloning by Mueckler. This structure is reproduced for all class 1 GLUTs but is slightly different in placement of the carbohydrate moiety on the exofacial loop in other GLUT types. In this model of GLUT1, an N-linked asparagine residue on the exofacial (upper) surface of the cell membrane has an attached carbohydrate moiety that in certain isoforms may alter the efficiency of transport function. N- and C-termini of the proteins reside in intracellular sites.

Table 1 The GLUT family (SLC2), with each member (except the related SMIT myoinositol transporter) listed and given its class, and some characteristics of tissue distribution and other features.

Common name	Class	Tissue distribution	Features/Comments
GLUT1	I	Brain microvessels, glia, erythrocytes, placenta, kidney	Widely expressed, synthesis induced by cell culture, growth factors, oncogenes, heat shock, cell stress, development
GLUT2	I	Liver, kidney, pancreatic β cells, small intestine	Low-affinity (high K_m) transporter, role in insulin release
GLUT3	I	Neurons, placenta, fetal skeletal muscle, platelets, leukocytes	High affinity (low K_m), expressed in glucose-dependent cells, regulated by development, metabolic stress
GLUT4	I	Skeletal muscle, heart, brain regions, vessels	Insulin responsive, translocates from intra-cellular compartment to plasma membrance stress hormone modulation
GLUT5	II	Testes, small intestine,	High affinity (low K_m) for fructose
GLUT6	II	Brain, spleen, leukocytes	Function ill defined, formerly GLUT9
GLUT7	III	Unknown	Homologous to GLUT5,? fructose transporter
GLUT8	II	Testes, brain, adrenal, liver spleen, fat, lung, blastocyst	High affinity for glucose, hormone/stress modulation
GLUT9	III	Kidney, liver	Transport activity unclear, GLUT5 homology
GLUT10	II	Heart, lung, brain, liver	High 2DG affinity
GLUT11	III	Liver, brain, lung, muscle	Low glucose affinity, multiple splice variants
GLUT12	II	Heart, muscle, fat, prostate	Substrate specificity not known

may occur as a result of stress hormones, such as glucocorticoids and epinephrine. In some tissues, these hormones have differing effects on expression of GLUTs or their transport activity, emphasizing their tissue-specific regulation. The effects of growth factors, physiological factors often involved in stress responses, increase GLUT1 transcription.

Stress Hormones and Glucose Transport

Stress hormone responses influence glucose transport in a tissue-specific and isoform-specific manner. Among the important influences on glucose transport are the stress hormones, particularly adrenal glucocorticoids. Another common stress hormone response that regulates glucose transport is the secretion of catecholamines, epinephrine and norepinephrine, by the adrenal medulla and the sympathetic nervous system. Glucocorticoid stress responses or exposure to synthetic glucocorticoid drugs, such as dexamethasone, regulates the expression of several glucose transporter isoforms. In cultured adipocytes and in skeletal muscle, which are both insulin-sensitive tissues, glucocorticoids downregulate glucose transport by decreasing the plasma membrane concentration of glucose transporters, particularly GLUT4, the insulin-sensitive glucose transporter. This was shown by several groups. This cellular redistribution of GLUT4 is opposite to the effects of insulin.

Kinase signaling may be important for glucose transport adaptations in response to stress hormones. In 3T3-L1 adipocytes, downregulation of GLUT4 activity has been found. The alteration is not from decreased PI3 kinase signaling, as might be expected, nor is it from downstream regulation in this insulin-responsive pathway. Instead, a decrease in p38 mitogen-activated protein (MAP) kinase phosphorylation occurs. This is caused by upregulation of MAP kinase phosphatases.

In adipocytes, glucocorticoids may stimulate the synthesis of GLUT1, however, consistent with tissue and isoform specificity of regulation. GLUT1 is also overexpressed in the small blood vessels of the brain (which comprise the blood–brain barrier) after *in vivo* dexamethasone treatment. β-adrenergic drugs and the stress hormone catecholamines may also reduce insulin-sensitive glucose transport via action of GLUT4 in tissues such as muscle and fat, although precise mechanisms are incompletely defined.

In the gut, GLUT2 may be downregulated as a result of stress. A complex effect of stress (restraint stress and uncontrolled diabetes have been studied) is seen with GLUT8 in the hippocampus. Short-term stress had no effect alone but normalized the increased GLUT8 mRNA levels resulting from diabetes. The GLUT8 protein shows no change in total protein, but instead a redistribution induced by stress in GLUT8 protein to high-density microsomal fractions occurs. Intriguingly, both uncontrolled diabetes and restraint stress lower GLUT8 protein in high-density microsomes, and the two combined reduce levels to a greater degree than either alone. These examples of stress hormone-mediated effects on glucose transport suggest the importance of tissue, stress, and isoform specificity when understanding the effects of stress on glucose transport. The net effect of such regulation may redistribute glucose to tissues such as the brain that most need it as a fuel. Tissues, such as muscle, during stress may utilize other fuels, e.g., fatty acids. Some of these stress responses are thus thought to be adaptive, although given the biphasic nature of some, there may also be maladaptive or deleterious aspects, particularly of combined stresses.

GLUT1 as a Stress-Related Protein

GLUT1, the ubiquitously expressed glucose transporter, which is constitutively expressed at low levels by most, if not all, cells, is regulated by cellular stress. A variety of cell stressors, including glucose starvation, mercaptoethanol, calcium ionophores, tunicamycin, and heat shock, upregulated glucose transport and GLUT1 expression in L8 muscle cells and in 3T3L1 fibroblasts in an isoform-specific fashion. Another glucose transporter, GLUT4, failed to respond similarly. The GLUT1 stress responses were regulated in a manner very similar to that seen for another cell stress protein, glucose-regulated protein 78 (GRP78), in these studies. Subsequently, other studies confirmed the stress-related increase in GLUT1 expression in a variety of tissues and cell types. GLUT1 is thus the prototypical stress-responsive GLUT isoform. Nonetheless, many other GLUT isoforms are regulatable by factors associated with stress.

Metabolic Stress and Glucose Transport

Hypermetabolism

One aspect seen frequently with cellular stress or injury is a transient hypermetabolism. Perhaps this hypermetabolism is used to provide biochemical energy in the form of ATP or its high-energy phosphate bond equivalents for restoration of ionic cellular equilibrium and energy-dependent repair processes. The increased energy requirements after stress or injury might exert regulatory effects on glucose transport and transporters through an energy intermediate in the metabolic pathways of glucose. A potential linkage to altered metabolism and glucose transport is the fuel sensor enzyme AMP kinase, which accelerates catabolic pathways such as glycolysis and fatty acid oxidation to restore the ATP/AMP ratio that may be depleted. Increased glucose transport can be seen in some tissues as a result of AMP kinase activation.

Mitochondrial Inhibitors

Metabolic stress may regulate glucose transport and transporters *in vivo* and *in vitro*. Inhibitors of mitochondrial oxidative phosphorylation have long been known to increase glucose transport *in vitro*, although the precise metabolic pathways and mechanisms are complex and only partly elucidated. This phenomenon was first described in cultured fibroblasts. Mitochondrial inhibitors may similarly affect GLUT proteins. Hypoxia and mitochondrial inhibitors or uncouplers of oxidative phosphorylation (dinitrophenol, antimycin, and azide) act similarly to hypoxia and increase both GLUT1 mRNA and protein expression *in vitro*. Increasing evidence supports the idea that GLUT3 may also respond to these stimuli, albeit through different mechanisms than GLUT1 or GLUT4.

Fuel Deprivation: Oxygen, Glucose, Ischemia

In a like manner, glucose transport is upregulated by fuel deprivation *in vitro* and *in vivo*. This deprivation may occur due to glucose lack, hypoxic conditions, or ischemia. Glucose deprivation induced upregulation of glucose transport has been shown in fibroblasts, in muscle cells, and in many other cell types. Some forms of feedback probably occur by metabolic intermediates in the metabolism of glucose and/or by feedback directly from the energy state of the cell, although the specific metabolic compound is not clear. Perhaps ATP levels or ATP/ADP ratios may be involved in mediating this increased glucose transport. Indeed, a substantial body of evidence suggests that the regulation of glucose transport in many tissues is influenced by the availability of the transport substrate itself, i.e., glucose. Altered blood flow, reduced oxygen, or glucose availability may increase transport. Hypoxia and hypoglycemia can exert their effects on glucose transport (GLUT1) at least partly through action of vascular endothelial growth factor (VEGF). In some situations this occurs through extension of the half-life of the mRNA for VEGF. Hypoxia and ischemia may also induce hypoxia-inducible factor 1 alpha (HIF-1α), which in turn may be involved in

upregulation also through AMP kinase, the previously mentioned fuel sensor enzyme.

Overall Effects of Transport Regulation

The net effect of GLUT regulation in stress is to redistribute glucose fuel to tissues that have an obligate requirement for this energy substrate. Glucocorticoids may upregulate GLUT1 protein expression in tissues such as the brain, resulting in increased availability of fuel for that tissue. A complex aspect of that upregulation, however, is that endothelial cells may also have a relatively acute effect to decrease transport activity of glucose as well, leaving the net effect to vary depending upon the balance of transport-inhibiting effects that are probably not related to GLUT expression and enhancing effects that probably are related to GLUT expression. In contrast to effects in the brain of glucocorticoids, in insulin-dependent tissues, which employ GLUT4 as their primary glucose transporter, an intracellular sequestration of this transporter may prevent draining of glucose fuel by muscle during stress responses.

Although there is controversy about this point in some tissues, evidence suggests that local energy metabolism may be affected by such stress-mediated regulation of glucose transporters and glucose transport. For example, with *in vivo* hypoglycemia, an upregulation of brain endothelial transport of glucose occurs in animal studies and in some human studies. At blood glucose levels of about 3 mM (equal to 56 mg/dl), brain dysfunction normally begins to occur and presumably is related to a lack of adequate glucose entry into the brain to support the rather rigid requirement for glucose by brain metabolism. With an adaptation of glucose transport that occurs within several days of repeated hypoglycemia (in this case produced *in vivo* by overdoses of exogenous insulin), there is maintenance of glucose-6-phosphate and brain creatine phosphate and ATP levels. Presumably, the increased transport efficiency, which appears to involve both brain vascular (GLUT1) and neuronal glucose transporters (GLUT3), effectively operates to shuttle a greater amount of glucose across the brain endothelial and neuronal cellular barriers. This helps feed starving neurons. Interestingly, although such an adaptation would seem to be an unalloyed benefit, it has been suggested that a reduced awareness of hypoglycemia also occurs as a result. This reduced awareness may actually increase the risk of subsequent hypoglycemia in those with insulin-treated diabetes, which might risk brain injury from fuel deprivation. Glucose sensing in the brain may occur in discrete neurons, which may be important in hypoglycemia responses and in feeding.

Signaling Cascades and Glucose Transport

Stress in cells and whole organisms is associated with a wide variety of hormonal and biochemical changes that induce cellular responses via many mechanisms. One mechanism for signal transduction in stress occurs via certain types of MAP kinase pathways, particularly the p38 and jun-kinase subtypes. The p38 kinases, mammalian homologs of osmotic stress kinases found in yeast, may help regulate both basal- and stress-activated expression of glucose transporters, including GLUT1 and GLUT3, according to work performed in cultured muscle cells. The fuel sensor kinase, AMP kinase, is able to stimulate GLUT expression in some tissues as well.

Summary

It is clear that stress can either activate or suppress glucose transport in many tissues. GLUT1, the widely expressed isoform, appears to be a prototype of the stress-activated glucose transporter isoform, but GLUT3 and GLUT4 may also increase or decrease in response to certain kinds of cellular stress. New data suggest that GLUT2 and GLUT8 show stress-related regulation as well. Less is known about the regulation of other GLUT isoforms. Hormones associated with stress response may be important for increasing or, in some instances, decreasing cellular glucose transport. The preservation of an adequate supply of glucose fuel to tissues is believed to be adaptive, but occasionally the redirection of glucose to certain tissues may also have adverse consequences. Adaptations of glucose transport and GLUT transporters are responsive to many signaling pathways activated by stress, including hormones, kinase signaling, fuel or oxygen or energy lack, and probably other pathways as yet incompletely delineated. Stress-mediated changes in glucose transporter amount or function probably act to redistribute this fuel to tissues such as the brain that have an obligate demand for it.

Acknowledgments

A.L.M. acknowledges support for laboratory research reported in part in this article from the National Institutes of Health (NINDS; NS22213, NS17493, NIDDK; DK 58006) and the Juvenile Diabetes Foundation International.

Further Reading

Bazuine, M., Carlotti, F., Tafrechi, R. S., Hoeben, R. C. and Maassen, J. A. (2004). Mitogen-activated protein kinase (MAPK) phosphatase-1 and -4 attenuate p38 MAPK during dexamethasone-induced insulin resistance in 3T3-L1 adipocytes. *Molecular Endocrinology* **18**(7), 1697–1707.

Bazuine, M., Carlotti, F., Rabelink, M. J., Vellinga, J., Hoeben, R. C. and Maassen, J. A. (2005). The p38 mitogen-activated protein kinase inhibitor SB203580 reduces glucose turnover by the glucose transporter-4 of 3T3-L1 adipocytes in the insulin-stimulated state. *Endocrinology* **146**(4), 1818–1824.

Joost, H. G., Bell, G. I., Best, J. D., et al. (2002). Nomenclature of the GLUT/SLC2A family of sugar/polyol transport facilitators. *American Journal of Physiology Endocrinology and Metabolism* **282**(4), E974–E976.

Klip, A., Tsakiridis, T., Marette, A. and Ortiz, P. (1994). Regulation of expression of glucose transporters by glucose: a review of studies in vivo and in cell cultures. *FASEB Journal* **8**, 43–53.

Kumagai, A., Kang, Y., Boado, R. and Pardridge, W. (1995). Upregulation of blood-brain barrier GLUT1 glucose transporter protein and mRNA in experimental chronic hypoglycemia. *Diabetes* **44**, 1399–1404.

Lee, M., Hwang, J. T., Lee, H. J., et al. (2003). AMP-activated protein kinase activity is critical for hypoxia-inducible factor-1 transcriptional activity and its target gene expression under hypoxic conditions in DU145 cells. *Journal of Biological Chemistry* **278**(41), 39653–39661.

Levin, B. E., Routh, V. H., Kang, L., Sanders, N. M. and Dunn-Meynell, A. A. (2004). Neuronal glucosensing: what do we know after 50 years? *Diabetes* **53**(10), 2521–2528.

Nordal, R. A., Nagy, A., Pintilie, M. and Wong, C. S. (2004). Hypoxia and hypoxia-inducible factor-1 target genes in central nervous system radiation injury: a role for vascular endothelial growth factor. *Clinical Cancer Research* **10**(10), 3342–3353.

Piroli, G. G., Grillo, C. A., Charron, M. J., McEwen, B. S. and Reagan, L. P. (2004). Biphasic effects of stress upon GLUT8 glucose transporter expression and trafficking in the diabetic rat hippocampus. *Brain Research* **1006**(1), 28–35.

Shepherd, E. J., Helliwell, P. A., Mace, O. J., Morgan, E. L., Patel, N. and Kellett, G. L. (2004). Stress and glucocorticoid inhibit apical GLUT2-trafficking and intestinal glucose absorption in rat small intestine. *Journal of Physiology* **560**(Pt 1), 281–290.

Simpson, I., Chundu, K., Davies-Hill, T., Honer, W. and Davies, P. (1994). Decreased concentrations of GLUT1 and GLUT3 glucose transporters in the brains of patients with Alzheimer's disease. *Annals of Neurology* **35**, 546–561.

Stein, I., Neeman, M., Shweiki, D., Itin, A. and Keshet, E. (1995). Stabilization of vascular endothelial growth factor mRNA by hypoxia and hypoglycemia and coregulation with other ischemia-induced genes. *Molecular and Cellular Biology* **15**(10), 5363–5368.

Taha, C., Tsakiridis, T., McCall, A. and Klip, A. (1997). Stress-activated pathways in the regulation of glucose transporters. *American Journal of Physiology Endocrinology and Metabolism* **273**, 68–76.

Uehara, Y., Nipper, V. and McCall, A. (1997). Chronic insulin hypoglycemia induces GLUT-3 protein in rat brain neurons. *American Journal of Physiology Endocrinology and Metabolism* **272**, E716–E719.

Weber, T., Joost, H., Kuroda, M., Cushman, S. and Simpson, I. (1991). Subcellular distribution and phosphorylation state of insulin receptors from insulin- and isoproterenol-treated rat adipose cells. *Cell Signaling* **3**, 51–58.

Glutamate *See:* Glucocorticoids – Adverse Effects on the Nervous System.

Glycobiology of Stress

G Lauc and M Flögel
University of Zagreb, Zagreb, Croatia

This article is a revision of the previous edition article by G Lauc and M Flögel, volume 2, pp 276–282, © 2000, Elsevier Inc.

Glycoconjugates Are Important Mediators of Many Physiological Functions

Glycoproteins in Stress

Lectins in Stress

Stress Affects the Activity of Glycosyltransferases

Model of Glycobiology of Stress

Glossary

Glyco-conjugate	A compound composed of an oligosaccharide linked to a protein or a lipid.
Glycolipid	A compound containing both lipid and oligosaccharide moieties.
Glycoprotein	A protein molecule containing one or more oligosaccharide attachments.
Glycosylation	The posttranslational modification of a protein by the addition of a carbohydrate moiety; catalyzed by specific enzymes called glycosyltransferases.
Glycosyltransferase (GT)	A group of enzymes that transfer monosaccharides to a growing oligosaccharide chain on glycoconjugates.
Lectin	A physiological receptor for carbohydrate structures attached to glycoconjugates.
Sialyltransferase	An enzyme that transfers sialic acid to a glycoconjugate.

The metabolic response to psychological stress is a very complex and demanding physiological process that involves numerous organs and organ systems. Although it is highly important for survival in an ever-changing environment, its excessive activation is associated with various detrimental effects. A number of epidemiological and experimental studies conducted during the past years have clearly demonstrated a link between stress and the development and course of many diseases, from simple virus infections and gastric ulcers to cardiovascular diseases and cancer. It is estimated that up to two-thirds of all visits to the physician's office are associated with stress.

Molecular mechanisms underlying the link between the response to stress and the development of disease appear to be exceedingly complex and are only partly understood. Although hormonal changes are key mediators of the physiological changes in stress, other factors appear to be decisive in the development of stress-associated disorders. Molecular response of a target cell appears to be defined not only by the incoming hormone but also by the current molecular situation within the cell itself. A good illustration of this principle is the way in which corticosteroids affect neurons in the hippocampus. If neurons are at rest, corticosteroids apparently have no effects. These effects become visible only when neurons are shifted from their basal condition by the action of neurotransmitters.

After more than 50 years of research, a lot is known about the endocrinology of the stress response, but the key molecular mechanism that explains how and why corticosteroids and other stress hormones cease to be beneficial and start to cause damage is still not known. One important link between stress and disease is the stress-induced decrease in the immune response, but the decrease in the immune response cannot explain all the effects of stress and other mechanisms have to be involved. Glycosylation appears to be involved, and the modification of glycoconjugate structures and their interaction with lectin receptors modulate at least some of these processes.

Glycoconjugates Are Important Mediators of Many Physiological Functions

Glycosylation is a very complex posttranslational modification that plays an important role in the integration of higher organisms. The surface of all cells is covered by oligosaccharide structures covalently attached to proteins and lipids (glycoproteins and glycolipids). Escalation in the extent and diversity of protein glycosylation correlates with the appearance of multicellular life, and apparently most of the interaction between cells and their surroundings include carbohydrate–protein recognition. An essential difference between proteins and the oligosaccharide structures attached to them is the fact that the carbohydrate part is not encoded in the DNA (**Figure 1**). Although genes unequivocally define the structure of each protein, there is no template for attached oligosaccharides. This makes them inherently sensitive to all changes within the cell, and glycan structures that are being produced at any individual moment actually mirror all relevant past events in the cell. In addition, the evolution of carbohydrate structures is much faster than the evolution of proteins, and often in different species we see significant differences in carbohydrate structures attached to nearly identical protein or lipid backbones.

Glycan parts of glycoconjugates are being synthesized by GTs that act in a sequence, and each

enzyme transfers specific monosaccharide to a specific acceptor contributing to the final glycan structure (**Figure 2**). It is estimated that over 300 specific enzymes (glycosidases and GTs) are involved in the synthesis of carbohydrate structures on glycoconjugates, and the whole process is very complex and energy expensive for the cell. Defects that disturb early phases of glycoconjugate synthesis are incompatible with multicellular life, whereas mutations in the end modifications of oligosaccharides result in specific physiological alterations. Because oligosaccharide structures are not encoded in genes, the final structure of a glycan is determined by the current cellular repertoire of expressed GTs (the expression, intracellular localization, and regulation of specific GTs that is commonly referred to as the glycosylation phenotype).

At the level of the individual molecule, from the structural point of view, there is no significant difference between the protein and carbohydrate parts. Glycoprotein is an entity composed of a protein and a carbohydrate part, and both parts have structural and functional roles that are specific to a given protein. Due to very high structural variability and the lack of adequate methods to analyze them, the carbohydrate parts of glycoconjugates were ignored by the most of the scientific community until very recently. However, thanks to the development of novel methods, in the last decade there has been an exponential increase in the knowledge about the physiological roles of carbohydrate structures. Now it is known that glycan part of glycoconjugates are crucial for many physiological processes from fertilization and development to regulation of hormonal activity and the formation of memory. Recent evidence has established differential glycan processing as a novel regulator of protein function, and the speculation that the invention of glycosylation was the key evolutionary step that enabled the development of multicellular organisms appears to be correct.

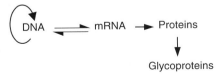

Figure 1 Central dogma of molecular biology amended with the biosynthesis of glycoproteins. Contrary to proteins, which all have their templates in the DNA, the carbohydrate structures attached to glycoproteins are not defined by genes. Their exact structures are determined by the regulation of expression, intracellular localization, and activity of various glycosyltransferases.

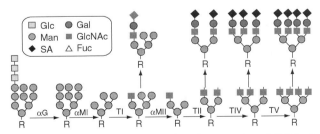

Figure 2 Schematic representation of processing of N-linked glycans. N-linked glycans are being synthesized by sequential action of numerous glycosyltransferases and glycosidases that add or remove specific monosaccharides to a growing oligosaccharide chain.

Glycoproteins in Stress

The influence of stress on glycosylation was first studied on gastric mucosa in rats. Mucosal cells of rats stressed by immersion in water were found to incorporate up to 50% less N-acetylgalactosamine than control animals. Subsequently, it was also shown that stress is associated with changes in the binding of lectins to gastric mucosa. Stress-induced alterations were found in the binding of several lectins, the most specific being changes detected with peanut agglutinin (PNA) lectin that specifically recognizes galactose β(1,3) linked to N-acetylgalactosamine. These studies were not continued, but they undoubtedly indicated that stress does have some influence on glycosylation. *Helicobacter pylori* (causative agent of most peptic ulcers) attaches to the gastric mucosa through specific interactions with carbohydrate structures, and the stress-induced changes in the expression of these structures might be one of the molecular mechanisms that explains the effects of stress on the development of gastric ulcers.

An indirect confirmation of the hypothesis that structures of glycoconjugates might change in stress came from the studies of acute-phase proteins in depression. For some time, it is known that depression can significantly influence the immune system, especially some positive acute-phase proteins such as haptoglobin or α_1-acid glycoprotein. Similar changes were detected in association with surgical stress, and recently it was shown that even a single episode of uncontrollable stress can activate acute-phase response in the experimental animals. Nearly all acute-phase proteins are glycosylated, and in addition to changes in the concentration of the whole proteins, depression is also associated with changes in the individual carbohydrate structures attached to acute-phase proteins. Specific changes in carbohydrate structures on glycoproteins also occur during inflammation and some diseases that are associated with stress. In their recent work, van Dijk and colleagues proposed that these changes might be associated with the regulation of the immune response.

The first indications that psychological stress can influence human glycoconjugates came from the studies of Flögel and colleagues in early 1990s. They used lectin-western blot to analyze changes in the glycosylation of proteins in sera of prisoners released from the Serbian concentration camps during the war in Croatia and Bosnia. Significant changes in glycosylation patterns were established with several different lectins, each recognizing specific segments of the oligosaccharide structure (**Table 1**).

Corticotropin releasing hormone (CRH) plays a crucial role in integrating the body's overall response to stress, including the integration of the response of the immune system to physiological, psychological, and immunological stressors. In addition to the hypothalamus, where it was initially identified, CRH, its receptors, and related ligands are present throughout the brain and periphery. By activating the glucocorticoid and catecholamine secretion, CRH from the central nervous system (CNS) mediates the suppressive effects of stress on the immune system. The action of CRH is exhibited through CRH receptors CRH1 and CRH2, which are differentially expressed on brain neurons located in neocortical, limbic, and brainstem regions of the CNS and on the pituitary corticotrophs. An intriguing aspect of both CRH receptors and CRH binding protein is their glycosylation pattern. CRH1 contains five potential N-glycosylation sites. Early studies showed that its glycosylation differs in different regions of the CNS, indicating potential functional roles for different glycoforms. The conversion of oligosaccharide chains to oligomannose structures by kifunensine (an inhibitor of mannosidase I that prevents the conversion of oligomannose to complex glycans) was reported not to change the ligand-binding properties of individual receptors, but mutation experiments have shown that the presence of at least three (out of five) oligosaccharide chains is required for normal CRH1 function.

Another system in which glycosylation might play an important role in the stress response is the cholinergic activation of the brain. It is generally accepted that in the CNS stress induces primarily cholinergic hyperactivation. Within several hours, the excess acetylcholinesterase (AChE) exerts a protective effect by retrieving cholinergic balance through enzymatic acetylcholine (ACh) hydrolysis. In addition to hydrolysis of ACh at the brain cholinergic synapses and neuromuscular junctions, AChE also affects cell proliferation, differentiation, and responses to various insults. Through alternative splicing of its 3′ end, AChE is considered to be one of the general stress-responding proteins, both in the brain and in the periphery. AChE

Table 1 Specificity of lectins[a]

Lectin	Source	Specificity
GNA	*Galanthus nivalis*	Man-α(1,3), Man-α(1,6); Man-α(1,2)-Man
SNA	*Sambucus nigra*	Sia-α(2,6)-Gal
MAA	*Maackia amurensis*	Sia-α(2,3)-Gal
PNA	Peanut	Gal-β(1,3)-GalNAc
DSA	*Datura stramonium*	Gal-β(1,4)-GlcNAc

[a]Lectins are physiological receptors for carbohydrate structures in animals and plants. Plant lectins are easy to isolate and they are commercially available as tools for specific recognition of the exactly defined segments of carbohydrate structures.

is glycosylphosphatidylinositol (GPI)-anchored protein, and efficient glypiation is necessary for proper localization and secretion. For more than 10 years, it has been known that differences in glycosylation affect the stability of the enzyme, but the functional consequences of altered glycosylation are still not understood. Pharmacokinetic profiling of the AChE glycoforms demonstrated a correlation between circulatory longevity and the number of attached N-glycans. Glycosylation of AChE was shown to be altered in breast cancer, but this was not studied in detail. Abnormally glycosylated forms of the enzyme also accumulate in the cerebrospinal fluid in some neurological disorders, and changes in AChE glycosylation were reported to be a potential diagnostic marker for Alzheimer's disease.

Contraception, which is a form of hormonal stress for the body, also affects glycosylation. Oral estrogen treatment induces an increase in the degree of branching and a decrease in fucosylation and sialyl Lewis x expression on α_1-acid glycoprotein compared to individuals receiving no estrogens or transdermal estrogen treatment. The effects of oral estrogens are identical in both males and females, and they can be reduced by the administration of progestagen. The effects of oral estrogens on glycosylation of α_1-acid glycoprotein are the opposite of those induced by inflammation, indicating that estrogens can modulate the glycosylation-dependent inflammatory actions of α_1-acid glycoprotein. Interestingly, estrogens that are applied transdermally do not exert this effect on hepatic glycosylation.

Lectins in Stress

Some glycans on glycoconjugates have only structural roles, but some also take part in specific recognition processes. One of the major mechanisms by which glycoconjugates perform their molecular functions is the interaction with their specific molecular receptors, lectins. Hundreds of endogenous lectins function as physiological receptors for oligosaccharides that interpret molecular information encoded in glycans. They take part in numerous physiological processes including folding, intracellular transport, fertilization, regulation of the inflammatory response, and brain plasticity.

The best-known example of lectin function is inflammation, in which the interaction between lectins called selectins and carbohydrate structures on glycoproteins represents the first decisive step leading to the adhesion of circulating lymphocytes to the endothelium at the site of inflammation. Carbohydrate–lectin interactions are very interesting because they can be inhibited with small oligosaccharides that are generally nontoxic and, using modern carbohydrate cycling technologies, are relatively inexpensive to prepare for therapeutic purposes.

The first indications that lectins might change in stress came from a study of a phenomenon only remotely associated with stress. Bardosi and colleagues were analyzing the influence of prolonged anesthesia on mannose receptor and some other lectins on murine peripheral blood polymorphonuclear leukocytes. They demonstrated reduced expression of mannose receptor and changes in the expression of receptors for several other sugars, indicating that prolonged anesthesia affects the regulation of lectin expression.

Evidence that psychological stress can influence lectins came from studies of Lauc and colleagues on lectins in livers of rats exposed to immobilization stress. Immobilization stress was found to influence galectin-3, a galactose-specific lectin, so that it binds to another nuclear lectin CBP67 (67-kDa carbohydrate binding protein). The formation of the complex from CBP67 and galectin-3 resulted in the binding of the galactose-specific galectin-3 to the glucose-affinity column, for which it shows no affinity under normal conditions. This is a very interesting effect because galectin-3 is involved in mRNA splicing and changes in its functions might have profound effects on the whole cell. However, whether this binding was mediated by protein–protein interactions or through lectinlike binding of galectin-3 to galactose residues on carbohydrate structures attached to CBP67 (as well as other details of this interaction) is not known.

Galectin-3 is a versatile galactoside-binding lectin that has been implicated in numerous cellular functions. It also appears to be affected by stress and, interestingly, different types of stress have exactly opposite effects on its expression. As shown by Dumić and colleagues in 2000, whereas exposure to UV light or transfer to *in vitro* conditions induces galectin-3 in cultured cells, immobilization stress *in vivo* results in a decrease in galectin-3 in mouse spleen and liver. The regulation of galectin-3 expression involves transcription factor nuclear factor (NF)-κB, which connects galectin-3 with corticosteroids (and CRH) and places its expression downstream from hormonal signals in the stress-response pathway.

A major problem in studying changes of lectin activity in different physiological processes is the lack of adequate methods for measuring lectin activity in complex biological samples. A new method (**Figure 3**) using photoaffinity glycoprobes labeled with digoxin was recently developed, and it is hoped that it will enable easier identification of changes in lectins in different diseases. Until now, only one new lectin was found to appear in stress. It was found

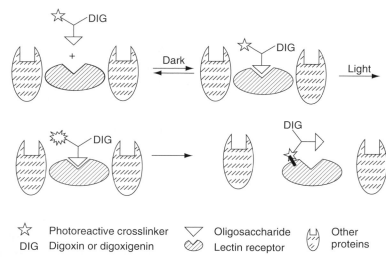

☆ Photoreactive crosslinker　　▽ Oligosaccharide　　⊔ Other
DIG Digoxin or digoxigenin　　◌ Lectin receptor　　⊔ proteins

Figure 3 Photoaffinity method for the detection of lectins. Photoaffinity glycoprobes containing target carbohydrate structures are incubated with biological samples to allow the formation of noncovalent complexes between the probe and lectin receptors in the sample. Illumination activates the photoreactive cross-linker, and it forms covalent bonds with neighboring molecules, mostly lectin receptors. The result is a lectin with a covalently incorporated digoxin tag (DIG) that can be easily identified with labeled antibodies against digoxin.

to bind to glucose-containing glycoprobes, and according to the electrophoretic mobility of the protein isolated from rat liver named CBP33.

Stress Affects the Activity of Glycosyltransferases

The carbohydrate parts of glycoconjugates are synthesized by sequential action of numerous GTs, enzymes that are specific for both the structure of the glycoconjugate acceptor and the monosaccharide that is being added. The appearance of novel or altered glycoconjugate structures in stress indicates that stress should somehow affect the activity of GTs, but the only GTs whose relation with stress have been studied up to now are the sialyltransferases (enzymes that transfer sialic acids to glycoproteins).

For some time it has been known that corticosteroids can change the activity of sialyltransferases *in vitro*. Breen and colleagues have shown that corticosteroids and other hormones from the adrenal gland significantly influence the activity of sialyltransferases *in vivo*. Adrenalectomy and the subsequent administration of corticosterone and/or aldosterone significantly influence the activity of sialyltransferases in various rat tissues. Whereas sialyltransferases in some tissues such as the kidney are apparently not influenced by adrenalectomy or by the addition of steroid hormones, sialyltransferases in the liver are under the negative control of corticosteroids. Adrenalectomy results in the increased activity of sialyltransferases in the liver that cannot be reverted to normal values by the administration of dexamethasone.

Enzymes that perform the same function in the brain react to same hormonal signals in the exactly opposite way. Adrenalectomy and the consequential lack of circulating corticosteroids lead to the decrease of total sialyltransferase activity in the brain. The subsequent administration of exogenous corticosteroids exhibits regional specificity, with the enzyme activities in the cortex, cerebellum, and brain stem being stimulated by both dexamethasone and aldosterone and enzyme activity in the hippocampus being stimulated only by aldosterone. Total sialyltransferase activity in some tissue does not represent the activity of a single enzyme but the sum of the activities of all enzymes that transfer sialic acids. Breen and colleagues also studied the effects of corticosteroids on two individual enzymes, $\alpha(2,3)$-sialyltransferase and $\alpha(2,6)$-sialyltransferase. Both enzymes transfer sialic acids, but they link them to different carbon atoms on the preceding sugar in the carbohydrate structure.

As shown by Dabelic and colleagues in 2004, immobilization stress affects sialyltransferase activity in different rat tissues. Acute and chronic stress have different effects, but, even more interesting, the same type of stress has opposite effects on sialyltransferase activity in different tissues. In general, stress induces sialyltransferase activity in extraneural tissues and suppresses the activity of the same enzymes in most brain tissues. The fact that same enzymes respond differently to the same hormonal signals depending on their cellular environment exemplifies the fact that the molecular setup of the targeted cell, and not hormonal signal by itself, is the decisive player in

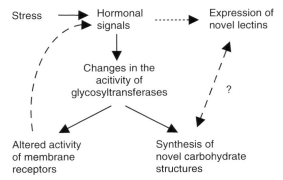

Figure 4 Hypothetical model of the glycobiology of stress. Hormones mediate numerous stress-associated changes, and among them alter the activity of different glycosyltransferases. Changed activity of glycosyltransferases results in the appearance of different carbohydrate structures on glycoproteins, which could either present a novel structures with potential to interact with specific endogenous lectins or modify the activity of various membrane receptors. Although this has yet to be proven, it could be one of the mechanisms explaining why prolonged stress has different effects than acute stress. In the same time, it is known that stress is associated with changes in composition and activity of endogenous lectins, but the exact mechanisms linking stress and changes in lectin activity are still not known.

determining the direction and consequences of the stress response.

Model of Glycobiology of Stress

At the moment only several fragments of the glyco-biological mechanisms involved in the physiological response to psychological stress are known, but the complete picture is slowly emerging (**Figure 4**). Stress causes numerous changes in the circulating hormones, and many molecular details of this process are known. It is also known that corticosteroids affect the activity of at least one GT both *in vitro* and *in vivo*. The altered activity of GTs results in different carbohydrate structures attached to glycoproteins, and these changes have been demonstrated both in humans and in experimental animals. A change in the carbohydrate structures attached to a glycoprotein is a well-established way to change its structural and functional properties, and recently this was shown

to be one of the mechanisms that control the activity of membrane receptors. Although this type of glyco-sylation-mediated receptor modulation in stress still has to be proven, it is a very interesting hypothesis. On the other hand, new glycoconjugate structures could also represent novel signals on the cell surface that could alter the interaction of the cell with neighboring cells in a process analogous to the selectin-mediated adhesion of lymphocytes. Stress is also known to be associated with the appearance of novel lectins, but the exact mechanism of this process is not known. These lectins could be receptors for either novel or normal glycoconjugate structures, translating their structures into molecular functions. Although most of this is still speculative, it is hoped that more will soon be known about the molecular role of glycoconjugates, their lectin receptors, and GTs in the physiological response to psychological stress.

Further Reading

Assil, I. Q. and Abou-Samra, A. B. (2001). N-glycosylation of CRF receptor type 1 is important for its ligand-specific interaction. *American Journal of Physiology, Endocrinology and Metabolism* **281**, E1015–E1021.

Axford, J. (2001). The impact of glycobiology on medicine. *Trends in Immunology* **22**, 237–239.

Chitlaru, T., Kronman, C., Velan, A., et al. (2002). Overloading and removalof N-glycosylation targets on human acetylcholinesterase: effects on glycan composition and circulatory residence time. *Biochemical Journal* **363**, 619–631.

Dabelic, S., Flogel, M., Maravic, G., et al. (2004). Stress causes tissue-specific changes in the sialyltransferase activity. *Zeitschrift fur Naturforschung* **59**, 276–280.

Lauc, G., Supraha, S., Lee, Y. C., et al. (2003). Digoxin derivatives as tools for glycobiology. *Methods in Enzymology* **362**, 29–37.

Nalivaeva, N. N. and Turner, A. J. (2001). Post-translational modifications of proteins: acetylcholinesterase as a model system. *Proteomics* **1**, 735–747.

Partridge, E. A., Le Roy, C., Di Guglielmo, G. M., et al. (2004). Regulation of cytokine receptors by golgi N-glycan processing and endocytosis. *Science* **306**, 120–124.

Golgi Complex *See:* Protein Synthesis.

Gonadotropin Secretion, Effects of Stress on

M Ferin
Columbia University, New York NY, USA

This article is a revision of the previous edition article by M Ferin, volume 2, pp 283–288, © 2000, Elsevier Inc.

Control of Normal Gonadotropin Secretion

The Gonadotropin Response to Stressors: Cross-Talk between the Hypothalamic-Pituitary-Adrenal and the Hypothalamic-Pituitary-Gonadal Axes

Central Pathways Mediating the Stress Response

Stressors and the Reproductive Cycle

Glossary

Amenorrhea	The absence of menstruation, denoting a silent hypothalamic-pituitary-ovarian endocrine axis.
Arginine vasopressin (AVP)	An adjunct neurohormone in control of the hypothalamic-pituitary-adrenal endocrine axis. It is colocated with and released together with CRH in response to stressors.
Corticotropin releasing hormone (CRH)	The main neurohormone in control of the hypothalamic-pituitary-adrenal endocrine axis. Its release from the hypothalamic paraventricular nucleus is activated by stressors. It stimulates the pituitary to secrete adrenocorticotropic hormone.
Estradiol	The main sex steroid secreted by the ovarian follicle.
Follicular phase	The first stage of the menstrual cycle, during which the process of folliculogenesis is completed through the maturation of the soon-to-be-ovulated dominant follicle.
Follicle stimulating hormone (FSH)	A gonadotropin that promotes the recruitment of a new cohort of follicles at the start of each follicular phase.
Gonadotropin releasing hormone (GnRH) pulse generator	The hypothalamic structure responsible for the pulsatile release of GnRH, in a process that is essential for the normal function of the reproductive process.
Gonadotropin	Two hormones, follicle stimulating hormone and luteinizing hormone, released by the anterior pituitary following stimulation by GnRH.
Luteal phase	The second stage of the menstrual cycle, when the ovulated follicle is transformed into a new structure, the corpus luteum, which secretes both estradiol and progesterone.
Luteinizing hormone (LH)	A gonadotropin that stimulates the release of estradiol from the maturing follicle and of progesterone from the corpus luteum.
Progesterone	The main sex steroid secreted by the corpus luteum. It prepares the uterus for the implantation of the fertilized egg.
Proopio-melanocortin (POMC)	The common precursor molecule to β-endorphin (an endogenous opioid peptide) and to α-melanocyte stimulating hormone. Both peptides modulate the gonadotropin response to stressors.

Control of Normal Gonadotropin Secretion

Hypothalamic Control: The Gonadotropin Releasing Hormone Pulse Generator

The hypothalamic-pituitary-gonadal (HPG) axis, which governs the reproductive system, is driven by the brain. Gonadotropin (FSH and LH) secretion by the anterior pituitary gland is controlled by the hypothalamus through the release of GnRH. GnRH, a 10-amino-acid peptide, is synthesized within several hypothalamic nuclei and released into the hypophysial portal circulation to stimulate the release of both gonadotropins. This direct vascular connection between the hypothalamus and the anterior pituitary allows for the rapid and undiluted transport of minute amounts of GnRH to its target, the pituitary gonadotroph. Gonadotropins, in turn, act on the gonads, the ovaries or testes, to induce specific morphological changes and to stimulate the release of gonadal steroids, such as testosterone, estradiol, and progesterone. Constant communication between the several levels of the HPG axis through the negative feedback loop is essential for normal function; estradiol or testosterone secreted by the ovaries or testes continuously feeds back to the hypothalamus and pituitary to adjust GnRH, LH, and FSH secretion. The interruption of this negative feedback loop, for instance, following castration, results in an increase of GnRH, FSH, and LH release.

Significantly, GnRH is released from the hypothalamus in a pulsatile fashion (the GnRH pulse generator), and thus tonic secretion of gonadotropins is pulsatile in nature. Each pulse of LH consists of an abrupt and brief release of the hormone followed by an exponential decrease according to its half-life. A pulsatile GnRH stimulus is required to increase the transcription of the gonadotropin subunit genes.

Pathological events that interfere with the function of the GnRH pulse generator disrupt the pituitary-gonadal axis. For example, the complete absence of GnRH pulsatility results in a dormant reproductive axis, whereas lesser abnormalities, such as a decrease in GnRH pulse frequency, may interfere with proper reproductive function.

Gonadotropins and the Reproductive Cycle

The reproductive cycle, estrous cycle (in rodent and sheep) or menstrual cycle (in nonhuman primate and human) involves a remarkable coordination of hormonal secretion and morphological changes within the HPG axis. In the primate, a rise in FSH at the start of the follicular phase promotes the recruitment of a cohort of antral follicles from which the dominant follicle destined for ovulation will be selected. Stimulated by the pulsatile release of the gonadotropins, the dominant follicle grows exponentially and releases estradiol in amounts proportional to its size. The maturity of the dominant follicle is marked by a high estradiol release, which when a threshold is reached activates the positive estradiol feedback loop; this induces the ovulatory LH surge and ovulation. After ovulation, the dominant follicle is transformed into the corpus luteum, which secretes both estradiol and progesterone when stimulated by LH. Substantial progesterone secretion promotes uterine differentiation in preparation for implantation of the fertilized egg.

A proper pattern of GnRH and gonadotropin pulsatile release is required for the normal reproductive cycle to occur. In the human, for example, an optimal GnRH–LH pulse frequency of approximately one pulse every 90 min is required for normal folliculogenesis to occur during the follicular phase. A pulse frequency that is too low may fail to bring the recruited follicle to a timely maturation, and a too rapid pulse frequency may result in pathology (such as polycystic ovary syndrome).

The Gonadotropin Response to Stressors: Cross-Talk between the Hypothalamic-Pituitary-Adrenal and the Hypothalamic-Pituitary-Gonadal Axes

Effects of Stressors on Tonic Gonadotropin Release

The activation of the hypothalamic-pituitary-adrenal (HPA) axis by several types of stressors, such as immune/inflammatory challenges as simulated by the administration of endotoxin or cytokines, temporary restraint, or insulin-induced hypoglycemia, results in an inhibition of tonic pulsatile LH release, mainly in the form of a decrease in LH pulse frequency. In women, psychogenic stress has also been related to lower basal tonic levels of FSH, LH, and estradiol compared to normal cycling women; these patients have reduced integrated 24-h LH and FSH concentrations, reduced LH pulse frequency, and increased LH interpulse interval.

Overall evidence suggests that this decrease in tonic pulsatile LH release is primarily related to a central action of stressors exerted through an inhibitory action on the hypothalamic GnRH pulse generator; a decline in the generator's ability to properly stimulate the gonadotroph, mainly through a reduction in the frequency of pulsatile GnRH release, appears to be the main mechanism involved. In addition, there is experimental evidence that stressors may also subtly influence the gonadotroph's responsiveness to GnRH and thereby decrease the amplitude of the gonadotropin response. This effect may reflect a pituitary action of adrenal corticosteroids released in response to the activation of the HPA axis by the stressor.

Effects of Stressors on the Surge Mode of Luteinizing Hormone Release

Data in the rodent and ewe also suggest that an immune/inflammatory challenge or restraint (and possibly other stressors) can also suppress the estradiol-induced ovulatory LH surge. In the rodent, this effect appears to be exerted at the level of GnRH perikarya, where the percentage of GnRH neurons expressing the c-fos protein and the GnRH primary transcript are significantly reduced by these stressors. The administration of a GnRH agonist concomitantly with the stressor completely restores the LH surge. In the ewe, endotoxin was shown to prevent the GnRH surge into the hypophysial portal circulation, also suggesting a central effect of the challenge. Significantly, this inhibitory action is seen only if the stressor acts quite ahead of the expected time of the LH surge, primarily at the initial time of activation of the estradiol positive feedback signal.

Stressors and an Early Short-Term Rise in Gonadotropins

In addition to the previously mentioned inhibitory action of stressors on gonadotropin release, investigators have also reported a very transient rise in LH in rodents within the first hour of the response to various stressors, such as handling; restraint; exposure to ether or to a novel environment; or visual, audiogenic, and thermal stressors. This rapid and transient stimulatory effect of stressors on tonic LH release has been reported mostly in the intact, but generally not in the castrated, male rat, and in men but not women.

The mechanisms behind this phenomenon and its role in the stress response remain to be elucidated.

Central Pathways Mediating the Stress Response

The Hypothalamic Paraventricular Nucleus

The paraventricular nucleus (PVN) plays a pivotal role in the response to stressors. The neuroendocrine activation of the HPA axis by stressors involves the release of two neuropeptides, corticotropin releasing hormone (CRH) and AVP, from discrete populations of hypophysiotrophic neurons in parvocellular areas of PVN. These two neuropeptides, which are colocalized within perikarya of PVN neurons and in secretory granules, play a complementary role in mediating the effects of stressors on the HPA axis (see **Figure 1**).

There is good experimental evidence for an active mediatory role by CRH in the inhibition of GnRH and gonadotropins that follow stressors. In the nonhuman primate, the administration of a CRH receptor antagonist or of a drug decreasing endogenous CRH activity prevents not only the cortisol increase but also the inhibition of pulsatile GnRH–LH release induced by stressors such as an immune/inflammatory challenge (**Figure 2a**) or insulin-induced hypoglycemia. Similar mediatory effects of a CRH antagonist or of CRH antiserum have been reported in the rodent after various stressors, except in the response to an inflammatory challenge. The latter is in a marked difference with the primate. The administration of

CRH also results in a rapid inhibition of pulsatile LH release and in a decrease in the frequency and duration of GnRH pulses. Data in the nonhuman primate suggest that this inhibitory action is not mediated by downstream activation of the pituitary-adrenal axis: indeed, the inhibitory effects of a CRH infusion on pulsatile LH release cannot be mimicked by adrenocorticotropic hormone (ACTH) infusion, are not reversed by treatment with metyrapone (an inhibitor of adrenal steroidogenesis), and persist following adrenalectomy.

Data in CRH-deficient male and female mice indicate that stressors such as restraint or food withdrawal can still inhibit tonic LH secretion or the proestrus LH surge, suggesting that molecules other than CRH may also play a role. Although there fewer data, AVP has also been shown to mediate the inhibitory action of certain stressors on the HPG axis and conceivably may take over in the CRH-deficient animal. In the ovx monkey, the inhibitory effects of a central infusion of interleukin (IL)-1 on pulsatile LH release are prevented by the co-administration of an AVP antagonist, even though the antagonist is without effect on the cortisol increase (**Figure 2b**). Some, but not all, investigators also report that the same antagonist prevents hypoglycemia-induced LH suppression in ovx and in male monkeys.

The Endogenous Opioid Peptides

There is substantial evidence to indicate that the inhibitory action of CRH and of most stressors on pulsatile GnRH–LH release occurs at suprapituitary sites that not only involve the neuroendocrine HPA axis but also mediation by endogenous opioid peptidergic pathways. Endogenous β-endorphin is known to be a powerful inhibitor of the GnRH pulse generator; for instance, during the luteal phase of the menstrual cycle of the human and nonhuman primate, there is a marked decreased in LH pulse frequency that parallels elevated endogenous β-endorphin activity and that is prevented by the administration of naloxone, a μ-opioid receptor antagonist. Hypothalamic β-endorphin activity is stimulated by CRH and by stressors. Naloxone administration also prevents the CRH- or AVP-mediated suppression of GnRH–gonadotropin release and restores pulsatile LH secretion (**Figure 3a**). This opioid antagonist also prevents the LH inhibition that follows several types of stressors, except for insulin-induced LH inhibition.

β-Endorphin derives from POMC, a large glycoprotein precursor molecule synthesized primarily in the hypothalamus and pituitary gland. Posttranslational processing of POMC is tissue-specific and in the hypothalamus yields not only β-endorphin but also α-melanocyte stimulating hormone (α-MSH).

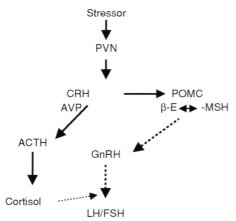

Figure 1 Main pathways mediating the inhibitory effects of stressors on pulsatile gonadotropin release. α-MSH, α-melanocyte stimulating hormone; β-E, β-endorphin; ACTH, adrenocorticotropic hormone; AVP, arginine vasopressin; CRH, corticotropin releasing hormone; FSH, follicle stimulating hormone; GnRH, gonadotropin releasing hormone; LH, luteinizing hormone; POMC, proopiomelanocortin; PVN, paraventricular nucleus.

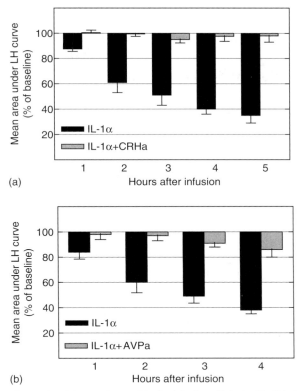

Figure 2 Reversal of the inhibitory effects of an intracerebroventricular infusion of interleukin (IL)-1 on luteinizing hormone (LH) release. a, By a CRH antagonist (CRHa); b, By a VP antagonist (AVPa). Reprinted with permission from (a) Feng, Y. J., Shalts, E., Xia, L., Rivier, J., Rivier, C., Vale, W., Ferin, M. (1991) An inhibitory effect of interleukin-1 on basal gonadotropin release in the ovariectomized rhesus monkey: reversal by a corticotropin-releasing factor antagonist, *Endocrinology* **128**, 2077–2082, Copyright 1991, The Endocrine Society; and (b) Shalts, E., Feng, Y. J., Ferin, M. (1992) Vasopressin mediates the interleukin-1α-indiced decrease in LH secretion in the ovariectomized rhesus monkey, *Endocrinology* **131**, 153–158, Copyright 1992, The Endocrine Society.

α-MSH has been shown to antagonize some of the actions of β-endorphin and may function as an endogenous opioid antagonist. In fact, α-MSH antagonizes the inhibitory action of exogenously administered β-endorphin on LH release and restores normal pulsatile LH release in ovx monkeys treated with CRH (**Figure 3b**) or subjected to an immune/inflammatory challenge. These data support the notion that post-translational processing of POMC may represent an important step in the response mechanisms to stressors and that the ratio of β-endorphin to α-MSH may be more significant than the absolute β-endorphin concentration in determining the ultimate effects of stressors on pulsatile LH release.

Stressors and the Reproductive Cycle

Stress and Amenorrhea

The reproductive cycle requires a remarkable coordination of hormonal secretion and morphological changes within all levels of the hypothalamic-pituitary-ovarian-uterine axis. Thus, it is not surprising that stressors can disrupt the normal estrous or menstrual cycle. If sufficiently intense or chronic, stressors can completely interrupt the cycle. In women, psychogenic stress, usually the result of overt or latent psychological disturbances, is known to interfere with normal reproductive function and thought to be a common cause of amenorrhea in a syndrome known as functional hypothalamic chronic anovulation (FHCA). When fully established, the syndrome is characterized by ovarian quiescence, amenorrhea, and infertility. Several studies in the human underscore the association among FHCA, increased HPA activity in the form of an amplified circadian cortisol excursion, and low basal tonic levels of FSH and LH coupled with reduced LH pulse frequency.

Stress and Menstrual Cycle Defects

Although the long-term consequences of chronic stress may include amenorrhea and infertility and result in the full-blown FHCA syndrome, more recent data also demonstrate that stressors that initially are

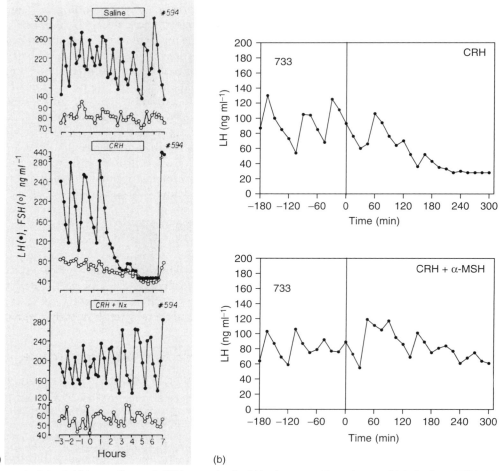

Figure 3 Reversal of the inhibitory effects of CRH on pulsatile LH release. a, By naloxone (Nx); b, By α-MSH. Reprinted with permission from (a) Gindoff, P. R., Ferin, M. (1987) Endogenous opioid peptides modulate the effect of corticotropin-releasing hormone (CRH) on gonadotropin release in the primate, *Endocrinology* **121**, 837–842, Copyright 1987, The Endocrine Society; and (b) Shalts, E., Feng, Y. J., Ferin, M., Wardlaw, S. L. (1992) α-Melanocyte-stimulating hormone antagonizes the neuroendocrine effects of corticotropin-releasing factor and interleukin-Ia in the primate, *Endocrinology* **131**, 132–138, Copyright 1992, The Endocrine Society.

of an insufficient intensity to induce amenorrhea may nevertheless produce temporary cyclic defects.

Prolongation of the follicular phase As shown in the ewe and monkey, endotoxin administration, mimicking an inflammatory/immune challenge, or exercise during the follicular phase results in a lengthening of the follicular phase and in the interruption of the normal follicular estradiol profile. The stressor prevents the development of high-frequency LH pulses that are the essential stimulus for the preovulatory increase in estradiol secretion; without these, the estradiol rise is curtailed and the preovulatory LH surge is delayed. Significantly, in the monkey, the delay in the resumption of a normal follicular phase greatly exceeds the duration of the stress challenge itself.

Inadequate luteal phase In the monkey, a short-term inflammatory/immune challenge or a psychogenic-like stress, whether confined to the follicular or luteal phase of the menstrual cycle, invariably result in reduced luteal function, as demonstrated by overall diminished progesterone and inhibin A secretion during the luteal phase (**Figure 4**). In many animals, these short-term stress challenges continue to interfere with normal luteal function through the first or two subsequent stressor-free cycles. The lower progesterone levels are related to the decrease in LH induced by the stressor. Inadequate luteal phases have also been reported during exercise, suggesting that this syndrome may well represent a general initial response to stressors and/or energy-related demands in the normal cyclic female.

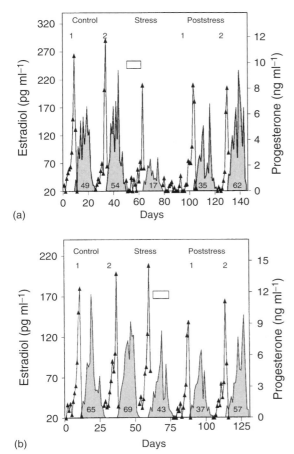

(a)

(b)

Figure 4 Inadequate luteal phase following a 10-day psychogenic-like stress. a, During the follicular phase; b, During the luteal phase. Illustrated are daily levels of estradiol during the follicular phase (triangles) and of progesterone during the luteal phase (shaded areas) throughout two control menstrual cycles, the stress cycle, and two poststress cycles. Luteal progesterone secretion is significantly decreased in the stress cycle and in the first of the two poststress cycles (numbers within the shaded areas are integrated luteal progesterone values). Reprinted with permission from Xiao, E., Xia-Zhang, L., Ferin, M. (2002) Inadequate luteal function is the initial clinical cyclic defect in a 12-day stress model that includes a psychogenic component in the Rhesus monkey, *Journal of Clinical Endocrinology & Metabolism* **87**, 2232–2237, Copyright 2002, The Endocrine Society.

Premature ovulatory luteinizing hormone surge
Studies in the primate have shown that the activation of the HPA axis by endotoxin or IL-1 in the mid- to late follicular phase (but not at other stages of the cycle) results in a large release of LH. Data in the monkey suggest that progesterone, which is released in small amounts by the adrenals in response to the stressor, may be responsible for this acute release of LH because this effect is prevented by a progesterone or CRH antagonist. Smaller increases in LH have also been reported in women following exercise during the mid-follicular phase.

The precise physiopathological significance of these three cyclic defects in response to a stressor during the menstrual cycle remains to be further studied in patients. The data, however, suggest that the HPG axis is closely monitored by the brain and that a stress challenge, even one not sufficient or extended enough to interrupt the cycle and to result in amenorrhea, may well induce endocrine changes too subtle to be appreciated in the clinical environment but nonetheless substantial enough to temporarily impact on fertility or to provide a temporary suspension of pregnancy in suboptimal conditions. For instance, decreased luteal progesterone secretion in response to a stressor may interfere with the process of implantation of a fertilized egg and result in spontaneous abortion by delaying the endometrial changes required for proper implantation. Prematurely elevated LH concentrations in the follicular phase may damage the maturing follicle and/or oocyte and desynchronize the ovulatory signal from a timely follicular maturation process and thereby result in early pregnancy loss.

See Also the Following Article

Reproduction, Effects of Social Stress on.

Further Reading

Battaglia, D. F., Brown, M. E., Krasa, H. B., et al. (1998). Systemic challenge with endotoxin stimulates corticotropin-releasing hormone and arginine vasopressin secretion into hypophysial portal blood: coincidence with gonadotropin-releasing hormone suppression. *Endocrinology* **139**, 4175–4181.

Berga, S. L. (1996). Functional hypothalamic chronic anovulation. In: Adashi, E. Y., Rock, J. A. & Rosenwaks, Z. (eds.) *Reproductive endocrinology, surgery, and technology*, pp. 1061–1075. Philadelphia: Lippincott-Raven.

Chrousos, G. P., Torpy, D. J. and Gold, P. W. (1998). Interactions between the hypothalamic-pituitary-adrenal axis and the female reproductive system: clinical implications. *Annals of Internal Medicine* **129**, 229–240.

Feng, Y. J., Shalts, E., Xia, L., et al. (1991). An inhibitory effect of interleukin-1 on basal gonadotropin release in the ovariectomized rhesus monkey: reversal by a corticotropin-releasing factor antagonist. *Endocrinology* **128**, 2077–2082.

Ferin, M. (1999). Clinical review 105: stress and the reproductive cycle. *Journal of Clinical Endocrinology & Metabolism* **84**, 1768–1774.

Ferin M. (2006). Stress and the reproductive system. In: Knobil, E. & Neill, J. (eds.) *The physiology of reproduction* (3rd edn., pp. 2627–2696). San Diego, CA: Elsevier.

Gindoff, P. R. and Ferin, M. (1987). Endogenous opioid peptides modulate the effect of corticotropin-releasing hormone (CRH) on gonadotropin release in the primate. *Endocrinology* **121**, 837–842.

Karsch, F. J., Battaglia, D. F., Breen, K. M., et al. (2002). Mechanisms for ovarian cycle disruption by immune/inflammatory stress. *Stress* 5, 101–112.

Rivest, S. and Rivier, C. (1995). The role of corticotropin-releasing factor and interleukin-1 in the regulation of neurons controlling reproductive functions. *Endocrine Review* 16, 177–199.

Shalts, E., Feng, Y. J. and Ferin, M. (1992). Vasopressin mediates the interleukin-1 alpha-induced decrease in luteinizing hormone secretion in the ovariectomized rhesus monkey. *Endocrinology* 131, 153–158.

Shalts, E., Feng, Y. J., Ferin, M., et al. (1992). α-Melanocyte-stimulating hormone antagonizes the neuroendocrine effects of corticotropin-releasing factor and interleukin-1 α in the primate. *Endocrinology* 131, 132–138.

Xiao, E., Xia-Zhang, L., Barth, A., et al. (1998). Stress and the menstrual cycle: relevance of cycle quality in the short- and long-term response to a 5-day endotoxin challenge during the follicular phase in the rhesus monkey. *Journal of Clinical Endocrinology & Metabolism* 83, 2454–2460.

Xiao, E., Xia-Zhang, L. and Ferin, M. (2002). Inadequate luteal function is the initial clinical cyclic defect in a 12-day stress model that includes a psychogenic component in the Rhesus monkey. *Journal of Clinical Endocrinology & Metabolism* 87, 2232–2237.

Xiao, E., Xia-Zhang, L., Thornell, D., et al. (1996). Interleukin-1 stimulates luteinizing hormone release during the midfollicular phase in the rhesus monkey: a novel way in which stress may influence the menstrual cycle. *Journal of Clinical Endocrinology & Metabolism* 81, 2136–2141.

Graves' Disease (Thyrotoxicosis)

W M Wiersinga
University of Amsterdam, Amsterdam, Netherlands

Introduction
Historical Observations
Association between Stress and Graves' Disease
Stress and Graves' Disease: A Causal Relationship?

Glossary

Autoimmunity	Immune response directed at self antigens (belonging to the body of the individual), giving rise to antibodies against these antigens.
Euthyroid	Normal thyroid function.
Graves' disease	A multisystem autoimmune disease characterized by hyperthyroidism, enlarged thyroid gland (goiter), and frequently eye changes.
Thyroid peroxidase (TPO)	An enzyme in the thyroid gland involved in thyroid hormone synthesis.
Thyrotoxicosis	A disease caused by an excess of thyroid hormones; also called hyperthyroidism.
Thyrotropin (TSH)	The thyroid-stimulating hormone, which after release from the pituitary stimulates the thyroid gland to synthesize and release thyroid hormone.

Introduction

Thyrotoxicosis is a syndrome characterized by the clinical and biochemical manifestations of thyroid hormone excess in the target tissues of thyroid hormone. The most prominent clinical features of thyrotoxicosis are weight loss despite increased appetite, palpitations and tachycardia, fine tremor of the fingers, heat intolerance, perspiration, and a warm moist skin, all readily explained from an increased metabolic rate induced by thyroid hormone excess. Many patients also suffer from nervousness, irritation, anxiety, or mood disturbances, especially depression. Thyrotoxicosis is a very prevalent disease, occurring more frequently in women than in men. The annual incidence rate is approximately 0.4 per 1000 women and 0.1 per 1000 men.

Thyrotoxicosis can be caused by various diseases such as Graves' disease, toxic multinodular goiter, toxic adenoma, and destructive thyroiditis. Most prevalent, however, is Graves' disease, which is present in 75–90% of all thyrotoxic patients. Its relative frequency is dependent on ambient iodine intake, being lower in iodine-deficient areas. The peak incidence of Graves' disease is between ages 20 and 50 years. Graves' disease is an autoimmune disease characterized by antibodies directed against the thyrotropin receptor (TSH-R) on the surface of follicular epithelial cells in the thyroid gland; these antibodies (called thyroid-stimulating immunoglobulins) after binding to the TSH-R stimulate the thyroid gland to synthesize and release thyroid hormone, thereby causing the clinical picture of thyrotoxicosis. The disease is referred to as Graves' hyperthyroidism (GH), a typical autoimmune thyroid disease. At the other end of the spectrum of autoimmune thyroid diseases is chronic lymphocytic thyroiditis, also called Hashimoto's disease, characterized by the presence of autoantibodies against thyroid peroxidase (TPO), an enzyme involved in thyroid hormone synthesis. Hashimoto's disease frequently results in hypothyroidism. TPO antibodies are also found in the majority of patients with Graves' hyperthyroidism.

Autoimmune thyroid disease frequently runs in families. The autoimmune reaction against thyroid antigens is thought to develop against a certain genetic background, provoked by environmental factors. Recent twin studies have indicated that genes are responsible for approximately 80% of the risk to get Graves' disease. Among these genes are HLA-DR3, CTLA-4, and PTPN-22, but their contribution is relatively small and most of the genes involved are still unidentified. It follows that 20% of the risk on Graves' disease is derived from the environment. Smoking is a clear risk factor for Graves' hyperthyroidism (especially for the eye changes in Graves' disease) but not for Hashimoto's hypothyroidism; smoking might even protect against the occurrence of TPO antibodies. Ever since the early descriptions of Graves' disease, stress has been implicated in its pathogenesis.

Historical Observations

In August 1803, Elizabeth S., a 21-year-old patient of Dr. Parry, became acutely frightened when she lost control of her wheelchair and careered downhill. Two weeks later she developed swelling of the thyroid gland, palpitations of the heart, nervous troubles, marked pulsation of the carotid arteries, and a small hard regular pulse of 96. Since Dr. Parry's description, the relation between stressful life events and the precipitation of clinical Graves' disease has been underlined by many other physicians, including Graves and von Basedow. In humans, a sudden fright may cause acute exophthalmos and thyroid enlargement with pulsating thrills (*Schreckbasedow*). The French refer to the thyroid as *la glande d'emotion*. An increase in the incidence of Graves' disease has been observed during every major war since the Franco-Prussian conflict, and the German term *Kriegsbasedow* reflects this association. Indeed, hospital admissions for Graves' disease increased fivefold in occupied Scandinavian countries during

World War II, returning to normal levels after liberation. Many textbooks in the second half of the twentieth century thus conclude that a period of severe emotional stress almost always precedes the onset of Graves' disease. The occurrence of Graves' hyperthyroidism in President George Bush, Sr., shortly after the Gulf War in 1991 apparently underlines this conclusion. The conclusion, however, is not supported by all studies. Environmental stress caused by the civil unrest in Northern Ireland was not associated with a higher incidence of thyrotoxicosis. Moreover, defining and quantifying stress is difficult. The death of a spouse is generally viewed as a stressful life event, highly distressing for the survivor after a long-standing marriage of mutual love and caring. But the death of an abusive wife-beating husband might come as a welcome relief to his widow. In addition, we may ask: which came first, the stress or Graves' disease? Increased anxiety and hyperreactivity to stressors might be an early manifestation of Graves' hyperthyroidism, preceding other symptoms and signs of the disease by months.

Association between Stress and Graves' Disease

Since the early 1990s there have been six case–control studies on the relation between stress and the onset of Graves' hyperthyroidism (see **Table 1**). The cases are well-documented patients with Graves' hyperthyroidism and were compared with controls who in general are reasonably well selected at random from a healthy population and matched for sex and age, although not always for marital and social status. Stress evaluation is standardized, applying either interviews or questionnaires, asking for stressful life events in the year prior to the diagnosis or prior to the first symptoms and signs of Graves' hyperthyroidism. The results have always been obtained in a retrospective manner, making all studies liable to recall bias. It has been argued that memory is differentially affected by mood, and, in particular, that negative events or memories are better recalled in the presence of a negative affect. Because hyperthyroid patients frequently have depressive symptoms, their negative affect could explain the increased reporting of negative life events in comparison with healthy controls. To avoid the effect of hyperthyroidism, some studies have chosen to perform the stress evaluation after the patient's thyroid function has been restored to normal levels; in doing so, the time interval for memorizing past events becomes longer, which by itself may increase recall bias. Evaluating stressful life events in the year prior to the first occurrence of hyperthyroid symptoms and signs is preferable to evaluating them

Table 1 Case–control studies on the relationship between stress and the onset of Graves' hyperthyroidism

Author (year)	Cases[a]		Controls[b]		Stress evaluation			Relation stress and Graves
	n	%	Matching criteria	Origin	Method[c]	Period	When done	
Winsa et al. (1991)	208	82	A, S	General population	1	1 year prior to diagnosis	Hyperthyroid; <2 wk after diagnosis	Yes
Sonino et al. (1993)	70	83	A, S, M, C	Advertisement, hospital staff	2	1 year prior to first signs	Euthyroid; 10 months (3–39) after first sign	Yes
Kung (1995)	95	84	A, S, M, C	Volunteers in community	1	1 year prior to diagnosis	Hyperthyroid; at referral	Yes
Radosavljevic et al. (1996)	100	93	A, S	Outpatients with other conditions	2	1 year prior to diagnosis	Not stated	Yes
Yoshiuchi et al. (1998)	228	80	A, S	Healthy controls from database	1	1 year prior to diagnosis	<1 month after diagnosis	Yes
Matos-Santos et al. (2001)	31	71	A, S, M, C	Preventive medicine appointments	1	1 year prior to first symptoms	Euthyroid after treatment	Yes

[a]All Graves'.
[b]A, age; C, social class; M, marital status; S, sex. Number of controls same as number of cases, except for Winsa (1991) study with 372.
[c]1 = Sarason's questionnaire Life-Event Survey, with modifications in Yoshiuchi study 5; 2 = Paykel's interview for Recent Life Events.

in the year prior to the time at which the diagnosis was made by the physician, but it cannot always be known with certainty when precisely the first symptoms and signs started. Nevertheless, all six studies observed more stressful life events in the patients with Graves' hyperthyroidism than in the controls.

Winsa et al. reported more negative stressful life events in patients than in controls (odds ratio, OR, 1.33; 95% confidence interval, CI, 1.20–1.48); the odds increased with increased scores attached to the negative life events, from OR 1.0 for a score of 0 points to OR 6.3 (95% CI 2.7–14.7) for a score of ≥ 5 points; the number of positive events was similar in both groups. The prevalence of divorce was higher and job satisfaction was lower in patients than in controls, but a score for mastery in life (apart from work) did not differ between the groups. Patients had type A behavior not more frequently than controls (28 vs. 18%, not significant). The effect of negative life events was similar in patients with or without familial occurrence of thyroid disease, implying different mechanisms for these two risk factors.

Sonino et al. also reported more life events in patients than in controls (1.51 vs. 0.54, $p < 0.001$); patients had more independent events (defined as not likely to be a consequence of the illness) and events with negative impact than controls, according to a blind rater.

Kung likewise observed a higher number of negative events in patients than in controls (0.94–1.54 vs. 0.38–0.88, $p = 0.003$) and higher negative event

scores (1.55–2.69 vs. 0.58–1.45, $p = 0.002$); the reporting of positive and neutral events was similar in both groups. Groups did not differ in coping ability, but Graves' patients experienced more daily hassles (12.11–17.05 vs. 6.36–11.00, $p = 0.001$) and higher hassle scores (17.55–25.34 vs. 8.92–15.87, $p = 0.001$).

Radosavljevic et al. reported a mean number of 3.18 stressful life events in patients versus 1.85 in controls ($p = 0.0001$). Life events that were significantly more prevalent in patients than in controls were change in time spent on work, unemployment, arguments at work, change in work conditions, increased arguments with spouse or fiancé, hospitalization of family member for serious illness, and moderate financial difficulties.

Yoshiuchi et al. found a lower score for problem-oriented coping skills and a higher prevalence of smoking but not of daily hassles in patients than in controls. After adjustment for these variables, stressful life event were significantly associated with the risk of Graves' disease in women but not in men; the relative risk was 7.7 (95% CI 2.2–27) for women with highest stress scores compared with lowest stress scores.

Matos-Santos et al. reported a significantly greater number and impact of negative stressful life events in patients with Graves' disease than in healthy controls.

Taken together, these six studies, despite their limitations, provide fair evidence for the association between negative stressful life events and the onset of Graves' hyperthyroidism. The lack of evidence for such an association in a previous study by Gray and Hoffenberg might be explained by the inclusion of thyrotoxic patients without Graves' disease.

Stress and Graves' Disease: A Causal Relationship?

The case–control studies do not provide conclusive evidence that stress plays a causative role in the immunopathogenesis of Graves' hyperthyroidism because of their retrospective nature. It would be ideal to have prospective studies with regular stress evaluation in euthyroid subjects at risk for developing Graves' disease to see whether the stress load is higher in subjects who become hyperthyroid than in subjects who remain euthyroid; such studies have not been done. But there have been two prospective studies in patients with Graves' hyperthyroidism who were investigated when euthyroid on antithyroid drug treatment. In both studies, Yoshiuchi and Fukao observed higher scores of daily hassles in patients who experienced recurrent hyperthyroidism after the discontinuation of antithyroid drugs than in patients who remained euthyroid.

Matos-Santos et al. evaluated stressful life events in Graves' hyperthyroid patients and controls and also in 31 patients with toxic nodular goiter – a nonautoimmune disease causing thyrotoxicosis. The number and impact of negative stressful life events were higher in patients with Graves' disease than in patients with toxic nodular goiter or controls, whereas the difference between patients with toxic nodular goiter and controls was not significant. The data suggest that hyperthyroidism itself is not responsible for more stressful life events preceding the diagnosis of thyrotoxicosis; the data, rather, support the view that stress precipitates autoimmunity.

There are almost no data on a putative relationship between stress and TPO antibodies, an early marker of autoimmune thyroid disease, except a study by Strieder et al., who compared euthyroid women with or without TPO antibodies. No difference was found between both groups in the number of stressful life events, the number of daily hassles, or the scores of negative and positive affect scales. Stress apparently seems more related to thyroid autoimmunity against the TSH receptor, causing Graves' hyperthyroidism. This is underlined by a significant increase in the incidence of Graves' disease in eastern Serbia during the civil war in former Yugoslavia. The specificity of this finding is indicated by the fact that during the same time period the incidence of toxic nodular goiter did not increase. Chiovato et al. did not find a single case of Graves' hyperthyroidism in patients with panic disorder; they hypothesize that failure to activate the hypothalamic-pituitary-thyroid axis by chronic endogenous stress due to panic disorder (as opposed to exogenous stress due to life events) might explain why panic disorder does not precipitate Graves' hyperthyroidism.

It can be concluded that the association between stressful life events and the onset of thyrotoxicosis is specific for Graves' hyperthyroidism and that stress probably is involved in the immunopathogenesis of Graves' disease. How stress contributes to the precipitation of the disease is presently poorly understood. The activation of the hypothalamus-pituitary-adrenal axis would be expected to cause immunosuppression rather than autoimmunity. Paradoxically, however, a surprising increase in Graves' disease was reported in patients with multiple sclerosis undergoing anti-T cell immunosuppressive therapy. Regulatory CD4+ CD25+ T-cells may be involved. These cells suppress autoimmune disease; if these cells are more sensitive to immunosuppression and slower to regenerate than other T cell subsets, this may explain the paradoxical observations.

Further Reading

Chiovato, L., Marino, M., Perugi, G., et al. (1998). Chronic recurrent stress due to panic disorder does not precipitate Graves' disease. *Journal of Endocrinological Investigation* 21, 758–764.

Dayan, C. M. (2001). Stressful life events and Graves' disease revisited. *Clinical Endocrinology* 55, 13–14.

Fukao, A., Takamatsu, J., Murakami, Y., et al. (2003). The relationship of psychological factors to the prognosis of hyperthyroidism in antithyroid drug-treated patients with Graves' disease. *Clinical Endocrinology* 58, 550–555.

Gray, J. and Hoffenberg, T. (1985). Thyrotoxicosis and stress. *Quarterly Journal of Medicine* 214, 153–160.

Kung, A. W. C. (1995). Life events, daily stresses and coping in patients with Graves' disease. *Clinical Endocrinology* 42, 303–308.

Matos-Santos, A., LacerdaNobre, E., Costa, J. G. E., et al. (2001). Relationship between the number and impact of stressful life events and the onset of Graves' disease and toxic nodular goitre. *Clinical Endocrinology* 55, 15–19.

Mizokami, T., Li, A. W., El-Kaissi, S., et al. (2004). Stress and thyroid autoimmunity. *Thyroid* 14, 1047–1055.

Paunkovic, N., Paunkovic, J., Pavlovic, O., et al. (1998). The significant increase in incidence of Graves' disease in Eastern Serbia during the civil war in the former Yugoslavia (1992 to 1995). *Thyroid* 8, 37–41.

Radosavljevic, V. R., Jankovic, S. M. and Marinkovic, J. M. (1996). Stressful life events in the pathogenesis of Graves' disease. *European Journal of Endocrinology* 134, 699–701.

Rosch, P. J. (1993). Stressful life events and Graves' disease. *Lancet* **342**, 566–567.

Sonino, N., Girelli, M. E. and Boscaro, M. (1993). Life events in the pathogenesis of Graves' disease: a controlled study. *Acta Endocrinologica* **128**, 293–296.

Strieder, T. G. A., Prummel, M. F., Tijssen, J. G. P., et al. (2005). Stress is not associated with thyroid peroxidase antibodies in euthyroid women. *Brain, Behavior, and Immunity* **19**, 203–206.

Winsa, B., Adami, H-O. and Bergström, R. (1991). Stressful life events and Graves' disease. *Lancet* **338**, 1475–1479.

Yoshiuchi, K., Kumano, H., Nomura, S., et al. (1998). Psychosocial factors influencing the short-term outcome of antithyroid drug therapy in Graves' disease. *Psychosomatic Medicine* **60**, 592–596.

Yoshiuchi, K., Kumano, H., Nomura, S., et al. (1998). Stressful life events and smoking were associated with Graves' disease in women, but not in men. *Psychosomatic Medicine* **60**, 182–185.

Grieving

A Ray
Harvard Medical School and Dana-Farber Cancer Institute, Boston, MA, USA

H Prigerson
Dana-Farber Cancer Institute, Harvard Medical School, and Brigham and Women's Hospital, Boston, MA, USA

This article is a revision of the previous edition article by S Noaghiul and H Prigerson, volume 2, pp 289–296, © 2000, Elsevier Inc.

Introduction
Diagnosis of Complicated Grief
Outcomes and Risk Factors of Complicated Grief
Treatment

Glossary

Complicated grief	The experience of debilitating grief symptoms 6 months postloss and beyond.
Separation anxiety	Fear and anxiety provoked by the threat of separation from a primary attachment figure.

Introduction

Grieving describes the emotional state associated with losing a person to whom one is attached. Bereavement is a natural part of life, and the normal process of grieving is self-limited and is most commonly not a cause for clinical concern. Despite this, research shows that bereavement is one of the most challenging life experiences and that bereaved people, as a group, have a higher risk of mortality and morbidity. This increased risk is largely a function of the significant minority for whom the process of grieving becomes overwhelming, causing distress and disruption for an unusually long period. In these cases of complicated grief, there is cause for clinical concern and appropriate interventions are required.

Normal Grief

The vast majority of bereaved individuals experience normal or uncomplicated grief. Although normal grieving is painful and disruptive initially, eventually bereaved survivors are able to accept the loss as a reality and move on with life. They are able to carry out daily functions and gradually begin to enjoy leisure activities.

One of the most commonly cited models of normal grief resolution among professionals and laypersons is Kubler-Ross's stage theory. This theory proposes orderly progression through the following stages: disbelief or shock, yearning, anger and protest, depressed mood, and ultimate acceptance of the loss. Recent research attempting to test this theory suggests that multiple stages may be present simultaneously. Instead of clear-cut stages, on average the bereaved person's distress gradually declines as acceptance increases.

For the first few months following the loss, the symptoms of uncomplicated grief are difficult to distinguish from complicated grief. After 6 months, however, the majority of bereaved individuals have reached some level of acceptance, are able to engage in productive and enjoyable activities, and can remain connected with others while developing new relationships. Bereaved survivors who are experiencing adjustment difficulties 6 months postloss, such as suicidal thoughts and gestures, major depressive disorder (MDD), or posttraumatic stress disorder (PTSD), and those who are experiencing persistent symptoms of grief are a cause for clinical concern.

Resilient Responses to Bereavement

Some bereaved people exhibit little or no distress postloss. Bereavement experts have debated the causes for this. Some have suggested that minor grief symptoms may signify a more superficial attachment to the deceased. Others have suggested that low distress levels following a significant personal loss are the sign of a maladjusted, emotionally distant person. The traditional view has been to see the lack of grief as denial or an inhibition of the normal grieving process. Thus, these bereaved people have been counseled to assist in the resolution of their latent grief. Studies have shown, however, that some of these subjects may have a healthy resilience to loss that allows them to recover with little disruption in functionality. By this view, resilient subjects have little to benefit from grief counseling because they show little evidence of struggling internally with the loss. Still, using the absence of grief as a marker for resilience is somewhat controversial. Because grief intensity is in direct proportion to the attachment to the deceased, the absence of grief is truly a mark of experienced resilience only if the attachment to the deceased was very strong. This is often difficult to assess. However, there is much to be gained in further understanding the resilient response so that individuals struggling with grief can adopt some of these successful coping strategies.

Diagnosis of Complicated Grief

Descriptive Features

The term complicated grief has been used interchangeably with pathological grief, abnormal grief, atypical grief, and pathological mourning. At one time traumatic grief was also used, but since the attacks on September 11, 2001, this term has been reserved for the psychological reaction following a traumatic event and for grief following the loss of a person during such an event. The term complicated grief is now primarily used to describe the experience of losing a person to natural causes.

Complicated grief can be described as a state of chronic mourning. The bereaved survivor cannot accept the reality of the loss and as a result is reluctant to make any adaptations to life. The psychological distress is characterized by intense yearning for the absent loved one. His or her constant focus on the absence of the deceased creates a barrier to maintaining and forging relationships. This simply heightens the sense of isolation the bereaved person feels. This state of grieving has been shown to be a risk factor for suicidal thoughts and ideation, over and above any confounding influences of diagnoses such as MDD.

Diagnostic Criteria

The proposed set of diagnostic criteria for complicated grief from the *Diagnostic and Statistical Manual of Mental Disorders* (5th edn.; DSM-V) is shown in **Table 1**. This diagnosis requires that the bereaved person be persistently yearning for the deceased in a manner that disrupts his or her daily life. In addition, four of the following eight symptoms must be experienced to a distressing and disruptive degree (i.e., several times a day, interfering with social or occupational functioning): trouble accepting the death, inability to trust others since the loss, excessive bitterness related to the death, feeling uneasy about moving on, detachment from formerly close others, feeling life is meaningless without the deceased, feeling that the future holds no prospect for fulfillment without the deceased, and feeling agitated since the death. Also, as mentioned earlier, the severity and number of symptoms must persist for at least 6 months, regardless of when those 6 months occur in relation to the loss. This allows both chronic and delayed types of grief to be included in the diagnosis.

There is evidence to support the 6-month delay in making a complicated grief diagnosis. It is important

Table 1 Criteria for complicated grief proposed for DSM-V[a]

Criterion A	Yearning, pining, and longing for the deceased; yearning must be experienced at least daily over the past month or to a distressing or disruptive degree
Criteria B	In the past month, the person must experience four of the following eight symptoms as marked, overwhelming, or extreme:
	Trouble accepting the death
	Inability to trust others since the death
	Excessive bitterness or anger about the death
	Feeling uneasy about moving on with his or her life (e.g., difficulty forming new relationships)
	Feeling emotionally numb or detached from others since the death
	Feeling life is empty or meaningless without the deceased
	Feeling the future holds no meaning or prospect for fulfilment without the deceased
	Feeling agitated, jumpy, or on edge since the death
Criterion C	The symptom disturbance causes marked dysfunction in social, occupational, or other important domains
Criterion D	The symptom disturbance lasts at least 6 months

[a]From Prigerson, H. G., Vanderwerker, L. C. and Maciejewski, P. K. (in press). Chapter 8. In: Stroebe, M., Hansson, R., Schut, H. & Stroebe, W. (eds.) *Handbook of bereavement research and practice: 21st century perspectives*. New York: American Psychological Association Press.

to allow time for the normal grieving symptoms to subside, in order to detect those who are unusually distressed. This allows for a more conservative threshold for diagnosing complicated grief, and we are less likely to include false-positive patients whose symptoms will eventually naturally resolve. Also, patients still experiencing symptoms at 6 months were found to be less likely to experience natural grief resolution and more likely to experience negative outcomes 13–23 months postloss.

Differential Diagnosis

Bereavement may be complicated by a number of other psychiatric disorders. Major depression is the primary reported disorder following the death of a loved one. However, complicated grief symptoms form a symptom cluster distinct from the depressive or anxiety-related symptom clusters. Depressive symptoms include depressed mood, psychomotor retardation, and decreased self-esteem; complicated grief is specifically associated with yearning, disbelief, detachment, bitterness, and anger related to the death. PTSD is another complication associated with bereavement, especially if the death was associated with a traumatic incident. Studies have shown, however, that unlike PTSD, complicated grief in response to a natural death is not accompanied by fears of violent harm to self and others, hypervigilance, or avoidance of a fear-inducing stimulus. Complicated grief may, of course, occur in conjunction with PTSD in the context of the violent death of a loved one. In fact, complicated grief does frequently occur in addition to MDD and/or PTSD; however, many cases of complicated grief are currently missed due to the reliance on guidelines for psychiatric diagnoses provided in the DSM-IV.

Other factors that set complicated grief apart from MDD and PTSD are the risk factors, outcomes, and responses to treatment.

Outcomes and Risk Factors of Complicated Grief

Physical and Psychological Outcomes

Bereaved subjects suffering from complicated grief have been found to suffer myriad negative consequences. Long periods of distress and dysfunction may be responsible for this. Complicated grief has been associated with heightened risks of cancer, hypertension, cardiac events, and suicidal ideation. It has also been associated with disability, functional impairment (social, familial, and occupational dysfunctions), hospitalization, and reduced quality of life. Those suffering from complicated grief are also more likely to engage in unhealthy behaviors such as alcohol and cigarette consumption. Psychologically, patients with complicated grief are more likely to develop comorbid conditions with depressive symptoms and major depressive episodes. The relative risks for negative health outcomes associated with complicated grief are summarized in **Table 2**.

Risk Factors

Given the negative outcomes of untreated complicated grief, the identification of at risk individuals should be a priority for clinicians. Several possible risk factors for the development of complicated grief have been identified in studies. One important risk factor is the closeness of the relationship between the bereaved and the deceased. Relationships that were dependent, confiding, and close led to the poorest bereavement adjustment. In fact, relationships that are conflicted at baseline result in lower rates of bereavement disorders. The belief that complicated grief is fundamentally an attachment disturbance is borne out by the identification of weak parental bonding in childhood as a risk factor for complicated grief. Bereaved people with a damaged sense of security due to childhood abuse or severe neglect have a higher risk of experiencing complicated grief as adults. Childhood separation anxiety was identified as a risk factor as well. Also, individuals who are generally averse to change of any kind (e.g. lifestyle changes) are more likely to experience complicated grief. Two factors that have been found to reduce the risk of complicated grief are advance preparation for the death and a strong support network.

Thus, in summary, patients who have attachment difficulties at baseline and who feel unprepared and unsupported during and after the death are at higher

Table 2 The relative risk of some negative health outcomes among bereaved individuals diagnosed with complicated grief at 6 months postloss[a]

Health outcome (incidence)	Relative risk	Confidence interval (95%)
High systolic blood pressure at 13 months post loss	1.11	1.02–1.20
Depression at 13 months post loss	2.72	0.84–8.81
Changes in smoking at 13 months post loss	16.7	0.86–320.4
Changes in eating at 13 months post loss	7.02	1.62–30.6
Heart trouble at 25 months post loss	1.15	1.04–1.27
Problems with alcohol at 25 months post loss	1.25	0.98–1.63

[a]From El-Jawahri, A. and Prigerson, H. G. (in review). Evidence-based guidelines for the diagnosis and treatment of complicated bereavement. *Journal of Palliative Medicine.*

risk of experiencing complicated grief. This indicates that interventions geared toward preparing caregivers for the impending death of a loved one, as well as promoting secure alternative engagements to others, would be helpful in the treatment of persistent grief symptoms.

Treatment

As previously mentioned, there is a strong connection between a lack of preparedness for the death of a loved one and the development of complicated grief postloss. Thus, it would seem that interventions administered preloss might prove promising at reducing bereaved survivors' risk of complicated grief. Clinicians who provide palliative care might extend their efforts to the caregivers of a dying patient, encouraging them to say goodbye and accept the impending loss. This would entail a greater comfort with prognosticating the end of life, an issue that is fraught with controversy and complexity.

Just as physician involvement and communication can increase the chances of caregivers being prepared for the death, similarly, hospice enrollment has been shown to reduce the risk of MDD. This is consistent because hospice enrollment usually requires acceptance that death will occur within 6 months, intimating caregiver preparedness. In the Netherlands, a study found that caregivers of cancer patients who died by euthanasia were less likely to experience disruptive grief symptoms than those whose loved ones died a natural death. This, too, is consistent, given that euthanasia implies a greater acceptance of the patient's prognosis on the part of the caregivers.

Concrete interventions to help caregivers prepare for the loss center around proactively assisting caregivers to "hope for the best, plan for the worst." Traditionally, getting one's affairs in order include making an effort to visit the patient and expressing appreciation, regrets, and reassurances before it is too late. In addition, health-care professionals should not hesitate to recommend hospice and palliative care services when their need becomes apparent. An earlier referral to a hospice has been shown to be beneficial in promoting a peaceful death and lessening distress for caregivers.

As noted earlier, after the loss, in most cases grief is manageable and resolves naturally, requiring no professional interventions. Bereavement interventions are more appropriate for those individuals who are particularly at risk or those who present with unremitting, severely disruptive grief symptoms six months postloss.

Research has shown that interventions such as nortriptyline and interpersonal psychotherapy, which were effective for the treatment of depressive symptoms, were not effective in treating grief symptoms. To date, there have been no randomized controlled trials of pharmacotherapies for the reduction of grief-symptom severity. Open trials of selective serotonin reuptake inhibitors have been conducted and suggest that these and similar agents show promise for the reduction of complicated grief symptom severity, but randomized placebo-controlled trials are needed before more definitive conclusions can be drawn about their efficacy for the amelioration of complicated grief symptomatology.

Future pharmacotherapeutic options may also evolve from ongoing studies of functional neuroanatomy. In one study, grieving subjects were exposed to visual and verbal stimuli to remind them of the deceased. The stimuli led to activation in the posterior cingulate cortex, cerebellum, and medial/superior frontal gyrus. Thus, grief is mediated through a complex network involving affect processing, visual imagery, autonomic regulation, memory retrieval, processing of familiar faces, and modulation/coordination of these functions. New insights into the long-term health consequences of grief may follow, as well as therapies to modulate the neurochemical response.

As mentioned previously, a lack of social support is a significant risk factor for the development of complicated grief. Thus, it follows that bereaved individuals who lack a social network may be helped greatly by group therapy and support groups. Studies show that the perception of social support leads to a reduction of depression, whereas group therapy for complicated grief leads to an increase in perceived support.

One therapy specifically developed for complicated grief is known as complicated grief treatment. This combines a number of different approaches, including psychoeducation about normal grief and complicated grief, a dual focus on adjusting to the loss and restoration of a satisfying life, and motivational therapy to create appropriate life goals. This therapy was found to be more effective in a shorter time than interpersonal psychotherapy in a population of complicated grief patients. However, given the eclectic nature of the treatment, it is difficult to discern which specific component is providing the main benefit. Using a model in which grief is conceptualized as trauma, the therapy also includes desensitization through imagined conversations with the deceased, retelling of the death scene, and viewing photographs of the deceased. For nontraumatic deaths, however, this aspect of the treatment may be less important than dealing with issues of attachment, separation, loss, and reattachment.

Further research will yield insight into the most effective therapies for bereaved people suffering from overwhelming grief symptoms. Most important, an understanding of complicated grief will encourage clinicians to help prepare caregivers of terminally ill patients for their loss. Providing appropriate resources before the loss will better facilitate normal grieving and grief resolution and ensure that survivors can more successfully adapt and resume a functional and joyful life.

Further Reading

Bowlby, J. (1980). *Attachment and loss. Vol. 3: Loss: sadness and depression*. New York: Basic Books.

Brown, G. W. and Harris, T. O. (1989). Depression. In: Brown, G. W. & Harris, T. O. (eds.) *Life events and illness*, pp. 49–94. New York: Guilford Press.

Clayton, P. J. (1990). Bereavement and depression. *Journal of Clinical Psychiatry* 51, 34–38.

El-Jawahri, A. and Prigerson, H. G. (in review). Evidence-based guidelines for the diagnosis and treatment of complicated bereavement. *Journal of Palliative Medicine*.

Freud, S. (1953–1974). Mourning, melancholia (1917). In: Strachey, J. (ed.) *Standard edition of the complete psychological works of Sigmund Freud*, (vol. 14), pp. 239–258. London: Hogarth Press and the Institute of Psychoanalysis.

Jacobs, S. (1993). *Pathologic grief: maladaptation to loss*. Washington, DC: American Psychiatric Press.

Kubler-Ross, E. (1969). *On death and dying*. New York: Macmillan.

Parkes, C. M. and Weiss, R. S. (1983). *Recovery from bereavement*. New York: Basic Books.

Prigerson, H. G., Bierhals, A. J., Kasl, S. V., et al. (1997). Traumatic grief as a risk factor for mental and physical morbidity. *American Journal of Psychiatry* 154, 616–623.

Prigerson, H. G., Frank, E., Kasl, S. V., et al. (1995). Complicated grief and bereavement-related depression as distinct disorders: preliminary empirical validation in elderly bereaved spouses. *American Journal of Psychiatry* 152, 22–30.

Prigerson, H. G. and Jacobs, S. C. (2001). Perspectives on care at the close of life. caring for bereaved patients: "all the doctors just suddenly go." *Journal of the American Medical Association* 286, 1369–1376.

Prigerson, H. G., Maciejewski, P. K., Reynolds, C. F., III, et al. (1995). Inventory of complicated grief: a scale to measure maladaptive symptoms of loss. *Psychiatry Research* 59, 65–79.

Prigerson, H. G,. Vanderwerker, L. C. and Maciejewski, P. K. (in press). Chapter 8. In: Stroebe, M., Hansson, R., Schut, H. & Stroebe, W. (eds.) *Handbook of bereavement research and practice: 21st century perspectives*. New York: American Psychological Association Press.

Shear, M. K., Frank, E., Houck, P., et al. (2005). Treatment of complicated grief: a randomized controlled trial. *Journal of the American Medical Association* 293, 2601–2659.

Zisook, S. and Shuchter, S. (1993). Uncomplicated bereavement. *Journal of Clinical Psychiatry* 54, 365–372.

Relevant Website

National Cancer Institute. http://www.nci.nih.gov.

Group Therapy

N Wong
Uniformed Services University of the Health Sciences, Bethesda, MD, USA

This article is a revision of the previous edition article by N Wong, volume 2, pp 297–301, © 2000, Elsevier Inc.

Rationale for Group Therapy
Therapeutic Elements of Group Therapy
Applications
Conduct of Group Therapy

Glossary

Abreaction	A process by which repressed material, particularly a painful experience or conflict is brought back into consciousness. In the process, the person not only recalls but relives the emotional situation and experiences the appropriate emotional response.
Catharsis	The verbalization of ideas, thoughts, and expressed material that is accompanied by an emotional response and that produces a state of relief to the individual.

Corrective recapitulation of the primary family group	The phenomenon that patients in a therapy group relate to the group leaders and other members in ways reminiscent of how they once interacted with their parents, siblings, or other significant figures as they grew up; also called family reenactment.
Counter-transference	Reactions evoked in the therapist in response to the patient. These feelings, conscious or unconscious, may be realistic or arise from unresolved pathology. They are regarded as analogs of the patient's transferences.
Group debriefing	An intervention and stress management technique in which the major elements of a trauma are reviewed by participants in an attempt to prevent or reduce the immediate or long-term adverse psychological changes. Although it is therapeutic, is conducted in a group setting, and employs many principles and techniques of group therapy, group debriefing is not truly group therapy. It may proceed to group therapy if the members request that meetings continue because of persistent symptomatology and both the leader and members agree to further sessions.
Group facilitator	A support or educational group leader who assists the group in maintaining its boundaries, keeps the group on task, and provides group feedback by sharing observations and summarizing the process of the group with its members. The intent of the facilitator is not to attempt individual personality changes but to encourage self-learning, attitudinal shifts, and stress reduction.
Group therapist/leader	The most important person in the group; responsible for selecting and preparing patients, forming the group, and conducting the group in a manner that models ideal group behavior and creates therapeutic group norms to enable its members to attain their therapeutic goals, which may involve personality and behavior changes.
Group therapy	A widely accepted psychiatric treatment modality that uses therapeutic forces within the group, constructive interactions between members, and interventions of a trained leader to change the maladaptive behavior, thoughts, and feelings of people with a psychiatric disorder.
Repression	The unconscious act of controlling and inhibiting an unacceptable impulse, emotion, or thought.
Suppression	The conscious act of controlling and inhibiting an unacceptable impulse, emotion, or thought.
Transference	In the classic sense, all aspects of a patient's feelings and behavior toward a therapist, including rational and irrational aspects that arise from unconscious sources; usually classified into positive and negative reactions. In the general sense, it includes real aspects of the relationship and the unconscious influences of parental or other meaningful figures early in the individual's development.
Universality	The experience by the patient in a group setting that he or she shares many similarities and features in common with others, that "We are all in the same boat."

Rationale for Group Therapy

Some of the principles of group therapy have been applied with success in the fields of business and education in the form of training, sensitivity, and encounter groups. Individuals participating in such groups are generally not regarded as having a psychiatric disorder. Group therapy is also used in the prevention of psychiatric illness, and some of its tenets are applied in debriefing formats for acute stress reactions. Because of the numerous forms of group therapy, it is more accurate to speak of the many group therapies. However, for the sake of simplicity, it should be understood that the generic term group therapy in this article is used to describe a wide array of treatments in a group setting with their particular requirements and different objectives and goals.

Treatment in groups is a proven and effective therapeutic modality for stress-related conditions. Historically, the group has served as a protector and nurturer of the individual and a purveyor of culture. Although originating in the United States in 1905, group methods were initially used by English psychiatrists who were under pressure to treat the vast number of psychiatric casualties suffering from stress and trauma during World War II. In the safe environment of the group, patients or members have the opportunity to interact with others in a setting reflective of society at large; to gain mutual support; to be exposed to new learning situations; to express and benefit from altruism, which in itself can be beneficial; and to find opportunities for multiple healthy identifications and catharsis. In the group, a here-and-now focus and interpersonal relationships are stressed more than in individual therapy.

Therapeutic Elements of Group Therapy

Numerous conceptual models of group therapy exist, but they share in common certain therapeutic elements or factors that have been studied and found to be curative for individuals in groups. More than 200 group process and therapeutic elements have been described in the literature to account for the curative changes that occur in group therapy. These can be classified into the broad categories of intellectual, emotional, and action factors. One of the most widely accepted classifications identifies 11 primary elements: the installation of hope, universality, the imparting of information, altruism, the corrective recapitulation of the primary family group, the development of socializing techniques, imitative behavior, interpersonal learning, group cohesiveness, catharsis, and existential factors. The therapeutic factors, are frequently interdependent and share similarities.

Not all of these curative or therapeutic factors need to be present for the group to be effective. Certain types of groups require the presence of particular elements. For example, in groups dealing with stress disorders arising from an acute or immediate traumatic event, emphasis is placed on imparting information, abreaction, catharsis, and universality. When the stress has been chronic and caused conditions of a chronic nature, there is a greater focus on interpersonal learning, the corrective recapitulation of the primary family group, and the development of socializing techniques, in addition to the aforementioned factors. In the latter setting, transference and countertransference are more likely to occur.

Types of Groups

Group therapy is used in inpatient and outpatient settings, institutional work, partial hospitalization units, halfway houses, community settings, and private practice. Open-ended groups exist for an indefinite time period, are open to new members, and pursue a variety of therapeutic goals. Closed-ended groups are time-limited, closed to new members, and focus on achieving a particular goal or purpose. Time-limited groups, or short-term groups, are commonly employed to treat people with acute stress-related disorders. The duration of treatment is ordinarily stated at the start of the group and rarely exceeds several months. Individuals exposed to a traumatic or catastrophic event may be seen for only one group session.

Placement in a long-term group is usually indicated for patients who have experienced chronic stress from underlying medical conditions or needing to reduce chronic stress that may contribute to the formation of physical or emotional illnesses. Long-term groups typically run for several months to several years and convene at regular and frequent intervals such as once or twice weekly.

Group Size

The size of the group varies considerably in the treatment of stress-related conditions. When a catastrophic or traumatic event involves a large number of people, debriefing groups may have as many as 100 or more people, whereas a therapy group for posttraumatic stress disorder (PTSD) patients usually consists of 5–10 members. Generally, smaller groups are more appropriate for an intensive and prolonged group therapy experience.

Group Composition

Individuals placed in a group setting for the treatment or prevention of psychiatric symptoms or illness in which stress plays a prominent role are admitted on the basis of their primary symptom (such as phobias, anxiety, or depression), an illness or diagnosis (such as PTSD; cancer; or human immunodeficiency virus, HIV), or an event (such as rape, surviving the Holocaust or a concentration camp, or a recent disaster). Although secondary considerations of age, gender, socioeconomic, and ethnic factors are of lesser importance in stress-related groups than in traditional group therapy, a compatible matching of these elements may ensure greater success for the individual and the group.

Applications

Group therapy is useful for people who have experienced a vast number of situations or medical conditions in which stress plays a major role. Some examples include PTSD patients, sexual or physically abused victims, concentration camp survivors and their families, bereaved people, cancer patients, and family members and caretakers of patients with chronic mental or physical illnesses. There are established groups for patients with HIV and acquired immunodeficiency syndrome (AIDS), with chronic fatigue syndrome, with ulcerative colitis, with heart disease, with diabetes, with obesity, with fibromyalgia, and on long-term dialysis. The list is varied and growing.

Conduct of Group Therapy

The basic principles of group therapy are observed in most therapy groups, although the approach varies with the type of group that has been formed in response to the specific situation. A few of the common approaches and indications for group treatment are described next.

Group Debriefing

Perhaps the most widely known and used intervention to treat individuals exposed to acute traumatic situations, the aims of group debriefing are to manage the immediate emotional distress and to prevent adverse long-term psychological changes. There are several debriefing protocols; one of the best known and most widely practiced is the critical incident stress format developed by J. Mitchell in 1981. The protocol consists of consecutive phases in which various aspects of a traumatic exposure are explored and worked through by the participants. The focus remains on the individual and not on the group. Members are encouraged to recall their personal experiences of the traumatic event to allow for ventilation and to attempt to understand and master the confusion and trauma. Education and the mobilization of social support are key elements in this approach, and symptomatic individuals are identified and referred for further treatment. Some of the goals of debriefing are to assist individuals to regain emotional and cognitive controls; reduce cognitive dysfunction; diminish traumatic conditioning; and reduce group scapegoating, projection, and nihilistic and antisocial attitudes that may arise in response to the trauma and to correct improper information about the event. Debriefing is usually conducted in naturally occurring groups, is considered short term, lasting at most only a few sessions. Because this approach has the potential to produce negative outcomes as well as positive results, it is essential that the leader or leaders be well trained in group work.

Cancer Groups and Groups for the Terminally Ill

Depending on the nature of the illness and prognosis, cancer and terminally ill patient support groups may be short or long term and open- or closed-ended. Breast cancer group therapy has been the best researched of the group approaches and in many studies it has been shown to increase the length and quality of patients' lives. Patients suffering from terminal cancer experience significant stress in attempting to deal with their anguish, loss of control over what is happening to them, physical pain and disability, and sense of uselessness while awaiting death. Through the group experience, they are afforded the opportunity to find meaning outside themselves and provided a sense of purpose as they support one another and share their life experiences.

Patients in the terminal stage of cancer frequently harbor irrational and rational anger toward their families, the helping professions, and society in general. The group experience often assists them to transcend their immediate plight to find a deeper meaning for their existence and to accept death with greater equanimity. Similarly, the caretakers of these patients who are members of cancer support groups derive emotional support and gain helpful information from others to reduce their stress levels and to deal with the resentment, guilt, and anger that may develop in the course of caring for terminally ill relatives.

The hypothetical 5-year waiting period during which no evidence of recurrence has been found and a cure is likely is a stressful time for many post-treatment cancer patients. Group therapy for these recovering patients may be long term and supportive in nature as individuals share medical information, personal setbacks, and coping strategies. For many members, it is a time for personal growth and maturation as they struggle with their illness and the impact it has had on their lives.

The main therapeutic elements present in successful cancer groups appear to be group cohesion, social support, enhancing communication skills with family and health-care workers, relaxation training, and the opportunity for emotional expressiveness.

Support Groups for Other Medical Conditions

Group therapy has been useful for a wide array of medical illnesses that are partially caused or aggravated by stress. In turn, stress may arise as a consequence of suffering with a medical illness. Most of these groups are open-ended, long term, and meet on a regular basis. Many of the therapeutic elements found in cancer support groups are also present in these groups. Major emphasis is placed on imparting information, learning coping skills, social support, the installation of hope, and dealing with here-and-now situations. Unlike those in cancer support groups, the patients in these groups may not face imminent death despite the chronicity and severity of their illnesses.

Posttraumatic Stress Disorder Groups

Group therapy is one of the most widely used treatments for patients with PTSD. Individuals diagnosed with acute PTSD, in which the symptoms have been present for less than 3 months, may be treated successfully in a time-limited or short-term group. Individuals showing symptoms of a chronic PTSD generally require long-term treatment.

In the various group therapies used for patients with these disorders, the goals and objectives are to contain their severe distress and suffering and to improve the quality of their lives. To attain these ends, a variety of group approaches are employed, ranging from a cognitive behavioral focus to the use of psychodynamically oriented psychotherapy. The behavioral model emphasizes the reduction of symptoms, the acquisition and maintenance of coping skills, and the systematic examination of the assumptions and misattributions that govern the patient's behavior, expectations, and appraisal of events (as described in the works of Foa and colleagues in the 1990s). Prominent in these groups are the mechanisms of group cohesiveness, imparting of information, imitative behavior, interpersonal learning, and installation of hope.

Since the 1970s, Horowitz and his colleagues have researched and firmly established that a psychodynamically oriented approach is successful in the treatment of PTSD. The goal for the traumatized patient is to reconcile the occurrence of the trauma with his or her personal concept and the world. The principal aim of this therapy is to assist individuals to integrate their traumatic experiences through the therapeutic reexperiencing of the events in a supportive environment. Attempts are made to gain insight into the conscious and unconscious meaning of the symptoms to enable patients to master the trauma and restore functioning. This approach acknowledges the influence of dispositional variables on the patients' response to the trauma and therapy and emphasizes the use of the corrective recapitulation of the primary family group, interpersonal learning, insight, and catharsis more than other types of group treatments for stress.

Staff and Caretaker Support Groups

Because of a heightened awareness of dementias, especially Alzheimer's disease, the increasing longevity of the world population, and the large numbers of the chronically mentally and physically ill, participation and interest in staff and caretaker groups have grown significantly. Typically, health-care providers and caretakers operate under high and sustained daily levels of stress, and they benefit from participation in a group. The emphasis on these groups is to enable individuals to provide better patient care and smoother functioning in their surroundings through improved staff well-being. The groups are usually conducted by a facilitator instead of a group therapist or leader, and the goals and objectives are to assist members in reducing stress rather than to explore personal conflicts or to attempt personality change. Group meetings may occur weekly, on an ad hoc basis, or for a set number of sessions in defined modules over the span of a year.

Benefits gained from participating in the group experience include decreased anxiety, reduced sense of isolation, more open communication between caregivers, increased self-esteem, improved adaptation in working with patients or ill family members, and greater group cohesion and teamwork.

Scapegoating and irrationality diminish, patient-care goals become more realistic, and staff members are better able to tolerate and accept pain and suffering in their patients without feeling excessive personal distress.

Concentration Camp and Torture Survivor Groups

A large number of Holocaust survivors exist in the world, with Israel alone housing over 250,000. In addition to Holocaust survivors, there are concentration camp survivors from the Bosnia-Herzegovina war and survivors of torture from Central and South America and nations in Africa. Many elderly Holocaust survivors manifest the survivor syndrome, typically, reporting anxiety, sleep disorders, affective disturbances, and survivor guilt. As these individuals age, their symptoms intensify because of economic and health problems and because of the constant reminder of their previous plight due to the unstable world situation with reports of internment camps, torture, terrorism, and serious religious and ethnic conflicts. Exiled survivors of torture must deal with the acute trauma, loss of family or close ones, often forced migration, and adaptation to a new culture.

Group therapy is supportive in nature and attempts to help survivors cope with the anxieties and painful memories that are still fresh or have been rekindled by disturbing world events, work through the mourning for lost relatives and their own personal losses, improve their mental equilibrium, and enhance their adaptation to their inner and outer worlds. A major objective is to create a sense of safety and well-being in the groups so patients can express themselves freely. Attempts are made early in therapy to create supportive group interpersonal relationships with active leader interventions to help members integrate their painful past with current joys and successes in the present. Many of these groups are open-ended both for membership and in duration because rarely are these individuals able to completely set aside what has happened to them and to successfully proceed in life without a periodic resurgence of disturbing symptoms.

Rape and Sexual Abuse Victims Groups

Victims of rape and sexual abuse typically experience effects on body image, identity, self-regulation, and interpersonal functioning. If the abuse has occurred in childhood and is ongoing, these areas may be affected profoundly. Victims experience both acute and chronic stress when reminded of the trauma, and they are frequently conflicted in their social and sexual relationships. Group therapy helps victims through the reenactment of the traumatic situation and abuse in the confines of a safe environment, increases their capacity for self-soothing, deals therapeutically with the shame, and teaches patients how to end the cycle of repeated victimization.

The therapeutic or curative factors of universality, interpersonal learning, catharsis, developing socializing techniques, and imparting information are prominent in the group processes. The groups may be short or long term, depending on the acuity of the situation. These groups are often open-ended to accommodate newcomers and to allow previous members to return for periodic reinforcement and support of their newly acquired knowledge and behaviors. Psychoeducation is provided in these groups to instruct patients about abuse effects, in developing problem-solving skills, and in becoming active in supportive topic-focused discussions.

In summary, group therapy or a group therapeutic approach is an effective modality in the treatment of acute and chronic stressful conditions. Indications for group therapy mirror those for individual approaches; but the group has as an advantage the presence of group therapeutic or curative factors not present in individual therapy. The group becomes a safe haven and laboratory where members learn from one another, practice new behaviors in a supportive setting, and are provided opportunities to show altruism, which in itself is a constructive healing force. The group serves as a microcosm of society from which members can venture forth again into the larger society with new knowledge and personal gains from the group experience.

Some individuals find it difficult, if not impossible, to develop sufficient trust and the sense of confidentiality in a group setting, and they may require an introductory period of individual care before introducing them to group therapy. In addition, individuals may benefit from a combination of concurrent individual and group approaches to test out new behaviors and learning.

Perpetrator Groups

Perpetrator groups are gaining in popularity with the increase in public awareness about sexual predators and about emotional and physical abuse in relationships. Common in institutional and court-directed settings, many are now present in both community and private locations. Individuals are afforded a safe environment for catharsis, to sense their impact on others with similar backgrounds, to gain understanding into their behavior, and to learn techniques to control and modify their destructive behavior. These groups tend to be long term and open-ended, and they may employ treatment principles found in alcohol and substance abuse groups. Anger management techniques and psychoeducation also play important roles.

See Also the Following Articles

Acute Stress Disorder and Posttraumatic Stress Disorder; Cancer Treatment; Holocaust Survivors, Experiences of; Posttraumatic Therapy; Reenactment Techniques.

Further Reading

Abramowitz, I. A. and Coursey, R. D. (1989). Impact of an educational support group on family participants who take care of their schizophrenic relatives. *Journal of Consulting and Clinical Psychology* 57, 232–236.

Allan, R. and Scheidt, S. (1998). Group psychotherapy for patients with coronary heart disease. *International Journal of Group Psychotherapy* 48, 187–214.

Baider, L. and De-Nour, A. K. (1989). Group therapy with adolescent cancer patients. *Journal of Adolescent Health Care* 10, 35–38.

Classen, C., Butler, L. D., Koopman, C., et al. (2001). Supportive-expressive group therapy and distress in patients with metastatic breast cancer: a randomized clinical trial. *Archives of General Psychiatry* 58, 494–501.

Forester, B., Kornfeld, D. S., Fleiss, J. L., et al. (1993). Group psychotherapy during radiotherapy: effects on emotional and physical distress. *American Journal of Psychiatry* 150, 1700–1706.

Foy, D. W., Ruzek, J. I., Glynn, S. M., et al. (2002). Trauma focused group therapy for combat-related PTSD: an update. *Journal of Clinical Psychology* 58, 907–918.

Freehill, K. M. (1992). Critical incident stress debriefing in health care. *Critical Care Clinics* 8, 491–500.

Gregurek, R. (1999). Countertransference problems in the treatment of a mixed group of war veterans and female partners of war veterans. *Croatian Medical Journal* 40, 493–497.

Kelly, J. A. (1998). Group psychotherapy for persons with HIV and AIDS-related illnesses. *International Journal of Group Psychotherapy* 48, 143–162.

Lansen, J. and Cels, J. P. (1992). Psycho-educative group psychotherapy for Jewish child-survivors of the Holocaust and non-Jewish child-survivors of Japanese concentration camps. *Israeli Journal of Psychiatry & Related Sciences* 29, 22–32.

Wallis, D. A. (2000). Reduction of trauma symptoms following group therapy. *Australian and New Zealand Journal of Psychiatry* 36, 67–74.

Wong, N. (2005). Group psychotherapy and combined individual and group psychotherapy. In: Sadock, B. J. (ed.) *Kaplan and Sadock's comprehensive textbook of psychiatry* (8th edn., pp. 2568–2583). Philadelphia: Lippincott Williams and Wilkins.

Yalom, I. D. (1995). The theory and practice of group psychotherapy. New York: Basic Books.

Gulf War Syndrome, Psychological and Chemical Stressors

H Soreq
Hebrew University of Jerusalem, Jerusalem, Israel

This article is a revision of the previous edition article by H Soreq, volume 2, pp 302–312, © 2000, Elsevier Inc.

Acute Psychological Stress and Exposure to Anticholinesterases Cause Similar Delayed Effects

The Blood–Brain Barrier Is Disrupted under Stress

Early Immediate Response Genes Modulate Acute Stress Signals

Hypothalamic-Pituitary-Adrenal Involvement in Acute Stress Responses

Poststress Changes Are Long-Lasting

Acetylcholinesterase Accumulation Confers Protection against Anticholinesterases

Acetylcholinesterase Gene Expression Associates with State and Trait Anxiety

Delayed Nervous System Deterioration under Persistent Acetylcholinesterase Overexpression

Retrospective and Prospective Implications

Glossary

Acetylcholinesterase (AChE) inhibitors	Chemical agents capable of preventing the enzyme acetylcholinesterase from performing its catalytic function, namely, the hydrolysis of acetylcholine. These inhibitors may vary in their chemical structure and include natural compounds, drugs, commonly used insecticides, and chemical warfare agents.
Alternative splicing	A molecular process through which a single gene may produce more than one protein with distinct properties.
Blood–brain barrier (BBB)	The complex structures and processes that prevent the free penetration of compounds into the brain (and free exit from it). It includes the epithelial cells lining the walls of blood vessels in the brain and the end foot of astrocytes surrounding these blood vessels. The tight junctions between endothelial cells in brain blood vessels are major players in this function, as are several proteins and active pumps controlling the move of compounds in and out of the brain.
Psychological stress	An emotional state of anxiety and hyperexcitation that may have various origins

and causes and that varies in intensity. It probably is important to ensure rapid, alert functioning under external insults; however, it may also cause delayed adverse consequences at different levels and functions.

Transgenic overexpression	The excessive production of a foreign protein in the cells and tissues of an organism that has been made transgenic by the introduction of foreign DNA into its genome. The transgene included in this DNA directs the production of its protein product in the host organism, leading to overexpression because it is produced in addition to the normal functioning of the host gene.

Acute Psychological Stress and Exposure to Anticholinesterases Cause Similar Delayed Effects

Posttraumatic stress disorder (PTSD) involves delayed cognitive deterioration, depression, irritability, and persistent deficits in short-term memory, as summarized by Robert Sapolsky in 2003. Stress-induced changes in nervous system structure and function appear in many diverse species, suggesting that they reflect an evolutionarily conserved adaptation to environmental insults. For example, magnetic resonance imaging (MRI) demonstrates reduced hippocampal volume in PTSD patients.

Surprisingly similar effects are often reported years after acute or chronic exposures to cholinesterase inhibitors. The use of the carbamate anticholinesterase (anti-AChE) pyridostigmine during the Gulf War for prophylactic protection under threat of chemical warfare emphasizes the importance of this topic, as does the increasing use of anti-AChE drugs for the treatment of Alzheimer's disease. **Table 1** summarizes these reports.

Neurophysiological stress events are initiated by millisecond-long bursts of neurotransmitter release, whereas the long-term, persistent brain changes occur at a very slow pace, sometimes over years. Moreover, stress responses primarily elicit hormonal modulations in peripheral tissues, and ACh controls inflammatory reactions. Yet, it is not clear how this imprints on brain structure and function in a long-delayed manner. Finally, the link between structural and functional properties in the brain itself calls for an

Table 1   Common outcomes of psychological stress and anticholinesterase exposure[a]

	Organism	Inducer
Neuropathological phenomena		
Excessive sprouting and retraction of neuronal processes	Mollusk	Variety of stressors
Decreased density of dendritic spines, where synaptic connections take place	Transgenic mice overexpressing AChE	Cage life
Atrophy of apical dendrite in the hippocampus region CA3	Tree shrews (primate)	Restraint stress
Reduced hippocampal volume	Humans (war veterans)	Acute traumatic war experience
Degenerative changes in the spinal cord	Hens	Low-level exposure to the organophosphate anti-AChE leptophos
Degeneration of the hippocampus	Rats	Low-level exposure to the organophosphate anti-AChE fenthion
Arrest of neuronal proliferation	Primates (rhesus)	Sociological stress
Impaired functioning		
Enhanced long-term depression of hippocampal activity	Rats	Mild behavioral stress
Enhanced long-term depression and suppressed long-term potentiation of hippocampal activity	Rats	Restraint stress and electric tail shock
Increased permeability of the blood–brain barrier	Mice	Forced swimming stress, transgenic AChE overexpression
Behavioral changes	Primates (*Callithrix jacchus jacchus*)	Psychological stress
Deficits in short-term memory, long-term psychopathologies	Humans	Combat-related stress, childhood abuse
Impaired firing of CA1 neurons in the hippocampus	Rabbits	Acute exposure to the organophosphate anti-AChE parathion
Suppressed long-term potentiation in the hippocampus	Rats	Acute exposure to the organophosphate anti-AChE soman
Memory impairments	Rats	Low-level exposure to the organophosphate anti-AChE DFP or phosphorodithioate
Increased permeability of the blood–brain barrier	Rats	Soman intoxication
Deficient cognitive performance	Rhesus monkeys	Soman intoxication
Progressive deterioration of memory and general cognitive decline	Humans	Organophosphate pesticide poisoning
Intensified traumatic memories	Mice	Immobilization stress

[a]Long-term consequences of psychological insults and anticholinesterase exposures in various evolutionarily remote species. Note the similarities in the nature of the changes observed in both the structural and functional properties of neurons. AChE, acetylcholinesterase; DFP, diisopropyl-fluorophosphonate.

in-depth study of the causal relationships leading to these changes.

The Blood–Brain Barrier Is Disrupted under Stress

Several studies have demonstrated enhanced penetration of the brain by anti-AChEs under psychological stress. This stress-induced disruption of the BBB can explain some of the nervous system-associated sequelae reported by Gulf War veterans. Soldiers at the Gulf were exposed to unknown doses and combinations of various harmful xenobiotics. For prophylactic protection from the anticipated chemical warfare agents, which would have irreversibly blocked acetylcholinesterase (AChE), Gulf War soldiers were administered pyridostigmine, a reversible carbamate cholinesterase inhibitor. Pyridostigmine includes a quaternary ammonium group that under normal circumstances prevents its crossing the BBB. Thanks to this property, it is used routinely to treat peripheral neuromuscular

junction deficiencies in patients with the autoimmune disease myasthenia gravis. During peacetime clinical tests that involved healthy volunteers, pyridostigmine caused mild, primarily peripheral side effects. In contrast, during the Gulf War, pyridostigmine in the same dosage caused a significant increase in reported central nervous system (CNS) symptoms. Friedman and colleagues showed, in animal experiments, that the dose of pyridostigmine required to block 50% of brain AChE was 100-fold lower in stressed mice.

The sudden need for energy in the stressed brain suggests that the disruption of the BBB may be beneficial when neurons are overactivated. Nevertheless, BBB disruption may also allow toxic agents and unneeded proteins to penetrate the brain, which may impair brain functioning under stress. However, the linkage between neuronal excitability and the nature of those impairments is still largely obscure. AChE inhibitors, which increase cholinergic signaling by preventing acetylcholine (ACh) hydrolysis, were reported to cause transient permeabilization of the

BBB. Revealing the molecular mechanisms underlying the links between cholinergic and other elements in BBB-associated cells should therefore contribute significantly toward our understanding of the mechanism(s) leading to BBB disruption under psychological stress. Because cholinergic neurotransmission is imbalanced following traumatic impacts, this question was addressed using transgenic mice overexpressing synaptic AChE. Diffusion-weighted MRI showed impaired water diffusion and BBB functioning, and DNA microarray analyses demonstrated the enhanced production of multiple ion channels and the water channel aquaporin 4. Thus, persistent cholinergic imbalance may by itself cause BBB malfunctioning.

Early Immediate Response Genes Modulate Acute Stress Signals

The similar symptoms reported for patients with PTSD and those exposed to anti-AChEs pointed to ACh as the common inducer of these delayed responses. Several pieces of evidence support this conclusion.

1. Robust elevations of ACh levels occur under both PTSD and anti-AChE intoxication.
2. ACh interaction with an ACh receptor(s) elevates intracellular Ca^{2+} levels, inducing the transcription of genes that have promoters with Ca^{2+} response elements (CRE motifs).
3. One of these Ca^{2+}-induced genes encodes the early immediate transcription factor c-*Fos*. Interestingly, c-*Fos* expression is elevated drastically within minutes under stress.

Both the choline acetyltransferase gene, *ChAT*, and the AChE gene, *ACHE*, are subject to stress-induced regulation. The first intron in the *ChAT* gene includes the coding sequence for the vesicular ACh transporter VAChT. Together they form the cholinergic locus. Therefore, these two mRNA transcripts are coregulated, and the early immediate gene (IEG) c-*Fos* can control both the initiation and the termination of cholinergic neurotransmission. This operates through regulating ACh production by *ChAT*, its vesicle packaging by VAChT, and its hydrolysis by AChE. Measurements of mRNA levels in conjunction with neurophysiology tests have indeed demonstrated the suppression within 3 h of the initial cholinergic hyperexcitation, most likely through the suppression of ACh synthesis (through decreases in ChAT and VAChT mRNA levels) and the enhancement of its hydrolysis (through increases in AChE mRNA levels) within 30 min postinsult. However, the association of stress processes with the bimodal suppression of the initial increase in released ACh does not tell us how

specific c-*Fos* dimers sort out their respective promoters to induce the observed opposing effects. Moreover, it is not clear how much of the increased intracellular Ca^{2+} is due to influx through specific channels in the plasma membrane and how much of it results from Ca^{2+} release from intracellular stores. In addition, other IEGs may also contribute to the observed phenomenon. For example, the activation of muscarinic cholinergic receptors induces multiple IEGs. Also, the time scale of the Ca^{2+}-induced transcriptional response should be refined. Most important, the initial phase of the feedback response probably leads to delayed cascades of the transcription of other relevant genes, and both the scope and the nature of these secondary phenomena are still unknown.

Hypothalamic-Pituitary-Adrenal Involvement in Acute Stress Responses

Stress-induced activation of the hypothalamic-pituitary-adrenal (HPA) axis enhances the release of adrenocorticotropic hormone (ACTH) from the hypothalamus and of corticosterone from the adrenals. Corticosterone, in turn, stimulates the production of several cytokines, among them interleukin (IL-)1, tumor necrosis factor (TNF), and IL-6. Tracey and colleagues have found that ACh controls the production of pro-inflammatory cytokines by tissue macrophages. This suggests that AChE overproduction and the resultant reduction in ACh levels induce an increase in the inflammatory reactions, as summarized in **Figure 1**. Thus, the capacity for AChE overproduction under stress affects both peripheral and brain-mediated responses. When produced in the brain, IL-1 interacts with IL-1 type I and type II receptors. This induces c-*Fos* overproduction, which further potentiates the peripheral production of steroid hormones. Therefore, many responses evoked by stress depend on the activation of the HPA axis, are prevented by adrenalectomy, and can be mimicked by exogenous corticosterone (or cortisol in humans). Glucocorticoids induce increases in intracellular Ca^{2+} within the hippocampal neurons, inducing neurotoxic effects in the brain, mainly atrophy and degeneration of hippocampal neurons that are enriched in glucocorticoid receptors. Brain endothelial cells also express IL-1 receptors, suggesting a link between this cytokine, the BBB, and the HPA axis.

Not all stress responses are totally dependent on adrenal functions. An example is the cholinergic feedback response to stress and anti-AChEs described earlier, which apparently includes an HPA-independent component. This is supported by the following:

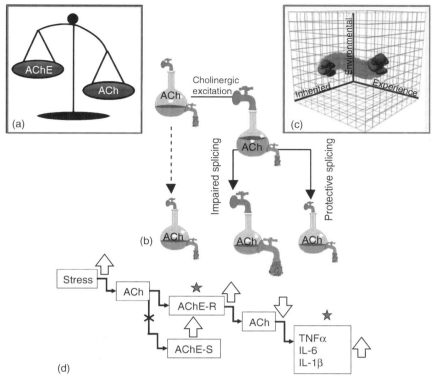

Figure 1 Cholinergic reactions to stress. a, Acetylcholinesterase (AChE) and acetylcholine (ACh) balance determines the cholinergic signaling status; b, cholinergic excitation modifies the alternative splicing of AChE-mRNA transcripts; c, origins of risk factors affecting stress reactions; d, links among stress, cholinergic signaling, and inflammatory reactions. In b, cholinergic synapses are presented as glass beakers, with ACh inflow shown as the top taps and ACh outflow as water streaming out. Impaired splicing (i.e., accumulated synaptic AChE-S) potentiates the outflow, whereas protective splicing (production of AChE-R) maintains balanced flow. When mimicked in transgenic mice, impaired splicing exacerbates stress neuropathology, whereas protective splicing ablates it. In c, a schematic graph shows inherited, experience-derived (e.g., increased body mass index), and environmental measures (e.g., insecticides exposure) affecting the level of risk for stress-induced damages. In d, stress induces ACh release, which induces a shift from synaptic AChE-S to the stress-induced AChE-R splice variant. The excess AChE reduces ACh, which relieves the control over production by tissue-residing macrophages of pro-inflammatory cytokines. Therefore, AChE-R levels are associated with those of pro-inflammatory cytokines (stars). AChE-R, readthrough variant of acetylcholinesterase; AChE-S, synaptic form of acetylcholinesterase; IL, interleukin; TNFα, tumor necrosis factor α.

1. Acute ACh release and its delayed suppression occurred in adrenalectomized rats.
2. Stress-induced overproduction of c-*Fos* mRNA occurs in adrenalectomized mice.
3. The transcriptional feedback response occurs in brain slices.
4. Transgenic mice with a cholinergic, but not HPA, imbalance show impaired BBB and stress neuropathology.

Altogether, this information calls for further research into the specific contributions of the HPA and internal brain processes to the cholinergic feedback response.

Poststress Changes Are Long-Lasting

Alternative splicing produces three AChE isoforms. Of these, the readthrough variant (AChE-R) encodes a hydrophilic enzyme form secreted as a globular monomer following stress events. The amphiphilic soluble properties of the stress-induced AChE isoform may provide easy accessibility to extracellular spaces flooded under stress with excess ACh. This form of the enzyme is therefore best suited for suppressing the activation of ACh receptors that is associated with stress or anti-AChE exposures.

Biochemical analyses of catalytically active AChE demonstrated that globular monomers are produced following treatment with diisopropylfluorophosphonate (DFP; a potent AChE inhibitor) and in the cerebrospinal fluid (CSF) of Alzheimer's disease patients.

In the nonstressed brain, AChE mRNA is positioned around the nucleus of cortical neuronal somata. Following stress or under anti-AChEs, AChE-mRNA appears throughout the cell body, extending to prolonged dendrites. Intracellular changes in the distribution of mRNAs are often associated with modified functions of their protein products. Therefore, Meshorer and coworkers postulated in 2002 that this altered localization may be physiologically significant.

The poststress accumulation of AChE takes place primarily in cholinoceptive brain regions involved in learning and memory, such as the cortex and the hippocampus. The accumulation of the enzyme in the hippocampus is relatively short-lived (a few hours). This suggests the cessation of the poststress AChE-mRNA transcription (or the enhanced degradation of AChE-mRNA or protein) in brain regions that extend cholinergic afferents to the hippocampus. In contrast, cortical AChE levels remain significantly elevated over 3 days poststress. This may reflect continuous local production in cortical cholinergic interneurons. The initiation of CNS stress responses can thus lead, within milliseconds and continuing for several days at least, to AChE excess in the mammalian cortex. Interaction of the stress-induced AChE with signaling kinases can explain the changes induced in neuronal functioning.

Acetylcholinesterase Accumulation Confers Protection against Anticholinesterases

The accumulation of brain AChE increases the concentration of binding sites for anti-AChEs. For example, Kaufer et al. demonstrated in 1998 that pyridostigmine doses that reduce body temperature in normal, untreated FVB/N mice have no effect when administered 24 h after stress treatment. Similarly, transgenic mice overexpressing AChE in their brain neurons also display resistance to the hypothermic response to pyridostigmine. This supports the conclusion that the stress-induced resistance to anti-AChEs is due to AChE accumulation because elevated AChE levels persist in the brains of these mice. Pyridostigmine protects against the lethal effects of chemical warfare agents that are anti-AChEs. The protection conferred by pyridostigmine may therefore be related, at least in part, to AChE overproduction that is induced by pyridostigmine during the first few hours following treatment.

Acetylcholinesterase Gene Expression Associates with State and Trait Anxiety

Recent genotype–phenotype interaction studies support the notion of AChE interactions with stress responses. In the U.S. population, volunteers with polymorphisms debilitating the functioning of the *ACHE* gene or the adjacent paraoxonase *PON1* gene on the long arm of chromosome 7 were found to display increased trait anxiety or the tendency for state anxiety, as shown in **Figure 2**.

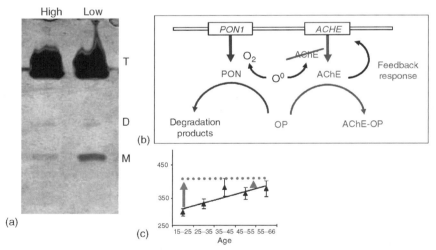

Figure 2 Association of AChE and PON variations with state and trait anxiety. a, Gel electrophoresis of serum samples from volunteers with high or low trait anxiety; b, the putative genomic link; c, age-dependent changes in the capacity for AChE overproduction ($R^2 = 0.73$). In a, note that subjects with low anxiety show more AChE monomers (M) than those with high anxiety, although tetramers (T) and dimers (D) remain unmodified ($N = 472$ volunteers). Thus, the alternative splicing process yielding AChE-R monomers links to trait anxiety. In b, the *ACHE* and *PON1* genes are positioned close to one another on the long arm of chromosome 7. Exposure of AChE to organophosphate inhibitors (OP) inhibits its activity by forming irreversible AChE–OP complexes. This induces a feedback response leading to AChE overproduction. However, paraoxonase (PON) degrades OPs, thus protecting the AChE protein. In addition, PON functions as a peroxidase, protecting blood proteins (AChE included) from oxidative stress. In c, blood AChE levels increase by over 25% between the ages 15 and 66, suggesting a progressive limitation in the capacity for stress-induced AChE overproduction (arrows).

Delayed Nervous System Deterioration under Persistent Acetylcholinesterase Overexpression

Apart from its capacity to hydrolyze ACh, the AChE protein possesses other, noncatalytic activities. These are apparently related to neurite extension in cholinergic as well as dopaminergic neurons and are fully sustained in genetically inactivated AChE. This suggests that the structural effects of AChE might also operate when the AChE protein is inactivated catalytically by anti-AChEs. The long-term outcome of neuronal AChE excess was studied in patients with the autoimmune disease myasthenia gravis and in rats with experimental autoimmune myasthenia. In both cases, the chronic overproduction of AChE-R was observed. Antisense oligonucleotide suppression of this excess enzyme improved neuromuscular functioning in treated rats. Parallel outcomes in clinical trials was reported at the U.S. Society of Neurology in 2004. In the neuromuscular junctions of AChE transgenic mice (the synapses connecting motor neurons with the innervated muscle), impaired neuromuscular transmission was observed. Similar phenomena were reported for patients with neurodegenerative or neuromotor syndromes associated with cholinergic malfunction, such as Down syndrome, Alzheimer's disease, and myasthenia gravis. Indeed, Farchi and co-workers reported the deterioration of the physiological responses of AChE transgenic muscle, reminiscent of those of myasthenia patients.

Exposure to agricultural insecticides, which serves as a case study for the risks involved in exposure to chemical warfare agents, also increases the risk of Parkinson's disease. It was known for several decades that this risk also involves predisposing genotype–phenotype elements. In a study performed in Israel, this increased risk was found to be associated with debilitating polymorphisms in the ACHE and the PON1 genes. Exposed patients showed an increased incidence of such debilitating polymorphisms, suggesting that an inherited interactive weakness of AChE and PON1 was the cause. These findings, reported by BenMoyal-Segal and co-workers, are schematically presented in Figure 3.

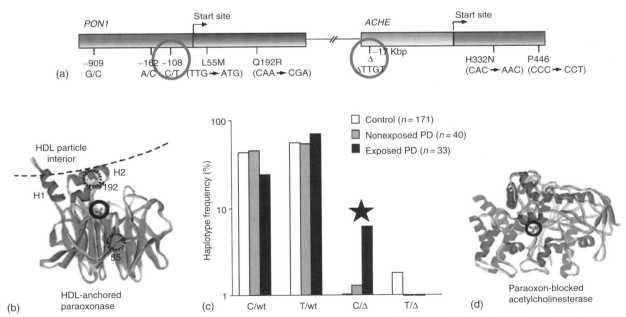

Figure 3 Risk-associated ACHE/PON1 polymorphisms are strongly overrepresented in exposed Parkinson's disease (PD) patients. a, The ACHE/PON1 locus; b, the PON1 protein and frequent polymorphisms; c, graphs of increased incidence of debilitating ACHE/PON1 haplotype in insecticide-exposed Parkinson's patients; d, the AChE protein and its interaction with paraoxon. In a, a diagram of the adjacent ACHE and PON1 genes is shown, with the tested nucleotide polymorphisms marked below. The two debilitating polymorphisms found frequently in patients with Parkinson's disease who were continuously exposed to agricultural insecticides are circled. In b, the crystal structure of paraoxonase is shown with the two frequent changes in it, in positions 55 and 192. Note that PON1 interacts with blood lipids (HDLs). The paraoxon binding site is circled. In d, the crystal structure of the AChE protein is shown. Paraoxon is circled in its deep-buried binding site, where its binding blocks AChE functioning irreversibly. Star indicates a statistically significant difference in the incidence of the debilitating ACHE/PON1 polymorphisms within insecticides-exposed Parkinson's disease patients. C/Δ, carriers of the robust PON1 and the debilitated AChE variant; C/wt, carriers of the two robust variants; HDL, high-density lipoprotein; T/Δ, carriers of the two debilitated variants; T/wt, carriers of debilitated PON1 and robust AChE.

Retrospective and Prospective Implications

The feedback response to acute stress and anti-AChEs apparently varies in its intensity with age, body mass index, gender, and ethnic origin. Homozygous carriers of mutations in the *ACHE* homologous *BCHE* gene, encoding serum butyrylcholinesterase (BCHE; e.g., the atypical variant), have anomalous responses to cholinergic drugs. In such individuals, relatively low doses of anti-AChEs may penetrate the brain quite effectively, which results in higher effective doses than intended. This creates a genetic predisposition to adverse responses to anti-AChEs. This inherited sensitivity, and the findings already summarized, raise a concern with regard to the long-term dangers of chronic exposure to household and agricultural insecticides because these are frequently organophosphate or carbamate anti-AChEs. Moreover, the partial symptomatic relief offered by the currently approved Alzheimer's disease anti-AChE drugs appears to be limited in its duration, suggesting that the feedback response to stressor anti-AChEs marks the initiation of progressive damage caused by the production of excess AChE. AChE, an important constituent of cholinergic neurotransmission, may thus cause neuropathological damage when it accumulates in the mammalian brain over long periods. Like many other essential proteins, AChE should be there at the right time and in the right amount or else it can initiate a vicious cycle of long-term harmful responses.

Acknowledgments

Writing this article would not have been possible without the contribution of my co-workers. Special thanks are due to Daniela Kaufer, Alon Friedman, Ella Sklan, and Noa Farchi for research contributions and to Eyal Soreq for artwork. Research was supported by grants from the Israel Science Fund, The Israel Ministry of Defense, and Ester Neuroscience, Ltd.

See Also the Following Articles

Combat Stress Reaction; Persian Gulf War, Stress Effects of; War-Related Posttraumatic Stress Disorder, Treatment of.

Further Reading

Benmoyal-Segal, L., Vander, T., Shifman, S., et al. (2005). Acetylcholinesterase/paraoxonase interactions increase the risk of insecticide-induced Parkinson's disease. *FASEB Journal* 19(3), 452–454.

Birikh, K., Sklan, E., Shoham, S., et al. (2003). Interaction of "readthrough" acetylcholinesterase with RACK1 and PKCbetaII correlates with intensified fear-induced conflict behavior. *Proceedings of the National Academy of Sciences USA* 100, 283–288.

Brenner, T., Hamra-Amitay, Y., Evron, T., et al. (2003). The role of readthrough acetylcholinesterase in the pathophysiology of myasthenia gravis. *FASEB Journal* 17(2), 214–222.

Darreh-Shori, T., Hellstrom-Lindahl, E., Flores-Flores, C., et al. (2004). Long-lasting acetylcholinesterase splice variations in anticholinesterase-treated Alzheimer's disease patients. *Journal of Neurochemistry* 88(5), 1102–1113.

Farchi, N., Soreq, H. and Hochner, B. (2003). Chronic acetylcholinesterase overexpression induces multilevelled aberrations in mouse neuromuscular physiology. *Journal of Physiology* 546(1), 165–173.

Friedman, A., Kaufer, D., Shemer, J., et al. (1996). Pyridostigmine brain penetration under stress enhances neuronal excitability and induces early immediate transcriptional response. *Nature Medicine* 2, 1382–1385.

Kaufer, D., Friedman, A., Seidman, S., et al. (1998). Acute stress facilitates long-lasting changes in cholinergic gene expression. *Nature* 393, 373–377.

Meshorer, E., Erb, C., Gazit, R., et al. (2002). Alternative splicing and neuritic mRNA translocation under long-term neuronal hypersensitivity. *Science* 295(5554), 508–512.

Meshorer, E., Biton, I., Ben-Shaul, Y., et al. (2005). Chronic cholinergic imbalances promote brain diffusion and transport abnormalities. *FASEB Journal* 19(8), 910–922.

Nijholt, I., Farchi, N., Kye, M., et al. (2004). Stress-induced alternative splicing of acetylcholinesterase results in enhanced fear memory and long-term potentiation. *Molecular Psychiatry* 9(2), 174–183.

Pollack, Y., Gilboa, A., Ben-Menachem, O., et al. (2005). Acetylcholinesterase inhibitors reduce brain and blood interleukin-1β production. *Annals of Neurology* 57(5), 741–745.

Sapolsky, R. (2003). Bugs in the brain. *Scientific American* 288(3), 94–97.

Sklan, E. H., Lowenthal, A., Korner, M., et al. (2004). Acetylcholinesterase/paraoxonase genotype and expression predict anxiety scores in Health, Risk Factors, Exercise Training, and Genetics study. *Proceedings of the National Academy of Sciences USA* 101(15), 5512–5517.

Soreq, H. and Seidman, S. (2001). Acetylcholinesterase – new roles for an old actor. *Nature Reviews Neuroscience* 2, 294–302.

Tracey, K. J. (2002). The inflammatory reflex. *Nature* 420(6917), 853–859.

Weinberger, D. R. (2001). Anxiety at the frontier of molecular medicine. *New England Journal of Medicine* 344(16), 1247–1249.

H

Headache *See:* Migraine.

Health and Socioeconomic Status

T Chandola and M Marmot
University College London, London, UK

This article is a revision of the previous edition article by M Marmot and A Feeney, volume 2, pp 313–321, © 2000, Elsevier Inc.

Socioeconomic Gradient in Health
Model
Explanations

Glossary

Psychosocial factors	Measurements of psychological phenomena that relate to specific social environments.
Social exclusion	People or areas that suffer from a combination of linked problems such as poor health, unemployment, inadequate skills, low incomes, poor housing, high crime rates, lack of educational opportunities, and family breakdown.
Socioeconomic gradient	The positive association between greater socioeconomic disadvantage and the amount of death, disability, and disease.
Socioeconomic status	An individual's rank or status in a social hierarchy, usually evaluated with reference to a person's access to and consumption of goods, services, and knowledge in a society.

Socioeconomic Gradient in Health

The association between health and socioeconomic status results in the socioeconomic gradient in health. In rich countries, people who are more socioeconomically disadvantaged have poorer health and higher levels of chronic and infectious diseases. In poor countries, there is a similar socioeconomic gradient in infectious diseases and an emerging socioeconomic gradient in chronic diseases such as obesity.

These observed socioeconomic gradients are not simply a question of poverty. **Figure 1** shows the infant mortality rate by levels of wealth in some of the poorest countries in the world. There is a strong socioeconomic gradient in infant mortality, with richer people, in the poorest countries of the world, having much lower rates of infant mortality compared to poorer people. It is not just the poor who have high infant mortality rates. Those who are not poor, but also not rich, have higher infant mortality rates compared to the richest groups in poor countries.

Furthermore, within rich countries, there is a socioeconomic gradient in health even among relatively well-off sections of society. One of the most famous examples of this comes from the Whitehall and Whitehall II studies of British civil servants. In the original Whitehall study, which started in 1960, the initial finding after 5 years of follow-up was that coronary heart disease mortality was higher in the lower employment grades of the British civil service. After 25 years of follow-up, there was a similar finding of an inverse gradient in mortality: the lower the grade, the higher the mortality. Data from the more recent Whitehall II study (1985–2004) shows a similar inverse gradient in all-cause mortality. In **Figure 2**, as we proceed lower down the civil service hierarchy of jobs, the risks of mortality increase for all-cause, cardiovascular, and coronary heart disease deaths. It is not just the poor who suffer from higher levels of mortality and disease. Those who cannot be described as being in poverty, such as clerical British civil servants, have poorer health than the people at the top of the socioeconomic hierarchy.

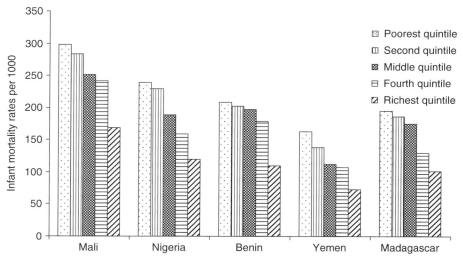

Figure 1 Infant mortality rates by wealth quintiles in Mali, Nigeria, Benin, Yemen and Madagascar. Data from Gwatkin et al. (2000).

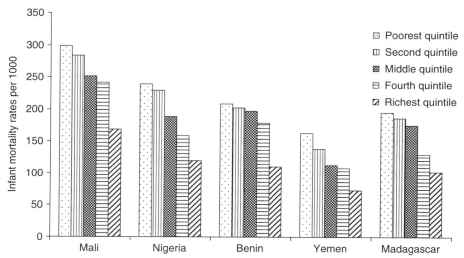

Figure 2 Percentage distribution of deaths by employment grade, adjusted for age and sex: Whitehall II cohort followed up for 19 years.

Socioeconomic status (SES) refers to an individuals' rank or status in a social hierarchy, usually evaluated with reference to a person's access to and consumption of goods, services, and knowledge in a society. A number of different measures have been used as proxy indicators of SES, including income, educational level, and occupational prestige. Although they all display similar socioeconomic gradients in health and disease, it is important to distinguish between different measures of SES, as they may affect health through different mechanisms and pathways. For example, education is likely to have indirect effects on health through positive effects on occupation and income as well as on other factors influencing health, including health-related behaviors such as smoking and diet.

Furthermore, measurements of SES need to specify which period of life they are meant to represent. Socioeconomic disadvantage can accumulate over a lifetime, from early childhood, to school level education, to work experiences and living conditions, and on to retirement. Each of these periods of socioeconomic disadvantage can have independent effects on health later on in life. Because being disadvantaged at an earlier period increases the risk of being disadvantaged later in life, measures of SES across the life course are usually correlated with each other. However, a measure of SES in mid-life may not adequately capture the specific risks for poor health that arise from living in disadvantaged socioeconomic circumstances in childhood.

Any explanation of the association between SES and health has to take account of the socioeconomic gradient. This is not just a question about a divide between those living in poverty and others. Explanations need to take account of the socioeconomic gradient in risk factors for disease and mortality and their distribution across the population. Furthermore, the challenge for explanations is not only to explain the socioeconomic gradient, but also to suggest how it is possible for everyone in the population to have the good health enjoyed by those at the top of the socioeconomic ranks. In order to progress toward eliminating socioeconomic gradients in health, we need to understand the causes of this gradient in health. For this, we need to have an appropriate model to describe how SES can get under our skin and affect health.

Model

It is not difficult to understand how poverty in the form of material deprivation – dirty water, poor nutrition, lack of medical care – can account for the poorer health and higher mortality of poor people. However, poverty alone cannot explain the socioeconomic gradient in health. First, dirty water, lack of calories, and poor medical care cannot account for why British civil servants who work in clerical jobs are over twice as likely to die compared to those in the top ranks of the civil service. Furthermore, the poverty-only model fails to take into account the fact that relief of such material deprivation is not simply a technical matter of providing clean water or better medical care – those resources are socially determined. Even among poorer sections of society, those who are relatively better off are more likely to take advantage of policy interventions to provide better material living conditions, thereby potentially perpetuating and increasing the socioeconomic gradient in health.

In order to reduce inequalities in health, we need to understand the mechanisms and pathways that link the socioeconomic circumstances to health. **Figure 3** presents a simplified model of how different causal factors link the social structure to cardiovascular disease outcomes. This helps us to understand the different mediators and pathways linking SES to health.

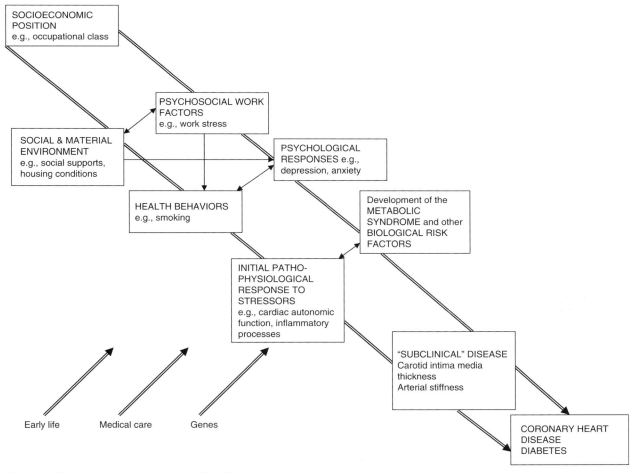

Figure 3 Model of social determinants of health.

This is not meant to be a complete model but a simplified representation. There are further causal factors that may be added to the model, and more causal arrows that may be drawn. This model, in particular, draws our attention to how potential causal factors in the work, social, living, and material environments relate to health behaviors or to more direct psychological processes that influence the psycho-neuro-endocrine-immune systems of the body.

This model helps us to understand how different causal factors interrelate, and it also provides a guide to potential points of intervention for reducing inequalities in health. For example, the metabolic syndrome is a risk factor for heart disease. Treatment of the metabolic syndrome through medical care may reduce heart disease, but may not reduce the socioeconomic gradient in heart disease if poorer people are less likely to have access to or get treated for the metabolic syndrome. Another potential point of intervention could be to change the health behaviors that influence the development of the metabolic syndrome. Getting more people to quit smoking may reduce the development of the syndrome, but telling people to quit smoking alone is not enough. The model suggests that there is a socioeconomic gradient in smoking that alerts us to the socioeconomic factors that underlie smoking behaviors. In order to reduce the socioeconomic gradient in the metabolic syndrome and consequently reduce heart disease, we need to understand the causes of the causes: the living, working, social, and material environmental contexts in which these health behaviors originate and operate. So if stressful work circumstances make it hard to give up smoking, we need to identify interventions that reduce stress at work. If being poor makes it hard to afford quitting smoking aids, then these aids need to be made freely available.

Explanations

The concept of multiple causal factors operating in conjunction with each other, as outlined in **Figure 3**, is not unique to the development of chronic diseases. Although the tubercle bacillus is the specific cause of tuberculosis, most people infected with the tubercle bacillus do not have clinical tuberculosis. Other factors, such as those associated with poverty and nutrition, influence susceptibility to the disease. In the case of tuberculosis, exposure to an infectious agent is not enough to cause a disease. The exposure, in conjunction with the socioeconomic circumstances, affects the development of the disease.

Similarly, we do not believe that the material, behavioral, psychosocial, and environmental causal

factors outlined in **Figure 3** operate in isolation. The division of explanations of the socioeconomic gradient in health into these categories often dismisses the interrelationships and interactions between all of them. So instead, the following sections highlight some of the broad groups of factors related to the social determinants of health, all of which encompass different dimensions and combinations of material, behavioral, psychosocial, and environmental factors.

Early Life

Research from observational and intervention studies shows that the foundations of adult health are laid in early childhood and even before birth. Slow growth, poor emotional support, and socioeconomic deprivation in childhood increase the risk of poor physical, emotional, and cognitive functioning in adulthood. There is a strong patterning of these childhood risk factors for poor adult health by SES.

A number of factors associated with pregnancy, such as nutritional deficiencies during pregnancy, maternal stress, maternal smoking, misuse of drugs and alcohol, insufficient exercise, and inadequate prenatal care, can lead to less than optimal fetal development, low birth weight, and subsequently to an increased risk of heart disease in adulthood. A mother living in poorer socioeconomic circumstances is much more likely to experience some of these risk factors for poor fetal development compared to a mother living in better circumstances.

Infancy is a particularly important period of time for the development of integrated biological systems with long-term consequences for adult health. Research shows that biological systems in infancy are highly malleable through cognitive, emotional, and sensory inputs into the brain. Insecure emotional attachment and poor stimulation in infancy can lead to problematic behaviors in childhood, and adolescence as well as low educational attainment. This in turn increases the risk of social marginalization in adulthood and the ability to obtain employment or steady jobs. Furthermore, health-promoting behaviors in adulthood, such as exercise, healthy diet, and not smoking, are influenced by such parental behaviors in childhood.

It has been argued that parental poverty starts a chain of social and biological risk. Parental poverty increases the risk of poor fetal development, stimulation, and emotional and cognitive inputs in infancy. This leads to slow growth in childhood, poor behavior and educational attainment at school, leading to a raised risk of unemployment, low-status jobs, and lower SES. All of these links in the chain have consequences for physical and mental health in adulthood and old age – some of them indirectly, through influencing the risks further down the chain, others more directly influencing adult health. However, it is also possible to break the links between the chains at critical periods of social and biological development. This is the area where interventions on reducing the socioeconomic gradient in health need to concentrate.

Social Exclusion

Absolute poverty, defined in terms of a lack of basic material necessities of life, continues to exist, even in the richest countries. The long-term unemployed, many ethnic minority groups, guest workers, disabled people, refugees, and homeless people are at risk of living in absolute poverty in rich countries. Homeless people living on the streets have the highest rates of premature death. In poorer countries, the proportion of people living in absolute poverty is much larger than in richer countries, and this contributes to the poorer health in these countries relative to richer countries.

However, absolute poverty alone does not explain all of the socioeconomic gradient in health. Relative poverty, often defined as living on less than 60% of the national median income, affects a greater proportion of people in a population than absolute poverty. It could deny people access to decent housing and jobs, education, transport, and other vital factors for full participation in social life.

The stresses of living in absolute and relative poverty are particularly harmful during pregnancy, to babies, and to the elderly, when people are particularly vulnerable. People move in and out of poverty during their lives, so the number of people who experience poverty and social exclusion during their lifetime is far higher than the number of socially excluded people at any one time.

Furthermore, poverty and social exclusion increase the risk of social isolation, influencing divorce and separation, disability, illness, and addiction. Social isolation affects individuals and communities. Communities and neighborhoods that experience high levels of unemployment, deprivation, poor housing, and limited access to services often have far poorer health outcomes than would be expected by aggregating the number of poor people living in those communities. Social isolation in such communities is hard to escape from, as social exclusion and social isolation are intertwined, often forming a vicious cycle.

Unemployment

Unemployed people and their families have substantially increased risks of premature death and poorer physical and mental health compared to those with stable employment. People who are long-term unemployed, in particular, have much poorer health than the employed. The health effects of unemployment are linked to both its psychological consequences and the financial problems it brings.

The health effects start when people first feel that their jobs are threatened, even before they become unemployed and before any change in their financial circumstances. Job insecurity has been shown to increase the risk of anxiety and depression, sickness absence, smoking, lack of exercise, and heart disease. Unsatisfactory jobs can be just as harmful to health as unemployment; merely having a job will not always protect physical and mental health. As job insecurity grows, it can act as a chronic stressor whose pernicious effects on health increase with the length of exposure.

Disability and ill health increase the risk of unemployment. So the association between unemployment and health could be a result of prior ill health (or selection) or the effects of unemployment on health. There is evidence for both causal models. Any interventions aimed at reducing the association between unemployment and health need to take account of the risk of unemployment through ill health as well as the risk of ill health through unemployment.

Addiction

Alcohol dependence, illicit drug use, and cigarette smoking are all closely associated with socioeconomic disadvantage. Addictions to these substances may help alleviate some of the stressors associated with socioeconomic disadvantage, but in turn, they can generate further problems as well as have long-term consequences on biological systems.

Some of the transitional economies of Central and Eastern Europe experienced great social upheaval following the end of Communist governments at the end of the twentieth century. In these countries, deaths linked to alcohol use – such as accidents, violence, poisoning, injury, and suicide – rose sharply in the 1990s. Some have argued that this sudden increase in alcohol-related deaths was due to the changed socioeconomic circumstances in these countries. In the Whitehall II cohort, a stressful work environment, measured by an imbalance between effort and rewards at work, was found to be a risk factor for alcohol dependence in men.

Smoking is a well-established and important cause of ill health and premature death. Socioeconomic disadvantage is associated with high rates of smoking and very low rates of quitting. Furthermore, smoking is a major drain on poor people's incomes, thereby contributing to further financial deprivation as well as increasing risks of ill health. Simply increasing the price of cigarettes, to decrease the rates of smoking, may actually increase the socioeconomic gradient in smoking. Tackling addictions requires attention to the social determinants of these addictions.

Food

A good diet and adequate food supply are central for promoting health and well-being. Shortage of food and lack of variety cause malnutrition and deficiency diseases, which in turn are causes of other infectious and chronic diseases. While food deficiency occurs in poorer countries, in richer countries, excess food intake contributes to cardiovascular diseases, diabetes, cancer, and obesity. Furthermore, food poverty can exist side by side with food abundance. Some developing countries are experiencing the double burden of obesity and malnutrition-related diseases.

Economic growth and improvements in housing and sanitation resulted in an epidemiological transition from infectious to chronic diseases, as well as a nutritional transition. Diets have changed to overconsumption of energy-dense fats and sugars, producing more obesity. In rich countries, as well as some developing poor countries, obesity is becoming more common among the poor than the rich. The main dietary difference between socioeconomic groups is the sources of nutrients. The poor tend to substitute cheaper processed foods for fresh food, with much higher levels of energy-dense fats and sugars. People on low incomes are least able to obtain key nutrients from their diets.

The important public health issue is the availability and cost of healthful, nutritious food. Telling people they should eat healthfully is of little use when they do not have access to healthful food, either because they cannot afford it or because they live in food deserts where shops sell processed foods that are inexpensive but unhealthful.

Exercise

As mechanization has reduced the exercise involved in jobs, housework, and commuting, people need to find new ways of building physical activity and exercise into their lives. Regular exercise protects against heart disease and diabetes by limiting obesity. It also promotes a sense of well-being and can protect older people from depression.

There is a strong socioeconomic gradient in leisure-time physical activity – people from lower socioeconomic positions exercise less. This may be because they have less time to spend on exercise, they do not have access to leisure sports facilities, or they live in an environment that does not encourage walking or cycling.

Social Support

Supportive relationships are important emotional and practical resources that contribute to health. Social support may buffer the effects of negative events in a person's life, helping them to cope better with the effects of unemployment or disability. Alternatively, social support may directly contribute to a person's health by making him or her feel cared for, esteemed, and valued. Belonging to a social network and having mutual obligations have a powerful protective effect on health.

Social isolation, or the absence of social networks, is associated with increased rates of premature death and poor chances of survival after a heart attack. People who get less social and emotional support from others are more likely to have depression, poorer well-being, and higher levels of disability from chronic diseases. In addition, negative aspects of support from close relationships can lead to poor mental and physical health. Poverty can contribute to social isolation and negative social support.

Social cohesion, defined as the quality of social relationships and the existence of trust, mutual obligations, and respect in communities, helps to protect people and their health. Some argue that social inequalities tend to corrode good social relations and destroy social cohesion. Societies with high levels of income inequality tend to have less social cohesion and more violent crime. The breakdown of social relations, which is linked to greater inequality, reduces trust and increases levels of violence. Declines in social cohesion in some communities have also been linked to increases in rates of heart disease.

Stress

Disadvantaged social and psychological circumstances can cause long-term stress. Continuing anxiety, insecurity, low self-esteem, social isolation, and lack of control over work and home life have powerful effects on health. Such psychosocial risks accumulate during life and increase the chances of poor mental health and premature death. People in lower socioeconomic groups are more likely to experience these psychosocial stressors.

Psychosocial and other stressors activate hormones and the nervous system by triggering the fight-or-flight response: raising the heart rate, mobilizing stored energy, diverting blood to muscles, and increasing alertness. This stress response diverts energy and resources away from many physiological processes important to long-term health maintenance. While biological stress responses to acute stressors are healthy, both the cardiovascular and immune systems may be affected if there are repeated exposures

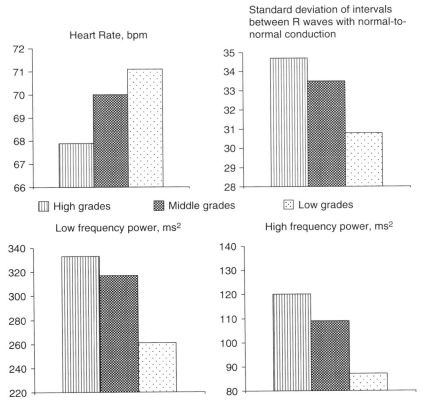

Figure 4   Heart rate variability by employment grade. Data from Hemingway et al. (2005).

to psychosocial stressors or if it goes on for too long. In the Whitehall II cohort, men from lower civil service grades had higher heart rates and lower heart rate variability, indicating poorer autonomic function (see **Figure 4**). In addition, those with low job control, an indicator of stress at work, were more likely to have impaired autonomic function.

Policy

Health policy was once thought to be about the provision and funding of medical care. This is now changing. While medical care can prolong survival and improve prognosis after some serious diseases, the socioeconomic conditions that make people ill in the first place are more important for the health of the population.

A review of policies in European countries identified several that took action on the social determinants of health, including policies on taxation, old age pensions, sickness benefits, maternity or child benefits, unemployment benefits, housing policies, labor markets, and community facilities. These policies may not be directly related to health, but the evidence suggests that they form part of the broader causes that indirectly influence health. The World Health Organization has set up an independent Commission on the Social Determinants of Health, with the mission to influence public policy, both national and global, to take into account the evidence on the social determinants of health and interventions and policies to address them.

Policies at all levels of government, and between national governments, need to take account of the evidence on the social determinants of health. Improving access to medical care is important for reducing the socioeconomic gradient in health. However, policies relating to poverty reduction, education, work stress, transport, unemployment, addiction, and social exclusion – policies that cut across the whole business of government – are also needed.

The evidence suggests that telling individuals what they should do to improve their health does not reduce socioeconomic gradients in health. Understanding the causes of the causes implies emphasizing the social determinants of these health-promoting behaviors and recommending social, political, and economic interventions leading to healthier behaviors and healthier outcomes.

See Also the Following Articles

Economic Factors and Stress; Psychosocial Factors and Stress; Social Networks and Social Isolation.

Further Reading

Adler, N., Marmot, M. and McEwen, B. (eds.) (1999). *Socioeconomic status and health in industrial nations: social, psychological and biological pathways* (vol. 896). New York: New York Academy of Sciences.

Bartley, M. (2004). *Health inequality*. Cambridge: Polity Press.

Berkman, L. F. and Kawachi, I. (eds.) (2000). *Social epidemiology*. New York: Oxford University Press.

Brunner, E. J. (1997). Socioeconomic determinants of health: stress and the biology of inequality. *British Medical Journal* 314, 1472–1476.

Gwatkin, D. R., Rustein, S., Johnson, K., Pande, R. and Wagstaff, A. (2000). *Socioeconomic differences in health, nutrition and population: health, nutrition and population discussion paper*. Washington, D.C.: World Bank.

Hemingway, H., Shipley, M., Brunner, E., Britton, A., Malik, M. and Marmot, M. G. (2005). Does autonomic function link social position to coronary risk? The Whitehall II Study. *Circulation* 111, 3071–3077.

Krieger, N. (2001). A glossary for social epidemiology. *Journal of Epidemiology & Community Health* 55, 693–700.

Kuh, D. and Ben-Shlomo, Y. (1997). *A life course approach to chronic disease epidemiology*. Oxford, UK: Oxford University Press.

Marmot, M. (2004). *The status syndrome*. New York: Henry Holt.

Marmot, M. (2005). Social determinants of health inequalities. *The Lancet* 365(9464), 1099–1104.

Marmot, M. and Wilkinson, R. (eds.) (2006). *Social determinants of health* (2nd edn.). Oxford: Oxford University Press.

Wilkinson, R. and Marmot, M. (eds.) (2003). *Social determinants of health: the solid facts* (2nd edn.). Copenhagen: World Health Organisation.

Health Behavior and Stress

A Steptoe
University College London, London, UK

This article is a revision of the previous edition article by A Steptoe, volume 2, pp 322–325, © 2000, Elsevier Inc.

Definition of Health Behavior
Importance of Links with Stress
Different Behavior–Stress Relationships
Health Behaviors as Coping Responses
Study Designs in the Investigation of Health Behavior
Conclusions

Glossary

Health risk behavior	An action carried out by people with a frequency or intensity that increases risk of disease or injury, whether or not the person is aware of the link between the activity and risk of disease or injury.
Positive health behavior	An action that may help prevent disease, detect disease and disability at an early stage, promote and enhance health, or protect from risk of injury.

Definition of Health Behavior

There are two broad classes of health-related behaviors: risk behaviors and positive health behaviors. A health risk behavior can be defined as an activity carried out by people with a frequency or intensity that increases risk of disease or injury, whether or not the person is aware of the link between the activity and risk of disease or injury. Common health risk behaviors include smoking, drinking and driving, drug abuse, and certain sexual practices. The definition of risk behavior recognizes that "dose" is important, as some activities carry no risk in moderation but are problematic when carried out at a high level (e.g., alcohol consumption).

Positive health behaviors are activities that may help prevent disease, detect disease and disability at an early stage, promote and enhance health, and protect from risk of injury. Such behaviors are defined by medical, scientific, and social consensus and are not immutable. As knowledge evolves and the nature of environmental risks is modified, different actions may come to be defined as positive health behaviors. Typical positive health behaviors are regular physical exercise, avoidance of dietary fat, consumption of fruit and vegetables, use of sunscreen protection, breast self-examination, regular dental care, and use of vehicle seat belts.

Importance of Links with Stress

Not all health behaviors are related to stress. Even when behaviors are linked with stress, there are typically many other influences on the frequency and intensity of the activity. Health behaviors are embedded within a complex sociocultural matrix, with factors such as tradition, legislation, taxation, income, and systems of provision all influencing lifestyle and health behavior. Thus, alcohol use is not only modified by stress, but also is related to religious and social traditions, costs relative to disposable income, family experiences and peer group influences, and individual attitudes and habits. Leisure-time physical activity can be used as a way of coping with stress, but is also affected by other motives such as interest in sport and concern about appearance and by availability of a safe place to exercise, cost, time constraints, health status, and cultural attitudes.

Nevertheless, stress does have a significant role in many health behaviors, and this can be important for understanding associations between stress and health. The reason is that if stress does increase the occurrence of a health risk behavior or decreases a positive health behavior, then these behaviors may mediate the influence of stress on health risk. Indeed, changes in behavior sometimes play a more important role in the stress–health relationship than neuroendocrine, autonomic, and immunological responses. For instance, one study evaluated the impact of work stress on the development of hypertension (high blood pressure) over a 5 year period among male air traffic controllers. Some 20% of the air traffic controllers who initially had normal blood pressure developed hypertension during the study. This might be assumed to have been the result of sustained neuroendocrine and autonomic activation elicited by working in this responsible and stressful job. However, it was found that alcohol consumption also rose in individuals who became hypertensive, and it was this factor that accounted for the increase in blood pressure. Thus, the association between work stress and cardiovascular disease was mediated by a health-related behavior rather than by activation of biological stress pathways.

Other examples can be found in the epidemiological literature on psychosocial factors and health risk. A study reported by Everson and colleagues of a large sample of middle-aged men in Finland explored associations between hostility and cardiovascular disease mortality over a 9 year period. It was found that high levels of hostility measured at the beginning of the study predicted cardiovascular mortality independently of known risk factors such as cholesterol and socioeconomic status. However, when smoking, alcohol consumption, body mass index, and physical activity were taken into account, the association between hostility and mortality was diminished substantially. This suggests that the influence of hostility was mediated not by neuroendocrine pathways, but rather by differences in health behaviors. The more hostile individuals were also those who smoked, drank alcohol excessively, and were overweight and physically inactive, which accounted for the increase in cardiovascular risk.

Health behaviors also influence links between stress and health outcomes in patients with medical conditions. One important health behavior in many illness states is adherence to medication and health advice. Low adherence can result in ineffective treatment and risk to future health. Poor adherence is affected by life stress and by states of subjective distress and depression. This might explain why, for instance, cardiac patients who suffer depression and distress following a myocardial infarction are at increased risk for recurrent cardiac events.

Thus, the relationship between health behavior and stress is of interest not only in itself, but also for its role in mediating health effects.

Different Behavior–Stress Relationships

The association between stress and health behavior can take several forms, which complicates systematic investigation, particularly in humans. The different possibilities are outlined in **Figure 1**. The first model (**Figure 1a**) shows that behavior change is one aspect of the psychobiological stress response. Just as stressful episodes elicit distress and physiological adjustments, they also stimulate changes in behavior. Stressful life events, for instance, may lead to increases in cigarette smoking or dietary fat intake, or an increased likelihood of drinking and driving, in the same way that they elicit upsetting emotions. The different elements of psychobiological stress responses are typically coupled only loosely. Hence, although changes in health behavior would be expected to correlate with an increased distress in response to stressful episodes, the association may be relatively weak.

The second possibility is that changes in health behavior are stimulated by the distress that people experience during a stressful episode in their lives (**Figure 1b**). For example, increased alcohol consumption may occur in response to family conflict in

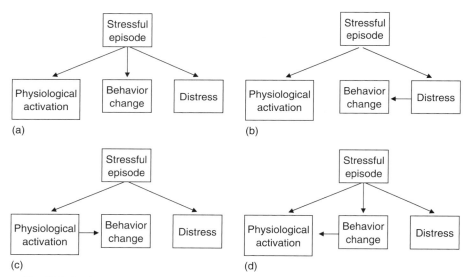

Figure 1   Stress and health behaviors.

individuals who become very depressed or anxious. Under these circumstances, the changes in health behavior arise not as a direct consequence of exposure to stressors, but indirectly as a result of mood change. If a person experiencing a threatening event does not become distressed or copes well with the event, there may be no change in behavior. A threshold of distress may exist below which no alteration in behavior will be measurable.

Third, the physiological adjustments that take place as part of the stress response may provoke changes in health behavior (**Figure 1c**). It has been proposed, for example, that elevated glucocorticoids in response to stress modulate the control of feeding and preference for foods high in fat and sucrose, and that these serve in turn to dampen adrenocortical and sympathetic nervous system responses. This pathway may contribute to the effects of stress on long-term fat consumption and hence on cardiovascular and metabolic disease risk. When such a process operates, the behavior change will take place only secondarily and not directly as part of the stress response.

Health behaviors can, in turn, influence the magnitude of the physiological adjustments that contribute to stress responses (**Figure 1d**). Alcohol consumption, smoking, and diet all have effects on immune function. If changes in these behaviors take place during stressful episodes, they may modulate the extent of immunosuppression during stress. Similarly, regular physical exercise has been shown in some studies to reduce the magnitude of cardiovascular and affective reactions to stress, whereas functional foods may alter physiological adjustments by increasing the bioavailability of neurotransmitter substrates.

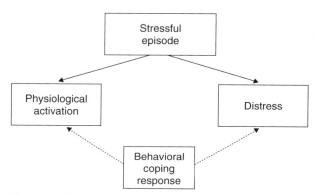

Figure 2   Health behavior change as a coping response.

Health Behaviors as Coping Responses

Thus far, changes in health behavior have been described as direct or indirect components of the stress response. A further possibility is that people change their health behavior in an effort to cope with distress and ameliorate their negative emotional states (**Figure 2**). Health behavior change may therefore not be part of the stress response, but may occur as one element of the way in which people attempt to manage stress responses. There are several familiar examples of health behavior changes as coping responses. Some people turn to comfort foods such as chocolate when upset, whereas others engage in vigorous physical exercise in order to improve their mood or distract themselves from the troubling situation. These health behaviors may be effective in managing stress. Thus, it has been found that vigorous physical activity in smokers who are trying to quit can help ameliorate sensations of craving. But in other cases, the beneficial effects of the behavior as a coping response may be more apparent than real. For instance, a large proportion of smokers believe that smoking helps relieve tension and manage stress. However, studies indicate that smoking is associated with poor well-being rather than positive states and that giving up smoking leads to reductions in perceived stress. While smoking may aid mental concentration by increasing alertness in the short term, there is little evidence that it is an effective coping behavior in most circumstances. In Western society, alcohol is sometimes used as a palliative; people drink to cope and disengage from their troubles. Unfortunately, this palliative also has adverse effects and may ultimately become a source of stress in itself.

These different associations between health behavior and stress are not mutually exclusive. An increase in alcohol consumption may, for example, be a direct response to stress (**Figure 1a**), as well as being a coping behavior (**Figure 2**). Links between stress and health behavior are therefore not straightforward, which in turn has implications for research designs.

Study Designs in the Investigation of Health Behavior

Experimental studies in animals and humans can be used to tease out associations between stress and health behavior. They allow antecedent conditions to be controlled carefully so that the impact of defined stimuli can be explored systematically. However, because much interest is focused on mental and physical health outcomes, observational studies of naturally occurring stressors are also essential. A major problem that has limited progress in the investigation of stress and health behavior has been the use of cross-sectional designs in naturalistic studies. These prevent conclusions from being drawn about causality. For example, a study of drug dependency might show that drug-dependent individuals frequently live in deprived conditions, experience a high frequency of adverse life events such as family disruption, divorce, and job loss, and have poor social supports. There is therefore an association between stress and drug dependency, but are these adverse social conditions the effects of drug dependence or did they stimulate drug use in the first place? Without longitudinal or prospective study designs, cause and effect cannot be distinguished.

Another design problem in some studies of health behavior is sample selection. A study that focuses on individuals with problems related to a particular behavior may produce results that are not broadly representative. Many studies of stress and alcohol use, for instance, have been carried out with samples of people suffering from alcohol-related problems. There may be other people in the population, however, who drink as much alcohol as the people in these samples without suffering from health problems. Studies of individuals with health problems will be biased toward observing stress-related effects that would not manifest with a population-based sampling frame.

Conclusions

Health risk and positive health behaviors show complex relationships with stress, as they can be both elements of the stress response and coping behaviors. A combination of research designs is needed to delineate these associations, and the inferences that can be drawn from cross-sectional studies are very limited. Health behaviors require detailed investigation in the context of stress research, as they contribute to many of the associations between stressful phenomena and health risk identified in the literature.

See Also the Following Articles

Alcohol and Stress: Social and Psychological Aspects; Diet and Stress, Non-Psychiatric; Exercise; Psychosocial Factors and Stress; Smoking and Stress.

Further Reading

Dallman, M. F., Pecoraro, N. C. and la Fleur, S. E. (2005). Chronic stress and comfort foods: self-medication and abdominal obesity. *Brain, Behavior and Immunity* **19**, 275–280.

DeFrank, R. S., Jenkins, C. D. and Rose, R. M. (1987). A longitudinal investigation of the relationships among alcohol consumption, psychosocial factors, and blood pressure. *Psychosomatic Medicine* **49**, 236–249.

Everson, S. A., Kauhanen, J., Kaplan, G. A., et al. (1997). Hostility and increased risk of mortality and acute myocardial infarction: the mediating role of behavioral risk factors. *American Journal of Epidemiology* **146**, 142–152.

Greeno, C. G. and Wing, R. R. (1994). Stress-induced eating. *Psychological Bulletin* **115**, 444–464.

Kassel, J. D. and Hankin, B. L. (in press) Smoking and depression. In: Steptoe, A. (ed.) *Depression and physical illness*. Cambridge, UK: Cambridge University Press.

Steptoe, A. and Ayers, S. (2004). Stress, health and illness. In: Sutton, S., Baum, A. & Johnston, M. (eds.) *Sage handbook of health psychology*, pp. 169–196, London: Sage.

Steptoe, A. and Wardle, J. (2004). Health behaviour: prevalence and links with disease. In: Kaptein, A. & Weinman, J. (eds.) *Health psychology*, pp. 21–51, Oxford: Blackwell.

Stewart, S. H. (1996). Alcohol abuse in individuals exposed to trauma: a critical review. *Psychological Bulletin* **120**, 83–114.

Ussher, M., West, R., McEwen, A., Taylor, A. and Steptoe, A. (2003). Efficacy of exercise counselling as an aid for smoking cessation: a randomized controlled trial. *Addiction* **98**, 523–532.

Ziegelstein, R. C., Fauerbach, J. A., Stevens, S. S., Romanelli, J., Richter, D. P. and Bush, D. E. (2000). Patients with depression are less likely to follow recommendations to reduce cardiac risk during recovery from a myocardial infarction. *Archives of Internal Medicine* **160**, 1818–1823.

Heart Disease/Attack

G J Baker, S Suchday and D S Krantz
Uniformed Services University of the Health Sciences, Bethesda, MD, USA

This article is reproduced from the previous edition article by G J Baker, S Suchday and D S Krantz, volume 2, pp 326–332, © 2000, Elsevier Inc.

Introduction
Overview of Pathophysiology
Psychosocial Risk Factors for Coronary Heart Disease
Individual Coronary Heart Disease Risk Factors
Cardiac Stress Management Interventions
Conclusion

Glossary

Atherosclerosis	A condition in which fatty plaques build up in the coronary arteries.
Cardiovascular reactivity	An excessive hemodynamic response to stressors.
Coronary heart disease	A usually symptomatic condition in which cardiac function is impaired (thought to result from atherosclerosis).
Myocardial infarction (MI)	A heart attack.
Myocardial ischemia	The inadequate supply of blood to cardiac tissue.

Introduction

Chronic cardiovascular diseases (CVD), including coronary heart disease (CHD), high blood pressure, and stroke, is the leading cause of death in developed countries. CVD is caused by the interaction of physiological, environmental, and behavioral variables, many of which are a function of individuals' lifestyles and can, to some extent, be controlled and modified by the individual.

Despite the decline in cardiovascular mortality, CVD continues to be the leading cause of death in the United States, and an increasing body of evidence suggests that exposure to chronic and acute psychological stress may play a role in the development and/or triggering of cardiovascular pathology. This article provides a selective overview of current knowledge regarding the role of acute and chronic stress as risk factors for coronary heart disease.

Overview of Pathophysiology

Coronary atherosclerosis, which is a precursor to symptomatic coronary heart disease, results from the formation of plaques (fatty deposits) on the arterial walls that obstruct blood flow to the heart. Myocardial ischemia results from this inadequate blood supply and is often accompanied by chest pain, also known as angina pectoris. The occurrence of frequent and severe myocardial ischemia increases the risk for cardiac-rhythm disturbances, which can result in sudden cardiac death. Prolonged or severe ischemia, or plaque rupture in the coronary arteries, which may result in complete blockage, can lead to more serious manifestations of CHD. These include death of cardiac tissue (MI), also known as a heart attack, and sudden cardiac death.

Current models of the effects of acute physical and mental stress on cardiac pathophysiology suggest that the activation of the autonomic nervous system induced by behavioral factors may increase the risk of cardiovascular events. **Figure 1** illustrates pathways through which acute mental stress is linked to myocardial ischemia and clinical coronary events such as heart attack or sudden death. These links are thought to exist in individuals with preexisting coronary artery disease or dysfunction, prior MI, or poor

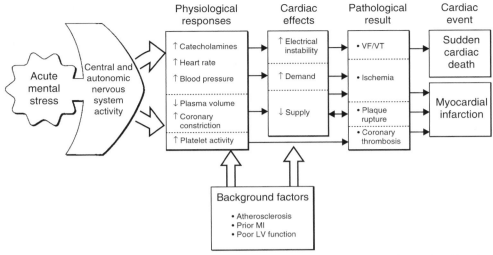

Figure 1 Pathophysiological model of the actions of acute stress as a trigger of myocardial infarction and sudden death in vulnerable individuals. Via its actions on the central and autonomic nervous system in patients with coronary artery disease, stress can produce a cascade of physiological responses that may lead to myocardial ischemia, ventricular fibrillation/tachycardia (VF/VT), plaque rupture, or coronary thrombosis (MI, myocardial infarction; LV, left ventricular). Reprinted from *Cardiology Clinics*, Volume 14(2), May 1996 with permission.

cardiac function, who are therefore at higher risk for these clinical events.

Psychosocial Risk Factors for Coronary Heart Disease

Psychosocial factors that have been implicated as risk factors for developing heart disease include individuals' accessibility to social and economic resources, the work environment, and stressful life circumstances. Animal model studies in primates also suggest that conditions involving psychological stress can promote the development of atherosclerosis. Each of these factors is discussed in the following sections.

Animal Model Studies

A series of studies involving cynomolgus monkeys has been conducted to examine the effects of mental stress on coronary disease. Monkeys not only have similar coronary disease pathology to humans, but they also exhibit many of the same behavioral characteristics that have been cited as potential risk factors, such as competition, aggression, and the formation of social hierarchies. Stressful situations were created for these monkeys by rearranging their social groups periodically, known as the unstable condition. Monkeys were then labeled as either dominant or subordinate based on their behavior patterns in the groups.

In one study, more coronary atherosclerosis developed in dominant male monkeys in the unstable social condition than in their subordinate counterparts. The differences in disease progression between dominants and subordinates in the stable social condition were less pronounced. Another study, using female monkeys, found more coronary artery disease in subordinate animals than in dominants. Reproductive function was also disrupted in many of the subordinate monkeys, which may have decreased the animals' resistance to coronary disease.

Low Social Support as a Coronary Heart Disease Risk Factor

Lack of social resources, particularly inadequate social support and social isolation, can increase the risk of CVD. Social resources can be categorized as social networks or as social support derived from those networks. Social support is defined as the instrumental, emotional, and informational aid obtained from an individual's social ties and community resources, and it exerts a mediating or moderating impact on health. A lack of supportive networks also impacts health by interfering with practical aid. Research indicates that people with access to strong social networks are at a relatively lower risk of developing CHD. Social networks also exert a beneficial impact on recovery after incidence of disease.

Industrial countries demonstrate a graded, inverse relationship between socioeconomic status (SES) and morbidity and mortality, with higher disease rates appearing in poorer populations. SES has typically been defined using standard measures, including education, income, occupation, or combinations of these three factors. Although it has been shown that the prevalence of standard CHD risk factors (e.g., high blood pressure and smoking) diminishes with increasing SES, that does not fully explain the increase in coronary mortality attributable to low SES. Regardless of other prognostic factors, social isolation and low household incomes predict an increased risk of cardiovascular death over a 5-year period. Presumably, psychological reactions to MI may be exacerbated by diminished social and economic resources.

Occupational Stress

Karasek and Theorell attempted to define specific characteristics of stressful occupations that promote risk of coronary disease. Specifically, high job strain (defined as conditions of high demand and few opportunities to control outcomes) predicted job stress-related illnesses, especially CHD. The Karasek job demand/control hypothesis explained cardiovascular disease and mortality in studies of Swedish workers and in studies of U.S. men and women.

A study of occupational stress and CHD in women also suggests that the relationship between conditions in the workplace and cardiovascular disease, at least in part, depends on family and work demands on the individual and the amount of control the individual has over these situations. The Framingham Heart Study, a major epidemiologic study of heart disease conducted by the National Institutes of Health, examined these issues. Haynes and Feinleib analyzed data from this study to address the question of whether the increase of women working outside the home has affected their cardiovascular health adversely. An 8-year follow-up of middle-age women in the mid-1960s examined the development of CHD in this population. Women who had been employed outside the home for more than half of their adult lives were compared with housewives and with men. The results indicated that generally there was not a significantly greater risk of subsequent heart disease in working women. However, there was a greater risk of CHD development in clerical workers, working women with children, and women whose bosses were unsupportive. It is thought that the increased risk in these groups is due to low job control, high family demands, or low job satisfaction. It is interesting to note that the risk of CHD increased linearly with the number of children for working women but not for housewives.

Acute Stress as a Trigger of Cardiovascular Symptoms

Research has also focused on the role of acute stress and of emotions as triggers of coronary disease symptomatology in individuals with preexisting disease. One early study observed that 40 out of 100 sudden cardiac death patients had experienced a stressful life event (i.e., death of a spouse) within the 24 h preceding their deaths and that loss events (e.g., death of a loved one) were more common in sudden death victims than in controls. These studies support the findings of previous research that observed increased mortality of widowers from cardiovascular events.

Research has also shown an increase in cardiovascular deaths and increased rates of MI following disasters and personal traumas. The Iraqi missile attacks on Israel during the initial days of the Gulf War have been the subject of studies that examined the effect of these attacks on fatal and nonfatal cardiac events among the population living close to Tel Aviv. The intensive care unit of a Tel Aviv medical center reported an increase in acute MI cases during the week following the missile attacks (January 17–25, 1991) compared with the week prior to the attacks and with a control period consisting of the same week a year earlier.

An increase in cardiac mortality has been attributed to acute psychological stress following earthquakes and other natural disasters. For example, during the 1994 Los Angeles earthquake, the incidence of critical-care admissions for acute MI reportedly increased (odds ratio 2.4). Unstable angina, however, did not increase in the week following the earthquake compared to the week prior to the disaster, especially for hospitals within 15 miles of the earthquake epicenter.

Psychologically stressful events have also been implicated as environmental triggers occurring prior to the onset of MI. In a study of patients with acute MI, nearly half reported one or more possible triggers, the most common of which was emotional distress. Mittleman and colleagues used a more sophisticated epidemiological methodology in which each patient's activities just prior to MI were compared to a control period defined as his or her own usual levels of activity in order to examine the most common physical and mental triggers of MI. This study of MI patients interviewed a median of 4 days after the MI revealed that 39 out of 1623 patients (2.4%) reported experiencing anger within the 2 h prior to MI onset. The relative risk of MI following an anger episode was more than twice the risk during nonanger periods.

Mental Stress as a Trigger of Ischemia

Although the most important end points for studies of cardiovascular disease are MI and sudden cardiac death, research has also focused on myocardial ischemia as an intermediate measure of the effects of stress on CHD. Studies of myocardial ischemia also have the benefit of being unconfounded by reporting biases because ischemia often occurs without symptoms that are known to the patient.

Using a structured diary method, Barry and colleagues observed that most of the episodes of daily life ischemia occurred during moderate or low levels of physical activity (e.g., talking on the phone, speaking with a friend, or clerical work). There was a graded relationship between the likelihood of ischemia and the intensity of both mental and physical activities, suggesting that as levels of physical and mental activity become more intense, they are increasingly likely to evoke transient daily life ischemia.

Gabbay and coworkers asked 63 subjects who were undergoing ambulatory electrocardiographic monitoring to fill out a more sophisticated diary. Results showed that ischemia occurred most often during moderately intense physical and mental activities. The amount of ischemic time (5%) was approximately equal for high-intensity physical and mental activities, as compared to only 0.2% of ischemic time in low-intensity activities. In summary, ambulatory electrocardiographic monitoring studies illustrate that various physical and mental activities are associated with the occurrence of ischemia during daily life. Both physical and mental activities can act as potent triggers. Thus, it seems that many features of daily life ischemia may be due to behavioral influences, including daily life stress.

Individual Coronary Heart Disease Risk Factors

Type A Behavior

The type A behavior pattern was originally described by cardiologists Friedman and Rosenman in the 1950s as a behavior pattern characterized by agitation, hostility, rapid speech, and an extremely competitive nature. The contrasting type B behavior pattern consists of a more laid-back style and a lack of the type A characteristics mentioned previously. A structured interview was developed to measure type A behavior based on behaviors such as speech characteristics and subjects' responses to various questions.

In the 1960s and 1970s, many studies were conducted to probe the relationship between type A behavior and heart disease. Most of the studies revealed a correlation between type A behavior and coronary heart disease in both men and women, which is comparable and independent of the effects of smoking and hypertension. For example, two major studies obtained results supporting the findings that type A behavior is a risk factor for heart disease. The Western Collaborative Group Study (WCGS) followed

initially healthy men for 8.5 years. The men were given questionnaires and took part in interviews to determine their type A status at the outset of the study. Those individuals who were identified as type A were more likely to have developed heart disease over the course of the 8.5 years of the study than the type B group. The Framingham Heart Study also showed that type A behavior was a predictor of CHD among white-collar men and women who worked outside of the home.

Since the 1980s, however, most studies have not corroborated the relationship between type A behavior and heart disease. The Multiple Risk Factor Intervention Trial (MRFIT) assessed whether interventions to reduce coronary risk factors, such as high blood pressure, smoking, or high cholesterol levels, decreased the potential for coronary disease in high-risk men and women. After 7 years, the results did not show a relationship between these measures of type A behavior and the incidence of the first heart attack. Further, there were reports from research that indicated that, after a heart attack, type B patients were more likely to die than type A patients. This finding could be explained as the result of healthier type A patients being the ones who initially survived their first heart attack. Regardless, however, this result certainly presented doubts about type A behavior as a coronary risk factor.

It is unclear why these studies resulted in such inconsistent findings. Some have suggested that type A behavior may be a risk factor for younger individuals rather than for older or high-risk individuals, such as the ones tested in the MRFIT study. Still, it seems that there are certain aspects of type A behavior, particularly anger and hostility, that remain correlated with coronary disease, even in studies in which overall type A behavior was not related to CHD.

Hostility and Anger

As noted earlier, it is possible that some particular characteristics of the multifaceted type A behavior are more pertinent risk factors for CHD than others, and perhaps the type A concept as a whole does not constitute increased risk. Factors that have been shown consistently to correlate with CHD are hostility, anger, certain speech characteristics drawn from the structured interview, and not expressing anger or irritation. For example, an analysis of WCGS data showed that the strongest predictors of CHD were, in fact, the potential for hostility, vigorous speech, and reports of frequent anger or irritation. The MRFIT study, which did not show a correlation between type A behavior and coronary disease, also demonstrated a relationship between hostility and an increased risk of CHD.

The Cook and Medley hostility inventory, a scale that measures certain attitudes such as cynicism and mistrust of others, has been shown to relate hostility to the occurrence of heart disease. In one study, a 25-year follow-up of physicians who completed the MMPI while attending medical school revealed that high Cook-Medley scores predicted not only the incidence of CHD but also mortality from all causes. This relationship was independent of the individual effects of other risk factor such as smoking, age, and the presence of high blood pressure. Evidence also suggests that low hostility scores are correlated with a decrease in death rates during the 20-year follow-up of the almost 1900 participants in the Western Electric Study. Research also illustrates that hostility scores are higher in low socioeconomic groups, men, and nonwhites in the United States, as well as being correlated positively with smoking prevalence. Therefore, it is possible to suggest that hostility may account for some of the socioeconomic and gender differences in death rates from cardiovascular diseases.

Depression and Exhaustion

Clinical depression, which includes symptoms such as fatigue, exhaustion, and dysphoric mood, is prevalent among patients with CHD and is associated with poor health outcomes in CHD patients. Studies have reported that nearly one in five cardiac patients can be diagnosed as clinically depressed. Depression among post-MI patients, however, goes largely untreated, despite its prevalence. In several studies, the presence of a major depressive episode in CHD patients is associated with poor psychosocial rehabilitation and increased medical morbidity.

Appels and colleagues identified a syndrome of fatigue or exhaustion called vital exhaustion, which overlaps with some of the symptoms of depression. Research indicates that vital exhaustion is predictive of the development or worsening of cardiovascular disease. Further, the predictive value of fatigue or exhaustion cannot be explained by the effects of illness on mood or energy levels. Studies are currently underway to assess whether risk of death and recurrence in post-MI patients can be lessened by treating the symptoms of depression.

Responsiveness (Reactivity) to Acute Stress

It has been known for some time that individual reactions to stress vary widely, and research suggests that physiological responses to stress may be implicated in the development of CHD and/or high blood pressure. Cardiovascular reactivity is measured by assessing changes in heart rate, blood pressure, or other cardiac measures in response to stress, as opposed to the sole measurement of resting levels of cardiovascular function. The magnitude of these responses varies widely from one individual to another. Some people are so-called hot reactors and display large increases to the challenging task, whereas others show very little or no increase at all. For example, evidence shows that behaviors present in type A individuals are often accompanied by the same types of responses that are believed to link psychosocial stress to CHD.

It may be possible that high levels of stress reactivity is a risk factor for CHD or a marker for other stress-related risk processes. Keys and coworkers followed a group of initially healthy men for 23 years and found that the magnitude of their diastolic blood pressure reactions in a cold pressor test (immersing the hand in very cold water) was a good predictor of subsequent heart disease; in fact, it was a better predictor than many of the standard risk factors. However, a later attempt to replicate these findings was unsuccessful.

Cardiac Stress Management Interventions

Evidence suggests that psychosocial interventions, when combined with the standard medical treatments for these patients and stress management, may be one way to reduce cardiac morbidity and mortality. For example, the Recurrent Coronary Prevention Project (RCPP) assessed the effects of modifying type A characteristics, such as anger, impatience, and irritability, on the recurrence of heart attacks and CHD-related deaths. Patients were divided into three groups: a cardiology counseling treatment group, a combined cardiology counseling and type A-behavior modification group, or a no treatment control group. After 4.5 years of follow-up, the type A-behavior modification group displayed significantly lower rates of heart attack recurrence than the cardiology counseling and control groups.

The Ischemic Heart Disease Life Stress Monitoring Program assigned heart attack patients to either a treatment or a control group. The treatment group was exposed to life stress monitoring and intervention, whereas the control group received only standard medical follow-ups. The results at the 1-year follow-up showed that cardiac deaths decreased by 50% and that this lower death rate persisted for 6 months beyond the end of the study.

Ornish and colleagues conducted an intervention study on 28 patients with documented coronary artery disease. Patients were assigned to either a usual care control group or a treatment group that was given a low-fat vegetarian diet, yoga-based stress management training, smoking cessation program, and aerobic exercise. After 1 year, the results demonstrated that the treatment group showed slightly less coronary artery blockage, whereas the controls showed a progression in disease. Further, the more compliant patients in the treatment group exhibited greater disease reduction and the least compliant patients showed less change.

Finally, Blumenthal and coworkers examined the effects of an exercise regimen and stress management on CHD. The Myocardial Ischemia Intervention Trial assigned patients to receive 4 months of stress management, 4 months exercise training, or simply their standard medical follow-up care. The patients in the stress management group showed a lower risk of cardiac events in the 38 months of follow-up than the control group. There was also a lower risk associated with the exercise training group, but this did not reach significant levels.

Conclusion

There are many physiological, environmental, and behavioral influences that affect the development of cardiovascular disease. Many of the standard CHD risk factors have behavioral components, and increasingly, evidence points to important psychosocial risk factors for CHD as well, including occupational stress, hostility, and physiological reactivity to stress. In cardiac patients, acute stress, low levels of social support, and depression also seem to have an impact on the development and progression of CHD. However, several studies suggest that stress management programs, when added to usual care medical treatments, can significantly lessen cardiac morbidity in cardiac patients. Thus, it is important to consider more than simply the physiological aspects of coronary disease when discussing treatment and prevention. Greater public awareness of the aspects of coronary disease that are under individuals' control may aid in the struggle to reduce cardiac morbidity and mortality in the United States; however, continued research is needed to examine and explain these phenomena further.

See Also the Following Articles

Anger; Atherosclerosis; Captivity, Recovery from; Eating Disorders and Stress; Sleep, Sleep Disorders, and Stress; Social Stress, Animal Models of; Trauma and Memory.

Further Reading

Barefoot, J. C. and Lipkus, I. M. (1994). The assessment of anger and hostility. In: Siegman, A. W. & Smith, T. W. (eds.) *Anger, hostility, and the heart*, pp. 43–66. Hillsdale, NJ: Lawrence Erlbaum.

Barry, J., Selwyn, A. P., Nabel, E. G., et al. (1988). Frequency of ST segment depression produced by mental stress in stable angina pectoris from coronary artery disease. *American Journal of Cardiology* **61**, 989–993.

Blumenthal, J. A., Wei, J., Babyak, M., et al. (1997). Stress management and exercise training in cardiac patients with myocardial ischemia: effects on prognosis and on markers of myocardial ischemia. *Archives of Internal Medicine* **157**, 2213–2223.

Carney, R. M., Freedland, K. C., Rich, M. W., et al. (1995). Depression as a risk factor for cardiac events in established coronary heart disease: a review of possible mechanisms. *Annals of Behavioral Medicine* **17**, 142–149.

Case, R. B., Moss, A. J., Case, N., et al. (1992). Living alone after myocardial infarction. *Journal of the American Medical Association* **267**, 515–519.

Cohen, S. and Wills, T. A. (1985). Social support and the buffering hypothesis. *Psychological Bulletin* **98**, 310–357.

Gabbay, F. H., Krantz, D. S., Kop, W. J., et al. (1995). Triggers of myocardial ischemia during daily life in patients with coronary artery disease: physical and mental activities, anger, and smoking. *Journal of the American College of Cardiology* **27**, 585–592.

Frasure-Smith, N. and Prince, R. (1987). The ischemic heart disease life stress monitoring program. *Psychosomatic Medicine* **5**, 485–513.

Friedman, M. and Rosenman, R. H. (1974). *Type A behavior and your heart*. New York: Knopf.

Haynes, S. B. and Feinleib, M. (1980). Women, work, and coronary disease: prospective findings from the Framingham Heart Study. *American Journal of Public Health* **700**, 133–141.

Kaplan, G. A. and Keil, J. E. (1993). Socioeconomic factors and cardiovascular disease: a review of the literature. *Circulation* **88**, 1973–1998.

Kaplan, J. R., Adams, M. R., Clarkson, T. B., et al. (1984). Psychosocial influences on female "protection" among cynomolgus macaques. *Atherosclerosis* **53**, 283–295.

Karasek, R. A. and Theorell, T. G. (1990). *Health, work, stress, productivity, and the reconstruction of working life*. New York: Basic Books.

Keys, A., Taylor, H. L., Blackburn, H., et al. (1971). Mortality and coronary heart disease among men studied for 23 years. *Archives of Internal Medicine* **128**, 201–214.

Kop, W. J., Appels, A. P. W. M., de Leon, C. M., et al. (1994). Vital exhaustion predicts new cardiac events after successful coronary angioplasty. *Psychosomatic Medicine* **56**, 281–287.

Krantz, D. S., Kop, W. J., Gabbay, F. H., et al. (1996). Circadian variation in ambulatory myocardial ischemia: triggering by daily activities and evidence for an endogenous circadian component. *Circulation* **93**, 1364–1371.

Krantz, D. S. and Manuck, S. B. (1984). Acute psychophysiologic reactivity and ride of cardiovascular disease: a review and methodological critique. *Psychological Bulletin* **96**, 435–464.

Matthews, K. A. and Haynes, S. G. (1986). Type A behavior pattern and coronary disease risk: update and critical evaluation. *American Journal of Epidemiology* **123**, 923–960.

Mittleman, M. A., Maclure, M., Sherwood, J. B., et al. (1995). Triggering of acute myocardial infarction onset by episodes of anger. *Circulation* **92**, 1720–1725.

Muller, J. E., Tofler, G. H. and Stone, P. H. (1989). Circadian variation and triggers of onset of acute cardiovascular disease. *Circulation* **79**, 733–743.

Ornish, D., Brown, S. E., Scherwitz, L. W., et al. (1990). Can lifestyle changes reverse coronary heart disease? *Lancet* **336**, 129–133.

Shumaker, S. A. and Cjakowski, S. M. (eds.) (1994). *Social support and cardiovascular disease*. New York: Plenum.

Tofler, G. H., Stone, P. H., Maclure, M., et al. (1990). Analysis of possible triggers of acute myocardial infarction (the MILIS study). *American Journal of Cardiology* **66**, 22–27.

Williams, R. B., Barefoot, J. C., Califf, R. M., et al. (1992). Prognostic importance of social and economic resources among medically treated patients with angiographically documented coronary artery disease. *Journal of the American Medical Association* **267**, 559–560.

Heart Failure, Stress Effects

M Alevizaki
Evgenidion Hospital and Alexandra Hospital, Athens University School of Medicine, Athens, Greece
G P Chrousos
Evgenidion Hospital and Athens University School of Medicine, Athens, Greece

Glossary

Apoptosis	(From the Greek words *apo* = from and *ptosis* = falling); one of the main types of programmed cell death.
Atrial natriuretic peptide (ANP)	Released by atrial cardiomyocytes and has a direct diuretic, natriuretic and vasodilator effect.
Cardiomyocytes	Striated muscle cells of the heart, deriving from cardiac myoblasts; they participate in the contraction of the heart.
Catecholamines	Biogenic amines produced mainly from the adrenal medulla and the postganglionic neurons of the sympathetic nervous system; they participate in the stress system, influencing heart rate, blood pressure and various metabolic parameters.
Cytokines	Polypeptides produced in a variety of tissues; mediators of the inflammatory and immune responses.
Nitric oxide synthase (NOS)	Enzyme responsible for the synthesis of nitric oxide (NO).
Norepinephrine (noradrenaline)	A catecholamine, released both from noradrenergic neurons of the sympathetic nervous system and from the medulla of adrenal glands.
Pheochromocytoma	Tumor arising from cells of neural rest origin of the medulla of the adrenal gland.
Renin–angiotensin–aldosterone system	Participates in the regulation of the extracellular fluid volume and the long-term arterial pressure, as well as in the maintenance of Na and K blood concentrations.

Heart failure is the end result of declining pumping capacity of the heart; it follows some initial injury to the heart, which may be of either an acute or progressive nature. In recent years, neurohormonal mechanisms that may be involved in the progression of heart failure have been proposed. These represent compensatory physiological responses activated to assist the heart and to slow down the deterioration of its pumping function. The increased secretion of catecholamines; release of various peptides with vasodilatory effects, such as the atrial natriuretic peptides; and production of the gas hormone nitric oxide all contribute in the assistance of the heart. Several cells from within the heart, however, produce other hormones, such as endothelin, with vasoconstrictive effects, which, when present at increased levels or when administered in excess, are able to partially reproduce the syndrome of heart failure in experimental animal models. These effects are generally reversible.

Stress is classically linked to elevated adrenergic activity. In the failing heart the original increase in adrenergic activity is beneficial because it facilitates an increase in the heart rate and contractility.

However, in the progress of heart failure, further increases in circulating norepinephrine occur, which may be detrimental to the myocardium. Elevated norepinephrine concentrations are positively correlated with the severity of heart failure, with the more elevated levels linked to a worse prognosis and higher mortality. Chronically elevated catecholamines may be cardiotoxic, and heart failure associated with pheochromocytoma is a well-recognized entity. Prolonged and excessive β-adrenergic receptor stimulation may result in intracellular calcium overload, which may promote cardiomyocyte apoptosis. Therefore, the effects of increased adrenergic stimulation are paradoxical and change as the disease progresses, starting as beneficial and ending as detrimental. Slowly, the failing heart may lose its ability to respond to catecholamines.

The use of antagonists of neurohormonal factors may reverse heart failure progression to some extent; thus, the use of both β-adrenergic blockade and of angiotensin-converting enzyme inhibitors partially reverse the progression of heart failure.

Stress is also associated with the production of pro-inflammatory cytokines. Recently, an important role of pro-inflammatory cytokines in the pathophysiology and progression of heart failure has been recognized. These cytokines may be produced under the influence of stress by cardiac myocytes independently of the activation of the immune system and have direct adverse effects on the cardiovascular system. Studies have specifically shown that tumor necrosis factor (TNF-)α, interleukin (IL)-2, and IL-6 exert immediate negative inotropic effects on the heart and, thus, aggravate heart failure. Increased circulating TNF-α levels are associated with more severe degrees of heart failure. It also appears that these molecules may have adverse effects on the remodeling of the cardiac cells and left ventricular structure through effects on apoptosis, as well as on the endothelium, by influencing the transcription of the NO synthase.

This knowledge has led to clinical trials studying the effects of TNF-α blockade on the progression of heart failure; these studies, however, have not shown encouraging results. Interestingly, the blockade of nuclear factor (NF-) κB activity, which is a ubiquitous transcription factor involved in the transcription of the pro-inflammatory cytokine genes, has also been associated with an improvement in heart failure. It has thus been suggested that NF-κB might be a promising target for future drug development for the treatment of heart failure. The current general view is that there is an interplay among catecholamines, the renin–angiotensin system, and pro-inflammatory cytokines that is involved in the pathophysiology of

heart failure. Thus, many conventional therapeutic modalities may be acting through their effects on the pro-inflammatory cytokines. One example is that angiotensin type I receptor antagonists reduce the level of circulating inflammatory mediators in patients with heart failure.

Another interesting observation linking hormones that help the body adapt to stress with heart failure was recently published. It was shown that corticotropin releasing hormone receptor 2 (CRH-R2)- and urocortin 2-deficiencies were associated with heart failure in an animal model and that the reversal of this abnormality was associated with improvement in cardiovascular function.

Finally, it was recently suggested that certain cases of cardiovascular disease may be linked to posttraumatic stress disorder (PTSD). This is not surprising because these conditions are characterized by increased sympathetic activity and elevated concentrations of circulating cytokines such as IL-6. PTSD has, indeed, been associated with heart-rate abnormalities and increased incidence of coronary artery disease; thus, although direct links of PTSD with heart failure have not been shown, the association of this disorder with coronary artery disease points in that direction.

See Also the Following Articles

Catecholamines; Depression and Coronary Heart Disease; Cardiovasular Disease, Stress and; Primate Models, Cardiovascular Disease; Stress Management and Cardiovascular Disease; Stress, NPY and Cardiovascular Diseases.

Further Reading

Bale, T. L., Hoshijima, M., Gu, Y., et al. (2004). The cardiovascular physiologic actions of urocortin II: acute effects in murine heart failure. *Proceedings of the National Academy of Sciences USA* 101, 2697–3702.

Bozkurt, B., Kribbs, S., Clubb, F. J., Jr., et al. (1998). Pathophysiologically relevant concentrations of TNFα promote progressive left ventricular dysfunction and remodeling in rats. *Circulation* 97, 1382–1391.

Cotter, G., Milo-Cotter, O., Rubinstein, D., et al. (2006). Posttraumatic stress disorder: a missed link between psychiatric and cardiovascular morbidity? *CNS Spectrums* 11, 129–136.

Deswal, A., Petersen, N. J., Feldman, A. M., et al. (2001). Cytokines and cytokine receptors in advanced heart failure: an analysis of the cytokine database from the versarinone trial (VEST). *Circulation* 103, 2055–2059.

Gurlek, A., Kilickap, M., Dincer, I., et al. (2001). Effect of losartan on circulating TNF alpha levels and left ventricular systolic performance in patients with heart failure. *Journal of Cardiovascular Risk* 8, 279–282.

Kapadia, S., Dibbs, Z., Kurrelmeyer, K., et al. (1998). The role of cytokines in the failing human heart. *Cardiology Clinics* **16**, 645–656.

Levine, B., Kalman, J., Mayer, L., et al. (1990). Elevated circulating levels of TNF in severe chronic heart failure. *New England Journal of Medicine* **223**, 236–241.

Mann, D. L. (2004). Activation of inflammatory mediators in heart failure. In: Mann, U. (ed.) *Heart failure: a companion to Brownwald's Heart Disease*, pp. 159–180. Philadelphia: Saunders.

Port, J. D., Linseman, J. V. and Bristow, M. R. (2004). Adrenergic receptor signaling in chronic heart failure. In: Mann, U. (ed.) *Heart failure: a companion to Brownwald's Heart Disease*, pp. 145–158. Philadelphia: Saunders.

Heart Rate

J R Jennings
University of Pittsburgh School of Medicine, Pittsburgh, PA, USA

This article is a revision of the previous edition article by J R Jennings, volume 2, pp 333–337, © 2000, Elsevier Inc.

Forms of Heart Rate Measurement
Heart Rate Assessment in Behavioral Medicine
Heart Rate Assessment in Psychological Science
Summary

Glossary

Baseline	A condition to which responses are compared. This can be a resting condition with no stimulation or a condition that has all the elements of the task or stressor condition except for the critical task or stress element.
Electrocardiogram	A changing voltage over time collected from the chest of a person using surface electrodes. The electrocardiogram's changing voltages show atrial contraction (p wave) followed by ventricular contraction (qrs wave) and then ventricular recovery (t wave). Because of its relatively large amplitude, the qrs wave is typically used as the marker for the computation of heart rate or interbeat interval, although the heartbeat is initiated by the atrial contraction (p wave).
Heart rate	The number of contractions (beats) of the heart expressed per unit time, typically the number of heartbeats per minute.
Interbeat interval	The time, typically expressed in milliseconds, between contractions of the heart.
Phasic response	A transient change in the rate of the heart (or other index) induced by an environmental or physiological stimulus. Phasic responses are typically compared to a baseline and last for a second or more but less than a minute.
Stressor/task	Any event that poses a challenge to an individual. Conditions that threaten to induce harm or pain or frustrate achievement of positive rewards are termed stressors. Conditions that pose a requirement to mentally or physically manipulate objects are typically termed tasks; these may or may not also be stressors.
Tonic response	A sustained change in the rate of the heart (or other index) induced by an environmental or physiological condition. Tonic responses are typically compared to a baseline and last for a minute or more.

Forms of Heart Rate Measurement

Clinical

The pulse, obtained by palpitation over an artery, is the basic means of obtaining heart rate in the medical clinic. The contractions of the heart are counted based on the mechanical sensation in the thumb or finger of the observer induced by the expansion of the artery due to cardiac contraction. The experience of the pulse during stress probably arises from a similar mechanism: mechanical sensations from the viscera induced by cardiac contraction – contractions that increase in force during stress. Collection of heart rate via palpitation requires the presence of another person and physical contact. The person must accurately sense the heartbeats and time the interval over which the counts are made. Use of palpated heart rate in studies of stress has been reduced due to the possibility of error in judgments of timing and beat occurrence as well as the likelihood that the presence of a person may alter any laboratory-induced stress. Heart rate derived by this technique is typically expressed as beats per minute.

Physiological

Heart rate in physiological studies is typically derived from measurements taken from the electrocardiogram. The number of qrs waves per unit time are counted or the time between these waves is measured. Time between waves (interbeat interval) can be translated to the rate of the heart for any pair of beats. For example, if the time between heartbeats is 1000 ms (1 s), then the corresponding heart rate would be 60 beats/min; that is, 60 of these intervals of 1000 ms would equal 60 000 ms, 60 s, or 1 min. Such detailed measurements permit the tracking of how the heart is reacting beat by beat (or second by second) to environmental and physiological stimuli.

Heart rate arises from the integration of an individual's intrinsic rate with the influences of the sympathetic and parasympathetic branch of the nervous system. The heartbeat is initiated in the sinus node of the heart, which is a patch of spontaneously active neural tissue located in the cardiac atrium. The sinus node discharge rate depends on a basic intrinsic or constitutional rate for that person as modulated by the speeding influences of sympathetic nervous system firing and the slowing influences of parasympathetic system (vagus nerve) firing upon the sinus node. Thus, a second-by-second recording of heart rate provides a second-by-second record of a balance between sympathetic and parasympathetic nervous system influences on the heart.

Psychological

The sensitivity of heart rate to nervous system activation provides the justification for its use as an index of psychological stress. Stress is typically assumed to activate the sympathetic nervous system and deactivate the parasympathetic nervous system. Direct influences of the sympathetic nervous system on the sinus node as well as indirect influences via circulating catecholamines (derived primarily from the endocrine gland, the adrenal medulla) will activate β-adrenergic receptors, resulting in a speeding of the heart rate and an increase in cardiac contractility. Both nervous and endocrine reactions are transient responses to stressors. Some individuals report being in stressful circumstances lasting a year or more; such circumstances are unlikely to be directly reflected in heightened heart rate or even adrenomedullary reactions because these are reactions that return to baseline values after a brief period. Specific stressors arising from stressful circumstances can induce tonic reactions or phasic reactions of heart rate. Reactions to stressor lasting minutes to hours can be detected by examining tonic reactions in which the average heart rate over periods of minutes can be demonstrated to be elevated relative to a baseline period. Acute reactions to specific stressors may induce transient nervous system responses lasting seconds rather than minutes. Such phasic responses are typically assessed by comparing heart rate (or interbeat interval) for the seconds after the stressor to that of the seconds just before the stressor. The rapidity with which heart rate returns to baseline can also be informative. Increased vagal activation or decreased sympathetic activation will return heart rate to baseline values. Psychological factors, such as rumination over the stressful incident, may prolong heart rate speeding in some individuals. Concurrently, physiological factors may play a role in the recovery of heart rate, e.g., some individuals may have rapid vagal activation after a stressor with consequently brief heart rate reactions to stress. In short, the measurement of heart rate as an index of stress must be gauged to the type of stress, most particularly its temporal duration.

Heart Rate Assessment in Behavioral Medicine

Cardiovascular Reactivity

Because of its influence on the cardiovascular system, stress may influence the course of cardiovascular disease. A general hypothesis, the reactivity hypothesis, states that the cardiovascular reactivity resulting from repeated stressful events might contribute to the development of hypertension, myocardial infarction, and stroke. Presumably certain individuals are predisposed to show consistent and large cardiovascular reactions to stress, or are placed in an environment in which stressors are frequent and repetitive, or both. This hypothesis has been widely investigated using both laboratory challenges to assess reactivity and the ambulatory monitoring of heart rate and blood pressure as individuals perform their usual activities. The consistency within an individual over time of heart rate responses to laboratory stress has been established. Heart rate also changes in response to daily events in ambulatory recordings.

The number and size of heart rate responses do not seem, however, to predict cardiovascular disease onset and course; blood pressure increases in response to stressors have proven more predictive. The extensive parasympathetic influence on heart rate may explain this difference in the predictive utility of heart rate and blood pressure.

Heart Rate Variability

Derived measures of heart rate related to nervous system function have been found to correlate positively with cardiovascular health. Parasympathetic influences on heart rate are exerted via the vagus nerve, which innervates the heart (along with innervation by the cardiac sympathetic nerves). The vagus is more important than the sympathetic nerves for most transient changes in heart rate. Vagal firing influencing the heart waxes and wanes with respiration; this results in heart rate increasing during inspiration and decreasing during expiration. The rhythmic changes in heart rate over time, heart rate variability, can then be used to measure vagal influence on the heart. Heart rate has been found to show rhythmic changes with lower frequencies than respiration as well. For example, a frequency of 0.1 Hz has been related in part to sympathetic activity related to blood pressure, and heart rate shows a 24-h rhythm related to the sleep–wake cycle. Variability at the respiratory rate has been shown to be due almost completely to vagal/parasympathetic activity. Variability at other frequencies is not as well defined. Relatively greater variability has in general, however, been associated with cardiovascular health. A related measure positively associated with cardiovascular health is baroreceptor sensitivity. The baroreceptors are sense organs in major arteries that sense pressure change and transmit this to the brain, which then alters sympathetic and parasympathetic control to return blood pressure to normal. Pressure increases induce a vagal activation reducing heart rate. Greater heart rate change per unit of heart rate change (baroreceptor sensitivity) is correlated with better cardiovascular health. The associations of cardiac variability and baroreceptor sensitivity with cardiovascular health have led to the hypothesis that cardiac variability, most specifically parasympathetically induced variability, may act to buffer the influence of stress on the cardiovascular system.

Heart Rate Assessment in Psychological Science

Motivation/Affect

A psychological analysis of stress typically suggests that the threat or stressor induces an affective reaction as well as influences a person's motivational state. Subsequently, coping with the stressor may require other psychological processes. Behavioral medicine investigations have not typically attempted to separate the different processes influenced by stress, but the psychological analysis raises the question of whether heart rate reactions are controlled by one or more of the different psychological processes. The inference of a psychological process that is not directly observable is difficult, and this difficulty is compounded when the processes are as complex and conceptually overlapping as categories of affect and motivation. Studies do show that heart rate increases with the induction of most emotions, with the exception of disgust. Similarly, cues for reward or punishment can induce heart rate increases, perhaps with stronger increases related to cues for reward. Interpretation is further complicated by the possibility that coping with the affect or acting upon the motivational cue may elicit other processes controlling heart rate. For example, the induction of affect with an imaged scenario that contains an action element appears to induce greater heart rate change than induction with a more passive scenario.

Attention/Cognition

Coping refers to a set of action and mental processes that permit the person to redefine the threat and/or develop a means of neutralizing the threat. Thus, a multitude of cognitions and actions may be elicited as coping. If heart rate responds to processes such as attention and memory processes, then the involvement of these processes in coping, or even in the initial evaluation of the stressor, may be the source of phasic heart rate changes after a stressor. Muscle activation is a strong metabolic stimulus that induces rapid increases in heart rate. Similarly, change in breathing patterns, e.g., breath holding, have rapid, large effects on heart rate. These changes can readily be demonstrated in the absence of a stressor, while it is difficult to ensure that reactions to a stressor do not include muscle tension changes or changes in breathing pattern. Of greater psychological interest is attentive waiting, which induces clear phasic changes in heart rate. Heart rate decreases during the anticipation of any significant task or task element. Conceptually, heart rate seems to decrease whenever an action must be chosen at a specific point in time and potentially competing actions must be inhibited. The heart slows reliably prior to a signal to respond, even when that signal is accompanied by an electrical shock. This slowing of the heart rate does not appear to be due to respiratory changes or the inhibition of the peripheral musculature. The relevance of this observation to behavioral medicine studies of reactivity is clear. Many studies have used as their stressor/challenge computer games with periods of anticipatory attention.

Interpretive Issues

Heart rate can serve as an index of stress, but its utility and validity can be increased by a few simple precautions. First, stress and stress reactions should be conceptualized. Should heart rate in response to an increase in muscle tension be considered a stress reaction or a muscle artifact? Second, the stressor and overall conditions of eliciting the stress reaction should be controlled or assessed so it is possible to separate heart rate changes due to motor activity, respiration, transient attention, and affect/motivation. If a tonic response is of greatest interest, than scoring of the heart rate should occur after transient changes related to attention, breath holding, and muscle tensing. Fortunately, many of these phasic changes disappear after the initial few seconds of a task or stimulus presentation. Care must be taken in interpretation to recognize all the possible sources – other than those defined as stress – of the observed change in heart rate.

Summary

Heart rate increases rapidly during stress. The response may be initiated by motivational threat, affect, or the thoughts and actions induced by the stressor. Separation of the cause of the heart rate change is difficult in both the laboratory and real life. The degree of heart rate increase in response to stress or psychological challenge has been less predictive of medically significant cardiovascular disease than degree of change of blood pressure. The degree of variability of heart rate over time has, however, been associated with relatively better cardiovascular health.

Acknowledgment

The author acknowledges the assistance in writing this article from the support of NIH grant HL57529.

See Also the Following Articles

Blood Pressure; Cardiovasular Disease, Stress and; Sympathetic Nervous System.

Further Reading

Bernston, G. G. and Cacioppo, J. T. (2000). Homestasic to allodynamic regulation. In: Cacioppo, J. T., Tassinary, L. G. & Bernston, G. G. (eds.) *Handbook of psychophysiology* (2nd edn., pp. 459–490). Cambridge, UK: Cambridge University Press.

Dekker, J. M., Crow, R. S., Folsom, A. R., et al. (2000). Low heart rate variability in a 2-minute rhythm strip predicts risk of coronary heart disease and mortality from several causes: the ARIC Study. Atherosclerosis risk in communities. *Circulation* **102**, 1239–1244.

Huikuri, H. V., Jokinen, V., Syvanne, M., et al. (1999). Heart rate variability and progression of coronary atherosclerosis. *Arteriosclerosis, Thrombosis, and Vascular Biology* **19**(8), 1979–1985.

Jennings, J. R., Berg, W. K., Hutcheson, J. S., et al. (1981). Publication guidelines for the heart rate studies in man. *Psychophysiology* **19**, 226–231.

Jennings, J. R., van der Molen, M. W., Somsen, R. J., et al. (2002). Vagal function in health and disease: studies in Pittsburgh. *Physiology and Behavior* **77**(4–5), 693–698.

Jennings, J. R., Kamarck, T. W., Everson-Rose, S. A., et al. (2004). Exaggerated blood pressure responses during mental stress are prospectively related to enhanced carotid atherosclerosis in middle-aged Finnish men. *Circulation* **110**(15), 2198–2203.

Kamarck, T. W., Jennings, J. R., Debski, T. T., et al. (1992). Reliable measures of behaviorally-evoked cardiovascular reactivity from a PC-based test battery: results from student and community samples. *Psychophysiology* **29**, 17–28.

Krantz, D. S. and Manuck, S. B. (1984). Acute psychophysiologic reactivity and risk of cardiovascular disease: a review and methodologic critique. *Psychological Bulletin* **96**, 435–464.

Lovallo, W. R. (2005). *Stress and health: biological and psychological interactions* (2nd edn.). Thousand Oaks, CA: Sage.

Noble, D. (1979). *The initiation of the heart beat*. Oxford, UK: Clarendon Press.

Task Force (1996). Heart rate variability: standards of measurement, physiological interpretation, and clinical use. *Circulation* **93**, 1043–1065.

Heat Resistance

A J L Macario and E Conway de Macario
New York State Department of Health and
The University at Albany (SUNY),
Albany, NY, USA

Published by Elsevier Inc.

Diversity of Life Forms and Habitats
Definition
Chaperones and Chaperonins
Thermoprotectants
Intrinsic Molecular Features
Cell Envelopes and Multicellular Structures
Spores
Applications

Glossary

Biofilm   A flat multicellular structure, one or very few cells thick, that consists of a single or several (consortium) species. The single-species variety appears during the normal life cycle of an organism or in response to stress. Most biofilms must adhere to a surface as a support for growth and are, like granules, more heat-resistant than are their individual components living outside the structure. Other biofilms, such as the lamina formed by the archaeon *Methanoarcina mazeii* S-6, do not need to adhere to a surface for growth.

Granule   A multicellular structure or consortium composed of two or more species of organisms; it is more resistant to stressors such as heat than are the free organisms outside it.

Heat resistance   The capacity to withstand temperatures higher than 37°C without a significant loss of function; also called thermotolerance. More specifically, a cell condition characterized by an increase in the capacity to withstand temperatures above the optimal for that cell's growth, whether 37°C, higher, or lower. The cell condition involves an active process with a differential regulation of gene expression and protein levels induced by the elevation of temperature above the optimal one (heat shock); also called acquired or induced heat resistance.

Hyper-thermophile   An organism with an optimal temperature for growth of 80°C or higher.

Packet   A globular multicellular structure, composed of only one species, formed by certain microbes (e.g., the archaeon *Methanosarcina mazeii* S-6) as part of their life cycles or in response to environmental stressors. The packet is more resistant to stressors, including heat shock, than are the individual cells living outside it.

Thermophile   An organism with an optimal temperature for growth of 50–70°C; it prefers temperatures higher than 37°C and has constitutive heat resistance, namely an inborn capacity to carry out all of its physiological functions at temperatures that are not optimal for (or will damage or kill) human cells.

Thermo-protectant   A nonprotein molecule that plays an active role in thermotolerance by protecting proteins, and perhaps other cellular components, from the damaging effects of elevated temperatures, whether during normal growth (thermophiles and hyperthermophiles) or on a sudden increase above the optimal temperature (heat shock). There are several thermoprotectants that have rather simple structures. They are different from molecular chaperones and chaperonins, which are proteins.

Diversity of Life Forms and Habitats

In nature, living cells and organisms are diverse, encompassing a wide range of species that thrive under very varied conditions. Temperature is one of the major conditions that significantly influence the life of cells. As a reference point, bear in mind that the normal body temperature of adult humans is 36.8 (±0.4)°C and that human cells grow well in laboratory cultures at 37°C. There are, however, very many organisms, both single- and multicelled, on our planet that have optimal temperatures for growth (OTGs) that differ from 37°C, either lower or higher and sometimes radically.

Organisms are classified, according to their OTGs, into the following groups: psychrophiles (OTG 15°C or lower), mesophiles (OTG 35–40°C), thermophiles (OTG 50–70°C), and hyperthermophiles (OTG 80°C or higher). Within the mesophiles, those that can still grow at 0–4°C are termed psychrotolerant; within the hyperthermophiles, those that have OTGs above 95°C are termed extreme thermophiles.

Although organisms grow best at their OTGs, they can also grow and multiply, albeit more slowly, within temperature ranges on either side of their optimum. For example, the mesophilic organism *Methanosarcina mazeii* S-6 displays its fastest growth rate at 37–40°C, but it is capable of growing and multiplying within the 25–45°C range. Likewise, the extreme thermophile *Pyrolobus fumarii* has an OTG of 106°C, but it can grow at temperatures between 90 and 113°C. Determinations of this sort have shown that the maximum temperature at which any given organism can grow is closer to its OTG than to the minimum that still allows its survival. This suggests that, as a general rule, organisms are more sensitive to overheating than to cooling. Excess heat may kill (lethal temperature), whereas a comparable excess of cold may only slow down the functions of the cell.

Cells exposed to an elevation of temperature above their OTGs are stressed, or heat shocked, and they mount a stress or heat shock response. This response is characterized by the activation of stress (heat shock) genes along with the slowing down or shutting off of many other genes. The stress genes produce stress (heat shock) proteins, some of which are molecular chaperones; the latter play a role in cell survival during stress and recovery after stress.

Definition

Heat resistance, also called thermotolerance, is a condition that makes the cell capable of withstanding a temperature excess. Because of this capability, the cell can survive a heat shock that would otherwise be lethal.

If we use as a reference point the OTG for human cells, 37°C, we can recognize two main types of thermotolerance: constitutive and acquired. The former pertains to organisms that normally grow at temperatures considered stressful or lethal for human cells, as exemplified by the thermophiles and hyperthermophiles.

Acquired thermotolerance, in contrast, is an experiential tolerance that an organism gains after a heat shock. The following experiment illustrates a typical case of acquired thermotolerance. Cells from a hyperthermophilic organism with an OTG of 80°C, but that can grow within the 60–86°C range, was heat-shocked when exposed to 88°C (sublethal temperature for this organism) for 1 h, but it was killed by exposure to 92°C (lethal temperature). Remarkably, cells that had been heat shocked at 88°C did not die when they were subsequently exposed to the lethal temperature. The heat-shocked cells had acquired

thermotolerance; the cells were able to survive a lethal temperature because they had been prepared (preconditioned) by preexposure to a sublethal, heat-shocking temperature.

Cross-Tolerance

Temperature excess is a cell stressor, but it is not the only one known. There are many cell stressors of mechanical (e.g., compression and shearing), physical (e.g., heat and ultraviolet radiation), or chemical (e.g., alcohol, hydrogen peroxide, high salinity, and lack of oxygen) nature that elicit a stress (heat shock) response in cells. Interestingly, stress tolerance induced by one stressor may also result in efficient resistance (i.e., cross-tolerance) to other stressors. Thus, thermotolerance induced by heat shock may also increase the resistance to a chemical stressor and vice versa. Cross-tolerance to stressors is of extraordinary potential value to fields such as medicine and surgery.

Mechanism

Heat resistance or thermotolerance is mediated by a variety of factors and mechanisms: stress proteins, molecular chaperones, chaperonins, thermoprotective compounds, innate characteristics of proteins that make them thermostable, cell-wall composition and architecture, formation of multicellular structures, and formation of spores.

One of the key harmful events in heat stress is protein denaturation. If the stress is too drastic (a heat-shocking temperature far above the OTG or very prolonged heat shock), the cellular proteins denature and aggregate. Cell death ensues. An illustrative example is the hard-boiled egg. There is no known way to restore a hard-boiled egg to a viable form so that the denatured, aggregated proteins disaggregate and regain their functional, native conformation. There are, however, many instances in which protein denaturation does not reach such extreme, irreversible levels. Milder stresses cause only partial denaturation, and the damage is reversible; the proteins can be restored to their functional form. The recovery is mediated by several mechanisms, one of which involves the molecular chaperones. These chaperones are also involved in preventing protein damage and in eliminating protein molecules damaged beyond repair.

Thermotolerance is based on various mechanisms and a key one is the presence and use of all the cellular molecules and mechanisms that prevent and cure protein denaturation and also those that eliminate irreversibly damaged and aggregated proteins before these reach levels that will clog the intracellular machinery.

Chaperones and Chaperonins

Chaperones and chaperonins belong to the large group of stress (heat shock) proteins, although not all of them are the product of stress-inducible genes. Their functions are to assist nascent polypeptides in folding correctly so that each can reach a functional configuration (its native conformation), to protect the polypeptides from aggregation during synthesis and during stress, and to refold them after partial unfolding (reversible denaturation) caused by stressors such as heat.

Thermoprotectants

Thermoprotectants are simple cellular components that confer resistance to other molecules, by mechanisms not yet fully elucidated. They are considered integral to thermotolerance because they have been found in hyperthermophilic organisms and because laboratory tests *in vitro* have indicated that they stabilize protein molecules, rendering them heat resistant.

Two thermoprotectants have been studied in some detail: di-*myo*-inositol phosphate (DIP), and cyclic diphosphoglycerate (cDPG). These molecules are believed to be important for the physiology of organisms living in high-temperature ecosystems (e.g., hot springs, hot pools and mud pots, solfataras and geysers, and hydrothermal vents at the bottom of the ocean) and for their survival when stressed by the variations in temperature, pH, and hydrostatic pressure that are characteristic of these extreme environments. Trehalose, a disaccharide, has also been implicated in the mechanism of heat resistance, either alone or in association with chaperones.

Intrinsic Molecular Features

Many proteins, including enzymes, of thermophilic and hyperthermophilic organisms withstand heat stress better than do their counterparts from mesophiles, even in the absence of thermoprotectants. They are believed to have built-in structural features that make them thermostable, but the nature of these features has not been determined. It has been proposed that innumerable subtle interactions occur among various points of the molecule that confer great stability, even in the face of stressors, and enhanced resistance to the denaturation induced by the latter. The identification and measurement of these interactions have proven elusive up to the present time.

Cell Envelopes and Multicellular Structures

Many organisms, particularly those living in extreme environments, are protected from harsh environmental factors by specialized cell envelopes that are resistant to the stressors (e.g., high temperature or salinity) that are inherent to their ecosystems. In addition, many species form multicellular structures that are more resistant to stressors than are single cells. In these structures, cells are held together either by an intercellular connective material, consisting of a flat sheet with a thickness of one or very few cells or in a globular conglomerate resembling a sphere (**Figure 1**). The former, flat structure is called a biofilm, and it is usually, but not always, attached to a supporting surface (e.g., rock in natural habitats or sand particles in methanogenic bioreactors).

The globular structures are of two types; they are formed either by a single species or by an association of two or more species. The multispecies type is called a granule, and it constitutes a microbial consortium that can live in both natural and manufactured ecosystems. Examples of manufactured ecosystems are the anaerobic methanogenic bioreactors used in waste-processing plants. In the granular consortium, various species of microorganisms cooperate with one another in a food web that bioconverts organic molecules while being shielded from the shearing and other stressors typical of bioreactors, such as temperature and pH variations. Indeed, the consortium is very resistant to these stressors, and it survives stresses that would kill its microbial components outside the granule.

The single-species type of globular multicellular structure is formed by a single species of organism as part of its life cycle or in response to stressors. An example of a single-species multicellular structure is that built by the methanogenic microorganism *Methanosarcina mazeii* S-6 in culture and in bioreactors (**Figure 1**). The globular morphotype, termed a packet, is considerably more resistant to mechanical, chemical, and thermal stressors than is the single-celled form of this archaeon.

Spores

Some microbes subjected to harsh environmental conditions, such as scarcity of nutrients, desiccation, and exposure to toxic substances, undergo sporulation. They form a very stress-resistant structure called a spore or endospore. The microbe becomes dehydrated, and its genetic material is enclosed in a thick coat with a special composition that is, most likely,

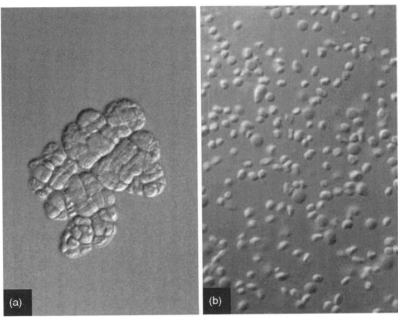

Figure 1 Archaeal microbe *Methanosarcina mazeii* S-6. (a) Cells growing in a packet, a globular, heat-resistant multicellular structure; (b) cells growing individually. The packet is composed of many cells joined together by an intercellular connective material that also enwraps the whole structure. From A. J. L. Macario and E. Conway de Macario (2001), *Frontiers in Bioscience* **6**, d262–d283, [online].

responsible for the extreme resistance of spores to stressors, including heat.

Because spores are produced by microbes that can cause disease in humans and animals (e.g., *Clostridium tetani* and *C. botulinum*), they are of special interest to the field of medicine and to the food industry, which must resort to sterilization and pasteurization (both involving heating) to prevent contamination and infection.

Applications

Stress resistance is a desirable attribute from the organism's perspective because confrontation with stressors, such as heat shock, is a frequent occurrence in the life of any cell or organism. However, as pointed out in the previous section, microbial stress resistance may be undesirable from the human perspective, when the organisms is pathogenic and must be destroyed.

In other circumstances, when stress resistance is a convenient attribute from the medical or industrial perspective, attempts at making certain cell types more resistant to stressors are not only justified but also are an attractive scientific and biotechnologic endeavor. Means are being developed at the present time to enhance cell survival during stress and to accelerate cell recovery after stress. Briefly, the idea is to provide a cell with those elements now known to

play (or that are suspected of playing) a key role in maintaining its normal array of proteins in working condition. These elements can help in restoring the functional conformation of damaged proteins or in degrading those damaged beyond repair during and after stress. Genetic engineering and preconditioning are two approaches to achieving this; they can be applied independently of one another or in combination. Essentially, in the genetic engineering approach, an extra set of genes encoding the proteins of interest (e.g., molecular chaperones or proteases) are grafted into the genome of the target cell whose stress resistance is to be increased. Alternatively, the extra set of genes is incorporated into the cytoplasm of the cell via a self-replicating extrachromosomal element such as a plasmid. In both instances, the expression of the foreign genes increases the levels of the stress proteins inside the cell, which in turn enhances the folding of newly formed, much needed polypeptides and also the refolding of partially denatured molecules. Of course, it is a possibility that secondary effects may also occur that are negative from the standpoint of the cell, tissue, or organism we are trying to protect from the consequences of stress. Because of this possibility, many tests with experimental models are necessary to certify the benefits of this type of anti-stress treatment before it is applied to valuable cells in bioreactors or to humans in a therapeutic context.

The preconditioning approach involves the use of mild stressors, for example, chemical compounds known to induce stress genes, to generate cross-tolerance to potent stressors or the use of a potent stressor at low doses to induce a stress response of low intensity. Both procedures confer a sort of cellular memory. When the cell is challenged with a potentially very damaging or lethal stressor against which a cross-tolerance was previously induced, the cell has increased chances of survival. Likewise, a cell preconditioned with low doses of a potent stressor also has increased chances of survival when challenged with the same stressor at doses that would be lethal for a nonpreconditioned cell.

These strategies and procedures are being applied and have a promising future in the biotechnology industry and in medicine and surgery. In the biotechnology field, bioreactors (also called fermentors) are used for a variety of purposes ranging from the large-scale production of useful molecules (e.g., hormones and antibiotics) to the bioconversion of wastes. However, a drawback is that the cells in bioreactors are susceptible to stressors generated by the process itself or received with the influent (e.g., wastes). Oscillations or abrupt changes in temperature, pH, and content of toxic chemicals are common events in bioconversion technology. These stressors cause frequent bioreactor malfunctions or failures because the bioprocessing cells suffer stress, malfunction, and even die. Obviously, the generation of resistant cells, capable of withstanding the stressors, will improve the efficiency and economic value of this technology.

Another obvious need for cells equipped with strong antistress mechanisms exists in surgery. Poor oxygenation, resulting in cell stress, occurs in many tissues; most important, it occurs in the brain and heart during large-scale surgical operations, particularly those necessitating blood exchange. It is, therefore, crucial to prevent brain- and heart-cell damage and to ensure the preservation of these vital tissues. To achieve this goal, a promising strategy is to induce stress tolerance. Stress proteins, specifically molecular chaperones, are being tested in experiments whose aim is to invigorate the cells. A stress protein or its gene is introduced into the tissue to confer resistance in a manner similar to that described for microbes in bioreactors that process wastes.

An alternative approach takes advantage of cross-tolerance. Heat resistance is induced in the cells of tissues targeted for protection from ischemia hypoxia (e.g., brain and heart tissues) by mild heat shock. This preparatory mild stress, or preconditioning, is relatively harmless, yet it is sufficient to elicit a heat shock response and heat resistance, which are efficient in counteracting the harmful effects of ischemia hypoxia during a surgical procedure.

Last, replacement therapy, genetic or otherwise, may be indicated in chaperonopathies – diseases in which deficient chaperones are the primary etiology of or significant contributors to the pathogenesis. In these instances, chaperone genes may be used in genetic engineering approaches, as described earlier, or purified molecular chaperones may be administered directly, as antibodies are sometimes provided to treat infections.

On the negative side, microbial heat resistance is an obstacle to the sterilization of surgical and laboratory instruments, plasticware and glassware, sera, solutions, culture media, and any other object or substance that must be freed from pathogenic organisms while avoiding a significant loss of biological or medicinal properties. The heat resistance of microbes also presents a problem for the food industry whenever it is necessary to improve the safety and preservation of edible products. Some very serious food-borne pathogens, such as *Clostridium botulinum*, form spores and can be in a dormant state for years until favorable environmental conditions induce their return to a vegetative, pathogenic status. The food industry must apply heat and other means to get rid of the pathogens, but only to the extent that the nutritional and sensory qualities of the product are not impaired significantly. The achievement of such a balance between killing or disarming the pathogens and preserving food quality is a major challenge for science and technology.

See Also the Following Articles

Chaperone Proteins and Chaperonopathies; Heat Resistance; Heat Shock Genes, Human; Heat Shock Response, Overview; Viral Virulence and Stress; Chaperonopathies; Proteases in the Eukaryotic Cell Cytosol; Proteases in Prokaryotes and Eukaryotic Cell Organelles.

Further Reading

Attfield, P. V. (1997). Stress tolerance: the key to effective strains of industrial baker's yeast. *Nature Biotechnology* 15, 1351–1357.

Beaucamp, N., Harding, T. C., Geddes, B. J., et al. (1998). Overexpression of *hsp70i* facilitates reactivation of intracellular proteins in neurons and protects them from denaturing stress. *FEBS Letters* 441, 215–219.

Blochl, E., Rachel, R., Burggraf, S., et al. (1997). *Pyrolobus fumarii*, gen. and sp. nov., represents a novel group of archaea, extending the upper temperature limit for life to 113 °C. *Extremophiles* 1, 14–21.

Conway de Macario, E. and Macario, A. J. L. (2003). Molecular biology of stress genes in methanogens:

potential for bioreactor technology. *Advances in Biochemical Engineering/Biotechnology* **81**, 95–150.

da Silva, R., Lucchinetti, E., Pasch, T., et al. (2004). Ischemic but not pharmacological preconditioning elicits a gene expression profile similar to unprotected myocardium. *Physiological Genomics* **20**, 117–130.

Dinh, H-K. B., Zhao, B., Schuschereba, S. T., et al. (2001). Gene expression profiling of the response to thermal injury in human cells. *Physiological Genomics* **7**, 3–13.

Gross, C. and Watson, K. (1997). Transcriptional and translational regulation of major heat shock proteins and patterns of trehalose mobilization during hyperthermic recovery in repressed and derepressed *Saccharomyces cerevisiae*. *Canadian Journal of Microbiology* **44**, 341–350.

Holden, J. F., Adams, M. W. W. and Baross, J. A. (2000). Heat-shock response in hyperthermophilic microorganisms. In: Bell, C. R., Brylinsky, M. & Johnson Green, P. (eds.) *Microbial biosystems: new frontiers* (vol. 2), pp. 663–670. Halifax, Canada: Atlantic Canada Society for Microbial Ecology and Acadia University Press.

Juneja, V. K., Klein, P. G. and Marmer, B. S. (1998). Heat shock and thermotolerance of *Escherichia coli* O157:H7 I in a model beef gravy system and ground beef. *Journal of Applied Microbiology* **84**, 677–684.

Kregel, K. C. (2002). Heat shock proteins: modifying factors in physiological stress responses and acquired thermotolerance. *Journal of Applied Physiology* **92**, 2177–2186.

Macario, A. J. L. and Conway de Macario, E. (2001). The molecular chaperone system and other anti-stress mechanisms in Archaea. *Frontiers in Bioscience* **6**, d262–d283. To see tables and figures go to: http://www.bioscience.org/2001/v6/d/macario/fulltext.htm

Madigan, M. T., Martinko, J. M. and Parker, J. (2003). *Brock biology of microorganisms* (10th edn.). Upper Saddle River, NJ: Prentice Hall.

Mestril, R. (2005). The use of transgenic mice to study cytoprotection by the stress proteins. *Methods* **35**, 165–169.

Mohsenzadeh, S., Saupe-Thies, W., Steier, G., et al. (1998). Temperature adaptation of house keeping and heat shock gene expression in *Neurospora crassa*. *Fungal Genetics and Biology* **25**, 31–43.

Nollen, E. A. A., Brunsting, J. F., Roelofsen, H., et al. (1999). In vivo chaperone activity of heat shock protein 70 and thermotolerance. *Molecular and Cellular Biology* **19**, 2069–2079.

Pedone, E., Bartolucci, S. and Fiorentino, G. (2004). Sensing and adapting to environmental stress: the archaeal tactic. *Frontiers in Bioscience* **9**, 2909–2926. To see tables and figures go to: http://www.bioscience.org/2004/v9/af/1447/fulltext.htm

Pespeni, M., Hodnett, M. and Pittet, J-F. (2005). *In vivo* stress preconditioning. *Methods* **35**, 158–164.

Piper, P. (1998). Differential role of Hsps and trehalose in stress tolerance. *Trends in Microbiology* **6**, 43–44.

Roberts, M. F. (2004). Osmoadaptation and osmoregulation in archaea: update 2004. *Frontiers in Bioscience* **9**, 1999–2019. To see tables and figures go to: http://www.bioscience.org/2004/v9/af/1366/fulltext.htm

Sabehat, A., Weiss, D. and Lurie, S. (1998). The heat-shock proteins and cross-tolerance in plants. *Physiologia Plantarum* **103**, 437–441.

Scandurra, R., Consalvi, V., Chiaraluce, R., et al. (2000). Protein stability in extremophilic archaea. *Frontiers in Bioscience* **5**, d787–d795. To see the complete article go to: http://www.bioscience.org/2000/v5/d/scan/scan.pdf

Sharp, F. R., Massa, S. M. and Swanson, R. A. (1999). Heat-shock protein protection. *Trends in Neuroscience* **22**, 97–99.

Takai, K., Nunoura, T., Sako, Y., et al. (1998). Acquired thermotolerance and temperature induced protein accumulation in the extremely thermophilic bacterium. *Rhodothermus obamensis*. *Journal of Bacteriology* **180**, 2770–2774.

Tolson, J. K. and Roberts, S. M. (2005). Manipulating heat shock protein expression in laboratory animals. *Methods* **35**, 149–157.

Weibezahn, J., Tessarz, P., Schlieker, C., et al. (2004). Thermotolerance requires refolding of aggregated proteins by substrate translocation through the central pore of ClpB. *Cell* **119**, 653–665.

Westerheide, S. D., Bosman, J. D., Mbadugha, B. N. A., et al. (2004). Celastrols as inducers of the heat shock response and cytoprotection. *Journal of Biological Chemistry* **279**, 56053–56060.

Heat Shock Genes, Human

A J L Macario and E Conway de Macario
New York State Department of Health and
the University at Albany (SUNY),
Albany, NY, USA

Published by Elsevier Inc.

Introduction

Molecular Phylogeny

Origins of the Human Cell

Microanatomic Components of the Human Cell

Stress Proteins in the Various Compartments
of the Human Cell

Stress Genes

The Human Genome

Perspectives

Glossary

Endoplasmic reticulum (ER)	A eukaryotic cell component consisting of a labyrinthine system of flat cavities delimited by a membrane that is continuous with the outer membrane bounding the nucleus. The ER is involved in the synthesis and transport of proteins and other molecules.
Genome	The complete set of genetic information carried by a cell (or organism), representing its entire hereditary complement.
Genomics	The cataloguing and large-scale investigation of the sequence, structure, and function of whole genomes, or of whole sets of genes and their interactions and expression patterns.
Mitochondrion	A eukaryotic cell organelle, evolutionarily related to gram-negative bacteria; it houses the cellular respiration apparatus and produces energy.
Molecular phylogeny	The science of classifying organisms through comparisons of molecular sequences. This type of classification reflects the evolution of individual molecules and shows evolutionary relationships between molecules and organisms.
Nucleolus	A relatively small region within the nucleus that contains the ribosomal RNA (rRNA) genes; this is where rRNA synthesis occurs.
Nucleus	The distinctive organelle of the eukaryotic cell (it is not present in prokaryotes), consisting mainly of packed genetic material (DNA) encased in a double membrane. Gene expression begins in
Proteomics	this organelle with transcription, which generates the messenger RNA (mRNA). The cataloguing and study of the full set of proteins encoded by a genome; also, the analysis of the set of proteins produced by a genome or a large group of genes (expression profile) under various circumstances, e.g., conditions of cell stress vs. basal conditions (no stress).

Introduction

Heat shock genes are also called stress genes. The latter is a more appropriate name, since these genes are induced not only by heat shock but also by other stressors. Hence, the term stress genes is given preference in this article.

A better understanding of human stress genes can be gained by examining them from the evolutionary standpoint rather than by studying them in isolation, without connection with the same genes in other species or with their evolutionary history. Modern molecular phylogeny has provided the means to look at genes and their proteins while taking into consideration their structural and evolutionary relations, at a level of resolution that was not attainable in the past. Furthermore, genome sequencing has now become a reality, expanding the possibilities for gene analysis and comparison beyond previously imaginable limits.

Molecular Phylogeny

Molecular phylogeny is a relatively new scientific discipline that involves the comparative analysis of the nucleotide sequences of genes and the amino acid sequences and structural features of proteins from which evolutionary histories and relationships, and in some cases also functions, can be inferred.

The basic classification of organisms furnished by molecular phylogeny is based upon the comparison of 16S/18S (small subunit) ribosomal RNA (rRNA) sequences. Thus, all living cells are divided into three main evolutionary branches or phylogenetic lines of descent termed domains: bacteria (eubacteria), archaea (archaebacteria), and eucarya (eukaryotes).

In addition to the small ribosomal subunit rRNA, other molecules such as stress (heat shock) proteins have been used for phylogenetic analyses. One of the most convenient targets for these analyses is the stress protein Hsp70(DnaK), for the following reasons. (1) It is long enough (about 600 amino acids on average, of which nearly 500 are conserved) to permit the occurrence of mutations at an observable level; (2) it is highly conserved, being present in virtually all organisms and cells with few exceptions, with an amino acid sequence that is very similar in all organisms; (3) it has segments that are more highly conserved than others, which allows for reliable alignments for comparative analyses of matching structural domains; and (4) it has distinctive structural features called motifs or signatures, some of which have a known function, that facilitate comparisons among molecules from different organisms, including functional comparisons without actually performing functional assays in the laboratory.

Origins of the Human Cell

Comparative analyses of sequences and sequence signatures have provided information on the evolution of organisms and consequently of their relationships (what or who is derived from what or whom). These analyses have also clarified the origins of the eukaryotic cell (including the human cell) as a whole, and those of its components.

With the preceding in mind, we can now add that a better understanding of human stress genes also requires familiarity with the components of the eukaryotic cell and their origins, as revealed by molecular phylogenetic analyses and studies of full genome sequences.

Microanatomic Components of the Human Cell

Human cells are composed of the cytoplasmic membrane that encloses the cytoplasm or cytosol in which the organelles reside. Examples of the latter are the nucleus with the nucleolus, mitochondria, Golgi apparatus, and endoplasmic reticulum (ER). Plant cells also have these various organelles, and in addition they have chloroplasts, in which photosynthesis takes place. Stress proteins are present in all the cellular compartments, whereas the genes that code for them are in the DNA of the nucleus.

Molecular phylogenetic analyses of nucleotide and amino acid sequences of various types of molecules, including stress genes and proteins, have revealed that the genes in the nuclear DNA are a mixed assemblage of bacterial and archaeal components side by side with typically eukaryotic constituents. Furthermore, it has been shown that mitochondria are derived from ancestors of modern gram-negative bacteria and that chloroplasts are descendants of the ancestors of today's cyanobacteria.

It has been concluded that the human cell is an assemblage of bacterial, archaeal, and eukaryotic components that coexist in a functional unit. This is the result of billions of years of genetic changes, exchanges, gains, and losses during evolution from the most primitive ancestral forms to today's *Homo sapiens*.

Stress Proteins in the Various Compartments of the Human Cell

A sample of stress proteins that have been studied in human cells and whose corresponding genes have been identified and characterized, at least partially, is given in **Table 1**, which classifies stress proteins based on molecular mass.

Comparative sequence analyses of the type mentioned in the previous sections have provided insights into the evolutionary origins of the stress proteins residing in the cytosol, nucleus, mitochondria, and ER. For instance, mitochondrial Hsp60 is derived from ancestors of modern gram-negative bacteria (it is equivalent to the GroEL chaperonin of extant bacteria), whereas the cytosolic Hsp60 is the homolog of the chaperonin subunits that compose the thermosome in modern archaea. The Hsp70(DnaK) in all compartments of the human cell is related to a gram-negative bacterial ancestor and is similar to the homologs of extant gram-negative bacteria but distinct from those of modern gram positives.

Stress Genes

Human stress genes and their proteins have been studied only to a limited extent compared to those from other eukaryotic organisms. A sample of the human cell types, cell lines, and tissues in which expression of the stress genes has been assessed is displayed in **Table 2**.

In general, constitutive (basal) gene expression was measured and compared with expression induced by a stressor, for instance, a temperature higher than optimal for cell growth (heat shock) or some other agent of medical significance, such as a heavy metal. Whenever possible, the levels of expression in pathological cells were compared with those in normal counterparts. Overall, the results showed alterations in the levels of expression in cells from diseased tissues, increases more often than decreases, as compared with normal controls. However, the physiopathological or pathogenic significance of these alterations could not be established with certainty in most instances. This deficiency is chiefly attributable to the difficulties in designing properly controlled experiments, including direct manipulation of cells or tissues, when performing research involving human subjects and clinical samples. Hence, many more data are available from experiments done with simple

Table 1 Examples of human stress (heat shock) and molecular chaperone proteins whose genes have been at least partially identified and characterized

Family		Locale of residence in the cell[a]		
Name(s)	Mass (kDa)	Cytosol/Nucleus	Mitochondria	Endoplasmic reticulum (ER)
Heavy; high molecular weight; Hsp100	100 or higher	Hsp110; Hsp105alpha; Hsp105beta		
Hsp90	81–99	Hsp90alpha (Hsp90; Hsp84) Hsp90beta (Hsc90; Hsp86)		Hsp90alpha (Hsp90; Hsp84); Hsp90beta; (Hsc90; Hsp86); Grp94
Hsp70; chaperones	65–80	Hsp70–1; Hsp70–2 (Hsc70); Hsp-Hom		Grp78 (BiP)
Hsp60 chaperonins group I chaperonins group II	55–64	Hsp60 CCT (TriC; TCP-1) 8–9 subunits	Cpn60(Hsp60)	
Hsp40; DnaJ	35–54	Hsp40; HDJ-1; HSJ-1; HSJ-2; HDJ-2; Hsc54		HDJ-1 (Hsp40); Hsp47
Other small Hsp; sHsp	34 or lower	Hsp27; alpha-crystallin family (HspB1–10)		
Miscellanea		PDIase; PPIase	Hsp23(GrpE); Cpn10(Hsp10)	PDIase

[a]The corresponding genes are in the nuclear DNA.

Table 2 Some human cell types, cell lines, and tissues in which expression of stress (heat shock) genes has been investigated[a]

Cells/lines/tissues	Gene
Cells	
Fibroblasts	hsp70i; hsc70(hsp73); HSP7OBρ; hsp60
Melanocytes	Hsp70
Lymphoid tumor cells	hsp72(hsp70i)
Macrophages	hsp70
Mononuclear cells from peripheral blood	hsp90; hsp70
Hepatocytes	hsp70–1; hsc70; hsp90
Unbilical vein endothelial cells	grp78
Wilms tumor cells	hsp70i
Cell line	
Breast cancer T47-D	grp94; grp78; hsp72
Embryonic kidney 293	hsp47
Erythroleukemia K562	hsp70; hsp70–1; hsp70–2; hsp70B'
RAJI	hsp70–1; hsp70–2; hsp70B'
HL60	hsp70–1; hsp70–2; hsp70B'
HeLa	hsp105; grp78; hsp70i(hsp72); hsc70(hsp73)
Human lung tumor HS24	hsc70-like or HSP24/p52
Melanoma	grp94; hsp90α; hsp90β; HSP70–1; HSP70–2; hsp27
Tissue	
Arterial intima	hsp70; hsp60
Jejunal epithelium	hsp60
Liver	hsp60
Lung	hsp73; hsp72; hsp60
Skeletal muscle	hsp90; hsp70
Stomach	hsp60
Retina	alpha-crystallin

[a]Constitutive (basal) and stressor (usually heat shock)-induced expression was studied in many cases, with pathologic cells or tissues compared to their normal counterparts whenever possible.

organisms (e.g., the bacterium *Escherichia coli*, the archaeon *Methanosarcina mazeii*, and the unicellular fungus *Saccharomyces cerevisiae*) and animal models (e.g., mice, rats, and gerbils) than are available from research carried out directly in human cells or tissues.

In animal models, it has been shown, for example, that the levels of stress proteins, especially Hsp70-(DnaK), are elevated in tissues damaged by ischemia-hypoxia. Research has focused on determining the presence of Hsp70(DnaK) in brain and heart tissues afflicted by ischemia-hypoxia. Around the dead, central zone of an infarct in the brain (stroke) or in the heart (cardiac attack), caused by occlusion of an artery and blood flow interruption, there are zones in which the brain or heart cells are not dead, but only injured. These zones are called penumbra in the brain and areas of stunned myocardiocytes in the heart. Cells in such zones are damaged mainly due to protein denaturation. The latter may be reversible, particularly with the help of stress proteins that, like Hsp70(DnaK), are molecular chaperones.

The Human Genome

The human genome has been sequenced, and the information is now being processed, with the data available at various websites (**Table 3**). It will take considerable effort over the coming years to process all the data and to complete the annotation, based on thorough analyses of each gene (genomics) and gene product (proteomics). A hint at the enormous complexity of the situation is provided, for instance, by the fact that at present there are more than 30 candidate genes that encode Hsp40(DnaJ)-related proteins and more than 20 that encode Hsp70(DnaK)-related

proteins. A similar situation holds true for all the other heat shock proteins and molecular chaperones.

Perspectives

A full view of the human species' stress gene candidates should become available when the sequence of the human genome has been more fully analyzed. In addition to identification of the genes through comparisons of their sequences – and those of the proteins encoded in them – with homologs of known functions from other organisms, experiments will be required to establish whether these genes are transcribed and translated and also to determine these genes' responses to various stressors. Based on the results, it should become possible to devise strategies for using the genes, their regulatory components and factors, and the proteins that they produce to both prevent and treat stress-induced lesions and diseases.

Also, a detailed phylogenetic analysis of each heat shock protein and molecular chaperone will be necessary if we are to understand their evolution and if we are to gain insight into their biological roles in organisms from the three phylogenetic domains. These analyses will also provide valuable information on the evolution and function of each protein's structural-functional domain and motif present in human heat shock proteins and molecular chaperones. In turn, this information will be instrumental for elucidating the nature of genes and gene products that are abnormal in genetic and acquired chaperonopathies; currently, only preliminary information is available for these disorders, suggesting that the affected molecules are chaperones.

See Also the Following Articles

Chaperone Proteins and Chaperonopathies; Chaperonopathies; Heat Resistance; Heat Shock Response, Overview; Viral Virulence and Stress; Proteases in the Eukaryotic Cell Cytosol; Proteases in Prokaryotes and Eukaryotic Cell Organelles.

Table 3 Human genome websites

Website	Chromosome
http://www.gdb.org	1–22, X, Y
http://www.ensembl.org	1–22, X, Y
http://www.ncbi.nlm.nih.gov/genome/guide/human/	122, X, Y
http://www.jgi.doe.gov	5, 16, 19
http://www.sanger.ac.uk/HGP/	1, 6, 9, 10, 11, 13, 20, 22, X
http://genome.ucsc.edu	1–22, X, Y
http://www.hgsc.bcm.tmc.edu	1–22, X, Y
http://www.ncbi.nlm.nih.gov/Sitemap/index.html#HumanGenome	1–22, X, Y
http://www-shgc.stanford.edu/finishing/human.html	5, 16, 19
http://www.nature.com/cgi-taf/DynaPage.taf?file=/nature/journal/v434/n7034/full/nature03466_fs.html	2, 4

Further Reading

Andley, U. P., Mathur, S., Griest, T. A. and Petrash, J. M. (1996). Cloning, expression, and chaperone-like activity of human alpha-crystallin. *Journal of Biological Chemistry* **71**, 31973–31980.

Bukach, O. V., Seit-Nebi, A. S., Marston, S. B. and Gusev, N. B. (2004). Some properties of human small heat-shock protein Hsp20 (HspB6). *European Journal of Biochemistry* **271**, 291–302.

Ellgaard, L. and Ruddock, L. W. (2005). The human protein disulphide isomerase family: Substrate interactions and functional properties. *EMBO Reports* **6**, 28–32.

Hansen, J. J., Bross, P., Westergaard, M., et al. (2003). Genomic structure of the human mitochondrial chaperonin genes: HSP60 and HSP10 are localised head to head on chromosome 2 separated by a bidirectional promoter. *Human Genetics* **112**, 71–77.

Hinton, A., Gatti, D. L. and Ackerman, S. H. (2004). The molecular chaperone, Atp12, from *Homo sapiens*. *Journal of Biological Chemistry* **279**, 9016–9022.

Ishihara, K., Yasuda, K. and Hatayama, T. (1999). Molecular cloning, expression and localization of human 105 kDa heat shock protein, hsp105. *Biochimica et Biophysica Acta* **1444**, 138–142.

Kappe, G., Franck, E., Verschuure, P., Boelens, W. C., Leunissen, J. A. M. and de Jong, W. W. (2003). The human genome encodes 10 alpha-crystallin-related small heat shock proteins: HspB1–10. *Cell Stress and Chaperones* **8**, 53–61.

Kleizen, B. and Braakman, I. (2004). Protein folding and quality control in the endoplasmic reticulum. *Current Opinion in Cell Biology* **16**, 343–349.

Leung, T. K. C., Rajendran, M. Y., Monfries, C., Hall, C. and Lim, L. (1990). The human heat shock protein family. *Biochemical Journal* **267**, 132–152.

Macario, A. J. L. (1995). Heat-shock proteins and molecular chaperones: implications for pathogenesis, diagnostics, and therapeutics. *International Journal of Clinical Research* **25**, 59–70.

Macario, A. J. L. and Conway de Macario, E. (1999). The archaeal molecular chaperone machine: Peculiarities and paradoxes. *Genetics* **152**, 1277–1283.

Macario, A. J. L. and Conway de Macario, E. (2002). Sick chaperones and ageing: a perspective. *Ageing Research Reviews* **1**, 295–311.

Macario, A. J. L. and Conway de Macario, E. (2004). The pathology of anti-stress mechanisms: a new frontier. *Stress* **7**, 243–249.

Macario, A. J. L., Grippo, T. M. and Conway de Macario, E. (2005). Genetic disorders involving molecular-chaperone genes: a perspective. *Genetics in Medicine* **7**, 3–12.

Meacham, G. C., Lu, Z., King, S., Sorscher, E., Tousson, A. and Cyr, D. M. (1999). The Hdj-2/Hsc70 chaperone pair facilitates early steps in CFTR biogenesis. *EMBO Journal* **18**, 1492–1505.

Nagai, N., Tetuya, Y., Hosokawa, N. and Nagata, K. (1999). The human genome has only one functional *hsp47* gene (CBP2) and a pseudogene (*pshsp47*). *Gene* **227**, 241–248.

Orchard, S., Hermjakob, H. and Apweiler, R. (2005). Annotating the human proteome. *Molecular and Cellular Proteomics* **4**, 435–440.

Snoeckx, L. H. E. H., Cornelussen, R. N., van Nieuwenhoven, F. A., Reneman, R. S. and van der Vusse, G. J. (2001). Heat shock proteins and cardiovascular pathophysiology. *Physiology Reviews* **81**, 1461–1497.

Won, K-A., Schumacher, R. J., Farr, G. W., Horwich, A. L. and Reed, S. I. (1998). Maturation of human cyclin E requires the function of eukaryotic chaperonin CCT. *Molecular and Cellular Biology* **18**, 7584–7589.

Heat Shock Proteins   *See:* Chaperone Proteins and Chaperonopathies; Heat Shock Response, Overview.

Heat Shock Proteins: HSP60 Family Genes

H Kubota
Institute for Frontier Medical Sciences, Kyoto University, Kyoto, Japan

This article is a revision of the previous edition article by H Kubota, volume 2, pp 347–349, © 2000, Elsevier Inc.

Introduction
Members of the HSP60 Family
Response to Heat Shock and Related Stress
Function in Protein Folding
Medical Aspects

Glossary

Chaperonin containing TCP-1 (CCT)   The HSP60 family member protein distributed in the eukaryotic cytosol and nucleus. CCT is also called TRiC or c-cpn.

Chaperonins   Alternative name for the HSP60 family, preferentially used by molecular biologists and biochemists. This term is often confused with chaperones, which refers to all molecular chaperones. The term chaperonin is also used for the 10-kDa co-chaperone of the HSP60 family. In this case, the HSP60 family and 10-kDa co-chaperone are called chaperonin 60 (Cpn60) and 10 (Cpn10), respectively.

GroEL   The HSP60 family member protein contained in *Escherichia coli* and related bacterial species.

Group II archaebacterial chaperonins   The HSP60 family member proteins contained in archaebacterial species.

Heat shock proteins (HSPs)   Proteins induced by heat shock and related stress.

HSP60 (60-kDa heat shock protein)   The HSP60 family member protein distributed in mitochondria.

Molecular chaperone   A group of proteins that associate with unfolded proteins and assist in their folding.

Protein folding   The process by which newly synthesized polypeptides or denatured proteins produce functional conformations.

Rubisco subunit binding protein   The HSP60 family member protein distributed in plastids.

Introduction

Heat shock proteins (HSPs) are a group of proteins induced by heat shock and related stress including heavy metals and amino acid analogs. Most HSPs were named according to their molecular mass in kilodaltons with the abbreviation HSP (such as HSP90, HSP70, and HSP60) in mammals. Proteins in the HSP60 family (also called the chaperonin family) form large complexes composed of subunits of approximately 60 kDa. Each complex contains 14–18

subunits and shows a double doughnut-like structure. HSP60 family proteins act as molecular chaperones, assisting in refolding of proteins denatured by heat and related stress and in folding of newly synthesized polypeptides. These proteins were found to be distributed in all organisms investigated to date and in most compartments of eukaryotic cells, including the cytosol, nucleus, mitochondria, and chloroplast. The ubiquitous distribution and chaperone activity of the HSP60 family proteins indicate that the HSP60 family proteins play fundamental roles in the survival of organisms by mediating production and recovery of functional conformations of proteins in the cell.

Members of the HSP60 Family

The HSP60 family includes GroEL of eubacteria, HSP60 of mitochondria, Rubisco subunit binding protein of plastids, the chaperonin containing TCP-1 (CCT, also called TRiC or c-cpn) of eukaryotic cytosol and nucleus, and archaebacterial chaperonins (e.g., TF55/56, thermosome). These proteins can be divided into two groups based on the amino acid sequence homology and structural similarities (**Table 1**). GroEL, HSP60, and Rubisco subunit binding protein are classified as group I, while CCT and archaebacterial chaperonins are classified as group II. GroEL is a major heat-inducible protein of *Escherichia coli* and plays a fundamental role in the stress response by assisting in the refolding of denatured proteins. GroEL is also important for the folding of newly synthesized proteins. HSP60 assists in refolding of mitochondrial proteins imported from the cytosol across the mitochondrial membrane, or after denaturation by heat and related stress. A considerable level of HSP60 is also found in the cytosol, although roles of the cytosolic HSP60 have not been clarified. Rubisco subunit binding protein mediates folding of ribulose-1,5-bisphosphate carboxylase/oxygenase

Table 1 Characteristics of HSP60 family proteins[a]

	Organism	Localization	Amino acid identity with		Rotational symmetry	Subunit species	Inducibility by stress
			GroEL	CCT			
Group I							
GroEL	Eubacteria	Soluble	–	<20%	7	1	+
HSP60	Eukaryotes	Mitochondria	60%	<20%	7	1	+
RSBP[b]	Plants	Plastids	60%	<20%	7	2	+
Group II							
CCT (TRiC, c-cpn)	Eukaryotes	Cytosol and nucleus	<20%	–	8	8–9	+
TF55/56	Archaebacteria	Soluble	<20%	40%	9	3	+
Thermosome	Archaebacteria	Soluble	<20%	40%	8	2	+

[a]MKKS and BBSIO show very weak homology to HSP60 family proteins.
[b]Rubisco subunit binding protein.

(Rubisco) in plastids. CCT is known to assist in the folding of newly synthesized actin, tubulin, and some other proteins in eukaryotic cytosol and is composed of eight different subunit species encoded by independent genes. Archaebacterial chaperonins are the major heat-inducible proteins and bind denatured proteins, although they do not always show refolding activity. Recently, a gene encoding novel mammalian chaperonin-like protein was discovered by chromosome mapping for the McKusick–Kaufman syndrome (MKKS) gene. The MKKS gene was also found to be the sixth locus for Bardet–Biedl syndrome (BBS6). The amino acid sequence of MKKS shows a weak identity to those of group II subfamily members. Although this protein distributes in the cytosol with a highly concentrated distribution in the centrosome when overexpressed in mammalian cells, its function and stress inducibility have not been determined. Very recently another BBS gene product (BBSIO) was found to show very weak identity to the HSP family, although no experimental information is currently available for the BBSIO protein.

Response to Heat Shock and Related Stress

GroEL is required during normal and stress conditions for the survival of *E. coli*. Expression of GroEL in *E. coli* is strongly induced by a variety of stressors such as heat shock, ethanol shock, heavy metals, and amino acid analogs. These treatments cause denaturation of proteins in the bacteria, and the denatured proteins require help from molecular chaperones to recover functional conformations. The heat shock response of GroEL is mediated by a transcription factor called σ32, which is the product of the *RpoH* gene. The translation of σ32 becomes more efficient at higher temperatures by structural changes of its mRNA, and the translated protein transiently becomes more stable after heat shock. The activity of σ32 is inhibited by GroEL but not by substrate-occupied GroEL, suggesting the presence of a transcription factor–chaperone network for sensing and controlling protein folding environment *in vivo*.

Mammalian HSP60 is constitutively expressed under normal conditions and upregulated under stress conditions. Heat shock and related stress induce HSP60 expression, and this response is regulated by a family of transcription factors called heat shock factors (HSFs) through the heat shock elements (HSEs) in the HSP60 gene promoter. In vertebrates, four members of this family (HSF1–4) are known, and HSF1 plays the most important role in controlling the heat shock response. HSF1 is activated by heat shock and related stress, and the HSF1 activity is controlled by HSP70 and HSP90 by monitoring the protein folding environment at least in part.

CCT is expressed at a basal level under normal growth-arrested conditions such as terminally differentiated cells *in vivo*. CCT expression is upregulated by growth stimulation. For example, CCT is highly expressed in embryos, tumors, and rapidly growing cultured cells. Under the rapidly growing conditions, CCT expression is upregulated by transcription factors whose expression and activity are highly dependent on growth stimulation. In addition, CCT is highly expressed in tissues that are abundant in substrate proteins. CCT expression is particularly high in testis to assist in the folding of tubulin, a major component of sperm tail. CCT is further induced by chemical stress including arsenite and proline analog treatments. As CCT gene promoters contain HSE-like sequences that are recognizable by HSF1 and HSF2, these factors may play a role in the chemical stress-induced expression of CCT. In contrast, CCT was not induced by heat shock as far as investigated. Thus, the mechanism of stress-induced regulation of CCT expression is probably somewhat different from that of typical HSPs.

In several archaebacterial species, chaperonins become the most major protein under stress conditions. This is considered to be due to severe environmental conditions. For example, thermophilic species grow at temperatures above 80°C.

Function in Protein Folding

The major contribution of HSP60 family proteins in the stress response is to assist in refolding denatured proteins. All the members bind denatured proteins but do not bind functional proteins that are completely folded. Most members of this family show ATPase activity and use it to obtain conformational changes that allow these proteins to release target proteins. Activity of group I members is modulated by co-chaperones of approximately 10 kDa, such as GroES and cpn-10, although homologs of the co-chaperone for group II members are not known. All HSP60 family members have back-to-back stacked double-ring-like structure composed of 14–18 subunits, although rotational symmetry differs between group I and II: group I members show sevenfold symmetry whereas group II members show eight- or ninefold symmetry. Denatured substrate protein is trapped in the central cavity of these cylinder-like molecules near their opening in the absence of ATP. In the case of GroEL, ATP and GroES are bound to the cylinder following trapping substrate. GroES acts as a lid of the GroEL cylinder, and the substrate is encapsulated in the GroEL–GroES cage. In this protected environment, the single substrate protein is allowed to fold properly without forming nonproductive aggregation. After ATP hydrolysis, the GroES lid and folded substrate are released from the GroEL cylinder. In contrast, group II members including CCT and archaebacterial chaperonins are able to produce cagelike structures for encapsulating substrate proteins in the absence of GroES-like co-chaperones.

The HSP60 family proteins are considered to cooperate with other molecular chaperones such as HSP70 and HSP40 (DnaJ homolog) family proteins. The HSP60 family proteins also play important roles in the folding of newly synthesized proteins with other molecular chaperones and co-chaperones. In this view, *E. coli* strains overexpressing GroEL can be used to produce some recombinant proteins efficiently.

Medical Aspects

It is known that HSP60 homologs in mycobacteria and related species are highly antigenic in mammals. Immune responses to these proteins and/or HSP60 itself are considered to be involved in several diseases mediated by the immune system, including reactive arthritis, juvenile chronic arthritis, rheumatoid arthritis, Lyme disease, Bechcet's disease, systemic lupus erythematosus and insulin-dependent diabetes mellitus.

Recently, SPG13, a dominant human gene responsible for hereditary spastic paraplegia, was mapped to the gene encoding mitochondrial HSP60. Hereditary spastic paraplegia is a genetically heterologous neurodegenerative disorder characterized by progressive spasticity and weakness of lower limbs. HSP60 carrying the V72I mutation that is found in the patient group cannot compensate for the function of GroEL when expressed in *E. coli*, whereas wild-type HSP60 can. These observations suggest that the chaperone function of HSP60 plays an important role in preventing diseases caused by protein misfolding, including neurodegenerative disease.

Although exact function of MKKS protein is unknown, its weak homology to the HSP60 family suggests that a particular function may be shared between MKKS and the HSP60 family proteins. Mutations in the MKKS gene cause human developmental anomalies including vaginal atresia with hydrometrocolpos, polydactyly, and congenital heart defects. MKKS also causes BBS, and provides more severe symptoms when mutated together with other BBS genes. BBS is a genetically heterogeneous disorder characterized by obesity, retinal dystrophy, polydactyly, mental retardation, renal malformations, and hypogenitalism. MKKS knockout mice show BBS-like phenotypes including retinal degeneration, failure of sperm flagella formation, photoreceptor

degeneration, obesity, and deficits in olfaction and social dominance. As MKKS and some BBS proteins are highly concentrated in the centrosome and/or basal body of cilia, MKKS protein function may be related to the activity of these organella and may work together for this activity. It is also possible that MKKS protein functions in protein transport, as suggested for other BBS proteins. As recently identified BBS10 also shows weak homology to the HSP60 family proteins, the function of this BBS protein may be related to that of MKKS.

See Also the Following Articles

Chaperone Proteins and Chaperonopathies; Genetic Factors and Stress; Heat Shock Genes, Human; Heat Shock Response, Overview.

Further Reading

Barral, J. M., Broadley, S. A., Schaffar, G. and Hartl, F. U. (2004). Roles of molecular chaperones in protein misfolding diseases. *Seminars in Cell and Developmental Biology* 15, 17–29.

Beales, P. L. (2005). Lifting the lid on Pandora's box: the Bardet-Biedl syndrome. *Current Opinion in Genetics & Development* 15, 315–323.

Bukau, B. (ed.) (1999). *Molecular chaperones and folding catalysts: regulation, cellular function and mechanisms.* New York: Harwood Academic Publishers.

Ellis, R. J. (ed.) (1996). *The chaperonins.* San Diego, CA: Academic Press.

Fares, M. A., Moya, A. and Barrio, E. (2004). GroEL and the maintenance of bacterial endosymbiosis. *Trends in Genetics* 20, 413–416.

Fenton, W. A. and Horwich, A. L. (2003). Chaperonin-mediated protein folding: fate of substrate polypeptide. *Quarterly Review of Biophysics* 36, 229–256.

Gething, M.-J. (ed.) (1997). *Guidebook to molecular chaperones and protein-folding catalysts.* Oxford, UK: Oxford University Press.

Gomez-Puertas, P., Martin-Benito, J., Carrascosa, J. L., Willison, K. R. and Valpuesta, J. M. (2004). The substrate recognition mechanisms in chaperonins. *Journal of Molecular Recognition* 17, 85–94.

Kubota, H. (2002). Function and regulation of cytosolic molecular chaperone CCT. *Vitamins and Hormones* 65, 313–331.

Latchman, D. S. (ed.) (1999). *Stress proteins, handbook of experimental pharmacology* (Vol. 136). Berlin: Springer-Verlag.

Morimoto, R. I., Tissieres, A. and Georgopoulos, C. (eds.) (1994). *The biology of heat shock proteins and molecular chaperones.* New York: Cold Spring Harbor Laboratory Press.

Prakken, B. J., Roord, S., Ronaghy, A., Wauben, M., Albani, S. and van Eden, W. (2003). Heat shock protein 60 and adjuvant arthritis: a model for T cell regulation in human arthritis. *Springer Seminars in Immunopathology* **25**, 47–63.

Spiess, C., Meyer, A. S., Reissmann, S. and Frydman, J. (2004). Mechanism of the eukaryotic chaperonin: protein folding in the chamber of secrets. *Trends in Cell Biology* **14**, 598–604.

Thomas, J. G., Ayling, A. and Baneyx, F. (1997). Molecular chaperones, folding catalysts, and the recovery of active recombinant proteins from *E. coli*: to fold or to refold. *Applied Biochemistry and Biotechnology* **66**, 197–238.

van Eden, W. and Young, D. (eds.) (1996). *Stress proteins in medicine*. New York: Dekker.

Young, J. C., Agashe, V. R., Siegers, K. and Hartl, F. U. (2004). Pathways of chaperone-mediated protein folding in the cytosol. *Nature Reviews Molecular and Cell Biology* **5**, 781–791.

Heat Shock Response, Overview

A J L Macario and E Conway de Macario
New York State Department of Health and the University at Albany (SUNY), Albany, NY, USA

Published by Elsevier Inc.

Heat Shock and Stress

Definition

Scope

Events

Characteristics

Mechanisms

Clearing the Rubble

Milestones

New Developments to 2005

Perspectives

Glossary

Heat shock gene	A gene inducible by heat shock or any other stressor; also called stress gene.
Microarray	A miniaturized collection of samples (e.g., cDNA made from the mRNAs present in a cell under specific experimental conditions), anchored in a predetermined spatial order to many microareas delimited on a support (e.g., microchip, glass slide, filter, or silicon wafer); this makes the samples available for reaction (e.g., cDNA–DNA hybridization) in a high-throughput mode with known, labeled probes (e.g., DNA with sequences of known genes).
Messenger ribonucleic acid (mRNA)	A molecule composed of bases in a sequence complementary to that of the coding region of a gene; it has the message to synthesize the protein encoded in the gene.
Protein	A molecule formed by amino acids in a sequence dictated by the sequence of bases in the corresponding mRNA.
Ribosome	A large, multimolecular structure present in the cytoplasm of all cells at which protein synthesis takes place according to the message encoded in the mRNA.
Stressor	An agent, which can mechanical, physical, psychological, or chemical, capable of causing cell stress and inducing a stress (heat shock) response. Although the term heat shock response may be used as synonym of stress response, it is more properly applied only to stress responses caused by the stressor heat.
Systems biology	Large-scale, computer-assisted analyses of genomic and proteomics data to elucidate intra- and intercellular gene and protein interactions as they might occur *in vivo*. The purpose of such analyses is ultimately to provide mathematical models and simulations of cellular pathways and networks and of their dynamics. An example is the pathways followed by each chaperoning system and the networks formed by two or more of these systems between them and/or between them and protein-degrading systems so as to maintain intracellular protein homeostasis.
Transcription	The process of synthesis of the mRNA, marking the initial main step of gene expression.
Transcriptome	The whole suite of mRNAs that can be transcribed from a genome; also, more specifically, the subset of mRNAs that are transcribed from a genome of a particular cell (or organism or tissue), at any given time, under specific conditions, for example, under conditions of cell stress

	or under basal, constitutive conditions (no stress).
Translation	The process of synthesis of a protein molecule on the ribosome, in which amino acids are linked in a linear non-branching chain that follows the order encoded in the corresponding mRNA.

Heat Shock and Stress

A heat shock response consists of the series of events occurring in a cell that are induced by heat stress (i.e., a sudden temperature elevation) and that reflect the cell's perturbed status compared with the status prior to the stressor's impact. Among all such events, only a few are considered in this article, whose focus is intracellular proteins produced by stress-inducible genes and the phenomena mediated by these proteins.

Many stressors other than a sudden increase in temperature can cause virtually the same series of events as does heat shock. Such cellular reactions are also called heat shock responses for historical reasons. To avoid confusion, the term stress response should be used regardless of the stressor, and the stressor should be mentioned in all cases. Examples of common cell stressors are listed in **Table 1**. In this article, the expressions stress response, stress gene, and stress protein are preferred over heat shock response, heat shock gene, and heat shock protein, respectively.

Definition

The shock (or stress) produced on an object by an abrupt temperature elevation is called heat shock or heat stress. Shock and stress are considered synonyms within the context of this article and may be defined as the impact – and its consequences – of an agent, such as heat, on an object. Stress is a perturbed status of the object generated by the impacting agent. The object may be inanimate (e.g., a piece of metal) or living (e.g., a cell or an organism made up of one or more cells). This article deals chiefly with cell stress.

Scope

Stress may be defined more specifically from several different standpoints, depending on the natures of the object and the stressor and on the particular field of knowledge being considered, materials, physical, mechanical, psychological, physiological, or medical sciences, just to name some representative examples.

This article deals with cellular stress caused by heat shock, or heat stress, and by other stressors that produce very similar effects, pertaining to biology in its broadest sense – that of all living organisms, whether uni- or multicelled. If the organism is unicelled, cellular and organismal stresses are synonymous. An illustrative list of organisms that have been used to study the stress response is in **Table 2**.

It must be borne in mind that although the effects of stressors on the cell are, on the whole, not specific, there are details of the cell's response to stress that vary according to the stressor.

Events

The stress response manifests itself in diverse cellular changes that affect many of the cell's components and properties, from gross morphology to the most

Table 1 Examples of cell stressors[a]

Type/group	Name/description
Physical	Heat (including fever), cold, irradiation (e.g., ultraviolet rays), magnetic fields
Mechanical	Compression, shearing, stretching
Nutritional	Starvation: multiple, specific (carbon, glucose, nitrogen, phosphate, nitrate)
pH	Alkalosis, acidosis, pH shift
Osmotic	Changes in the concentration of salt, sugars, other osmolytes (hyper- and hypoosmotic shocks)
Antibiotics	Puromycin, tetracycline, nalidix acid
Alcohols	Ethanol, methanol, butanol, propanol, octanol
Oxygen	Oxygen-derived free radicals (ROS), hydrogen peroxide, anaerobiosis to aerobiosis shift (e.g., reperfusion), hypoxia/anoxia (ischemia)
Biological	Infection, inflammation, fever
Psychological	Emotions, conflicts; hormonal imbalance (HPA axis, autonomic nervous system)
Metals	Cadmium, copper, chromium, zinc, tin, aluminum, mercury, lead, nickel
Other	Desiccation, benzene and derivatives, phenol and derivatives, teratogens, carcinogens, mutagens, arsenite, arsenate, amino acid analogs, nicotine, anesthetics,; insecticides, pesticides

[a]These agents cause stress not only in human and other (e.g., mouse and rat) eukaryotic cells but also in prokaryotic (e.g., bacterial) cells. HPA, hypothalamic-pituitary-adrenal; ROS, reactive oxygen species. Modified from Macario, A. J. L. and Conway de Macario, E. (2000), Stress and molecular chaperones in disease, *International Journal of Clinical and Laboratory Research* **30**, 49–66, with permission from the copyright owner.

Table 2 Examples of organisms whose cells and tissues have been used as experimental models to study cell stress and the stress (heat shock) response

Type	Name
Prokaryote	
Bacterium	*Agrobacterium tumefaciens, Anabaena* sp., *Bacillus subtilis, Borrelia burgdorferi, Bradyrhizobium japonicum, Campylobacter jejuni, Clostridium acetobutylicum, Escherichia coli, Lactococcus lactis, Rhodothermus obamensis, Shewanella oneidensis, Staphylococcus aureus, Streptomyces coelicolor, Synecoccus* sp.
Archaeon	
Methanogen	*Methanosarcina mazeii, Methanosarcina thermophila, Methanococcus voltae*
Extreme halophile	*Halobacterium halobium, Haloferax volcanii*
Thermophile	*Thermoplasma acidophilum*
Hyperthermophile	*Archaeoglobus fulgidus, Pyrodictium occultum, Sulfolobus shibatae*
Eukaryote	
Unicelled	*Arxiozyma telluris, Mrakia frigida, Saccharomyces cerevisiae* (yeasts)
	Tetrahymena thermophila (protozoan)
	Euglena gracilis (alga)
Multicelled	*Neurospora crassa* (fungus)
	Schistosoma mansoni, Caenorrabditis elegans (worms)
	Crassostrea gigas (oyster)
	Drosophila melanogaster (insect)
	Salmo gairdnerii [rainbow trout], *Danio rerio* [zebrafish] (fishes)
	Arabidopsis thaliana [wall cress], *Lycopersicon esculentum* [tomato] (plants)
	Gallus gallus [chicken] (bird)
	Mus musculus [mouse], *Rattus norvegicus* [rat], *Meriones ungiculatus* [gerbil], *Homo sapiens* [human] (mammals)

detailed biochemical and molecular mechanisms. A list of cellular components and properties affected by stressors such as heat shock and the methods used to study the cell's response or reaction to stressors are shown in **Table 3**.

Characteristics

The stress response is characterized by a decrease in the levels of many proteins and a concurrent increase in the levels of others. In addition, a series of proteins appear that were not detectable prior to the stressor's impact. The proteins that increase or appear as a consequence of stress are the stress proteins. The subset of these proteins that are the product of genes induced by heat shock are called heat shock proteins (Hsps). However, for historical reasons the same name Hsp is also used to designate proteins encoded in genes that are inducible by any stressor. An illustrative sample of stress proteins, including Hsps, is presented in **Table 4**. In this table, some molecules (thermoprotectants) that are not proteins but that, like the stress proteins, function to counteract the effects of stressors are also mentioned. These nonproteinic antistress compounds are mentioned to convey the idea that the cell possesses a variety of antistress mechanisms beyond the stress proteins and also to draw attention to

the fact that all the proteins (e.g., enzymes) that participate in the production and trafficking of these antistress compounds must work during the stress response and that, therefore, they are part of the antistress mechanisms, too.

Mechanisms

Many genes are downregulated or shut off as a consequence of stress. If the affected genes are ones that produce proteins, their protein products decrease or disappear. In contrast, other genes are upregulated or induced *de novo* by stress. These are the heat shock or stress genes *sensu lato*. Among them, there is a group that belongs to the category of protein producers. Their products are the heat shock or stress proteins, some of which are important for cell survival during stress and for cell recovery after stress. A subset of heat shock proteins are molecular chaperones; they assist other proteins to fold correctly during synthesis and to refold if they have been partially denatured by stress. One of the best-known molecular chaperones is the stress protein Hsp70(DnaK), which interacts with at least two others, Hsp40 (DnaJ) and GrpE in prokayotes (or BAG-1, or HspPB1 in eukaryotes), to bring about protein folding or refolding.

Table 3 Cellular components and properties affected by heat shock and methods used to study the stress (heat shock) response of the cell

Component/property	Method
Viability, growth rate	Cell counts
Morphology (size; shape; formation of multicellular structures or spores)	Various types of light and electron microscopies
	Biochemical and immunochemical analyses of cell envelopes and intercellular connective materials
	Histochemistry
	Immunohistochemistry
Proteins	
General contents	One- and two-dimensional electrophoresis
Synthesis, general	Incorporation of radioactively labeled amino acids followed by quantification of radioactive fractions resolved by electrophoresis or other fractionation methods (e.g., chromatography)
	DNA microarray-proteomics (two-dimensional electrophoresis plus other methods, e.g., western blotting, mass spectrometry, microsequencing) to determine the exact nature of the proteins synthesized in response to stress
	Two-hybrid method to detect protein–protein interactions followed by bioinformatics (systems biology, neural networks)
Synthesis, specific	Separation and/or quantification of target stress proteins using specific antibodies (immunoprecipitation, western blotting)
	Identification of protein complexes by electron microscopy combined with immunochemistry and functional assays (e.g., determination of ATPase activity and capacity to assist protein folding or refolding)
	Microsequencing
Genes[a]	Measurement of transcript (mRNA) for stress proteins: quantity, size (length), transcription initiation and termination sites (northern blotting, primer extension, S-1 nuclease protection, reverse PCR)
	DNA microarray-transcriptomics and proteomics (two-dimensional electrophoresis plus other methods, e.g., northern and western blottings, mass spectrometry, microsequencing) to determine the exact nature of the proteins synthesized in response to stress and, thus, identify genes involved
	Systems biology, neural networks

[a]Presence or absence of genes is determined by genome sequencing; cloning and sequencing; and Southern, northern, and western blottings. PCR, polymerase chain reaction.

Table 4 Some stress (heat shock) proteins proven or believed to play a role during the stress (heat shock) response and in cell recovery after stress[a]

Group	Examples
1	Molecular chaperones and chaperonins, Hsp70(DnaK), Hsp40(DnaJ), GrpE, GroEL, GroES, Hsp90, Hsp104, sHsp
2	Regulators of stress (heat shock) genes: sigma factors (e.g., σ^{32}, σ^E, σ^B), positive regulators or activators (e.g., HSF), negative regulators (e.g., HrcA, HspR)
3	Proteins that constitute the intercellular connective material of multicellular structures formed as a response to stress
4	Transport proteins: e.g., archaeal TrkA
5	Proteases: Clp family, Lon/La, HtrA, proteasome components
6	Enzymes and cofactors involved in the synthesis of other stress proteins (listed in the preceding groups 1–5) and other molecules, such as thermoprotectants (trehalose; di-*myo*-inositol phosphate; cyclic diphosphoglycerate)
7	All proteins, enzymes, cofactors, and gene-regulatory factors involved in sporulation

[a]HSF, heat shock factor; Hsp, heat shock protein. Modified from Macario, A. J. L. and Conway de Macario, E. (2000), Stress and molecular chaperones in disease, *International Journal of Clinical and Laboratory Research* **30**, 49–66, with permission from the copyright owner.

A balanced set of proteins, each in its native functional conformation and at its physiological concentration, is key to cell survival. Heat shock and other stresses alter the cellular proteins. These tend to lose their functional shapes; they denature. Protein denaturation is a central harmful factor for the cell during stress. Thus, the mechanisms for preventing protein denaturation, and for reversing it when it is still reversible, are major survival tools for the cell. Among these tools, the stress proteins, including the molecular chaperones, are prominent. Therefore, it is not surprising that the levels of these proteins are maintained or augmented in response to stress, whereas many other proteins decrease or become undetectable.

There are several ways for the cell to readjust the concentration of stress proteins when it has been affected by a stressor. One way is to upregulate the genes that produce the useful proteins, and another is to diminish the degradation of the latter. All cellular proteins undergo a cycle of birth, maturation, function, and degradation (equivalent to death). By postponing the degradation of stress proteins, the cell enhances the chances of its survival in the face of stress.

Another mechanism for increasing the levels of useful proteins during stress is to facilitate their synthesis from their mRNAs. This may be achieved in various ways. One way is to increase the life span of the mRNAs that encode stress proteins (mRNAs are usually short-lived). If the stability of the mRNA increases, the same mRNA molecules can reach the ribosome and be translated more than just once, avoiding delays due to the unavailability of newly synthesized mRNA molecules. Furthermore, translation itself may be enhanced, so mRNA is decoded more rapidly and more mRNA molecules are translated per ribosome.

In summary, gene activation, involving both an initiation of the transcription of genes inactive in the absence of stress and an increase in the rate of transcription of genes already active before stress, is not the only mechanism that brings about the increase of heat shock proteins. Prolongation of the life span of mRNAs and of the stress proteins themselves also plays a role in building up the cellular defenses against the ravages of stress.

Clearing the Rubble

The rescue of proteins partially damaged by stress is a key mechanism for cell survival, as explained earlier. However, many molecules may be damaged irreversibly and cannot be rescued. These denatured proteins tend to aggregate and to form relatively large precipitates. These may be toxic, and they may also obstruct other cellular components. This is the reason why the cell has a battery of enzymes that digest seriously damaged, useless proteins. These enzymes are called proteases, and some of them are considered stress proteins because they handle the key task of removing stress-damaged proteins to clear the way for the trafficking and functioning of other, viable molecules essential for survival. Furthermore, the degradation products generated by the action of proteases on their substrates serve as building materials

for the synthesis of other molecules necessary for mounting a stress response.

In summary, a series of mechanisms are set in motion by stress. The main objective of the cell is to maintain a range of functionally competent proteins at the concentrations required for survival. The production of nonessential proteins is stopped, the synthesis of required proteins is started or increased, and damaged or useless molecules are eliminated.

Milestones

The heat shock response has been the focus of research efforts for at least 4 decades. If we bear in mind the current division of living organisms into three major lines of descent or phylogenetic domains – Eucarya (eukaryotes), Bacteria (eubacteria), and Archaea – it is possible to see that the chronology of specific contributions proceeded from the Eucarya to Bacteria, and only considerably later reached the Archaea. Currently, organisms from the three domains are used as experimental models, but those from the Archaea are still in the minority.

In 1962 it was reported that a temperature elevation induced distinct puffing patterns in the chromosomes of the salivary gland of the fly *Drosophila buschii*. These puffs were transient but reproducible, and they always affected the same chromosomal regions (bands). Puffing occurred when the fly larvae were moved out of their optimal temperature for growth (i.e., 25°C) and into a temperature of 30°C and kept there for 30 min. The same results were obtained with another fly species, *D. melanogaster*, which is much used for research.

At the time, these results were interpreted to represent gene activation induced by a change in the environmental temperature, which as we know now is what constitutes a heat shock response. Similar effects were obtained with 2–4 dinitrophenol and salicylate, two compounds that today we would call chemical cell stressors (see **Table 1**). These observations established that heat shock activates some genes, always the same ones in a defined location in the chromosome, and that similar gene activation can be induced by agents other than heat. The conclusion was that heat shock and other stressors induce gene transcription with production of new mRNAs.

That these mRNAs were actually the precursors of new proteins, whose synthesis was set in motion by heat shock, was demonstrated in 1974, once again in the salivary glands of *D. melanogaster* and also in other tissues. The results showed a correlation between the typical heat shock-induced puffing patterns, mRNA synthesis, and the appearance of several new proteins in the tissues of the fly.

The new proteins were visualized by one-dimensional gel electrophoresis. At this time, it became clear that heat shock induces the synthesis of proteins that are not present at detectable levels under normal physiological conditions. It also became clear that gene activation and protein synthesis are not restricted to a single tissue or organ (e.g., the salivary glands) but are more generalized.

The main characteristics of the heat shock response were in fact defined by these early studies with the fruit fly. These characteristics are the transient activation of a restricted, defined group of genes by an abrupt temperature upshift with the synthesis of a set of mRNAs and proteins, occurring in all types of tissues and cells. Similar effects can be produced by other agents or stressors.

Thus, the field of heat shock or stress response was opened for further investigations at the biochemical, molecular, and genetic levels by these pioneering studies on a eukaryotic organism, an insect. Several years passed before knowledge of the stress response of prokaryotes began to emerge. The prokaryotic organism most used for research in the field has been the bacterium *Escherichia coli*. Investigations with this model system were reported from the beginning of the 1980s. A number of stress genes and proteins were identified, and many of them have been characterized thoroughly, including detailed structure–function determinations by very sophisticated techniques such as crystallography, electron microscopy, and computer-assisted imaging analysis. Also, considerable progress has been made toward the elucidation of the mechanisms that regulate stress genes, addressing the following questions. How are these genes instructed to start transcription, and to stop it, according to the cell's needs? How does the cell sense the temperature or other environmental changes (stressors) around it and transmit from its surface the orders for activity or inactivity to the genes?

Over the years, since the time of the initial studies with *E. coli*, other bacterial species have been added to the list of model systems used for studying the stress response. These species include representatives from many of the known bacterial groups, such as gram positives and gram negatives; mesophiles, thermophiles, and hyperthermophiles; and pathogens and nonpathogens (see **Table 2**). In parallel, eukaryotes other than *Drosophila* have also been used to study the stress response and the stress genes and proteins. Examples are the single-celled fungus *Saccharomyces cerevisiae*, known also as baker's yeast, and several other organisms representing the major groups of eukaryotes (see **Table 2**).

These studies with members of the domains Bacteria and Eucarya proliferated in the 1980s and 1990s, not only because they helped to advance our understanding of important cellular functions and mechanisms under physiological conditions and during and after stress (see **Table 3**) but also because some of the organisms are pathogens for humans and for animals valued by humans. Hence, it was pertinent to examine the role of the stress response in health and disease. In addition, other model organisms have existing or potential industrial applications and are, therefore, of commercial interest.

While the research activities mentioned so far were ongoing, the identification and characterization of the third evolutionary domain, the Archaea, proceeded steadily since the late 1970s. However, it was only in 1991 that a heat shock gene, *hsp70(dnaK)*, was first identified by cloning and sequencing in an organism of the domain Archaea, the mesophilic methanogen *Methanosarcina mazeii*. In the same year, the chaperonin complex called the thermosome was visualized in another member of the Archaea, a hyperthermophile. Both findings opened the doors to exciting new territories for exploration. Research with archaeal organisms has progressed, driven by the same motivations that propelled research on organisms of the other two domains. Archaeal species are attractive to the scientist because they possess a series of characteristics that are unique to them and that were unknown before these organisms were discovered. Some of these characteristics are extreme compared with what is known for the more familiar, and better studied, eukaryotes and bacteria. In addition, there are archaeal species and molecules from Archaea that have potential in the biotechnology industry, including the development of clean and efficient means for waste treatment with the generation of useful or harmless by-products. In a variety of these applications, the stress response and the stress genes and proteins play a key role. Consequently, their manipulation is a promising way to improve extant technology and develop better alternatives than those currently available.

Currently, research continues on organisms of the three domains. The goals are to discover other stress genes, to characterize more thoroughly the mechanisms that bring about the stress response and the mechanisms involved in the regulation of the stress genes, and to design strategies and procedures to manipulate these genes and their protein products to prevent or cure lesions caused by stressors in plants and animals (see **Table 4**).

New Developments to 2005

Recent developments pertain to (1) stress genes in the Archaea; (2) chaperones and disease; (3) genomics and automated methods by which sequenced genomes can be studied and by which large amounts of information about expressed genes (including stress genes), their regulatory networks, and the interactions of their protein products in the cell can be obtained and analyzed; (4) high-throughput technology to measure gene transcription at the level of the entire genome and to determine the full range of proteins present in a cell or tissue at any given time; and (5) techniques to measure the presence of stressors in environmental samples such as wastewaters, soil, food, paints, and construction materials.

Stress genes in Archaea proved to have a distribution unexpected from what was known from bacteria and eukaryotes. For example, the molecular chaperone machine Hsp70(DnaK)-Hsp40(DnaJ)-nucleotide exchange factor, which is present in all bacteria and eukaryotes tested, was not found in several archaeal species. Furthermore, the chaperonin system group I, which had been considered to be exclusive to bacteria and bacterial-related eukaryotic organelles, was discovered in some species of Archaea. Two new chaperonin group II subunits were discovered in an archaeal species. This finding elevated the total number of subunits in the Archaea to five (the maximum known before was three), approaching a total number of eight, which is characteristic of eukaryotes.

The concept that defective molecular chaperones can contribute to pathogenesis not only as auxiliary factors but also as primary etiological agents was developed, and a number of diseases were identified as examples of this newly recognized pathological entity, chaperonopathy. The negative impact of chaperonopathies on stress responses, on survival in the face of protracted stress, and on recovery after stress remains to be evaluated. This will most likely be an area of intensive research in the first decades of the twenty-first century.

High-throughput automatic technologies with relatively low turnaround times were developed for sequencing genomes, which increased considerably the information available in databases. In parallel, similar, automated methods were standardized for mining genome sequences for stress genes and their regulatory genes and DNA elements, and to obtain clues on the multiple interactions of stress proteins and molecular chaperones with other proteins and cell components (systems biology and cellular neural networks) and with foreign compounds. The results of these genomic, computer-assisted searches will be instrumental in guiding laboratory experiments, focusing on a few selected genes and proteins for elucidating their functions, regulation, and interaction *in vitro* and *in vivo*.

Also, microarray technology has radically changed the analysis of gene expression profiles at the whole genome level. Microarray analysis provides enormous quantities of data for the comparison of different tissues from healthy and sick organisms or of cells under basal conditions (constitutive gene expression) and cells affected by stressors (stress-induced gene expression). This approach has shown that the number of genes induced by stressors is relatively large considering the total number of genes in any given genome, encompassing not only the genes that encode the classic Hsps and chaperones but also many others whose products have a variety of other roles. Thus, it has become clear beyond doubt that there are many stress genes and proteins but that only a fraction of them belong to the Hsp and chaperone families. Likewise, it is clear that not all molecular-chaperone genes are induced by stressors and, therefore, not all chaperones can be classified as Hsps.

The increasing concerns about the contamination of the environment and food with toxic compounds (i.e., cell stressors) have given impetus to the development of novel assays for measuring the potency of these compounds for causing cell stress.

Perspectives

In addition to the stressors discussed in the preceding sections, psychological stress due to professional, financial, social, and family pressures and obligations also cause cell stress via the hormonal and biochemical imbalances inherent in this unpleasant condition. The list of stressors becomes longer and longer as new compounds are isolated from natural sources or are synthesized in the laboratory and released into the environment (added to water, foods, fuels, paints, building materials, clothing, etc.). The hole in the ozone layer of the atmosphere and the greenhouse effect add another dose of stressors (radiation and overheating) on top of all the others already alluded to. No doubt plants and animals – including humans – will have to face stress as the scourge of our time. The more that is known about the heat shock (stress) response, the easier it will be to find ways to counteract the effects of stressors. Research in this field promises to be vigorous in the near future and will most likely attract many scientists. The topic should also be of interest to virtually everybody, regardless of educational level or profession. The public at large ought to know, at least in a general way, what can cause cell stress and how to avoid stressors and abate their deleterious effects. For these purposes, the usual means of using good hygiene and common sense should be helpful, along with efforts to promote legislation aimed at reducing the number and quantities of stressors.

The malfunctioning of antistress mechanisms has recently come into prominence as a new field of medicine. For example, abnormalities in chaperone molecules have an impact on the chaperoning systems throughout the organism and have been implicated in various genetic and acquired pathological disorders. This new medical field will no doubt attract the attention of more and more scientists and practitioners to improve diagnostics, therapeutics, and prevention.

See Also the Following Articles

Chaperone Proteins and Chaperonopathies; Heat Resistance; Heat Shock Genes, Human; Viral Virulence and Stress; Chaperonopathies; Proteases in the Eukaryotic Cell Cytosol; Proteases in Prokaryotes and Eukaryotic Cell Organelles.

Further Reading

Abdollahi, M., Ranjbar, A., Shadnia, S., et al. (2004). Pesticides and oxidative stress: a review. *Medical Science Monitor* 10, RA141–RA147.

Bomholt, S. F., Harbuz, M. S., Blackburn-Munro, G., et al. (2004). Involvement and role of the hypothalamo-pituitary-adrenal (HPA) stress axis in animal models of chronic pain and inflammation. *Stress* 7, 1–14.

Conway de Macario, E., Maeder, D. L. and Macario, A. J. L. (2003). Breaking the mould: Archaea with all four chaperoning systems. *Biochemical and Biophysical Research Communications* 301, 811–812.

Gao, H., Wang, Y., Liu, X., et al. (2004). Global transcriptome analysis of the heat shock response of *Shewanella oneidensis*. *Journal of Bacteriology* 186, 7796–7803.

Gash, A. P., Spellman, P. T., Kao, C. M., et al. (2000). Genomic expression programs in the response of yeast cells to environmental changes. *Molecular Biology of the Cell* 11, 4241–4257.

Gibney, E., Gault, J. and Williams, J. (2004). A novel immunocytochemistry technique to measure Hsp70 induction in L929 cells exposed to cadmium chloride. *Biomarkers* 9, 353–363.

Helman, J. D., Wu, M. F., Kobel, P. A., et al. (2001). Global transcriptional response of *Bacillus subtilis* to heat shock. *Journal of Bacteriology* 183, 7318–7328.

Hickey, A. J., Conway de Macario, E. and Macario, A. J. L. (2002). Transcription in the Archaea: basal factors, regulation, and stress-gene expression. *Critical Reviews in Biochemistry and Molecular Biology* 37, 537–599.

Holden, J. F., Adams, M. W. W. and Baross, J. A. (2000). Heat-shock response in hyperthermophilic microorganisms. In: Bell, C. R., Brylinsky, M. & Johnson Green, P. (eds.) *Microbial biosystems: new frontiers* (vol. 2), pp. 663–670. Halifax, Canada: Atlantic Canada Society for Microbial Ecology and Acadia University Press.

Krone, P. H., Blechinger, S. R., Evans, T. G., et al. (2005). Use of fish liver PLHC-1 cells and zebrafish embryos in cytotoxicity assays. *Methods* 35, 176–187.

Macario, A. J. L. and Conway de Macario, E. (2000). Stress and molecular chaperones in disease. *International Journal of Clinical and Laboratory Research* 30, 49–66.

Macario, A. J. L. and Conway de Macario, E. (2004). The pathology of anti-stress mechanisms: a new frontier. *Stress* 7, 243–249.

Macario, A. J. L., Lange, M., Ahring, B. K., et al. (1999). Stress genes and proteins in Archaea. *Microbiology and Molecular Biology Reviews* 63, 923–967.

Macario, A. J. L., Malz, M. and Conway de Macario, E. (2004). Evolution of assisted protein folding: the distribution of the main chaperoning systems within the phylogenetic domain Archaea. *Frontiers in Bioscience* 9, 1318–1332.

Maeder, D. L., Macario, A. J. L. and Conway de Macario, E. (2005). Novel chaperonins in a prokaryote. *Journal of Molecular Evolution* 60, 409–416.

Schoffl, F., Prandl, R. and Reindl, A. (1998). Regulation of the heat-shock response. *Plant Physiology* 117, 1135–1141.

Stintzi, A. (2003). Gene expression profile of *Campylobacter jejuni* in response to growth temperature variation. *Journal of Bacteriology* 185, 2009–2016.

Thakurta, D. G., Palomar, L., Stormo, G. D., et al. (2002). Identification of a novel *cis*-regulatory element involved in the heat shock response in *Caenorhabditis elegans* using microarray gene expression and computational methods. *Genome Research* 12, 701–712.

Traustadottir, T., Bosch, P. R. and Matt, K. S. (2005). The HPA axis response to stress in women: effects of aging and fitness. *Psychoneuroendocrinology* 30, 392–402.

Voellmy, R. (2005). Dominant-positive and dominant-negative heat shock factors. *Methods* 35, 199–207.

Weber, H., Polen, T., Heuveling, J., et al. (2005). Genome-wide analysis of the general stress response network in *Escherichia coli*: sigma S-dependent genes, promoters, and sigma factor selectivity. *Journal of Bacteriology* 187, 1591–1603.

Zhao, R., Davey, M., Hsu, Y-C., et al. (2005). Navigating the chaperone network: an integrative map of physical and genetic interactions mediated by the Hsp90 chaperone. *Cell* 120, 715–727.

Relevant Websites

http://www.bioscience.org/current/special/macario.htm

Hemostasis and Stress

Roland von Känel
University Hospital Berne, Berne, Switzerland

Historical Perspective
Hemostasis Pathways
Hemostasis Factors and Cardiovascular Disease
Acute Stress
Chronic Stress
Conclusions and Future Directions

Glossary

Blood coagulation	Physiological process as part of hemostasis in which liquid blood is changed into a blood clot of platelet aggregates and fibrin.
Endogenous anticoagulants	Proteins produced by the body to regulate thrombin activity during blood coagulation.
Fibrinolysis	Physiological process of hemostasis in which the fibrin clot is broken down.
Hemostasis	Physiological process in which bleeding is halted in a damaged blood vessel requiring the combined regulated activity of vascular, platelet, and plasma factors.
Hyper-coagulability	A shift in the hemostatic balance favoring formation and maintenance of a clot.
Platelets	Small anuclear blood cells that adhere to sites of blood vessel injury, where they become activated and aggregate with each other.
Thrombosis	Pathological process in which a blood clot forms in the lumen of a blood vessel.

Historical Perspective

The possible influence of stress and stress hormones on blood coagulation and fibrinolysis has attracted researchers for more than a century. As early as 1903, Vosburgh and Richards observed that epinephrine added to the surface of the pancreas and injected into the abdominal cavity of dogs hastened the coagulation time of whole blood, in some cases to as much as four-fifths the coagulation time of control animals. In 1911, von den Velden reported a similar decrease in coagulation time in humans after subcutaneous injection of epinephrine. Only a few years later, Walter Cannon and his co-workers demonstrated in a series of carefully conducted experiments that stimulation of the splanchnic nerve, pain, fear, and enragement all shortened blood clotting in the cat. They noted that rapid coagulation did not occur if adrenals had been removed or were exhausted because of previous excitement, when cats had been caged near dogs. These observations prompted Cannon to state that "rapid coagulation may reasonably be considered as an instance of adaptive reaction serviceable to the organism in the injury which may follow the struggle that fear or rage may occasion."

Patients with hemophilia A lack substantial activity of clotting factor VIII (FVIII:C) such that severe bleeding occurs with minor traumas or even spontaneously. In search of treatment options for this bleeding disorder, systematic investigations in the 1960s and 1970s found that parenteral administration of epinephrine evoked a dose-dependent increase in plasma levels of antihemophilic FVIII:C with concomitant shortening of the clotting time of whole blood. Electric brain stimulation evoked an increase in plasma FVIII:C and a corresponding decrease in the clotting time in dogs. Plasma FVIII:C also rose after air inflation in the skull during a diagnostic procedure in humans. In terms of fibrinolysis, anecdotal reports from the 1940s observed fibrinolytic activation by epinephrine and by a variety of acute naturalistic stressors eliciting a fear response, e.g., planned surgery, air raid warning, and exams.

These earlier studies suggested what has become consensus today, namely, that in a healthy organism, acute stress concomitantly activates the coagulation and fibrinolysis part of hemostasis to result in net hypercoagulability. Clearly, this supports Cannon, who argued that thickening of blood in response to an acute and potentially life-threatening stressor is actually physiological and provided our ancestors with an evolutionary benefit. Indeed, we can readily imagine that hunters who were injured and women who gave birth increased their odds of surviving if hypercoagulability constrained excessive bleeding. Equally exciting, some of this early research can be viewed as first evidence for a regulatory mechanism of hemostasis by the brain involving the sympathomedullary axis and catecholamines.

Hemostasis Pathways

The scheme in **Figure 1** simplifies complex and closely intertwined hemostasis pathways. Activation of hemostasis results in a sequential interaction between

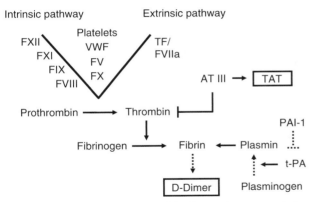

Figure 1 Hemostasis pathways. The figure shows coagulation steps in solid lines and fibrinolysis steps in dashed lines with the symbol → meaning activation of a step and the symbol —| meaning inhibition of a step. Hypercoagulability markers thrombin-antithrombin (AT) III compex (TAT) and D-dimer are depicted in boxes. Von Willebrand factor (VWF), platelets, and clotting factor V (FV) and X (FX) are involved in both coagulation pathways. FXII, FXI, FIX, and FVIII are components of the intrinsic pathway, and tissue factor (TF) and FVII belong to the extrinsic pathway of blood coagulation. PAI-1, plasminogen activator inhibitor-1; t-PA, tissue-type plasminogen activator. Cf. text for details of activation steps.

enzymes and inhibitors of the coagulation and fibrinolysis cascades, of platelets, and of the von Willebrand factor (VWF). Two pathways of blood coagulation are commonly distinguished. Whereas the intrinsic pathway is initiated by FXII, the extrinsic pathway is triggered when tissue factor becomes exposed to the bloodstream at sites of tissue damage, e.g., on material of a ruptured atherosclerotic plaque. Tissue factor instantly binds to circulating FVII. Both pathways result in activation of several clotting factors in a sort of cascade, and eventually converge in a common activator complex. This complex converts prothrombin to thrombin, which, in turn, converts fibrinogen to fibrin. Together with platelet aggregates, fibrin forms a blood clot that, e.g., may critically occlude a coronary artery to result in myocardial infarction. Circulating VWF mediates adherence of platelets to sites of blood vessel injury where platelets are activated and aggregate with each other through fibrinogen bridges. Negatively charged phospholipids on activated platelets catalyze activation of circulating clotting factors.

Termination of clot formation involves several anticoagulant steps, e.g., binding of antithrombin III to thrombin. This step neutralizes thrombin, a potent activator of several clotting factors and platelets, in a thrombin/antithrombin III (TAT) complex. Fibrinolysis is initiated by tissue-type plasminogen activator (t-PA) converting plasminogen into fibrin-cleaving plasmin. The breakdown of cross-linked fibrin chains yields soluble fibrin fragments such as D-dimer. The antifibrinolytic enzyme plasminogen activator

inhibitor-1 (PAI-1) is the main inhibitor of t-PA, neutralizing t-PA in a t-PA/PAI-1-complex.

TAT and D-dimer are viewed as coagulation activation markers because they combine several coagulation steps leading to thrombin and fibrin formation, respectively. In addition, TAT and D-dimer are hypercoagulability markers indicating exaggerated coagulation activity. It is important to note that, unlike individual clotting and fibrinolysis factors, D-dimer indicates activation of the entire hemostatic system, i.e., fibrin formation by the coagulation system and fibrin degradation by the fibrinolytic system.

Hemostasis Factors and Cardiovascular Disease

Since the mid-1980s, numerous large-scale and prospectively designed epidemiological studies have been published suggesting that numerous components of the hemostatic system may predict cardiovascular disease. Most of this research has investigated the predictive value of hemostasis factor for coronary artery disease (CAD) and acute myocardial infarction, while a minor proportion of previous work has addressed the role of hemostasis factors in cerebrovascular and peripheral arterial disease. Meta-analyses have shown CAD risk factor status for fibrinogen, D-dimer, and VWF, whereas FVII:C, FVIII:C, TAT, PAI-1, t-PA, and platelet activity were risk factors of CAD and myocardial infarction across a series of individual investigations.

Remarkably, hemostasis factors not only predicted recurrent cardiac events in patients with cardiovascular diseases but also prospectively predicted the cardiovascular disease risk in individuals who were in apparently good health at study entry. Moreover, many studies showed that the prospective relationship between hemostasis factors and coronary events was independent of sociodemographic factors, lifestyle factors, and the established cardiovascular risk factors of smoking, diabetes, hypertension, and obesity, all of which may affect hemostasis. Altogether, this abundant epidemiological research challenges the view of some researchers that hemostasis factors are mere risk markers of cardiovascular disease and do not actively contribute to atherosclerosis.

It is assumed that a procoagulant milieu, as reflected by increased activity of clotting factors, coagulation activation markers, platelets, and the VWF on the one hand and impaired fibrinolysis on the other, will gradually contribute to atherosclerosis progression over many decades by promoting fibrin deposits in the atherosclerotic vessel wall and inflammation. In addition, upon rupture of a vulnerable atherosclerotic plaque, a procoagulant milieu may accelerate and enhance intravascular thrombus growth and critical occlusion of a coronary artery. Chronic low-grade systemic activation of coagulation processes with chronic stress and repetitive hypercoagulability in response to daily hassles, for example, thus provide one psychobiological pathway through which stress might accelerate atherosclerosis progression. Moreover, the stress procoagulant response is exaggerated in atherosclerotic vessels because the endothelium has become dysfunctional and partially deprived of its anticoagulant properties. Therefore, an exaggerated stress procoagulant response could enhance thrombus formation at times of plaque rupture triggered by acute stress-induced blood pressure peaks.

Acute Stress

Summary of Findings

Table 1 summarizes findings from well-conducted and standardized laboratory studies on acute stress effects on hemostasis factors in apparently healthy subjects reaching beyond individual findings. Different types of speech tasks, mental arithmetic, the mirror star tracing task, and the Stroop color-word conflict test were regularly applied as mental stressors in these studies. This research suggests that acute stress elicits a significant increase both in procoagulant factors (i.e., FXII:C, FVII:C, FVIII:C, fibrinogen, VWF, platelet activity) and in profibrinolytic t-PA. However, the finding of an increase in coagulation activation markers TAT and D-dimer suggests that the concomitant activation of virtually all hemostasis components with acute stress results in net hypercoagulability compatible with the evolution paradigm of Cannon. Unlike changes in blood pressure and cortisol, changes in the coagulation system do not adapt in response to the same stressor (i.e., combined speech task and mental arithmetic) applied three times on healthy subjects within an interval of

Table 1 Changes in hemostasis factors with stress

Hemostasis factor	Acute stress	Chronic stress
FVII:C	↑	↑
FXII:C	↑	
FVIII:C	↑	
Fibrinogen	↑	↑
Thrombin/antithrombin III complex	↑	—
D-dimer	↑	↑
von Willebrand factor	↑	↑ / —
Platelet activity markers	↑	
Plasminogen activator inhibitor-1	—	
Tissue-type plasminogen activator activity	↑	↓

↑, increases with stress; ↓, decreases with stress; —, no response to stress.

1 week. Apparently, evolution empowered humans to mount the same hypercoagulability any time we might potentially be injured independently of whether or not we perceive the situation as threatening.

Modulators of the Procoagulant Stress Response

Certain diseases, psychological states, and life circumstances have been shown to exaggerate the acute stress procoagulant response. In particular, it has been shown that D-dimer formation is increased and fibrinolytic activation is attenuated in acutely stressed patients with cardiovascular disease. Also, recovery of platelet activity after stress was delayed in patients with CAD as compared to those without. Anxiety, depression, and poor coping strategies (i.e., low problem solving and low personal mastery) have been shown to be associated with greater D-dimer formation and antifibrinolytic activity with acute stress in elderly subjects who were caregivers for a spouse with Alzheimer's disease. These caregivers also experienced greater acute procoagulability to stress when they experienced relatively more negative life events in the preceding month and if their spouse showed relatively more severe dementia. In accordance with the stress reactivity paradigm, these findings suggest that the stress procoagulant response, because of being hyperactive, might embed potential cardiovascular harm in certain individuals with certain diseases and at certain times of their life.

However, hemostatic effects of negative affect are not straightforward and may differ between elderly individuals, many of whom have cardiovascular disease, and healthy individuals. In the latter, an inverse relationship was found between levels of different domains of negative affect (e.g., anxiety and depression) and the magnitude of coagulation changes with acute stress. We may assume that endothelial dysfunction in the elderly might interact with negative affect to promote acute hypercoagulability. In contrast, greater hypercoagulability with less negative affect might still reflect normal physiology in healthy individuals preparing the organism for fight or flight.

Physiological Mechanisms

Molecular studies in *in vitro* and *in vivo* studies in animals and humans convincingly demonstrate that the sympathetic nervous system (SNS) regulates hemostatic activity. Much of this knowledge derives from human studies in which adrenergic compounds, particularly the stress hormones epinephrine and norepinephrine, had been infused together, with or without previous blockade of adrenergic receptors by various drugs. Table 2 summarizes adrenergic receptors and mechanisms assumed to be involved

Table 2 Adrenergic receptors and hemostasis regulation

Hemostasis factor	Adrenergic receptors (ARs)	Mechanisms
FVIII	Endothelial β2-AR	Release from endothelial cells and the liver
VWF	Endothelial β2-AR	Release from endothelial cells
t-PA	Endothelial β2-AR	Release from endothelial cells
	(β1- and) β2-adrenergic stimulation	Increases t-PA clearance
	α1-adrenergic stimulation	Reduces t-PA clearance
Platelets	Platelet α2-AR	Platelet activation
	Platelet β2-AR	Inhibition of platelet activation
PAI-1	β1- and/or β2-adrenergic stimulation	PAI-1 mRNA expression

FVIII, clotting factor VIII, VWF, von Willebrand factor, t-PA, tissue-type plasminogen activator; PAI-1, plasminogen activator inhibitor-1.

in hemostasis regulation. Via stimulation of vascular endothelial β2-adrenergic receptors, catecholamine surge releases preformed FVIII, VWF, and t-PA from endothelial storage pools into the circulation. This phenomenon takes place within minutes and shows dose dependency. Catecholamines also stimulate release of FVIII from the liver and affect hepatic clearance of t-PA. In addition, platelets are activated by stimulation of their α2-adrenergic receptors, with platelet β2-adrenergic receptors likely exerting an inhibitory effect on platelet activation by catecholamines. Greater sensitivity of the β2-adrenergic receptor was associated with greater thrombin formation in response to acute stress.

Stress-induced hemoconcentration was not associated with acute stress-induced changes in coagulation factors and activities. This suggests that coagulation activation during stress is an active phenomenon and does not merely reflect a passive increase of factors due to stress-induced plasma volume contraction. To date, there is little evidence for a significant effect of the hypothalamic-pituitary adrenal (HPA) axis and cortisol activity on the acute stress procoagulant response. Conceivably, evolution wanted the blood to clot instantly after injury as mediated by the SNS. In contrast, the HPA axis peaks its activity only 15 to 30 min after stress and, therefore, is a system likely too slow to critically limit bleeding.

Chronic Stress

Summary of Findings

Table 1 shows that, as with acute stress, chronic stress leads to an increase in procoagulant factors, namely, FVII:C, fibrinogen, and D-dimer, while data for VWF are conflicting. Notably, effects of chronic stress on fibrinolytic activity are distinctly different from those observed with acute stress. Chronic stress impairs the fibrinolytic activity such that the balance between procoagulant factors and profibrinolytic factors is shifted toward hypercoagulability to an extent that

exceeds the physiological net hypercoagulable changes seen with acute stress in healthy individuals.

These findings derive from investigations on hemostasis factors in subjects with high job strain, with low socioeconomic status, and who are caregivers of a demented spouse. In these studies, job strain was mainly defined as a mismatch between job demands and decision latitude and an imbalance between effort spent and reward obtained, moderated by a personality trait of overcommitment to work. Although relationships between various job strain variables and elevated plasma levels of FVII:C, fibrinogen, and PAI-1 on the one hand and decreased t-PA activity on the other were independent, most of the association between low socioeconomic status and hypercoagulability became insignificant when statistics controlled for health habits.

The number of negative life events in the preceding month correlated positively with plasma D-dimer in Alzheimer caregivers. In another study, chronically stressed dementia caregivers had higher D-dimer levels than age- and gender-matched noncaregiving controls, even when controlling for cardiovascular diseases and risk factors, lifestyle, and medication. Increased D-dimer was also observed in elderly hypertensive subjects in the weeks after they had experienced catastrophic stress. A fairly consistent line of research suggests that a state of excessive exhaustion ensuing from long-term psychological strain is associated with elevated PAI-1. Therefore, an antifibrinolytic effect could help explain the observation that profound feelings of fatigue may precede an acute myocardial infarction.

Physiological Mechanisms

The pathophysiological underpinnings of the link between chronic stress and hemostatic changes are far from clear, though gene regulation, the SNS, and the HPA axis could all be involved. This seems particularly true in terms of PAI-1. In accordance with the observed decrease in PAI-1 with chronic stress, restraint stress and injection of nonselective β-adrenergic substances in animals (i.e., epinephrine, isoprenalin) both resulted in upregulation of PAI-1 mRNA (**Table 2**) with a concomitant increase of PAI-1 activity in tissue homogenates. Moreover, homozygote carriers of the 5G allele of the PAI-1 4G/5G gene polymorphism who were exhausted had higher PAI-1 levels than homozygote 5G allele carriers who were not exhausted. In contrast, homozygote 4G carriers and heterozygote 4G/5G carriers did not differ in their PAI-1 levels in relation to their state of exhaustion.

When controlling for a whole range of possible confounders, greater overnight catecholamine secretion predicted higher morning levels of fibrinogen and D-dimer, while overnight cortisol excretion was not independently related to morning PAI-1 levels in a working population. However, research on the role of the HPA axis and endogenous cortisol activity on hemostasis in situations of chronic stress is too scarce to make a definite statement. Notably, patients with Cushing's disease, which is characterized by high production of endogenous cortisol, have an increased risk of thrombosis. In addition, subjects who received exogenous glucocorticoids either experimentally or as treatment manifested a hypercoagulable state.

Conclusions and Future Directions

More than a century of research on stress effects on hemostasis strongly suggests that, in response to acute stress, healthy individuals show a hypercoagulable state that is physiological and that has served the human species to enhance the odds of surviving fight-and-flight situations. However, this evolutionary benefit could be harmful today in an environment characterized by comparably longer lasting psychological stressors than those encountered in ancient times when humans either were killed or could escape. Daily hassles experienced in a rapidly changing society, years of marital stress, and job strain, as well as becoming a caregiver for a loved one, may elicit repetitive and sustained hypercoagulability that has lost its protective nature, thereby contributing to atherosclerosis and eventually myocardial infarction.

There is good evidence to assume that, of the stress-mediating systems, it is the sympathomedullary system that plays a major role in hemostasis regulation. However, data on the role of the HPA axis are rare, and the effect of the parasympathetic nervous system on hemostasis has not been explored. Although there is preliminary evidence that the brain transforms perceived stress into a physiological stress response resulting in rapid hemostatic activation further downstream in the peripheral blood and gene expression of hemostasis molecules, much research needs to be done to better elucidate these pathways. Also, we lack prospective studies investigating whether increased stress procoagulant reactivity has any impact on hard cardiovascular endpoints later in life. Often in the same large cohort, researchers reported that both hemostasis factors and stress predicted cardiovascular endpoints. However, none of these studies has investigated an additive or even multiplicative effect of stress and hemostasis on endpoints. If stress interacts with hypercoagulability in predicting cardiovascular disease, carefully conducted intervention studies on effects of stress management in its broadest sense on hemostatic function seem warranted. We could learn from these studies whether individuals with hypercoagulability exceeding its physiological magnitude could profit from, e.g., cognitive-behavioral stress management for better cardiovascular health.

See Also the Following Articles

Acute Stress Response: Experimental; Atherosclerosis; Beta-Adrenergic Blockers; Cardiovascular System and Stress; Caregivers, Stress and; Catecholamines; Corticosteroids and Stress; Fibrinogen and Clotting Factors; Genetic Factors and Stress; Heart Disease/Attack; Sympathetic Nervous System; Cardiovasular Disease, Stress and.

Further Reading

Brydon, L., Magid, K. and Steptoe, A. (2006). Platelets, coronary heart disease, and stress. *Brain, Behavior, and Immunity* 20, 113–119.

Cacioppo, J. T., Berntson, G. G., Malarkey, W. B., et al. (1998). Autonomic, neuroendocrine, and immune responses to psychological stress: the reactivity hypothesis. *Annals of the New York Academy of Science* 840, 664–673.

Camacho, A. and Dimsdale, J. E. (2000). Platelets and psychiatry: lessons learned from old and new studies. *Psychosomatic Medicine* 62, 326–336.

Cannon, W. B. and Mendenhall, W. L. (1914). Factors affecting the coagulation time of blood IV. The hastening of coagulation in pain and emotional excitement. *American Journal of Physiology* 34, 251–261.

Cannon, W. B. (1953). *Bodily changes in pain, hunger, fear, and rage. An account of recent researches into the function of emotional excitement* (2nd edn.). Boston, MA: Charles T. Branford Company.

Folsom, A. R. (2001). Hemostatic risk factors for athero-thrombotic disease: an epidemiologic view. *Thrombosis and Haemostasis* 86, 366–373.

Lee, K. W. and Lip, G. Y. (2003). Effects of lifestyle on hemostasis, fibrinolysis, and platelet reactivity: a systematic review. *Archives of Internal Medicine* 163, 2368–2392.

Loscalzo, J. and Schafer, A. I. (eds.) (2003). *Thrombosis and haemorrhage* (3rd edn.) Philadelphia, PA: Lippincott Williams & Wilkins.

Markovitz, J. H. and Matthews, K. A. (1991). Platelets and coronary heart disease: potential psychophysiologic mechanisms. *Psychosomatic Medicine* **53**, 643–668.

Preckel, D. and von Känel, R. (2004). Regulation of hemostasis by the sympathetic nervous system – any contribution to coronary artery disease? *Heart Drug* **4**, 123–130.

von Känel, R. and Dimsdale, J. E. (2000). Effects of sympathetic activation by adrenergic infusions on hemostasis in vivo. *European Journal of Haematology* **65**, 357–369.

von Känel, R. and Dimsdale, J. E. (2003). Hemostatic alterations in patients with obstructive sleep apnea and the implications for cardiovascular disease. *Chest* **124**, 1956–1967.

von Känel, R. and Dimsdale, J. E. (2003). Fibrin D-dimer: a marker of psychosocial distress and its implications for research in stress-related coronary artery disease. *Clinical Cardiology* **26**, 164–168.

von Känel, R., Mills, P. J., Fainman, C. and Dimsdale, J. E. (2001). Effects of psychological stress and psychiatric disorders on blood coagulation and fibrinolysis: a biobehavioral pathway to coronary artery disease? *Psychosomatic Medicine* **63**, 531–544.

von Känel, R., Preckel, D., Zgraggen, L., et al. (2004). The effect of natural habituation on coagulation responses to acute mental stress and recovery in men. *Thrombosis and Haemostasis* **92**, 1327–1335.

von Känel, R., Kudielka, B. M., Preckel, D., et al. (2005). Opposite effect of negative and positive affect on stress procoagulant reactivity. *Physiology & Behavior* **86**, 61–68.

Herpes Simplex *See:* Herpesviruses.

Herpesviruses

D A Padgett, M T Bailey and J F Sheridan
The Ohio State University, Columbus, OH, USA

This article is a revision of the previous edition article by D A Padgett and J F Sheridan, volume 2, pp 357–364, © 2000, Elsevier Inc.

Introduction
Virology
Immunobiology and Recurrent Disease
Stress and Herpesvirus Reactivation
Conclusion

Glossary

Capsid	The protein coat or shell that contains the nucleic acid genome of the virus particle.
Capsomeres	The individual morphological units (or sides) on the surface of the capsid.
Envelope	The lipid-containing outer membrane that surrounds the entire virus particle. The envelope arises from budding of mature herpesvirus particles through the nuclear membrane.
Icosohedron	Geometric shape with 20 equal sides or capsomeres (similar to a soccer ball). The herpesvirus capsid is an icosohedron.
Latent infection	When the virus persists in a quiescent (occult or cryptic) form most of the time with very little viral replicative activity. Herpesviruses are characterized by intermittent flare-ups of clinical disease.
Nucleocapsid	Includes the capsid and the enclosed nucleic acid.

Introduction

The Herpesviridae represent a large group of viruses that are pathogenic for many vertebrates. To date, there are more than 130 identified herpesviruses, nine of which are classified as human herpesviruses. These include herpes simplex virus type 1 (HSV-1), HSV-2, human cytomegalovirus (HCMV), varicella-zoster virus (VZV), Epstein–Barr virus (EBV), and human herpesviruses 6A, 6B, 7, and 8. The name herpesvirus is derived from the Greek word *herpein*, which means to creep. Such a name is quite appropriate, as this family of viruses is characterized by chronic, latent, and recurrent infections that appear to creep or crawl across the skin.

The pattern of infection with a herpesvirus depends on the portal of entry, and the site of viral replication is restricted by the surface proteins expressed by each species of virus. The herpesvirus family members cause a range of diseases, including infectious mononucleosis, chicken pox, shingles, gingivostomatitis (i.e., fever blisters and cold sores), genital herpes, and Kaposi's sarcoma. The severity of disease is chiefly dependent upon the immune status of the host. For example, in newborns or in immunocompromised adults, infection by HSV can be severe, resulting in encephalitis and possibly death. In contrast, healthy adults resolve the primary infection, and the virus becomes latent. In fact, several members of the herpesvirus family cause lifelong infections in humans that are characterized by periods of quiescence interrupted by reactivation and expression of clinical symptoms.

The type of cell in which a herpesvirus can become latent is specific to each herpesvirus. For HSV, the development of latency means that virions reside quietly in neural tissues without causing disease. In contrast, EBV establishes latency in B lymphocytes. In each case, periodic reactivation of the latent virus is frequently accompanied by clinical symptoms, production of infectious virus, and the development of herpetic lesions.

Virology

Characteristic Structure

Herpesviruses are large DNA viruses that share similar architectural details; they are morphologically indistinguishable from one another. Each member has a double-stranded DNA genome arranged in what has been described as a toroid core; in such a core, the DNA is spooled around a cylinder of proteins. The herpesvirus's toroid core is encapsulated within an icosahedral capsid. The capsid is composed of 162 capsomeres and is itself packaged within a lipid envelope. This envelope is formed from the nuclear membrane of an infected cell from which progeny viruses bud. Within this nuclear-lipid envelope are virus-encoded glycoproteins, or spikes, about 8 nm long. An additional feature of the herpesvirus family is a tegument, which is an amorphous, asymmetrical structure located between the capsid and envelope. The entire virion measures 120–200 nm, and the naked capsid is approximately 100 nm in diameter.

Characteristic Genome

The genome of herpesviruses is double-stranded linear DNA ranging from 120 to 250 kilobase pairs. The variation in size of the DNA genome among herpesvirus family members is due to a characteristic arrangement of their DNA sequences. Their genomes have terminal and internal repeat sequences that are bounded by a unique long (UL) and a unique short (US) region. These repeats allow some members of the family to undergo genomic rearrangement of their unique regions, giving rise to different genomic isomers. In addition, because of the high incidence of rearrangement, spontaneous deletions occur, and defective viral particles are common. Within the herpesvirus family, there is little DNA homology among the different species, with a few notable exceptions to this generality. Specifically, HSV types 1 and 2 share 50% sequence homology and herpesvirus 6 and 7 share 30–50% homology. However, because of the low homology among the herpesviruses, digestion of the genome with restriction endonucleases will yield a characteristic fragment pattern specific for each family member. This allows for rapid epidemiologic tracing of a given strain.

The genome of the typical herpesvirus is large and encodes for at least 100 different proteins, many of which (>35) are structural in nature. Additionally, all herpesviruses encode for a number of virus-specific enzymes that are involved in nucleic acid metabolism. These can include DNA polymerase, thymidine kinase, dUTPase, ribonucleotide reductase, helicase, and primase. It is important to note that none of these enzymes are packaged within the mature virus particle. They are expressed only during replication within the host cell.

Subclassification

More than 130 different herpesviruses have been identified, including nine human isolates. The herpesviruses are subdivided into three subclasses without regard to DNA sequence homology. Assignment to one of the three subfamilies, the alpha-, beta- and gammaherpesviruses, is based on biological properties, with emphasis given to host-range restriction and cellular tropism.

Alphaherpesviruses Alphaherpesviruses have a broad host range; they replicate rapidly in many types of cells. Although these are highly lytic viruses, members of this subclass can establish latency in neurons and glial cells. This group includes human HSV-1 and HSV-2, human VZV, and bovine herpesvirus type 1 (BHV-1).

Betaherpesviruses Betaherpesviruses have a restricted host range and grow slowly in tissue culture. Infection typically causes cells to enlarge, which is termed cytomegalia. These members can establish latency in hematopoietic progenitor cells and can cause persistent infections of epithelial and glandular cells. This group includes human and murine cytomegaloviruses (CMV), human herpesvirus 6, and human herpesvirus 7.

Gammaherpesviruses Gammaherpesviruses have a restricted host range. These viruses can replicate in epithelial cells and establish long-term latency in lymphocytes. In addition, some of these viruses can transform or immortalize their host cell. This group includes EBV and Kaposi's sarcoma-associated human herpesvirus (also called human herpesvirus type 8).

Virus Replication

Viruses are obligate intracellular parasites; as such, members of the Herpesviridae family must enter a host cell to undergo replication. Entry is a multistep process beginning with weak association of the virus envelope with the sugar moieties of cell membrane-associated proteoglycans (i.e., heparan sulfate and chondroitin sulfate). The second step of entry involves specific binding of the virus to a surface receptor. For example, EBV recognizes complement receptor 2 (CD21 or CR2) and HLA class II molecules. Human cytomegalovirus recognizes β_2-microglobulin, while HSV-1 binds to a member of the tumor necrosis factor/nerve growth factor receptor family. In addition to these common receptors, other glycoproteins have also been implicated in herpesvirus recognition of host target cells, and the group of receptors has been termed herpes virus entry mediators (HVEMs). Distribution of HVEMs determines the tropism of herpesvirus for specific cell types. After binding, the virus enters the host cell by fusion with the cell membrane. After entry, the viral envelope remains part of the cell's plasma membrane, but the capsid is transported through the cytoplasm to a nuclear pore. At the pore, the DNA is released from the capsid through the pore and into the nucleus. Once inside the nucleus, the viral DNA immediately circularizes.

Expression of the viral genome is tightly regulated and sequentially ordered in a cascade fashion. Immediate-early genes are expressed, yielding alpha proteins (alpha proteins are those that are produced in the absence of prior virus gene transcription). The alpha genes contain promoters that are recognized by the host cell's own transcription factors and are, therefore, turned on as soon as the viral DNA enters the nucleus of the cell. During a productive herpesvirus infection, the host cell's enzymes are hijacked

for the good of the virus. For example, herpesviruses are dependent upon the host cell's RNA polymerase II for all viral gene transcription. Even though the cell's own enzymes are used by the virus during replication/infection, normal cellular DNA and protein synthesis virtually stop as viral replication begins. Synthesis of the immediate-early alpha proteins promotes the expression of the next set of genes, or early genes, which are translated into beta proteins.

Beta proteins are those that are expressed before DNA replication begins but require alpha gene expression. Synthesis of the beta proteins represents the telltale sign that viral DNA synthesis has begun. It is believed that the beta proteins include the enzymes that are required to replicate the herpesvirus genome (i.e., DNA polymerase, thymidine kinase, dUTPase, ribonucleotide reductase, helicase, and primase). Because it circularizes when it enters the nucleus, herpesvirus DNA is synthesized by a rolling circle or concatameric mechanism that appears seemingly endless. The length of the replication cycle varies from about 18 h for herpes simplex virus to over 70 h for cytomegalovirus.

As viral DNA replication begins, late transcripts are produced that give rise to gamma proteins (gamma proteins are those that are expressed after DNA synthesis). While many of the alpha and beta proteins are enzymes or DNA-binding proteins, the gamma proteins are structural in nature and are the proteins of the tegument, toroid core, capsid, and envelope. In other words, synthesis of the gamma proteins is necessary for assembly of infectious virus progeny. Of interest, the virus's capsid is assembled before the newly synthesized viral DNA is inserted. This occurs in the cell nucleus. After encapsidation (i.e., DNA insertion into the capsid), maturation of infectious progeny occurs by budding of nucleocapsids through the inner nuclear membrane. Enveloped viral particles are then released from the cell through the plasma membrane by a poorly defined mechanism. The host cell that produces infectious progeny does not survive.

Overview of Diseases Caused by the Herpesviridae

As there are over 130 different types of herpesviruses, it is not surprising that they cause a wide variety of diseases. As their subclassification into alpha-, beta-, and gammaherpesviruses suggests, primary infection and possible latency may involve different cell types and present a widely different set of symptoms and clinical disease.

Herpes simplex viruses Herpes simplex viruses (HSV) are extremely widespread in the human population and exhibit an ability to replicate in many host tissues. They also infect other animals. There are two main forms of the herpes simplex viruses, human herpes viruses (HHV)-1 and -2, which are also known as HSV-1 and HSV-2. Both viruses grow rapidly and are extremely cytolytic. Typically, these viruses infect epithelial cells found in mucosal tissue and establish latent infections in peripheral neurons. HSV-1 has been classically associated with oropharyngeal lesions characterized by recurrent fever blisters. HSV-1 is spread by contact, usually involving infected saliva. HSV-2 has been associated with recurrent genital herpes and is usually transmitted sexually or from mother to neonate during vaginal birth. Both viruses can cause neurologic disease, with HSV-1 being the leading cause of sporadic encephalitis in the United States. Both HSV-1 and HSV-2 can cause severe primary infections in newborns. Latent infection followed by recurrent disease is the hallmark of these viruses. HSV-1 and HSV-2 reside in latently infected ganglia in a nonreplicating state with only a few viral genes being expressed; infectious virus cannot be isolated during latency. Persistence of the viral genome within a latently infected cell lasts for the lifetime of the host. Following a reactivating stimulus, the virus follows axons back to the peripheral site and replication proceeds in the epithelial cells. Spontaneous reactivation occurs despite HSV-specific immunity. More than 80% of the human population harbors HSV-1 in a latent form, but only a small percentage experience reactivation. Neither the cellular nor the molecular basis for reactivation is completely understood.

Varicella-zoster virus   Varicella-zoster virus (VZV or human herpesvirus 3) is highly contagious and is a very common virus. Like the HSVs, VZV is an alphaherpesvirus. The typical route of infection for VZV is the mucosa of the upper respiratory tract. After primary replication in the mucosal epithelium, the virus enters the circulation and eventually localizes to the skin, where it causes two distinct syndromes. Upon primary infection, usually in children, it causes chicken pox (also called varicella), which is characterized clinically by a generalized vesicular eruption of the skin and mucous membranes. However, VZV subsequently establishes a latent infection, and upon reactivation, the virus causes shingles (also called zoster). Shingles is a sporadic, incapacitating disease of adults or immunocompromised individuals that is clinically characterized by a rash limited in distribution to the skin innervated by a single sensory ganglion. The lesions are similar to varicella.

Epstein–Barr virus   Epstein–Barr virus (EBV or human herpesvirus 4) causes infectious mononucleosis and is latent in most adults. EBV is commonly transmitted by infected saliva (hence the nickname the kissing disease). Primary infection involves epithelial cells of the oropharynx and parotid gland. Viral shedding occurs for weeks to months after infection. Following replication in epithelial cells, EBV infects B cells and quickly becomes latent. Latent EBV is a factor in the development of nasopharyngeal carcinoma, Burkitt's lymphoma, and other lymphoproliferative disorders in immunocompromised individuals. As it has been known for years that cells in tissue culture could be immortalized by EBV, we now realize that EBV is the prototypic gammaherpesvirus and is oncogenic in humans.

Cytomegalovirus   Cytomegalovirus (CMV or human herpesvirus 5) infects respiratory epithelial cells or epithelial cells within salivary glands or the kidneys. CMV is believed to infect a majority of the human population worldwide, often without symptoms of overt disease. However, CMV infection causes congenital defects and mental retardation in more than 5000 infants in the United States per year. CMV is the largest herpesvirus, with a genome of approximately 240–250 kilobase pairs. Infection is characterized by massive enlargement of infected cells. Human CMV is the prototypical betaherpesvirus. Primary CMV infections in immunocompromised hosts are more severe than in normal hosts. Therefore, organ transplant recipients on immunosuppressive therapy and individuals with AIDS are predisposed to life-threatening infections by CMV.

Human herpesvirus 6 and human herpesvirus 7   Human herpesvirus 6 (HHV-6) and human herpesvirus 7 (HHV-7) were first recognized in 1986 and 1990, respectively. Both viruses were isolated from cultures of peripheral blood cells from patients with lymphoproliferative disorders involving T cells. Both have been classified as betaherpesviruses, as infection results in the formation of giant cells. HHV-6 and HHV-7 share significant sequence homology; however, they are antigenically and immunologically distinct. HHV-6 has been further subclassified into HHV-6A and HHV-6B based on distinct cellular tropism. Although HHV-6B is associated with roseola or exanthema subitum, HHV-6A and HHV-7 have not been associated with any known human disease.

Human herpesvirus 8   Human herpesvirus 8 is also known as Kaposi's sarcoma-associated herpesvirus; it was originally isolated in the mid-1990s from an AIDS patient with Kaposi's sarcoma. It is present in all forms of Kaposi's sarcoma, in primary B-cell effusion lymphomas, and in some forms of Castleman's disease, each of which is more prevalent in immuno-compromised patients. As each of these diseases is a form of cancer, HHV-8 has been characterized as a human tumor virus or gammaherpesvirus. HHV-8 expresses a number of cellular regulatory genes that the virus appears to have acquired from mammalian cells as a way of defeating host defense mechanisms.

B virus B virus is highly pathogenic for humans, although transmissibility of the virus from its normal host to humans is limited. Typically, B virus infects Old World monkeys and is enzootic in rhesus, cyno-molgus, and other macaque monkeys. B virus infections in the natural host seldom cause overt disease, but latency is established and B virus is easily reactivated under stressful conditions. Infection of humans usually results from monkey bites and is associated with a high rate of mortality due to an acute, ascending myelitis and encephalomyelitis.

Immunobiology and Recurrent Disease

The course or natural history of a herpes viral infection is influenced by the site of viral entry and host defenses. Primary infection with a herpesvirus induces both innate and adaptive immune responses, which result in the termination of viral replication and cessation of clinical symptoms. However, unlike acute viral infections, in which a successful immune response leads to elimination of the virus, infection with herpesviruses frequently leads to latency and thus the opportunity for episodic recurrent disease.

Innate Immunity

All mammals are born with a genetically inherited resistance to infectious microbes termed innate or natural resistance. Expression of natural resistance does not require previous exposure to the viral antigen (as does the adaptive immune response). Recent evidence suggests that toll-like receptor (TLR)-2 and TLR-9, which are pattern recognition receptors, are the first to detect that the host has been infected with herpesvirus. Activation of the TLR pathway initiates the innate immune response, which is aimed at restricting the early spread and replication of the virus without regard to the type of virus. Macrophages, natural killer (NK) cells, and killer cells mediating antibody-dependent cellular cytotoxicity (ADCC) all have roles in restricting the early spread of the virus. Infection by members of the Herpesviridae family is also accompanied by the expression of genes encoding the type I interferons that impart resistance to uninfected cells surrounding an infected cell.

Adaptive Immunity

Most infections with members of the Herpesviridae result in the induction of virus-specific humoral (antibody) and cell-mediated immune responses. In contrast to innate immunity, it takes several days for these herpesvirus-specific adaptive immune responses to be generated. A primary infection with HSV, whether asymptomatic or symptomatic, results in the production of virus-specific antibodies (both binding and neutralizing). These antibodies play multiple roles in mediating resolution of the primary infection through direct viral neutralization and through lysis of the infected cells by an ADCC mechanism. Virus-specific T cells are also very important during infection; individuals with cell-meditated immunodeficiency suffer severe herpetic disease. Clearance of virus correlates with the presence of CD8+ T cells with virus-specific cytolytic activity. Immunological memory in both the B cell and T cell compartments also follows primary infection. However, neither the successful termination of virus replication during primary infection nor the establishment of immunological memory prevents reactivation of latent virus and the development of recurrent lesions.

Recurrent Disease

Whether the time to reactivation of latent virus is weeks to months (as is the case for HSV) or years to decades (as is the case for VZV), it is apparent that immune memory, which results from the resolution of a primary infection with these viruses, offers little protection against recurrent disease. The development of recrudescent lesions is a two-step process. The first step occurs at the cellular/molecular level and involves the regulation of viral and host transcription factors influencing the state of expression of the latent viral genome. The balance between positive and negative transcription factors determines whether the genome will be reactivated, and this process is mediated by numerous hormonal and growth factor signals. These signals may result from many different stimuli. Psychological stress, physical trauma, UV irradiation from a sunburn, and hormonal fluctuations of the menstrual cycle have all been associated with reactivation of latent virus.

The period of time in which the reactivated virus gets to replicate, and thus cause clinical symptoms, is immunologically limited (and represents the second step in the process). Healthy adults generally limit clinical symptoms during a recurrence to a couple of days or less, whereas individuals with diminished cell-mediated immunity, as seen in AIDS, often develop severe disease that lasts much longer.

Stress and Herpesvirus Reactivation

The capacity of latent herpesviruses to reactivate and replicate is essential for completion of the viral life cycle. In the case of HSV-1 latency, reactivation of herpesvirus from ganglia results in the appearance of infectious virus at the site of the initial primary infection – typically the lips or gingiva. During the latent phase of any herpesvirus infection, viral gene expression is highly restricted; latency-associated transcripts (LATs) are among the few viral genes routinely detected during latency. It is believed that LAT gene expression establishes and maintains latency as mutations in LAT or its promoter limit herpesvirus latency.

The factors that lead to reactivation are even less clear. The limited knowledge of the pathogenesis of herpesvirus reactivation has been generated from studies in laboratory animals including mice, guinea pigs, and rabbits. In these models, reactivating stimuli range from mechanical and pharmacological to immunological alterations of cells and surrounding tissues. It is known that the first viral genes that are expressed during reactivation are the herpesvirus alpha, or immediate-early, genes whose promoter regions contain sequences that are similar to the host's cells own promoters. Reactivating stimuli may drive transcription of cellular genes whose promoter regions share homology with the promoters of the herpesvirus alpha genes. Thus, it is thought that the alpha genes are transcribed by the host cell's own transcription factors. The virus is then triggered for reactivation.

It is commonly thought that physical and psychological stress may be contributing factors to reactivation of herpesvirus. The impact of psychological stress on immune function is well documented in the literature and supports the hypothesis that psychological stress can reactivate latent virus. Several studies have shown that reactivation of latent HSV infections is more frequent in individuals who experience traumatic life events such as the death of a family member, the stress of interpersonal problems, or work-related difficulties. Similar relationships between psychosocial stress and reactivation of other herpesviruses, including EBV and VZV, have also been reported. It is thought that the physiologic alterations that ensue during stress alter the cellular and molecular microenvironment and serve as reactivators of latent herpes infections.

In mammals, stressors typically activate a specific set of core stress responses, including the hypothalamic-pituitary-adrenal (HPA) axis and sympathetic nervous system (SNS). Activation of the HPA axis results in increases in glucocorticoids such as cortisol, while activation of the SNS results in increases in circulating and tissue levels of catecholamines such as epinephrine and norepinephrine. Each of these alterations in host physiology has been linked to herpes reactivation. For example, a model for *in vivo* reactivation has been established in the rabbit eye. Epinephrine induces reactivation and shedding of mature infectious virus in the rabbit's tears. Glucocorticoids have also been implicated in reactivation. For example, cortisol can drive viral replication in primary cell cultures established from latently infected mouse trigeminal ganglia. Other experimental stressors (e.g., UV irradiation and transient hyperthermia), in a variety of animal models, can also cause recrudescence. However, the events that occur between stress and production of infectious herpesvirus are incompletely understood *in vivo*. Therefore, important biological knowledge remains unknown concerning reactivation.

Conclusion

The herpesviruses represent a diverse group of viruses that have evolved unique relationships with their hosts. Members of this viral group have been associated with diverse disease manifestations ranging from malignant transformation to latency and reactivation. Herpes infections occur from the cradle (neonatal HSV encephalitis) to the grave (shingles caused by reactivation of VZV in the later decades of life). They affect healthy individuals (e.g., CMV and mononucleosis) and immunodeficient individuals (e.g., human herpes virus type 8 which causes Kaposi's sarcoma in AIDS patients). Reactivation of the latent members of the herpesvirus family has been associated with multiple forms of stress (from physical stressors such as UV irradiation to psychological stress such as social conflict). Unfortunately, detailed knowledge of the molecular steps that trigger reactivation is lacking. Additional research is needed to gain a better understanding of these mechanisms and to help develop new prevention and treatment strategies that limit the replication, spread, and reactivation of the Herpesviridae.

See Also the Following Articles

Disease, Stress Induced; HIV Infection/AIDS.

Further Reading

Brooks, G. F., Butel, J. S. and Ornston, L. N. (2004). Herpesviruses. In: Jawetz, E., Melnick, J. L. & Adelberg, E. A. (eds.) *Medical Microbiology* (23rd edn., pp. 429–453). McGraw-Hill Companies.

Enright, A. M. and Prober, C. G. (2004). Herpesviridae infections in newborns: varicella zoster virus, herpes simplex virus, and cytomegalovirus. *Pediatric Clinics of North America* 51, 889–908.

Knipe, D. M. and Howley, P. M. (eds.) (2001). *Fields virology* (4th edn.). Philadelphia, PA: Lippincott Williams & Wilkins.

Mitchell, B. M., Bloom, D. C., Cohrs, R. J., Gilden, D. H. and Kennedy, P. G. (2003). Herpes simplex virus-1 and varicella-zoster virus latency in ganglia. *Journal of Neurovirology* 9, 194–204.

Moore, P. S. and Chang, Y. (2003). Kaposi's sarcoma-associated herpesvirus immunoevasion and tumorigenesis: two sides of the same coin? *Annual Review of Microbiology* 57, 609–639.

Hippocampal Neurons

R L Spencer and S T Bland
University of Colorado, Boulder, CO, USA

This article is a revision of the previous edition article by R D Brinton and T W Berger, volume 2, pp 364–371, © 2000, Elsevier Inc.

Overview

Hippocampal Formation

Laminar Organization of Dentate Gyrus and Hippocampus

Lammelar Organization (Trisynaptic Circuit) of Dentate Gyrus and Hippocampus

Principal Neurons

Interneurons

Intrinsic and Extrinsic Neural Connections

Neurochemistry

Neuroplasticity

Hippocampal Function

Glossary

Adenylyl cyclase	A protein enzyme that when activated, for example by a G-protein, catalyzes the formation of an intracellular second-messenger molecule, cyclic adenosine monophosphate (cAMP).
Cation channel	A protein complex embedded in a cell's membrane that allows positively charged ions (e.g., Na^+, K^+, or Ca^{2+}) to pass through the membrane.
G-proteins	Guanine nucleotide (guanosine triphosphate, GTP, and guanosine diphosphate, GDP) binding proteins that associate with the intracellular portion of metabotrobic receptors. G-protein alterations are the first step in a cascade of intracellular molecular changes triggered by neurotransmitter or hormone (ligand) binding of metabotropic receptors at the membrane surface.
Neuropil	Brain region that consists primarily of neuronal processess (dendrites and axons) rather than neuronal cell bodies.
Spatial learning	Learning tasks in which optimal performance requires that the organism has learned the relative spatial relationship between objects in the environment. Spatial learning can be demonstrated by tasks in which the organism is able to select the most direct route to a location that it has been to before or, alternatively, by tasks in which the organism avoids revisiting places that it has been to before.

Overview

The hippocampal formation consists of the hippocampus and the closely associated dentate gyrus and subiculum. The hippocampal formation first attracted attention as a primitive region of the cortex that had an architecturally simple and orderly cellular organization. Strikingly detailed drawings of the microscopic organization of the hippocampal formation were provided by Ramón y Cajal in the late 1800s (**Figure 1**). This structure is dominated by the orderly alignment of two principal neuronal cell types: pyramidal cells and granule cells. Moreover, the principal cells of the hippocampal formation were found to be interconnected in such a way as to produce a simple intrinsic neurocircuit (the trisynaptic circuit). Interest in the hippocampal formation intensified when, based on human amnesic cases, it was found to be essential for the formation of new episodic memories and the acquisition of declarative facts. The intense study of the hippocampus has yielded the first characterized cellular functional response (long-term potentiation) believed to reflect the fundamental neuroplasticity underlying memory formation.

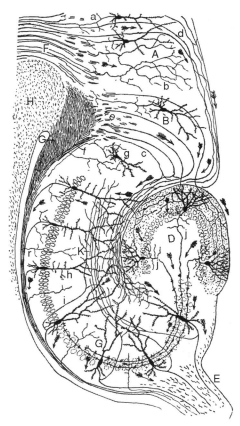

Figure 1 Drawing of a transverse section of the hippocampal formation highlighting the principal cells (e.g. B, D, G, h), their interconnections and presumed flow of neural impulses (arrows). Drawing by S. Ramón y Cajal, first published in 1911 (Ramón Y Cajal, Histologie du systeme nerveux de lHomme et des Vertebres. Paris: A. Maloine, 1911).

Subsequent study of the hippocampus has revealed a range of neuroplasticity phenomena that include dynamic changes in neuronal arborization, spine density, and synapse formation. Investigations in recent years have determined that neurogenesis is a routine feature of the adult dentate gyrus portion of the hippocampal formation. The characterization of these forms of hippocampal neuroplasticity has revolutionized recent neuroscience with the discovery that these neuroplastic changes are not restricted to critical developmental periods or recovery from brain injury but are a normal daily occurrence that persists throughout the life span.

Hippocampal Formation

Each of the components of the hippocampal formation is characterized by a single principal cell body layer sandwiched between two zones of neuropil, yielding a simplified version of cortex with only three distinct layers. Extensively associated with the hippocampal formation, in terms of interconnections, is the adjacent six-layer entorhinal cortex. The hippocampus and its interleaved partner, the dentate gyrus, are two phylogenetically primitive cortical structures that are buried underneath the cortical mantle. In the human brain, these two enfolded sheets of rudimentary cortex are located within the temporal lobe (**Figure 2**). In the rodent brain, these structures extend more dorsal-anteriorly. The dorsal portion of the hippocampus is located immediately beneath the corpus callosum and has an anterior extension that approaches the septal region (**Figure 3**). The most caudal extent of the hippocampus is located in the ventral half of the caudal portion of rodent forebrain.

Dissected out of a rat brain, the combined dentate gyrus and hippocampus are somewhat banana-shaped. The longitudinal axis of this structure is often referred to as the septal-temporal axis of the hippocampus and dentate gyrus. The rostral approximately two-thirds of this structure is known as the dorsal hippocampus, and the caudal third is known as the ventral hippocampus. This structure is usually studied and depicted in the tranverse/cross-sectional plane (**Figure 3**). The cellular organization of the hippocampus and dentate gyrus in mammals is remarkably consistent throughout its longitudinal extent. Recent anatomical studies, however, have demonstrated important differences in intrinsic and extrinsic connections within the dorsal and ventral hippocampus. These differences may have important functional significance. For example, there is some evidence that the dorsal hippocampus is more important for spatial learning and memory and that the ventral hippocampus selectively contributes to fear and other emotion-dependent behaviors and learning.

Laminar Organization of Dentate Gyrus and Hippocampus

The principal cell body layer of the hippocampal formation consists primarily of pyramidal cell bodies (hippocampus and subiculum) or granule cell bodies (dentate gyrus). The surrounding neuropil zones primarily comprise the proximal principal cells' dendrites and axons and the nerve terminals of extrinsic and intrinsic afferents. This laminar organization can be easily visualized when examining microscopically a transverse section of dentate gyrus and hippocampus (**Figure 4a**). Anatomists have subdivided the neuropil zones into different strata, based primarily on microscopic differences in the principal cell processes and the afferents and efferents present within each strata (**Figure 4b**). Note that each of these cortical

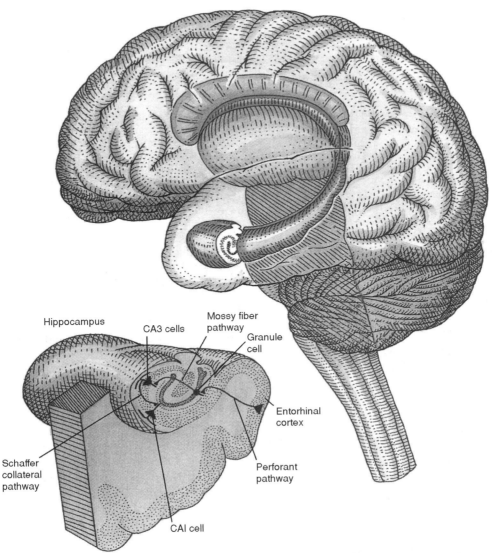

Figure 2 Relative location of hippocampal formation in human brain. The hippocampus and its interleaved partner, the dentate gyrus, reside beneath the cortical surface in the temporal lobe. An enlarged transverse slice of the hippocampus and dentate gyrus is depicted in the lower left portion of the figure. From Squire, L. R. and Kandel, E. R. (2000), *Memory, from mind to molecules,* New York: Scientific American Library.

sheets has been folded in half along its longitudinal axis. Therefore, when we view a cross section of this structure in the rat brain, the orderly aligned principal cell bodies form a C-shaped (hippocampus) or V-shaped (dentate gyrus) formation. As is evident when we view a horizontal cross section of ventral hippocampus, one edge of the hippocampal sheet is adjacent to the subiculum and entorhinal cortex (**Figure 4c–d**). The other edge of the hippocampal sheet is tucked inside the two folds of the dentate gyrus. The C-shaped formation of pyramidal cell bodies in the hippocampus is subdivided into three subfields based on morphological and interconnection distinctions. These subfields are designated CA1, CA2, and CA3 (drawing on the Latin name for the hippocampus, *cornus Ammonus,* Ammon's horn). The CA3 region is adjacent to the dentate gyrus, and the CA1 region is adjacent to the subiculum. The smaller CA2 region has morphological, phenotypical, and connectional features that overlap with those of the CA3 and CA1 subregions, but in combination makes for a clearly distinct functional zone of cells. The granule cells in the dentate gyrus are relatively uniform throughout the V-shaped formation in terms of morphology, innervation, and projections. The two folds of dentate gyrus giving rise to the V-shaped formation are commonly referred to as the enclosed and free blades, or the

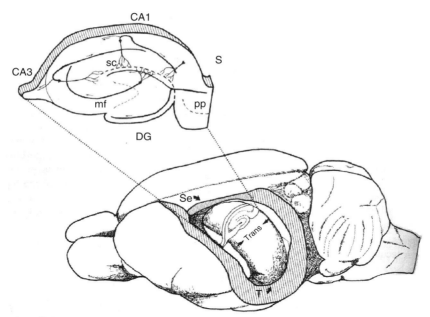

Figure 3   Relative location of hippocampal formation in rat brain. The hippocampus (including CA1 and CA3 subregions) and dentate gyrus (DG) form a banana-like structure with one end of the longitudinal axis located dorsal-rostrally near the septal (Se) region and the other end located ventral-caudally near the temporal (T) pole of the rat forebrain. An enlarged transverse slice is depicted in the upper portion of the figure. mf, mossy fiber; pp, perforant path; sc, Schaffer collateral; S, subiculum. From Amaral, D.G. and Witter, M.P. (1989) The three-dimensional organization of the hippocampal formation: a review of the anatomical data. *Neuroscience* **31**, 571–591.

suprapyramidal and infrapyramidal blades, of the dentate gyrus. Recent studies indicate that there are some clear differences in the relative afferent connections to the two blades of the dentate gyrus as well as discriminable tendencies in their projection to CA3 subregions. The intervening space between the two granule cell body-forming blades of the dentate gyrus is known as the hilus or polymorphic region of the dentate gyrus.

Lammelar Organization (Trisynaptic Circuit) of Dentate Gyrus and Hippocampus

Significantly, many of the intrahippocampal neural connections are maintained within a narrow cross-sectional area (lammelae). A simple unidirectional trisynaptic connection among the components of the hippocampal formation was deduced by Ramón y Cajal based on microscopic architecture (**Figure 1**). Around 1970, Andersen and colleagues provided electrophysiological evidence to support a predominantly lammelar organization of hippocampal function. This trisynaptic circuit (**Figure 5a**) begins with pyramidal neurons predominantly localized in layer II of entorhinal cortex. These cells project (perforant pathway) to both blades of the dentate gyrus

and form synapses on granule neuron dendrites (synapse 1). The granule neurons project (mossy fiber pathway) to CA3 and form synapses on the apical dendrite of CA3 pyramidal neurons within the stratum lucidum (synapse 2). A collateral axonal branch of the CA3 pyramidal neurons projects (Schaffer collateral) to CA1 and forms synapses on basilar and apical dendrites of CA1 pyramidal neurons (synapse 3). The primary output from this circuit, and from the hippocampus overall, proceeds from CA1 neurons to the adjacent subiculum and entorhinal cortex as well as to subcortical structures.

More recent investigations have determined that there is considerable divergence and convergence within the longitudinal plane of connections between the entorhinal cortex and the dentate gyrus and between CA3 pyramidal neurons and other CA3 and CA1 cells. Only the mossy fiber connections between the dentate gyrus and CA3 are predominantly restricted to a cross-sectional lammelae. Nevertheless, a fairly thin cross section of the dentate gyrus and hippocampus contains a number of intact cells of each trisynaptic circuit component. Therefore, the hippocampal formation is ideally suited for *ex vivo* study, in which a 250- to 500-μm cross-section of this structure contains an electrophysiologically functional trisynaptic circuit. Consequently, with appropriate bath conditions for

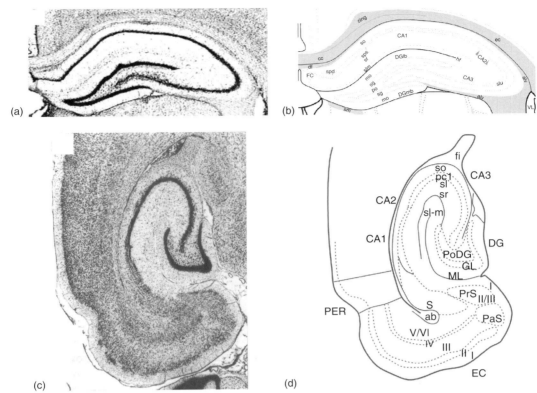

Figure 4 Laminar organization of rat hippocampal formation. a, Photomicrograph of histologically stained tissue of transverse section of the dorsal hippocampus (coronal plane); b, corresponding line drawing; c, photomicrograph of histologically stained tissue of transverse section of the ventral hippocampus (horizontal plane); d, corresponding line drawing. The strata of the hippocampus shown are stratum oriens (so), pyramidal cell body layer (spd, sps, or pcl), stratum lucidum (sl), stratum radiatum (sr), and stratum lacunosum-moleculare (slm). The strata of the dentate gyrus shown are the molecular layer (mo), granule cell body layer (gl or sg), and the hilus or polymorphic region (po). The tightly packed and orderly aligned pyramidal and granule cell bodies result in a darkly stained C- or V-shaped formation in the hippocampus or dentate gyrus, respectively. ab, angular bundle; alv, alveus; cc, corpus callosum; cing, cingulum; DGlb, dentate gyrus lateral or enclosed blade; Dgmb, dentate gyrus medial or free blade; EC, entorhinal cortex (layers I–VI); fi, fimbria of fornix; hf, hippocampal fissure; PaS, parasubiculum; PER, perirhinal cortex; PrS, presubiculum (layers I–III); S, subiculum; VL, lateral ventricle. Panels a and b from Swanson. L. W. (2004), *Brain maps: structure of the rat brain* (3rd edn.), Amsterdam: Elsevier Academic Press.; panels c and d from Witter, M. P. and Amaral, D. G. (2004), Hippocampal formation, In: Paxinos, G. (ed.) *The rat nervous system* (3rd edn.), pp. 635–704. Amsterdam: Elsevier Academic Press.

neuronal survival, a cross-sectional brain slice of the hippocampus and dentate gyrus maintains many functional features of an intact hippocampal circuit. The *ex vivo* electrophysiological study of hippocampal slices has been instrumental in deciphering the cellular and molecular correlates of hippocampal-dependent learning (**Figure 5b**).

Principal Neurons

All the principal cells of the hippocampal formation (pyramidal and granule cells) are believed to be glutamatergic. Pyramidal cells have a distinctly pyramid or tear-drop shape. Pyramidal cells in CA3 and CA2 have larger cell bodies (approximately 25 µm in diameter) than those in CA1 (approximately 15 µm in diameter) (**Figure 6**). Separate multibranching dendritic trees emerge from the apex and base of

each cell. The base of the cell is defined by the surface from which the axon emerges, and the separate dendritic trees are referred to as apical and basilar dendrites, with each cell having one or two apical dendrites and several basilar dendrites. All hippocampal pyramidal cells are aligned in the same orientation, with the apical dendritic trees radiating toward the center of the C-shaped semicircle of cells (filling the stratum radiatum). The basilar dendrites extend in the opposite direction (filling the stratum oriens). Hippocampal pyramidal cell axons penetrate the stratum oriens and travel as part of the alveus to distal hippocampal or subcortical targets.

Granule cells of the dentate gyrus have small spherical or ovoid-shaped cell bodies (approximately 8–15 µm in diameter). One moderately complex dendritic tree (filling the stratum moleculare) is attached to the pole of the cell opposite from where

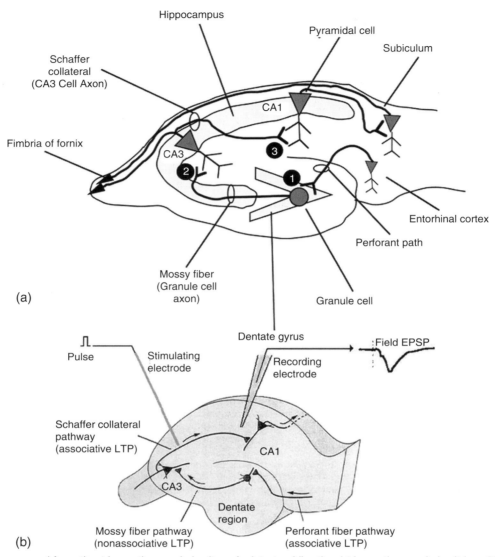

Figure 5 Hippocampal-formation trisynaptic neural circuit. a, An intact unidirectional trisynaptic neural circuit in a 250- to 500-μm transverse section of rat hippocampal formation (lamellae); b, *ex vivo* stimulation of a transverse slice of hippocampal formation placed in a chamber containing a solution of artificial cerebrospinal fluid to assess the electrophysiological activity in one component of the trisynaptic circuit. In (a) representative pyramidal cells (present in the entorhinal cortex, CA3, CA1, and subiculum) and a granule cell (in the dentate gyrus) that participate in the circuit are depicted. The three featured synapses of the circuit are numbered in the temporal order in which they are engaged by neural activity, starting with pyramidal neurons in the entorhinal cortex. In (b) a stimulating and recording electrode is applied to the tissue slice in order to assess electrophysiological activity within one component of the trisynaptic circuit. EPSP, excitatory postsynaptic potential; LTP, long-term potentiation. Adapted from Squire, L. R. and Kandel, E. R. (2000), *Memory, from mind to molecules,* New York: Scientific American Library.

the axon emerges and projects. There is also a population of large-diameter cells in the hilus region of the dentate gyrus called mossy cells that also appear to be glutamatergic. These cells receive input from the mossy fibers and project back to the dentate gyrus granule cells. Interestingly, mossy cells preferentially project bilaterally to granule cells at other levels of the longitudinal axis than that in which they reside.

The dendritic trees of hippocampal formation principal cells are densely covered with bulbous spines

(**Figure 6**). The head of these spines form the postsynaptic site for much of the excitatory input to these cells. There are especially large prominent spines on CA3 neurons and mossy cells called thorny excrescences, which form the postsynaptic site for the mossy fiber input from the dentate gyrus. Inhibitory synapses, largely arising from γ-aminobutyric acid (GABA)ergic interneurons, are mostly localized to the soma, dendritic shafts, and axonal initial segments of the principal cells.

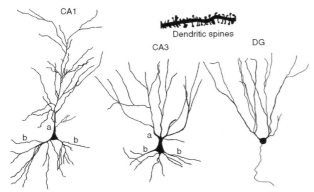

Figure 6 Hippocampal formation principal cells. Camera lucida tracings of representative CA1 and CA3 pyramidal cells in the hippocampus and a granule cell in the dentate gyrus (DG) from rat brain are shown. All three representative cells are oriented such that the axon emerges from the bottom of the cell body (an axon is clearly evident for the granule neuron). Multibranched apical (a) and basilar (b) dendritic trees are attached to the pyramidal cell body. The dendritic trees for the granule cell are attached to the upper portion of the cell body. A camera lucida tracing of an enlarged portion of a CA1 apical dendrite is also included. This tracing illustrates the dense presence of spines that cover the dendrites of these principal cells. Adapted from Gould, E., Woolley, C.S., Frankfurt, M., et al. (1990), Gonadal steroids regulate dendritic spine density in hippocampal pyramidal cells in adulthood. *Journal of Neuroscience* 10, 1286–1291. © 1990 by the Society for Neuroscience.

Interneurons

There are various types of interneuron cell bodies scattered throughout all strata of the dentate gyrus and hippocampus. Most of these interneurons are presumed to be GABAergic, and they have been further categorized by the differential expression of various neuropeptides and calcium-binding proteins. Many of these interneurons have extensive axon collaterals and arborization that extend fairly long distances within both the longitudinal and transverse plane and form numerous synaptic contacts with principal cells. Although there are substantially fewer hippocampal interneurons than principal cells (probably totaling less than 1% of all hippocampal neurons), this pattern of connectivity allows them to have substantial effects on overall hippocampal function. Two of the better-characterized types of inhibitory interneurons are the basket cells and the chandelier or axoaxonic cells. The basket cells are so named because their multibranched axons form an extensive interwoven contact with the cell body of target pyramidal cells. The chandelier cells form strong synaptic contacts on the initial axonal segment of pyramidal cells. It should also be noted that there are many synaptic contacts between inhibitory interneurons as well as axodendritic contacts from principal cells. Thus, the interneurons are interconnected in such a way as to mediate complex feedforward and feedback inhibition and disinhibition within the hippocampal formation.

Intrinsic and Extrinsic Neural Connections

A major source of neural input to the dentate gyrus, as previously described, is from the entorhinal cortex and constitutes the first component of the trisynaptic circuit. There are considerable reciprocal connections of the entorhinal cortex with other regions of neocortex, most notably the adjacent perirhinal cortex and the nearby postrhinal and piriform cortex. There are also substantial direct interconnections with the medial prefrontal, insular, and retrosplenial cortex. Thus, the entorhinal cortex is believed to provide the dentate gyrus and hippocampus with the rich multimodal sensory content of ongoing experience. In addition to the extensive input to the dentate gyrus, the entorhinal cortex also provides (via the temporal-ammonic pathway) direct monosynaptic parallel input to the CA3 region of the hippocampus, as well as direct input to CA1 pyramidal cells. Thus, both CA3 and CA1 neurons are in the position to integrate or compare direct and processed information from the entorhinal cortex. The projection of CA1 neurons back to the entorhinal cortex, either directly or via the subiculum, makes the entorhinal cortex the principal bidirectional interface between the hippocampal formation and various neocortical regions.

In addition to the trisynaptic circuit, there are extensive commissural and longitudinal associational connections within the hippocampus. The major source of these additional associational connections are provided by the non-Schaffer collateral branch of CA3 pyramidal cell axons, with additional contribution from CA2 pyramidal cells and mossy cells of the hilus.

There are other important neural inputs to the dentate gyrus and hippocampus from various populations of biogenic amine-containing neurons that may primarily modulate the general excitatory tone and neural synchronization within this structure. In addition, the CA1 region receives direct excitatory input from basal nuclei of the amygdala and midline nuclei of the thalamus. Interestingly, the amygdala input to the hippocampus is largely restricted to the ventral hippocampus.

The major output neurons of the hippocampal formation are pyramidal cells in CA1, subiculum, and deep layers of the entorhinal cortex. CA1 and subiculum pyramidal cells provide a large subcortical projection via the fornix to the septum and hypothalamus, with minor contribution from CA3 pyramidal cells. There are also strong direct connections of the

CA1 and subiculum with the medial prefrontal cortex. However, as previously indicated, there are more extensive indirect connections of the CA1 and subiculum with the prefrontal and other cortical areas via the entorhinal cortex.

Neurochemistry

Amino Acid Neurotransmitters

The excitatory neurotransmitter, glutamate, is released from hippocampal-formation principal cells and is therefore the neurotransmitter used by the perforant path, mossy fibers, and Schaffer collaterals. Glutamate receptor subtypes include the ionotropic receptors (iGluRs), which directly gate cation channels and are named after the ligands that preferentially bind to them: N-methyl-D-aspartate (NMDA), α-amino-3-hydroxy-5-methyl-4-isoxazolepropionic acid (AMPA), and kainate. All the iGluRs are present in the excitatory pathways of the hippocampus. AMPA and kainate receptors mediate fast excitatory postsynaptic potentials (EPSPs), and NMDA receptors mediate slower EPSPs. All the iGluRs open Na^+ and K^+ channels. NMDA as well as some AMPA and kainate receptors are also permeable to Ca^{2+}. The NMDA receptor is unique in that channel permeability is both ligand- and voltage-dependent.

There is also a family of metabotropic glutamate receptors (mGluRs) that are coupled to guanine nucleotide-binding proteins (G-proteins). mGluRs have both pre- and postsynaptic localization and can coexist in the postsynaptic density with iGluRs. Postsynaptically, mGluR regulate synaptic transmission by stimulating specific second-messenger cascades and generating slow synaptic responses. When expressed presynaptically, mGluR activation can modulate transmitter release.

The inhibitory neurotransmitter GABA can also act on both ionotropic and metabotropic receptors. $GABA_A$ receptors are ionotropic and gate ion channels that are permeable to the anion Cl^-. GABA also binds a metabotropic receptor, $GABA_B$, which is coupled to a G-protein that, when activated, opens K^+ channels. When expressed postsynaptically, $GABA_B$ receptor activation leads to a slow hyperpolarization. When expressed presynaptically, $GABA_B$ receptor activation reduces neurotransmitter release.

Biogenic Amines

The major cholinergic input to the hippocampus is from the medial septal nucleus. Acetylcholine (ACh), similar to glutamate and GABA, can act on both ionotropic (nicotinic receptors) and metabotropic (muscarinic) receptors, both of which are expressed in the hippocampus. Nicotinic ACh receptors are ligand-gated ion channels that mediate fast excitatory transmission via an influx of Na^+ and Ca^{2+}. Nicotinic receptors are expressed on both excitatory and inhibitory interneurons in the hippocampus and can be expressed pre- and postsynaptically. Muscarinic receptors are very densely expressed in the hippocampus, and different subtypes are differentially expressed on specific populations of neurons: M_1/M_3 on principal cells and M_2/M_4 on interneurons. The actions of muscarinic receptor activation can be excitatory or inhibitory, depending on the type of G-protein to which the receptor is coupled: M_1/M_3 are coupled to G_q (which stimulates phospholipase C), and M_2/M_4 are coupled to $G_{i/o}$ (which can inhibit adenylyl cyclase or activate a K^+ channel). Muscarinic receptor activation potentiates NMDA receptor activity, probably by the activation of the M_1 subtype. M_2 can be expressed as autoreceptors on cholinergic terminals. Acetylcholine is also known to regulate the release of dopamine, serotonin, and neuropeptides by the activation of presynaptic nicotinic and muscarinic receptors.

Cholinergic neurons that project to the hippocampus from the medial septal nucleus and the nucleus of the diagonal band of Broca contribute to the synchronous discharge of principal cells reflected by the prominent theta frequency hippocampal electroencephalograph (EEG). Theta is observed both during voluntary movement (Type 1, 8–12 Hz) and during alert immobility (Type 2, 4–6 Hz), although only Type 2 theta is sensitive to cholinergic manipulations.

Dopamine afferent terminals are observed in the ventral subiculum, in all strata of CA1, in the stratum oriens of CA3, and in the hilus of the dentate gyrus. The source of hippocampal dopamine comes from the midbrain ventral tegmentum and substantia nigra and there is some evidence for different populations of dopaminergic cells innervating dorsal and ventral hippocampal formations. Dopamine receptors comprise two types, D1-like (D1 and D5) and D2-like (D2, D3, and D4), and all are metabotropic. D5 is the most prominent D1-like receptor in the hippocampus and is coupled to G_s (which stimulates adenylyl cyclase). D5 receptors are expressed on pyramidal cells and can enhance NMDA- and AMPA-mediated currents. Dopamine D4 is the most prominent D2-like receptor in the hippocampus. D4 receptors are densely expressed on pyramidal neurons in CA1, on granule cells in the dentate gyrus, and on GABA interneurons. D4 receptors are coupled to $G_{i/o}$ and decrease NMDA-mediated excitatory transmission.

Norepinephrine innervation of the hippocampus arises primarily from the locus ceruleus, and the hippocampus contains one of the highest densities of norepinephrine-containing terminals in the brain. Receptors for norepinephrine (adrenergic receptors) have been divided into two classes: α and β, which are further subdivided based on the specific G-proteins to which they are coupled. β-adrenergic receptors are coupled to G_s, while $α_1$ types are coupled to G_q and $α_2$ types to G_i. Electrical stimulation of the locus ceruleus produces an inhibition of hippocampal pyramidal neuron firing, followed by a transient increase in firing. The inhibition appears to be mediated by $α_2$ and the excitation by β receptors.

Serotonin (5HT) input to the hippocampus derives almost exclusively from the median raphe nucleus. Serotonin receptors in the hippocampus are preferentially expressed on calbindin-positive GABA interneurons, and the specific subtypes expressed include $5HT_{1A}$, which is coupled to $G_{i/o}$; $5HT_{2A}$, which is coupled to G_q; and $5HT_3$. The $5HT_3$ receptor is an ionotropic receptor, the activation of which opens a nonspecific cation channel, resulting in fast depolarization. The activation of $5HT_3$ receptors can thus inhibit the firing of pyramidal neurons by a GABA interneuron-mediated mechanism. There are also autoreceptors of the $5HT_{1B/D}$ subtype on serotonergic terminals that inhibit the release of serotonin. Intracellular recording studies show that the most prominent effect of serotonin application to the hippocampus is hyperpolarization of pyramidal neurons caused by an increase in K^+ conductance.

Histamine projections arise from the tuberomammillary nucleus of the hypothalamus. Histamine H_2 receptors are dense in CA1 and CA3 and are primarily located on pyramidal cell dendrites, but are also found on granule cells in the dentate gyrus. H_2 receptors are coupled positively to adenylyl cyclase, and the activation of these receptors causes strong excitation. Histamine H_1 receptors are mostly found in CA3, where their activation causes hyperpolarization. The H_1 receptor is coupled to stimulation of phospholipase C via $G_{q/11}$. H_3 receptors are also inhibitory (coupled to $G_{i/o}$) and are located on perforant path terminals in the dentate gyrus, where their activation can suppress glutamate secretion.

Other Neuromodulators

The hippocampus is rich in other neuromodulators, including neuropeptides, growth factors, cytokines, and endocannabinoids as well as their receptors. Neuropeptides are typically coreleased with classical neurotransmitters. Neuropeptides expressed in hippocampal neurons include cholecystokinin, somatostatin, neuropeptide Y, leptin, galanin, corticotropin releasing hormone, and the opioid peptides β-endorphin, enkephalin, and dynorphin. Receptors for the

gonadal and adrenal steroid hormones and thyroid hormone are also expressed in the hippocampus. Growth factors that are abundant in the hippocampus include brain-derived growth factor (BDGF), nerve growth factor (NGF) and fibroblast growth factor (FGF). Growth factors perform neurotrophic and neuroprotective functions and are critically involved in development and neuroplasticity. Cytokines regulate intercellular communication, including glial-to-neuronal and immune-to-neuronal communication. Cytokine ligands and their receptors found in the hippocampus include interleukin-1, tumor necrosis factor, and fractalkine. Eicosanoids are metabolites of arachidonic acid, which is derived from dietary linoleic acid. Several of the eicosanoids, including anandamide (arachidonylethanolamine) and arachidonoylglycerol, are known as endocannabinoids because they act on the cannabinoid receptor CB1. High levels of CB1 expression are found throughout the hippocampus.

Neuroplasticity

Long-term potentiation (LTP) reflects a cellular model of learning and memory, first described in rabbit hippocampus in 1973. LTP is induced by applying a brief high-frequency electrical stimulus to an excitatory synaptic pathway, such as the hippocampal Schaffer collateral pathway, the perforant pathway, or the mossy fiber pathway (**Figure 5b**). For periods of hours (*in vitro*) to weeks (*in vivo*) after this conditioning stimulus, a test stimulus can subsequently provoke an increased synaptic response that is 50–200% above baseline. In the Schaffer collateral–CA1 synapse and the perforant path–dentate gyrus synapse, LTP is dependent on the activation of the NMDA receptor and subsequent Ca^{2+} influx (associative LTP), whereas in the mossy fiber–CA3 synapse, LTP appears to be dependent on kainate receptors (nonassociative LTP).

LTP has four basic characteristics that resemble features of learning and memory:

1. Temporal specificity: the presynaptic cell must fire before the postsynaptic cell.
2. Cooperativity: many synapses must be active to induce LTP.
3. Associativity: a strong input can induce potentiation at a weakly activated, adjacent synapse on the same postsynaptic cell.
4. Input specificity: potentiation is only induced at the synapses that received the conditioning stimulation.

In contrast to the potentiation caused by brief high-frequency stimulation, prolonged low-frequency stimulation of a pathway induces a long-term depression

(LTD) of the synaptic response to a test stimulus. Like the typical LTP found in most pathways (but not the mossy fiber pathway), LTD is also dependent on the activation of the NMDA receptor. It is thought that different patterns of Ca^{2+} influx produced during LTP and LTD induction determine the differential responses to these stimuli; high-frequency stimulation results in a large Ca^{2+} elevation and activation of the Ca^{2+}/calmodulin-dependent protein kinase (CaMK) cascade, whereas the smaller but more prolonged Ca^{2+} elevation produced by low-frequency stimulation leads to activation of a phosphatase cascade.

Hippocampal Function

The hippocampal formation appears to play a uniquely pivotal role in the brain's ability to form rapid and long-lasting associations between environmental stimuli in a way that allows for the learning of new concrete and abstract factual information (declarative memory) and detailed recall and recognition of events and places (episodic memory). The hippocampus in rodents appears to have an especially important role in learning the spatial configuration of places. Many CA1 and CA3 pyramidal cells behave as place cells; on initial exposure to a new environment, these cells acquire within several minutes the ability to increase their neuronal firing rate whenever the rat returns to a particular place in that environment.

The role of the hippocampus in stress response is less clear. As part of the limbic system, the involvement of the hippocampus in the generation of a stress state has often been presumed, but its anatomical neighbor, the amygdala, appears to play a much more important role than the hippocampus in this process. The cells of the hippocampus, however, appear to be especially sensitive to the effects of various stressors, perhaps in part due to their high expression of adrenal steroid receptors. Although the hippocampus may not be directly involved in the generation of a stress state, in the rat its more ventral regions contribute regulatory influences on hypothalamic-pituitary-adrenal (HPA) axis activity. Whether the primate hippocampus also has direct modulatory effects on the HPA axis remains to be determined.

See Also the Following Articles

Glucocorticoids – Adverse Effects on the Nervous System; Hippocampus, Corticosteroid Effects on; Hippocampus, Overview; Learning and Memory, Effects of Stress on; Memory and Stress; Neurogenesis; Steroid Hormone Receptors; Glucocorticoid Effects on Memory: the Positive and Negative.

Further Reading

Amaral, D. G. and Witter, M. P. (1989). The three-dimensional organization of the hippocampal formation: a review of anatomical data. *Neuroscience* 31, 571–591.
Andersen, P. (1975). Organization of hippocampal neurons and their interconnections. In: Isaacson, R. L. & Pribram, K. H. (eds.) *The hippocampus Vol. 1: Structure and development*. New York: Plenum Press.
Andersen, P., Bliss, T. V. P. and Skrede, K. (1971). Lamellar organization of hippocampal excitatory pathways. *Experimental Brain Research* 13, 222–238.
Bland, B. H. and Oddie, S. D. (2001). Theta band oscillation and synchrony in the hippocampal formation and associated structures: the case for its role in sensorimotor integration. *Behavioral Brain Research* 127, 119–136.
Bliss, T. V. and Lomo, T. (1973). Long-lasting potentiation of synaptic transmission in the dentate area of the anaesthetized rabbit following stimulation of the perforant path. *Journal of Physiology* (London) 232, 331–356.
Eichenbaum, H. and Otto, T. (1992). The hippocampus – what does it do? *Behavioral and Neural Biology* 57, 2–36.
Freund, T. F. and Buzsaki, G. (1996). Interneurons of the hippocampus. *Hippocampus* 6, 347–470.
Joels, M. (2001). Corticosteroid actions in the hippocampus. *Journal of Neuroendocrinology* 13, 657–669.
Gould, E., Woolley, C. S., Frankfurt, M., et al. (1990). Gondadal steroids regulate dendritic spine density in hippocampal pyramidal cells in adulthood. *Journal of Neuroscience* 10, 1286–1291.
Johnston, D. and Amaral, D. G. (2004). Hippocampus. In: Shepherd, G. M. (ed.) *The synaptic organization of the brain* (5th edn., pp. 455–498). Oxford: Oxford University Press.
Malenka, R. C. and Bear, M. F. (2004). LTP and LTD: an embarrassment of riches. *Neuron* 44, 5–21.
O'Keefe, J. and Nadel, L. (1978). *The hippocampus as a cognitive map*. Oxford: Oxford University Press.
O'Reilly, R. C. and Rudy, J. W. (2001). Conjunctive representations in learning and memory: principles of cortical and hippocampal function. *Psychological Review* 108, 311–345.
Ramón y Cajal, S. (1968). The structure of Ammon's horn. Original publication in Spanish, 1893. Kraft, L. M. (trans.). Springfield, IL: Charles C. Thomas.
Risold, P. Y. and Swanson, L. W. (1996). Structural evidence for functional domains in the rat hippocampus. *Science* 272, 1484–1486.
Squire, L. R. and Kandel, E. R. (2000). *Memory, from mind to molecules*. New York: Scientific American Library.
Swanson, L. W. (2004). *Brain maps: structure of the rat brain* (3rd edn.). Amsterdam: Elsevier Academic Press.
Witter, M. P. and Amaral, D. G. (2004). Hippocampal formation. In: Paxinos, G. (ed.) *The rat nervous system* (3rd edn., pp. 635–704). Amsterdam: Elsevier Academic Press.

Hippocampus, Corticosteroid Effects on

M Joëls and H Karst
University of Amsterdam, Amsterdam, Netherlands

This article is a revision of the previous edition article by M Joëls and H Karst, volume 2, pp 372–378, © 2000, Elsevier inc.

Mechanism of Corticosteroid Action

Targets for Corticosteroid Action

Changes in Network Properties

Cellular Effects after Chronic Hypo- or Hypercorticism

Glossary

Extracellular recording	A method for recording of electrical activity on the outside of neurons; often applied *in vivo* when recording the collective response of a group of neurons to the stimulation of afferents (i.e., the field response).
Hippocampal slice	A transversal slice of the hippocampal formation (~350 μm thick) kept alive *ex vivo*, in which the main synaptic pathways are still intact.
Intracellular recording	A method for recording of electrical activity in which the cell is impaled with a sharp electrode; generally used to record the potential or resistance over the entire membrane and changes thereof in the presence of neurotransmitters.
Ion currents	Ion fluxes over the neuronal membrane through specific ion channels. The activation of many of these channels depends on the membrane potential. In addition, some channels become inactive in a voltage-dependent manner.
Long-term potentiation (LTP)	Prolonged strengthening of synaptic contacts by patterned stimulation of afferent fibers; thought to play an important role in memory processes.
Long-term depression (LTD)	Prolonged weakening of synaptic contacts by patterned stimulation of afferent fibers; thought to play an important role in memory processes.
Neuro-transmitter response	Neurotransmitters change the electrical properties of neurons either through activation of ligand-gated ion channels or G-protein-coupled receptors, which, via the intermediate effects of G-proteins and/or second messengers, act on a specific type of ion channel. Electrophysiological methods record only the final change in electrical activity, (i.e., the neurotransmitter response).
Patch clamp recording	A method in which a very tight seal between an electrode and the cell membrane is established, allowing the recording of currents through single ion channels. If the membrane patch under the electrode is disrupted, the recording of potentials or currents over the whole cell is possible.

Corticosteroid hormones affect cellular and network properties in the hippocampus in a slow but persistent manner. The nature of the effects depends on the relative participation of mineralocorticoid and glucocorticoid receptors.

Mechanism of Corticosteroid Action

Corticosteroid hormones, which are secreted from the adrenal gland in particularly high amounts after stress, enter the brain and bind to specific receptors. Two main types of receptors have been recognized: the high-affinity mineralocorticoid receptor (MR) and the lower-affinity glucocorticoid receptor (GR). Both receptor types are expressed abundantly in the hippocampal formation. In fact, most principal neurons in the hippocampal subfields (**Figure 1a**) coexpress the two receptor types. This has raised the question of how the activation of the two corticosteroid receptor types affects cellular properties in the hippocampus. One of the premises of initial studies was that the activation of MRs may affect hippocampal cell properties in a different way than GR activation. This has proven to be correct.

For neurons that coexpress MRs and GRs, the relative participation of the two receptor types in cellular effects depends on several factors. First, the relative amounts of the two receptor types are important. Even within the hippocampus, the amounts vary among the different subfields. For instance, pyramidal neurons in the CA1 region and granule cells in the dentate gyrus (see **Figure 1a**) express high amounts of both MRs and GRs. Pyramidal neurons in the CA3 region, however, have relatively low amounts of the GR. Second, the affinity of the receptor for the natural ligand, in combination with the availability of the ligand, plays an important role. The bio-availability in the hippocampus is not only determined by adrenal release of corticosterone, but also by factors such as the passage over membranes in which p-glycoproteins play a major role as well as the presence of converting

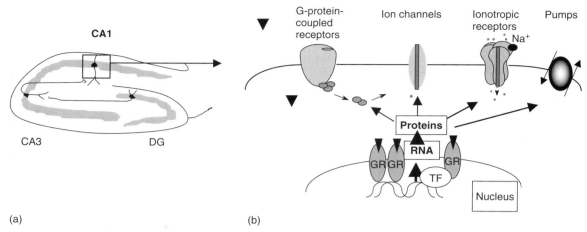

Figure 1 Corticosteroid effects on hippocampal cells. a, Representation of a hippocampal slice showing the main cellular subfields and the synaptic contacts between these subfields; b, Gene-mediated actions of corticosteroid hormones affecting the properties of hippocampal cells, aiming at various targets: ion channels, ionotropic receptors, G-protein-coupled receptors, and ion pumps. Intracellular corticosteroid receptors affect gene transcription either as homodimers binding directly to specific sequences in responsive genes or as monomers interacting with other transcription factors. CA1, cornus ammoni 1; CA3, cornus ammoni 3; DG, dentate gyrus; TF, transcription factor.

enzymes such as 11β-hydroxysteroid dehydrogenase. Low levels of the ligand activate MRs extensively due to their high affinity, whereas the lower-affinity GRs are only partly occupied. GRs are fully activated only when corticosteroid levels are very high. These two factors are not static entities but are prone to regulation, for example, during prolonged periods of exposure to stress.

Once corticosteroids are bound to their receptor, the steroid–receptor complex dissociates from attached proteins and translocates to the nuclear compartment. Rapid cellular effects of corticosteroids that are not gene-mediated have recently been described in hippocampus, but are not discussed here. Classically, it was thought that all gene-mediated corticosteroid actions, including those in the brain, involve binding of receptor homodimers to hormone response elements in the DNA (**Figure 1b**). Indeed, all functional effects studied so far in hippocampal cells appear to require DNA-binding of GR homodimers. However, molecular investigations – including microarray surveys in the hippocampus – indicate that effects can also take place via the interactions of steroid receptor monomers with other transcription factors. A third possible mode of action, via the heterodimerization of MR and GR molecules, has been suggested based on studies in transfected cells in which (among other things) protein–protein interactions were examined. It is still undecided whether MR–GR heterodimers play a major role in the development of corticosteroid actions in the hippocampus.

Over the past years, much more has become known about the genes that form a target for corticosteroid action in the hippocampus, as surveyed with serial

analysis of gene expression, microarrays, and single-cell RNA amplification of material from identified hippocampal cells. Thus, MR and GR activation each leads to altered expression of some 70–100 genes, of which roughly 50% was found to be upregulated and one-third were responsive to both receptor types. The hormone coordinates the expression of genes underlying aspects of energy metabolism, cell adhesion, synaptic transmission, oxidative stress, neurogenesis, cell cycle and structural plasticity. These transcriptional effects are likely to underlie cellular changes that have been observed, although the entire pathway has not yet been resolved for any of these. The functional data are in line with the molecular observations and indicate too that steroid-responsive genes may be involved in very diverse aspects of cellular function, such as cell structure and growth, energy metabolism, and membrane properties involved in signal transduction. Part of these cellular effects are summarized next.

Targets for Corticosteroid Action

Ion Channels

Under resting conditions, (passive) membrane properties of hippocampal CA1 and CA3 pyramidal cells are not affected by corticosteroid hormones. However, when the membrane potential of the cells is shifted from its resting level toward more depolarized or hyperpolarized levels (e.g., in response to a neurotransmitter), clear corticosteroid effects can be observed. These effects are generally slow in their onset and very persistent, which is in line with a gene-mediated mechanism of action. Patch clamp and intracellular studies have shown that some, although not all, of the ionic conductances in hippocampal cells are modulated by MR or GR activation. This underlines that the hormone actions are pleiotropic but nevertheless show a distinct degree of selectivity.

Three types of ion conductances have been investigated with regard to corticosteroid sensitivity: potassium (K^+), sodium (Na^+), and calcium (Ca^{2+}). Of these, voltage-dependent Ca^{2+} conductances are clearly most sensitive to corticosteroid receptor activation. It was found that low levels of corticosteroids resulting in a predominant MR activation are associated with small Ca^{2+} currents. If activation of GRs occurs in addition to MRs (e.g., after stress exposure) this results in an increased amplitude of Ca^{2+} currents compared to the situation in which mostly MRs are occupied. Several types of Ca^{2+} channels contribute to the overall Ca^{2+} currents in hippocampal cells. The steroids affect at least L-type Ca^{2+} channels, which cause the sustained current seen with large depolarizations of the cell, such as happen during an action potential. Only the amplitude of the currents and not the kinetic properties or voltage dependency is altered by corticosteroid treatment. Interestingly, in the absence of corticosterone, Ca^{2+} current amplitudes are also large, pointing to a U-shaped corticosteroid dose-dependency (see **Figure 2**). These data indicate that MR activation is necessary to retain Ca^{2+} currents within certain limits (a situation that is preferable for a neuron), whereas GR activation in addition to MR activation increases the Ca^{2+} influx into the hippocampal cells.

Steroid modulation of Ca^{2+} influx indirectly affects the slow Ca^{2+}-dependent K^+ conductance, which is extremely sensitive to the intracellular Ca^{2+} concentration. This conductance is slowly activated when neurons are depolarized for a considerable period of time (>100 ms) and causes accommodation of the firing frequency during depolarization; because the channels are also slowly deactivated, a lingering after-hyperpolarization (AHP) of the membrane is seen after the depolarizing influence is terminated. Both accommodation and AHP suppress the transmission of excitatory input to the hippocampal cells. In agreement with the small Ca^{2+} influx seen with predominant activation of MRs, it was found that accommodation and AHP under those conditions are relatively small, which promotes the transmission of excitatory input. With additional GR activation, accommodation and AHP are increased, leading to a temporary suppression of excitatory signals. Thus, hippocampal CA1 neurons in which mostly MRs are activated effectively transmit excitatory signals without being exposed to large intracellular Ca^{2+} levels. The large Ca^{2+} influx seen with additional

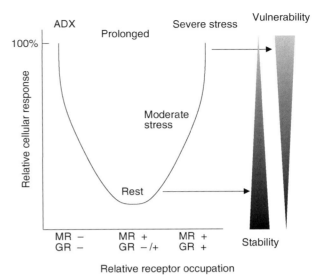

Figure 2 Many hippocampal cell properties, such as calcium currents, are large in the absence of adrenal steroids (adrenalectomy, ADX) or when both corticosteroid receptor types are extensively activated and are small with predominant MR activation. This results in a U-shaped corticosteroid dose-dependency, similar to what has been found for the potency to induce long-term depression versus long-term potentiation in the hippocampus. The relative MR and GR activation is indicated below the dose–response curve. Cellular responses associated with predominant MR occupation induce a situation of stability and resistance to degeneration. Additional GR activation (e.g., after a moderate stress) generally results in a temporary suppression of hippocampal cell activity, in agreement with the adaptive and normalizing role of this receptor in the stress response. The instability linked to GR activation can become deleterious when GR activation occurs concurrently with other challenging situations for the tissue, such as ischemia. Under these conditions, cellular vulnerability is increased if the relative GR to MR activation is high.

GR activation is normally restrained because Ca-dependent K^+ conductances prevent large-scale depolarization. However, when GR activation is associated with extensive depolarization of neurons, such as occurs during epileptic or ischemic insults, cells are at high risk of being exposed to very high Ca^{2+} levels. This may partly explain why hippocampal cells show a more profound loss of function and integrity after hypoxia-ischema or epileptic seizures when corticosteroid levels are persistently elevated.

The K^+ and Na^+ conductances that were investigated appeared to be far less sensitive to corticosteroid receptor activation. Relatively minor effects were observed on the properties of the inwardly rectifying K^+ conductance I_h and on the fast, tetrodoxin (TTX)-sensitive Na^+ conductance. Other K^+ conductances, such as the delayed rectifier or transient A current, showed no steroid dependency at all in the hippocampus. Although the effects on voltage-dependent Na^+ and K^+ conductances are thus relatively small, they could still result in an altered shape of the action potential.

Neurotransmitter Responses

Based on chemical structure, three classes of neurotransmitters are recognized that affect the cellular function of hippocampal cells: amino acids, biogenic amines, and neuropeptides. Of these, the responses to biogenic amines appear to be most sensitive to corticosteroid receptor activation. Corticosteroid effects on amino acid-mediated transmission seem to be diverse and only partly gene-mediated. Neuropeptide actions have largely not been investigated in this respect.

The responses to serotonin (5-hydroxytryptamine, 5-HT) are strongly modulated by corticosteroid receptor activation. Serotonin can bind to several types of receptors on CA1 pyramidal neurons, including the 5-HT$_{1A}$ receptor. The activation of this receptor leads, through G-protein-coupling, to the opening of K$^+$ channels, which results in a hyperpolarization of the membrane. With intracellular recording, it was found that the 5-HT$_{1A}$ receptor-mediated hyperpolarization is small under conditions of predominant MR activation. This may be due to a MR-dependent downregulation of 5-HT$_{1A}$ receptor mRNA expression, as was observed in the dentate gyrus and in some studies also in the CA1 region. The activation of GRs in addition to MRs (e.g., after exposure to a physical stressor) induces large 5-HT$_{1A}$ receptor-mediated responses. The molecular mechanism underlying these large responses is unclear because 5-HT$_{1A}$ receptor expression and binding are not increased after GR activation. Potential targets for steroid modulation downstream of the 5-HT$_{1A}$ receptor are probably also not modulated because steroid actions on the G-protein function or the K$^+$ channel opened by the G-proteins cannot explain the changes in 5-HT$_{1A}$ response. In addition to modulation of 5-HT$_{1A}$ receptor-mediated responses, corticosteroids also affect responses or expression of 5-HT$_4$ and 5-HT$_7$ receptors.

Depolarizing responses mediated via muscarinic acetylcholine receptors appear to have a similar steroid dependency. Because both serotoninergic and cholinergic responses are relatively large in the absence of corticosteroid hormones, there seems to be a U-shaped dose-dependency for the transmitter responses, as in the case of Ca^{2+} conductances (see **Figure 2**). This may signify the existence of a common denominator underlying all these steroid effects. It is possible that corticosteroid receptor activation results in the altered activity of kinases or phosphatases, which affect several membrane components in a comparable way through posttranslational modifications. This does not exclude the development of steroid actions aiming at specific genes. This is supported by the observation that responses to norepinephrine, mediated by β1-adrenoceptors, show an inverse linear steroid dose-dependency rather than the U-shape.

Whereas the steroid modulation of biogenic amine responses is slow in onset, persistent, and requires *de novo* protein synthesis, steroid effects on amino acid-mediated responses seem to have different features. This was mostly investigated by examining the steroid modulation of synaptically evoked responses in the CA1 hippocampal region. The stimulation of Schaffer/commissural fibers in this region leads to a subsequent activation of glutamatergic AMPA and NMDA receptors. It was found that the administration of very high amounts of corticosterone, resulting in concomitant MR and GR occupancy, suppresses field responses mediated by glutamate receptors. With these very high doses of corticosterone a rapid onset of effects is seen and the effects are very prominent when extracellular Ca^{2+} concentrations are high. Moreover, the steroid effects are particularly evident after the repeated stimulation of the afferent pathway. The data suggest that under these circumstances energy-dependent processes in the signal transduction and cellular integrity may be impaired. When glutamate transmission is recorded under more physiological conditions (i.e., comparable to the design used to study effects on ion currents and aminergic responses), a slow GR-mediated enhancement rather than impairment of the responsiveness to synaptic stimulation becomes apparent.

Inhibitory responses mediated by GABA$_A$ receptors are affected only by extreme (and probably physiologically not relevant) doses of corticosterone. GABA$_B$ receptor-mediated responses were found to be stable with predominant MR activation, but declined rapidly with repeated stimulation both in the absence of steroids and in the presence of very high amounts of corticosterone.

Changes in Network Properties

The corticosteroid effects on the properties of individual hippocampal cells or small groups of cells clearly alter the function of hippocampal networks in which these cells participate. In addition, corticosteroid hormones could change network properties that depend critically on the connections and associative contacts between cells in a network.

Examples of processes that depend both on the characteristics of individual hippocampal cells and on the connections between cells are LTP and LTD. The former refers to the situation in which the high-frequency stimulation of afferents results in a prolonged strengthening of synaptic contacts. The fact that LTP is induced rapidly in hippocampal subfields, persists for hours to days, and involves associativity of inputs has led to the hypothesis that LTP may be the neurobiological substrate for learning and memory, although a direct link is still disputed. Stimulating hippocampal pathways at a lower frequency can lead to LTD, the weakening of synaptic contacts. The processes of LTP and LTD each require specific intracellular signaling cascades, phosphorylation targets, and Ca^{2+} levels. In nonstressed animals, LTP can be induced easily with high-frequency stimulation, whereas homosynaptic LTD is relatively hard to obtain.

Many studies over the past decade have demonstrated that MR and GR activation largely affect the likelihood to evoke LTP and LTD. Both in the dentate gyrus and in the CA1 region, conditions that result in the near-complete activation of MRs and only partial activation of GRs are associated with a very efficient induction and maintenance of LTP. When GRs are activated extensively, it becomes hard to evoke LTP, whereas LTD induction is promoted. In the absence of corticosteroid hormones, LTP induction is also suppressed. The degree of potentiation therefore shows an inverted U-shaped steroid dose-dependency, which points to an underlying process that may be common to and perhaps evolve from the steroid actions on Ca^{2+} influx and responses to neurotransmitters such as serotonin.

These observations, generally obtained by administering exogenous corticosterone or selective agonists or antagonists for the corticosteroid receptors, can be extended to behaviorally relevant situations. Thus, several studies have shown that the exposure of animals to stressors that are unpredictable and out of the context of a learning experience suppresses the likelihood of inducing LTP and instead allows the induction of LTD. Even less extreme situations, such as the subjection of animals to a novel environment out of the context of a learning experience, led to a similar suppression of LTP and promotion of LTD. Stress effects on LTP and LTD are sometimes quite rapid in onset and not always associated with extensive changes in GR activation. This indicates that a shift in the likelihood of evoking LTP depends not only on the actual MR–GR occupation but also on other factors, such as the recent history of the postsynaptic cells, which may be influenced by other stress hormones as well, such as norepinephrine and corticotropin releasing hormone (CRH). In the intact organism, the effects of corticosteroids on synaptic plasticity are also determined by the degree to which multiple brain regions, such as the prefrontal cortex and amygdala nuclei, are involved, which in turn depends on the nature of the stressor.

Cellular Effects after Chronic Hypo- or Hypercorticism

The corticosteroid effects on cellular properties and network function described previously, are generally observed over a period of several hours after a change in MR/GR occupation. It is therefore very likely (and this has indeed been demonstrated in several cases) that these effects on hippocampal function take place shortly after exposure to an acute stressful situation. Increased corticosterone levels after stress, resulting in GR activation on top of already activated MRs, evokes an array of effects, most of which temporarily suppress the transmittal of excitatory signals (see **Table 1**). These GR-mediated events may help restore hippocampal function following stress, which is in accordance with the normalizing and adaptive mode by which GRs participate in the stress response.

Although large variations in MR activation probably do not take place under physiological conditions, data nevertheless show that MRs play an important role in hippocampal function. First, MRs seem to be important for the full development of GR-mediated events (and vice versa). Second, MR activation is essential for maintaining a basal level of hippocampal activity (see **Table 1**). And MR activation is even a prerequisite for neuronal viability. This is most evident in granule cells of the dentate gyrus. Dentate granule cells proliferate from progenitor cells even in adulthood and after some time die through apoptosis. There is a continuous balance between the incorporation of newly formed cells and the removal of old cells. When rats are adrenalectomized, this balance is disturbed, so that 3 or more days after adrenalectomy proliferation is increased but also more cells

Table 1 Cellular effects observed with predominant MR activation or with concurrent MR and GR activation[a]

	Excitability ↑	Excitability ↓
MR activation	Accommodation/AHP ↓	Carbachol responses ↓
	5-HT$_{1A}$ receptor response ↓	
	Glutamatergic response ↑	
	LTP ↑	
MR + GR activation	GABA$_B$ response ↓	Accommodation/AHP ↑
	Glutamate release (?)↑	5-HT$_{1A}$ receptor response ↑
	Carbachol responses ↑	β-Adrenergic response ↓
		Glutamate response ↓
		LTD ↑, LTP ↓

[a]AHP, after-hyperpolarization; GR, glucocorticoid receptor; LTD, long-term depression; LTP, long-term potentiation; MR, mineralocorticoid receptor.

undergo apoptosis. In adrenalectomized rats undergoing apoptosis, the synaptic transmission as well as the plasticity between the entorhinal cortex and the dentate gyrus is impaired. The functional impairment most likely occurs prior to and independent of the change in cell turnover and may in fact form a trigger for an overall synaptic reorganization in the dentate. The impaired synaptic function, as well as the changes in cell turnover, can be prevented by treating animals with MR ligands. The fate of an individual cell also appears to be determined by its specific gene expression pattern. The data indicate that relatively young dentate cells can increase the expression of proteins that will help them survive, whereas older cells fail to do so, explaining why destabilizing factors such as enhanced calcium influx or impaired synaptic communication, seen in the absence of corticosterone, can become deleterious. Collectively, normal MR function in the dentate gyrus seems to be important in preserving the delicate balance between viability and cell death.

Although prolonged deprivation of corticosteroids is a threat for dentate granule cell survival, chronic overexposure of the hippocampus to corticosteroid hormones is also potentially harmful. Exposure of rats to 3 weeks of restraint stress causes atrophy of apical dendrites in CA3 pyramidal neurons. Under these conditions, both the presynaptic nerve terminals and the postsynaptic spine density in the CA3 area are altered. Chronic stress also decreases proliferation in the dentate gyrus and in fact may slow down the entire cell cycle for a considerable period of time, possibly by changing the expression of endogenous factors involved in the cell cycle. In addition to (or perhaps related to) the morphological effects, other hippocampal properties are also altered after chronic stress. Glutamate transmission is enhanced both in the CA3 area and dentate gyrus. Conversely, LTP is markedly impaired in all hippocampal subareas. Interestingly, 5-HT_{1A} receptor-mediated responses become gradually attenuated after chronic stress or prolonged overexposure to corticosterone. This may be one explanation for the increased risk of mood disturbances after prolonged hypercortisolemia.

The mechanisms underlying the changes in hippocampal morphology and cell turnover after chronic stress exposure are largely unknown. The observed enhancement in glutamate transmission may be a causative factor, but clearly sequential regulation of many gene targets, including genes encoding for corticosteroid receptors and chaperones, enzymes, structural proteins, cell cycle factors, and growth factors, in concert determines the outcome of the process. Understanding this sequence of events will be one of the challenges for the future. It is already clear that the cellular actions induced by repeated overexposure to corticosterone are not a simple extrapolation of the effects seen after an acute rise in corticosteroid level. Also, in the hippocampus there is no evidence for steroid resistance – generally effects are strongest when chronic stress is combined with an acute rise in the level of corticosterone. Insight into these fundamental processes as well as the potential to intervene with pharmacological treatment (e.g., by applying antiglucocorticoids) will be essential for novel treatment strategies of stress-related disorders involving hippocampal dysfunction.

See Also the Following Articles

Corticosteroid Receptors; Hippocampal Neurons; Hippocampus, Overview; Neurogenesis.

Further Reading

Datson, N. A., van der Perk, J., de Kloet, E. R., et al. (2001). Identification of corticosteroid-responsive genes in rat hippocampus using serial analysis of gene expression. *European Journal of Neuroscience* **14**, 675–689.

De Kloet, E. R., Joëls, M. and Holsboer, F. (2005). Stress and the brain: from adaptation to disease. *Nature Reviews Neuroscience* **6**, 463–475.

Gould, E. and Tanapat, P. (1999). Stress and hippocampal neurogenesis. *Biological Psychiatry* **46**, 1472–1479.

Karst, H., Karten, Y. J., Reichardt, H. M., et al. (2000). Corticosteroid actions in hippocampus require DNA binding of glucocorticoid receptor homodimers. *Nature Neuroscience* **3**, 977–978.

Kim, J. J. and Diamond, D. M. (2002). The stressed hippocampus, synaptic plasticity and lost memories. *Nature Reviews Neuroscience* **3**, 453–462.

Kole, M. H., Swan, L. and Fuchs, E. (2002). The antidepressant tianeptine persistently modulates glutamate receptor currents of the hippocampal CA3 commissural associational synapse in chronically stressed rats. *European Journal of Neuroscience* **16**, 807–816.

Korz, V. and Frey, J. U. (2003). Stress-related modulation of hippocampal long-term potentiation in rats: involvement of adrenal steroid receptors. *Journal of Neuroscience* **23**, 7281–7287.

Maroun, M. and Richter-Levin, G. (2003). Exposure to acute stress blocks the induction of long-term potentiation of the amygdala-prefrontal cortex pathway *in vivo*. *Journal of Neuroscience* **23**, 4406–4409.

McEwen, B. S. (1999). Stress and hippocampal plasticity. *Annual Review of Neuroscience* **22**, 105–122.

Shakesby, A. C., Anwyl, R. and Rowan, M. J. (2002). Overcoming the effects of stress on synaptic plasticity in the intact hippocampus: rapid actions of serotonergic and antidepressant agents. *Journal of Neuroscience* **22**, 3638–3644.

Hippocampus, Overview

M J Meaney and S J Lupien
McGill University, Montreal, Quebec, Canada

This article is reproduced from the previous edition article by M J Meaney and S J Lupien, volume 2, pp 379–385, © 2000, Elsevier Inc.

Glossary

Feedback inhibition	A process whereby the end product of the system is able to inhibit the activity of higher order, stimulating events. In the case of the hypothalamic-pituitary-adrenal axis, the adrenal glucocorticoids inhibit corticotropin-releasing factor synthesis in hypothalamic neurons.
Plasticity	The ability of neurons to establish new contacts with other neurons through the formation of synaptic connections. The process can also refer to the strengthening of established connections.

Hippocampal Regulation of Hypothalamic-Pituitary-Adrenal (HPA) Activity

Under most conditions, the hypothalamic-pituitary-adrenal (HPA) axis lies under the dominion of specific releasing factors secreted by neurons located in paraventricular nucleus (PVN) of the hypothalamus, notably corticotropin-releasing factor (CRF) and arginine vasopressin (AVP). Neurons of the PVN project extensively to the portal capillary zone of the median eminence, furnishing a potent excitatory signal for the synthesis and release of adrenocorticotropic hormone (ACTH) from the anterior pituitary, and thus the means by which neural activity associated with the stressor is transduced into endocrine signals. Elevated ACTH levels, in turn, increase the synthesis and release of glucocorticoids from the adrenal (in primates the primary glucocorticoid is cortisol, whereas in rodents it takes the form of corticosterone).

The responsivity of the HPA axis to stress is in part determined by the ability of the glucocorticoids to regulate ACTH release (i.e., glucocorticoid negative feedback). Circulating glucocorticoids act on pituitary and specific brain regions to inhibit the synthesis and secretion of releasing factors from hypothalamic neurons and pituitary ACTH. In addition to pituitary and hypothalamic sites, there is now considerable evidence of the importance of the limbic system, the hippocampus, and the front cortex in the regulation of HPA activity.

Circulating glucocorticoids bind with high affinity to two corticosteroid receptor subtypes: the mineralocorticoid receptors (MRs) and the glucocorticoid receptors (GRs). Both receptor subtypes have been implicated in mediating glucocorticoid feedback effects. Interestingly, ligand-activated MRs and GRs act as a common DNA-binding site (the corticosteroid receptor response element), but the receptors differ in their ability to interact with intracellular proteins (i.e., protein–protein actions).

Lesions to the hippocampus in the rat or the primate result in elevated corticosterone levels under basal and poststress conditions, whereas glucocorticoid implants into the hippocampus normalize ACTH levels in adrenalectomized rats. Hippocampectomized animals show a reduced suppression of HPA activity following exogenous glucocorticoid administration. Finally, hippocampectomy results in increased CRH mRNA levels in the parvocellular region of the PVN (a region that contains neurons whose axons terminate in the median eminence and increased portal concentrations of ACTH secretagogues). The negative feedback effects of glucocorticoids at the level of the hippocampus appear to involve both corticosteroid receptor subtypes. Implants of RU28318, an antagonist selective for the mineralocorticoid sites, and/or RU38486, an antagonist selective for the glucocorticoid site, increase basal and poststress HPA activity (i.e., antagonize endogenous glucocorticoid negative feedback). Levels of GR occupancy in the hippocampus and hypothalamus are correlated negatively with portal concentrations of CRH and AVP. Finally, both MR and GR agonists with selective antagonists underscore the state-dependent influence of these receptors. MR antagonists implanted into the hippocampus elevate basal as well as stress-induced HPA activity, whereas GR antagonists affect stress-induced activity. In humans, both mineralocorticoid and GR antagonists have been found to increase plasma ACTH levels, and, as in the rat, the effects of MR and GR blockade depend on the time of day. These roles are consistent with corticosteroid receptor pharmacology, as modest basal steroid levels serve to occupy largely MRs. Dynamic variations in GR levels occur only under conditions of elevated steroid levels, such as with the circadian peak or during periods of stress.

Naturally occurring and experimentally induced variations in hippocampal corticosteroid receptor levels produce effects of HPA activity that are consistent with this formulation. In the rat, postnatal handling increases hippocampal GR but not MR expression, and the effect is largely unique to the hippocampus. Predictably, animals handled in early life show dampened stress-induced HPA activity as adults, whereas there is no effect on basal activity. Likewise, increased maternal licking/grooming during early life increases hippocampal GR expression, resulting in enhanced glucocorticoid negative feedback sensitivity, decreased hypothalamic CRF mRNA expression, and more modest HPA responses to stress. Lewis rats exhibit increased hippocampal MR levels and show lower basal and stress-induced activity in comparison to the parent Wistar strain. Thus, both MR and GR activation can potentially alter both basal and stress-induced HPA activity; under normal circumstances, the low corticosteroid levels prevailing under basal conditions selectively activate MRs. GR activation normally occurs during the peak in the circadian cycle or during periods of stress, and it is at this time that the GR influence on HPA activity is apparent.

Glucocorticoid Regulation of Hippocampal Activity

Glucocorticoids have been known for some time to regulate the excitability of hippocampal neurons, and more recent studies using models of long-term potentiation (LTP) have helped clarify the relevant mechanisms of action. LTP can be induced by the brief tetanic stimulation of glutaminergic afferents to either the CA1 or dentate gyrus region of the hippocampus and is defined by the enhanced synaptic response to subsequent stimulation. This LTP is thought to model the processes of synaptic plasticity that mediate learning. The magnitude of the hippocampal LTP response in the rat is decreased with adrenalectomy, and this effect is reversed with low levels of corticosterone replacement that affect largely MR occupancy. However, higher levels of corticosterone, which serve to occupy both MR and GR sites, reverse this effect, and with increasing GR activation, there is an even further suppression of LTP well beyond the effect of ADX, resulting in an inverted U-shaped relationship between circulating glucocorticoid levels and

hippocampal LTP. The mechanism underlying this effect involves the corticosteroid regulation of intracellular Ca concentrations. Following a prolonged sequence of stimulation, hippocampal neurons exhibit a slow, enduring afterhyperpolarization (AHP) that is mediated by a slow Ca-dependent K conductance, serving to decrease hippocampal excitability. Ca influx through voltage-gated channels, and thus the strength of AHP, is modest under conditions of MR occupancy and is increased substantially with the occupation of GRs. Elevated corticosterone levels increase mRNA levels for several Ca channels, whereas MR activation has the opposite effect.

There are also relevant corticosteroid effects on neurotransmitter systems. Glutaminergic transmission drives hippocampal LTP and is enhanced under conditions of MR activation and suppressed with increasing GR activation. Norepinephrine acts via cAMP-coupled β-adrenoreceptors to attenuate the magnitude of the AHP and thus enhance hippocampal excitability, an effect that is diminished under conditions of elevated corticosterone levels, which activate GRs. Serotonin (5-HT) acts via 5-HT1A receptors to produce a hyperpolarization and thus a decrease in hippocampal excitability. This effect is enhanced through GR activation. Finally, GR activation can also serve to metabolically compromise the function of hippocampal neurons through effects on glucose transport.

These findings are consistent with the idea that hippocampal excitability and LTP formation are facilitated under conditions of low basal corticosterone levels that result in MR activation. As corticosterone levels rise, such as under conditions of stress, there is greater GR activation, which serves to increase AHP, dampen glutaminergic transmission, attenuate noradrenergic facilitation of excitability, and increase serotonergic inhibition. Taken together, these findings are consistent with the inverted U relationship between circulating corticosterone levels and hippocampal LTP. Importantly, steroid pharmacology is also consistent with the findings that stress impairs hippocampal LTP formation.

Chronic Stress and Hippocampal Function

Exposure to chronically elevated glucocorticoid levels further compromises hippocampal function to the point of endangering neuronal integrity and survival. The story again focuses, at least in part, on corticosteroid effects on Ca homeostasis. Chronic stress in rodents and primates produces a reversible regression of apical dendrites. The effect is mimicked by high doses of corticosterone and is blocked by corticosterone synthesis inhibition or by Ca channel blockers. Interestingly, these effects parallel changes in the expression of a hippocampal-derived neurotrophic factor, brain-derived neurotrophic factor (BDNF). Chronic stress or chronically elevated corticosterone levels decrease BDNF mRNA expression as well as that for trkB, the BDNF receptor.

Elevated glucocorticoid levels compromise not only the maintenance of the existing synaptic form, but also synaptic sprouting. This finding is consistent with the GR-mediated effects on LTP, which appear to involve synaptic plasticity. Partial deafferentation in selected regions of the adult brain results in a sequence of compensatory events involving both the remaining afferent fibers and denervated dendrites, culminating in a reorganization of the circuitry in the denervated area. These events include sprouting of the remaining afferent fibers, restoration of spine density and length, and replacement of vacated synaptic contacts. One of the best examples of such reactive synaptogenesis occurs in the dentate gyrus of the hippocampus in animals following entorhinal cortex lesions. Entorhinal cortex lesions disrupt the perforant path, resulting in nearly 60% loss of synaptic input to the granule cells of the dentate gyrus. However, beginning as early as a few days after the lesion, new synapses are formed, and within 2 months virtually all the lost inputs are replaced. Following fimbria-fornix lesions, synaptic replacement occurs as a result of the growth of fibers from the adrenergic neurons in the superior cervical ganglion into the denervated region. In the case of entorhinal damage, the new synapses originate from the cholinergic cells of the medial septum, from glutaminergic commissural-associational pyramidal cells, and, to a lesser extent, from neurons of the contralateral entorhinal cortex.

Glucocorticoids suppress hippocampal sprouting in young animals in a dose-related manner. High glucocorticoid levels reduce hippocampal sprouting significantly following lesions of either the fimbria-fornix or the entorhinal cortex. This effect appears to be mediated by glucocorticoid effects on the expression of genes involved in synaptic repair, such as cellular receptor systems involved in cholesterol scavenging and microtubule-associated proteins.

The degree of glucocorticoid exposure appears to be a determinant of hippocampal pathology after neurological insult, as well as during the aging process. In humans, poststroke damage is correlated positively with circulating cortisol levels. In brief, Sapolsky's studies have shown that glucocorticoids endanger hippocampal neurons by (1) limiting the availability of energy substrates, thus rendering neurons metabolically compromised, and (2) increasing

extracellular glutamate concentrations by reducing glutamate uptake by glial cells. Both corticosteroid actions are GR mediated. These effects appear to be most apparent under conditions of insult associated with hyperexcitation and metabolic challenge. In contrast, MR activation appears to be neuroprotective under these same conditions.

Data from the laboratories of Sloviter and McEwen have illustrated another dimension to the corticosteroid regulation of neuronal survival in the hippocampus. In these studies, long-term adrenalectomized animals showed a profound decrease in neuron density in the dentate gyrus, a hippocampal subregion. In this case, the absence of glucocorticoid stimulation in adult animals resulted in neuron loss. Interestingly, the effects were observed uniquely in the granule cells of the dentate gyrus. Pyramidal cell density in Ammon's horn (CA1–CA4) was completely unaffected. In contrast, chronic exposure to elevated glucocorticoid levels results in the loss of pyramidal neurons in Ammon's horn, whereas the dentate is unaffected. Landfield's group reported that long-term adrenalectomized animals maintained under conditions of low corticosterone replacement showed no changes in neuron density in the dentate gyrus. The key here is the low level of corticosterone replacement. McEwen's group found that low levels of corticosterone or aldosterone replacement are sufficient to block the effects of adrenalectomy on neuron density in the dentate gyrus; both treatments selectively target the hippocampal MR. In contrast, Sapolsky's group showed that the loss of pyramidal neurons in Ammon's horn in the presence of elevated glucocorticoid levels is mediated by the GR. Thus, glucocorticoid potentiation of the neurotoxic effects of excitatory amino acids on hippocampal neurons is mimicked by RU28362, a GR agonist, and blocked by RU38486. In an interesting parallel, Meaney and Lupien showed that during the early postnatal period, an active period of hippocampal development, there are high, adult-like levels of MRs and very low levels of GRs. In essence, low levels of corticosteroid stimulation are necessary for the maintenance of hippocampal granule neurons, and chronically elevated glucocorticoid levels are hazardous for the integrity and survival of pyramidal neurons. The ideal state is one of tight titration around low basal glucocorticoid levels, an important argument for efficient glucocorticoid negative feedback.

Glucocorticoids and Hippocampal Function

Corticosteroid treatment has been known for some time to induce a reversible psychotic condition (so-called steroid psychosis) in certain individuals. This condition also includes logical thinking. A dementia-like syndrome (including attentional deficits and memory impairments) occurs frequently in a group of patients given high doses of corticosteroids for disorders not related to the central nervous system and who did not show evidence of psychosis. These findings are consistent with studies of Cushing's patients, in which cortisol levels are elevated profoundly. Cushing's patients consistently show attentional deficits and memory impairments, and the magnitude of the impairments correlates with plasma cortisol levels. Interestingly, the older subjects (>45 years) were affected more seriously; these subjects showed significantly greater memory impairments than younger subjects. Importantly, these deficits were reversible; surgical intervention to correct the hypercortisolemic state resulted in normalized cortisol levels and improved cognitive performance.

In addition, cognitive impairments, including attentional deficits and verbal and visual memory impairments, are often associated with clinical depression and are correlated with increased cortisol levels. Again, both the increase in plasma cortisol and the magnitude of the cognitive disturbances are more severe in elderly patients, often resulting in a condition of so-called pseudodementia. Importantly, in hypercortisolemic patients (especially dexamethasone-resistant patients) the cognitive disturbances are more pronounced. Results showed that subjects who received hydrocortisone treatment presented an impaired performance in the declarative memory task but not in the nondeclarative memory task, thus suggesting that cortisol interacts with hippocampal neurons to induce cognitive deficits. Another study reported comparable deficits in declarative memory in response to higher cortisol levels associated with major stress.

Depression is also associated with hippocampal atrophy, and is commonly associated with increased cerebrospinal levels of CRF and adrenal hypertrophy, suggesting a degree of glucocorticoid feedback insensitivity. Considering the evidence for hippocampal atrophy in this propulsion, it is tempting to speculate on the potential involvement of the hippocampus dysfunction as a source of this feedback insensitivity and the hypercorticoid state. The problem is that the hippocampus can be seen as both victim and villain in this conspiracy. It is both a source of feedback regulation over HPA activity and a primary target for elevated glucocorticoid levels. It also appears to be a target for therapeutic intervention. Antidepressant drugs increase hippocampal expression of both MR and GR, enhance glucocorticoid negative feedback sensitivity, and reduce hypothalamic CRF expression.

Among aged rats, increased hippocampal GR levels are associated with enhanced feedback inhibition of HPA activity and reduced evidence of hippocampal aging.

While the results of the clinical studies have been largely correlative, there is considerable evidence for the idea that the exogenous administration of corticosteroids impairs cognitive function. The oral administration of 10 mg of hydrocortisone leads to a significant decrease in memory performance as tested 60 min after hydrocortisone intake. In this study, declarative and nondeclarative memory performance was measured in order to assess the influence of corticosteroids on the hippocampal formation process. The logic for the inclusion of this amnesic dissociation is due to the fact that studies report that the hippocampus is essential for a specific kind of memory, notably declarative, while it is not essential for nondeclarative memory. Declarative memory refers to the conscious or voluntary recollection of previous information, whereas nondeclarative memory refers to the fact that experience changes the facility for the recollection of previous information without affording conscious access to it (priming). Thus, this somewhat specialized role of the hippocampus serves as the basis for specific hypotheses regarding the effects of acute administration of corticosteroids on human cognition. The results showed that subjects who received hydrocortisone treatment presented an impaired performance in the declarative memory task but not in the nondeclarative memory task, thus suggesting that cortisol interacts with hippocampal neurons to induce cognitive deficits.

Although most of the effects of exogenous administration of glucocorticoids on human psychophysical and cognitive processing have been found using hydrocortisone as a compound, some other studies have used other compounds and reached different conclusions. Poor performance (errors of commission; incorrectly identifying distractors as targets) on verbal memory tasks occurs in normal volunteers following the administration of prednisone (80 mg/day for 5 days). The general cognitive deficit described in this study involved the relative inability to discriminate previously presented relevant information (target) from irrelevant information (distractors) in a test of recognition memory. The authors concluded that exogenous administration of corticosteroids may diminish the encoding of meaningful stimuli and impair selective attention (i.e., reducing the ability to discriminate relevant from irrelevant information).

It appears that medium–high levels of circulating glucocorticoids may first affect the process of selective attention, thus impairing further explicit acquisition of information, whereas high–very high levels of circulating corticosteroids may affect explicit memory. This suggestion has been confirmed by a dose–response hydrocortisone infusion study in normal controls in which a 300 µg/kg/h infusion of hydrocortisone impaired selective attention capacity, whereas a 600 µg/kg/h infusion impaired both selective attention and explicit memory.

The results of these studies suggest that in humans, as in rodents, elevated glucocorticoids serve to compromise hippocampal function and promote cognitive impairments. This hypothesis was tested in a population of elderly, generally healthy human subjects in a study that examined cognitive function in relation to individual differences in HPA activity and hippocampal integrity. Basal cortisol levels were correlated inversely with impairments, including deficits in spatial learning and memory, and were associated with the degree of hippocampal loss. These findings are consistent with those using rodent populations. Prolonged exposure to elevated glucocorticoid levels can serve to compromise hippocampal integrity and certain forms of learning and memory. There is an impressive level of functional equivalence between the rodent and human model of hippocampal aging and the apparent role of corticosteroids in promotion degeneration.

Conclusions

The assumption drawn from earlier rodent studies is that all of this is entirely irreversible. However, more recent studies have emphasized the role of dendritic atrophy as a major component of the loss of hippocampal volume associated with a prolonged exposure to elevated corticosteroid levels. Neuron loss may be a more minor component of the earlier phases of hippocampal degeneration than was originally thought. Second, more recent studies have underscored the very dynamic effects of elevated circulating glucocorticoid levels on cognitive process, suggesting that attentional impairments that culminate in learning and memory deficits need not necessarily be seen as arising only under circumstances in which prolonged corticosteroid exposure has led to rampant structural damage. Rather, the processes by which glucocorticoids impair cognition can be dynamic.

The central question for human studies, then, is whether in at least some cases the functional impairments associated with elevated glucocorticoid exposure are reversible. Rodent studies suggest that stress-induced hippocampal atrophy is reversible. The critical question is whether it can be reversible in an elderly human population. As has so often been the case, the seminal experiment on this issue comes from the Landfield laboratory, which showed that the

effects of chronic stress on hippocampal function were more serious and enduring in older than in younger animals. It might well be that this scenario emerges from a conspiracy between the endangering effects of glucocorticoids against a background of aging, which involves a more limited level of trophic support and thus a decreased ability to repair the damage associated with the stressor. In our minds, the question of reversibility is critical.

See Also the Following Articles

Cushing's Syndrome, Medical Aspects; Cushing's Syndrome, Neuropsychiatric Aspects; Hippocampal Neurons; Hippocampus, Corticosteroid Effects on; Neurogenesis.

Further Reading

Bodnoff, S. R., Humphreys, A., Lehman, J., Diamond, D. M., Rose, G. M. and Meaney, M. J. (1995). Enduring effects of elevated glucocorticoid levels on spatial memory deficits, dampened long-term potentiation, and hippocampal neuron loss in mid-aged rats. *Journal of Neuroscience* **15**, 61–69.

Dallman, M. F., Akana, S. F., Bradbury, M. J., Strack, A. M., Hanson, E. S. and Scribner, K. A. (1994). Regulation of the hypothalamo-pituitary-adrenal axis during stress: feedback, facilitation and feeding. *Seminars in Neuroscience* **6**, 205.

de Kloet, E. R. (1991). Brain corticosteroid receptor balance and homeostatic control. *Frontiers in Neuroendocrinology* **12**, 95.

DeKosky, S., Scheff, S. and Cotman, C. (1984). Elevated corticosterone levels: A possible cause of reduced axon sprouting in aged animals. *Neuroendocrinology* **38**, 33.

Duman, R. S., Heninger, G. and Nestler, E. (1997). A molecular and cellular theory of depression. *Archives of General Psychiatry* **54**, 597–606.

Francis, D. and Meaney, M. J. (1999). Maternal care and the development of stress responses. *Current Opinion in Neurobiology* **9**, 128–134.

Issa, A., Gauthier, S. and Meaney, M. J. (1990). Hypothalamic-pituitary-adrenal activity in aged cognitively impaired and cognitively unimpaired aged rats. *Journal of Neuroscience* **10**, 3247.

Joels, M. and de Kloet, E. R. (1989). Effect of glucocorticoids and norepinephrine on excitability in the hippocampus. *Science* **245**, 1502.

Kerr, D. S., Campbell, L. W., Hao, S.-Y. and Landfield, P. W. (1989). Corticosteroid modulation of hippocampal potentials: Increased effect with aging. *Science* **245**, 1505.

Kirschbaum, C., Wolf, O. T., May, M., Wippich, W. and Hellhammer, D. H. (1996). Stress and drug-induced elevation of cortisol levels impair explicit memory in healthy adults. *Life Science* **58**, 1475.

Landfield, P., Baskin, R. K. and Pitler, T. A. (1981). Brain-aging correlates: Retardation by hormonal-pharmacological treatments. *Science* **214**, 581.

Lupien, S., DeLeon, M., DeSanti, S., et al. (1998). Longitudinal increase in cortisol during human aging predicts hippocampal atrophy and memory deficits. *Nature (Neuroscience)* **1**, 59–65.

Martgnoni, E., Costa, A., Sinforiani, E., et al. (1992). The brain as a target for adrenocortical steroids: cognitive implications. *Psychoneuroendocrinology* **17**, 343–354.

McEwen, B. S. (1999). Stress and hippocampal plasticity. *Annual Review of Neuroscience* **22**, 105–122.

Meaney, M. J., Aitken, D. H., Bhatnagar, S., van Berkel, C. and Sapolsky, R. M. (1988). Postnatal handling attenuates neuroendocrine, anatomical, and cognitive impairments related to the aged hippocampus. *Science* **239**, 766.

Newcomer, J. W., Craft, S., Hershey, T., Askins, K. and Bardgett, M. E. (1994). Glucocorticoid-induced impairment in declarative memory performance in adult humans. *Journal of Neuroscience* **14**, 2047.

Newcomer, J. W., Selke, G., Melson, A. K., et al. (1999). Decreased memory performance in healthy humans induced by stress-level cortisol treatment. *Archives of General Psychiatry* **56**, 527.

Poirer, J., May, P. C., Osterburg, H. H., Geddes, J., Cotman, C. and Fince, C. E. (1989). Selective alterations of RNA in rat hippocampus after entorhinal cortex lesioning. *Proceedings of the National Academy of Sciences USA* **87**, 303.

Reul, J. M. H. M. and deKloet, E. R. (1985). Two receptor systems for corticosterone in rat brain; microdistribution and differential occupation. *Endocrinology* **117**, 2505.

Roy-Byrne, P. P., Weingartner, H., Bierer, L. M., Thompson, K. and Post, R. M. (1986). Effortful and automatic cognitive processes in depression. *Archives of General Psychiatry* **43**, 265.

Rubinow, D., Post, R., Savard, R. and Gold, P. (1984). Cortisol hypersecretion and cognitive impairment in depression. *Archives of General Psychiatry* **41**, 279.

Sapolsky, R. M. (1992). *Stress, the aging brain, and the mechanisms of neuron death.* Cambridge, MA: MIT Press.

Sloviter, R., Valiquette, G., Abrams, G., Ronk, E., Sollas, P., Paul, L. and Neubort, F. (1989). Selective loss of hippocampal granule cells in the mature rat brain after adrenalectomy. *Science* **243**, 535.

Smith, M. A., Makino, S., Kvetnansky, R. and Post, R. M. (1995). Stress and glucocorticoids affect the expression of brain-derived neurotrophic factor and neurotrophin-mRNAs in the hippocampus. *Journal of Neuroscience* **15**, 1768–1777.

Starkman, M. N., Gebarski, S. S., Berent, S. and Schteingart, D. E. (1992). Hippocampal formation volume, memory dysfunction, and cortisol levels in patients with Cushing's syndrome. *Biological Psychiatry* **32**, 756.

Varney, N. R., Alexander, B. and MacIndoe, J. H. (1984). Reversible steroid dementia in patients without steroid psychosis. *American Journal of Psychiatry* **141**, 369.

Wolkowitz, O. M., Weingartner, H., Rubinow, D. R., et al. (1993). Steroid modulation of human memory: biochemical correlates. *Biological Psychiatry* **33**, 744.

Hiroshima Bombing, Stress Effects of

R J Lifton
Harvard Medical School and Cambridge Health Alliance, Cambridge MA, USA

Published by Elsevier Inc.

I was recently told that a prominent Zen Buddhist leader in this country has made a vow to himself that, in any conversation he enters into, he must bring up the subject of nuclear threat. That includes – so the story goes – the most casual social conversations, talks with taxi drivers, brief exchanges with strangers, whatever. The vow did not sound strange to me. Without being quite aware of it, I had, in effect, made a similar, if much more modest, vow to myself: that in any public statement I make on nuclear threat, I will bring up the subject of Hiroshima.

My strong impulse is to convey to everyone Hiroshima's indelible impact upon me. And I also have come to sense, as both psychiatrist and antinuclear activist, the special power of specific Hiroshima or Nagasaki images for those able to receive them. Images that extreme are best described in relatively quiet, understated tones that encourage reflection on our contemporary situation. The themes put forward in this article (originally from a chapter of mine in a book co-authored with Richard Falk, *Indefensible Weapons*) are meant to portray Hiroshima not as an event of the past, but as a source of necessary knowledge for the present and the future.

Those Hiroshima images continue their insistent claim on me: the searing details of survivors' experiences; the moving scenes, collective pain, and ultimate inadequacy of the 6 August day of commemoration; our own bittersweet family celebration, with a few Hiroshima friends, of our son's first birthday. Put most simply, the 6 months spent in Hiroshima in

1962 have formed in me a special constellation of truth that, when I am wise enough to draw upon it, informs everything I have to say about nuclear threat and much else.

I arrived in Hiroshima in the early spring of 1962. I intended no more than a brief visit. But very quickly I made a discovery that I found almost incomprehensible. It had been 17 years since the dropping of the first atomic weapon on an inhabited city – surely one of the tragic turning points in human history – and no one had studied the impact of that event. There had of course been research on the physical aftereffects of the bomb, and there had been brief commentaries here and there on the behavior of some of the survivors at the time of the bomb and afterward. But there had been no systematic examination of what had taken place in people's lives, of the psychological and social consequences of the bomb.

I came to a terrible, but I believe essentially accurate, rule of thumb: the more significant an event, the less likely it is to be studied. Again, there are reasons. One reason, certainly relevant to Hiroshima, has to do with the fear and pain the event arouses – the unacceptable images to which one must, as an investigator, expose oneself. To this anxiety and pain I can certainly attest.

But another source of avoidance is the threat posed to our traditional assumptions and conventional ways of going about our studies. We would rather avoid looking at events that, by their very nature, must change us and our relation to the world. We prefer to hold on to our presuppositions and habits of personal and professional function. And we may well sense that seriously studying such an event means being haunted by it from then on, taking on a lifelong burden of responsibility to it.

I was able to stay in Hiroshima and conduct interview research with people there over a 6-month period. The best way I know to describe a few of my findings that might be of use to us now is to look at the Hiroshima experience as taking place in four stages.

The first stage was the immersion in the sea of dead and near-dead at the time the bomb fell. This was the beginning of what I have called a permanent encounter with death. But it was not just death: it was grotesque and absurd death, which had no relationship to the life cycle as such. There was a sudden and absolute shift from normal existence to this overwhelming immersion in death.

Survivors recalled not only feeling that they themselves would soon die but experiencing the sense that *the whole world was dying*. For instance, a science professor who had been covered by falling debris and temporarily blinded remembered: "My body seemed all black. Everything seemed dark, dark all over.

Then I thought, 'The world is ending.'" And a Protestant minister, responding to scenes of mutilation and destruction he saw everywhere, told me: "The feeling I had was that everyone was dead. The whole city was destroyed. . . . I thought all of my family must be dead. It doesn't matter if I die. . . . I thought this was the end of Hiroshima, of Japan, of humankind." And a writer later recorded her impressions:

> I just could not understand why our surroundings changed so greatly in one instant. . . . I thought it must have been something which had nothing to do with the war, the collapse of the earth, which was said to take place at the end of the world, which I had read about as a child. . . . There was a fearful silence, which made me feel that all people . . . were dead. (Lifton, 1982 [1967] pp. 22–23.)

As psychiatrists, we are accustomed to look upon imagery of the end of the world as a symptom of mental illness, usually paranoid psychosis. But here it may be said that this imagery is a more or less appropriate response to an extraordinary external event.

In referring to themselves and others at the time, survivors described themselves as "walking ghosts", or, as one man said of himself: "I was not really alive." People were literally uncertain about whether they were dead or alive, which was why I came to call my study of the event *Death in Life* (1968).

Indicative of the nature of the event is the extraordinary disparity in estimates of the number of people killed by the bomb. These vary from less than 70, 000 to more than 250, 000, with the City of Hiroshima estimating 200, 000. These estimates depend on whom one counts and how one goes about counting, and can be subject at either end to various ideological and emotional influences. But the simple truth is that nobody really knows how many people have been killed by the Hiroshima bomb, and such was the confusion at the time that nobody will ever know.

The second stage was associated with what I call "invisible contamination". Within hours or days or weeks after the bomb fell, people – even some who had appeared to be untouched by the bomb – began to experience grotesque symptoms: severe diarrhea and weakness, ulceration of the mouth and gums with bleeding, bleeding from all of the body orifices and into the skin, high fever; extremely low white blood cell counts when these could be taken; and later, loss of scalp and body hair – the condition often following a progressive course until death. These were symptoms of acute radiation effects. People did not know that at the time, of course; and even surviving doctors thought it was some kind of strange epidemic. Ordinary people spoke of a mysterious "poison."

But the kind of terror experienced by survivors can be understood from the rumors that quickly spread among them. One rumor simply held that everyone in Hiroshima would be dead within a few months or a few years. The symbolic message here was: none can escape the poison; the epidemic is total – all shall die. But there was a second rumor, reported to me even more frequently and with greater emotion: the belief that trees, grass, and flowers would never again grow in Hiroshima; that from that day on, the city would be unable to sustain vegetation of any kind. The meaning here was that nature was drying up altogether. Life was being extinguished at its source – an ultimate form of desolation that not only encompassed human death but went beyond it.

These early symptoms were the first large-scale manifestation of the invisible contamination stemming from the atomic particles. The symptoms also gave rise to a special image in the minds of the people of Hiroshima – an image of a force that not only kills and destroys on a colossal scale but also leaves behind in the bodies of those exposed to it deadly influences that may emerge at any time and strike down their victims. That image has also made its way to the rest of us, however we have resisted it.

The third stage of Hiroshima survivors' encounter with death occurred not weeks or months but years after the bomb fell, with the discovery (beginning in 1948 and 1949) that various forms of leukemia were increasing in incidence among survivors sufficiently exposed to irradiation. That fatal malignancy of the blood-forming organs became the model for the relatively loose but highly significant term "A-bomb disease." Then, over decades, there have been increases in various forms of cancer – first thyroid cancer, and then cancer of the breast, lung, stomach, bone marrow, and other areas. Since the latent period for radiation-induced cancer can be quite long, and since for many forms it is still not known, the results are by no means in. Researchers are still learning about increases in different cancers, and the truth is that the incidence of virtually *any* form of cancer can be increased by exposure to radiation.

An additional array of harmful bodily influences have been either demonstrated, or are suspected, to be caused by radiation exposure – including impaired growth and development, premature aging, various blood diseases, endocrine and skin disorders, damage to the central nervous system, and a vague but persistently reported borderline condition of general weakness and debilitation. Again, the returns are not in. But on a chronic level of bodily concern, survivors have the feeling that the bomb can do anything, and that anything it does is likely to be fatal. Moreover,

there are endless situations in which neither survivors themselves nor the most astute physicians can say with any certainty where physical radiation effects end and psychological manifestations begin. There is always a "nagging doubt". For instance, I retain a vivid memory of a talk I had in Hiroshima with a distinguished physician who, despite injuries and radiation effects of his own, had at the time of the bomb courageously attempted to care for patients around him. He spoke in philosophical terms of the problem of radiation effects as one that "man cannot solve"; but when I asked him about general anxieties he smiled uneasily and spoke in a way that gave me the strong sense that a raw nerve had been exposed:

> Yes, of course, people are anxious. Take my own case. If I am shaving in the morning and I should happen to cut myself very slightly, I dab the blood with a piece of paper – and then, when I notice that it has stopped flowing, I think to myself, 'Well, I guess I am all right.' (Lifton, 1982[1967] p. 54).

Nor does the matter end with one's own body or life. There is the fear that this invisible contamination will manifest itself in the next generation, because it is scientifically known that such abnormalities *can* be caused by radiation. There is medical controversy here about whether genetic abnormalities have occurred: they have not been convincingly demonstrated in studies on comparative populations, but abnormalities in the chromosomes of exposed survivors have been demonstrated. People, of course, retain profound anxiety about the possibility of transmitting this deadly taint to subsequent generations. For instance, when I revisited Hiroshima in 1980, people said to me: "Well, maybe the next generation is okay after all, but what about the third generation?" The fact is that, scientifically speaking, no one can assure them with certainty that subsequent generations will not be affected. Again, nobody knows. So there is no end point for possible damage, or for anxiety.

No wonder, then, that a number of survivors told me that they considered the dropping of the bomb to be a "big experiment" by the United States. It was a new weapon; its effects were unknown; American authorities wanted to see what those effects would be. Unfortunately, there is more than a kernel of truth in that claim, at least in its suggestion of one among several motivations. More important for us now is the idea that any use of nuclear warheads would still be, in a related sense, "experimental."

The fourth stage of the Hiroshima experience is its culmination in a lifelong identification with the dead – so extreme in many cases as to cause survivors to feel "as if dead" and to take on what I spoke of as an "identity of the dead." Hiroshima and Nagasaki survivors became, in their own eyes as well as in those of others, a tainted group, one whose collective identity was formed around precisely the continuous death immersion and the invisible contamination I have been discussing. The identity can include what we may think of as paradoxical guilt – the tendency of survivors to berate themselves inwardly for having remained alive while others died, and for not having been able to do more to save others or to combat the general evil at the time of the bomb. In connection with the latter, the sense of "failed enactment" (Lifton, 1983 [1979] p. 174) can have little to do with what was possible at the time or with what one actually did or did not do.

More than that, survivors underwent what can be called a second victimization in the form of significant discrimination in two fundamental areas of life: marriage and work. The "logic" of the discrimination was the awareness of potential marriage partners (or families and go-betweens involved in making marriage arrangements) and prospective employers that survivors are susceptible to aftereffects of the bomb, making them poor bets for marriage (and healthy children) and employment. But the deeper, often unconscious feeling about atomic bomb survivors was that they were death-tainted, that they were reminders of a fearful event people did not want to be reminded of, that they were "carriers," so to speak, of the dreaded "A-bomb disease."

At the end of my study of these events, I spoke of Hiroshima, together with Nagasaki, as a last chance, a nuclear catastrophe from which one could still learn. The bombs had been dropped, there was an "end of the world" in ways I have described, yet the world still exists. And precisely in this end-of-the-world quality of Hiroshima lie both its threat and its potential wisdom.

Is Hiroshima, then, our text? Certainly as our *only* text, it would be quite inadequate. We know well that what happened there could not really represent what would happen to people if our contemporary nuclear warheads were used. When the Hiroshima and Nagasaki bombs were dropped, they were the only two functional atomic bombs in the world. Now there are approximately 50,000 nuclear warheads, most of them having many times – some a 100 or a 1000 or more times – the destructive and contaminating (through radiation) power of those first "tiny" bombs. While those early bombs initiated a revolution in killing power, we may speak of another subsequent technological revolution of even greater dimensions in its magnification of that killing power. The scale of Hiroshima was difficult enough

to grasp; now the scale is again so radically altered that holding literally to Hiroshima images misleads us in the direction of extreme understatement.

Yet despite all that, Hiroshima and Nagasaki hold out important nuclear-age truths for us. The first of these is the *totality of destruction*. It has been pointed out that Tokyo and Dresden were decimated no less than was Hiroshima. But in Hiroshima it was one plane, one bomb, one city destroyed. And the result of that single bomb was incalculable death and suffering.

A second Hiroshima truth for us is that of the weapon's *unending lethal influence*. Radiation effects were (and are) such that the experience has had no cutoff point. Survivors have the possibility of experiencing delayed but deadly radiation effects for the rest of their lives. That possibility extends to their children, to their children's children, indefinitely into the future – over how many generations no one knows. And we have seen how the physical and psychological blend in relation to these continuing effects.

A third truth, really derived from the other two, has to do with Hiroshima and Nagasaki survivors' identification of themselves as *victims of an ultimate weapon* – of a force that threatens to exterminate the species. This sense had considerable impact on Hiroshima survivors, sometimes creating in them an expectation of future nuclear destruction of all of humankind and most of the earth.

And there is still something more to be said about Hiroshima and Nagasaki regarding our perceptions of nuclear danger. The two cities convey to us a sense of *nuclear actuality*. The bombs were really used there. We can read, view, and, if we will allow ourselves, *feel* what happened to people in them. In the process we experience emotions such as awe, dread, and wonder (at the extent and nature of killing, maiming, and destruction) – emotions surely appropriate to our current nuclear threat. Such emotions can transform our intellectual and moral efforts against nuclear killing into a personal mission – one with profound ethical, spiritual, and sometimes religious overtones. Hiroshima, then, is indeed our text, even if in miniature.

The argument is sometimes extended to the point of claiming that this sense of nuclear actuality has prevented full-scale nuclear war; that, in the absence of the restraining influence of Hiroshima and Nagasaki, the United States and the Soviet Union would have by now embarked upon nuclear annihilation. The claim is difficult to evaluate; and while I feel some of its persuasiveness, I do not quite accept it. In any case, one must raise a countervailing argument having to do with another dimension of Hiroshima and Nagasaki's nuclear actuality: namely, the legitimation of a nation's using atomic bombs on human populations under certain conditions (in this case, wartime). Once a thing has been done, it is psychologically and in a sense morally easier for it to be done again. That legitimation can then combine with an argument minimizing the effects of the Hiroshima bomb: the claim that one has unfortunately heard more than once from American leaders that Hiroshima's having been rebuilt as a city is evidence that one can fight and recover from a limited nuclear war.

Here I may say that part of Hiroshima's value as a text is in its contrasts with our current situation. One crucial contrast has to do with the existence of an outside world to help. Hiroshima could slowly recover from the bomb because there were intact people who came in from the outside and brought healing energies to the city. Help was erratic and slow in arriving, but it did become available: from nearby areas (including a few medical teams); from Japanese returning from former overseas possessions; and, to some extent, from the American Occupation. The groups converging on Hiroshima in many cases contributed more to the recovery of the city as such than to that of individual survivors (physically, mentally, or economically). But they made possible the city's revitalization and repopulation.

In Hiroshima there was a total breakdown of the social and communal structure – of the web of institutions and arrangements necessary to the function of any human group. But because of the existence and intervention of an intact outside world, that social breakdown could be temporary.

Given the number and power of our current nuclear warheads, can one reasonably assume that there will be an intact outside world to help? I do not think so.

Like any powerful text, Hiroshima must be read, absorbed, and recreated by each generation searching for its own truths.

Further Reading

Lifton, R. J. (1982 [1967]). *Death in life: the survivors of Hiroshima.* New York: Basic Books.

Lifton, R. J. and Mitchell, G. (1995). *Hiroshima in America: fifty years of denial.* New York: Grosset/ Putnam Books.

Lifton R. J. and Falk, R. (1982). *Indefensible weapons: the political and psychological case against nuclearism.* New York: Basic Books.

Lifton, R. J. (1987). *The future of immortality and other essays for a nuclear age.* New York: Basic Books.

Lifton, R. J. (1983 [1979]). *The broken connection: on death and the continuity of life.* New York: Basic Books.

Lindqvist, S. (2001). *A history of bombing.* New York: The New Press.

HIV Infection/AIDS

B W Dixon
University of Pittsburgh School of Medicine and Allegheny County Health Department, Pittsburgh, PA, USA

This article is reproduced from the previous edition article by B W Dixon, volume 2, pp 386–389, © 2000, Elsevier Inc.

Stress Associated with Initial Testing for HIV
Stress Associated with the Presence of HIV Disease
Stress for Family and Friends of HIV-Infected Individuals
Stress for the Health-Care Team

Glossary

Acquired immuno-deficiency syndrome (AIDS)	A clinical state of severe immune compromise associated with HIV infection, characterized by opportunistic infections, malignant tumors (especially Kaposi sarcoma), or a CD4 lymphocyte count of less than 200.
CD4 cell	A specialized cell of the T portion of the immune system, also referred to as a helper T lymphocyte. This cell is responsible for maintaining immune competence and is one of the cells infected selectively with the HIV virus and destroyed as a consequence of viral replication. As the body's ability to

Human immunodeficiency virus (HIV)	replenish CD4 cells fails, the CD4 cell count number falls. This is one predictor of worsening disease. One of a group of RNA-containing retroviruses, a specific causative agent of AIDS. Similar but distinct retroviruses appear to be fairly widely disseminated in nature and are responsible for such diverse illnesses as feline leukemia, a simian AIDS-like illness, and, rarely in humans, a T-cell lymphoma.

Perhaps no disease in history – ancient or modern – has evoked such strong emotional and societal reaction as has HIV infection. Certainly the major infectious pandemics – plague of the Middle Ages, cholera of Victorian England, and influenza of 1918 – have had higher attack rates and greater mortality. Those diseases, however, were limited geographically and communication was primitive, so news of their occurrence was not disseminated readily. In contrast, HIV is of worldwide occurrence, and its end result, AIDS, which was first described in the early 1980s, was initially associated with a very high mortality rate. HIV infection in an asymptomatic state may persist for years and may respond well to newer treatments, resulting in a chronic rather than acutely fatal disease. Because, however, of the earlier picture of AIDS, many people still equate HIV infection with a rapidly progressive fatal disease. Those perceptions result in stress for the HIV-infected individual, for his or her family and friends, and for noninfected individuals who have no behaviors to put them at risk but who harbor unrealistic fears concerning the transmission of HIV. Although fear seems to be the biggest psychological stress associated with HIV, the reactions to fear are varied and include anxiety, guilt, anger and frustration, denial, and obsessive disorders. Whereas most individuals are able to handle their stress in an appropriate way, a number of people have psychological, psychosomatic, or physiological symptoms as a result of the stress associated with HIV.

Stress Associated with Initial Testing for HIV

Many emotional factors go into the decision to obtain a test for HIV. The need to acknowledge behaviors that participants have engaged in, either episodically or consistently, but with which they are uncomfortable, influences the decision. Fear of rejection by family and peers, should they be infected, appears to be important. Incomplete knowledge of the significance of a positive test for HIV antibodies and feelings of hopelessness at being able to deal with the

consequences, such as loss of future, loss of employment, isolation, and pain, have been reported. Fears of discrimination in housing, in the workplace, and in society are not uncommon. Proponents of anonymous testing point out that anonymous testing has a tendency to allay those fears. It is clear that some individuals, having mustered their courage to get a test, do not return for results. Some members of the health community who feel an obligation to ensure that individuals, particularly those who test positive, are counseled appropriately argue against anonymous testing. The role of anonymous testing in reducing stress is thus not clear.

Some home-based HIV antibody test kits have been marketed. They have a certain appeal to individuals who are concerned with privacy to a degree that they will not otherwise be tested. If the test is positive, however, individuals may not seek or may delay appropriate medical care and avoid the necessity of dealing with the stresses that result from a positive test or deal with them in inappropriate ways.

The test that is performed most commonly involves sequential testing, first by enzyme-linked immunosorbent assay (ELISA) fluorescent antibody testing and a confirmatory chromatographic (western blot) test. Although the ELISA test may be performed quite rapidly (results usually available within a matter of 24 h), the western blot test takes somewhat longer and, in most laboratories, is not run with great frequency. Because it is important to have a confirmatory western blot test in every presumptively positive ELISA test and because there may be a considerable delay between obtaining blood and receiving results, there is tremendous anxiety during the interval between obtaining blood and obtaining the results. Although some practitioners report negative ELISA test results within 24 h to reduce that anxiety, the consequence is that people who do not have their test returned in a short period of time assume (although it is not necessarily true) that their test is positive. For that reason, most testing centers have an interval of 5–7 days between obtaining blood and giving results to all individuals. At the initial encounter, it is important that the counselor or phlebotomist take extra precautions, particularly in individuals at risk for HIV, to explain the consequences of a positive test and to explain the testing procedure to reduce fears about being tested.

Stress Associated with the Presence of HIV Disease

Individuals newly diagnosed with HIV infection go through the entire spectrum of behaviors from denial to bargaining to acceptance, as occurs in many chronic and serious diseases. These reactions have been well documented by Kubler-Ross and are not covered here. The initial denial of infection may be a barrier to obtaining care because, on initially being told of the presence of HIV infection, many people do not hear or integrate further information at that session. Thus, many health practitioners bring patients back repeatedly over a short period of time and provide easy access to someone skilled in dealing with the emotional responses to a serious life-threatening disease. Many individuals rationalize that, although they are HIV infected, at least they do not have AIDS. This is a beneficial coping mechanism during early infection.

Soon after the detection of HIV infection, analyses of viral load and CD4 count are often obtained, and this information is used in predicting not only the course of the disease in an individual but also in arriving at a plan for therapeutic intervention. Individuals who have a normal CD4 count and low viral load, in most instances, progress very slowly over a period of years. This allows sufficient time to deal with the potential psychological issues that arise. Despite the best intentions of the practitioner, a small number of people have committed self-destructive acts, including suicide, on learning of HIV infection. It is important that practitioners be aware of these potential adverse affects and allow for continuing support. For individuals with more advanced disease who meet the case definition of AIDS and for people continuing to show deterioration of immune function, modern therapies have been able to reverse or at least stabilize the disease, and numerous authors have pointed out that a positive outlook is associated with longer survival and less frequent adverse consequences, including opportunistic infections.

Unfortunately, as the disease progresses, the HIV infection itself may be associated with symptoms that can be confused with psychosomatic illness. Paresthesia in the limbs, abdominal pain, dysphasia, and changes in mental outlook and functioning may all be a result of HIV infection, its therapy or secondary infections, or neoplastic disease. Similar symptoms, however, may result on a purely psychosomatic basis without any organic cause. The challenge to the practitioner is to discern which symptoms are organic and which are psychosomatic and to deal with them by appropriate intervention. Continuity of care from a multifaceted health-care team, including physicians, social workers, advocates, and individuals who are themselves HIV-infected, appears to be important in reducing the psychological stress associated with HIV.

Whereas the stress associated with HIV infection does not appear to vary with specific racial, ethnic, or behavioral factors, individuals who acquire this infection through intravenous drug use have a separate set of stressors because of the drug use. This must be dealt with, either prior to or concomitantly with the evaluation and treatment of the HIV infection, to maximize outcome. It is clear that treating individuals who remain active drug users with potent antiviral medications is, more often than not, fraught with failure and the development of antiviral-resistant organisms. A small but well-documented group of individuals have expressed anger at finding they are HIV-infected and have purposely tried to infect other members of society with HIV. An even larger group of individuals do not understand the infectiousness of a nonsymptomatic transmissible disease and continue to expose others by persistent risk-taking behavior. On learning that they have been the source of infection for a loved one – a sexual partner or other close societal member – they experience significant guilt.

In addition to the psychological and psychosomatic stresses exhibited by individuals who are HIV-infected, physiological changes occur as a result of HIV infection. It is well documented that stress factors of a nonspecific type have a depressant effect on the immune system and may hasten the onset of symptomatic HIV disease and reduce life expectancy. Diurnal and stress-related changes in CD4 cell count and immune function are well known. There seems to be general agreement that a fall in natural killer cell numbers and $CD8^+$ lymphocytes, both of which are present in high numbers with heightened immune activity, may occur in the presence of stress. Their mechanisms of falling are not clear but may be mediated by glucocorticoids and endorphins. A similar relationship of stress to the recurrence of herpes simplex viral infections is well described, hence the term cold sore or fever blister, the symptom that occurs when a concomitant stressful situation, including infection, causes the herpes virus to reactivate. Individuals addicted to crack or cocaine in any form, which seems to have a direct immuno-suppressive effect, have a shortened life expectancy.

Stress for Family and Friends of HIV-Infected Individuals

The stresses imposed on the families of people who are HIV-infected are enormous. In many instances, because of the behaviors that resulted in the individuals becoming HIV-infected (particularly sex with members of the same gender and drug use), adult individuals who have moved some distance from the family will return home when the diagnosis of HIV is made or when symptomatic AIDS occurs. The family is often unaware of the behaviors that resulted in the individuals becoming HIV-infected, and the family members are left with the consequences of dealing with or accepting behaviors with which they are not comfortable, as well as the grief from the potential fatal outcome of AIDS. Fears concerning acceptance by relatives, neighbors, and friends add to family stress.

In the case of parents, many are aged and unable to understand adult children and the behaviors that have led to HIV. The physical stress of moving individuals or caring for them when they become weakened from disease is physically and emotionally taxing. For many parents, dealing with the potential death of a child prior to their own demise is stressful, and they may require professional help. In areas where there is a high prevalence of HIV, children may be born HIV-infected as a result of pre- or perinatal transmission, and there are many well-documented instances of parents abandoning a child on learning that he or she is HIV-infected. This may add grief and guilt to the psychological stress of the family.

Stress for the Health-Care Team

As HIV infection becomes a much more chronic disease, a variety of stresses have become more apparent in the health-care team. The difficulties of dealing with a generally young population that is losing weight and becoming physically impaired and dependent have been severe. The short natural history of the infection in the past allowed people to cope with this deterioration in health. As the disease becomes chronic, health practitioners, particularly volunteers

and people who themselves may be at risk for HIV, have become increasingly frustrated with their inability to deal with the disease over the long term. In some instances, anger has replaced sympathy, leading to depression and other stress-related symptoms in the health-care team.

See Also the Following Articles

AIDS; Herpesviruses; Immune Suppression.

Further Reading

Antoni, M. H., August, S., LaPerriere, A., et al. (1990). Psychological and neuroendocrine measures related to functional immune changes in anticipation of HIV-1 serostatus notification. *Psychosomatic Medicine* **52**, 496–510.

Burack, J. H., Barrett, D. C., Stall, R. D., et al. (1993). Depressive symptoms and CD4 lymphocyte decline among HIV-infected men. *Journal of the American Medical Association* **270**, 2568–2573.

Glaser, R. and Kiecolt-Glaser, J. (1987). Stress-associated depression in cellular immunity: implications for acquired immune deficiency syndrome (AIDS). *Brain, Behavior, & Immunity* **1**, 107–112.

Hedge, B. (1991). Counselling the HIV-positive patient. *Practitioner* **235**, 436–438.

Kubler-Ross, E. (1970). *On death and dying*. New York: Macmillan.

Lyketsos, C. G., Hoover, D. R., Guccione, M., et al. (1993). Depressive symptoms as predictors of medical outcomes in HIV infection. *Journal of the American Medical Association* **270**, 2563–2569.

Holocaust Survivors, Experiences of

P Valent
Victoria, Australia

This article is a revision of the previous edition article by P Valent, volume 2, pp 396–398, © 2000, Elsevier Inc.

Cultural Background to Holocaust Experiences
Overview of Stress and Trauma Experiences in Different Traumatic Situations
Stress and Trauma Experiences on the Moral and Spiritual Levels
Mitigating Factors and the Truth

Glossary

Holocaust	The genocidal extermination of Jews during World War II.
Stressors	Noxious events that actually or potentially interfere with survival or the fulfillment of life's goals.
Survivor	A person who has lived through traumas, in this case the Holocaust.
Trauma	A state of irretrievable loss of a life promoting equilibrium.
Traumatic stressors	Situations that lead to trauma.

The experiences of the Holocaust have become a benchmark of suffering in stress and trauma situations. This was the result of the vast Nazi machinery of the day having directed all political, military, industrial, psychological, and bureaucratic resources to the unrelenting persecution and extinguishing of the culture, dignity, spirituality, and physical lives of all Jewish people. The extent and severity of the persecution resulted in every possible stress and trauma consequence occurring in large numbers and sharp relief, and, unlike in other genocides, they have been extensively recorded from both the perpetrators' and victims' standpoints. Further, the Holocaust has been a moral watershed that has not only tortured survivors but challenged our civilization. For all these reasons, the Holocaust is worth studying in its own right, in addition to being used as a source that can inform other traumatic situations.

The word experiences ambiguously subsumes events as well as subjective responses to them. This article concentrates on descriptions of stress and trauma inducing events (technically, stressors or traumatic stressors) of the Holocaust. (For the experiential consequences of the events, see **Holocaust, Stress Effects of.**) In what follows, first the cultural backdrop and the traumatic situations of the Holocaust are overviewed. Next, attacks on the morality and spirituality of the victims, including ultimate perversities and evil, are examined. Last, mitigating experiences are examined.

Cultural Background to Holocaust Experiences

The rise of Nazism ruptured an uneasy anti-Semitic equilibrium that had been present to varying degrees over the centuries in Europe, including Germany. The Nazis drew both on this anti-Semitism and on primitive tribal, religious, and ideological myths to demonize, dehumanize, and scapegoat Jews. Thus, Jews were portrayed variably as predatory monsters, subhuman parasites sucking German blood, and superhuman world conspirators.

To the Jews, many of whom had fought for their various countries, including Germany, and who were frequently at the forefront of local culture, the authorities' portrayals of them were an incredible betrayal. Persecution based on the false propaganda shattered their assumptions about a moral and just world. The total attacks on the deeper humanity and spiritual fiber of the victims made the physical attacks on their survival much harder to bear. The following two sections deal with the events that threatened physical and spiritual survival.

Overview of Stress and Trauma Experiences in Different Traumatic Situations

Wartime Situations

Some traumatic events, such as bombing and evacuation ahead of invading armies, were shared with the general population. Such events were felt to be far less noxious than the additional intentional sufferings for which Jews were earmarked.

The precursors to genocide were the following. In Germany and occupied territories, Jews had to display yellow stars on their clothes. Their identification cards indicated their Jewishness. Laws forbade their entry into public areas, segregated them in ghettoes, and appropriated their means of livelihood and property. Jewish children were not allowed to attend schools.

In Germany, Krystallnacht in November 1938 broke the taboo on violence and killing. At government instigation, Jewish synagogues and property were smashed and burned, and Jews were killed. According to the new model of justice, Jews were blamed and collectively fined for the events.

As genocidal plans were ever more intensely implemented, segregation, robbery, and killing were accelerated. In occupied countries, within hours of entering villages and towns, Jews were rounded up and killed by firing squads, burned in synagogues, or beaten to death. Alternately, they were slowly killed by starvation and disease in ghettoes.

Extermination camps with gas chambers and crematoria were established to increase the efficiency of killing great numbers of people. Entering such places was like entering hell. The only respite from being killed was temporary slavery, with harsh conditions and cruelty.

Some Jews escaped the Nazis to other countries in the early years. Others hid in forests, cellars, and holes. Some pretended to be non-Jews, which was called open hiding. The tension of hiding could be worse than being caught. Many were either caught or denounced and handed over.

Totality of attacks   It should be emphasized that these attacks on Jews were total, relentless, and without mercy. Because the criterion for punishment was having 25% or more Jewish genes, there was no way out, such as conversion. Neither the elderly nor children were spared anything. Indeed, children were a prime target as the carriers of future genes. One and a half million children (90%) in Nazi-occupied Europe were murdered.

For the Nazis, physical and genetic extinction were not enough. Schools, culture (e.g., anything written by Jews), and even cemeteries were destroyed. No evidence or memory of Jews was to survive.

Postwar

For those who survived the Holocaust, many postwar experiences were extremely stressful. Survivors had to come to terms with having lost most or all their relatives, friends, communities, property, and way of life. Dreams of reunion, taking up life where it had been disrupted, hopes that had sustained victims during their worst times, were now shattered. Worse, some local populations rejected returning Jews, withheld returning their property, expressed anti-Semitic views, and in some cases even killed the survivors.

In such circumstances, survivors had to hide their wounds and cope with the new survival challenges of oppression, political persecution, uprootings, and emigrations. The children who had survived had to cope with all these adult stressor events, as well as with their changed and stressed parents.

Stress and Trauma Experiences on the Moral and Spiritual Levels

In order to put the huge Nazi-inspired killing machine into action, it was essential to deprive Jews of human status. If they were deemed to not be human, then the principles of justice and law would not apply to them any more than they did to cattle or vermin and they could be killed without guilt like such animals. The Nazi machine therefore consciously used every means to first kill their victims' humanity in preparation for their physical killing.

Unrestricted and unabashed propaganda was used to portray the monstrous, parasitic, and demonic conspiracy nature of Jews. Their religion, culture, and values were attacked through constant lies. Personal humiliation and stripping of dignity were important conscious precedents and justifications to personal robbery, damage, and killing. Examples of public humiliations included cutting off old men's beards, public mocking, beating, and being made to perform menial tasks. Laws equated Jews with dogs. "No Jews or dogs allowed" signs appeared in public places. Jews were transported in cattle cars like cattle to their places of slaughter. Degradation during transportation was effected through lack of food and drink, forced lack of privacy, and having to excrete in crowded conditions. On arrival in the concentration camps, the dehumanization continued. Prisoners were herded by dogs and whips, were cursed and beaten, and were branded with numbers. Those not slaughtered immediately had all control taken away. They had to work like animals, had to obey trivial orders and routine on the pain of death, and had their most intimate human functions such as of ingestion and excretion governed by guards. Even their deaths were undignified. Prisoners were stripped naked, beaten, and herded into communal impersonal killing machines. In other words, in addition to the constant threats to their lives, Jews had to contend with forces that were meant to strip them of their humanity, identity, and everything they cherished and loved, their very spiritual and existential meanings. Their souls were attacked as much as their bodies.

Some attacks were particularly cruel and perverse. They included the forced separation of families. When attempts were made to keep family members together, such as when mothers chose to stay with their babies, this love was punished by killing both the mothers and children. Victims were forced to make perverse choices, sacrificing some in order for all not to be killed. For instance, communities were forced to give up their old and young so that all would not to be killed. Compounding this perversity, prisoners were forced to take part in the killing and the body-looting process. Worse, victims had to suppress their emotions in order to survive.

Thus, in addition to being the targets of physical sadism and abuse of unlimited power, victims were forced to shed civilized values, relinquish what they held dear, and even turn against what had made their lives meaningful. Mengele, who like the Angel of Death chose with a motion of his finger who was to live and who to die, became a symbol of the victims' powerlessness. The meaninglessness of the slaughter was highlighted by the banality of the industrialization and bureaucratization of the killing process, which used and parodied all the achievements of modern civilization, including the use of psychological knowledge to inure the killers to continuous killing.

Mitigating Factors and the Truth

In the midst of genocide, there was no lack of devotion and courage among Holocaust victims, who risked and helped one another whenever possible. Sometimes kindness and bravery were shown by outsiders at the risk of their lives. The truth of Holocaust experiences can often be absorbed against the background of survival, courage, and victory of goodness, as in Steven Spielberger's film *Schindler's List*. But the truth is that redemptive experiences were far outweighed by the suffering and pain, ineffectiveness of bystanders, meaningless deaths of millions, and long-term moral and existential wounds of the survivors.

See Also the Following Article

Holocaust, Stress Effects of.

Further Reading

Friedrich, O. (1982). *The kingdom of Auschwitz.* New York: HarperCollins.
Gilbert, M. (1986). *The Holocaust; the Jewish tragedy.* London: Collins.
Levi, P. (1987). *If this is a man.* London: Abacus.

Holocaust, Stress Effects of

P Valent
Melbourne, Australia

This article is a revision of the previous edition article by P Valent, volume 2, pp 390–395, © 2000, Elsevier Inc.

Stress Effects during the Holocaust
Stress Effects Soon after the Holocaust
Stress Effects over the Years
Stress Effects in Recent Times
Lessons and Challenges Regarding Stress Effects from the Holocaust

Glossary

Holocaust	The genocidal extermination of Jews during World War II.
Stress effects	Biological, psychological, and social responses to stressors; they can form the constituents of traumas and illnesses.
Stressors	Noxious events that actually or potentially threaten life and its fulfillment.
Survivor	A person who has lived through traumas, in this case, the Holocaust.
Trauma	A state of irretrievable loss of a life-promoting equilibrium.
Traumatic stressors	Stressors that lead to trauma.
Traumatic situations	Situations that often lead to trauma.

Just as the experiences of Holocaust survivors (see **Holocaust Survivors, Experiences of**) can serve as a benchmark for the stressor nature of Holocaust traumatic situations, so the range and depth of the consequent stress effects of Holocaust experiences can serve as a standard against which stress effects from other traumatic situations can be compared. Further, because Holocaust stress effects have been well documented for over 60 years, the progression of stress effects – biological, psychological, and social – can be examined over an individual's life cycle, as well as down the generations.

Stress Effects during the Holocaust

Adults

Although, understandably, not scientifically researched in an extensive manner, reports indicate a wide variety of biological, psychological, and social stress responses associated with roundups and deportation, segregation into ghettoes, concentration camps, and being in hiding.

Roundups and deportation During roundups and deportations, severe anxiety and reactive depressions were ubiquitous and were perceived as understandable rather than pathological. However, panic attacks, severe depressions, suicide attempts and completed suicides, and the new development of angina and hypertension in these situations, although still understandable, were indistinguishable from physical and psychiatric illnesses.

The sense in many of the neurotic and psychotic symptoms that also occurred can easily be discerned. For instance, agoraphobia developed in response to the danger of going outside. Hysterical symptoms to avoid deportation and paranoid delusions, such as of the gas man, are also quite understandable. The abeyance of prior neuroses and the development of new ones seemed to be dictated by survival needs.

Ghettoes and hiding Anecdotal evidence indicates that stress effects in ghettoes overlapped those of the roundups, deportations, and concentration camps. Hiding in some ways was more stressful than being caught because people had to cope with constant isolation in hostile circumstances and the fear of being caught could be worse than actually being caught.

Concentration camps On entering the camps, psychic shock (see **Disaster Syndrome**) was often described subjectively as apathy, exhaustion, and emotional blunting. When apathy and total exhaustion continued, they contributed to the 20–50% who just died without obvious disease soon after entering concentration camps. Older and middle-class people were more prone to such shock. Many of them also committed suicide.

In the psychiatric ward in the concentration camp Teresienstadt, all psychiatric diagnostic categories were reported to occur well above expected rates. The diagnoses included schizophrenia and manic-depression. Reports from other concentration camps also described not infrequent cases of depressions, phobias, paranoias (such as of being poisoned), hallucinations, and psychotic reactions. Most psychiatrically ill prisoners died or were shot if their behavior did not conform to strict rules. Some psychoneuroses and psychosomatic illnesses disappeared, and new ones appeared. In some cases, psychosomatic illnesses that went into abeyance during internment reappeared after liberation.

Most prisoners in concentration camps who were not actively murdered, succumbed to the just-as-lethal extermination process, which included starvation, cold, physical assaults, and disease. Physical symptoms such as stomach cramps, diarrhea, dizziness, and headaches due to a variety of diseases were frequent, although some may have been psychophysiological.

Coping and defenses Most people did what they could to help others and themselves. Mostly nothing could be done except to obey orders, resign oneself to circumstances, and maintain hope deep inside.

The most potent factor in survival was luck. But, in addition, to survive victims had to have a strong desire to live no matter what. Other factors that helped them to survive were the suppression of feelings, dissociation and detachment, and living in small stretches of time. Some were helped by intellectual curiosity, others by magical beliefs, humor, and art. Socially, younger people, those who paired to help one another, and those who had strong beliefs had better chances of survival. Religious beliefs helped some but hindered survival for others. However, hope was essential for everyone. The sudden loss of hope was deadening and could lead to a fast demise through infections such as typhus.

Children

Stressors were larger for children, and their responses to stress were frequently insufficient, especially among the youngest children. Children were often the first to succumb to starvation, cold, and disease,

and they had the highest mortality rates – 90% of Jewish children died in Nazi-occupied Europe. The surviving children's responses were shaped by their developmental phases.

Younger children The younger children's worlds fragmented easily. Stress effects frequently included somatic symptoms such as stomachaches, diarrhea and asthma and uncontained emotions and behavior. Younger children tended also to have relatively more vivid, concrete, and phantastic interpretations of events. For instance, human persecutors were admixed with images of monsters, and separations from parents were interpreted as punishment for being bad.

Older children The older children, especially those beyond the age of seven, experienced dread, fear, grief, despair, anger, and guilt akin to the adults. Their capacities and ingenuity sometimes saved adults.

Few children survived the concentration camps; however, in a relatively privileged part of Bergen-Belsen, children were noted to suffer night anxieties, enuresis, and phobias; to be irritable and aggressive; and to form gangs akin to civilian wayward youth.

Coping and defenses Especially when children felt themselves to be under their parents' protective shields, they could interpret the frightening events in part according to their normal developmental phases. For instance, they could see deportation as an adventure.

From about the age of four on, children's psychological defenses resembled increasingly those of adults in their abilities to dissociate and freeze their emotions and the meanings of events. In addition they had amazing capacities for obedience and discerning that life was at stake. For instance, they separated silently from their parents, were docile with strange caretakers, and kept silent when hidden, even when alone and in the dark for long periods. They assumed and lived out a series of false identities and arranged their psyches as desired.

Children also owed their survival to luck, an inner drive to live, suppressing feelings, and maintaining hope. The latter was often through a tenacious clinging to objects and memories representing loving parents. Being appealing, evoking caring impulses, and being plastic when making various adjustments also helped their survival.

Stress Effects Soon after the Holocaust

Adults

At liberation The joy of liberation was mitigated by continued physical debilitation, which in some cases led to death. Unfortunately, too, many died of eating food that their frail digestive systems could not handle.

Mental debility from camp life could continue after liberation. For instance, in Bergen-Belsen concentration camp, over 40 schizophrenic and several hysterical survivors maintained the psychiatric symptoms that had helped them to survive hunger, death, and torture during their incarceration. Many of the survivors continued to suffer dulled and blunted affect and decreased memory. Others developed reactive despair and paranoid delusions only after liberation.

Postwar Many postwar stressors were worse than the wartime ones. The reality of murdered families, empty communities, and hostile countrymen shattered the dreams that had kept survivors going. Many let go now and took ill. Some died. The rates for suicide and schizophrenic illnesses rose. Some became chronically depressed. Others developed psychosomatic pains, dizziness, and weight-gain problems, all of which often became chronic. Amenorrhea, dysmenorrhea, abortions, and premature babies were not infrequent.

Coping and defenses Most victims resumed their survivor modes. They cut off emotions and memories, labored for today, and hoped for the future. Many married quickly and had children. Many started to achieve financial security, imbued with new hopes in their children and new countries.

Children

Children also enjoyed their freedom, but came to despair when their parents did not materialize or had changed from those in their dreams. Others grieved at having to leave their foster families. Many children were now treated for tuberculosis and other neglected illnesses, and this could mean further separation from their parents. Many exhibited neurotic symptoms and nonsocial behaviors. On the whole, the children coped, like the adults, by suppressing their emotions and memories and by concentrating on establishing their school and social lives.

Stress Effects over the Years

Adults: The Survivor Syndrome

The wide-ranging and marked biological, psychological, and social effects of the Holocaust came to be recognized only slowly and reluctantly. Psychiatry had to invent diagnostic labels to designate the salient image of the shuffling corpse, and the pervasively psychologically scarred survivor with numerous symptoms. Survivor syndrome became the most commonly accepted label for these symptoms. Its features, described next, subsumed the many biological, psychological, and social symptoms and illnesses, which occurred in many fluctuating combinations and permutations.

Physical sequelae Research on ex-concentration camp prisoners (the same probably applies to other Holocaust survivors) found that they suffered excessive mortality and morbidity from a great variety of illnesses for decades compared to control populations. Illnesses included tuberculosis and other infections, cancer, hypertension, coronary heart disease, stomach ulcers, digestive disorders, hyperthyroidism, and accidents. Premature aging and arteriosclerosis were also noted.

Survivors also suffered excessive autonomic nervous system psychophysiological symptoms. Common sympathetic (fight-or-flight) symptoms were tension, muscle pains, and digestive and cardiovascular symptoms, parasympathetic symptoms included tiredness, dizziness, lassitude, and exhaustion. In addition survivors relived symptoms such as stomach cramps, diarrheas, and headaches along with other wartime memories or (in somatization) as symbolic substitutes for them. Finally, any of these symptoms could be used hypochondriacally to signal anxieties directly or indirectly related to Holocaust fears.

Psychosocial and psychiatric sequelae Psychosocial sequelae include mainly negative emotions, cognitions, defenses, psychiatric illnesses, and spiritual and existential dilemmas. They, in turn, affected relationships and worldviews.

• Emotions. Anxiety, fear, and terror were the most common emotions, followed by depression. The latter was often associated with suppressed grief and was often complicated by survivor guilt (see **Survivor Guilt**).

• Cognitions. Holocaust events could present as hypermnesias or amnesias. In the hypermnesias, the past events were relived vividly in dreams, nightmares, flashbacks, thoughts, and fantasies. The relived events might not be distinguished from the original ones. They could be especially set off by cues reminiscent of the initial Holocaust events; such cues could act as phobias, which survivors might avoid strenuously. The amnesias, on the other hand, were the consequences of avoidance and a variety of defenses such as dissociation, repression, regression, splitting, and projection. The tension between reliving and avoidance (the two main features of posttraumatic stress disorder, PTSD) was noted to lead to restlessness, decreased concentration, sleeplessness, memory disturbances, moodiness, emotional lability, irritability, and physiological lability.

• **Psychiatric sequelae.** As in the physical arena, Holocaust stresses led to a wide variety of psychiatric symptoms and illnesses. They could be present from early on or could develop after a latent period (even decades later). Most commonly, anxiety and depression intensified into a range of anxiety and depressive disorders, the latter again associated with unresolved mourning. Dissociative defenses were associated with dissociative symptoms such as depersonalization, projection, and displacement, with suspiciousness, persecutory delusions, nighttime hallucinations, schizophreniform psychoses, and schizophrenia. All of these constellations could emerge years later and usually had Holocaust-laden content.

• **Spiritual and existential sequelae.** Survivors were ubiquitously plagued with moral, identity, spiritual, and existential problems, often causing more distress than the physical and psychological problems. Survivor guilt torments included "Why am I alive, when my family/such good people died?" and "Why did I acquiesce to go left, when my mother was sent right to her death?" Other questions included "How could such injustices occur?" "Where was the world/God?" "What does it all mean?" "Who am I now?" and "What purpose can my life have now?" Survivors could become cynical, lacking confidence in the world and themselves, always ready for further wounds.

Coping and defenses Many survivors did well financially due to their single-minded efforts, and their wives helped in their businesses and ran spotless homes. These were scotomized areas of fulfillment because they were intermingled with insecurity.

Survivors achieved meaning by having children to defeat Hitler's genocide, bear witness, and execute missions of remembrance. Israel was the political answer to vulnerability. Many survivors found purpose by trying to prevent suffering in others. Thus, survivors provided more than their share of moral leadership, philanthropy and cultural accomplishments.

Children

Like their parents, child survivors also suffered excessive mortality and morbidity rates from all types of illnesses, including psychoses and suicides. Child survivors, unlike their parents, often could not remember the events that still plagued them. This was because of their young age at the time and the strong desire of adults that the children not remember. Thus,

they lived their unhappiness as a saturated solution of unacknowledged turmoil, out of which could crystallize clearer symptoms and illnesses. Child survivors coped, like their parents, by concentrating on survival, the future, their own children, and ameliorating suffering in the world.

Only in the 1980s, in their forties and fifties, were child survivors recognized, and they recognized themselves. They explored their identities and memories beyond the molds that had been arranged by others.

Second-Generation Holocaust Survivors

Instead of making sure that their post-Holocaust children's experiences were linked to a normal external world, Holocaust survivors often linked their children's experiences to the Holocaust that still dominated them. The children then became unconsciously attuned to their parents' Holocaust experiences. For instance, a child was spanked for hopping happily in the park because to the parent this was an affront to all the dead; this child grew up to be a sad adult, pervaded by death, without knowing why. Children also absorbed unconscious roles, such as substituting for dead parents and prior children.

Second-generation children often felt overburdened, overprotected, and frustrated with parents who did not recognize them, yet felt unable to be angry with their fragile parents who themselves craved care and understanding. The children developed both symptoms due to identifying with their parents and symptoms resulting from their own attachment problems and unintegrated identities. These children often copied their parents' means of coping, such as being devoted to their own children and being prominent in humanist and healing occupations.

Stress Effects in Recent Times

Adult Survivors

As Holocaust survivors reach the ends of their lives, it can be seen that the effects of stress and trauma are lifelong. Retirement, the illnesses of old age, diminished brain function, and helplessness can intensify memories, and, for instance, doctors and nurses may be experienced by survivors as Nazis whose injections kill the sick.

On the other hand, survivors enjoy seeing the generations flourish, and this can reconnect them with their pre-Holocaust memories. It is never too late to resolve guilt and integrate frozen meanings. For instance, many survivors have recently given testimonies to the Spielberg Shoah Foundation and have broken their silence with their children.

Child Survivors

Child survivors, having been recognized and having discovered their own identities, have emerged from hiding, which in a sense they had been in since the Holocaust. Although still suffering, some with increased symptoms like their parents, for many it is more important to retrieve their memories clearly, integrate their Holocaust traumas, and make meaning of their lives. To these retrieve memories, many have visited the places of their traumas and have broken the conspiracy of silence. Once they have regained their identity and memories, they trauma pains can be integrated and new meanings can be forged.

Child survivors have formed local, national, and international groups. They have also given testimonies and feel the special privilege and responsibilities associated with being the last witnesses of the Holocaust.

Second and Subsequent Generations

The integration of the Holocaust by second-generation children has been harder because their Holocaust-derived culture has been pervasive and ego-syntonic. Nevertheless, many have come to realize the sources of their problems and have attempted to resolve them with their parents, including going with them to the places of their suffering. Alternately, they have attempted to work out in psychotherapy who they were and why.

Lessons and Challenges Regarding Stress Effects from the Holocaust

If Holocaust stress and trauma effects are seen a kind of benchmark, what principles can be abstracted from them?

1. **Biopsychosocial nature of stress effects.** Holocaust stress effects indicate that a wide variety of biological, psychological, and social stress effects may occur in many combinations and are subsumed in a great variety of symptoms and illnesses.

2. **Diagnostic categories arising from stress effects.** This great variety of symptoms and illnesses challenges us to adopt a nonlinear model in which trauma is like the big bang at the center and the symptoms and illnesses freeze out at different points on different ripples emanating from such a center. Survivor syndrome and PTSD may then be conceptualized as generic entities that subsume stress-derived symptoms and illnesses.

3. **Multidimensional nature of stress effects.** In addition to the rippling of stresses and traumas into symptoms and illnesses, the Holocaust, especially, indicates that trauma disrupts the human dimension, including morality, meaning, spirituality, identity, and purpose. The Holocaust further alerts us that stress effects take place in individuals, families, communities, and nations; in children and adults; and across generations.

4. **Adaptive as well as maladaptive stress effects.** During the Holocaust, many responses were adaptive and later could be elaborated into adaptive concerns that benefited large sections of the population. This must be remembered but not idealized – the suffering far outweighed any beneficial results of the traumatic events.

In conclusion, the stress effects of the Holocaust are very varied, deep, and intense. The sense of the overwhelming nature of the effects and the despair about being able to do anything about them parallels our general avoidance of trauma and despair about being able to treat it. Yet the fear is excessive, and helpful recognition of even the greatest traumas can be very beneficial and rewarding to both survivors and to those in contact with them.

See Also the Following Articles

Concentration Camp Survivors; Disaster Syndrome; Holocaust Survivors, Experiences of; Survivor Guilt; War-Related Posttraumatic Stress Disorder, Treatment of.

Further Reading

Bergman, M. S. and Jucovy, M. E. (eds.) (1982). *Generations of the Holocaust.* New York: Columbia University Press.

Dwork, D. (1991). *Children with a star; Jewish youth in Nazi Europe.* New Haven, CT: Yale University Press.

Krell, R. and Sherman, M. I. (eds.) (1997). *Medical and psychological effects of concentration camps on Holocaust survivors; genocide: a critical bibliographic review.* New Brunswick, NJ, and London: Transaction Publishers.

Krystal, H. (ed.) (1968). *Massive psychic trauma.* New York: International Universities Press.

Marcus, P. and Rosenberg, A. (eds.) (1989). *Healing their wounds; psychotherapy with Holocaust survivors and their families.* New York: Praeger.

Niederland, W. G. (1968). Clinical observations on the "survivor syndrome." *International Journal of Psychoanalysis* 49, 313–315.

Valent, P. (1998). *From survival to fulfillment; a framework for the life-trauma dialectic.* Philadelphia: Brunner/Mazel.

Valent, P. (2002). *Child survivors of the Holocaust.* New York and London: Brunner-Routledge.

Homeostasis

B S McEwen
Rockefeller University, New York, NY, USA

This article is a revision of the previous edition article by B S McEwen, volume 2, pp 399–400, © 2000, Elsevier Inc.

Characteristics of Homeostatic Systems

Problems with the Concept of Homeostasis and Alternative Terminology

Glossary

Homeostasis	The ability of an organism to maintain the internal environment of the body within limits that allow it to survive; self-regulating processes that return critical systems of the body to a set point, or range of operation, consistent with survival of the organism.

Characteristics of Homeostatic Systems

Homeostasis is highly developed in warm-blooded animals living on land, which must maintain body temperature, fluid balance, blood pH, and oxygen tension within rather narrow limits while at the same time obtaining nutrition to provide the energy to maintain homeostasis. This is because maintaining homeostasis requires the expenditure of energy. Energy is used for locomotion as the animal seeks and consumes food and water, for maintaining body temperature via the controlled release of calories from the metabolism of food or fat stores, and for sustaining cell membrane function as it resorbs electrolytes in the kidney and intestine and maintains neutral blood pH.

Homeostasis also refers to the body's defensive mechanisms. These include protective reflexes against inhaling matter into the lungs, the vomiting reflex as a protection to expel toxic materials from the esophagus or stomach, the eye blink reflex, and the withdrawal response to hot or otherwise painful skin sensations. Also included is the defense against pathogens through innate and acquired immunity.

According to Cannon, "Bodily homeostasis . . . results in liberating those functions of the nervous systems that adapt the organism to new situations, from the necessity of paying routine attention to the management of the details of bare existence. Without homeostatic devices we should be in constant danger of disaster, unless we were always on the alert to correct voluntarily what normally is corrected automatically. With homeostatic devices, however, that keep essential body processes steady, we as individuals are free from such slavery – free to enter into agreeable relations with our fellows, free to enjoy beautiful things, to explore and understand the wonders of the world about us, to develop new ideas and interests, and to work and play, untrammeled by the anxieties concerning our bodily affairs."

The body has a considerable redundancy or margin of safety when it comes to many of these mechanisms. There are two kidneys and adrenal glands in case one fails, and the digestive tract is able to function adequately for food absorption even if intestinal length is shortened. Moreover, individuals are able to survive with one lung. And the cardiovascular system has a number of devices to maintain blood pressure after considerable blood loss. Finally, as Cannon notes, the body displays considerable resilience in the face of injury and after surgery to compensate for lost function.

Problems with the Concept of Homeostasis and Alternative Terminology

Yet there are paradoxes and problems with the notion of a set point that is always maintained. In discussing obesity, Cannon states, "What leads to the storage of fat in large amounts – sometimes in grotesquely large amounts – in some persons, and in slight amounts in others, is not well-understood." This and other aspects of pathophysiology, particularly in response to stress, has forced a reevaluation of the processes that reestablish homeostasis in the face of a challenge and that, under some circumstances, exacerbate disease (see **Allostasis and Allostatic Load**).

Another problem with homeostasis is that, taken literally, it is a rather static concept, akin to the notion of equilibrium in classical thermodynamics; in real life, an organism experiences changing set points around which it maintains stability over a finite period of time. Moreover, unlike the closed systems of classical thermodynamics, a living organism is an open system in which energy and matter flow in and out, with equilibrium being replaced by a steady state. Cannon recognized this and used the term steady state; he even suggested that homeodynamics might be a better term than homeostasis.

The same problem was also recognized by a number of other authors. Nicolaides introduced the term homeorheusis in 1977; here stasis is replaced by rheusis, meaning "something flowing." Mrozovsky introduced the term rheostasis in 1990, "a condition or state in which, at any one instant, homeostatic defenses are still present but over a span of time there is a change in the regulated level, or set point of a system." He considered this concept advantageous in explaining how organisms adjust to changing environments such as the seasons of the year by storing body fat or changing reproductive physiology, and he believed that rheostasis allows for the kinds of physiological plasticity that is involved in evolution.

See Also the Following Articles

Allostasis and Allostatic Load; Feedback Systems.

Further Reading

Cannon, W. B. (1929). Organization for physiological homeostasis. *Physiological Reviews* **9**, 399–431.
Cannon, W. B. (1939). *The wisdom of the body.* New York: W. W. Norton.
Mrosovsky, N. (1990). *Rheostasis: the physiology of change.* New York: Oxford University Press.
Nicolaides, S. (1977). Physiologie du comportement alimentaire. In: Meyer, P. (ed.) *Physiologie humaine,* pp. 908–922. Paris: Flammarion Medecine-Sciences.

Homosexuality, Stress and

J Drescher
New York, NY, USA

Heterosexism
Gender Beliefs and Gender Stress
Homophobia
Moral Condemnations of Homosexuality
Antigay Violence
The Stress of Being in the Closet

Glossary

Being in the closet	Psychological and behavioral activities intended to keep one's homosexuality a secret.
Coming out	Admitting one's homosexuality to oneself or revealing it to others.
Dissociation	A psychological mechanism that allows individuals to keep unwanted or anxiety-producing information out of their awareness.
External homophobia	The irrational fear and hatred that heterosexuals feel toward gay people.
Gay bashing	Physical violence directed at people because they are gay.
Gender beliefs	Cultural ideas about what constitutes the essential qualities of men and women.
Gender identity	An individual's psychological sense of being either a man or a woman.
Heterosexism	A belief system that naturalizes and idealizes heterosexuality and either dismisses or ignores a gay subjectivity.
Internal/ internalized homophobia	The self-loathing gay people feel for themselves.
Moral condemnations of homosexuality	Beliefs that regard homosexual acts as intrinsically harmful to the individual, to the individual's spirit, and to the social fabric.
Outing	The unwanted revelation of an individual's homosexuality to others by a third party.
Sexual orientation	A person's attraction to members of either the same sex (homosexual), the other sex (heterosexual), or to both sexes (bisexual).
Sodomy laws	Legislation that criminalizes homosexual behavior, ruled unconstitutional by the United States in 2003 by the Supreme Court.

Throughout the life cycle, gay, lesbian, and bisexual (GLB) individuals experience significant stressors that are a consequence of society's antihomosexual attitudes. Some of those attitudes and the stresses they engender are discussed here.

Heterosexism

Those with GLB identities are routinely stressed by cultural expectations that each individual have a heterosexual identity. This is known as heterosexism, a belief system that naturalizes and idealizes heterosexuality and either dismisses or ignores a gay subjectivity.

Heterosexism does not necessarily imply malice or ill will toward GLB individuals; idealizing oneself does not necessarily require denigrating those who are different. However, heterosexist ideology typically frames its antihomosexual arguments in terms of the normal, the natural, or the traditional. Such arguments, sometimes implicitly and at other times explicitly, tend to equate identities that are not conventionally heterosexual with immorality and can rationalize condemnations of same-sex feelings and behaviors. Heterosexist attitudes are pervasive in many cultures, and they inevitably place gay people in the awkward and often stressful position of either (1) keeping their homosexuality a secret (being in the closet) or (2) having to reveal they are gay (coming out) to disprove cultural myths and assumptions about homosexuality. The most dramatic example of this stressful dilemma can be seen in the U.S. military's Don't Ask, Don't Tell policy, under which either revealing oneself to be gay or being found out to be gay can lead to a discharge.

In Western culture, most books, plays, movies, and print and television ads contain naturalized depictions of heterosexuality. "Boy meets girl, boy loses girl, boy gets girl" are the common elements of a heterosexist script. Heterosexism renders gay lives so invisible that at the time of writing this chapter, there is enormous media attention and controversy over *Brokeback Mountain,* a film in which the two male leads fall in love. Many heterosexual people have openly stated either their reluctance or opposition to seeing two men kiss on the silver screen.

Common expressions of heterosexism include valuing heterosexual relationships above homosexual ones, unquestioned opposition to gay parenting regardless of a gay parent's actual qualities as a parent, and the belief that lesbians and gay men are unsuited to teach small children, to serve in government, or to practice medicine. Heterosexist assumptions lead to separating men and women from one another in locker rooms. Yet gay teenagers may be stressed by having to hide any possible arousal they may experience on seeing naked peers in the locker room's ostensibly asexual environment. Similarly, a heterosexist world may make it difficult for elderly gay couples to openly live together in either retirement communities or assisted living programs.

A decade ago, marriage was implicitly assumed to be a ritual reserved for heterosexual couples. As a result of lawsuits initiated by gay couples in the 1990s and following the 2003 decision to allow same-sex marriage in Massachusetts, many other states rewrote their constitutions to specifically state that marriage should only be between a man and a woman. The stated impetus for these constitutional changes is often termed the "defense of marriage." Yet laws ostensibly written to preserve heterosexual relations inevitably create stress for gay couples and their families. The U.S. General Accounting Office has computed over 1000 rights, privileges, and benefits accrued through marriage. Consequently, the heterosexist denial of legal marriage to long-term, committed gay couples adds to the latter's stress by denying them and their families basic needs, including clearly defined inheritance rights, pension benefits, survivor death benefits, custody rights in cases of divorce, and health benefits, just to name a few. A growing literature also indicates increased psychological resilience in those who marry; denying legal marriage to same-sex couples denies them marriage's psychological benefits as well.

Gender Beliefs and Gender Stress

Any discussion of antihomosexual stressors necessitates some discussion of both scientific and popular heterosexist beliefs about gender and sexuality. Modern sexology distinguishes a person's gender identity, or the sense that one is a man or a woman, from the person's sexual orientation, whether one is attracted to members of the same sex (homosexual), the other sex (heterosexual), or to both sexes (bisexual). However, the general culture uses conventional heterosexuality as an organizing frame of reference and frequently conflates the categories of gender identity and sexual orientation. These common but mistaken gender beliefs include the notion that an attraction to men is a female trait or that gay men feel and act like girls. Although such mundane gender beliefs can be stressful because they misrepresent GLB people, GLB individuals are not alone in having to contend with them. Gender beliefs also include ideas about the kind of shoes men should wear (construction boots rather than spike heels) and the kind of career a woman should choose (becoming a nurse rather than a doctor). In other words, gender beliefs are not confined to the realm of sexuality; they concern themselves with many aspects of day-to-day life.

Gender beliefs play an important role in the development of gender identity. One may be born with an anatomical gender, but one's psychological gender is a later acquisition that has both cognitive and affective elements. How one's gender identity actually develops is not precisely known, although empirical data suggest it is a long and complex process. Clinical work shows that a person's sense of being a man or a woman can involve processes that are entirely dependent on attitudes from the external environment over extended periods of time. Children must learn a psychological construct of gender that is based not solely on anatomy but also on myriad cultural and familial clues (e.g., boys like to play ball or girls are made of sugar and spice). Consequently, the meanings of, for example, aggression in girls or a lack of athletic interests in boys can be internalized along a family or cultural model that codes these attributes as gender-specific. From this developmental perspective, a gender identity can be thought of as the accretion of experiences or interactions with the external and internalized gender-coding environment. That is to say, a person's gender is an activity occurring in a relational matrix.

For children who grow up to be heterosexuals, conformity to conventional gender beliefs and norms can sometimes offer a sense of comfort. However, gender beliefs can be stressful to heterosexuals as well. Real men and real women are powerful cultural ideals against which all men and women may unfavorably compare themselves. However, GLB individuals must contend with the dissonance created by early same-sex attractions and their learned cultural beliefs about the relationship between homosexuality and gender. Consequently, in some children who grow up to be gay, their developing gender beliefs about the meanings of their homoerotic feelings may lead them to question their own gender identities.

Seen from this perspective, children who grow up to be gay may be gender stressed. This is a process that can occur over a protracted period of time as early homoerotic feelings become linked to other gender-nonconforming interests and as these children come to realize that they are failing to meet the cultural and social expectations of their assigned gender. This is commonly seen in gay men who were effeminate boys, often denigrated for being sissies. However, even gay men who were more conventionally masculine as children recall gender stresses in their attempts to integrate their same-sex feelings into a male identity. Sometimes gender stress can lead to gender confusion. Clinically, gender confusion can be expressed as "If I am attracted to boys, I must be like a girl." But it might also include responses such as "I am depraved," "I will be alone," or "I have sinned." These are common and stressful gender beliefs associated with transgressing gender boundaries.

Homophobia

George Weinberg is generally credited with coining the term homophobia. He defines external homophobia as the irrational fear and hatred that heterosexuals feel toward gay people and internal (or internalized) homophobia as the self-loathing gay people feel for themselves. Weinberg suggests several origins of homophobia: the religious motive, the secret fear of being homosexual, repressed envy, and the threat to values. In fact, plethysmographic studies demonstrate that in some men, homophobic attitudes may defend against unwanted homoerotic feelings.

Weinberg's early work has been followed by an ever-expanding literature devoted to studying intolerance of homosexuality. Other factors thought to contribute to homophobic attitudes include (1) rare contact with GLB people, (2) a lack of homosexual experiences of one's own, (3) perceiving that one's own community does not accept homosexuality, (4) living in communities where homosexuality is unacceptable, (5) being older, (6) being less educated, (7) identifying oneself as religious or as belonging to a conservative religion, (8) being less permissive about sexuality in general, and (9) expressing high levels of authoritarianism.

In 1954, the U.S. Supreme Court ruled in *Brown v. The Board of Education* that racial segregation was unconstitutional. In support of that decision, the justices cited the psychological literature of the time that demonstrated how stressful and harmful racism was to the self-esteem of black children. Just as one cannot grow up black in America without internalizing racism, one cannot grow up gay without internalizing homophobic and other antihomosexual attitudes. Self-hatred is extremely stressful. In the clinical setting, internalized homophobia can present as low self-esteem, difficulty in sustaining relationships, estrangement from one's family of origin, work difficulties, or self-medication with drugs or alcohol to reduce stress-induced anxieties.

Homophobia is often expressed in the association of male homosexuality with effeminacy. Sissies of all ages are regularly targets of homophobia. The low social status accorded to sissies leads some parents, fearful that their children will grow up to be gay, to seek professional treatment to change the behaviors of their effeminate sons. However, when mental health professionals and parents join the social chorus of derision, presumably for a child's own good, being labeled effeminate at an early age can entail great stress and suffering.

Although some gay men are effeminate, assuming that all gay men are effeminate falls under the rubric of stereotyping. In addition to disdain for effeminacy, homophobia can be expressed in other stereotypes, clichés, or caricatures of sexual identities. Common stereotypes of gay men describe them as being sexually promiscuous or compulsive, having a talent for the arts, being mama's boys, or lacking in courage. Common stereotypes of gay women label them as being man-haters, tomboys, overly aggressive, or physically unattractive. Both gay men and women have been stereotyped as sexual predators or being fated to lead single lives of loneliness. Clinical experience has demonstrated that it is extremely stressful for GLB individuals to have to constantly prove to heterosexual families, friends, employers, and co-religionists – and sometimes to themselves – that these are just stereotypes.

Moral Condemnations of Homosexuality

People who morally condemn homosexuality regard homosexual acts as intrinsically harmful to the individual, to the individual's spirit, and to the social fabric. Those who morally condemn same-sex activities believe that the tradition of philosophical, legal, and religious opposition to homosexuality is, in and of itself, sufficient reason to forbid the open expression of homosexuality in the modern world. Although critics of these condemnations attribute them to homophobia, antihomosexuality stemming from moral beliefs is often more complex. For example, religious and secular social conservatives who morally condemn homosexuality claim they do so out of love or concern for something else. In today's culture wars, such individuals and groups actively and vocally oppose gay and lesbian civil rights at the municipal, state, and federal level. Their political activities, which arise from their moral condemnations, are an ongoing source of stress for the GLB community.

The most severe forms of moral condemnation are embodied in laws that criminalize homosexual behavior, once referred to as sodomy laws. In the mid-twentieth century, homosexuality was illegal in all 50 states. By 2003, only 13 states still had such laws. Although rarely enforced, they were often a source of stress for GLB populations. Selective enforcement of sodomy laws allowed antihomosexual law enforcement communities to harass and discriminate against gay citizens. Furthermore, it was routinely argued in states with sodomy laws that gay couples, as potential criminals, should not be allowed to adopt their foster children. Obviously, criminalizing the sexual behaviors felt to be part of one's normal sexuality is extremely stressful to those so charged. In 2003, however, the U.S. Supreme Court ruled in the case of *Lawrence and Garner v. Texas* that all state sodomy laws were unconstitutional.

Moral condemnations of homosexuality hampered the early public health response to the AIDS epidemic and, in the process, added significantly to the losses and stress of the GLB community. Initially – and incorrectly – perceiving AIDS to be primarily a disease of gay men, public health systems were unprepared to talk frankly about either homosexuality or the kind of sexual practices that transmitted the virus. In 1987, 6 years after the initial cases were identified, President Reagan first mentioned the word "AIDS." Although teaching safe sex practices to sexually active individuals was important in slowing the spread of the epidemic, moral disapproval of homosexuality made federal funding of such educational efforts illegal. Even though most global AIDS cases have been transmitted heterosexually, many still argue, usually in a condemnatory way, that homosexuality causes AIDS rather than unsafe sexual practices that spread the virus. After experiencing thousands of preventable deaths, it is not unsurprising that many in today's GLB community feel their own government does not value their lives.

In their more subtle forms, moral condemnations of homosexuality include an attitude known as love the sinner, hate the sin. In earlier historical eras, religious authorities condemned sodomites to eternal damnation, to prison, and sometimes even physical torture. However, science and medicine's redefinition of homosexuality, as well as the growing number of openly gay and lesbian voices, had an enormous impact on religious attitudes. Consequently, religious groups were forced to integrate the accumulating scientific data regarding the presumptive etiologies and naturalness of homosexuality.

Today's religious authorities find themselves having to contend with the spiritual needs of a growing number of gay people, as well as those of their families. Some religious denominations (i.e., Episcopalians and the United Church of Christ) have adopted an accepting model of homosexuality and openly embrace lesbian and gay worshipers. Some denominations even admit openly gay men and women as priests, rabbis, and ministers. However, acceptance has not been the majority approach.

Many religious authorities have instead chosen to embrace the homosexual but not the homosexuality. Contrary to mainstream scientific findings, antihomosexual religious authorities believe one chooses to be a homosexual despite the prohibitions against it – "choice" being a charged word in moral debates about homosexuality. In recent years, antihomosexual groups have been publicizing so-called sexual conversion or reparative therapies intended to change homosexuals. Rather than excluding gay people, they invite them back into the religious fold if they change their ways. However, the overstated claims surrounding conversion therapies have generated much interpersonal stress in many religious GLB individuals, particularly when family members pressure them to undergo the process. The public relations effort promoting these treatments is worrisome because (1) their efficacy is questionable, (2) the etiological theories on which they are based are not supported by current scientific research, (3) the practitioners of these treatments incorrectly label homosexuality as a mental disorder, (4) there is sparse documentation of the cure rates and when the rates are documented they are quite low (27–35%), (5) long-term results are rarely validated, (6) there are an increasing number of anecdotal reports that these treatments may cause harm, and (7) the false hopes raised in offering such treatments often delay individuals or their family members from accepting them as gay. In fact, the American Psychiatric Association has issued a position statement asking ethical practitioners to refrain from such practices and to do no harm.

Religious beliefs that disapprove of homosexuality constitute substantive, ongoing stressors in the lives of gay people, particularly for those who had strict, fundamentalist, or orthodox religious upbringings. Because they may no longer be participating in religious activities, they are often estranged from their communities where family, social, and religious activities are deeply intertwined. The social isolation that ensues from gay people's fear of moral condemnation can also be stressful.

Antigay Violence

In 1990 the federal government passed a law ordering a study of hate crimes, including attacks on gay men and women, the first time a federal civil rights law covered sexual orientation. In one common presentation of gay-bashing, gangs of young men descend on neighborhoods where gay people meet. Armed with bats, clubs, or other weapons, they attack anyone they believe to be gay.

Since the much-publicized beating to death of Matthew Shepard in 1998, there has been increased awareness and documentation of antigay violence and gay-bashing incidents. Publicized cases have also led to the open articulation of previously unspoken cultural beliefs, for example, the belief that violence is an excusable response to an unwanted sexual advance from a gay man. Termed the "gay panic defense," no court has yet accepted it as justification for antigay violence. Its underlying rationale is that gay victims are responsible for provoking the violence against them. Others, however, argue that antigay violence is the inevitable outgrowth of unexamined and unstated beliefs implicit in homophobia, heterosexism, and moral condemnation. They argue that not everyone can distinguish the sinner from the sin and that those who marginalize homosexuality are either directly or indirectly responsible for the brutality against gay men and women.

Leaving the unanswered question of antigay violence's origins aside, most GLB people have legitimate concerns about it. Holding one's partners hand in public or a chaste kiss may provoke a physical attack.

Furthermore, antigay violence is believed to be an underreported phenomenon because its victims are often reluctant to come forward. Victims often blame themselves for being in the wrong place at the wrong time. Even gay people who have never been assaulted are sensitive to the ways in which members of the dominant culture, both in positions of authority or on its margins, can make threats and do as they please.

The Stress of Being in the Closet

In their developmental histories, gay men and lesbians often report periods of difficulty in acknowledging their homosexuality, both to themselves and to others. Children who grow up to be gay rarely receive family support in dealing with antihomosexual prejudices. On the contrary, beginning in childhood – and distinguishing them from racial and ethnic minorities – gay people are often subjected to the antihomosexual attitudes of their own families and communities. Consequently, gay men and lesbians may spend long periods of their lives unable to acknowledge their homosexuality, either to themselves or to others. Throughout childhood and the life cycle, even the suspicion of being gay can lead to teasing, ridicule, family censure, or even violence. Consequently, many gay people come to regard their homosexuality as an unpleasant fact they would rather not know about themselves, let alone admit to others; their homosexuality must be kept out of their awareness and separated from their public persona. The psychological means by which they accomplish this separation is called dissociation.

Dissociation, of course, is not limited to gay men and lesbians. Almost everyone is capable of pushing unwanted knowledge out of one's awareness. However, given some of the consequences of being openly gay – estrangement from family, loss of employment, loss of home, loss of child custody, loss of opportunity, loss of status and even blackmail – dissociation may seem a viable option for survival. Some closeted gay people can reflexively speak without revealing the gender of the person being discussed or without providing any gendered details of his or her personal life. Some closeted gay people marry and, on the surface, live their lives as if they were typical heterosexuals. Although some closeted gay men and women may not act on their homosexual feelings, others may develop secret sexual lives. In fact, through dissociation, a whole double life can be lived and yet never be acknowledged.

This psychological effort to solve one problem, however, creates others. It is stressful to continuously hide significant aspects of the self or to vigilantly separate aspects of the self from others. Constantly hiding creates difficulties in accurately assessing other people's perceptions of oneself as well as recognizing one's own strengths. Dissociation's impact on self-esteem can also make it difficult to feel one's actual accomplishments as reflections of one's own abilities. Hiding takes its toll, particularly because the psychological effort needed to maintain a double life often leads to errors in judgment that further add to one's stress. Maintaining a heterosexual identity while engaging in secret homosexual activity may inevitably lead a closeted individual into compromising situations.

Those who find this psychological split untenable may come out as either gay, lesbian, or bisexual. Coming out involves putting into words the feelings and ideas that previously had no acceptable form of open expression. Calling oneself gay or lesbian is an effort to reach some measure of self-acceptance. The process is not just about revealing oneself to others. It is a realization that previously unacceptable homosexual feelings or desires are actually part of one's self. Coming out is fraught with danger because of the social stigma attached to homosexuality due to antihomosexual attitudes in the culture. Given the difficulties associated with revealing a gay identity, it may seem a wonder that anyone comes out at all.

For some, coming out may be against their will, precipitated by an act of malice. In such cases of outing, a hidden homosexual identity is exposed by those seeking revenge, political advantage or financial gain. Fear of being outed is a major stressor in the lives of many closeted GLB individuals. However, those who come out of their own accord describe the experience positively, as "a switch being turned on," "coming home," or "discovering who I really am." For them, as stressful as it may be to come out, it may be even more stressful to stay in the closet.

Further Reading

Adams, H. E. (1996). Is homophobia associated with homosexual arousal? *Journal of Abnormal Psychology* 105(3), 440–445.

Cabaj, R. P. and Stein, T. S. (eds.) (1996). *Textbook of homosexuality and mental health*. Washington, DC: American Psychiatric Press.

Drescher, J. (1998). *Psychoanalytic therapy and the gay man*. Hillsdale, NJ: The Analytic Press.

Drescher, J., Stein, T. S. and Byne, W. (2005). Homosexuality, gay and lesbian identities, and homosexual behavior. In: Sadock, B. & Sadock, V. (eds.) *Kaplan and Sadock's comprehensive textbook of psychiatry* (8th edn., pp. 1936–1965). Baltimore, MD: Williams and Wilkins.

Drescher, J. and Zucker, K. J. (2006). *Ex-gay research: analyzing the Spitzer study and its relation to science, religion, politics, and culture*. New York: The Haworth Press.

Herek, G. (1984). Beyond homophobia: a social psychological perspective on the attitudes toward lesbians and gay men. *Journal of Homosexuality* 10, 1–21. (Reprinted in DeCecco J. (ed.) (1985). *Bashers, baiters & bigots: homophobia in American society*, pp. 1–21. New York: Harrington Park Press.)

Hoffman, L. G., Hevesi, A. G., Lynch, P. E., et al. (2000). Homophobia: analysis of a "permissible" prejudice; a public forum of the American Psychoanalytic Association and the American Psychoanalytic Foundation. *Journal of Gay & Lesbian Psychotherapy* 4(1), 5–53.

Kohlberg, L. (1966). A cognitive-developmental analysis of children's sex role concepts and attitudes. In: Maccoby, E. (ed.) *The development of sex differences*, pp. 82–172. Stanford, CA: Stanford University Press.

Shilts, R. (1987). *And the band played on: politics, people and the AIDS epidemic*. New York: St. Martin's Press.

Sullivan, A. (ed.) (1997). *Same-sex marriage: pro and con*. New York: Vintage Books.

Weinberg, G. (1972). *Society and the healthy homosexual*. New York: Anchor Books.

Hostility

L H Powell and K Williams
Rush University Medical Center, Chicago, IL, USA

This article is a revision of the previous edition
article by L H Powell, volume 2, pp 407–412,
© 2000, Elsevier Inc.

History of the Concept
Conceptualization
Assessment
Link to Physical Disease in Longitudinal Studies
Mechanisms of Association
Intervention

Glossary

Anger	An unpleasant emotion, ranging in intensity from irritation or annoyance to fury or rage, that is an emotional expression of hostility.
Cynicism	A component of hostility characterized by the belief that others are motivated by selfish concerns.
Hostile interactional style	A style of interaction characterized by the tendency to challenge, evade questions, and become easily irritated.
Hostility	A general cognitive personality trait including a devaluation of others' worth and motives, an expectation of wrong-doing in others, an oppositional approach to others, and a desire to see others harmed.
Mistrust	A component of hostility characterized by the belief that others are likely to be provoking and hurtful.
Type A behavior pattern	The early conceptualization of coronary-prone behavior that featured two key components: excessive time urgency and free-floating hostility.

History of the Concept

In the 1960s, the concept of the type A behavior pattern was introduced by cardiologists Meyer Friedman and Ray Rosenman to describe individuals who possessed excessive time urgency and free-floating hostility and who, by virtue of this behavior pattern, were believed to be coronary-prone. This conceptualization fostered hundreds of investigations in the 1970s and 1980s aimed at replicating early associations with coronary disease, refining its measurement, and understanding its physiological underpinnings.

In 1980, a classic paper was published by Williams and his colleagues that suggested that the hostility component of the type A behavior pattern was its toxic core (**Figure 1**). Angiography patients were divided by gender, type A behavior, and hostility, and these classifications were related to occlusive disease. For both males and females, hostility was a better predictor of $\geq 75\%$ occlusion than type A behavior. This seminal investigation was subsequently replicated in a large number of studies using a variety of subjects and study designs and resulted in a shift in thinking away from type A behavior toward hostility as a key coronary-prone behavior.

Conceptualization

Hostility is a negative attitude toward others consisting of enmity, denigration, and ill will. It is a stable personality trait with stability coefficients of 0.85 over 1 or 4 years, 0.67 over 5 years, and 0.40 over 24 years. Hostility appears to be a multidimensional trait with from two to four factor analyzed components. There is general agreement that the two key components are cynicism, or the belief that others are motivated by selfish concerns, and mistrust, or the belief that others are likely to be provoking and hurtful. Other components include such things as a hostile attributional style, which is the tendency to construe the actions of others as involving aggressive intent, and a hostile interactional style characterized by the tendency to challenge others, evade questions, and become easily irritated. Smith has argued for a transactional view of hostility, which includes aspects of both the person and the environment. When both hostility and social support are considered jointly, three distinct components emerge: (1) nonhostile and high socially supported healthy individuals, (2) highly hostile and low socially supported submissive individuals, and (3) highly hostile and high socially supported aggressive individuals.

Although hostility is often linked to the risk factors of anger and aggression, it is distinct from them in that it refers to a cognitive personality trait. Anger is an emotion that includes reactions ranging from mild irritation to intense anger and can be a transitory feeling state or an enduring predisposition. Aggression is a behavior defined as attacking or hurtful actions toward others, whether the harm is physical or verbal. Correlations among these characteristics are moderate, suggesting that they are related, but nonetheless distinct.

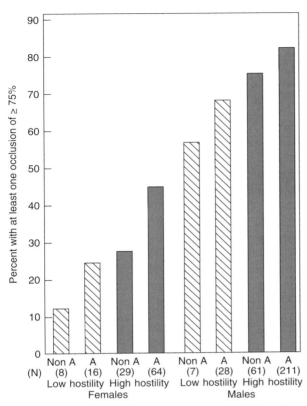

Figure 1 Relation of type A behavior pattern, hostility, and gender to presence of significant coronary occlusions. From Williams, R. B., et al. (1980). *Psychosomatic Medicine* **42**, 539–549, with permission.

Studies that have examined the sociodemographic correlates of hostility have found that it increases with age, is higher in men than in women, is higher in minorities than in Caucasians, and is higher in individuals of lower than in those of higher socioeconomic status. Moreover, there is consistent evidence that hostility is associated with smoking, elevated body mass index, and heavy alcohol consumption. Since these correlates are, in themselves, risk factors for disease, they can serve as confounders for any association between hostility and disease. Confounding in this case would be making the mistake that the true association is between hostility and coronary disease, when in fact the true association is actually between one or more of these established coronary risk factors (which are linked to hostility) and coronary disease. It is important to control for these potential confounders in the design or analysis of studies assessing the health impact of hostility.

Assessment

There are three popular assessment measures of hostility, all of which have subscales. Two of these are self-report questionnaires and the third is a behavioral rating. **Table 1** presents selected items from these scales.

The Cook-Medley Hostility Scale

The Cook-Medley Hostility Scale is a subscale of the Minnesota Multiphasic Personality Inventory

Table 1 Selected items from the most popular hostility assessment scales

SELF-REPORT QUESTIONNAIRES
Cook-Medley Hostility Scale: Mark each item as "true" or "false"

Cynicism	I think most people would lie to get ahead
	Most people are honest chiefly through fear of being caught
Mistrust/hostile attributions	It is safer to trust nobody
	I tend to be on guard with people who are somewhat more friendly than I had expected
Hostile affect	Some of my family have habits that bother and annoy me very much
Aggressive responding	I have at times had to be rough with people who were rude or annoying

Buss-Durkee Hostility Inventory: Mark each item as "true" or "false"

Expressed hostility	I lose my temper easily but get over it
	When people yell, I yell back
	I raise my voice when arguing
Experiential hostility	I don't seem to get what's coming to me (resentment)
	I know that people tend to talk about me behind my back (suspicion)
	My motto is "Never trust strangers" (mistrust)

BEHAVIORAL RATINGS
Interpersonal Hostility Assessment Technique: Behavioral ratings from a structured interview, based upon style of interaction

Direct challenges	Direct or explicit challenge of the question or the interviewer
Indirect challenges	Implication that the answer was obvious or the interviewer was stupid for having asked it
Hostile withholding or evasion	Avoidance or refusal to answer a question, associated hostile tone and intent not to answer
Irritation	Irritated tone, impatience, exasperation with the interview or interviewer, aroused reliving of negative events, condescension or snide remarks, harsh generalizations, punched words with angry emphasis

(MMPI) that is composed of 52 true–false items. Several factor analyses of this scale have produced slightly different solutions ranging from two to four factors. The two-factor solution includes the components of cynicism and mistrust/hostile attributions. The four-factor solution includes the components of cynicism, mistrust/hostile attributions, hostile affect, and aggressive responding. Studies of hostility as a risk factor have used the entire scale, the cynicism subscale, or the Abbreviated Cook-Medley (ACM) with the four subscales. The major limitation of the Cook-Medley scale is that it correlates consistently with depression and anxiety, characteristics that may be outside of the conceptual domain of hostility.

The Buss-Durkee Hostility Inventory

The Buss-Durkee Hostility Inventory is composed of 66 true–false items that are grouped into seven subscales: assault, indirect hostility, irritability, negativism, resentment, suspicion, and verbal hostility. In factor analytic studies, it has been consistently shown to assess two correlated dimensions, expressive hostility and experiential hostility. Expressive hostility assesses verbal and physical aggressiveness and is more highly correlated with antagonism than with neuroticism. Experiential hostility assesses the subjective experience of resentment, suspicion, mistrust, and irritation and is more highly correlated with neuroticism than with antagonism.

The Interpersonal Hostility Assessment Technique (IHAT)

The IHAT is an evolution of the structured interview for type A behavior in which the focus is on behavioral ratings of a hostile interpersonal style. It provides more objective criteria for assessing hostility than the subjective judgments that have characterized past interview ratings. Four types of hostile behaviors are rated from type A interview scripts, including direct challenges to the interviewer, indirect challenges to the interviewer, irritation, and hostile withholding of information or evasion. IHAT ratings have been correlated ($r = 0.32$) with potential for hostility ratings from the structured interview for type A behavior and have been shown to be stable over a 4-year period ($r = 0.69$).

Link to Physical Disease in Longitudinal Studies

Figure 2 summarizes the longitudinal studies that have examined a link between hostility and physical disease. Approximately half of all longitudinal studies have found the expected association.

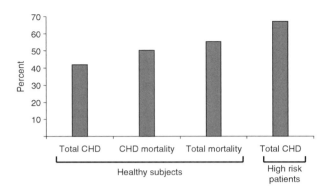

Figure 2 Percentage of prospective studies that have found a positive link between hostility and physical health.

Coronary Heart Disease in Healthy Subjects

To date there have been 12 longitudinal studies that have examined the role of hostility on the incidence of coronary heart disease (coronary mortality or myocardial infarction), six longitudinal studies that have examined the role of hostility on coronary heart disease (CHD) mortality, and two longitudinal studies that have examined the role of hostility on subclinical cardiovascular disease. Positive associations were found in five (41.7%) of the CHD studies, three (50%) of the CHD mortality studies, and two (100%) of the subclinical cardiovascular disease studies. Evidence exists that hostility is equally predictive in men and women, older and younger subjects, African American and Caucasian subjects, and the total scale and the abbreviated subscales.

Since hostility is embedded in a behavioral complex of other risk factors for coronary disease that includes lower education, higher body mass index, current smoking, and heavy alcohol consumption, these risk factors must be controlled for in multivariate analyses to avoid the problem of confounding. When the prospective studies that showed significant associations were examined for the adequacy of their control for these confounders, none of the studies controlled for all of these factors and most controlled only one or two of them. In one study, direct adjustment for these potential confounders eliminated a prior positive association. This suggests that any link between hostility and CHD may not be independent of standard risk factors but instead may be mediated by them.

Total Mortality in Healthy Subjects

There have been nine prospective studies of the link between hostility and total mortality. Of these, five (55.6%) found a positive association. The positive findings included both men and women and included both the total Cook-Medley scale and an abbreviated version. None of these studies controlled for education, and very few controlled for body mass index. Thus, the bulk of the evidence suggests that an association exists. It is not known, however, whether this association is independent of, or mediated by, established risk factors.

Coronary Heart Disease in High-Risk Subjects

There have been nine prospective studies of hostility and clinical CHD outcomes in patients with evidence of existing coronary disease. Of these, six (66.5%) found a positive association. These studies are characterized by inadequate control for confounding, with one exception. In a study of postmenopausal women with existing CHD from the Heart and Estrogen/Progestin Replacement Study (HERS) cohort, both the total Cook-Medley scale and the cynicism subscale predicted total CHD events after excellent controls for demographic and CHD risk factor confounders in multivariate analyses. Thus, the evidence is slightly stronger that an association, which is independent of the risk incurred by established risk factors, exists between hostility and CHD in high-risk patients than in their healthy counterparts.

Mechanisms of Association

There are three key mechanisms by which hostility may be associated with physical disease. The first is a direct mechanism whereby hostility triggers neuroendocrine pathogenic mechanisms for physical disease. The second is an indirect association whereby hostility fosters elevations in established risk factors and these risk factors increase risk for physical disease. The third suggests that hostility is embedded in a constellation of psychosocial risk factors, which together increase the psychosocial burden and, concomitantly, the risk of physical disease. Literature on potential mechanisms is growing rapidly, particularly evidence for a direct physiological link between hostility and disease.

Physiological

There is consistent evidence that hostility exerts a direct effect on CHD and total mortality through the mechanisms of amplified cardiovascular reactivity and neuroendocrine responses to stressors. Evidence exists for an association between hostility and such pathophysiological mechanisms as heart rate and blood pressure reactivity, increased platelet aggregation, vasoconstriction of atherosclerotic arteries, silent ischemia, decreased ejection fraction, decreased threshold for ventricular fibrillation, and decreased heart rate

variability. There also is evidence that hostility activates the sympathetic branch, and/or suppresses the parasympathetic branch, of the autonomic nervous system, mediated through epinephrine, norepinephrine, testosterone, and serotonin. Recent research suggests other possible physiological mechanisms involving the metabolic syndrome and inflammatory processes. Hostility has been associated with the metabolic syndrome of high levels of plasma lipids, insulin resistance, visceral body fat, and elevated blood pressure. Hostility has also been associated with inflammatory processes, specifically pro-inflammatory cytokines, tumor necrosis factor-α, and interleukin-6.

Health Behaviors

Evidence is accumulating that hostility is associated with smoking, heavy alcohol consumption, a sedentary lifestyle, obesity and overweight, elevated blood pressure, and lowered HDL cholesterol. Moreover, hostile individuals may be more likely to ignore health warnings and fail to comply with medical regimens. Two studies exist that have directly tested this model by examining the association between hostility and CHD before and after adjusting for established risk factors. One found that the association was maintained after adjustment; the other found that the association was eliminated. Thus, there is evidence from one study to support this mechanism.

Psychosocial Vulnerability

Hostile individuals not only may be hostile but also may have other psychosocial characteristics that have been observed to be coronary prone, including depression, anxiety, low social support, and/or general distress. Correlations between measures of hostility and these other psychosocial risk factors are between 0.25 and 0.30. Thus, it may not be the hostility alone but the overall adverse psychosocial risk factor profile that is associated with physical disease. For example, one study found that general distress was a better predictor than hostility of 6-month recurrence in patients with myocardial infarction. Another study found that although hostility is related to lower social support, when it is available, it provides fewer physiological benefits to hostile persons.

Intervention

Intervention for hostility can take one of two forms. Pharmacological interventions focus on blocking the impact of key physiological mechanisms on cardiac targets. Behavioral interventions focus on altering the cognitive, behavioral, and emotional concomitants of hostility as a way to reduce the frequency and intensity with which the physiological pathways are mobilized.

Pharmacological

β-adrenergic blocking drugs block the impact of increased sympathetic tone on the heart, triggered by hostility, and thereby reduce the hemodynamic response that may lead to plaque disruption. With this therapy, hostile individuals may construe the stressor as threatening, but the concomitant sympathetic arousal has little, if any, impact on heart rate or blood pressure. Aspirin has antiplatelet properties and thus may prevent sympathetically induced platelet aggregation that leads to thrombus formation. Estrogen therapy in women with existing coronary disease does not weaken the ability of hostility to predict recurrent coronary events.

Behavioral

Effective behavioral interventions for hostility must begin with the development of sensitivity to signs and symptoms of hostility in the individual him- or herself. This is a difficult task because hostility tends to be well rationalized, based upon real or perceived insults from the social environment. Interventions are most effective when they focus on the development of skills and competencies in all of the domains of hostility. Relaxation therapies help the individual to develop the skill to switch from sympathetic arousal to parasympathetic relaxation. Assertiveness training can help individuals to replace hostile interactional styles with less arousing and more effective alternatives. Cognitive therapy can help individuals to identify cognitions, such as blaming others, that are associated with arousal and to replace them with alternatives that are more rational and less arousing. The development of efficacy in controlling emotional arousal in response to environmental challenges has the effect of improving self-esteem, improving interpersonal effectiveness, and producing more positive feedback from the social environment. Progressively, as skills develop, the enhanced interpersonal effectiveness can challenge core cynical and mistrusting beliefs.

See Also the Following Articles

Aggression; Anger; Heart Disease/Attack; Type A Personality, Type B Personality.

Further Reading

Barefoot, J. C., Dodge, K. A., Peterson, B. L., Dahlstrom, W. G. and Williams, R. B., Jr. (1989). The Cook-Medley hostility scale: item content and ability to predict survival. *Psychosomatic Medicine* **51**, 46–57.

Buss, A. H. and Durkee, A. (1957). An inventory for assessing different kinds of hostility. *Journal of Consulting Psychology* **21**, 343–349.

Chaput, L. A., Adams, S. H., Simon, J. A., Blumenthal, R. S., Vittinghoff, E., Lin, F., et al. (2002). Hostility predicts recurrent events among postmenopausal women with coronary heart disease. *American Journal of Epidemiology* **156**, 1092–1099.

Cook, W. W. and Medley, D. M. (1954). Proposed hostility and pharisaic virtue scales for the MMPI. *Journal of Applied Psychology* **38**, 414–418.

Haney, T. L., Maynard, K. E., Houseworth, S. J., et al. (1996). Interpersonal hostility assessment technique: description and validation against the criterion of coronary artery disease. *Journal of Personal Assessment* **66**, 386–401.

McEwen, B. S. and Stellar, E. (1993). Stress and the individual. Mechanisms leading to disease. *Archives of Internal Medicine* **153**, 2093–2101.

Miller, T. Q., Smith, T. W., Turner, C. W., Guijarro, M. L. and Hallet, A. J. (1996). A meta-analytic review of research on hostility and physical health. *Psychiatric Bulletin* **119**, 322–348.

Siegman, A. W. and Smith, T. W. (1994). *Anger, hostility, and the heart*. Hillsdale, NJ: Lawrence Erlbaum.

Smith, T. W., Glazer, K., Ruiz, J. M. and Gallo, L. C. (2004). Hostility, anger, aggressiveness, and coronary heart disease: an interpersonal perspective on personality, emotion, and health. *Journal of Personality* **72**, 1217–1270.

Suarez, E. C. (2003). Joint effect of hostility and severity of depressive symptoms on plasma interleukin-6 concentration. *Psychosomatic Medicine* **65**, 523–527.

Suls, J. and Wan, C. K. (1993). The relationship between trait hostility and cardiovascular reactivity: a quantitative review and analysis. *Psychophysiology* **30**, 615–626.

Williams, R. and Williams, V. (1993). *Anger kills. Seventeen strategies for controlling the hostility that can harm your health*. New York: Times Books, Random House.

HPA Alterations in PTSD

R Yehuda
Mount Sinai School of Medicine, New York, NY, USA

Glossary

Hypothalamic-pituitary-adrenal (HPA) The HPA system is one of the major two neuroendocrine stress response systems of the body. Stress stimulates the release of the hypothalamic neurohormonal peptides, corticotropin releasing hormone and arginine vasopressin, that stimulate secretion of the pituitary adrenocorticotropic hormone (ACTH), which in turn stimulates the secretion of adrenal corticosteriods. In addition to its role in the stress response, the HPA system plays a role in and serves as a biomarker of mental disorders and especially depression and posttraumatic stress disorder (PTSD).

Introduction

The study of the neuroendocrinology of posttraumatic stress disorder (PTSD) has presented an interesting paradox – some of the alterations described have not historically been associated with pathological processes. In particular, initial observations of low cortisol levels in a disorder precipitated by extreme stress directly contradicted the emerging and popular formulation of hormonal responses to stress, the glucocorticoid cascade hypothesis, which posited that stress-related psychopathology involves hypercortisolism as either a cause or consequence of disorder. It is now clear that insufficient glucocorticoid signaling may produce detrimental consequences as robust as those associated with glucocorticoid toxicity.

With respect to PTSD, the majority of studies demonstrate alterations consistent with an enhanced negative feedback inhibition of cortisol on the pituitary and/or an overall hyperreactivity of other target tissues (adrenal gland and hypothalamus). Findings of low cortisol and increased reactivity of the pituitary in PTSD are also consistent with reduced adrenal output, although it is more difficult to fully explain cortisol elevations in response to stress and neuroendocrine challenge with this model.

Insofar as there have been discrepancies in the literature with regard to basal hormone levels, investigators more recently theorized that models of enhanced negative feedback, increased hypothalamic-pituitary-adrenal (HPA) reactivity, and reduced adrenal capacity may explain different facets of the neuroendocrinology of PTSD, including preexisting risk factors that may be related to certain types of early experiences, at least in certain people who develop PTSD. Notwithstanding that some aspects of HPA alterations may predate exposure to a traumatic event that precipitates PTSD, alterations associated with enhanced negative feedback inhibition also appear to develop over time in response to the complex biological demands of extreme trauma and its aftermath. Moreover, the findings of increased HPA reactivity may sometimes reflect a more nonspecific response to ongoing environmental challenges associated with having chronic PTSD. Certainly the absence of cortisol alterations in some studies imply that the alterations associated with low cortisol and enhanced negative feedback are present only in a biological subtype of PTSD. The observations in the aggregate, and the alternative models of pathology or adaptation suggested by them, must be clearly understood when using neuroendocrine data in PTSD to identify targets for drug development.

Basal Cortisol Levels in Posttraumatic Stress Disorder

The majority of the evidence supports the conclusion that cortisol levels in PTSD are different from those observed in acute and chronic stress and in major depression; that is, they are lower, rather than higher, compared to normal. However, it should be noted that there have been many reports that failed to observe low cortisol levels and (although fewer) that have reported cortisol increases in PTSD. This discrepancy may be due to the fact that basal alterations of cortisol in PTSD are subtle. That is, even when cortisol is reported to be significantly lower in PTSD, levels fall within the normal endocrinological range. There are numerous other sources of potential variability in such studies related to the selection of subjects and comparison groups, adequate sample size, and inclusion/exclusion criteria, as well as considerations that are specific to the methods of collecting and assaying cortisol levels, that can explain the discrepancies in the findings. However, the simplest explanation for the disparate observations is that cortisol levels may not represent stable trait markers and are likely to fluctuate, making it difficult to consistently observe group differences.

There is better agreement in studies of circadian rhymicity of cortisol in PTSD, although these are fewer in numbers. The advantage of these studies is that plasma samples can be obtained continuously throughout the 24-h cycle under controlled conditions. Thus, not only is it possible to confirm overall mean cortisol release but also to determine the times of day at which alterations are most likely to be present and note changes in circadian rhythm parameters. Indeed, it appears that the major difference between PTSD and non-PTSD groups is that cortisol levels are lower in the late night and remain lower for a longer period of time in PTSD during hours when subjects are normally sleeping.

Even in cases in which there is failure to find group differences in cortisol levels, there are often correlations within the PTSD group with indices of PTSD symptom severity or trauma exposure. Most often, investigators have reported negative correlations between cortisol levels (particularly integrated mean 24-h cortisol levels) and PTSD symptoms in combat veterans. Low cortisol levels have also been negatively correlated with duration since trauma, implying that low cortisol is associated with early traumatization. In fact, in some recent studies, cortisol levels were inversely related to childhood traumatic experiences, including emotional abuse, even in the absence of PTSD.

Cortisol levels have also been correlated with findings from brain imaging studies in PTSD. In one report, there was a positive relationship between cortisol levels and hippocampal acetylaspartate (NAA), a marker of cell atrophy presumed to reflect changes in neuronal density or metabolism, in subjects with PTSD, suggesting that, rather than having neurotoxic effects, cortisol levels in PTSD may have a trophic effect on the hippocampus. Similarly, cortisol levels in PTSD were negatively correlated with medial temporal lobe perfusion, whereas anterior cingulate perfusion and cortisol levels were positively correlated in PTSD but negatively correlated in trauma survivors without PTSD. These inverse correlations may result from an augmented negative hippocampal effect secondary to increased sensitivity of brain

glucocorticoid receptors, which would account for the inverse correlation in PTSD despite equal cortisol levels in both the PTSD and non-PTSD groups. On the other hand, the positive correlation between regional cerebral blood flow in the frontocingulate transitional cortex and cortisol levels in PTSD may reflect unsuccessful attempts of the frontocingulate transitional cortex to terminate the stress response, which has also been linked with low cortisol.

Cortisol may be related to specific or state-dependent features of the disorder, such as comorbid depression or the time course of the disorder. There is a long and rich tradition in psychosomatic medicine underscoring the importance of examining intrapsychic correlates of individual differences in cortisol levels in PTSD, reflecting emotional arousal and opposing antiarousal disengagement defense mechanisms or other coping styles. Finally, recent evidence also suggests that cortisol levels further decrease over time and in old age in trauma survivors.

Cortisol Levels in Response to Stress

Although cortisol levels may be lower at baseline, they may actually be elevated in PTSD relative to comparison subjects when challenged by physiological or psychological stressors. In particular, subjects with PTSD appear to show more anticipatory anxiety to laboratory stressors, which is reflected by increased cortisol levels. These studies provide at least some evidence that the adrenal is capable of producing ample cortisol levels at baseline and in response to stress. In fact, transient increases in cortisol levels are consistent with the notion of a more generalized HPA axis reactivity in PTSD, as reflected by enhanced negative feedback inhibition.

Basal Corticotropin Releasing Hormone and Adrenocorticotropic Hormone Levels in Posttraumatic Stress Disorder

Interestingly, all published reports examining the concentration of corticotropin releasing hormone (CRH) in cerebrospinal fluid (CSF) in PTSD have concluded that levels of this peptide are increased in PTSD. The assessment of CSF CRH does not necessarily provide a good estimate of hypothalamic CRH release but, rather, an estimate of both the hypothalamic and extrahypothalamic release of this neuropeptide. Nonetheless, that there is increased CRH release is somewhat of a paradox considering the lower cortisol levels. With respect to adrenocorticotropic hormone (ACTH), the majority of studies have reported no detectable differences in ACTH levels between PTSD and comparison subjects even when cortisol levels obtained from the same sample were found to be significantly lower.

Lower cortisol levels in the face of normal ACTH levels can reflect a relatively decreased adrenal output. Yet, under circumstances of classic adrenal insufficiency, there is usually increased ACTH release compared to normal levels. Thus, in PTSD, there may be an additional component of feedback on the pituitary acting to depress ACTH levels so that they appear normal rather than elevated. Indeed, elevations in ACTH are expected not only from a reduced adrenal output but also from increased CRH stimulation. On the other hand, the adrenal output in PTSD may be relatively decreased but not enough to substantially affect ACTH levels. In any event, the normal ACTH levels in PTSD in the context of the other findings suggest a more complex model of the regulatory influences on the pituitary in this disorder than reduced adrenal insufficiency.

Glucocorticoid Receptors in Posttraumatic Stress Disorder

Type II glucocorticoid receptors (GRs) are expressed in ACTH- and CRH-producing neurons of the pituitary, hypothalamus, and hippocampus and mediate most systemic glucocorticoid effects, particularly those related to stress responsiveness. Low circulating levels of a hormone or neurotransmitter can result in increased numbers of available GRs to improve response capacity and facilitate homeostasis. However, alterations in the number and sensitivity of both type I (mineralocorticoid) and type II GRs can also significantly influence HPA axis activity and, in particular, can regulate hormone levels by mediating the strength of negative feedback. In PTSD, there is evidence for both an increased number of GRs (measured in lymphocytes) and increased responsiveness of the GR.

Observations regarding the cellular immune response in PTSD are also consistent with enhanced GR responsiveness in the periphery, as indicated by increased beclomethasone-induced vasoconstriction and enhanced delayed-type hypersensitivity of skin test responses. Because immune responses, like endocrine ones, can be multiply regulated, these studies provide only indirect evidence of GR responsiveness. However, when considered in the context of the observation that PTSD patients showed an increased expression of the receptors in all lymphocyte subpopulations, despite a relatively lower quantity of intracellular GRs, as determined by flow cytometry, and in the face of lower ambient cortisol levels, the findings more convincingly support an enhanced sensitivity of the GRs to glucocorticoids. Furthermore, there appears to be an absence of alterations of the mineralocorticoid receptor in PTSD, as investigated by examining the cortisol and ACTH response to spironolactone following CRH stimulation.

With respect to increased glucocorticoid responsiveness, this was recently determined using an *in vitro* paradigm in which mononuclear leukocytes were incubated with a series of concentrations of dexamethasone (DEX) to determine the rate of inhibition of lysozyme activity. Subjects with PTSD showed evidence of a greater sensitivity to glucocorticoids as reflected by a significantly lower mean lysozyme median inhibitory concentration of DEX ($IC_{50\text{-DEX}}$; in nanomoles per liter). The lysozyme $IC_{50\text{-DEX}}$ was significantly correlated with age at exposure to the first traumatic event in subjects with PTSD. The number of cytosolic GRs was correlated with age at exposure to the focal traumatic event.

The Dexamethasone Suppression Test in Posttraumatic Stress Disorder

In contrast to observations regarding ambient cortisol levels, results using the dexamethasone suppression test (DST) present a more consistent view of reduced cortisol suppression in response to DEX administration. The DST provides a direct test of the effects of GR activation in the pituitary on ACTH secretion, and cortisol levels following DEX administration are thus interpreted as an estimate of the strength of negative feedback inhibition, provided that the adrenal response to ACTH is not altered. Using 0.50 mg DEX, most investigators have found a more dramatic reduction in plasma cortisol levels. This exaggerated cortisol suppression in response to DEX has been observed in PTSD related to people with combat exposure, survivors of childhood sexual abuse, Holocaust survivors, children exposed to disaster, women exposed to domestic violence, and mixed groups of trauma survivors.

The Metyrapone Stimulation Test

Metyrapone prevents adrenal steroidogenesis by blocking the conversion of 11-deoxycortisol to cortisol, thereby unmasking the pituitary gland from the influences of negative feedback inhibition. If a sufficiently high dose of metyrapone is used, such that an almost complete suppression of cortisol is achieved, this allows a direct examination of pituitary release of ACTH without the potentially confounding effects of differing ambient cortisol levels. When metyrapone is administered in the morning when HPA axis activity is relatively high, maximal pituitary activity can be achieved, facilitating an evaluation of group differences in pituitary capability. The administration of 2.5 mg metyrapone in the morning resulted in a similar and almost complete reduction in cortisol levels in both PTSD and normal subjects (i.e., removal of negative feedback inhibition) but in a higher increase in ACTH and 11-deoxycortisol in combat Vietnam veterans with PTSD, compared to nonexposed subjects. In the context of low cortisol levels and increased CSF CRH levels, the findings supported the hypothesis of a stronger negative feedback inhibition in PTSD. Both pituitary and adrenal insufficiency are not likely to result in an increased ACTH response to the removal of negative feedback inhibition because the former is associated with an attenuated ACTH response and reduced adrenal output would not necessarily affect the ACTH response. To the extent that ambient cortisol levels are lower than normal, an increased ACTH response following the removal of negative feedback inhibition implies that, when negative feedback is intact, it is strong enough to inhibit ACTH and cortisol. The increased ACTH response is most easily explained by increased suprapituitary activation; however, a sufficiently strong negative feedback inhibition would account for the augmented ACTH response even in the absence of hypothalamic CRH hypersecretion.

Evidence of increased ACTH was not observed when a lower dose of metyrapone was used, administered over a 3-h period at night (750 mg at 7:00 a.m. and 10:00 a.m.). However, interestingly, the manipulation produced a more robust suppression of cortisol in comparison subjects. Using a similar methodology, the effects of metyrapone was used to evaluate CRH effects on sleep. ACTH and cortisol levels were increased in the PTSD group relative to the controls the next morning, suggesting that the same dose of metyrapone did not produce the same degree of adrenal suppression of cortisol synthesis. Under these conditions, it is difficult to evaluate the true effect on ACTH and 11-deoxycortisol, which depends on achieving complete cortisol suppression, or at least the same degree of cortisol suppression, in the two groups. The endocrine response to metyrapone in this study do not support the model of reduced adrenal capacity because this would have yielded a large ratio of ACTH-to-cortisol release, yet the mean ACTH/cortisol ratio prior to metyrapone was no different in the PTSD subjects and the controls. On the other hand, the mean ACTH/cortisol ratio postmetyrapone was lower, although not significantly, suggesting, if anything, an exaggerated negative feedback rather than reduced adrenal capacity.

The Corticotropin Releasing Hormone Challenge Test and Adrenocorticotropic Hormone Stimulation Test in Posttraumatic Stress Disorder

The infusion of exogenous CRH increases ACTH levels and provides a test of pituitary sensitivity. A blunted ACTH is classically thought to reflect a reduced sensitivity of the pituitary to CRH, reflecting a downregulation of pituitary CRH receptors secondary to CRH hypersecretion. The results of studies in PTSD subjects using this challenge have also been mixed. Some studies have demonstrated a blunted ACTH response to PTSD; however, insofar as this blunting did not occur in the presence of hypercortisolism, as in depression, the attenuated ACTH response may reflect an increased negative feedback inhibition of the pituitary secondary to increased GR number or sensitivity. This explanation supports the idea of CRH hypersecretion in PTSD and explains the pituitary desensitization and resultant lack of hypercortisolism as arising from a stronger negative feedback inhibition. An augmented ACTH response to CRH has also been reported, which the authors interpreted as reflecting increased reactivity of the pituitary, although here too there was no evidence for increased cortisol levels.

Findings of Cortisol in the Acute Aftermath of Trauma

Recent data provided some support for the idea that low cortisol levels may be an early predictor of PTSD rather than a consequence of this condition. Low cortisol levels in the immediate aftermath of a motor vehicle accident predicted the development of PTSD in a group of accident victims consecutively presenting in an emergency room in two studies. In a sample of people who survived a natural disaster, cortisol levels were similarly found to be lowest in those with highest PTSD scores at 1 month posttrauma; however cortisol levels were not predictive of symptoms at 1 year. In the acute aftermath of rape, low cortisol levels were associated with prior rape or assault, themselves risk factors for PTSD, but not with the development of PTSD *per se*.

These findings imply that cortisol levels might have been lower in trauma survivors who subsequently developed PTSD even before their exposure to trauma and might therefore represent a preexisting risk factor. Consistent with this, low 24-h urinary cortisol levels in adult children of Holocaust survivors were specifically associated with the risk factor of parental PTSD. Interestingly, the risk factor of parental PTSD in offspring of Holocaust survivors was also associated with an increased incidence of traumatic childhood antecedents. In this study, both the presence of subject-rated parental PTSD and scores reflecting childhood emotional abuse were associated with low cortisol levels in offspring. Thus, it may be that low cortisol levels occur in those who have experienced an adverse event early in life and then remain different from those not exposed to early adversity. Although there might reasonably be HPA axis fluctuations in the aftermath of stress, and even differences in the magnitude of such responses compared to those not exposed to trauma early in life, HPA parameters would subsequently recover to their (abnormal) prestress baseline.

Low cortisol levels may impede the process of biological recovery from stress, resulting in a cascade of alterations that lead to intrusive recollections of the event, avoidance of reminders of the event, and symptoms of hyperarousal. This failure may represent an alternative trajectory to the normal process of adaptation and recovery after a traumatic event.

One of the most compelling lines of evidence supporting the hypothesis that lower cortisol levels may be an important pathway to the development of PTSD symptoms are the results of studies showing that the administration of stress doses of hydrocortisone prevents the development of PTSD and traumatic memories and attenuate these symptoms once present. These findings support the idea that low cortisol levels may facilitate the development of PTSD in response to an overwhelming biological demand, at least in some circumstances.

Conclusion

Cortisol levels are most often found to be lower than normal in PTSD subjects, but can also be similar to or greater than those in comparison subjects. Findings of changes in circadian rhythm suggest that there may be regulatory influences that result in a greater dynamic range of cortisol release over the diurnal cycle in PTSD. Thus, although cortisol levels may be generally lower, the adrenal gland is certainly capable of producing adequate amounts of cortisol in response to challenge.

The model of enhanced negative feedback inhibition is compatible with the idea that there may be transient elevations in cortisol, but suggests that, when present, these increases are shorter-lived due to a more efficient containment of ACTH release as a result of enhanced GR activation. An increased negative feedback inhibition results in reduced cortisol levels under ambient conditions. In contrast to other models of endocrinopathy, which identify specific and usually singular primary alterations in endocrine organs and/or regulation, the model of enhanced negative feedback inhibition in PTSD is in large part descriptive and currently offers little explanation of why some individuals show such alterations of the HPA axis following exposure to traumatic experiences and others do not.

The wide range of observations observed in the neuroendocrinology of PTSD underscores the important observation that HPA response patterns in PTSD are fundamentally in the normal range and do not reflect endocrinopathy. In endocrinological disorders, in which there is usually a lesion in one or more target tissue or biosynthetic pathway, endocrine methods can usually isolate the problem with the appropriate tests and then obtain rather consistent results. In psychiatric disorders, neuroendocrine alterations may be subtle, and therefore, when using standard endocrine tools to examine these alterations, there is a high probability of failing to observe all the alterations consistent with a neuroendocrine explanation of the pathology in tandem or of obtaining disparate results within the same patient group owing to a stronger compensation or reregulation of the HPA axis following challenge.

The next generation studies should aim to apply more rigorous tests of neuroendocrinology of PTSD based on the appropriate developmental issues and in consideration of the longitudinal course of the disorder and the individual differences that affect these processes. No doubt such studies will require a closer examination of a wide range of biological responses, including the cellular and molecular mechanisms involved in adaptation to stress, and an understanding of the relationship between the endocrine findings and other identified biological alterations in PTSD.

Acknowledgments

This work was supported by MH 49555, MH 55-7531, and MERIT review funding.

See Also the Following Articles

Depression and Manic-Depressive Illness; Depression Models; Depression, Immunological Aspects; Dexamethasone Suppression Test (DST); Hypocortisolism and Stress; Neuroendocrine Systems.

Further Reading

Baker, D. G., West, S. A., Nicholson, W. E., et al. (1999). Serial CSF corticotropin-releasing hormone levels and adrenocortical activity in combat veterans with posttraumatic stress disorder. *American Journal of Psychiatry* **156**, 585–588[errata] 986.

Bremner, J. D., Vythilingma, M., Vermetten, E., et al. (2003). Cortisol response to a cognitive stress challenge in posttraumatic stress disorder related to childhood abuse. *Psychoneuyroendocrinology* **28**, 733–750.

Boscarino, J. A. (1996). Posttraumatic stress disorder, exposure to combat, and lower plasma cortisol among Vietnam veterans: findings and clinical implications. *Journal of Consulting and Clinical Psychology* **64**, 191–201.

Delahanty, D. L., Raimonde, A. J. and Spoonster, E. (2000). Initial posttraumatic urinary cortisol levels predict subsequent PTSD symptoms in motor vehicle accident victims [in process citation]. *Biological Psychiatry* **48**, 940–947.

Holsboer, F. (2000). The corticosteroid receptor hypothesis of depression. *Neuropsychopharmacology* **23**, 477–501.

Raison, C. L. and Miller, A. H. (2003). When not enough is too much: the role of insufficient glucocorticoid signaling in the pathophysiology of stress related disorders. *American Journal of Psychiatry* **160**, 1554–1565.

Schelling, G., Briegel, J., Roozendaal, B., et al. (2001). The effect of stress doses of hydrocortisone during septic shock on posttraumatic stress disorder in survivors. *Biological Psychiatry* **50**, 978–985.

Yehuda, R. (2002). Status of cortisol findings in PTSD. *Psychiatric Clinics of North America* **25**, 341–368.

Yehuda, R., Boisoneau, D., Lowy, M. T., et al. (1995). Dose-response changes in plasma cortisol and lymphocyte glucocorticoid receptors following dexamethasone administration in combat veterans with and without posttraumatic stress disorder. *Archives of General Psychiatry* **52**, 583–593.

Yehuda, R., Halligan, S. L. and Grossman, R. (2001). Childhood trauma and risk for PTSD: relationship to intergenerational effects of trauma, parental PTSD and cortisol excretion. *Development and Psychopathology* **2001**, 733–753.

Yehuda, R., Levengood, R. A., Schmeidler, J., et al. (1996). Increased pituitary activation following metyrapone administration in post-traumatic stress disorder. *Psychoneuroendocrinology* **21**, 1–16.

Yehuda, R., Shalev, A. Y. and McFarlane, A. C. (1998). Predicting the development of posttraumatic stress disorder from the acute response to a traumatic event. *Biological Psychiatry* **44**, 1305–1313.

Yehuda, R., Teicher, M. H., Trestman, R. L., et al. (1996). Cortisol regulation in posttraumatic stress disorder and major depression: a chronobiological analysis. *Biological Psychiatry* **40**, 79–88.

HPA Role in Depression   *See:* HPA Alterations in PTSD; Depression and Manic-Depressive Illness; Depression Models; Dexamethasone Suppression Test (DST).

HSF (Heat Shock Transcription Factor)   *See:* Chaperone Proteins and Chaperonopathies; Heat Shock Response, Overview.

Hurricane Katrina Disaster, Stress Effects of

C Piotrowski
University of West Florida, Pensacola, FL USA

Calamity
Hurricane Katrina
Methodological Issues
Impact on Human Populations

Glossary

Chaos theory	A scientific paradigm that suggests that chaos and complexity are inherent to explaining phenomena; it aids in the understanding of how organizations respond, adapt, change, function, and renew.
Direct-contact victims	Emergency and rescue workers who searched for survivors and dead bodies, as well as morgue personnel.
Disaster mental health	A competency-bases intervention model, based on disaster-related psychopathology, that addresses a community's mental health needs.
First-responders	All emergency personnel that aid in the immediate aftermath of a disaster, such as police, firefighters, rescue workers, medical staff, and special response units.
Hurricane Andrew	The costliest hurricane to hit the United States prior to Hurricane Katrina; it caused $44 billion in damage in 1992.
Mass-casualty event	An event that involves multidimensional stressors that may result in differential patterns of posttraumatic reactions, both short and long term.

| Northeast quadrant | The storm quadrant with the strongest winds and rain (because hurricanes circulate counterclockwise). In Hurricane Katrina, this meant that the areas east of New Orleans, for 160 miles, received the brunt of the storm's wrath. |
| Self-efficacy | An individual's belief that his or her actions and behavior will produce the desired outcomes; coined by personality theorist Albert Bandura. |

Calamity

Without a doubt, Hurricane Katrina (August 29, 2005) was the most destructive and costly natural disaster in U.S. history. Months after the storm, the total destruction, including the human toll, is still being calculated. Perhaps as a key indicator of the enormity of the devastation, 6 months after the disaster news accounts on every aspect of the tragedy still appear each night on the national news networks, the number of deaths are provided as an estimate, and over 100 of the deceased victims have not yet been identified. The numbers, to date, allow an appreciation of the impact:

- Deaths: ~1500, either during or immediately after the storm.
- Homeless residents: 800,000.
- Victims left unemployed: ~550,000.
- Displaced people: 2 million.
- Homes destroyed: 350,000.
- Penetration of the storm surge along the Louisiana, Mississippi, and Alabama coast was measured in miles not feet.
- Property losses: ~$35 billion.
- Estimates for reclamation: 2 years to clear 22 million tons of waste and debris.
- Small businesses not in operation: 50%.
- Cars submerged under water: 200,000.
- Residents of the greater New Orleans area who may have to relocate permanently: ~75%.
- Area of the city of New Orleans that was flooded: ~70%.
- Evacuees separated from their pets: ~80%.
- Estimate of total economic costs and damage: varies widely, but will probably reach $200 billion.

Hurricane Katrina

Hurricane Katrina was both an immensely powerful and a large storm. Initial forecasts estimated winds of 145 mph at landfall, but revised figures from the National Hurricane Center in Miami reported maximum sustained winds of approximately 125 mph; officially, the storm was a high category 3 hurricane.

Hurricane-force winds (>74 mph) extended 160 miles out from the eye of the storm. Unbelievably, the city of Waveland, Mississippi, was struck by a 28-ft storm surge. Several hours after the eye of the storm passed New Orleans, the levee system that protected the city was either breached or undermined in three strategic areas; within hours, approximately two-thirds of the city was submerged under up to 12 ft of water. Many residents drowned, and thousands sought higher ground.

The initial governmental response, particularly that of the Federal Emergency Management Agency (FEMA), can be regarded as a complete debacle; however, many regular citizens, volunteers, and health-care personnel extended themselves to save lives. Unfortunately, most residents were left to fend for themselves for almost a week before basic necessities arrived. The result was untold human suffering. Small coastal cities along the gulf coast from Port Sulphur, Louisiana, to Mobile, Alabama, were hard hit by high winds, torrential rain, and a destructive storm surge; some small towns on the Mississippi and Alabama coast were literally wiped off the map.

Outside of the impact area, the country felt the residual impact of the calamity: anger over government malaise, a sense of national shame, and high energy prices. Undoubtedly, the social consciousness of the public was severely tested, particularly with regard to the racial issues and poverty that were brought to the forefront in the aftermath of the storm. In this regard, Hurricane Katrina will always be considered both a natural and human-made disaster.

Methodological Issues

Although the United States suffered several devastating natural disasters in its history (e.g., the San Francisco earthquake, the Galveston hurricane, and Mississippi River floods), the calamity of Hurricane Katrina has no precedent with regard to human suffering, social displacement, structural damage, and financial cost. Summarily, a continuous stretch of 200 miles of the U.S. coast was adversely impacted, including a population of approximately 3.6 million residents. At the time of this writing (6 months postdisaster), there is limited empirical research on the storm, although many articles have appeared in general media publications. Because I am a disaster researcher, I can attest to the fact that there are a plethora of research studies underway, particularly at universities in the New Orleans area.

Researchers should be cautioned about several unique features of investigating this disaster. First and foremost, Hurricane Katrina was not a unitary impact event; that is, from a methodological perspective, not all regions (and populations) were impacted in the same manner or experienced the same level or type of disaster. For example, New Orleans basically experienced a flood event and was not greatly impacted by hurricane winds (the city lay west of the eye of the storm). However, smaller coastal communities to the east of the eye (coastal Louisiana, Mississippi, and Alabama) felt the full brunt of hurricane-force winds and devastating storm surge. Some residents had recoverable property damage, whereas others were completely wiped out. Some residents evacuated to safety, whereas others rode out the storm. Many victims evacuated temporarily, whereas others were displaced to cities throughout the United States and many in this latter group will probably not return to their home areas. Moreover, there was a great disparity in the amount of governmental support and financial assistance that individuals received, commensurate with the amount of damage, need for shelter, and sustenance needs. Therefore, researchers need to be cognizant of these factors when studying select populations and be aware that not everyone experienced Hurricane Katrina in the same way. Green reviewed some of the difficulties encountered in designing sound disaster research studies, and several investigators have considered the heterogeneous nature of studying the effects of hurricanes on different cohort groups. Furthermore, due to the overwhelming nature of the disaster and its aftermath, Hurricane Katrina, for many victims, was a multiple traumatic loss: that is, a loss of loved ones, pets, residence, job, security, and the future.

Impact on Human Populations

Flooding

Much of New Orleans was severely flooded due to the failure of levee structures. Both natural and human-made disasters can result in flooding, for example, the Buffalo Creek dam collapse in 1972 and the Great Midwest Mississippi floods in 1993. The effects of extensive flooding were studied in the aftermath of Hurricane Floyd, which struck North Carolina in 1999. Emotional exhaustion, grief reactions and depression, posttraumatic stress disorder (PTSD) symptomotology, and somatic complaints were identified as the major sequela in several studies. The aged seemed to be the most affected.

Health Issues

The health consequences of natural disasters have been a major research area. For example, in the 1983 South Australian bush fires, Japan's 1995 Hanshin–Awaji earthquake, and California's 1994 Northridge earthquake, impacted populations were found to be vulnerable to a host of medical maladies, particularly stress-related conditions such as hypertension, gastrointestinal disorders, diabetes, and mental illness. Non-stress-related conditions were typically not affected. Most conditions were found to improve within 15 months postdisaster. Investigators have reported on the impact of immunological changes after natural disasters and found that adaptive coping to stress effects mediated immunological responses in affected populations.

Mental Health Symptoms

Psychiatric morbidity, particularly stress-related conditions, have been extensively studied in both natural and human-made disasters. Specifically, PTSD, depression, and substance abuse disorders have been reported to significantly increase following large-scale disasters. Researchers caution that acute stress disorder is prognostically important as a marker for the development of moderate or full PTSD symptoms in the long term. One study on mental health symptomotology following Hurricane Andrew reported that 36% of the sample had PTSD, 30% experienced major depression, and 20% showed signs of anxiety disorders. In fact, 56% had significant symptoms persisting beyond 6 months posthurricane. Due to the high prevalence of mental health problems experienced in the wake of hurricanes, researchers point to the critical importance of coping self-efficacy perceptions as a mediator between acute stress response and long-term distress following natural disasters.

Because geographical relocation was a major aspect of the Katrina disaster, it should be an area of particular research focus. Prior studies in this area concluded that displaced individuals in natural disasters exhibit more intense levels of psychopathology, particularly depression. Perhaps, this is the result of unresolved grief on the part of victims who were not only relocated but also lost their homes and needed to start over elsewhere. Moreover, in a study of family life following Hurricane Hugo in 1989, researchers found the divorce rate increased. In this regard, there have been recent media ad campaigns across the impacted Gulf Coast areas that address post-Hurricane Katrina family stress issues such as child and wife abuse.

Recovery Issues

There are a number of governmental recovery plans in place across the Gulf Coast, although their implementation seems to be progressing slowly. Research following Hurricane Andrew in 1992 indicated that disruption during rebuilding phases contributed to the exacerbation of mental health symptoms. In recent years, social scientists have advocated disaster mental health-planning initiatives via national organizations such the American Psychological Association to address preparedness planning, mitigation, agency coordination, and community resource development. Particularly in the context of the complexity of disasters, interagency cooperation and coordination are crucial to meeting the social and psychological needs of victims posthurricane.

By all accounts, the governmental response in the immediate aftermath of Katrina and the subsequent lethargic recovery efforts can only be described as appalling. This unfortunate state of affairs can only impede individual and collective efforts at achieving some sense of normality among the affected population. Instead, much of the goodwill and recovery assistance to the affected population came from local church groups and organizations such as the Red Cross. Indeed, this is also what occurred after the double hit of Hurricanes Erin and Opal in Pensacola, Florida.

Special Populations

It is incumbent that researchers pay particular attention to population groups such as the aged, health-delivery workers, children, the disabled, first-responders, and impoverished citizens. Unique populations cope with stressors in diverse ways, and stress reactions tend to be heterogeneous. This was the finding of a study on children following the Oklahoma City bombing. Furthermore, the critical function of denial in both child and adult populations has received theoretical support in prior research studies. Last, there has been much media attention given to race and poverty issues in the aftermath of Katrina; this will be an important factor in ongoing research, although recent research findings on this issue are equivocal.

See Also the Following Articles

Acute Stress Disorder and Posttraumatic Stress Disorder; Earthquakes, Stress Effects of; Floods, Stress Effects of; Refugees, Stress in; Life Events and Health; Neurosis; Posttraumatic Stress Disorder – Clinical.

Further Reading

Benight, C. and Harper, M. (2002). Coping self-efficacy perceptions as a mediator between acute stress response and long-term distress following natural disasters. *Journal of Traumatic Stress* **15**, 177–186.

David, D., Mellman, T. A., Mendoza, L. M., et al. (1996). Psychiatric morbidity following Hurricane Andrew. *Journal of Traumatic Stress* **9**, 607–612.

Elliot, J.R. and Pais, J. (2006). Race, class, and Hurricane Katrina: social differences in human responses to disaster. *Social Science Research* **35**, 295–321.

Green, B. L. (1991). Evaluating the effects of disasters. *Psychological Assessment* **3**, 538–546.

Jones, R. T., Frary, R., Cunningham, P., et al. (2001). Psychological effects of Hurricane Andrew on ethnic minority and Caucasian children and adolescents: a case study. *Cultural Diversity & Ethnic Minority Psychology* **7**, 103–108.

McMillen, C., North, C., Mosley, M., et al. (2002). Untangling the psychiatric comorbidity of posttraumatic stress disorder in a sample of flood survivors. *Comprehensive Psychiatry* **43**, 478–485.

Myers, D. and Wee, D. F. (2005). *Disaster mental health services*. New York: Brunner-Routledge.

Najarian, L. M., Goenjian, A., Pelcovitz, D., et al. (2001). The effect of relocation after a natural disaster. *Journal of Traumatic Stress* **14**, 511–526.

Norris, F., Friedman, M. J. and Watson, P. J. (2002). 60,000 disaster victims speak. II: Summary and implications of the disaster mental health research. *Psychiatry* **65**, 240–260.

Norris, F., Perilla, J. L. and Murphy, A. D. (2001). Postdisaster stress in the United States and Mexico: a cross-cultural test of the conceptual model of posttraumatic stress disorder. *Journal of Abnormal Psychology* **110**, 553–563.

Piotrowski, C. (2006). Hurricane Katrina and organization development: part 1, implications of chaos theory. *Organization Development Journal* **24**(3), 10–19.

Piotrowski, C. and Armstrong, T. (1998). Satisfaction with relief agencies during Hurricanes Erin and Opal. *Psychological Reports* **82**, 413–414.

Piotrowski, C., Armstrong, T. and Stopp, H. (1997). Stress factors in the aftermath of Hurricanes Erin and Opal: data from small business owners. *Psychological Reports* **80**, 1387–1391.

Piotrowski, C. and Dunham, F. (1983). Locus of control orientation and perception of "Hurricane" in fifth graders. *Journal of General Psychology* **109**, 119–127.

Rotton, J., Dubitsky, S., Milov, A., et al. (1997). Distress, elevated cortisol, cognitive deficits, and illness following a natural disaster. *Journal of Environmental Psychology* **17**, 85–98.

Solomon, G. F., Segerstrom, S., Grohr, P., et al. (1997). Shaking up immunity: psychological and immunologic changes after a natural disaster. *Psychosomatic Medicine* **59**, 142–143.

Hydrocortisone   *See:* Corticosteroids and Stress; Glucocorticoids, Overview.

11β-Hydroxysteroid Dehydrogenases

J R Seckl
Edinburgh University, Edinburgh, UK

This article is a revision of the previous edition article by J R Seckl, volume 2, pp 413–420, © 2000, Elsevier Inc.

Definition: 11β-Hydroxysteroid Dehydrogenase

The Mineralocorticoid Receptor Paradox

11β-Hydroxysteroid Dehydrogenase Type 2 in the Adult Central Nervous System

11β-Hydroxysteroid Dehydrogenase Type 2 in the Developing Central Nervous System

11β-Hydroxysteroid Dehydrogenase Type 2 and Fetal Programming

Programming the Hypothalamic-Pituitary-Adrenal Axis and Behavior

11β-Hydroxysteroid Dehydrogenase Type 1 in the Brain

11β-Hydroxysteroid Dehydrogenase Type 1 and the Hypothalamic-Pituitary-Adrenal Axis

11β-Hydroxysteroid Dehydrogenase Type 1 and Brain Aging

Conclusion

Glossary

11β-Hydroxysteroid dehydrogenase (11β-HSD)	An enzyme that catalyzes the interconversion of active cortisol (corticosterone in rats and mice) and inert cortisone (11-dehydrocorticosterone).
11β-HSD type 1 (11β-HSD1)	An isozyme that predominantly catalyzes the reduction of inert cortisone to active cortisol in intact cells and organs.
11β-HSD type 2 (11β-HSD2)	An isozyme that catalyzes the rapid dehydrogenation of active cortisol to inert cortisone.
Aromatase	The enzyme that catalyzes the conversion of androgens to estrogens.
Carbenoxolone	A nonselective 11β-HSD inhibitor.
Cushing's syndrome	The generic description of the phenotype observed with circulating glucocorticoid excess, due either to endogenous overproduction of cortisol or adrenocorticotrophic hormone (ACTH) or to exogenous pharmacotherapy.
Glucocorticoid receptor (GR)	Intracellular receptor for active cortisol.
Intracrine	The process whereby intracellular enzymic transformations of steroids alter their access to nuclear receptors.
Metabolic syndrome	The co-association of risk factors for atheromatous disease (insulin resistance, type 2 diabetes, dyslipidemia, and hypertension) and abdominal (visceral) obesity.
Mineralocorticoid receptor (MR)	Intracellular receptor for active cortisol, selectivity for aldosterone *in vivo* generated by 11β-HSD2.
Syndrome of apparent mineralocorticoid excess	A congenital syndrome of hypertension, hypernatremia, and hypokalemia due to inappropriate MR activation by glucocorticoids because of deleterious mutations of the 11β-HSD type 2 gene and hence lack of the enzyme in the kidney.

Definition: 11β-Hydroxysteroid Dehydrogenase

Elevated plasma cortisol or glucocorticoid pharmacotherapy has myriad adverse effects ranging from obesity, diabetes, and hypertension to depression and memory impairments. Glucocorticoid action is classically believed to be determined by the product of circulating glucocorticoid levels and the tissue density of corticosteroid receptors (GR and MR). However, recent discoveries suggest a key role for local enzymic tissue metabolism of glucocorticoids in determining receptor activation. The main enzymes involved are the 11β-hydroxysteroid dehydrogenases (11β-HSDs). These catalyze the interconversion of active cortisol (in humans and most mammals) and corticosterone (in rats and mice) and inert 11-keto forms (cortisone, 11-dehydrocorticosterone) (**Figure 1**). The roles of these enzymes in determining glucocorticoid actions in the central nervous system (CNS) and periphery are now becoming apparent.

The Mineralocorticoid Receptor Paradox

Purified MR binds aldosterone, cortisol, and corticosterone with equal and high affinity *in vitro*, but *in vivo*

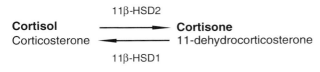

ACTIVE   **INERT**

Figure 1 11β-Hydroxysteroid dehydrogenases. Type 1 acts as a ketoreductase, regenerating active cortisol (corticosterone), whereas type 2 acts as a dehydrogenase, rapidly inactivating these physiological glucocorticoids.

only aldosterone binds to MR in the kidney, although there is much more glucocorticoid in the circulation. In resolution of this paradox, in 1988 groups in Edinburgh and Melbourne reported that 11β-HSD was a prereceptor enzymic mechanism that bestowed aldosterone selectivity on the intrinsically nonselective MR *in vivo*. The 11β-HSD activity associated with MR in the distal nephron acted as a dehydrogenase, rapidly inactivating physiological glucocorticoids (cortisol, corticosterone) to their inert 11-keto forms. Such 11β-HSD activity forms an intracellular barrier to glucocorticoids, preventing the occupation of MR. When the enzyme is congenitally deficient in the syndrome of apparent mineralocorticoid excess or is inhibited by liquorice, glucocorticoids inappropriately access MR, causing sodium retention, hypertension, and hypokalemia. Although an NADP(H)-associated 11β-HSD activity (now called 11β-HSD1) and its encoding cDNA were isolated from rat liver by Monder and colleagues in the mid-1980s, this was shown not to be responsible for renal MR selectivity: its encoding gene HSD11B1 was intact in patients with the syndrome. Subsequently a second 11β-HSD isozyme (11β-HSD2) was cloned from the kidney and placenta in a variety of species. This isozyme is a high-affinity 11β-dehydrogenase, which uses NAD as cofactor and is highly expressed in the distal nephron and placenta. Patients with the syndrome of apparent mineralocorticoid excess were homozygous or compound heterozygous for deleterious mutations in the HSD11B2 gene, and 11β-HSD2 knockout mice faithfully recapitulated the syndrome. This work underlined the fundamental principle that steroid access to nuclear receptors *in vivo* is regulated by prereceptor metabolism. Other examples include 5- and 5′-monodeiodinases (thyroid hormone receptors), 5α-reductase (androgen receptor), and aromatase (estrogen receptors).

11β-Hydroxysteroid Dehydrogenase Type 2 in the Adult Central Nervous System

Although the vast majority of MR in the CNS are nonselective and bind glucocorticoids (cortisol,

corticosterone) *in vivo*, it is anticipated that any selective effects of aldosterone in the CNS will require MR gated by local 11β-HSD2. In this regard, aldosterone mediates the central regulation of blood pressure and salt appetite. Thus, aldosterone infused intracerebroventricularly (ICV) elevates blood pressure in the rat, whereas the same dose given peripherally is ineffective, demonstrating a specific central action. Corticosterone ICV does not reproduce this action, and indeed antagonizes aldosterone hypertension. Similarly, aldosterone exerts central actions on salt appetite that cannot be reproduced by corticosterone. 11β-HSD2 action in the CNS is therefore inferred. This is supported by ICV infusion of the 11β-HSD inhibitor carbenoxolone, which increases blood pressure in the rat, an effect reversed by an MR antagonist, suggesting central 11β-HSD2 prevents access of glucocorticoids to central MR. Although 11β-HSD2 mRNA is only found in a few discrete sites in the adult rat brain, these loci also express MR and are believed to underlie the selective central effects of aldosterone to increase blood pressure (nucleus tractus solitarius, NTS), and modulate salt appetite (ventromedial hypothalamus, subcommissural organ, and central nucleus of the amygdala). In the mouse there is an even more limited distribution of 11β-HSD2, with expression confined to the NTS. 11β-HSD2 was not found in the human forebrain, although the brain stem has not been investigated. Thus, there is very little 11β-HSD2 in the adult brain, located appropriately for the few CNS actions specifically ascribed to this hormone.

11β-Hydroxysteroid Dehydrogenase Type 2 in the Developing Central Nervous System

Prenatal glucocorticoid administration reduces brain weight at birth; delays the maturation of neurons, glia, and cerebral vasculature; and retards CNS myelination. Given such widespread effects, it is unsurprising that GR and MR are highly expressed in the developing brain. However, whether these receptors are occupied by endogenous glucocorticoids until late gestation is uncertain because there is also plentiful 11β-HSD2 in the CNS at midgestation in rodents and humans. This presumably functions to protect vulnerable developing cells from premature glucocorticoid action. Strikingly, 11β-HSD2 expression is dramatically switched off in a CNS at the end of midgestation, coinciding with the terminal stage of brain nucleus development. This appears to be an exquisitely timed system of cellular protection from circulating glucocorticoids.

11β-Hydroxysteroid Dehydrogenase Type 2 and Fetal Programming

Human epidemiological studies show that low birth weight at term is associated with an increased later occurrence of cardiovascular (hypertension and ischemic heart disease) and metabolic disorders (type 2 diabetes) in adult life. In rodents, sheep, and humans, excessive exposure to glucocorticoids during gestation, either bypassing of fetoplacental 11β-HSD2 with nonsubstrate glucocorticoid such as dexamethasone or using 11β-HSD inhibitors such as carbenoxolone, reduces birth weight. Although in such models, the weight deficit is regained soon after birth, the adult offspring show increased blood pressure and serum insulin and glucose levels. These effects are underpinned by an increased tissue sensitivity to glucocorticoids via increased GR density in key metabolic loci such as the liver and visceral adipose tissue depots.

Programming the Hypothalamic-Pituitary-Adrenal Axis and Behavior

Prenatal 11β-HSD2 inhibition or bypass with the nonsubstrate dexamethasone permanently increases basal plasma corticosterone levels in the offspring in rats. The density of GR and MR in the hippocampus are reduced in this model, which is anticipated to reduce hypothalamic-pituitary-adrenal (HPA) axis feedback sensitivity. Moreover the glucocorticoid excess may drive, at least in part, the hypertension and hyperglycemia observed in such prenatal programming models. Maternal undernutrition also lowers placental 11β-HSD2 and alters adult offspring metabolic, cardiovascular, and HPA axis function, suggesting that HPA programming may be a common outcome of prenatal environmental challenge. Overexposure to glucocorticoids *in utero* also leads to alterations in adult behavior to produce a phenotype reminiscent of anxiety. Prenatal glucocorticoid exposure also affects the developing dopaminergic system with clear implications for proposed developmental contributions to schizo-affective, attention-deficit hyperactivity and extrapyramidal disorders. Mechanistically, prenatal dexamethasone or 11β-HSD inhibition increases corticotropin-releasing hormone (CRH) mRNA levels specifically in the central nucleus of the amygdala, a key locus for the effects of the neuropeptide on the expression of fear and anxiety. Intriguingly, fetoplacental 11β-HSD inhibition also permanently increases GR and MR in the offspring amygdala. A direct relationship between brain GR levels and anxiety behaviors is supported by transgenic mice with selective loss of GR in the forebrain, which exhibit reduced fearfulness.

Intriguingly, low-birth-weight humans also exhibit HPA hyperactivity in adult life.

11β-Hydroxysteroid Dehydrogenase Type 1 in the Brain

So what was the role of Monder's original 11β-HSD (type 1), highly expressed in liver, adipose tissue and the brain? Studies in intact cells from liver, fat, lung, and other sites have shown that 11β-HSD1, although bidirectional in tissue homogenates, is a predominant 11β-ketoreductase in intact cells. This reaction regenerates active glucocorticoids from inert 11-keto forms. A similar directional predominance is seen in the intact liver *ex vivo* and in rodents and humans *in vivo*. In the brain, 11β-HSD1-like immunoreactivity and mRNA are widespread. Fetal rat hippocampal cells in culture express 11β-HSD1 but no 11β-HSD2. Intact hippocampal cells show only 11β-reductase activity. This reaction direction increases intracellular glucocorticoid levels. In searching for functions, it was noted that licorice-derived 11β-HSD inhibitors given to rats alter hypothalamic secretagogs in pituitary portal blood *in vivo* and activate a series of regions of the CNS, including the hippocampus, a key glucocorticoid target with high GR and MR density where glucocorticoids act to suppress HPA activity and to modulate cognitive functions.

11β-Hydroxysteroid Dehydrogenase Type 1 and the Hypothalamic-Pituitary-Adrenal Axis

11β-HSD1 is expressed in the hippocampus, paraventricular nucleus of the hypothalamus (PVN) and pituitary, key sites of glucocorticoid negative feedback. 11β-HSD1 knockout (11β-HSD1$^{-/-}$) mice have hypertrophied adrenals and elevated basal adrenocorticotropic hormone (ACTH) and corticosterone levels at the nadir of the rhythm. These effects are compatible with the requirement for increased glucocorticoid production from the adrenal cortex in this mouse secondary to increased metabolic clearance of corticosterone because of the lack of glucocorticoid regeneration, notably in the liver. Unexpectedly, basal plasma corticosterone levels are also elevated in 11β-HSD1$^{-/-}$ mice, suggesting reduced glucocorticoid feedback on the HPA axis and increased forward drive on the HPA system. Altered central drive is rather unlikely because CRH mRNA levels in the PVN are unaltered. In contrast, some findings suggest that 11β-HSD1$^{-/-}$ mice have attenuated negative feedback because they show less suppression of corticosterone to exogenous cortisol 2 h prior to restraint stress. Interestingly, recent data show that obese Zucker rats have reduced 11β-HSD1 in the hippocampus, which may explain why this strain has reduced HPA feedback sensitivity and hence has increased corticosterone levels. Altered brain 11β-HSD1 has been reported in pregnancy, when the HPA axis becomes refractory to stressful stimulation. Interestingly, 11β-HSD1 activity is selectively increased in the PVN in pregnancy, so locally increased 11β-HSD1 may further amplify glucocorticoid feedback and hence attenuate HPA activity.

11β-Hydroxysteroid Dehydrogenase Type 1 and Brain Aging

A subgroup of aged rodents and humans shows the association of cognitive decline with a chronic elevation of plasma corticosterone levels. If glucocorticoids are maintained at low levels in rats, by adrenalectomy and low-dose corticosterone replacement, age-related impairments are reduced. The hippocampus requires glucocorticoids for neuronal function and survival but is especially vulnerable to the adverse effects of chronic glucocorticoid excess, which causes atrophy of dendrites and cognitive dysfunction. Therefore, chronic glucocorticoid overexposure has been implicated in the pathogenesis of age-related decline in hippocampus-associated cognitive functions.

In primary cultures of hippocampal cells, 11β-HSD1 potentiates kainic acid-induced neurotoxicity, not only by corticosterone but equally by intrinsically inert 11-dehydrocorticosterone, an effect prevented by carbenoxolone. 11-Dehydrocorticosterone increases kainic acid hippocampal toxicity in vivo, an effect also blocked by carbenoxolone. Crucially, old 11β-HSD1$^{-/-}$ mice learn as well as young mice in hippocampus tasks and avoid the cognitive decline seen in the majority of aged wild-type mice. This cognitive protection in aged 11β-HSD1$^{-/-}$ mice is associated with reduced intrahippocampal corticosterone levels, indicating the potency of intracellular metabolism by 11β-HSDs in determining effective glucocorticoid action on target receptors. In situ hybridization studies in postmortem human brain material show high expression of 11β-HSD1 mRNA in the hippocampus, prefrontal cortex, and cerebellum, mirroring rodent findings. In two small randomized double-blind placebo-controlled cross-over studies, the administration of the 11β-HSD inhibitor carbenoxolone improved verbal fluency after 4 weeks in ten healthy elderly men and improved verbal memory after 6 weeks in 12 elderly patients with type 2 diabetes. Plasma cortisol was unaltered, suggesting that 11β-HSD1 does not modulate HPA axis feedback

in humans, at least at the morning peak. Intriguingly, 11β-HSD1 may play a role in pathogenesis because rare haplotypes of the HSD11B1 gene are associated with a risk of Alzheimer's disease.

Conclusion

11β-HSDs interconvert active glucocorticoids and inert 11-keto forms. This seemingly obscure reaction is important in peripheral tissues and the CNS, determining glucocorticoid access to nuclear receptors and hence biological effects in health and disease. 11β-HSD1 is an 11β-ketoreductase that amplifies intracellular glucocorticoid levels. Studies in 11β-HSD1$^{-/-}$ mice show a role in HPA feedback. Deficiency of 11β-HSD1 reduces intracerebral glucocorticoid levels and prevents the emergence of cognitive deficits with aging. 11β-HSD2 is a potent 11β-dehydrogenase, which is little expressed in the adult CNS but which plays an emerging role in preventing premature glucocorticoid actions on the developing nervous system. The maintenance of fetoplacental 11β-HSD2 and the inhibition of 11β-HSD1 have therapeutic potential.

Further Reading

De Kloet, E. R. (2004). Hormones and the stressed brain. Stress: current neuroendocrine and genetic approaches. Annals of the New York Academy of Sciences 1018, 1–15.

Diaz, R., Brown, R. W. and Seckl, J. R. (1998). Ontogeny of mRNAs encoding glucocorticoid and mineralocorticoid receptors and 11β-hydroxysteroid dehydrogenases in prenatal rat brain development reveal complex control of glucocorticoid action. Journal of Neuroscience 18, 2570–2580.

Edwards, C. R. W., Benediktsson, R., and Lindsay, R. (1993). Dysfunction of the placental glucocorticoid barrier: a link between the foetal environment and adult hypertension? Lancet 341, 355–357.

Harris, H. J. Kotelevtsev, Y. and Mullins, J. J. 2001. 11β-hydroxysteroid dehydrogenase type 1 null mice have altered hypothalamic-pituitary-adrenal axis activity: a novel control of glucocorticoid feedback. Endocrinology 142, 114–120.

Kotelevtsev, Y., Holmes, M. C. and Burchell, A. (1997). 11β-hydroxysteroid dehydrogenase type 1 knockout mice show attenuated glucocorticoid inducible responses and resist hyperglycaemia on obesity or stress. Proceedings of the National Academy of Sciences USA 94, 14924–14929.

Kotelevtsev, Y., Brown, R. W. and Fleming, S. (1999). Hypertension in mice lacking 11β-hydroxysteroid dehydrogenase type 2. Journal of Clinical Investigations 103, 683–689.

Liu, D., Dioria, J. and Tannenbaum, B. (1997). Maternal care, hippocampal glucocorticoid receptors, and hypothalamic-pituitary-adrenal responses to stress. *Science* **277**, 1659–1662.

Matthews, S. G. (2002). Early programming of the hypothalamo-pituitary-adrenal axis. *Trends in Endocrinology and Metabolism* **130**, 373–380.

McEwen, B. S. (1999). Stress and hippocampal plasticity. *Annual Review of Neuroscience* **22**, 105–122.

Moisan, M.-P., Seckl, J. R. and Edwards, C. R. W. (1990). 11β-hydroxysteroid dehydrogenase bioactivity and messenger RNA expression in rat forebrain: localization in hypothalamus, hippocampus and cortex. *Endocrinology* **127**, 1450–1455.

Mune, T., Rogerson, F. M. and Nikkilä, H. (1995). Human hypertension caused by mutations in the kidney isozyme of 11β-hydroxysteroid dehydrogenase. *Nature Genetics* **10**, 394–399.

Phillips, D. I. W., Walker, B. R. and Reynolds, R. M. (2000). Low birth weight predicts elevated plasma cortisol concentrations in adults from 3 populations. *Hypertension* **35**(6), 1301–1306.

Rajan, V., Edwards, C. R. W. and Seckl, J. R. (1996). 11β-hydroxysteroid dehydrogenase in cultured hippocampal cells reactivates inert 11-dehydrocorticosterone, potentiating neurotoxicity. *Journal of Neuroscience* **16**, 65–70.

Roland, B. L., Li, K. X. Z. and Funder, J. W. (1995). Hybridization histochemical localization of 11β-hydroxysteroid dehydrogenase type 2 in rat brain. *Endocrinology* **136**, 4697–4700.

Sandeep, T., Yau, J., MacCullich, A., et al. (2004). Effects of 11beta-hydroxysteroid dehydrogenase inhibition on cognitive function in healthy elderly men and patients with type 2 diabetes. *Proceedings of the National Academy of Sciences USA* **101**, 6734–6739.

Seckl, J. R. (2004). 11β-hydroxysteroid dehydrogenases: changing glucocorticoid action. *Current Opinions in Pharmacology* **4**, 597–602.

Seckl, J. R. (2004). Prenatal glucocorticoids and long-term programming. *European Journal of Endocrinology* **151**, U49–U62.

Seckl, J. R. and Walker, B. R. (2004). 11beta-hydroxysteroid dehydrogenase type 1 as a modulator of glucocorticoid action: from metabolism to memory. *Trends in Endocrinology and Metabolism* **15**, 418–424.

Stewart, P. M. and Krozowski, Z. S. (1999). 11 beta-hydroxysteroid dehydrogenase. *Vitamins and Hormones* **57**, 249–324.

Weaver, I., Cervoni, N., Champagne, F., et al. (2004). Epigenetic programming by maternal behavior. *Nature Neuroscience* **7**, 847–854.

Welberg, L. A. M., Seckl, J. R. and Holmes, M. C. (2000). Inhibition of 11β-hydroxysteroid dehydrogenase, the feto-placental barrier to maternal glucocorticoids, permanently programs amygdala glucocorticoid receptor mRNA expression and anxiety-like behavior in the offspring. *European Journal of Neuroscience* **12**, 1047–1054.

Yau, J. L. W., Noble, J., Kenyon, C. J., et al. (2001). Lack of tissue glucocorticoid reactivation in 11β-hydroxysteroid dehydrogenase type 1 knockout mice ameliorates age-related learning impairments. *Proceedings of the National Academy of Sciences USA* **98**, 4716–4721.

Hyperreactivity (Cardiovascular)

A Georgiades
Duke University Medical Center, Durham, NC, USA

This article is a revision of the previous edition article by A Georgiades and M Fredrikson, volume 2, pp 421–424, © 2000, Elsevier Inc.

Cardiovascular Reactivity and Disease
Physiological Parameters
Assessments
Stress Tasks
Stability
Generalizability
Risk Factors and Hyperreactivity
Conclusion

Glossary

Blood pressure (BP)	The pressure of the circulating blood on the walls of the arteries and veins. BP is usually measured with a sphygmomanometer in millimeters of mercury (mmHg).
Coronary heart disease (CHD)	A disease associated with insufficient blood flow to the heart muscle, including myocardial infarction and angina pectoris.
Diastolic blood pressure (DBP)	The lowest BP within a cardiac cycle.
Hypertension	Elevated levels of arterial BP. According to Joint National Committee criteria of 2003, hypertension is systolic blood pressure levels over 140 and/or DBP levels over 90. Individuals in the prehypertensive range of 130–139 and/or 80–89 are at twice the risk of developing

	hypertension compared to those with lower values.
Mental stress testing	A method used to elicit cardiovascular stress reactivity in a laboratory setting through the administration of engaging, challenging, or aversive stimuli (stressors).
Risk factor	An attribute of individuals that is associated with an increased likelihood for developing a specific disease compared to individuals without the attribute.
Systolic blood pressure (SBP)	The peak blood pressure within a cardiac cycle.

Cardiovascular reactivity is defined as an individual's propensity to display cardiovascular reactions of greater or lesser magnitude compared to a baseline value when encountering stimuli or situations experienced as engaging, challenging, or aversive.

Cardiovascular Reactivity and Disease

It has been suggested that exaggerated cardiovascular reactivity plays an etiological role in cardiovascular disorders such as hypertension and CHD. Folkow suggested that the repeated elicitation of the defense reaction, which is associated with enhanced BP and heart rate (HR), translates into sustained hypertension by causing vascular hypertrophy in genetically susceptible or hyperreactive individuals. Because the normal outlet of the defense reaction (physical work) is inhibited during psychological stress, disruption of bodily homeostasis occurs. Through the repeated surges in arterial pressure and overperfusion of inactive muscles, lasting changes of the peripheral vascular resistance and a resetting of the baroreceptor set point may occur. Stress may further hamper adequate BP regulation by increasing renal vascular resistance, causing antinatriuresis with sodium retention, a decrease in the glomelural filtration rate, and the stimulation of renin release. Thus, it has been proposed that the development of high BP is stress-related.

Cardiovascular hyperreactivity has also been linked to the occurrence of CHD events. It has been hypothesized that exaggerated BP responses can cause endothelial injury, leading to accumulating atheroma, increasing the risk for cardiac arrhythmia. The adverse effects of stress are believed to be mediated by the autonomic nervous system, mainly enhanced sympathetic activity and subsequent physiological responses. For example, high plasma levels of norepinephrine and epinephrine that are associated with hyperreactivity may, in combination with cortisol, be toxic to the coronary vasculature, constituting an additional mechanism mediating the adverse effects of stress on the cardiovascular system.

A number of cross-sectional studies show that cardiovascular hyperreactivity is more prominent among individuals at an increased risk of developing hypertension and CHD. In addition, mental stress is a potent trigger of myocardial ischemia both in the laboratory and in the ambulatory state among cardiac patients. Also, results from prospective studies show that cardiovascular reactivity may be a risk factor in cardiovascular disease progression. Although the evidence is not conclusive, studies have found that cardiovascular responses to standardized mental stress testing can predict the development of hypertension, left ventricular mass, and atherosclerosis. Excessive BP increases during exercise have also been suggested as a marker of future hypertension and to be associated with an increased risk of cardiovascular mortality.

Because growing evidence suggests that exaggerated cardiovascular responses are a risk factor or marker for the development of cardiovascular disease, research on cardiovascular stress reactivity has focused on characterizing the determinants of hyperreactivity and identifying possible ways of modifying it.

Physiological Parameters

The most commonly measured variables during mental stress reactivity testing are BP and HR. In general, noninvasive BP measurements during laboratory testing require multiple measurements made at frequent intervals (e.g., every 1–2 min). Automatic or semiautomatic devices are preferred, using a variety of available methods, such as Korotkoff sounds, oscillometry, and ultrasound.

HR recordings are usually derived from interbeat interval information available from recording the electrocardiogram (EKG) via electrodes adhered to the chest. Automated BP monitors often include measurements of HR from either EKG signals or arterial pulse detection. Holter monitoring records the EKG waveform over 24 h and involves several algorithms to describe patterns associated with the underperfusion of the heart muscle.

For continuous noninvasive BP monitoring, spectral analysis can be used, allowing the computation of short-term BP variability and baroreflex sensitivity. Newer noninvasive techniques such as impedance cardiography make it possible to document a more complete hemodynamic pattern of the stress response, including measurements of cardiac contractility, cardiac output, and vascular resistance. These measures add important new information to the area of cardiovascular reactivity research.

Assessments

Reactivity testing in the laboratory typically consists of an initial rest (baseline) period followed by a period during which the subject is exposed to a stressor. During baseline, the individual should be stimulated minimally by external events, that is, be in a relaxed state. Reactivity is quantified as a change score, calculated as the difference between resting baseline levels and mean or peak levels during stress. To increase reliability, two or more measurements should be taken and averaged for each condition. Because reactivity scores are sometimes correlated with baseline levels, residualized change scores may be calculated to eliminate baseline effects on the calculated change scores.

Stress Tasks

Stimuli (stressors) used in laboratory stress testing have different characteristics. One distinction is made between psychological stressors and physical stressors. Some widely used and well-characterized psychological stressors with emotional and/or cognitive challenging components are mental arithmetic, mirror tracing, anger interview, public speech, video games, and the Stroop test. Physical stressors commonly used are isometric handgrip, dynamic exercise, and the cold pressor test. Another distinction has been made between passive and active tasks, with the cold pressor being an example of the former and mental arithmetic an example of the latter. In addition, various stressors elicit different hemodynamic patterns, reflecting β- or α-adrenergic receptor activity. For example, cold pressor predominantly activates α receptors, whereas mental arithmetic is considered to be a β-adrenergic task.

Stability

Because there are profound individual differences in both the magnitude and the patterning of cardiovascular responses to stress, it is of importance to establish the stability of the response magnitude and patterning to a given stressor. Numerous studies suggest the BP and HR reactivity show acceptable test–retest reproducibility measured over both the short and long term. In general, the highest stability coefficients have been found for SBP and HR levels and for SBP and HR reactivity scores during standardized mental stress testing, with a somewhat lower stability for DBP levels and reactivity scores. Studies also indicate that the higher test reliability can be achieved by aggregating measurements across multiple stimuli and by aggregating over multiple tasks administrated on multiple occasions. Thus, evidence suggests that BP and HR reactivity in the laboratory constitute a stable individual trait.

Generalizability

The reactivity definition discussed so far refers to individual differences in the response magnitude to a given stimulus on a particular occasion. The underlying assumption is that hyperreactivity to laboratory stressors is a generalized individual propensity and that the individual response pattern elicited by laboratory-induced stress can be generalized to responses in the natural setting during encounters with everyday stress. Noninvasive ambulatory blood pressure (ABP) monitoring provides the opportunity to study the relationship between cardiovascular responses in the laboratory and in natural settings, and several studies have examined the relationship between cardiovascular measurements in the laboratory and during everyday life using automated ABP recordings. Most studies have found a strong positive relationship between ABP levels and laboratory BP levels, whereas the relationship between laboratory-induced BP reactivity and ambulatory levels or variability seems less consistent.

Risk Factors and Hyperreactivity

A number of cross-sectional data show that cardiovascular hyperreactivity is more prominent among individuals at an increased risk of developing hypertension and CHD. Individual differences in cardiovascular reactivity to stress are, in part, mediated genetically. Also, male gender, family history of CHD, borderline hypertension, African American ethnicity, and type A behavior and depression have all been associated with an increased risk for CHD, and these high-risk group have independently shown exaggerated cardiovascular reactivity in several studies. In addition, smoking status, serum cholesterol levels, fasting insulin levels, left ventricular hypertrophy, and carotic artery atherosclerosis are all important independent risk factors for cardiovascular disease. A number of studies have investigated the relationship between these risk factors and cardiovascular hyperreactivity.

1. Gender. Sex differences exist in resting baseline and HR levels, with women having higher HR and men, in general, having higher BP levels (until the age of 60). In general, men are more SBP reactive than women, whereas there are small or no differences in DBP reactivity. Studies on HR reactivity are inconsistent, with men and women having an equal likelihood of displaying augmented HR reactivity.

2. Hypertension. In a meta-analysis of published reactivity studies related to hypertension, it was concluded that the majority of studies have shown that individuals with a positive family history of hypertension and individuals with borderline hypertension display enhanced BP reactivity compared to individuals without a family history of hypertension and to normotensive controls.

3. Ethnicity. African Americans have enhanced cardiovascular hyperreactivity compared to Caucasians. Studies also show that African Americans display increased total peripheral resistance during mental stress testing in the laboratory compared to Caucasians.

4. Type A behavior. Individuals with type A behavior (i.e., showing enhanced hostility, time urge, and competitiveness) have increased sympathetically mediated reactivity compared to type B individuals. It has been suggested that it is the hostility component in the type A behavior pattern that is most closely related to enhanced cardiovascular reactivity.

5. Depression. Accumulating evidence show that depressive symptoms are related to cardiovascular morbidity and mortality. Studies evaluating the association between depression and hyperreactivity have so far only shown moderate support for a link between depressive symptoms and enhanced cardiovascular reactivity.

6. Smoking. Evidence is accumulating that smoking, in combination with psychological stress, may be particularly harmful, both because smoking increases in stressful situations and because the cardiovascular effects of smoking combined with those of psychological stress may be synergistic. Nicotine itself has acute effects on the activity of the cardiovascular system, leading to an increase of both BP and HR, but smoking status per se (being a smoker or a nonsmoker) does not seem to affect the magnitude of the stress response. Nicotine administration has been found to enhance HR reactivity, but there is no conclusive evidence that nicotine enhances cardiovascular reactivity in general.

7. Lipids. Several studies have reported an association between serum lipid levels and cardiovascular reactivity to laboratory stressors, but findings are equivocal. Associations have been found to be lower or completely absent in youngsters but evident among older adults, which suggests an age-dependent association. Some evidence suggests that an enhanced cardiac responsiveness is associated positively with low-density lipoprotein levels but is related inversely with high-density lipoproteins.

8. Insulin resistance. Insulin resistance is part of the metabolic syndrome associated with hypertension and cardiovascular alternations. One mechanism through which insulin may be linked to hypertension is through the stimulation of sympathetic nervous activity. Thus, insulin concentrations may be correlated with indices of sympathetic activity such as hyperreactivity even before it affects resting BP. Fasting insulin concentrations have been associated with cardiovascular reactivity to exercise. There are also studies indicating that insulin resistance may be more closely related to BP levels during mental stress testing than during rest.

9. Left ventricular mass. Left ventricular hypertrophy is an important target-organ consequence of hypertension and an independent risk factor for cardiovascular morbidity and mortality. Several studies have shown that left ventricular mass is poorly related to casual clinic BP levels, whereas some studies have shown stronger associations to daytime ambulatory BP levels and variability and to BP levels during mental stress testing. Left ventricular mass (index) has also been found to be associated with a vasoconstrictive response pattern among children and adolescents. A few studies have found cardiovascular reactivity to predict the development of left ventricular mass over time. However, further evidence is needed to establish the association between stress-induced cardiovascular reactivity and left ventricular mass.

10. Atherosclerosis. Carotic intima-media thickness is an important preclinical measure of atherosclerotic vascular disease and has been strongly associated with the development of CHD. BP responses to mental stress have been found to be associated to intima-media thickness as well as plack height. Although studies have also shown reactivity to mental stress to be prospectively related to intima-media thickness, further evidence is required to establish the relationship between cardiovascular hyperreactivity and atherosclerosis.

11. Inflammation. Atherosclerosis is considered an inflammatory disease. In the atherosclerotic process, proinflammatory cytokines, derived from excess adipose tissue, increase the expression of adhesion molecules that promote the sticking of blood leukocytes to the inner surface of the arterial wall. Recent studies report that acute psychological stress in humans significantly increases the serum concentrations of proinflammatory cytokines such as interleukin-6 (IL-6) and the IL-1 receptor antagonist (IL-1Ra), suggesting that stress reactivity may affect the atherosclerotic process by eliciting an activation of the inflammatory response system.

Conclusion

Cardiovascular hyperreactivity is associated with several risk factors for cardiovascular morbidity and mortality, and, although the mechanisms are not fully established, there is evidence suggesting that heightened cardiovascular reactivity may independently contribute to the development of CHD and hypertension.

See Also the Following Articles

Ambulatory Blood Pressure; Beta-Adrenergic Blockers; Cardiovascular System and Stress; Heart Disease/ Attack; Heart Rate; Hypertension; Type A Personality, Type B Personality.

Further Reading

Folkow, B. S. (1982). Physiological aspects of primary hypertension. *Physiological Reviews* **62**, 374–504.

Fredrikson, M. and Matthews, K. A. (1990). Cardiovascular responses to behavioral stress and hypertension: a meta analytic review. *Annals of Behavioral Medicine* **12**, 17–29.

Kamarck, T. W. and Lovallo, W. R. (2003). Cardiovascular reactivity to psychological challenge: conceptual and measurement considerations. *Psychosomatic Medicine* **65**, 9–21.

Linden, W., Gerin, W. and Davidson, K. (2003). Cardiovascular reactivity: status quo and a research agenda for the new millennium. *Psychosomatic Medicine* **65**, 5–8.

Lovallo, W. R. and Gerin, W. (2003). Psychophysiological reactivity: mechanisms and pathways to cardiovascular disease. *Psychosomatic Medicine* **65**, 36–45.

Schneiderman, N., Weiss, S. M. and Kaufmann, P. G. (1989). *Handbook of research methods in cardiovascular behavioral medicine*. New York: Plenum Press.

Schwartz, A. R., Gerin, W., Davidson, K. W., et al. (2003). Toward a causal model of cardiovascular responses to stress and the development of cardiovascular disease. *Psychosomatic Medicine* **65**, 22–35.

Steptoe, A., Ruddel, H. and Neus, H. (1985). *Clinical and methodological issues in cardiovascular psychophysiology*. New York: Springer-Verlags.

Treiber, F. A., Kamarck, T., Schneiderman, N., et al. (2003). Cardiovascular reactivity and development of preclinical and clinical disease states. *Psychosomatic Medicine* **65**, 46–62.

Turner, J. R. (1994). *Cardiovascular reactivity and stress: patterns of physiological response*. New York: Plenum Press.

Hypertension

A Steptoe
University College London, London, UK

This article is a revision of the previous edition article by A Steptoe, volume 2, pp 425–430, © 2000, Elsevier Inc.

Prevalence
Etiological Factors
Experimental Evidence
Psychological Characteristics
Lifestyle and Adverse Life Experience
Stress Management and Quality of Life

Glossary

White-coat hypertension	Blood pressure that is elevated when measured in the clinic by a physician or nurse but normal when measured in other situations.
Hypertension	Sustained elevated blood pressure.
Left ventricular hypertrophy	The enlargement of the left ventricle of the heart, one of the adverse effects of hypertension.
Normotension	Blood pressure below the criteria for hypertension.

Prevalence

Hypertension is the condition of sustained elevated arterial blood pressure. The criteria for defining hypertension are somewhat arbitrary because the distribution of blood pressure level in the population is continuous. The current definition of hypertension is a systolic blood pressure ≥ 140 mmHg and diastolic pressure ≥ 90 mmHg. Most authorities regard a blood pressure in the range 130–139/85–89 mmHg as high-normal, although the Joint National Committee on Prevention, Detection, Evaluation, and Treatment of High Blood Pressure has defined levels of 120–139/80–89 mmHg as prehypertensive. Risk of coronary heart disease and stroke is directly related to blood pressure level, so hypertension defines those individuals who are at an especially elevated risk.

The prevalence of hypertension in the United States is approximately 29% in men and 30.5% in women. Recent figures from the United Kingdom indicate that approximately 37% of men and 34% of women are hypertensive. However, blood pressure tends to rise with age, so these overall figures disguise the substantial increase in hypertension in middle age. Thus, in the United States, the prevalence rises from 8.1% in men and 2.7% in women ages 20–34 years to 44.9% and 53.9% in those ages 55–64 years. There are also striking ethnic variations, with high rates in African Americans and in African Caribbean people in the United Kingdom.

Between one-third and one-half of hypertensives are not diagnosed and are unaware of their condition. Because hypertension is not consistently associated with symptoms, it is frequently identified only during routine screening, so it may continue for many years before detection. The number of diagnosed hypertensives who are not treated is substantial, whereas as many as 50% of patients who are prescribed antihypertensive medication do not have their blood pressure controlled adequately. The problem of hypertension is therefore considerable.

Etiological Factors

The etiology of hypertension is complicated. In a minority of cases, high blood pressure is associated with a specific pathological abnormality such as pheochromocytoma or a renovascular disorder. However, in most cases there is no single identifiable cause, and the condition is regarded as multifactorial. This condition was once known as essential hypertension because an elevated pressure was considered necessary to drive blood through partially blocked arteries. Now, cases without a single cause are sometimes called primary hypertensives to distinguish them from individuals whose hypertension is secondary to another disease. Hypertension typically develops over many years, with blood pressure gradually increasing until it reaches threatening levels. The most consistent predictors of future hypertension are a positive family history, a blood pressure in childhood or early adult life that is above average, and elevated body weight. High salt and alcohol intake also contribute.

The primary reason for considering stress to be an etiologic factor relates to the influence of the autonomic nervous system and neuroendocrine factors in hypertension. There is clear evidence of increased sympathetic nervous system activity in hypertension, as documented through raised levels of plasma norepinephrine. Microneurographic studies have shown elevated sympathetic nervous traffic to muscle. Hypothalamic activation may be responsible for these sympathetic responses, which in turn lead to inhibition of baroreceptor reflex sensitivity, peripheral vasoconstriction, and alterations of renal blood flow. Reduced parasympathetic activity may also be associated with the etiology of hypertension, together with the impairment of opioid-mediated counterregulatory processes. Abnormalities of adrenocortical function have been described in some cases of hypertension, and pro-inflammatory processes may contribute as well.

The hypothesis underlying much research on this topic is that the stress-induced activation of sympathetic and other pathways occurs repeatedly over months and years in susceptible individuals, leading to hemodynamic adjustments that increase hypertension risk. Evidence relevant to this hypothesis derives from several sources, including animal and human experimental studies and investigations of the impact of adverse life experiences, chronic stressors, and psychological characteristics.

Experimental Evidence

Animal Studies

Evidence that permanently elevated blood pressure can be produced with behavioral stress in animals is controversial. Although it is clear that acute hypertensive episodes can be induced, the development of sustained hypertension is more elusive. Aversive conditions such as restraint stress, unpredictable shock, and approach–avoidance conflict produce chronic hypertension in some studies but not others. Effects vary across species and are more prominent in the presence of risk factors such as a genetic predisposition and heightened salt sensitivity. Some of the most compelling evidence comes from studies carried out by Henry and co-workers on the effects of social conflict in CBA mice. Male mice raised in isolation were placed in complex colonies that encouraged conflict. There were immediate blood pressure increases that reverted to control levels after their removal from the colony. However, irreversible hypertension developed with prolonged exposure to conflict, accompanied by alterations in catecholamine synthesis and myocardial fibrosis and degeneration. Species differences are apparent in primates as well, although hypertension can be induced by prolonged shock avoidance in rhesus monkeys.

Cardiovascular Reactivity to Acute Behavioral Stress in Humans

Blood pressure increases acutely in response to a variety of behavioral stressors in humans, ranging from problem-solving tasks and emotionally laden interviews to painful stimuli such as the cold pressor test. The increase in blood pressure is typically accompanied by tachycardia, inotropic stimulation of the heart, vasodilatation in skeletal muscle and adipose tissue, and reduced blood flow to the kidneys, skin, and viscera.

The issue of whether these responses are involved in hypertension has been the subject of much research, stimulated in the 1950s by Jan Brod. Compared with normotensives, hypertensives typically show enhanced blood pressure responses to acute behavioral stress, accompanied by greater renal vasoconstriction and increased norepinephrine turnover. However, it is possible that this exaggerated cardiovascular responsivity is the result of the complex physiological adjustments that occur in hypertension and is not primary. Attention has therefore shifted to people with normal blood pressure who are at increased risk, for example, because of genetic factors. Results have again been variable, but a meta-analysis of this literature suggests that a proportion of people with a positive family history of hypertension are more reactive to tasks involving active behavioral responses (e.g., difficult problem solving) than are those without family histories. Young people with positive family histories may also have elevated blood pressure during their everyday lives, as assessed using automated ambulatory monitoring techniques.

Longitudinal studies have also been reported, testing the hypothesis that high reactivity to behavioral stress predicts future rises in blood pressure over 5–10 years. Most trials have found evidence in favor of this hypothesis. Impaired poststress recovery in blood pressure has also been shown to predict future increases. But such effects are not always observed, probably for two reasons. First, the investigation of acute responses to behavioral stress is complex and requires the careful standardization of procedures. Different types of stimuli elicit different patterns of physiological response. For instance, some tasks such as mental arithmetic elicit blood pressure responses that are primarily sustained through increased myocardial contractility and cardiac output, whereas others predominantly elicit increases in peripheral vascular resistance. These response profiles may not all be equally relevant to hypertension. Second, the nature of the hypothesized relationship between stress responsivity and hypertension should be considered. **Figure 1** outlines the presumed sequence of events. Heightened cardiovascular responses to acute stress *per se* will not increase the risk of hypertension. Such responses are relevant only if they are representative of the individual's experience during daily life. Stress-related factors are most likely to contribute to hypertension if reactive individuals are exposed over months or years to environments that elicit damaging patterns of intense response. This interaction has only

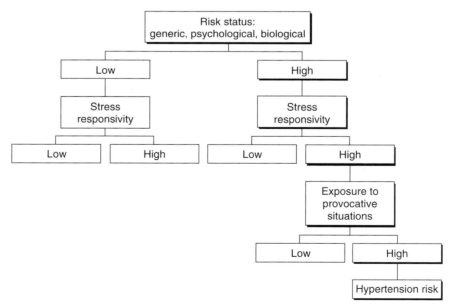

Figure 1 Schematic outline of the way in which acute cardiovascular and neuroendocrine stress responsivity might contribute to hypertension risk. Highlighted boxes indicate the highest risk group. The combination of high risk status, high stress responsiveness, and prolonged exposure to situations that provoke appropriate physiological responses is necessary.

been evaluated in a few studies to date. It should also be kept in mind that stress is only one of many factors contributing to hypertension and does not affect all those at risk in the same fashion.

Psychological Characteristics

The many comparisons that have been made between hypertensive patients and controls in terms of personality typically suffer from two limitations. First, the diagnostic label of hypertension may cause psychological distress and lead to changes on psychological tests. Second, because much hypertension is not diagnosed, any differences observed may be restricted to those who seek medical attention. Population-based studies involving measurements of blood pressure and psychological factors are therefore required.

Some population studies have shown prospective associations between tension or anxiety and future hypertension, but effects are small and inconsistent. A more persuasive body of evidence has linked hypertension with the ways that people cope with angry and hostile feelings. This notion was stimulated in the mid-1970s by research on hypertension and urban stress in Detroit. It was found that hypertension was more prevalent and that blood pressure was generally higher among black men living in high-stress areas (defined by population density, crime rate, and family instability) who also inhibited anger expression. Subsequent research has supported the link between anger inhibition and high blood pressure in a number of populations. However, it has also been found that the expression of anger is related to blood pressure, so perhaps the appropriateness of anger display and hostility management is more critical.

Hypertension is associated with mild deficits of cognitive function, as assessed by measures of memory, attention, and abstract reasoning. These effects vary with age, education, and whether blood pressure is being treated. The extent to which these impairments affect the performance of daily activities is not known. They may be the result of central nervous system neurophysiological sequelae of high blood pressure.

Lifestyle and Adverse Life Experience

What types of real-life stressful experience are likely to be associated with hypertension? If the inferences from laboratory studies are correct, they are experiences that are repeated or sustained over years and elicit active efforts to cope and maintain control. Acute traumatic events would not be expected to stimulate appropriate long-term cardiovascular and neuroendocrine responses, and indeed there is little

evidence that acute life events are associated with the development of hypertension. In contrast, some forms of chronic stress are associated with sustained increases in blood pressure. Experiences such as caring for demented relatives, marital conflict, and the experience of racism in ethnic minorities have been related to increased blood pressure. Interesting results have emerged from studies of migrants from traditional, isolated, rural cultures to modernized, developing and developed societies. For example, increases in blood pressure have been recorded among young adults from the Luo tribe in western Kenya who migrated to Nairobi. The blood pressure rise was associated with a higher salt intake and greater body weight, but stress-related increases in the sympathetic nervous stimulation may also have been involved. Similarly, studies of migrants from the isolated Pacific Tokelau islands to New Zealand have shown that blood pressure increases are greater among those who establish extensive contact with non-Tokelauans compared with individuals who maintain traditional ethnic affiliations.

Blood pressure has been shown in several studies to be associated inversely with the size of social networks and the extent of social support. A striking illustration of the protective effects of a tranquil lifestyle and supportive environment is illustrated in **Figure 2**. This shows results from a long-term study of Italian nuns in a secluded order compared with nonsmoking, age-matched women living in local communities. It can be seen that the typical age-related increases in blood pressure were attenuated among the nuns, which was coupled with a significantly lower incidence of fatal and nonfatal cardiac events.

Work and Hypertension

Some types of work might be expected to have the characteristics that would lead to acute stress-induced increases in blood pressure and sympathetic activation, thereby heightening the risk of hypertension. An important early study by Cobb and Rose of air traffic controllers demonstrated an increased incidence and earlier onset of hypertension among men working in this highly demanding occupation compared with controls. Subsequently, an automated ambulatory recording apparatus has been used to measure blood pressure repeatedly as people go about their everyday lives. Blood pressure is typically higher at work than at home, and it is elevated in people who work in high-demand, low-control jobs. For instance, in the Work Site Blood Pressure Study in New York City, job strain (high demand, low control) was an independent predictor of hypertension after controlling for age, body mass index, type A behavior, 24-h sodium

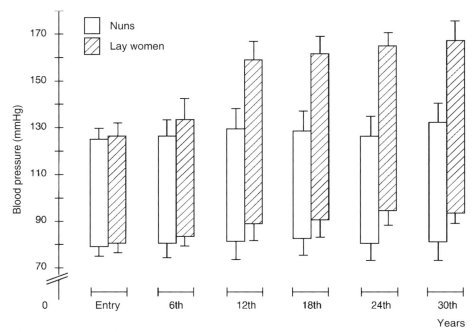

Figure 2 Results from a 30-year longitudinal study of 144 nuns from a secluded Catholic order and 138 age-matched nonsmoking women from the local community. The absence of age-related increases in blood pressure in the nuns is clear. Reproduced with permission from Timio et al. (1997). Blood pressure trend and cardiovascular events in nuns in a secluded order: a 30-year follow-up study. *Blood Pressure* **6**, 81–87. © Scandinavian University Press.

excretion, physical activity at work, education, smoking, and alcohol consumption. Longitudinally, individuals exposed to more years of high job strain had higher blood pressure. This is consistent with the evidence that lack of control over challenging situations is associated with heightened physiological activation.

White-Coat Hypertension

White-coat hypertension is the phenomenon of transiently raised blood pressure during measurement in the clinic by a physician or nurse compared with blood pressure as recorded at home or using an ambulatory recording apparatus. The definition of white-coat hypertension is somewhat arbitrary, but one study found that 20% of patients referred with a diagnosis of hypertension, whose diastolic pressure remained in the range of 90–104 mmHg on several occasions in the clinic, were normotensive during ambulatory monitoring. The phenomenon is clearly stress-related, in that it is dependent on physiological responses to the threatening clinical situation. People who exhibit white-coat effects do not have unusual psychological profiles, but do show heightened blood pressure responses to stressful behavioral tasks. There is also limited evidence that white-coat hypertension is associated with the secondary effects of hypertension such as left ventricular hypertrophy. However,

the boundaries and the significance of the problem remain poorly understood.

Stress Management and Quality of Life

Despite research over the past quarter of a century, the use of stress management in hypertension remains controversial. A number of well-controlled trials have shown that stress management involving relaxation training (sometimes accompanied by biofeedback) can reduce the blood pressure and medication needs of hypertensives. Problems have arisen, however, in establishing genuine pretreatment levels of blood pressure against which to measure the effects of stress management. Blood pressure may fall progressively with repeated measurement due to adaptation and the habituation of white-coat effects, and these phenomena may be confused with the effects of stress management. The evidence for specific techniques such as transcendental meditation reducing the blood pressure of hypertensives is inconclusive.

The pharmacological treatment of hypertension is a complex and continuously developing field. Older treatments, such as β-adrenergic blockade and diuretics, have been joined by calcium antagonists and angiotensin-converting enzyme inhibitors. Some hypertensive medications have side effects that lead to impairments in the health-related quality of life. Stress management may play a role in particular types of cases. One is the individual whose blood pressure is only mildly elevated (e.g., 170/100 mmHg), who might be able to reduce blood pressure without recourse to lifetime medication. The second is the established hypertensive who is already medicated but who wishes to try alternative methods to reduce drug intake or because their blood pressure is poorly controlled. Other behavior changes also benefit hypertensives, including weight loss, increased physical exercise, and restriction of salt and alcohol intake. Stress management should therefore be applied in the context of these other aspects of behavior modification.

See Also the Following Articles

Ambulatory Blood Pressure; Control and Stress; Demand–Control Model; Hypotension, Hypovolemia, and Septic Shock; Metabolic Syndrome and Stress; Stress Management and Cardiovascular Disease; War Stress in the Former Yugoslavia.

Further Reading

Chobanian, A. V., Bakris, G. L., Black, H. R., et al. (2003). The seventh report of the Joint National Committee on Prevention, Detection, Evaluation, and Treatment of High Blood Pressure: the JNC 7 report. *Journal of the American Medical Association* **289**, 2560–2572.

Eisenberg, D. M., Delbanco, T. L., Berkey, C. S., et al. (1993). Cognitive behavioral techniques for hypertension: are they effective? *Annals of Internal Medicine* **118**, 964–972.

Henry, J. P. and Stephens, P. M. (1977). *Stress, health, and the social environment.* New York: Springer-Verlag.

Muldoon, M. F., Terrell, D. F., Bunker, C. H., et al. (1993). Family history studies in hypertension research: review of the literature. *American Journal of Hypertension* **6**, 76–88.

Pickering, T. G., James, G. D., Boddie, C., et al. (1988). How common is white coat hypertension? *Journal of the American Medical Association* **259**, 225–228.

Rutledge, T. and Hogan, B. E. (2002). A quantitative review of prospective evidence linking psychological factors with hypertension development. *Psychosomatic Medicine* **64**, 758–766.

Steptoe, A. (1997). Behavior and blood pressure: implications for hypertension. In: Zanchetti, A. & Mancia, G. (eds.) *Handbook of hypertension – pathophysiology of hypertension*, pp. 674–708. Amsterdam: Elsevier Science.

Timio, M., Lippi, G., Venanzi, S., et al. (1997). Blood pressure trend and cardiovascular events in nuns in a secluded order: a 30-year follow-up study. *Blood Pressure* **6**, 81–87.

Waldstein, S. R. and Elias, M. F. (2001). *Neuropsychology of cardiovascular disease.* Mahwah, NJ: Lawrence Erlbaum.

Williams, D. R., Neighbors, H. W. and Jackson, J. S. (2003). Racial/ethnic discrimination and health: findings from community studies. *American Journal of Public Health* **93**, 200–208.

Hyperthermia

J Roth
University of Giessen, Giessen, Germany

This article is a revision of the previous edition article by J Roth, volume 2, pp 431–438, © 2000, Elsevier Inc.

Thermal Balance and Body Temperature
Physiological Responses to Heat Stress
Brain Function in Hyperthermia
Adaptation to Heat
Malignant Hyperthermia

Glossary

Adaptation	A change that reduces the physiological strain produced by stressful components of the total environment. This change may occur within the lifetime of an organism (phenotypic) or be the result of genetic selection in a species (genotypic).
Conductive heat transfer	The net rate of heat transfer by conduction down a thermal gradient, within an organism or between an organism and its external environment.
Convective heat transfer	The net rate of heat transfer by convection between an organism and its external environment or the transfer of heat with the bloodstream from the thermal core through the thermal shell to the heat-dissipating body surface.
Evaporative heat transfer	The loss of heat energy from the body to the ambience by evaporation of water from the skin and the surface of the respiratory tract.
Metabolic heat production	The rate of transformation of chemical energy into heat in an organism.

Radiant heat exchange	The net rate of heat exchange by radiation between an organism and its environment.
Temperature regulation	Maintenance of the temperature of a body within a restricted range under conditions involving variable internal or external heat loads.
Thermal stress	Any change in the thermal relation between a temperature regulator and its environment that, if uncompensated by temperature regulation, would result in hyper- or hypothermia.
Thermo-effector	An organ and its function that affect heat balance in a controlled manner as part of the process of temperature regulation.

Thermal Balance and Body Temperature

If body temperature is to be maintained at a constant level, there has to be a thermal equilibrium. This means that heat production or heat gain and heat loss must be equal. Under resting conditions, basal metabolic heat production, which occurs due to muscle contractions, to biosynthesis of molecules within the body, and to the activity of ion pumps, is predominantly counteracted by so-called dry heat loss. Dry heat loss consists of radiation, convection, and conduction of heat from the body to the surroundings and is dependent on and proportional to the temperature difference between body and surroundings. This means that a dry heat loss would be equal to zero at an ambient temperature of 37°C for a human subject; at lower temperatures it would increase and at higher temperatures the body would even gain dry heat from the surroundings. However, dry heat loss from the body also depends on the conduction and convection of heat within the body and thus on peripheral blood flow. Vasoconstriction of skin vessels prevents heat flow from the body core to the surface, and the activation and recruitment of additional (to the basal) heat production can be delayed to a lower ambient temperature. As a consequence, there is a so-called thermoneutral zone, a range of ambient temperatures in which heat loss can be matched to resting heat production by vasomotor adjustments. For humans, the range of the thermoneutral zone is between ambient temperatures of 28 and 32°C in nonmoving air. Beyond the lower limit of the thermoneutral zone, body temperature can be kept constant only if regulatory mechanisms increase thermogenesis in proportion to heat loss. In humans, heat production, predominantly due to the activation of shivering, can be increased as much as three to five times the basal metabolic rate. At an ambient temperature, which requires more than the maximum of

available heat production to keep the body core temperature constant, the lower limit of the thermoregulatory range is reached. When this limit is passed, hypothermia develops, which results in cold death. Beyond the upper limit of the thermoneutral zone, thermal balance is achieved by an additional heat loss mechanism, the evaporation of sweat (wet heat loss in contrast to the dry heat loss mentioned earlier). To a small degree of about 20% of the total heat loss, evaporative heat transfer also contributes to the heat loss under thermoneutral conditions. This is achieved by evaporation of water that has diffused either to the skin or from membranes of the respiratory tract; this is called insensible perspiration. Evaporation of water from the skin depends on the difference of vapor pressure between skin and surrounding air. This means that evaporative heat loss is difficult under conditions of high relative humidity. At an ambient temperature higher than 37°C and saturated vapor pressure of the surrounding air (e.g., the situation after a tropical rain on a very hot day), evaporative heat loss can become impossible.

At the upper limit of the thermoneutral zone, additional (to the insensitive) evaporative heat loss is achieved by activation of glandular water loss via sweat glands. When the ambient temperature exceeds that of the body, evaporation of sweat remains the only mechanism of the body to keep the temperature constant. The high effectiveness of thermoregulatory sweat secretion is based on the high amount of heat that is lost by evaporated water (2400 kJ/l). In humans, sweating rates of more than 2 l of water per hour can be observed under thermal stress. This means that an amount of heat can be dissipated by the evaporation of sweat that corresponds to seven times the basic metabolic heat production. At an ambient temperature that requires more than the maximum of available heat dissipation to keep the body temperature constant, the upper limit of the thermoregulatory range is reached. When this limit is passed, hyperthermia develops, which can result in heat death. A schematic diagram illustrating thermal balance within and beyond the zone of normothermy is shown in **Figure 1**.

Hyperthermia develops at ambient temperatures higher than the upper limit of the thermoregulatory range (see **Figure 1**). Also, during exercise, the rate of heat production increases above its level at rest mainly due to skeletal muscle contractions. The exercise-induced increase in heat production occurs immediately at the onset of exercise so that the rate of heat production exceeds the rate of heat dissipation. Therefore, body temperature is already rising during the early stage of exercise. When core temperature rises, heat-dissipating mechanisms (predominantly evaporation of

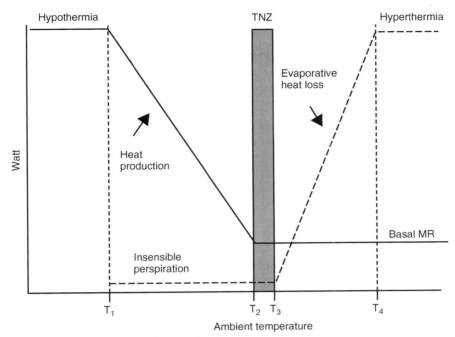

Figure 1 Schematic diagram illustrating thermal balance. Within the range of ambient temperatures between T_1 and T_4 there is an equilibrium between heat production and heat loss. Below T_1, more heat is lost than can be produced (hypothermia develops). Above T_4, production and influx of heat exceed the capacity for evaporative heat loss (hyperthermia develops). Between T_2 and T_3 (thermoneutral zone), heat loss can be matched to resting heat production by vasomotor adjustments. At T_2 there is a maximum of peripheral vasoconstriction, whereas at T_3 there is a maximum of peripheral vasodilation. MR, metabolic rate; TNZ, thermoneutral zone. Modified from Brück (1983), with permission from Springer-Verlag.

sweat) are activated, and the core temperature rises further with a smaller slope. Especially under conditions of high ambient temperature and/or high relative humidity, exercise can cause severe hyperthermia. During prolonged, exhausting exercise such as marathon running, rectal temperatures of higher than 41°C have been measured.

Physiological Responses to Heat Stress

During exposure to external heat or during production of additional internal heat, a number of vital homeostatic functions are influenced or even impaired. Important changes in cardiovascular responses, body fluid balance, endocrine responses, and responses of the immune system are described. In part, these adjustments serve to prevent or limit a developing hyperthermia.

Cardiovascular Responses

When the body has to counteract an increased heat load, it must direct enhanced blood flow to the skin, first to transport heat from the body core to the surface for dry heat loss (radiation, convection, conduction) and, second, to supply the water and electrolytes that are necessary for sweat formation.

Cardiovascular adjustments to whole body heating in humans can be summarized as follows. During an aggressive heating of the whole body surface with water-perfused suits, the skin temperature rises from 35 to 40.5°C and the blood temperature increases from 36.7 to 39.1°C. These body temperature changes are accompanied by a continuous rise of cardiac output from 6.4 to 13 l/min. The doubling of cardiac output is, to a large degree, driven by an increased heart rate (rise of about 30 beats per minute per degree increase of core temperature), whereas stroke volume changes little. Increased cardiac output during heat stress is accompanied by a regional redistribution of blood. Despite the doubled cardiac output, splanchnic, renal, and muscle blood flows are reduced by 1.2 l/min during the heating period. Thus, skin blood flow can approach about 8 l/min during external heat stress (6.6 l/min additional cardiac output plus 1.2 l/min redistributed blood). The dramatic increase in skin blood flow during heat stress occurs over the entire body surface and is distributed between two general vessel types: capillaries and arteriovenous anastomoses (AVAs). AVAs are shunt vessels between arterioles and venoles. Opening AVAs accelerates blood flow and thereby heat flux substantially. AVAs are concentrated on the so-called acral sites of the skin (tips of extremities, nose, ears, tongue, and lips); there is a lack of AVAs in nonacral sites (torso, forearms, upper arms, and legs). The major mechanisms by which skin blood flow is increased during heat stress are (1) a reduced activity in sympathetic vasoconstrictor nerves, (2) an increased activity of a sympathetic active vasodilator system, and (3) direct local vasodilative effects of elevated skin temperature. Cardiac output and distribution/redistribution of blood under resting conditions and during heat stress are summarized in **Figure 2**.

It has to be noted that the increase of thermoregulatory skin blood flow is limited by the demands of the working muscles during hyperthermia induced by physical exercise.

Effects on Body Fluid Balance

Maintenance of body fluid volume and composition is strongly impaired by heat stress. Exposure to heat species specifically results in sweating, panting, or saliva spreading to increase evaporative heat transfer to the environment. As a consequence, the constancy of total body water is disturbed by its considerable decrease. In humans sweating heavily, water loss from the body can exceed 2 l/h. All body fluid compartments and intracellular fluid, as well as extravascular and intravascular extracellular fluid, contribute to the water loss in heat stress. Without fluid replacement, a thermal dehydration results in hypovolemia (reduced intravascular compartment size) and hyperosmolality (increased plasma osmolality). Hypovolemia and hyperosmolality have adverse effects on thermoregulatory responses to heat stress. The rate of evaporative water loss is reduced in dehydrated humans and animals. As a consequence, heat stress results in faster onset and a stronger increase of body temperature in dehydrated subjects. Under conditions of restricted fluid supply, conservation of water is essential for survival. Therefore, the dehydrated organism tolerates an elevation of body temperature under conditions of heat stress to avoid a further loss of water by evaporation. This phenomenon is demonstrated impressively in the camel living at an ambient temperature of 34°C in the morning and 41°C in the afternoon. In the fully hydrated camel, which is watered every day, body temperature varies by about 2°C, between 36 and 38°C. When the camel is deprived of drinking water, however, daily body temperature fluctuations may increase to as much as 7°C, between 34 and 41°C. For a dehydrated camel, the amount of heat that is stored by this mechanism during the day equals a saving of 5 l of water. These interactions between water balance and body temperature control under the conditions of high external heat load are shown in **Figure 3**.

Corresponding observations are made under conditions of high internal heat load (exercise). At ambient temperatures higher than 30°C, an exercising man who is dehydrated responds with a strong increase of core temperature, while water replacement allows

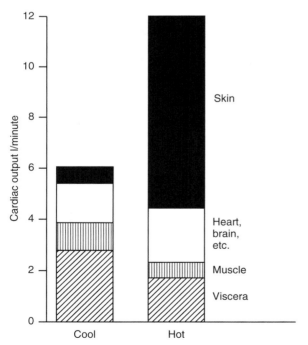

Figure 2 Distribution of human cardiac output between the skin and other major organs. The left column illustrates the conditions at rest in normothermia and the right column shows the conditions during severe hyperthermia when core temperature is higher than 39°C. From Rowell (1983), with permission from the American Physiological Society.

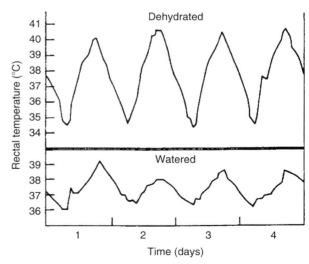

Figure 3 Daily body temperature fluctuations in a well-watered camel (about 2°C, bottom) and in a dehydrated camel deprived of drinking water (about 7°C, top). Modified from Schmidt-Nielsen et al. (1957), with permission from The American Physiological Society.

sustained sweating under the same external conditions so that the core temperature is maintained at a constant level. Sweating is thus inhibited by dehydration. In other words, the development of hyperthermia due to external or internal heat stress is accelerated if there is a strong demand for water conservation to avoid a pronounced deviation in the body fluid balance. Hypovolemia and hyperosmolality inhibit evaporative water loss in many species. It thus seems to be an evolutionary strategy to try to maintain body fluid balance during thermal dehydration with the consequence of a temporally developing hyperthermia.

Endocrinological Responses

Circulating levels of numerous hormones or amounts of hormones excreted with the urine change significantly under conditions of heat stress. As pointed out earlier, there are close interactions between heat defense strategies and the conservation of body fluid in hyperthermic conditions. Even a moderate level of dehydration by heat exposure or exercise affects the circulating levels of hormones that are involved in fluid and electrolyte homeostasis. Increasing dehydration is correlated with increments in arginine vasopressin, plasma renin activity, and aldosterone, hormones involved in the retention of water and electrolytes. In contrast, the secretion of atrial natriuretic peptide, which stimulates the excretion of sodium, is decreased by dehydration. Circulating levels of prolactin and adrenocorticotropic hormone, which both belong to the so-called stress hormones, are elevated during heat stress. Apparently, whenever thermal stress (heat or cold) induces marked discomfort or physiological strain, the hypothalamic-pituitary-adrenal axis is activated significantly.

Acute heat stress reduces serum thyroid-stimulating hormone. Further, decreased thyroid activity during chronic exposure to heat is indicated by attenuated circulating levels of thyroxine (T_4) and triiodothyronine (T_3). Finally, activity of the sympathoadrenomedullary system is also altered under hyperthermic conditions. The effects of acute and chronic heat exposure have to be differentiated. In most reports dealing with this question, an acute exposure to heat results in a rise of circulating epinephrine (E), whereas increases, no changes, or even decreases of norepinephrine (NE) can be observed depending on the experimental conditions, especially the intensity of the imposed heat stress. Long-term acclimation to heat is accompanied more constantly by a reduced excretion of NE, as long as the acclimation temperature is not excessively high. In summary, if the physiological strain evoked by acute heat stress is sufficient, an elevation of circulating or excreted A and NE is observed. Long-term exposure to heat may be accompanied by an attenuation of sympathetic activity. The most important endocrinological responses to heat stress are summarized in **Table 1**.

Immunological Responses

The thermal effects of fever, an evolutionarily conserved component of the acute phase response, has been associated with better survival and a shorter duration of disease in cases of infection. A possible explanation for this classical observation derived from a number of studies in which a whole body hyperthermia was induced in humans or experimental animals and various components of the innate and the specific immune defense mechanisms were analyzed under hyperthermic conditions. The benefits of heat for the immune system include enhanced neutrophil

Table 1 Endocrinological responses to heat stress[a]

Hormone	Stimulus	Direction of change	Species
AVP ACTH PRA ANG II ALD	Acute heat exposure or severe heat stress in a sauna bath or exercise	Increase in plasma	Human
AVP	Acute heat exposure	Increase in plasma	Rat
TSH	Acute heat exposure	Decrease in serum	Rat
T_3 T_4	Long-term heat acclimation	Decrease in plasma	Rat, chicken, guinea pig
E	Acute heat exposure or exercise	Increase in plasma	Human, dog, rat
NE	Long-term heat acclimation	Decrease in plasma or urine	Human, guinea pig

[a]Data compiled from Zeisberger and Roth (1988) and Fregly and Blatteis (1996). AVP, arginine vasopressin; ACTH, adrenocorticotropic hormone; PRA, plasma renin activity; ANG II, angiotensin II; ALD, aldosterone; TSH, thyroid-stimulating hormone; T_3, triiodothyronine; T_4, thyroxine; E, epinephrine; NE, norepinephrine.

and monocyte motility and emigration, enhanced phagocytosis, increased production and activity of interferon, increased T helper cell activation and antibody production, and induction of cytoprotective heat shock proteins in host cells. These effects of hyperthermia are thought to improve the pathogen-eliminating capacity by hindering the spread of local infection. The ability to warn the immune system distant from the site of primary infection suggests that hyperthermia or infectious fever has a messenger role for the immune system.

Brain Function in Hyperthermia

The Heat Stroke Syndrome

During prolonged hyperthermia, with a body temperature of 41°C or even higher, the brain suffers severe damage, which leads frequently to death. Alterations in microvascular permeability cause the development of cerebral edema. Postmortem findings further show microhemorrhages, tissue softening, and destruction of neurons. The victim exhibits disorientation, delirium, and convulsions. This syndrome is referred to popularly as heat stroke. Heat stroke can develop in response to severe external heat exposure. The heat illness syndrome can also be caused by exercise or work in hot environments. Perhaps the most famous example of heat stroke is the traditional 7-day pilgrimage to Mecca (Saudi Arabia), the so-called Makka Hajj. During the Hajj pilgrimage of 1982, high ambient temperatures (35–50°C), in addition to the large radiant heat load of the thermal environment resulting from the presence of a large number of human bodies in a very restricted area, caused more than 1500 cases of heat stroke. About 1100 people were treated successfully, whereas several hundred died. The use of molecular techniques has provided the basis for a number of pathophysiological changes in the heat-stressed brain.

Molecular Changes in the Heat-Stressed Brain

The expression of a number of molecules is upregulated in the brain under conditions of hyperthermia. Representative examples of these molecular changes are introduced briefly in the following sections. The role of these molecules in the hyperthermic brain, especially in the manifestation of detrimental effects, is the subject of current investigation. Knowledge about mechanisms by which all these molecules, which are induced in the hyperthermic brain, contribute to the heat stroke syndrome is still incomplete. Research is focusing on the roles of these molecules in the disturbance of microvascular permeability,

formation of edema, and cell injury within the hyperthermic brain.

Heat shock proteins Exposure of cells and tissues to stressful stimuli results in a rapid induction and synthesis of a specific set of proteins. These proteins are called heat shock proteins (HSPs) because their induction was originally discovered under hyperthermic conditions. However, because these proteins are also synthesized under the influence of nonthermal noxious stimuli, they are also called stress proteins. In the hyperthermic brain, the induction of HSPs is closely related to damaged brain areas and can thus be used as markers of cell injury. However, after induction of HSPs by a moderate hyperthermia, the brain becomes more resistant to a subsequent severe hyperthermia. HSPs may therefore have some neuroprotective properties. Experimental studies demonstrated that there is a correlation between the induction of HSPs and the breakdown of the blood–brain barrier in hyperthermia.

Glial fibrillary acidic protein Hyperthermic brain injury is accompanied by an activation of glial cells as indicated by the expression of the glia cell marker protein glial fibrillary acidic protein (GFAP). Under normal conditions, this protein is predominantly expressed in astrocytes. Under pathophysiological conditions, such as heat stress, increased induction of this protein is associated with a breakdown of the blood–brain barrier and vasogenic edema. The increased synthesis of GFAP is a part of the reactive response to almost any type of central nervous system (CNS) injury. Following injury, glia cells are activated to accomplish metabolic and structural roles in the CNS.

Cytokines Activation of the immune system during infection or inflammation is characterized by the expression of cytokines in the brain. Interleukin-1 (IL-1) is regarded as the most important cytokine to cause modifications of brain-controlled functions during infection. Evidence shows that the increased expression of IL-1 within the CNS is associated with brain injury. Heat stroke-induced cerebral ischemia and neuronal damage are accompanied by an increased production of IL-1 in the damaged brain. Because the survival time of rats after experimentally induced heat stroke can be prolonged by treatment with an IL-1 receptor antagonist, a role of IL-1 (and possibly other cytokines) in the manifestation of the heat stroke syndrome is indicated.

Prostaglandins A role of prostaglandins in fever is well established. Inhibition of cyclooxygenases, the enzymes responsible for prostaglandin formation, suppresses fever. Also, the hyperthermic response to heat stress is reduced slightly by treatment with cyclooxygenase inhibitors. In addition, the hyperthermia-induced formation of edema and cellular damage in the brain are reduced by inhibitors of prostaglandin synthesis. Thus, prostaglandins seem to contribute to the detrimental effects that are induced by hyperthermia in the brain.

Nitric oxide and carbon monoxide Nitric oxide (NO) and carbon monoxide (CO) are novel chemical messenger molecules that are involved in physiological and pathophysiological processes within the brain. NO and CO are produced by specific enzymes: NO synthases and heme oxygenases. Both of these enzymes are upregulated in the brain under conditions of heat stress. In the brain, the products of these enzymes seem to contribute to the disturbance of microvascular permeability in hyperthermia.

Adaptation to Heat

Adaptation has been defined as a set of modifications within organisms that take place during prolonged or repeated actions of an environmental stimulus, a so-called stressor. The process of adaptation improves the ability to cope with stressor-induced disturbances that interfere with the homeostasis of an organism. Such disturbances (i.e., repeated or continuous exposure to heat) evoke specific and nonspecific responses and can finally lead to functional and morphological modifications that counteract the disturbance. As a nonspecific response to various stressors, including heat, central nervous circuits are activated that lead to the stimulation of the sympathicoadrenal system and the hypothalamic-pituitary-adrenal axis. This nonspecific response or emergency reaction usually decreases in its intensity in response to repeated or prolonged actions of the same stressor. Specific adaptive responses to the stressor heat may lead to changes in the capacity of the effector systems that are predominantly activated in hyperthermia and to modifications of the regulatory characteristics of the control system being responsible for the thermal homeostasis under conditions of heat stress. The most profound heat-adaptive response of the thermoeffector system in humans is the increase of the sweat rate capacity, which nearly doubles during heat acclimation. This kind of adaptation to heat develops in response to repeated exposures to heat and to repeated severe exercise. Using this mechanism, a heat stress of the same intensity leads to much smaller hyperthermia at the end of the process of heat adaptation. The second component of the stressor-specific adaptive response

to heat concerns the modifications of the regulatory characteristics. Usually, sweating is activated when the mean body temperature rises to a certain value, the so-called threshold temperature for the onset of sweating. This sweating threshold is shifted to a lower mean body temperature after repeated exposures to external heat or to repeated exercise, which includes heat load such as marathon running. This means that the heat-adapted subject starts to sweat earlier and thereby delays or even prevents the developing hyperthermia. A different type of heat adaptation is observed in residents of areas with tropical climate. Here, the onset of sweating occurs at a higher body temperature than in controls. This kind of heat adaptation can be called tolerance adaptation, meaning that the subject tolerates an increase of body temperature before sweating is activated. This observation corresponds to the physiological response of the dehydrated camel (see **Figure 3**) and may be regarded as an avoidance of sweating (i.e., a loss of water) when living continuously in a hot climate.

Malignant Hyperthermia

Malignant hyperthermia is caused by a rare, genetically fixed defect in the transport of calcium within the sarcoplasmatic reticulum. This defect has been identified as a mutation of the ryanodine receptor (calcium release channel) in the membrane of the sarcoplasmatic reticulum. Some inhalation anesthetics such as halothane or isoflurane cause excessive release of calcium from the sarcoplasmatic reticulum in genetically susceptible subjects. Also, the muscle relaxant succinylcholine can act as a triggering agent for malignant hyperthermia. As a consequence, uncoordinated muscle contractions with a tremendous rise in oxygen consumption and metabolic rate induce a severe hyperthermia that is accompanied by acidosis, tachycardia, or cardiac arrhythmias. After its initiation by one of the triggering substances, malignant hyperthermia leads frequently to death.

See Also the Following Articles

Critical Thermal Limits; Heat Resistance; Hypothermia; Prostaglandins; Thermal Stress; Thermotolerance, Thermoresistance, and Thermosensitivity.

Further Reading

Adolph, E. F. (1956). General and specific characteristics of physiological adaptations. *American Journal of Physiology* **184**, 18–28.
Blatteis, C. M. (1997). Thermoregulation: tenth international symposium on the pharmacology of thermoregulation.

Annals of the New York Academy of Sciences **813**, 111–116.

Blatteis, C. M. (2004). Fever: pathological or physiological, injurious or beneficial? *Journal of Thermal Biology* **28**, 1–13.

Brück, K. (1983). Heat balance and regulation of body temperature. In: Schmidt, R. F. & Thews, G. (eds.) *Human physiology*, pp. 531–547. Berlin: Springer.

Brück, K. and Zeisberger, E. (1990). Adaptive changes in thermoregulation and their neuropharmacological basis. In: Schönbaum, E. & Lomax, P. (eds.) *Thermoregulation: physiology and biochemistry*, pp. 255–307. New York: Pergamon Press.

Fregly, M. J. and Blatteis, C. M. (1996). *Handbook of physiology* (vol. 1, sect. 4). New York: Oxford University Press.

IUPS Thermal Commission. (2001). Glossary of terms for thermal physiology. *Japanese Journal of Physiology* **51**, 245–280.

Khogali, M. and Hales, J. R. S. (1983). *Heat stroke and temperature regulation*. Sydney: Academic Press.

Rothwell, N. J. and Relton, J. K. (1993). Involvement of cytokines in acute neurodegeneration in the CNS. *Neuroscience and Biobehavioral Reviews* **17**, 217–227.

Rowell, L. B. (1983). Cardiovascular adjustments to thermal stress. In: Shepard, J. T. & Abboud, F. M. (eds.) *Handbook of physiology* (vol. III), pp. 967–1023. Baltimore, MD: Waverly Press.

Schmidt-Nielsen, K., Schmidt-Nielsen, B., Jarnum, S. A. and Houpt, T. P. (1957). Body temperature of the camel and its relation to water economy. *American Journal of Physiology* **188**, 103–112.

Selye, H. (1950). *The physiology and pathology of exposure to stress*. Montreal: Acta Inc. Medical.

Sharma, H. S. and Westman, J. (1998). *Progress in brain research: brain function in hot environments* (vol. 115). Amsterdam: Elsevier.

Zeisberger, E. and Roth, J. (1989). Changes in peripheral and central release of hormones during thermal adaptation in the guinea pig. In: Malan, A. & Canguilhem, B. (eds.) *Living in the cold*, pp. 435–444. London: John Libbey Eurotext Ltd.

Zeisberger, E. and Roth, J. (1996). Central regulation of adaptive responses to heat and cold. In: Blatteis, C. M. & Fregly, M. J. (eds.) *Handbook of physiology* (vol. I), pp. 579–595. New York: Oxford University Press.

Hyperthyroidism

I M Lesser and D L Flores
Harbor-UCLA Medical Center, Torrance, CA, USA

This article is a revision of the previous edition article by I M Lesser, volume 2, pp 439–440, © 2000, Elsevier Inc.

Causes of Hyperthyroidism
Behavioral and Neuropsychiatric Aspects of Hyperthyroidism
Association between Psychological Stress and Hyperthyroidism
Proposed Mechanism of Action Linking Stress and Hyperthyroidism

Glossary

Graves' disease	A type of hyperthyroidism thought to be an autoimmune disease.
Hyperthyroidism	Excessive functional activity of the thyroid gland leading to increased metabolism and symptoms such as weight loss, fatigue, anxiety, tremor, and increased heart rate.
Hypothalamic-pituitary-thyroid (HPT) axis	Regulatory feedback loop between the brain (hypothalamus and pituitary gland) and the thyroid gland.
T4 and T3	Circulating thyroid hormones (thyroxin and triiodothyronine, respectively) that have widespread effects throughout the body.

Causes of Hyperthyroidism

There are multiple causes of hyperthyroidism, all leading to a state of hypermetabolic activity. As a final common pathway, all have an increase in circulating thyroid hormones (free thyroxine [T4] and free triiodothyronine [T3]), which in turn lead to a variety of symptoms: increased heart rate, weight loss, tremulousness, fatigue, anxiety, weakness, and increased tolerance to cold. The most commonly occurring type of hyperthyroidism is Graves' disease, first described in the 1830s and now known to be an autoimmune disorder. Other causes of hyperthyroidism include toxic nodular goiter, thyroid adenomas, and several types of thyroiditis (inflammatory conditions).

Each may have a different clinical presentation, but they share many of the same symptoms as well. Diagnosis is made by clinical history, laboratory determinations, and imaging studies of the thyroid gland.

Behavioral and Neuropsychiatric Aspects of Hyperthyroidism

Behavioral and psychological symptoms may be the presenting and most prominent aspects of hyperthyroidism. Patients complain of being anxious, restless, agitated, irritable, dysphoric, emotionally labile, and angry; having poor concentration and at times trouble thinking; feeling weak and fatigued; and having insomnia. More serious, and more rarely, paranoid thinking or frank psychosis can occur. The most common group of psychiatric disorders, in which the presenting symptoms may be similar, are the anxiety disorders, specifically, generalized anxiety disorder and panic disorder. Less often, there may be some symptoms overlapping with depression, but the full depressive syndrome usually is not present in the hyperthyroid individual. Even more rarely, manic symptoms may occur. Because of these symptoms, it is not uncommon for patients with Graves' disease to be prescribed psychotropic medication prior to recognition and work-up of their thyroid illness.

Association between Psychological Stress and Hyperthyroidism

The association of stress with hyperthyroidism dates back to the original case reports of the early 1800s. In 1825, Parry described the onset of a hyperthyroid state in a young woman who became symptomatic after falling down the stairs in a wheelchair. In 1835, Graves described the disease, which now bears his name, and implied that there was an innate mental disposition to the disorder. Since then, the association between stress and hyperthyroidism has been recognized, although the universality of this finding has been questioned. The majority of studies (but not all) have shown that stressful events, both negative and positive, in the year prior to the onset of the illness are more commonly seen in patients with Graves' disease than in patients with other forms of thyroid disease and in control subjects without thyroid illness. There also have been reports of an increased prevalence of Graves' disease in people under severe stress, such as refugees from German concentration camps and from the civil war in the former Yugoslavia, where there was a fivefold increase in disease incidence.

Proposed Mechanism of Action Linking Stress and Hyperthyroidism

The mechanism by which stress may lead to hyperthyroidism or, more specifically, to Graves' disease is not clear. Because Graves' disease is an autoimmune disorder, hypotheses have been made regarding the link between stress and the immune system. It has been shown that stress can affect a number of neurohormones that modulate the immune response, specifically decreasing the efficacy of this response. Stress affects the function of the hypothalamic-pituitary-thyroid (HPT) axis by suppressing the secretion of pituitary thyroid-stimulating hormone (TSH) and blunting its response to thyrotropin-releasing hormone. Furthermore, the HPT axis has feedback loops with the hypothalamic-pituitary-adrenocortical (HPA) axis, which also is very involved in response to stress. It is possible that individuals with a genetic predisposition to thyroid disease could, if their immune responsiveness is compromised, develop Graves' disease. Stress, and its effects upon immune function, could be one of the intervening variables involved in the cascade of events leading to this disorder. This theory has not been proven with any certainty, but remains a testable hypothesis.

See Also the Following Articles

Autoimmunity; Graves' Disease (Thyrotoxicosis); Hypothyroidism; Thyroid Hormones.

Further Reading

Braverman, L. E. and Utiger, R. D. (eds.) (1996). *Werner and Ingbar's the thyroid* (7th edn.) Philadelphia, PA: Lippincott-Raven.

Dayan, C. M. (2001). Stressful life events and Graves' disease revisited. *Clinical Endocrinology* 55, 13–14.

Graves, R. J. (1835). Newly observed affection of the thyroid gland in females. *London Medical Surgery Journal* 7, 516–517.

Harris, T., Creed, F. and Brugha, T. S. (1992). Stressful life events and Graves' disease. *British Journal of Psychiatry* 161, 535–541.

Kung, A. W. (1995). Life events, daily stresses and coping in patients with Graves' disease. *Clinical Endocrinology* 42, 303–308.

Lesser, I. M., Rubin, R. T., Lydiard, R. B., et al. (1987). Past and current thyroid function in subjects with panic disorder. *Journal of Clinical Psychiatry* 48, 473–476.

Mizokami, T., Li, A. W., El-Kaissi, S., et al. (2004). Stress and thyroid autoimmunity. *Thyroid* 14, 1047–1055.

Parry, C. H. (1825). *Collections from the unpublished writing of the late C. H. Parry* (vol. 2). London: Underwoods.

Paunkovic, N., Paunkovic, J., Pavlovic, O., et al. (1998). The significant increase in incidence of Graves' disease in eastern Serbia during the civil war in the former Yugoslavia (1992–1995). *Thyroid* **8**, 37–41.

Sonino, H., Girelli, M., Boscaro, M., et al. (1993). Life events in the pathogenesis of Graves' disease: a controlled study. *Acta Endrocrinology* **128**, 293–296.

Stern, R. A., Robinson, B., Thorner, A. R., et al. (1996). A survey study of neuropsychiatric complaints in patients with Graves' disease. *Journal of Neuropsychiatry and Clinical Neurosciences* **8**, 181–185.

Weisman, S. A. (1958). Incidence of thyrotoxicosis among refugees from Nazi prison camps. *Annals of Internal Medicine* **48**, 747–752.

Winsa, B., Adami, H., Bergstrom, R., et al. (1991). Stressful life events and Graves' disease. *Lancet* **338**, 1475–1479.

Whybrow, P. C. (1996). Behavioral and psychiatric aspects of thyrotoxicosis. In: Braverman, L. & Utiger, R. D. (eds.) *Werner and Ingbar's the thyroid* (7th edn., pp. 696–700). Philadelphia, PA: Lippincott-Raven.

Hyperventilation

C Bass
John Radcliffe Hospital, Oxford, UK

This article is a revision of the previous edition article by C Bass, volume 2, pp 441–445, © 2000, Elsevier Inc.

Physiology

Causes

Clinical Features

The Hyperventilation Syndrome

Establishing the Diagnosis of Hyperventilation

Hyperventilation and Its Relation to Anxiety and Panic

Chronic Hyperventilation

Hyperventilation, Panic, and Asthma

Management of Hyperventilation

Breathing Exercises and Asthma

Glossary

Alveolar PCO₂ (PACO₂)	The partial pressure of carbon dioxide in alveolar space.
Arterial PCO₂ (PaCO₂)	The partial pressure of carbon dioxide in arterial blood.
Dysfunctional breathing	An abnormal pattern of breathing causing breathlessness, chest tightness, and other nonrespiratory symptoms that may not be associated with hyperventilation but that may respond to breathing retraining.
End-tidal PCO₂ (PetCO₂)	An uninvasive measure of CO_2 that is very close to arterial CO_2.
Hyperventilation provocation test (HVPT)	The patient is asked to hyperventilate for up to 3 min in an attempt to reproduce symptoms.
Hypocapnia	The reduction of CO_2 in the body that is the result of hyperventilation.
Respiratory alkalosis	A drop in PCO_2 with an arterial pH above 7.40 caused by hyperventilation.
Tetany	An abnormal increase in the excitability of nerves and muscles resulting in muscular spasms.

Physiology

Hyperventilation (HV) is a physiological term implying breathing in excess of metabolic requirements, thus producing arterial hypocapnia. The approach to HV requires a clear understanding of the physiological background of respiratory control. If carbon dioxide production remains constant and ventilation increases, there is an increased washout of carbon dioxide (i.e., hypocapnia) from the alveolar space with a consequent fall of alveolar PCO_2 ($PACO_2$) and arterial PCO_2 ($PaCO_2$). Stated another way, $PaCO_2$ below the normal range is invariably associated with a raised alveolar ventilation and excessive respiratory drive (see **Figure 1**). HV cannot be present without hypocapnia. Increases in ventilation without hypocapnia, respiratory tics, and other disorders of respiratory pattern are not HV. Following 15–20 min of voluntary hyperventilation to below 20 mmHg, hypocapnia can be maintained with only an occasional large breath, but even chronic persistent HV is associated with at least a 10% increase in ventilation. The cause or causes of this increased drive to breathe must always be sought in any individual with a HV-related disorder.

Hypocapnia and respiratory alkalosis develop rapidly after the onset of HV. If hypocapnia is sustained, renal compensation occurs through increased renal excretion of bicarbonate, but this is probably unimportant in humans. Tetany is often thought to be due

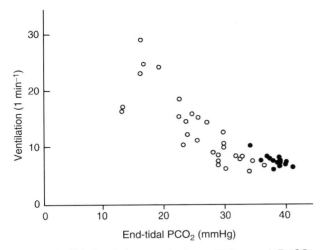

Figure 1 Relation between minute ventilation and PetCO$_2$ during resting breathing in eight normal subjects (closed symbols) and 16 patients with chronic hyperventilation (open symbols; two runs per subject). Each symbol is the mean of 40–100 breaths. From Gardner, W. N. (1996), The pathophysiology of hyperventilation disorders, *Chest* **109**, 516–534.

to a fall in serum calcium, but this has never been confirmed. There is, however, a rapid and consistent fall in the serum phosphorus level, and this provides a more likely explanation for the increase in neuronal excitability. Hypocapnic alkalosis is associated with a reduction in cerebral blood flow, which is probably due to a change of pH rather than PCO$_2$, and is associated with significant cerebral hypoxia. Cerebral blood flow is linearly related to PaCO$_2$, and there is a 2% reduction of arterial blood flow for each 1 mmHg decline in PaCO$_2$. This means that severe HV leading to profound hypocapnia of 15–20 mmHg can reduce the cerebral circulation by approximately 50%. Hypocapnia can also cause abnormal esophageal motility and increases in tone in the muscles in the colon. Patients with known coronary vasospasm with or without significant fixed coronary artery obstructions can develop coronary vasospasm and reduced coronary perfusion following hypocapnia; this may be associated with the development of angina and ischemic electrocardiographic changes. Electroencephalographic recordings during HV often reveal paroxysmal or continuous high-voltage slow-wave activity of approximately 2–5 cycles s^{-1}.

Causes

HV can be caused by a number of factors, which often overlap and interact. Organic causes include a variety of factors such as drug effects (aspirin overdose), the early stages of alcohol withdrawal, respiratory disease such as asthma and pulmonary embolus, central nervous system disorders, and chronic pain. Physiological causes include altitude acclimation, heat, and exercise. HV is also induced by speech, and progesterone in women reduces PaCO$_2$ by up to 8 mmHg in the second half of the menstrual cycle and even lower during pregnancy. Psychological factors include anxiety, depression, and panic attacks, but the relationship between anxiety and breathlessness is not simple.

Clinical Features

HV is clinically significant only if it results in physical complaints that are distressing or disabling. The way in which these symptoms are produced and interpreted is important in understanding why HV becomes a problem for some patients. A knowledge of the physiology suggests that the clinical manifestations of HV may be diverse and can involve almost any system in the body. For this reason, HV is said to have replaced syphilis as the great mimic in medical practice. No symptoms are truly specific for HV, but certain patterns are discernible. Common neurological complaints include dizziness, syncope, and tingling of the hands and feet (paresthesia), which may be unilateral and mimic a stroke; respiratory complaints include sensations of breathlessness or the inability to take a satisfactory breath (air hunger); cardiovascular manifestations are commonly chest pains often mimicking angina, palpitations, and racing pulse; gastrointestinal complaints include air swallowing (aerophagy) resulting in a bloated sensation, flatulence, and heartburn; musculoskeletal symptoms include muscle aches (a consequence of increased muscle tone with muscular tightness) and tetany (extremely rare); and general symptoms may include chronic and easy fatigability, weakness, the sensation of feeling cold, and poor concentration.

Although symptoms can be described in terms of organs and systems, it is probably more useful to divide them into those due to an increase in neuronal excitability; those due to a constriction of the blood vessels, especially in the cerebral, coronary, and skin circulations; and those of uncertain cause.

The Hyperventilation Syndrome

The term hyperventilation syndrome, first proposed in the 1930s, came under attack in the 1990s, and it was recommended that it be abolished. The reasons for this proposal were that (1) there were no established valid criteria, (2) the HV provocation test (designed to reproduce symptoms in patients with the syndrome) was found to be unreliable, (3) it is often impossible to establish the diagnosis in the absence of demonstrated hypocapnia, and (4) the link between panic attacks and HV was found to be tenuous. Because most symptoms reported by patients did not require a fall in $PaCO_2$, other terms such as dysfunctional breathing were suggested as an alternative. This umbrella term allows the inclusion of patients with and without HV, and it moves the focus of attention from physiological hypocapnia to a more pragmatic clinical approach.

Patients with dysfunctional breathing have an unsteadiness of breathing in response to stimuli such as exercise and a period of voluntary overbreathing, increased respiratory rate, abnormal orthostatic increases of respiratory gas exchange, predominantly intercostal respiratory effort, and frequent sighing. But not all patients with dysfunctional breathing hyperventilate or have hypocapnia.

The diagnosis of dysfunctional breathing can be difficult because the overbreathing aspect of the symptom complex may be episodic and difficult to demonstrate. The characteristic symptoms are common to other diseases, and there is no standard diagnostic test. This may lead to the underrecognition of the effects of abnormal breathing patterns, and symptoms may be wrongly attributed to other causes, resulting in inappropriate investigations and ineffective treatment, specially in patients with coexisting lung disease.

Establishing the Diagnosis of Hyperventilation

HV can coexist with other disorders, and it is important to decide which, if any, of the patient's symptoms could be due to HV. In particular, HV should be considered in any patient with a long history of unexplained physical symptoms involving a number of different organ systems.

Acute HV may be obvious from the fast rate and increased depth of breathing accompanied by the constellation of symptoms of hypocapnia. Because the disorder may be intermittent, however, a low $PaCO_2$ is not diagnostic; spot arterial or end-tidal samples may be normal. Conversely, making the measurement can induce overbreathing. Ambulatory transcutaneous measurement of PCO_2 for continuous monitoring is not yet responsive enough to be clinically useful, but it has led to important findings in recent research studies of *in vivo* panic attacks. End-tidal PCO_2 is sometimes measured uninvasively by capnograph sampling from a nostril as part of lung function testing; the reduction of PCO_2 at rest, or during or after various provocations such as exercise, may suggest that symptoms are related to HV.

A commonly employed test is the HV provocation test (HVPT); the patient is asked to hyperventilate for 3 min (with concomitant monitoring of end-tidal PCO_2) and to keep PCO_2 below 20 mmHg for at least 1 min. After 3 min, the patient completes a checklist of symptoms experienced during overbreathing. Although this test has limitations (as previously mentioned), it is often used as a diagnostic aid and has some clinical utility, especially when the physician is attempting to help the patient reattribute physical symptoms to HV (and not some imagined sinister disease). Because there is no widely accepted and reliable diagnostic test, the incidence of HV has probably been underestimated.

Hyperventilation and Its Relation to Anxiety and Panic

Similarities have long been noted between the symptoms of panic attacks and HV. It has recently been established that CO_2 inhalation (and to a lesser extent HV) causes more anxiety and panic in patients with panic disorder than in normal controls. One theory proposed to explain this phenomenon is that the respiratory drive in panic disorder patients is controlled by abnormally sensitive CO_2 receptors in the central nervous system. Klein suggested that panic disorder patients possess an abnormal suffocation detector that processes asphyxia-related causes. According to Klein, HV among panic disorder sufferers is a result of the body's adaptive attempts to reduce panicogenic CO_2. That is to say, chronic HV and sighing may adaptively keep PCO_2 below a depressed suffocation alarm threshold. The nature of the specific respiratory abnormality in panic disorder remains controversial, however, and investigators disagree on the interpretation of recent experimental data. Whereas some authors have interpreted biological challenge data as supporting a biological etiology for panic disorder, other investigators have argued that psychological factors (e.g., perceived safety, perceived control, or proximity to a safe person in the laboratory) mediate patients' responses to these challenges and that cognitive theories of panic disorder can account for these findings.

Recent work with ambulatory monitoring of CO_2 has failed to confirm the view that HV is a necessary factor for panic to occur. Although hypocapnia has been demonstrated to occur during a spontaneous panic attack in the laboratory, in a recent study there was a decrease in PCO_2 in only 1 of the 24 registered panic attacks that lasted 3 min, and even during this attack the degree of HV was not impressive. It is not possible, however, to discount a role for HV in the production of symptoms experienced during panic attacks. The crucial link between HV (when it occurs) and panic may be cognitive; panic attacks occur when the bodily and mental sensations accompanying HV are interpreted as signs of impending personal catastrophe, such as madness or heart attack (see **Figure 2**).

Chronic Hyperventilation

An initial attack of HV caused by a combination of physiological, psychological, and possibly pathological factors could create a vicious circle and lead to increasing anxiety and further HV. The patient may misattribute the first attack of HV to serious disease and then perpetuate the disorder by becoming more anxious and breathing more deeply to relieve chest discomfort. CO_2 homeostasis is then reset at a lower level. Such a sequence could rapidly lead to invalidism and chronic HV. In these patients, PCO_2 is either chronically low at rest and throughout a number of provocations or only mildly reduced at rest but precipitated into prolonged reduction by either exercise or voluntary overbreathing.

Hyperventilation, Panic, and Asthma

The prevalence of anxiety disorders (including panic) is above expected levels in patients with asthma, and asthma is more common in people with psychiatric illness. The relationship appears strongest in those with severe asthma and those with severe anxiety. Panic and anxiety can directly exacerbate asthma symptoms through HV.

In a recent longitudinal study, it was found that active asthma predicted subsequent panic disorder and that panic disorder predicted subsequent active asthma, this effect being stronger in women and in subjects younger than 30 years old. This relationship between physiological and psychological factors in asthma offers opportunities for research.

Management of Hyperventilation

The main aim of treatment is to reassure patients that they do not have a serious life-threatening illness and then to treat the underlying cause of the HV. If no cause is found or the cause is untreatable, it is often possible to teach patients to understand and adjust to the symptoms.

First, organic causes for the presenting symptoms (e.g., asthma or pulmonary embolus) should be excluded. Two of the main treatments used in the management of patients with HV-related symptoms in recent years have been breathing retraining and cognitive reattribution of physical symptoms to HV. Breathing retraining involves encouraging the patient to breathe in a slow regular fashion using the diaphragm; reattribution is aimed at helping the patient

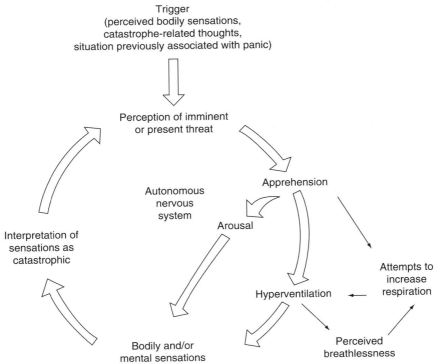

Figure 2 Principal components of the cognitive model of panic attacks in which hyperventilation is involved in the production of symptoms.

to ascribe the physical symptoms to anxiety and at explaining the relationship between stress and HV. In practice, however, it is very difficult to determine the relative contributions of these two therapeutic components to outcome.

Recent research supported the view that training in controlled breathing is not of specific benefit in patients identified as hyperventilators by the provocation test. Indeed, breathing retraining has been referred to as a rational placebo that is effective not by restoring levels of CO_2 but by inducing relaxation, providing a structured task and distraction, and giving the patient a sense of control and mastery. This may distract the patient from feelings of anxiety and promote self-reliance.

Breathing Exercises and Asthma

It has been reported that up to 30% of adults with asthma in the community may have symptoms suggestive of functional breathing disorders, and there is some evidence of a role for breathing exercises in the treatment of asthma complicated by these abnormal breathing patterns. A review of psychotherapeutic interventions for adults with asthma found conflicting evidence, however, with some positive studies but with insufficient data to draw firm conclusions.

Further Reading

Bass, C. (1997). Hyperventilation syndrome: a chimera? *Journal of Psychosomatic Research* **42**, 421–426.

Gardner, W. N. (1996). The pathophysiology of hyperventilation disorders. *Chest* **109**, 516–534.

Garssen, B., de Ruiter, C. and van Dyck, R. (1992). Breathing retraining: a rational placebo? *Clinical Psychology Review* **12**, 141–153.

Hasler, G., Gergen, P., Kleinbaum, D., et al. (2005). Asthma and panic in young adults; a 20 year prospective community study. *American Journal of Respiratory and Critical Care Medicine* **171**, 1224–1230.

Klein, D. F. (1993). False suffocation alarms, spontaneous panics, and related conditions. *Archives of General Psychiatry* **50**, 306–317.

Salkovskis, P. (1988). Hyperventilation and anxiety. *Current Opinion in Psychiatry* **1**, 76–82.

Thomas, M. (2003). Breathing exercises and asthma. *Thorax* **58**, 649–650.

Thomas, M., McKinley, R., Freeman, E., et al. (2001). Prevalence of dysfunctional breathing in patients treated for asthma in primary care: cross sectional survey. *British Medical Journal* **322**, 1098–1101.

Thomas, M., McKinley, R., Freeman, E., et al. (2003). Breathing retraining for dysfunctional breathing in asthma: a randomized controlled trial. *Thorax* **58**, 110–115.

Hypnosis

W G Whitehouse, E C Orne and M T Orne
University of Pennsylvania School of Medicine, Philadelphia, PA, USA

This article is a revision of the previous edition article by M T Orne and W G Whitehouse, volume 2, pp 446–452, © 2000, Elsevier Inc.

Historical Background
Induction of Hypnosis
Hypnotizability Assessment and the Phenomena of Hypnosis
Hypnotic Interventions for Stress Management
Conclusion

Glossary

Hypnotic induction	A series of suggestions that focus attention and bring about the transition from ordinary waking experience to hypnosis.
Hypnotizability	The potential to experience hypnosis; a relatively stable trait that varies from person to person and that can be assessed by standardized test procedures.
Nonspecific effect	A therapeutic outcome (e.g., symptom relief) that follows a hypnotic procedure but that occurs regardless of the patient's ability to experience deep hypnosis.

Historical Background

Special healing properties have been ascribed to trancelike conditions throughout civilizations and time. Some of the earliest examples can be traced back 4000 years to ancient Egypt and by the 5th century BC to the Greek empire. The priests of these times established healing sanctuaries or sleep temples, where people suffering from mental or physical problems could seek relief. In exchange for some sacrifice or atonement, the priest or priestess performed incantations and rituals designed to heighten suggestibility and promote a trancelike sleep, during which the individual's dreams could be affected by healing communications from the gods. Similarly, witchcraft practiced during the Middle Ages, exorcisms to alleviate demonic possession, Afro-Caribbean voodoo rituals, and faith-healing in relatively modern times each appear to involve elements of what is today subsumed by the term hypnosis.

Historically, explanations for the effectiveness of many of these practices appealed to supernatural or metaphysical causes. More modern perspectives arose from controversies surrounding the work of the Austrian physician, Franz Anton Mesmer (1734–1815) and his followers. Working in France at the time of the American Revolutionary War, Mesmer observed that some patients derived benefit from the passing of magnets over their bodies. In due time, Mesmer concluded that he, himself, possessed the critical animal magnetism, a putative fluid within the body that, in combination with certain accoutrements, could be transferred to others as needed to heal them. This claim expressly identified the source of the healing power as a property of the magnetizer. Indeed, one of Mesmer's students, the Marquis de Puysegur, claimed to have successfully magnetized a tree on his estate, where some of his peasant workers obtained relief from their ailments. Eventually, de Puysegur found that he could influence the behavior of mesmerized patients merely by talking with them, much the same way that hypnosis is used today. The fluid theory of animal magnetism was soon discredited, however, in a series of investigations conducted by such scientific luminaries as Benjamin Franklin and Antoine-Laurent Lavoisier (1784). Nevertheless, the therapeutic effects – at first dismissed as the products of imagination and suggestion – were too striking to be ignored for very long.

By the 1840s, the current term hypnosis had been coined by James Braid, a surgeon from Edinburgh, Scotland, who conceptualized the process as one of focusing attention, leading ultimately to a state of artificial sleep. Subsequently, demonstrations of its analgesic uses in surgery – many by James Esdaile, a physician employed by the East India Company in Calcutta – were being documented in British medical periodicals. It was not long before hypnosis was adopted for use in the treatment of psychiatric and neurological disorders following a number of celebrated cases by such renowned academics and physicians as Hippolyte Bernheim, Jean-Martin Charcot, Sigmund Freud, Pierre Janet, and Morton Prince. Today, hypnosis is commonly employed in clinical practice as an adjunctive psychological technique for the management of a variety of conditions, both acute and chronic, such as pain, anxiety, addiction, mood disturbance, dissociative disorders, and stress-related disorders.

Induction of Hypnosis

A typical hypnotic induction begins with the establishment of rapport between the hypnotist (sometimes referred to as the operator) and the to-be-hypnotized person (the subject). This serves not only to assure the subject of the hypnotist's competence and trustworthiness, but also to create a favorable expectation for a positive response to hypnosis (i.e., by explaining how hypnosis will be used with the subject and correcting any misconceptions about the procedure the individual may have). After this, the subject is invited to relax and be comfortable and to pick some target on which to fix his or her gaze. The hypnotist then exhorts the subject to experience a growing feeling of relaxation and proceeds to direct attention to simple, suggested perceptual changes (e.g., "Your eyelids are becoming heavier and heavier.... they will soon shut of their own accord...."). The specific suggestions are often designed to take advantage of normal bodily responses to the situation, such as the strain and fatigue associated with prolonged visual fixation. Because most individuals readily share such experiences and respond successfully, judiciously selected suggestions of this sort may also serve to enhance expectations for further responsiveness to hypnosis. Once eye closure has been accomplished, the hypnotist will often test whether the subject is truly beginning to experience the condition of hypnosis or is merely complying. Thus, the hypnotist may suggest that it is becoming increasingly difficult, perhaps impossible, for the subject to lift his or her hand. The majority of subjects who pass this challenge (i.e., fail to lift their hand) are indeed usually capable of positive responses to a number of ensuing hypnotic suggestions, provided they are administered in a generally graded sequence of increasing difficulty.

Often early suggestions attempt to promote subjective alterations involving sensory and motor responses, such as the hand growing lighter and lighter and beginning to float upward from the armrest of the subject's chair. Coupled with complementary remarks that as the hand rises the subject will sink deeper and deeper into hypnosis, such a relatively easily experienced suggestion is but one of several deepening techniques intended to shift the subject's awareness from the subject's ambient surroundings to a nearly exclusive focus on experiencing the hypnotist's suggestions. At this point, a suitable subject may experience marked distortions of perception, memory, and mood in response to carefully and methodically linked suggestions that are appropriate to the individual's level of hypnotic skill.

Hypnotizability Assessment and the Phenomena of Hypnosis

Contrary to the view, espoused by the eighteenth-century mesmerists and many modern-day stage hypnotists, that the power of hypnosis resides in the influence of the hypnotist, the scientific evidence is compelling that only a subset of people are capable of experiencing the full range of phenomena that constitute the domain of hypnosis. Thus, it is clear that the ability to respond to hypnosis is determined, in large part, by the individual about to undergo the procedure.

Formal attempts to measure hypnotic ability and to quantify aspects of hypnotic experience began in the United States in the 1930s. The most popular hypnotizability scales in use worldwide today were derived from efforts by Andre Weitzenhoffer and Ernest Hilgard of Stanford University in 1959. A tape-recorded adaptation of their Stanford Hypnotic Susceptibility Scales (SHSS), suitable for use with groups of individuals, was published in 1962 by Ronald Shor and Emily Carota Orne of Harvard University and is known as the Harvard Group Scale (HGS). The general design of these instruments includes a standardized induction and order of administration of hypnotic suggestions that is characterized by increasing difficulty over the course of 12 items. A person's hypnotizability is determined by the number of suggestions (which can range from 0 to 12) that evoke positive behavioral responses as judged by the hypnotist (SHSS) or by the subject (HGS). With the development of standardized scales for hypnotizability assessment, researchers have been able to identify three distinct clusters of hypnotic phenomena.

1. Ideomotor responses. One type of hypnotic response that nearly all individuals can experience to some degree is the tendency for vividly imagined bodily movement to produce corresponding physical movement on a seemingly involuntary basis. Such is the case, for example, when a subject responds to suggestions that his or her "forearm is beginning to feel lighter ... as if a large helium-filled balloon is attached to the wrist and is gently lifting the arm ... allowing it to float effortlessly upward and upward...." Response

to ideomotor suggestions can also occur in the absence of prior hypnotic induction, indicating that some degree of suggestibility may also operate under normal waking conditions. However, although waking suggestibility is moderately correlated with hypnotic responsivity, evidence shows that the hypnotic induction procedure contributes to hypnotic outcomes. Thus, it is exceedingly rare for an individual to respond to suggestions in the waking condition and fail to respond following induction; on the other hand, many individuals' responsiveness to suggestion is substantially increased following an appropriate hypnotic induction.

2. Challenge suggestions. Challenge items are intended to create a contradictory subjective experience involving the inability to carry out one's own will. For instance, the hypnotized subject might be told to "interlock your fingers tightly ... so tightly that they will be impossible to separate. In a moment, you may wish to try to separate your fingers, but you will find that you are unable to do so. Go ahead ... try ... just try to pull your fingers apart." If successfully passed (e.g., in this case, the fingers do not separate), challenge suggestions provide a compelling impression of external control over the individual's behavior – an impression that is often shared by the hypnotized person and onlookers.

3. Cognitive/perceptual alterations. Among the more difficult hypnotic suggestions are those designed to induce some kind of perceptual hallucination and those intended to alter the ability to remember personal experiences from the immediate or remote past. Hallucinatory suggestions can be either positive, in which a nonexistent stimulus is introduced by the hypnotist (e.g., it is suggested that a mosquito is buzzing annoyingly around the subject's face), or negative, in which an actual physical stimulus loses its perceptibility (e.g., the subject is told that he or she will be unable to smell anything, after which an open bottle of ammonia is passed under the nose). Suggested amnesia is an example of a commonly administered cognitive suggestion, whereby the subject is instructed that, on awakening, he or she will have no recollection of the events that transpired during the hypnotic proceedings. Similarly, posthypnotic suggestions are sometimes given during hypnosis with the intent that, following termination of hypnosis, the subject will perform a specific behavior in response to a prearranged cue but will not remember being told to do so. When properly used with suitable patients, amnesia and posthypnotic suggestions can be important clinical tools that may extend therapeutic gains outside the therapist's office.

In addition to delineating the general factor structure of hypnosis into ideomotor, challenge, and cognitive domains, the use of standardized assessment scales has resulted in a great deal of information about hypnotizability in general. One important feature, from both clinical and research perspectives, is the manner in which hypnotizability is distributed in the general population. Hilgard and his associates found that hypnotizability, like many other human skills, follows a normal or bell-shaped pattern, in which the majority of people have the capacity to experience most hypnotic phenomena to some degree, 15–20% are generally unresponsive, and an approximately equal percentage of people are highly responsive. Recognition of such individual differences in the ability to respond to hypnotic procedures is an important consideration for its use clinically, particularly when treatment is predicated on a successful response to difficult cognitive suggestions, such as to experience analgesia (a negative hallucination) for either acute (e.g., dental) or chronic (terminal-stage cancer) pain.

Although scores on standardized assessment scales prove useful in predicting the types of hypnotic suggestions that individuals are most likely to experience, they are not absolute prognosticators of hypnotic potential. This is because, for individuals with scores in the moderately hypnotizable range, various combinations of passed items from different realms of difficulty are possible. The hypnotizability score is determined merely by the sum of items that are passed, not by their classification as ideomotor, challenge, or cognitive (which corresponds roughly to their difficulty level). Thus, although there is virtual assurance that a subject with a score of 2 (out of a possible 12 points) will be unable to experience a positive hallucination, the same cannot be said of a subject with a score of 5 or 6. Modifications of the original SHSS have been published to identify and characterize individual hypnotic profiles, but their use has been limited primarily to research purposes.

A final yet particularly important observation made possible by the availability of standardized scales of hypnotic ability is the general stability of an individual's hypnotic potential over time. This has been confirmed in numerous laboratories throughout the world using correlations among scores obtained for the same participants at varying test–retest intervals, in some cases spanning several decades. Although some research suggests that environmental circumstances can occasionally increase a subject's responsiveness to hypnotic suggestion (e.g., situations involving extreme sensory deprivation or explicit training in the skills necessary to respond positively to specific suggestions), the overall consensus of the evidence is that hypnotizability is one of several relatively enduring characteristics of an individual's personality.

Hypnotic Interventions for Stress Management

Although hypnosis is widely regarded as an effective cognitive-behavioral method for alleviating stress, there is surprisingly little formal research on this issue. There are, however, numerous clinical and experimental studies concerned with specific problems that are often regarded as stressors. From this kindred literature, we can extrapolate conclusions pertaining to the effectiveness of hypnotic techniques in reducing stress. Before doing so, however, it seems prudent to characterize the type of stress to which we refer.

Conceptualizations of stress vary widely. Some investigators have identified stress primarily as a stimulus in which some aspect of the physical or psychological environment exacts a toll on individuals and/or society; others view stress as the psychological or physiological response to such hostile environmental provocation; and still others embrace a more dynamic view whereby the individual's appraisal of the specific environmental pressures, his or her own coping resources, and available options all converge to determine the nature and extent of the stressful experience. From the perspective of scientists and practitioners concerned with the use of hypnotic interventions for stress management, each of these variant emphases holds viability. This is because hypnosis is one of the few psychological techniques that, given an appropriately responsive individual, can be introduced at various points to modify the experience of stress. Thus, it has the potential to mitigate the stimulus impact of a stressor by altering perceptual experience. It can also be enlisted to modify cognitive and affective factors that influence a subject's appraisal of the stressor and his or her ability to cope. In addition, hypnosis may provide specific relief of symptoms precipitated or maintained by exposure to stress.

Pain Control

The use of hypnosis to suppress pain provides dramatic evidence of the technique's value for stress management. Although the widespread availability and safety of chemical anesthetic agents today obviates the use of hypnosis as a general method of surgical anesthesia, there are numerous documented cases in which hypnotic techniques were effectively employed as the sole anesthetic for surgery (e.g., limb amputations, temporal lobectomy, cardiac surgery, tooth extractions, appendectomies, and cesarean sections, among others). An important caveat, however, is that the effectiveness of hypnosis in blocking instances of acute pain is often correlated with the patient's ability to be hypnotized. This has been demonstrated in both clinical samples of patients undergoing painful medical procedures (e.g., bone marrow aspirations, lumbar punctures, and debridement and dressing of burn wounds) and experimental studies involving painful laboratory stressors (e.g., prolonged immersion of the hand in ice water). Another feature that may contribute to the efficacy of hypnosis in the control of acute pain in hypnotically responsive people is the use of direct suggestions delivered in a heterohypnotic or self-hypnotic context.

Hypnosis is decidedly less helpful in the management of certain forms of chronic pain, particularly those with a psychogenic component. Two issues are relevant here. The first concerns the impracticality of heterohypnotic treatments based on direct suggestion in blocking the experience of persistent chronic pain, most of which occurs outside the therapist's office. The alternative strategy, training in self-hypnosis, often requires regular contact with the therapist to reinforce its continued use by the patient in his or her daily life. The more formidable problem, however, concerns the powerful reinforcing value that pain behavior can acquire among family, friends, and other important members of the community. Thus, the sympathy and support provided by others – the so-called secondary gains – may serve to maintain the individual's pain and undermine the incentive to practice hypnotic techniques that otherwise might be helpful in bringing about relief. The most promising prognosis for patients suffering from functional pain of this nature is achieved by a combination of behavior therapeutic principles aimed at extinguishing pain behavior and the implementation of hypnotic or self-hypnotic approaches to minimize pain-related discomfort.

For other forms of chronic pain that do not involve a substantial functional component (e.g., pain from shingles, trigeminal neuralgia, and many types of cancer), hypnosis and self-hypnosis have proven useful as an adjunct to long-term pain management programs. Hypnosis, even self-hypnosis, derives much of its benefit from the interpersonal relationship between patient and therapist, which, among other consequences, tends to shape expectations for therapeutic improvement. In an appropriately supportive context, therefore, hypnotic techniques may prove beneficial without particular regard to the patient's overall ability to respond to hypnosis. For example, we have observed significant improvement among children and adolescents during the course of an 18-month intervention involving regular group training in self-hypnosis to control unpredictable episodes of pain associated with sickle-cell disease. Prior to the intervention, many of the children experienced frequent absences from school, occasionally for weeks

at a time, and the only treatments available included analgesics, narcotic medications, and hospitalization. Although the participants were enrolled in the study based on their expressed wish to help identify an effective nonpharmacological treatment for the disease and without regard to hypnotic ability, our findings indicated that, in this case, the ability to respond to hypnotic suggestion was not an overriding factor in determining how often self-hypnosis was practiced nor how beneficial it proved to be. Apparently, self-hypnosis training, along with consistent reinforcement of the technique during the regular group sessions, provided a much-needed coping skill; the group treatment sessions themselves were critical to maintaining motivation and providing a forum for the patients to share their common fears, misunderstandings, and concerns, which were not being adequately addressed by conventional medical management systems. For the group as a whole, the combination of these therapeutic approaches led to increased school attendance, improved nighttime sleep, less dependence on medication, and fewer bouts of pain, although the more severe episodes of pain still required nonhypnotic supplements for pain management.

Anxiety and Stress Disorders

Stress is inextricably linked to anxiety states, whether they are circumscribed by some anticipated source of realistic concern (e.g., impending open-heart surgery), are more persistent but specific fears (e.g., of elevators or spiders), or are unrelenting and pervasive hindrances to normal functioning (e.g., agoraphobia or social phobia). Hypnotic techniques have proven extremely effective in treating anxiety conditions. Available evidence suggests that there may be two distinct mechanisms responsible for the high success rate. The first, which is nonspecific to hypnosis, is the tendency for hypnotic induction to promote a profound state of relaxation and comfort in many individuals, regardless of their hypnotic capacity. As Joseph Wolpe demonstrated in his development of a behavior therapeutic approach to the treatment of anxiety disorders, relaxation is incompatible with fear. Thus, the cultivation of extreme relaxation, whether accomplished with hypnosis, self-hypnosis, or some other cognitive-behavioral technique (e.g., autogenic training, meditation, or progressive relaxation), will tend to inhibit symptoms of anxiety. The second mechanism is directly related to the ability to experience hypnotic-like conditions and applies to some of the more severe forms of anxiety and trauma-related disorders. Fred Frankel (Harvard Medical School) has compiled extensive data from case studies, which suggest that high hypnotizability may be a risk factor for the development of phobic anxiety. The same positive association involving hypnotizability has been found for acute stress disorder, posttraumatic stress disorder, and dissociative disorders following traumatic experiences. Although such evidence appears to suggest that highly hypnotizable people may be more vulnerable to developing severe anxiety and stress-related conditions pursuant to adverse life events, the picture is far from clear. To date, the majority of studies that report such a relationship have employed cross-sectional designs, meaning that hypnotizability is measured only at the time (or shortly after) the patient is diagnosed with a particular disorder. Thus, it is unknown whether high hypnotizability constitutes a predisposition to anxiety and dissociative symptoms in the aftermath of trauma or whether it is one of several consequences of the stressful experience. In support of the latter possibility, several studies have shown that hypnotizability may be enhanced under adverse conditions, such as sensory deprivation or restricted environmental stimulation. Only studies that adopt a prospective, longitudinal design, in which hypnotizability assessments occur both before and after a stressful life event, can determine the role of hypnotizability in the causal sequence leading to stress-related psychopathology. Nevertheless, and most important, the same highly hypnotizable people who may appear to exhibit a propensity to develop anxiety and stress-related disorders also benefit markedly from psychotherapy that involves the use of hypnosis and training in self-hypnosis as a coping strategy. Similarly, hypnotic methods have been successful in treating survivors of trauma whose symptoms of hyperarousal, emotional numbing, and avoidance are maintained by uncontrollable intrusive flashbacks and recurrent nightmares. In the treatment of posttraumatic stress disorders, hypnosis is most effectively employed as an adjunctive technique, secondary to pharmacotherapy and/or supportive psychotherapy. On a cautionary note, however, the heightened suggestibility and vividness of the imaginings that hypnotized individuals often experience have been associated with a corruption in the accuracy of recollections obtained during hypnotic interviews, whereas their confidence that such memories are veridical tends to be increased. Thus, current evidence warrants that clinical professionals carefully evaluate how hypnosis should be used in the treatment of victims who claim full or partial amnesia for details of past traumatic experiences. As a relaxation technique, hypnosis and self-hypnosis can be highly beneficial; as a tool for recovering memories of past life events, hypnosis elevates the risk that believed-in, false memories may emerge.

Psychophysiological Disorders and Psychoneuroimmunology

Stressors trigger specific neuroendocrine and sympathetic nervous system responses, which, if prolonged, can lead to a number of clinical manifestations linked to parasympathetic inhibition, including dysregulation of respiratory, cardiovascular, digestive, eliminative, and sexual functions. An abundance of case studies attests to the value of hypnotic and self-hypnotic procedures in the treatment of such conditions as asthma, tension headache, irritable bowel syndrome, Crohn's disease, and insomnia. However, there is a paucity of controlled studies in which the distinctive contributions of hypnotic responsiveness and placebo factors to clinical improvement can be evaluated. The available evidence suggests that hypnosis may be as effective as related methods (e.g., biofeedback and progressive relaxation) aimed at countering sympathetic arousal in the treatment of psychophysiological disorders. The mechanism of action appears to involve the induction of a profoundly relaxed condition, which can be achieved in a majority of individuals regardless of their capacity to respond to hypnotic suggestion.

Recent molecular and pharmacological studies have identified intricate patterns of communication between the immune system and the central nervous system, which gives substance to the long-held belief that stress can precipitate illness. Hypnosis is a versatile psychological approach that can alter the perception, evaluation, or symptoms of stress and that might therefore prove effective in the management of infectious or malignant disease. Many studies have found that hypnosis is beneficial in reducing stress symptomatology, which may result in a corresponding improvement in immune function, but the benefit is often only weakly correlated with subjects' hypnotizability, suggesting that any immune enhancement related to hypnosis may be due to nonspecific effects. However, in one study conducted by our laboratory, we were able to confirm a relation between ratings of the depth of relaxation and increases in both the number and cytotoxic capacity of natural killer cells from whole-blood samples from medical students trained to manage stress using self-hypnosis. Other investigators have reported findings that suggest a relationship between the practice of hypnotic methods and indices of humoral and cellular immunity. In addition, recent studies by Gruzelier and colleagues in Great Britain have identified a positive association between hypnotizability and several indices of immunocompetence, which was most evident when hypnotic procedures included guided imagery that specifically addressed immune system dynamics.

At present, we can conclude only that hypnotic techniques appear to be effective in promoting well-being and reducing reactivity to stress, which might otherwise impair immunity to disease. The development of optimal strategies for the use of hypnosis to counteract stress-related immune compromise continues to be informed by further investigation.

Conclusion

As with any clinical intervention, hypnosis can lay claim to the efficacy of both specific and nonspecific components. Because the benefit from hypnotic therapy is a function of the treatment itself, as well as the patient's ability to experience hypnosis, several processes may operate independently or synergistically to determine therapeutic outcome. For individuals who are able to profoundly experience hypnotic suggestion, the stimulus, evaluation, or symptom features of a stressor can be directly addressed in treatment, and the same individuals may be able to avail themselves of the additional benefits that accrue from generalized relaxation and positive expectancies. For individuals of lesser hypnotic capacity, the noncognitive aspects of hypnosis, particularly relaxation, clearly provide an effective technique for inhibiting sympathetic arousal. Finally, because hypnosis requires the establishment of a strong and trusting therapeutic alliance between the therapist and patient, mutual expectations regarding milestones for improvement, coupled with regular contact, may serve to enhance motivation sufficiently to assure adherence to treatment protocols. For some instances of stress, the ability to experience hypnosis may be paramount to effective coping, whereas, for other stressors, simply the subject's belief in his or her ability to benefit from the exercise may prove helpful. It must be emphasized, however, that individuals seeking treatment with hypnosis should consult with a qualified physician, psychologist, or dentist who, in addition to advanced training and practice in one of these health-care specialties, has skills in the adjunctive therapeutic use of hypnotic techniques. When properly applied, hypnotic methods can have a beneficial role in the prevention and treatment of stress-related disorders.

See Also the Following Articles

Stress Management and Cardiovascular Disease; Stress Management, CAM Approach.

Further Reading

Bowers, K. S. (1983). *Hypnosis for the seriously curious.* New York: Norton.

Crasilneck, H. B. and Hall, J. A. (1985). *Clinical hypnosis: principles and applications.* Orlando, FL: Grune & Stratton.

Frankel, F. H. (1979). *Hypnosis: trance as a coping mechanism.* New York: Plenum.

Gruzelier, J. H. (2002). A review of the impact of hypnosis, relaxation, guided imagery and individual differences on aspects of immunity and health. *Stress* 5, 147–163.

Hilgard, E. R. (1965). *Hypnotic susceptibility.* New York: Harcourt, Brace & World.

Orne, M. T. and Dinges, D. F. (1989). Hypnosis. In: Wall, P. D. & Melzack, R. (eds.) *Textbook of pain* (2nd edn., pp. 1021–1031). London: Churchill Livingstone.

Patterson, D. R. and Jensen, M. P. (2003). Hypnosis and clinical pain. *Psychological Bulletin* 129, 495–521.

Hypocortisolism and Stress

C M Heim and U M Nater
Emory University School of Medicine, Atlanta, GA USA

What is Hypocortisolism?

Clinical Findings of Hypocortisolism

Stress and Hypocortisolism

Potential Mechanisms of Hypocortisolism

Effects of Hypocortisolism on Disease Vulnerability

Clinical Implications

Glossary

Cortisol	Glucocorticoid hormone synthesized and secreted from the adrenal cortex in primates. Cortisol is secreted in a diurnal rhythm, and its secretion is increased in response to acute stress. Cortisol controls hypothalamic-pituitary-adrenal axis activity through negative feedback inhibition and exerts metabolic, immune-regulatory, and behavioral effects that adapt the organism to stress.

Functional somatic syndromes	The presence of multiple physical symptoms that manifest without identifiable physical signs or medical abnormalities. Specific symptoms or symptom patterns are used to define syndromal disorders, such as chronic fatigue syndrome, fibromyalgia, irritable bowel syndrome, and chronic pelvic pain.
Glucocorticoid receptors	Intracellular receptor molecules through which cortisol exerts its effects on target cells. There are two types of receptors, the mineralocorticoid receptors (MRs) and the glucocorticoid receptors (GRs). MRs are mainly located in the hippocampus, whereas GRs are widely distributed throughout the brain and periphery. During stress, MRs and GRs in concert control hypothalamic-pituitary-adrenal axis activity.
Hypothalamic-pituitary-adrenal (HPA) axis	Neuroendocrine cascade that controls the secretion of glucocorticoids during stress. Corticotropin releasing hormone from the paraventricular nucleus of the hypothalamus stimulates the secretion of adrenocorticotropic hormone from the anterior pituitary, which in turn stimulates the production and secretion of glucocorticoids (corticosterone in rodents, cortisol in primates) from the adrenal cortex.
Negative feedback inhibition	A decrease in HPA axis activation in response to increasing levels of circulating glucocorticoids, and vice versa, mediated through glucocorticoid receptors at the hippocampal, hypothalamic, and pituitary levels. The feedback sensitivity of the pituitary can be determined by measuring cortisol suppression in response to the synthetic glucocorticoid dexamethasone. Standard doses of dexamethasone detect nonsuppressors (feedback resistance), whereas low doses detect hypersuppressors (increased feedback sensitivity).
Posttraumatic stress disorder (PTSD)	An anxiety disorder that manifests secondary to the experience of a traumatic event and that is characterized by symptoms of reexperiencing of the event, avoidance of reminders of the event, and hyperarousal. Symptoms must last 1 month or longer and must be associated with significant impairment in work, family, or social functioning.
Stress	A state caused by real or perceived challenge to homeostasis, which is accompanied by a hormonal response.
Trauma	A stressful experience that involves actual or threatened death or serious injury or a threat to the physical integrity of the person or others and a response of intense fear, helplessness, or horror.

Since the seminal studies by Hans Selye in 1936, stress has been associated with the activation of the hypothalamic-pituitary-adrenal (HPA) axis, ultimately resulting in the increased secretion of cortisol from the adrenal glands. The physiological effects of cortisol help the organism to maintain homeostasis under conditions of stress. The association between stress and increased cortisol secretion has been consolidated over the past decades to such an extent that stress and increased cortisol secretion nearly have become synonyms in the literature and, moreover, the presence of cortisol hypersecretion has been used to define states of stress. However, representing a major challenge for current concepts in stress research, an increasing number of studies have now provided convincing evidence that the adrenal gland can be hypoactive in some stress-related states. The landmark studies in the 1990s by Rachel Yehuda and her group on neuroendocrine dysregulation in posttraumatic stress disorder (PTSD) have catapulted the phenomenon of hypocortisolism into the center of neuroendocrine stress research. The phenomenon of hypocortisolism has since received growing attention. In fact, hypocortisolism does not merely represent a specific correlate of PTSD but has also been observed in response to severe acute, chronic, and developmental stress in both animal models and studies of human subjects. In addition, hypocortisolism has been observed in patients with chronic fatigue syndrome, fibromyalgia, and chronic pelvic pain, among other functional somatic syndromes. All these disorders are arguably related to stress and frequently coincide with mood and anxiety disorders, including PTSD. Although hypocortisolism appears to be a frequent and widespread phenomenon, its precise definition and epidemiology as well as its underlying mechanisms and physiological relevance remain speculative. It is also unknown whether there are independent or interactive genetic contributions to the manifestation of hypocortisolism in stress and illness. It has been suggested that hypocortisolism is causally involved in the pathophysiology of stress-related disorders; the persistent lack of the regulatory effects of cortisol may promote an increased vulnerability for the development of a spectrum of stress-related disorders characterized by fatigue, pain, stress sensibility, and anxiety. This model has important implications for the prevention and treatment of disorders related to hypocortisolism. This article summarizes current knowledge on the phenomenon of hypocortisolism in stress research.

What is Hypocortisolism?

There is no consensus on the definition of relative hypocortisolism in the published literature. In clinical endocrinology, the normal physiological range of urinary cortisol excretion is 20–90 µg day^{-1}. Thus, medical disorders of adrenal insufficiency, such as Addison's disease, are defined as an abnormal cortisol excretion below the normal physiological range, with endocrine challenge testing performed to elucidate the source of the insufficiency. Interestingly, adrenal insufficiency is related to fatigue, weakness, and pain. However, the stress-related phenomenon of hypocortisolism that is the focus of this article does not necessarily encompass cortisol secretion below the normal physiological range. Rather, reports of hypocortisolism in the stress literature refer to relative decreases of mean cortisol secretion in a defined study group compared to controls, with mean cortisol levels usually in the physiologically normal range. Thus, relative hypocortisolism as observed in stress-related conditions reflects subtle changes in HPA axis regulation that are uncovered when comparing groups. Consequently, to date, there are no diagnostic methods or normative values that allow us to decide whether an individual exhibits such relative hypocortisolism, independent of comparison subjects. When defining relative hypocortisolism, we must decide whether decreased cortisol levels should be measurable under basal conditions, during pharmacological dynamic testing, during stress challenge, or in all of these.

The most stringent definition of hypocortisolism might refer to decreased 24-h urinary cortisol excretion. On the other hand, certain tests, such as the adrenocorticotropic hormone (ACTH)$_{1-24}$ stimulation test, the corticotropin releasing hormone (CRH) test, or the low-dose dexamethasone suppression test, have the potential to be more sensitive to detect relative hypocortisolism by directly targeting the potential mechanisms of dysregulation, such as adrenocortical sensitivity and enhanced negative feedback sensitivity. However, blunted cortisol responses in a CRH stimulation test might not be readily interpreted as hypocortisolism, given that pituitary responses might be low due to elevated circulating glucocorticoid feedback and/or CRH receptor downregulation. Therefore, the identification of relative hypocortisolism usually requires the consideration of a pattern of neuroendocrine results across various conditions. The development of economic, reliable, and valid methods for detecting hypocortisolism as well as normative data is an important task for future research.

In sum, hypocortisolism may reflect many facets of neuroendocrine dysregulation, which may differ within and across populations, ultimately causing a lack of cortisol effects in the organism. For the purposes of the following literature overview, hypocortisolism refers to a deficiency of cortisol, including (1) reduced basal cortisol secretion, (2) reduced adrenocortical sensitivity or capacity to challenge, or (3) enhanced negative feedback inhibition of the HPA axis. Reduced glucocorticoid signaling may also occur due to increased clearance or binding of free cortisol, as well as a reduced glucocorticoid sensitivity of target cells as a consequence of receptor abnormalities.

Clinical Findings of Hypocortisolism

Hypocortisolism has mainly been described in patients suffering from PTSD, chronic fatigue syndrome, fibromyalgia syndrome, and other functional somatic syndromes. Hypocortisolism also occurs in subsyndromal states of exhaustion and chronic pain.

Posttraumatic Stress Disorder

Because the development of PTSD by definition is related to extreme stress experiences, changes in neurobiological systems that participate in the mediation of the stress responses have been extensively studied in these patients. Paradoxically, initial studies demonstrated that basal cortisol concentrations, measured in urine or blood, were markedly reduced in combat veterans with PTSD compared to healthy controls. This finding has been replicated for Holocaust survivors with PTSD as well as for patients with abuse-related PTSD. Low basal cortisol secretion has been hypothesized to reflect hyperregulation of the HPA axis in the context of increased negative feedback sensitivity, as uncovered using low-dose dexamethasone suppression and metyrapone testing, although mild adrenal insufficiency might also play a role. In addition, findings of increased glucocorticoid receptor binding and function support the assumption of the increased negative feedback sensitivity of the HPA axis in PTSD. In the central nervous system (CNS), marked and sustained elevations of cerebrospinal fluid (CSF) concentrations of CRH have been reported in PTSD patients. Significantly, a circuit connecting the amygdala and the hypothalamus with the locus coeruleus, in which CRH and norepinephrine (NE) are the major neurotransmitters, participates in the regulation of vigilance, anxiety, and fear and in the integration of endocrine and autonomic responses to stress. Patients with PTSD exhibit markedly elevated CSF NE concentrations. Cortisol is known to inhibit the NE–CRH feedforward loop. Therefore, we might speculate that reduced cortisol availability leads to sensitization of the central stress responses, with increased negative feedback acting at the pituitary level. Enhanced CRH and NE activation probably contribute to core symptoms of PTSD, such as sleep disruption, increased autonomic arousal, imprinted emotional memories, and enhanced startle reactivity. It must be noted that the finding of hypocortisolism has not been replicated in all PTSD studies, with both normal and elevated cortisol levels reported. Differences in type and timing of the trauma, symptom patterns, and comorbidity, among other factors, might contribute to this inconsistency. However, even normal cortisol output reported in some studies may be inappropriately low in the face of markedly elevated CRH–NE concentrations.

Chronic Fatigue Syndrome and Burnout

A large number of studies have investigated HPA axis alterations in chronic fatigue syndrome (CFS). Several independent studies reported decreased 24-h urinary free-cortisol excretion in patients with CFS. Although some studies failed to detect decreased cortisol secretion in CFS patients, a recent meta-analysis confirmed a moderate overall effect size for reduced 24-h urinary cortisol excretion in CFS. Studies of serial basal cortisol measures in saliva or blood over time have provided inconsistent findings. However, several chronobiological studies demonstrated lower amplitudes of cortisol in CFS patients when controlling for diurnal rhythm changes. CFS patients also exhibit decreased salivary cortisol awakening responses. In addition, decreased adrenal gland volume was reported for hypocortisolemic patients with CFS. In order to identify the origins of decreased adrenocortical activity in CFS, several studies have evaluated alterations in the sensitivity of the adrenal cortex to low doses of ACTH. Results are conflicting, with increased, normal, and decreased sensitivity reported. Inconsistent findings have also been obtained using pituitary or centrally acting challenge tests, such as the CRH challenge test and the insulin tolerance test. The only study that evaluated integrated HPA axis response to a psychosocial stressor found lower ACTH responses in CFS patients. In addition, there is one study suggesting the increased suppression of the HPA axis by a low dose of dexamethasone, although the effect was not confirmed at the pituitary level. Glucocorticoid receptor studies in CFS patients suggest decreased functionality. Taken together, although there is relatively solid evidence for relative hypocortisolism in CFS, results regarding the contributing mechanisms are inconclusive. Based on the concatenation of available findings, it has been suggested that hypocortisolism in CFS originates from the CNS rather than reflecting a primary adrenal dysfunction.

Regardless of its origin, hypocortisolism in CFS has been proposed to be directly linked to aberrations in the control of immune regulators, possibly leading to the characteristic symptom complex of fatigue, pain, cognitive disturbance, and sleep disruption.

Findings of hypocortisolism were also reported in nurses with burnout syndrome. In addition, a study of teachers with burnout syndrome, low morning cortisol, and hypersuppression of cortisol in response to a low-dose dexamethasone suppression test was reported. Such relative hypocortisolism was associated with physical complaints.

Fibromyalgia and Other Chronic Pain Syndromes

A series of studies have provided evidence for hypocortisolism in fibromyalgia syndrome (FMS). Three independent studies report reduced 24-h urinary cortisol excretion in patients with FMS relative to controls. Neuroendocrine challenge studies provided evidence for a primary adrenocortical impairment in FMS, although findings are conflicting. Patients with FMS also demonstrate reduced adrenocortical reactivity in the CRH stimulation test, with ACTH responses being either normal or increased. Several investigators have applied a standard dexamethasone suppression test to patients with FMS. Although two studies reported increased rates of nonsuppressors among FMS patients, several other studies revealed strikingly low rates of nonsuppressors in this patient population, rates that are even lower than nonsuppressor rates in healthy individuals. Nonsuppression seems to occur only in patients with comorbid depression. Based on these findings, we may expect that FMS is related to increased negative feedback sensitivity, similar to PTSD, although the hypothesis has not yet been directly tested. Despite the pronounced suppression of cortisol by dexamethasone, reduced glucocorticoid receptor affinity has recently been measured in the lymphocytes of patients with FMS, suggesting reduced regulatory effects of already low cortisol on target cells in the immune system, which might contribute to the increased perception of pain.

Findings of hypocortisolism have also been reported in women with chronic pelvic pain (CPP). In a series of studies of HPA axis function, women with CPP with no identified organic correlate demonstrated normal to low diurnal salivary cortisol levels. In response to CRH stimulation, normal plasma ACTH but reduced salivary cortisol concentrations were observed. These patients also exhibited an enhanced suppression of salivary cortisol to a low dose of dexamethasone, suggesting enhanced negative feedback sensitivity of the HPA axis. These same women had an increased rate of sexual and physical abuse experiences in addition to

PTSD and high levels of chronic stress. Interestingly, similar findings for women with CPP and verified pelvic adhesions were obtained. Evidence for relative hypocortisolism was also reported in other groups with chronic pain syndromes, such as patients with chronic headaches and children with recurrent abdominal pain. In addition, patients who had chronic sciatic pain 8 weeks after disk surgery exhibited decreased cortisol secretion after awakening, which was negatively correlated with pro-inflammatory cytokine activity. Significantly, a recent prospective study suggests that preoperative hypocortisolism predicts the development of persistent pain after disk surgery, as well as decreased pain threshold, increased NE activity, and pro-inflammatory cytokine production, in failed back syndrome (FBS) patients compared to patients who did not develop persistent pain and to healthy controls.

Other Somatic Disorders Related to Hypocortisolism

Relative hypocortisolism has also been reported for several other somatic disorders. Children and adults with asthma or atopic dermatitis exhibit decreased cortisol responses to psychosocial stress. Patients with rheumatoid arthritis have decreased basal cortisol levels, concordant with the assumption of hyperimmune activation in hypocortisolism. Basal hypocortisolism has been reported for atypical depression, which is characterized by lack of energy and predominantly somatic symptoms, closely resembling CFS. Finally, there is some evidence for low basal cortisol levels with blunted ACTH and cortisol responses to CRH challenge in patients with functional gastrointestinal disorders, such as irritable bowel syndrome (IBS). In IBS, the lack of cortisol effects might lead to the increased activation of CRH–NE systems, which in turn exert direct effects on gastrointestinal function, potentially leading to bowel symptoms.

Is There a Spectrum of Hypocortisolism-Related Disorders?

Hypocortisolism has been identified in diverse stress-related bodily disorders, although the potential mechanisms of hypocortisolism and its causal relationship in the pathophysiology of these disorders have not been sufficiently studied. Nevertheless, given the accumulating evidence for hypocortisolism in many patients suffering from diverse stress-related disorders, we may speculate that these disorders represent a spectrum of related disorders with common pathophysiological pathways. Interestingly, there is symptom overlap and high rates of comorbidity among all the disorders related to hypocortisolism. There are also reports that cases with PTSD are at elevated risk for developing fatigue and pain over time. In addition, all these disorders share common risk factors, such as certain personality styles, chronic stress, and early adverse experience. Interestingly, the symptoms of all the disorders discussed so far are frequently triggered by acute or chronic stresses. Moreover, childhood abuse has been identified as a risk factor for the development of PTSD (after additional trauma in adulthood) as well as for CFS, FMS, CPP and functional gastrointestinal disorders. Although chronic stress and developmental stress have marked influences on the HPA axis, there are virtually no integrative studies assessing stress history and psychopathology together with HPA axis function in patients with bodily disorders. It is likely that stress experiences contribute to hypocortisolism in bodily disorders and might be linked to comorbid emotional problems. We next discuss whether there is preclinical evidence for an association between stress and hypocortisolism.

Stress and Hypocortisolism

Hypocortisolism does not seem to be an exclusive correlate of stress-related pathology; it has also been reported for healthy subjects living under ongoing stress as well as for healthy people with early developmental stress. In addition, some animal models of chronic and early-life stress have reported findings of decreased adrenocortical activity, particularly in nonhuman primates.

Studies in Humans

A small number of studies in humans suggest reduced adrenocortical activity or reactivity in states of chronic stress; some of these studies date back to the 1960s and 1970s. With increasing evidence for hypocortisolism in stress-related disorders, these early findings have regained attention in stress research. For example, decreased urinary excretion of the cortisol metabolite 17-hydroxycorticosterone (17-OHCS) was measured over several months in the parents of fatally ill children. Many of these parents demonstrated decreased 17-OHCS excretion below their initial baseline, even in phases of acute medical complications in their children. Lower than normal 17-OHCS excretion was also observed in soldiers of a special team in Vietnam who had been warned to expect an enemy attack; interestingly, 17-OHCS levels dropped even further on the day when the attack was anticipated. In another study, the same authors measured 17-OHCS excretion in helicopter medics in Vietnam. These medics demonstrated a stable pattern of decreased 17-OHCS excretion whether they were flying or not. On flying days, some medics even demonstrated lower 17-OHCS levels than on their days off. Similar findings were obtained in civilian paramedics who demonstrated lower cortisol levels on work days compared to their days off. More recently, decreased plasma cortisol concentrations were measured in Bosnian prisoners of war, in white-collar employees with high work loads, and in chronically stressed teachers. Finally, evidence for marked hypocortisolism under basal conditions has been reported in severely neglected children, such as Romanian orphans. Maltreated children exhibit flat cortisol cycles throughout the day, particularly on high-conflict days. Interestingly, greater numbers of work hours for employed mothers and greater numbers of children in the household are also associated with lower morning cortisol levels and a flat cortisol cycle across the day in children. Decreased basal cortisol secretion and mild adrenocortical insufficiency in response to maximal ACTH stimulation has also been reported in adult women with histories of childhood sexual or physical abuse, particularly in the absence of depression. There are also findings of hypocortisolism in healthy subjects with early loss experiences. Taken together, these findings suggest that hypocortisolism does occur in humans as a function of severe chronic or early-life stresses. The physiological meaning of hypocortisolism is unclear; it might reflect a physiological state of preparedness in threatening situations, a state of exhaustion after chronic stress, and/or a state of adaptive counterregulation to hyperactive central stress response systems.

Animal Studies

The increasing evidence for the phenomenon of hypocortisolism in clinical and preclinical human research is not paralleled by an equal focus on hypocortisolism in animal models. Indeed, there exist only very few published studies that found low glucocorticoid secretion in animal models of stress. The most conclusive reports to date are studies in nonhuman primates. For example, when tested as adults, nonhuman primates exposed to prolonged periods of maternal or social deprivation exhibit marked behavioral, physiological, and neurobiological changes, including fearfulness and anxiety, social dysfunction, anhedonia, and changes in immune and autonomic function. In terms of HPA axis function, basal and stress-induced cortisol secretion has been reported to be either increased or reduced. Squirrel monkeys exposed to repeated social separations demonstrate markedly reduced cortisol responses to later separation stress and

increased glucocorticoid feedback sensitivity. Similarly, decreased morning cortisol excretion was recently reported for marmoset monkeys exposed to repeated maternal separation. Another paradigm in nonhuman primates involves the exposure of bonnet macaque mothers with infants to unpredictable conditions with respect to food access for 3 months, resulting in a diminished perception of security and a reduction of maternal care for the infants. When tested as adults, bonnet macaques reared under these conditions demonstrated elevated CSF CRH concentrations, sensitization of the NE system, and behavioral sensitization to fear stimuli. However, their cortisol levels were markedly decreased. Thus, early-life stress appears to result in decreased adrenocortical activity in several nonhuman primate models, closely paralleling findings in PTSD patients.

Although there now are a number of reports of hypocortisolism in nonhuman primates, very few studies on hypocortisolism in rodent models of stress have been published. In one study, social isolation resulted in a reduction of plasma corticosterone levels, both under basal and stress-stimulated conditions. Prenatal exposure to dexamethasone also resulted in decreased HPA axis activity in rat offspring. In rats, a single session of prolonged severe foot shock stress induced enhanced negative feedback sensitivity compared to stress-naïve animals. However, when the rats were stressed again 2 weeks later, no differences in stress responses were observed. Interestingly, one study showed that chronically stressed rats that initially demonstrated lower corticosterone levels developed higher acoustic startle responses and gastrointestinal damage than rats with initially higher levels, suggesting a causal role of relative hypocortisolism for promoting high central stress/fear responses and physical symptoms.

It should be noted that there are numerous reports that adult rats that were subjected to early handling (3–15 min daily) exhibited lower HPA responses to stress and generally better adaptation and health than nonhandled rats. However, it was found that the handling procedure induces increased maternal care after the reunion, probably reflecting a nurturing early environment, whereas the nonhandled rats were more deprived and therefore had relatively increased stress reactivity. This hypothesis was confirmed when directly tested in rats with high and low maternal care.

Potential Mechanisms of Hypocortisolism

As already mentioned, relative hypocortisolism has been described in a multitude of stress-related conditions that share common symptoms and frequently manifest in comorbidity. Different mechanisms may contribute to decreased cortisol output under various conditions, and different facets of hypocortisolism have been emphasized for different study groups. For example, increased negative feedback inhibition has been emphasized for PTSD, adrenocortical dysfunction has been suggested for FMS, and central origins of hypocortisolism have been suggested for CFS. Clearly, to date, all of the possible contributing mechanisms have not been sufficiently studied in all of the disorders that appear to be related to hypocortisolism. It might well be that there is heterogeneity within diagnostic groups that might reflect different pathways to illness. Future studies should systematically scrutinize each of these disorders in terms of multiple potential mechanisms. Potential mechanisms include (1) reduced biosynthesis or depletion at several levels of the HPA axis (CRH, ACTH, and cortisol); (2) CRH hypersecretion and adaptive downregulation of pituitary CRH receptors, resulting in lower than normal ACTH and cortisol secretion once a stressor stops and CRH secretion returns to normal levels; (3) increased feedback sensitivity of the HPA axis; and (4) morphological changes (i.e., decreased adrenal gland volume). Lack of cortisol effects may also result from relative glucocorticoid resistance of target cells due to receptor changes; decreased availability of free, biologically active cortisol due to alterations in binding proteins; changes in enzyme activity (i.e., 11-β-hydroxysteroid dehydrogenase) that metabolizes glucocorticoid hormones on entry into the cell; and changes in the multidrug resistance pump, which extrudes cortisol but not corticosterone from the target cell.

It should be noted that superimposed factors, such as the nature or timing of the stressor, coping styles, personality, sex, and genetic variations probably contribute to hypocortisolism and might influence the specific mechanisms of its manifestation in relation to stress. For example, the timing of stress during development influences the direction of HPA axis changes in nonhuman primates. Passive-avoidant coping and alexithymic personality appear to be linked to hypocortisolism. Women generally have lower free-cortisol responses to psychosocial stress then men. Basal cortisol levels and HPA axis responses to stress have been shown to be influenced by genetic factors in twin studies. Finally, polymorphisms in genes involved in the stress response, such as the glucocorticoid receptor (GR) gene, have been shown to markedly moderate neuroendocrine responses to stress. In addition to these factors, it has been suggested that hypocortisolism might reflect

different symptom constellations or phases during the course of illness. Taken together, integrative longitudinal research approaches are needed to address the mechanisms of hypocortisolism, together with contributing factors and illness characteristics, in the future.

Effects of Hypocortisolism on Disease Vulnerability

There are several avenues through which the lack of cortisol might lead to characteristic symptoms of pain, fatigue, and anxiety/stress sensitivity. First, glucocorticoids secreted during stress induce gluconeogenesis, mobilize free fatty acids, and reduce the use of amino acids for protein synthesis, thereby increasing the organism's energy supplies. Altered metabolism during stress due to hypocortisolism might lead to exhaustion and fatigue.

Second, glucocorticoids exert inhibitory effects on the secretion of pro-inflammatory cytokines, such as interleukin (IL)-6 and tumor necrosis factor (TNF)-α, during stress and help return these cytokines to baseline levels after stress. These cytokines regulate cellular immunity and mediate pain. Increased or prolonged cytokine activity in the brain leads to impaired cognitive function and mood and anxiety symptoms through the stimulation of CRH–NE systems. Thus, the lack of glucocorticoid effects probably promotes the disinhibition of pro-inflammatory cytokines during stress, resulting in increased vulnerability to developing chronic fatigue, chronic pain, allergies, asthma, and emotional disorders. Interestingly, elevated pro-inflammatory cytokine levels have been reported for PTSD and several functional somatic syndromes, although the findings are inconsistent. Patients with adrenal insufficiency also have elevated levels of pro-inflammatory cytokines, such as IL-6, as well as symptoms of fatigue and pain.

Third, cortisol exerts direct effects on the brain and behavior. Thus, glucocorticoids exert negative feedback effects on the CRH-induced activation of the locus ceruleus NE cells. Relatively decreased cortisol output may have permissive effects toward an increased and sustained activation of the feedforward cascade between the CRH and NE systems, perhaps in concert with elevated cytokine responses. CRH and NE are implicated in enhanced encoding of traumatic emotional memories, facilitation of fear conditioning, and increased vigilance and arousal, including increased startle responses, leading toward the three symptom clusters of PTSD. Enhanced CRH–NE activation might further stimulate the immune system, promoting fatigue and pain, and might promote gastrointestinal disturbance. This model suggests that hypocortisolism indeed might occur as a preexisting (genetic or stress-related) risk factor that promotes the development of a spectrum of emotional and somatic disorders. In support of this hypothesis, increased autonomic activity and low cortisol secretion directly after the trauma are significant predictors of the development of PTSD. Low cortisol levels presurgery predict the development of ongoing pain and immune–NE hyperactivation after surgery in FBS patients.

Clinical Implications

If hypocortisolism indeed is causally involved in the development of certain stress-related disorders, reflecting a preexisting risk factor, this has seminal clinical implications. Once normative values are established, hypocortisolism could be measured in healthy subjects to predict the risk of developing PTSD or functional somatic disorders should severe or ongoing stress occur. Consequently, the substitution of hydrocortisone should have preventive effects. In fact, the administration of hydrocortisone during trauma has been shown to effectively prevent PTSD in humans in several studies. In addition, it was recently demonstrated that hydrocortisone treatment, simulating normal circadian cortisol rhythm, is effective in the treatment of PTSD. Randomized controlled clinical trials, furthermore, showed that some (but not all) patients with CFS benefit from hydrocortisone treatment.

In conclusion, given the high prevalence of disorders related to hypocortisolism, the development of studies aiming to describe the mechanisms of hypocortisolism across and within disorders, to scrutinize the effects of hypocortisolism in target cells of the immune system and CNS, and to reverse these effects surely is a promising and exciting area of future research.

See Also the Following Articles

Acute Stress Disorder and Posttraumatic Stress Disorder; Adrenal Cortex; Adrenal Insufficiency; Adrenocorticotropic Hormone (ACTH); Allostasis and Allostatic Load; Animal Models (Nonprimate) for Human Stress; Arthritis; Asthma; Burnout; Child Abuse; Childhood Stress; Chronic Fatigue Syndrome; Corticosteroids and Stress; Corticotropin Releasing Factor (CRF); Cytokines; Dexamethasone Suppression Test (DST); Disease, Stress Induced; Endocrine Systems; Fatigue and Stress; Gastrointestinal Effects; Glucocorticoid Negative Feedback; Glucocorticoids, Effects of Stress on; Glucocorticoids, Overview; Glucocorticoids, Role in Stress; Hypothalamic-Pituitary-Adrenal; Immune Response; Immune Suppression; Neuroendocrine Systems; Pain; Pharmacological Treatments of Stress; Posttraumatic Stress Disorder, Neurobiology of; Salivary Cortisol; Somatic Disorders; Stress Effects, Overview; Stress, Definitions and Concepts of.

Further Reading

Adler, G. K. and Geenen, R. (2005). Hypothalamic-pituitary-adrenal and autonomic nervous system functioning in fibromyalgia. *Rheumatic Disease Clinics of North America* **31**, 187–202.

Clauw, D. J. and Chrousos, G. P. (1997). Chronic pain and fatigue syndromes: overlapping clinical and neuroendocrine features and potential pathogenic mechanisms. *Neuroimmunomodulation* **4**(3), 134–153.

Chrousos, G. P. and Gold, P. W. (1992). The concepts of stress and stress system disorders: overview of physical and behavioral homeostasis. *Journal of the American Medical Association* **267**, 1244–1252.

Cleare, A. J. (2004). The HPA axis and the genesis of chronic fatigue syndrome. *Trends in Endocrinology and Metabolism* **15**(2), 55–59.

Fries, E., Hesse, J., Hellhammer, J., et al. (2005). A new view on hypocortisolism. *Psychoneuroendocrinology* **30**(10), 1010–1016.

Geiss, A., Rohleder, N., Kirschbaum, C., et al. (2005). Predicting the failure of disc surgery by a hypofunctional HPA axis: evidence from a prospective study on patients undergoing disc surgery. *Pain* **114**, 104–117.

Gunnar, M. R. and Vazquez, D. M. (2001). Low cortisol and a flattening of expected daytime rhythm: potential indices of risk in human development. *Developmental Psychopathology* **13**(3), 515–538.

Heim, C., Ehlert, U. and Hellhammer, D. H. (2000). The potential role of hypocortisolism in the pathophysiology of stress-related bodily disorders. *Psychoneuroendocrinology* **25**(1), 1–35.

McEwen, B. S. (1998). Protective and damaging effects of stress mediators. *New England Journal of Medicine* **338**(3), 171–179.

Raison, C. L. and Miller, A. H. (2003). When not enough is too much: the role of insufficient glucocorticoid signaling in the pathophysiology of stress-related disorders. *American Journal of Psychiatry* **160**, 1554–1565.

Sapolsky, R. M., Romero, L. M. and Munck, A. U. (2000). How do glucocorticoids influence stress responses? Integrating permissive, suppressive, stimulatory, and preparative actions. *Endocrine Reviews* **21**(1), 55–89.

Sternberg, E. M. (2001). Neuroendocrine regulation of autoimmune/inflammatory disease. *Journal of Endocrinology* **169**(3), 429–435.

Yehuda, R. (2002). Current status of cortisol findings in post-traumatic stress disorder. *Psychiatric Clinics of North America* **25**(2), vii, 341–368.

Hypoglycemia

B M Frier
Royal Infirmary of Edinburgh, Edinburgh, UK

This article is a revision of the previous edition article by B M Frier, volume 2, pp 453–459, © 2000, Elsevier Inc.

Physiological Responses to Hypoglycemia
Effects on Cerebral Function
Causes and Investigations

Glossary

Autonomic reaction	Physiological manifestations of acute activation of the sympathetic (sympatho-adrenal) division of the autonomic nervous system, through the autonomic neural stimulation of end organs and secretion of catecholamines.
Awareness of hypoglycemia	The subjective perception of the onset of symptoms generated by a decline in blood glucose.
Cognitive dysfunction	The impairment of intellectual and mental activities as a consequence of interference with cerebral function.
Counter-regulation	The process that promotes the secretion of hormones that oppose the actions of insulin, provoking metabolic changes that elevate blood glucose.
Gluconeo-genesis	The production of new glucose from three carbon precursors, principally in the liver and kidney.
Glucose homeostasis	The metabolic maintenance of blood glucose within a narrow range by regulatory mechanisms. The main factors controlling this are the intake of nutrients, the rates of gastric emptying and intestinal absorption, the hepatic production of glucose, and the secretion of insulin and counter-regulatory hormones.
Glycemic threshold	The blood glucose concentration at which a specific event is triggered during the development of hypoglycemia (e.g., onset of symptoms).
Glycogenolysis	The breakdown of hepatic glycogen into glucose, which is released into the circulation.
Neuro-glycopenia	The direct effect of glucose deprivation on neurons in the central nervous system.

Hypoglycemia (low blood glucose) is a biochemical abnormality that can be arbitrarily defined by a low blood glucose concentration. In a person with diabetes, a blood glucose below 3.5 mmol l^{-1} (61 mg dl^{-1}) is considered to represent hypoglycemia; in a nondiabetic person, a blood glucose below 2.2 mmol l^{-1} (38 mg dl^{-1}) is almost always pathological. Hypoglycemia *per se* is not a clinical diagnosis, and a cause for the low blood glucose should be sought.

Physiological Responses to Hypoglycemia

The human brain requires a continuous supply of glucose as its principal source of energy and malfunctions rapidly if deprived of this substrate. To protect the brain and prevent a dangerous fall in blood glucose, multiple counterregulatory mechanisms have evolved to maintain glucose homeostasis. These include the secretion of counterregulatory hormones including glucagon, epinephrine (adrenaline), cortisol, and growth hormone; the centrally activated release of various neurotransmitters; and simultaneous inhibition of endogenous insulin secretion. Hepatic autoregulation can release glucose during profound hypoglycemia. The secretion of pancreatic glucagon occurs independently of the activation of counterregulatory mechanisms within the brain. In contrast, epinephrine is secreted secondary to the stimulation of the sympathetic division of the autonomic nervous system following the activation of autonomic centers within the hypothalamus. The other counterregulatory hormones are released through the activation of the hypothalamic-pituitary-adrenal axis. These hormones promote the breakdown of glycogen to glucose within the liver (hepatic glycogenolysis) and the production of three carbon precursors from proteolysis and glycogenolysis in the skeletal muscle that are used for glucose formation (gluconeogenesis) within the liver and kidney. The oxidation of free fatty acids, produced by lipolysis, provides energy for gluconeogenesis.

Hypoglycemia generates symptoms (1) as a direct consequence of glucose deprivation of neurons in the brain (neuroglycopenia) and (2) secondary to acute autonomic stimulation. Symptoms are idiosyncratic and age-specific, varying considerably among individuals, both in nature and intensity. Common autonomic symptoms are sweating, trembling, pounding heart, hunger, and anxiety; neuroglycopenic symptoms include inability to concentrate, drowsiness, confusion, difficulty with speech, and incoordination. Common nonspecific symptoms include nausea, tiredness, and headache. The recognition of the early onset of the symptoms of hypoglycemia is essential for people with diabetes who are treated with insulin so that a correction of the low blood glucose can be made.

Symptomatic hypoglycemia is usually associated with the activation of the autonomic nervous system and a rise in plasma catecholamines of similar magnitude to that observed during major vascular events such as acute myocardial infarction and subarachnoid hemorrhage. Hypoglycemia can therefore represent a severe form of stress, which provokes major pathophysiological consequences. Catecholamines provoke hemodynamic changes through their direct effects on the cardiovascular system, causing changes in regional blood flow, and the effects on various organs induce physiological changes that are identified as autonomic symptoms (**Figure 1**). This is sometimes described as an autonomic reaction. A transient rise in heart rate is accompanied by an elevation in systolic blood pressure and a decline in diastolic blood pressure, with increased myocardial contractility and cardiac output. Blood flow is increased to the brain, heart, liver, gut, retina, and skeletal muscles, but is decreased to organs such as the kidney and spleen. Hypoglycemia also provokes significant hemostatic and hemorheological changes (mainly through hormonal action), which can affect the microcirculation.

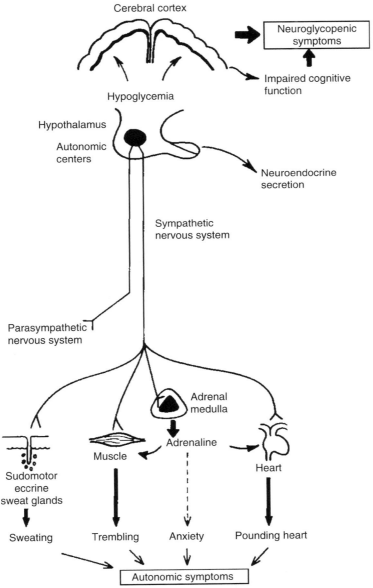

Figure 1 Autonomic neural pathways involved in the generation of the peripheral physiological manifestations and symptoms during insulin-induced hypoglycemia.

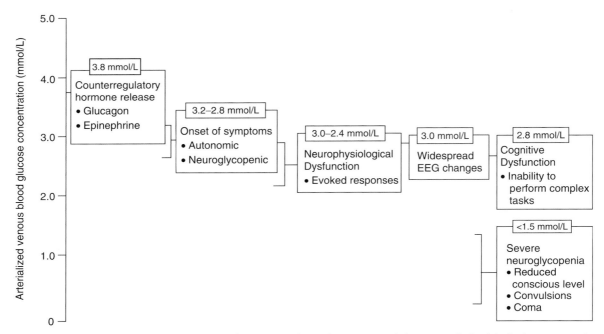

Figure 2 Glycemic thresholds for the secretion of counterregulatory hormones and the onset of physiological, symptomatic, and cognitive changes in response to acute hypoglycemia in nondiabetic adults. Glycemic thresholds are shown in relation to glucose values in arterialized venous blood. Reproduced from Frier, B. M. and Fisher, B. M. (eds.) (1999), *Hypoglycaemia and clinical diabetes,* Chichester, UK: John Wiley. Copyright 1999 John Wiley & Sons Limited. Reproduced with permission.

Effects on Cerebral Function

A progressive decline in blood glucose triggers a hierarchy of events that occur at individual glycemic thresholds (**Figure 2**). Counterregulation is stimulated when arterial blood glucose falls below 3.8 mmol l^{-1}, and impairment of cognitive function commences below 3.0 mmol l^{-1}. Early changes are subtle, and progressively greater cognitive impairment occurs around 2.6 mmol l^{-1}, with deteriorating performance evident in tests of several cognitive domains. Some of the neuroglycopenic symptoms of hypoglycemia are subjective manifestations of impaired cognitive function. Hypoglycemia also induces noncognitive changes in mood and behavior, including feelings of tense tiredness, unhappiness, fear, despondency, and, in some individuals, anger. Autonomic symptoms commence around 3.0 mmol l^{-1}, and the effects on neurophysiological function (sensory-evoked potentials and electroencephalographic abnormalities) become more prominent as blood glucose falls further. If the condition is untreated, confusion and drowsiness will progress to loss of consciousness and coma. The comatose state may be complicated by convulsions. Significant brain damage is rare and occurs only if the neuroglycopenia is protracted, leading to brain death. Thus, hypoglycemia can vary significantly in severity, ranging from asymptomatic biochemical hypoglycemia to profound coma. In people with insulin-treated diabetes, severe hypoglycemia is defined by the need of the individual for external assistance for recovery, in which situation acute neuroglycopenia is interfering with the individual's capability for self-treatment. Severity is not determined by the intensity of the symptomatic response or the development of coma.

Glycemic thresholds are not fixed, can vary among individuals, and, in people who have diabetes, can be influenced by recurrent exposure to hypoglycemia. In some people with insulin-treated diabetes, their symptom profile alters with time, the perception of the onset of symptoms becomes diminished, and they may develop a degree of impaired awareness of hypoglycemia. This is a major risk factor for severe hypoglycemia. With the increasing duration of insulin-treated diabetes, deficiencies of counterregulatory hormonal secretion often develop as an acquired defect, and this also increases the risk of severe hypoglycemia. This problem co-segregates with impaired awareness of hypoglycemia. In affected individuals, the glycemic thresholds for the onset of autonomic symptoms and for counterregulatory hormonal secretion are reset at a lower blood glucose than usual, allowing neuroglycopenia to supervene and interfere with the patient's ability to self-treat hypoglycemia. These acquired abnormalities are associated with strict glycemic control (particularly when glycated hemoglobin is within the nondiabetic range) and with repeated exposure to episodic (antecedent) hypoglycemia, and they occur in other conditions that cause chronic or recurrent hypoglycemia, such as insulin-secreting tumors (e.g., insulinoma). These changes represent an adaptation by the brain to allow it to function during glucose deprivation.

Although total cerebral blood flow is increased during hypoglycemia, the regional changes in blood flow within the brain vary considerably, being increased to frontal areas (including the cerebral cortex) and reduced in posterior regions of the brain. Localized changes in cerebral blood flow may provoke some of the neurological manifestations of hypoglycemia such as transient hemiplegia. However, the rate-limiting factor in protecting the brain against neuroglycopenia is the transport of glucose across the blood–brain barrier. Glucose transporters can be upregulated in response to chronic hypoglycemia, but this process is relatively slow and it takes time (hours to days) for the human brain to adapt and be able to function at low concentrations of blood glucose. Such a modification is essentially maladaptive because the warning symptoms of impending neuroglycopenia are obtunded, reducing the time available to detect the falling blood glucose and increasing the risk of progressing to severe hypoglycemia.

Hypoglycemic coma is associated with the release of excitatory amino acids, including glutamate and aspartate, which activate subtypes of excitatory amino acid receptors including N-methyl-D-aspartate receptors. Membrane depolarization occurs and leads to neuronal necrosis. The brain is affected in a rostrocaudal direction, with the cerebral cortex and hippocampus being most sensitive to neuroglycopenia; the brain stem and spinal cord are much more resistant. In fatal cases of hypoglycemic coma, the neuropathology of the brain is variable, but the laminar necrosis of neurons occurs in the third to fifth layers of the cerebral cortex. Survivors of severe protracted hypoglycemic coma develop cortical and hippocampal atrophy, with ventricular enlargement, often associated with a chronic vegetative state. The cumulative effects of recurrent severe hypoglycemia may cause intellectual impairment in the developing brain of infants and young children, but in adults (principally those with insulin-treated diabetes) the effect on cognitive impairment appears to be modest, with occasional anecdotal exceptions. Progression to severe intellectual impairment and dementia is rare, although a few cases have been described, particularly in patients exposed to chronic neuroglycopenia of long duration, for example in association with an undiagnosed insulin-secreting tumor. Although repeated exposure of people with insulin-treated diabetes to severe hypoglycemia may induce modest cognitive impairment, this may primarily be caused by other co-existing morbidities, such as hypertension, chronic hyperglycemia (poor glycemic control), and cerebrovascular disease, and underlies the concept of a diabetic encephalopathy.

Causes and Investigations

Multiple causes of hypoglycemia are recognized in humans, but most are rare. In the nondiabetic population, hypoglycemia is most commonly associated with excessive alcohol consumption. However, by far the most common cause is iatrogenic, resulting from the inadvertent use of insulin or drugs that promote insulin secretion (mostly sulfonylureas), which are used for the treatment of diabetes. Occasionally, hypoglycemia is the presenting feature of an illness or occurs as an important epiphenomenon, and it is then considered to be spontaneous. The classification of hypoglycemia can be based on etiology (see **Table 1**) or, alternatively, on whether insulin is detectable. Subdivision into "fasting" and "reactive" types of hypoglycemia is no longer used. The spectrum of causes of hypoglycemia varies between hospital and community practice. In hospitalized patients, hypoglycemia is associated with diabetic therapies, chronic renal failure, infections, liver disease, shock, pregnancy, neoplasia, and burns. In the community, excessive alcohol consumption and therapies for treating diabetes predominate as the main causes.

Hypoglycemia is usually episodic, but the symptoms that are commonly experienced with acute insulin-induced hypoglycemia may be absent in people who present with spontaneous hypoglycemia. A low blood glucose level should be suspected in people who present as an acute medical emergency with collapse, altered consciousness, convulsions, abnormal neurological findings, or confusion. A suspicion of underlying hypoglycemia should be considered even when an obvious cause of cerebral abnormality is apparent, such as hemiplegic stroke, alcoholic intoxication, or cerebral malaria. An accurate and reliable history may be difficult to obtain from the patient, and an objective account from witnesses may be valuable. Where subacute neuroglycopenia presents with deteriorating cognitive function over months or years, psychiatric features may be prominent, and such patients may have been referred to a neurologist or psychiatrist for investigation of funny turns, feeling faint, odd behavior, paresthesiae, or convulsions. In some cases, the only indication that hypoglycemia is responsible is the finding of a low blood glucose level on routine biochemical screening.

Tumor-induced hypoglycemia may occur as a pre-terminal feature of an advanced malignancy,

Table 1 Causes of hypoglycemia in adults

Type	Causes
Toxic hypoglycemia	Therapeutic hypoglycemic agents: insulin, sulfonylureas
	Alcohol
	Drugs, e.g. quinine, salicylates, propranolol, pentamidine
	Poisons, e.g. certain types of mushroom
Pancreatic	Insulinoma: benign, malignant, multiple and microadenomatosis
	Islet hyperplasia with functional hyperinsulinism
Extrapancreatic neoplasms	Mesenchymal tumors
	Hemangiopericytoma
	Primary hepatic carcinoma
	Various other tumors
Liver and kidney disease	Hepatocellular disease; cirrhosis
	Advanced renal failure
	Congestive cardiac failure
Endocrine disease	Pluriglandular syndrome
	Pituitary insufficiency
	Adrenocortical insufficiency
	Selective hypothalamic insufficiency
Autoimmune hypoglycemia	Autoimmune insulin syndrome
	Anti-insulin receptor antibodies
Inborn errors of metabolism	Adult glycogenolysis (liver glycogen disease)
	Hereditary fructose intolerance
Miscellaneous	Sepsis; burns
	Prolonged starvation; anorexia nervosa
	Dialysis
	Excessive, strenuous exercise
	Diseases of the nervous system
	Falciparum malaria

particularly in patients with extensive hepatic metastases and also with some very large tumors such as fibrosarcoma. Some tumors secrete substances with insulin-like activity; malignancies involving the liver disrupt hepatic gluconeogenesis and the maintenance of glucose homeostasis. Insulinomas are pancreatic islet cell tumors that secrete insulin and usually cause recurrent fasting hypoglycemia. They are rare (one to two cases per million population per year) but are one of the commonest causes of spontaneous hypoglycemia in nondiabetic individuals. Symptoms may occur before meals or during exercise and are relieved by the consumption of food or a glucose drink. The tumors are usually small (0.5–5 mm in diameter) and may occur in any part of the pancreas. Approximately 10% are malignant.

A firm diagnosis of hypoglycemia is usually based on Whipple's triad:

- Symptoms are associated with fasting or exercise.
- Symptoms are relieved by glucose.
- Low blood glucose is demonstrated by biochemical analysis.

In the investigation of suspected hypoglycemia, low blood glucose should be confirmed by laboratory analysis of venous or capillary blood glucose. Hypoglycemia is often associated with inappropriately elevated plasma insulin concentrations. Blood should be collected during the emergency presentation, and the plasma frozen and stored, both for immediate confirmation of hypoglycemia and for additional analyses (e.g., for hormones, alcohol, and drugs), which may identify a cause. This can avoid subsequent unnecessary investigations and is of forensic and medical-legal importance in cases of attempted suicide or deliberate poisoning.

The nature and timing of blood samples for the measurement of glucose are important in the evaluation of the causes of hypoglycemia. The possible development of a large arteriovenous difference after glucose absorption precludes the use of glucose tolerance tests that require an oral glucose load because the arterial plasma glucose concentration is 15% higher than that estimated from whole venous blood. Provocative tests for investigating suspected hypoglycemia include prolonged fasting with or without exercise and the infusion of intravenous insulin to induce hypoglycemia to see whether C-peptide (an index of endogenous insulin secretion) is suppressed. Plasma concentrations of insulin, C-peptide, pro-insulin, and other hormones such as insulin-like growth factor (IGF)-1 may also be measured during confirmed hypoglycemia. Characteristic patterns of plasma glucose and insulin are associated with different causes of hypoglycemia, and a diagnosis of endogenous hyperinsulinism depends on evidence of inappropriate insulin and/or C-peptide secretion in the presence of hypoglycemia. With an insulinoma, a mesenchymal tumor, and a sulfonylurea overdose, the fasting plasma insulin is usually inappropriately high for the prevailing blood glucose and endogenous insulin secretion is not suppressed. This can be demonstrated by elevated plasma C-peptide during insulin-induced hypoglycemia. Factitious hypoglycemia is characteristically associated with elevated plasma insulin and absent plasma C-peptide in nondiabetic individuals, indicating that an overdose of exogenous insulin has been administered.

True reactive hypoglycemia may occur in patients who have had previous gastric surgery or who have gastrointestinal motility disorders. However, some individuals describe symptoms suggestive of, but without biochemical evidence of, hypoglycemia that occur 1–2 h after food. This is called the postprandial syndrome, and such patients should be evaluated with ambulatory blood glucose measurements or by serial measurements of plasma glucose and insulin after a standard mixed meal, plus recording of symptoms and dietetic assessment.

The emergency treatment of acute hypoglycemia should not be withheld to await a confirmatory biochemical diagnosis. In diabetic patients, self-treatment of mild hypoglycemia requires the ingestion of a glucose drink or food. More severe hypoglycemia can be treated with intravenous glucose or intramuscular glucagon. In noniatrogenic causes of hypoglycemia, treatment depends on the specific diagnosis. Tumor-induced hypoglycemia may require prolonged therapy if surgical resection is not possible or the tumor cannot be located. Treatment with diet (regular intake of oral carbohydrate) and drugs that inhibit insulin secretion (e.g., diazoxide), thiazide diuretics, and somatostatin analogs (e.g., octreotide) may be beneficial. Patients with true reactive hypoglycemia usually respond to dietary measures such as the exclusion of highly refined sugars and the consumption of frequent regular meals that are high in fiber content; the α-glucosidase inhibitor acarbose may be beneficial.

Further Reading

Cryer, P. E. (2002). Hypoglycaemia: the limiting factor in the glycaemic management of type I and type II diabetes. *Diabetologia* 45, 937–948.

Cryer, P. E. and Frier, B. M. (2004). Hypoglycaemia. In: De Fronzo, R. A., Ferrannini, E., Keen, H. & Zimmet, P. (eds.) *International textbook of diabetes mellitus* (3rd edn., pp. 1079–1100). Chichester, UK: John Wiley.

Frier, B. M. and Fisher, B. M. (eds.) (1993). *Hypoglycaemia and diabetes: clinical and physiological aspects*. London: Edward Arnold.

Frier, B. M. and Fisher, B. M. (eds.) (1999). *Hypoglycaemia and clinical diabetes*. Chichester, UK: John Wiley.

Marks, V. (2001). Spontaneous hypoglycaemia. *CPD Clinical Biochemistry* 3, 67–71.

Marks, V. and Teale, J. D. (1998). Tumours producing hypoglycaemia. *Endocrine-Related Cancer* 5, 111–129.

Service, F. J. (1995). Hypoglycemic disorders. *New England Journal of Medicine* 332, 1144–1152.

Service, F. J. (1999). Hypoglycemic disorders. *Endocrinology and Metabolism Clinics of North America* 28, 467–661.

Hypotension, Hypovolemia, and Septic Shock

A Beishuizen and A B Johan Groeneveld
VU University Medical Center, Amsterdam,
The Netherlands
I Vermes
Medical Spectrum Twente, Enschede, The Netherlands

This article is a revision of the previous edition article by A Beishuizen, I Vermes and C Haanen, volume 2, pp 460–467, © 2000, Elsevier Inc.

Introduction
Neuroendocrine Regulation in Hypotension and
   Hypovolemia
Septic Shock

Glossary

Aldosterone	A mineralocorticoid hormone produced by the zona glomerulosa of the adrenal cortex and a key regulator of potassium balance where it induces sodium and water retention.
Angiotensin II	An octapeptide which acts to increase peripheral arterial resistance, raising blood pressure, and stimulates aldosterone biosynthesis.
Atrial natriuretic peptide (ANP)	A polypeptide hormone mainly synthesized in the cardiac atrium, released following atrial dilatation or increased intravascular volume, and involved in natriuresis and the regulation of blood pressure and volume homeostasis.
Circulatory shock	A generalized inadequacy of blood flow throughout the body, to the extent that the tissues are damaged because of too little flow, especially too little delivery of oxygen to tissue cells.
Cytokines	Polypeptide cell regulators, mainly produced by cells of the immune system, which all affect in some way the function of the immune system and have the ability to act as communication signals.
Hypotension	A systolic blood pressure of <90 mmHg or a reduction of ≥40 mmHg from baseline.
Hypovolemia	An abnormal decrease in blood (plasma) volume.
Multiple organ dysfunction syndrome	The presence of altered organ dysfunction in an acutely ill patient such that homeostasis cannot be maintained without intervention.

Renin	A glycoprotein hormone and proteolytic enzyme produced by the juxtaglomerular cells of the kidney in response to hypovolemia and hypotension and it cleaves its substrate angiotensinogen into angiotensin I.
Sepsis	The systemic response to infection.
Septic shock	Sepsis-induced hypotension, despite adequate fluid resuscitation along with the presence of perfusion abnormalities which may include, but are not limited to, lactic acidosis, oliguria, or an acute alteration in mental status.
Sympatho-adrenal system	An anatomical and physiological unit of the adrenal medulla and the sympathetic nervous system.
Vasopressin	A polypeptide hormone produced in the hypothalamus and stored in the posterior pituitary from which it is secreted upon osmotic and hemodynamic stimuli. Once released, it induces vasoconstriction and promotes free water clearance. Also known as antidiuretic hormone.

Introduction

The survival of multicellular organisms is exquisitely dependent on the continuous provision of all body cells with fluid, oxygen, minerals, nutrients, and the uninterrupted elimination of metabolic waste products in order to provide the cells and tissues with the essential circumstances necessary for life. To ensure these vital conditions an intact vascular and microvascular blood flow is a primary prerequisite. Any serious failure of the circulatory system to maintain the cellular perfusion and a fluid homeostasis causes a syndrome of clinical symptoms due to abnormal cellular metabolism, membrane dysfunction, and cell death in tissues and organs throughout the body, eventually ending up in death of the whole organism.

The main symptoms of circulatory failure include hypotension and tachycardia and the patient may show profuse perspiration, the extremities are cool and mottled, and peripheral pulses are weak or impalpable. Due to inadequate perfusion of the brain, a shock state can be demonstrated by restlessness, anxiety, confusion, somnolence, and unconsciousness up to deep coma. In cases of mild shock, there is a decreased perfusion of nonvital organs, such as skin, adipose tissue, skeletal muscle, and bones. The mental state is unimpaired; the urine output may be slightly decreased. In moderate shock, the perfusion of liver, gastrointestinal tract, and kidneys is decreased, but that of the heart and brain is still intact. Urine production is diminished and metabolic acidosis is present. In severe shock, the perfusion of heart and brain is inadequate with severe acidosis and an altered mental state. Finally, the cardiac output diminishes, which further compromises the blood pressure, and respiratory failure will develop.

Circulatory shock is characterized by a failure to maintain adequate tissue perfusion and an impaired oxygen delivery which will ultimately lead to anaerobic metabolism and adenosine triphosphate (ATP) depletion and mitochondrial dysfunction. In general, three stages of shock can be distinguished: early (non-progressive), progressive, and irreversible. The most frequent causes of shock can be divided in cardiogenic, distributive (such as sepsis or anaphylaxis), hypovolemic, and obstructive shock (**Table 1**).

Septic shock is more life threatening than hypovolemic or cardiogenic shock, because it is always accompanied by microcirculatory dysfunction and cellular membrane injury, which can lead to multiple organ dysfunctions. This severe stress state involves cardiac dysfunction, acute renal failure, adult respiratory distress syndrome, and hepatic failure.

Table 1 Classification and etiology of circulatory shock

Hypovolemic shock
  Decreased preload and subsequently decreased cardiac output
  Hemorrhage (external or internal)
  Fluid loss (diarrhea, vomiting, heat stroke, inadequate repletion of insensible losses, burns, and "third spacing" (which can occur in intestinal obstruction, pancreatitis, and cirrhosis)
Cardiogenic shock
  Pump failure (infarction, cardiomyopathy, myocarditis)
  Arrhythmias (both atrial and ventricular)
  Mechanical abnormalities (acute valvular insufficiency, rupture ventricular wall)
Distributive (vasodilatatory) shock
  Severe decrease in systemic vascular resistance, often associated with an increased cardiac output
  Septic shock
  Activation of the systemic inflammatory response (pancreatitis, burns, or multiple traumatic injuries)
  Toxic shock syndrome
  Anaphylaxis and anaphylactoid reactions
  Addisonian crisis
  Myxedema coma
  Neurogenic shock
  Post-cardiopulmonary bypass
Obstructive shock
  Massive pulmonary embolism
  Tension pneumothorax
  Severe constrictive pericarditis
  Pericardial tamponade
  Severe pulmonary hypertension producing Eisenmenger's physiology

Neuroendocrine Regulation in Hypotension and Hypovolemia

Because hypotension and/or hypovolemia compromise the distribution of essential nutrients to body tissue, they represent a threat to homeostasis. Homeostatic systems such as blood and tissue oxygen, acid–base status, and body temperature must be maintained within narrow ranges. Accordingly, hypovolemia- and/or hypotension-induced hormonal responses are part of the well-orchestrated defense mechanisms of the three major central systems of the individual: the nervous, endocrine, and immune system. Acute changes in the hormonal functions are primarily adaptive and provide optimal conditions of the organism for the fight, including optimal intravascular volume and perfusion pressure. Under physiological conditions the acute reaction of the body to these challenges is twofold, turning on defense mechanisms that initiate a complex adaptive pathway (adaptive phase), and then shutting off this response when the threat is past (recovery phase). However, there are limits to the ability of the hormonal system to compensate adequately when the inappropriate hormonal response can contribute to the breakdown of the body tissue (catabolic phase). Hormonal changes during or following hypotension and/or hypovolemia are summarized in **Table 2**. Salt and water balance is largely determined by factors regulating fluid and electrolyte intake and, more importantly, the ability of the kidney to regulate sodium and water excretion. Vasopressin, the renin-angiotensin-aldosterone (RAA) axis and the sympatho-adrenal system are the key players in the regulation of volume and water during stress (**Figure 1**).

Critical illness such as shock is characterized by striking alterations in the hypothalamic-anterior-pituitary-peripheral hormone axes, the severity of which is associated with a high risk of morbidity and mortality. There appears to be a biphasic neuroendocrine response to critical illness. The acute phase is characterized by an actively secreting pituitary, but most peripheral hormones are decreased, partly due to the development of target-organ resistance. This is considered to be beneficial, at least for short-term survival. In prolonged illness, uniform (hypothalamic) suppression of the neuroendocrine axes contributes to low levels of the target-organ hormones. These alterations are considered to be maladaptive and contribute to the catabolism and wasting.

Hypothalamo-Posterior Pituitary System

Vasopressin is a peptide hormone that is synthesized in the hypothalamic nuclei and transported to the posterior pituitary where it is stored. It is released

Table 2 Neuroendocrine changes during hypotension and hypovolemia

Hormone	Acute phase	Chronic phase	Recovery phase
HPA axis			
CRH	⇑	⇑	⇓
ACTH	⇑	⇓	N
Cortisol	⇑⇑⇑	⇑	⇑/N
DHEA(S)	⇓⇓	⇓⇓	N
CBG	⇓⇓	⇓	N
RAA system			
Renin	⇑	⇑	⇓/N
Angiotensin II	⇑	⇑	⇓/N
Aldosterone	⇑	⇓	⇓/N
Vasopressin	⇑/N	⇑	N
ANP	⇑	⇑⇑⇑	N
Sympatho-adrenergic system			
Epinephrine	⇑⇑⇑	⇑/N	N
Norepinephrine	⇑	⇑/N	N
Prolactin	⇑	?	N
Insulin	⇓	⇑	⇓
Glucagon	⇑	⇑	⇑
GH	⇑	⇓	⇑/N
IGF-I	⇓	⇓	⇑/N
IGFBP3	⇓	⇓	N
Pituitary-thyroid axis			
TSH	N	⇓	⇓/N
TT4	N	⇓	N
TT3	⇓	⇓	N
rT3	⇑	⇑	N
FT4	N	⇓	N
FT3	⇓	⇓	⇓/N
TBG	?	?	?

⇓, decrease; ⇑, increase; ?, unknown; ACTH, adrenocorticotropic hormone; ANP, atrial natriuretic peptide; CBG, cortisol-binding globulin; CRH, corticotropin-releasing hormone; FT3, free triiodothyronine; FT4, free thyroxine; GH, growth hormone; HPA, hypothalamic-pituitary-adrenal; IGF-I, insulin-like growth factor I; IGFBP3, insulin-like growth factor binding protein-3; N, number; RAA, renin-angiotensin-aldosterone; rT3, reverse triiodothyronine; TBG, thyroxine-binding globulin; TSH, thyrotropin; TT3, total triiodothyronine; TT4, total thyroxine.

into the circulation upon stimulation by increased plasma osmolality or as a baroreflex response to decreases in blood volume or blood pressure. Vasopressin exerts antidiuretic, hemostatic, and vasoconstrictive effects via stimulation of V_1- and V_2-receptors. Furthermore, vasopressin serves as a key secretagogue in the body's complex endocrinologic orchestra (**Figure 1**). The physiological effect of vasopressin is to promote free water clearance by altering the permeability of the renal collecting duct to water. This effect is mediated by renal V_2-receptors that are coupled to adenylyl cyclase and the generation of cyclic adenosine monophosphate (cAMP). Vasopressin is also capable of causing vasoconstriction and increasing blood pressure. In fact, vasopressin is a more potent vasoconstrictor than norepinephrine and is capable of

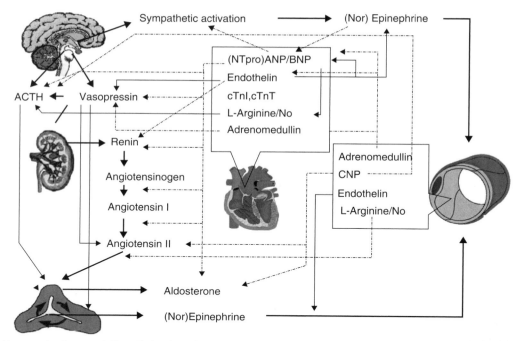

Figure 1 Neuroendocrine regulation of shock and hypotension. Thick lines represent positive feedback mechanisms. Thin lines represent less pronounced positive feedback regulation. Interrupted lines stand for negative feedback. ACTH, adrenocorticotropic hormone; ANP, atrial natriuretic peptide; BNP, brain (B type) natriuretic peptide; CNP, C-type natriuretic peptide; cTnI, troponin I; cTnT, cardiac troponin T; NO, nitric oxide; NTpro, N-terminal pro.

increasing systemic vascular resistance in doses less than those required to produce antidiuresis. Conversely, vasopressin is a relatively weak pressor agent because it resets the cardiac baroreflex to a lower pressure. These actions are mediated via V_1-receptors which are coupled to phospholipase C and increased intracellular Ca^{2+} concentration. Aside from the corticotropin-releasing hormone (CRH), vasopressin is known to be the most potent stimulator of adrenocorticotropic hormone (ACTH) and, consequently, cortisol release. Additionally, vasopressin exerts stimulatory effects on prolactin and endothelin-1 release, and it modulates atrial natriuretic peptide (ANP) and angiotensin II secretion.

Increased vasopressin release is, therefore, a key part of the hypotension- and/or hypovolemia-induced neuroendocrine stress adaptation. Low plasma vasopressin concentration during stress is a sign of the inappropriate autonomic adaptation which has been described in patients with septic or hypovolemic shock. However, it is unclear if this relative vasopressin deficiency has clinical relevance or therapeutic consequences.

Renin-Angiotensin-Aldosterone System

The RAA system plays a pivotal role in the control of cardiovascular homeostasis (**Figure 1**). Renin is a glycoprotein hormone produced by the renal juxtaglomerular cells in response to hypovolemia and hypotension, but is not a vasoactive substance. Its primary action is to cleave angiotensinogen into the decapeptide, angiotensin I. In the pulmonary circulation, angiotensin-converting enzyme (ACE) removes two more amino acids from angiotensin I to produce angiotensin II, which is the active hormone with a direct strong vasoconstrictor effect (40 times more potent than norepinephrine) and an effect on the adrenal cortex to stimulate aldosterone production. Aldosterone is the key regulator of the potassium balance and induces sodium and water retention. The appropriate response of the RAA axis to hypotension and hypovolemia is renin release, which, via angiotensin II, induces aldosterone secretion by the adrenal cortex, resulting in hyperreninemic hyperaldosteronism, which is a state of secondary hyperaldosteronism often caused by depletion of extracellular fluid and reflected by metabolic alkalosis and hypokalemia. Stress-induced ACTH and vasopressin release also induces aldosterone secretion independently of volume status. An elevated plasma-renin concentration accompanied by inappropriately low aldosterone level is present in some seriously ill patients with hypovolemia and hypotension, and is a sign of the insufficient adaptation of the RAA axis (hyperreninemic hypoaldosteronism, a transient and reversible syndrome characterized by a dissociation of plasma renin activity and aldosterone production (20–30% of critically ill patients) possibly due to a transient diffuse impairment of the zona glomerulosa of the kidney. Activation of the RAA system occurs during any type of pump failure or shock.

The family of natriuretic peptides consists of ANP, brain (B type) natriuretic peptide (BNP) and C-type natriuretic peptide. ANP is a 28-amino acid polypeptide hormone synthesized in the heart and released into the circulation in response to stretch of the heart chambers, fluid loading, and congestive heart failure. ANP works to oppose the function of the RAA axis via inhibiting the secretion and effects of renin, the effects of angiotensin II, and the adrenal secretion of aldosterone (**Figure 1**). ANP acts on the kidney to increase sodium excretion and glomerular filtration rate to antagonize renal vasoconstriction. In the cardiovascular system, ANP antagonizes vasoconstriction and shifts fluid from the intravascular to the interstitial compartment. The diuretic and blood pressure lowering effect of ANP may be partially due to adrenomedullin.

BNP and N-terminal pro-brain natriuretic peptide (NTproBNP) are mainly produced in the human ventricle and are cleaved from their inactive precursor proBNP. Both ANP and BNP levels are elevated in a variety of conditions in the critically ill, such as sepsis, trauma, and shock and have prognostic value.

Sympatho-Adrenal System

The sympatho-adrenal response to severe stress is marked, rapid, and transient and plays an important role in the early metabolic changes during the acute phase of a stress response (**Figure 1**). Epinephrine is secreted from the adrenal medulla in direct response to increased sympathetic tone; however, the majority of the circulating norepinephrine is released from the sympathetic nerve endings. Both catecholamines support blood pressure, heart rate, myocardial contractility, cardiac output, respiration, and bronchial tone. Epinephrine is an important catabolic hormone, inducing lipolysis, glycogenolysis, and gluconeogenesis, and stimulates glucagon release and inhibits insulin release. A high level of plasma catecholamines has been found during the acute phase of a stress response, but the measurements of plasma catecholamine concentrations have limited value as an index of the sympathetic nervous system activity because of their extremely short half-life.

Hypothalamo-Pituitary-Adrenal Axis

The hypothalamic-pituitary-adrenal (HPA) axis does not follow a simple activation response but rather demonstrates a biphasic process during hypotension and/or hypovolemia. There is a prompt, dramatic, and sustained increase in both cortisol and ACTH concentration in blood. This activation is accompanied by a loss of circadian rhythm, ACTH pulsatility, and CRH sensitivity of the pituitary. During the second catabolic phase the high plasma cortisol level is accompanied by paradoxically low ACTH levels. Vasoactive peptides such as vasopressin, endothelin, ANP, or calcitonin gene-related peptide (CGRP) are implicated in the adrenal activation in this stage. The degree of cortisol elevation correlates with the degree of homeostatic disturbances.

Neuropeptides

In addition to these classical stress hormones, several other hormones are augmented in response to hypotension and/or hypovolemia. There is no doubt that prolactin and growth hormone (GH) are released during this stress response but the biological meaning is much less clear. However, there are experimental observations that neuropeptides may play a causal role in the hypotension and/or hypovolemia-induced cardiovascular responses. There is now appreciable evidence that one such group of neuropeptides, the endogenous opioids, exert a major influence on cardiovascular responses as a counter-stressor system. In canine hemorrhagic shock models, administration of the opioid antagonist naloxone significantly improved mean arterial pressure without change in heart rate and total peripheral resistance; increased cardiac contractility and cardiac output; and reduced mortality. In patients with hemorrhagic shock, infusion of opiate antagonist resulted in improvement in hemodynamic status via a significant fall in heart rate together with improvement in stroke volume without reduction in cardiac output, and reduction in vasopressor requirements. Based on these observations, it has been suggested that although hypovolemic shock is best treated in the human by volume repletion, in an emergency situation, an opioid antagonist might stabilize the patient until the institution of conventional therapy. In addition to endogenous opiates, the endogenous release of the potent vasoconstrictor neuropeptide Y (NPY) is increased in hypovolemic shock. NPY co-exists and is co-released with norepinephrine, and causes direct vasoconstriction and potentiates norepinephrine-induced vasoconstriction in a complex manner. NPY plays a relatively minor role in the minute-to-minute maintenance of cardiovascular homeostasis; its role being one of a second line of defense that comes into play in situations of greater or more prolonged stress. However, the role of CGRP, the most potent vasodilatator and hypotensive agent yet tested, has been also suggested as a causal factor in hypotension-induced stress response. Plasma CGRP levels are related to hemodynamic changes and there is a correlation between the initial CGRP plasma level and the severity of the shock. It is possible that neuropeptides, especially endogenous opiates, represent a physiological buffer of the cardiovascular response to stress, namely as a major counter-stressor system exerting significant influence on cardiovascular responses to both physiological and pathophysiological stresses in animals and humans.

Septic Shock

Septic shock is the most common cause of death in intensive care units. The terms sepsis, severe sepsis, and septic shock are used to identify the continuum of the clinical response to infection. However, the definition of sepsis appears to be very complicated because of the nonhomogenous nature of the patient population studied and the underlying conditions related to sepsis. Septic shock is hypoperfusion with organ dysfunction in a septic patient. Sepsis represents a severe threat to homeostasis and it is related to a systemic inflammatory host response to an inciting event. In general terms, sepsis is a severe stress stimulus which disturbs the milieu interne and induces homeostatic responses specific to the stimulus and generalized responses when the disturbances are severe. Regulation of fluid and volume status is of critical important to survival. Multiple mechanisms exist to maintain normovolemia and adequate blood pressure in sepsis, and when they fail septic shock arises. Septic shock is often characterized by massive systemic vasodilatation with low vascular resistance, and increased cardiac output. The relative lack of effective pharmacologic interventions highlights the complex pathophysiologic events involved in sepsis. In this paragraph we focus on the pathogenesis, and neuroendocrine–immune interactions (**Figure 2**).

Pathogenesis

The clinical manifestations of septic shock are the result of an excessive host response to an (usually bacterial) infection. Although host defense mechanisms are usually beneficial and designed to localize and neutralize invading micro-organisms, remove dead and damaged cells, and repair tissue damage, excessive activation may be detrimental. The inflammatory response to infection or injury is a highly conserved and regulated reaction of the organism. Immediately, the organism produces several soluble and lipid pro-inflammatory molecules that activate cellular defenses and then produces similar anti-inflammatory molecules to attenuate and halt the pro-inflammatory

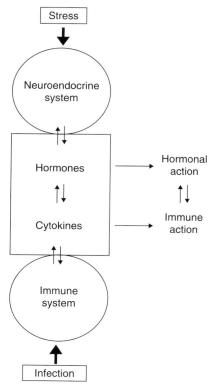

Figure 2 Bidirectional interactions between the neuroendocrine and immune systems during critical illness.

response. The complex interaction of these stress mediators can be seen as a cascade. The initial inflammatory response is kept in check by downregulating production and counteracting the effects of cytokines already produced. These mediators initiate overlapping processes that influence the endothelium, cardiovascular, hemodynamic, and coagulation systems directly. The release of many of these vasoregulators is often local, as part of the total septic-response picture. The overproduction of nitric oxide (NO), a potent vasodilator, has been held responsible for the hemodynamic and metabolic consequences of sepsis and endotoxemia. High levels of nitrite and nitrate, the stable end-products of NO metabolism, are found in patients with septic shock and these levels correlate with vasodilatation and the degree of shock.

The duration of illness also may alter the mix of mediators, leading to a state of metabolic disorders in which the body has no control over its own inflammatory response. If the balance cannot be established and homeostasis is not restored, a massive pro-inflammatory reaction (sepsis inflammatory response syndrome; SIRS) or a compensatory anti-inflammatory reaction (compensatory anti-inflammatory response syndrome, CARS) will ensue.

Bone and colleagues have proposed five stages in the development of septic shock and ultimately multiple organ dysfunction:

1. The local reaction at the site of injury or infection: the initial response is to induce a pro-inflammatory state in which mediators (TNF, IL-1, IL-6, interferon-γ, platelet-activating factor) have multiple overlapping effects designed to limit new damage and to ameliorate whatever damage has already occurred. They destroy damaged tissue, promote the growth of new tissue, and combat pathogenic organisms. A compensatory anti-inflammatory response soon ensures that the effects of these pro-inflammatory mediators do not become destructive. IL-4, IL-10, IL-11, IL-13, soluble TNF receptors, IL-1 receptor antagonists, and others work to diminish monocytic major histocompatibility complex class II expression, impair antigen presenting activity, and reduce the ability of cells to produce inflammatory cytokines. Local levels of these mediators can be much higher than are later found systemically.

2. The initial systemic response: if the original insult is severe enough, first pro-inflammatory and later anti-inflammatory mediators will appear in the systemic circulation. The pro-inflammatory mediators help recruit neutrophils, T cells and B cells, platelets, and coagulation factors to the site of injury or infection. Few significant clinical signs are produced.

3. Massive systemic inflammation: the loss of regulation of the pro-inflammatory response results in a massive reaction manifested as the systemic inflammatory response with (a) progressive endothelial dysfunction, (b) platelet sludging blocking the microcirculation, (c) activation of the coagulation system and (d) profound vasodilatation, fluid transition, and maldistribution of blood flow may result in severe shock.

4. Excessive immunosuppression: this 'immune paralysis' or 'compensatory anti-inflammatory response syndrome' is a result of an inappropriate anti-inflammatory reaction.

5. Immunologic dissonance: this is the final stage of MODS, an inappropriate, out-of-balance response of the immunomodulatory system. Sometimes, monocyte deactivation has been shown.

Basic and clinical science continues to reveal the molecular picture for the etiology and pathophysiology of sepsis, however, sepsis continues to puzzle and challenge physicians. Recent discoveries have shown that not only microbial products but also endogenous molecules can trigger Toll-like receptors (TLR), which are held responsible for the stimulation of widespread inflammation. TLR-4, the endotoxin receptor, is constitutively suppressed and the first step in sepsis could be the release of TLR-4 from suppression.

Neuro-Immuno-Endocrine Interactions

The endocrine and immune systems are interrelated via a bidirectional network through which hormones and neuropeptides affect immune function and, in turn, immune responses are reflected in neuroendocrine changes (**Figure 2**). Apparently, there is constant interaction between neuroendocrine and internal immunoregulatory mechanisms that assures the fine tuning of both the neuroendocrine and the immune system so that both are able to preserve homeostasis during severe and life-threatening illnesses. Evidence shows that inflammatory cytokines are produced in the brain and endocrine glands and that these organs have cytokine receptors. This suggests that paracrine mechanisms mediated by locally produced cytokines play certain roles in causing endocrine changes in inflammation or sepsis. Similarly, various neuropeptides, including GH and PRL, are produced in immunocompetent cells and neuropeptide receptors are present on these cells.

Many cytokines, such as IL-1 and TNF, can activate the HPA axis, when given by systemic routes. These cytokines seem to act through the hypothalamus via release of CRH, which is the most important regulator of ACTH. IL-1, IL-2, IL-6, and TNF act directly on the adrenal cortex to enhance biosynthesis of glucocorticoids, possibly contributing to the persisting hypercortisolism, present in critical illness. Injection of bacterial lipopolysaccharide (LPS) into healthy volunteers increases plasma TNF within 90 min followed by increases of plasma ACTH and cortisol levels. Plasma IL-6 also increases 2–3 h after LPS injection, but IL-1 and IFN-γ remain unchanged. IL-6, synthesized through increases of IL-1 and TNF plays a pivotal role in activating the HPA axis. Interestingly, IL-6 suppresses IL-1 production indicating a negative feedback regulation within the cytokine cascades. Cytokines are also produced locally in a variety of tissues, including in the brain. Both IL-1 and IL-6 are involved in activation of the HPA-axis. Various stimuli, for example LPS, lead to the production of cytokines in the anterior pituitary gland, acting through a paracrine or autocrine mechanism to modulate ACTH secretion and to regulate growth of pituitary cells. Cytokines can also be produced in the adrenocortical or medullary cells, with a modulating function in steroid hormone production.

Recent studies have led to the discovery of a mediator that acts as an endogenous counter-regulator of glucocorticoid action within the immune system: macrophage migration inhibitory factor (MIF) produced by the anterior pituitary gland, macrophages and T cells in response to inflammatory stimuli and upon incubation with low concentrations of glucocorticoids. Once secreted, MIF overrides the anti-inflammatory and immunosuppressive effects of steroids on macrophage and T cell cytokine production. Patients with sepsis show elevated MIF levels, which are correlated with poor prognosis. Anti-MIF antibodies protect animals from septic shock.

In conclusion, it appears that the acute response of the HPA axis is mediated by cytokines in inflammatory foci. Since cytokine levels in the brain or endocrine organs under unstimulated conditions are very low, the action of cytokines locally produced by LPS requires a certain latent period. Therefore, the paracrine mechanisms may become significant under prolonged stimulation by infectious agents. Metabolic alterations induced by TNF are considered to be dependant on tissue TNF levels, but not on systemic levels. This suggests the importance of locally produced cytokines. As a result of the activation of the HPA axis, glucocorticoids are finally produced and act on the immune system to inhibit the overshoot of cytokine production and to enhance the defense mechanism of the organism. Thus, there exists a feedback mechanism over the immune and endocrine systems; glucocorticoids inhibit cytokine-induced CRH release and also production of certain cytokines in endocrine organs. Another feedback mechanism may exist in cytokine cascades too. Both IL-1 and IL-1 receptor antagonist are produced by the same cells, probably with a different time course, to modulate overstimulation by IL-1. Complex interactions seem to exist also among inflammatory cytokines. These feedback mechanisms are involved in maintaining homeostasis in inflammatory processes and sepsis.

Sepsis may not only be attributable to hyperactivation of the immune system (uncontrolled hyperinflammation) but systemic anti-inflammatory responses might dominate the body's stress response. The immune system may be severely compromised and unable to eradicate pathogens. Future therapy may be directed at enhancing or inhibiting the patient's immune response.

Further Reading

Annane, D., Bellisant, E. and Cavaillon, J. M. (2005). Septic shock. *Lancet* **365**, 63–78.

Beishuizen, A., Hartemink, K. J., Vermes, I., et al. (2005). Circulating and cardiovascular markers and mediators in the critically ill: an update. *Clinica Chimica Acta* **354**, 21–34.

Beishuizen, A. and Thijs, L. G. (2004). The immunoneuroendocrine axis in critical illness: beneficial adaptation or neuroendocrine exhaustion? *Current Opinion in Critical Care* **10**, 461–467.

Besedovsky, H. O. and Del Rey, A. (1996). Immune-neuroendocrine interactions: facts and hypotheses. *Endocrine Reviews* **17**, 64–102.

Bone, R. C., Grodzin, C. J. and Balk, R. A. (1997). Sepsis: a new hypothesis for pathogenesis of the disease process. *Chest* **112**, 235–243.

Buckingham, J. C. (1998). Stress and the hypothalamopituitary-immune axis. *International Journal of Tissue Reactions – Experimental and Clinical Aspects* **20**, 23–34.

Calandra, T. and Bucala, R. (1997). Macrophage migration inhibitory factor (MIF): a glucocorticoid counterregulator within the immune system. *Critical Reviews in Immunology* **17**, 77–88.

Chrousos, G. P. and Gold, P. W. (1992). The concept of stress and stress system disorders. Overview of physical and behavioral homeostasis. *JAMA* **267**, 1244–1252.

Espiner, E. A. (1987). The effects of stress on salt and water balance. *Baillière's Clinical Endocrinology and Metabolism* **2**, 375–390.

Little, R. A., Kirkman, E. and Ohnishi, M. (1998). Opioids and the cardiovascular response to haemorrhage and injury. *Intensive Care Medicine* **24**, 405–414.

Hotchkiss, R. S. and Karl, I. E. (2003). The pathophysiology and treatment of sepsis. *New England Journal of Medicine* **348**, 138–150.

Riedemann, N. C., Guo, R-F. and Ward, P. A. (2003). The enigma of sepsis. *Journal of Clinical Investigation* **112**, 460–467.

Van den Berghe, G., de Zegher, F. and Bouillon, R. (1998). Acute and prolonged critical illness as different neuroendocrine paradigms. *Journal of Clinical Endocrinology and Metabolism* **83**, 1827–1834.

Vanhorebeek, I., Langouche, L., and Van den Berghe, G. Endocrine aspects of acute and prolonged illness. *Nature Clinical Practice* **2**, 20–31.

Vermes, I., Beishuizen, A., Hampsink, R. M., et al. (1995). Dissociation of plasma adrenocorticotropin and cortisol levels in critically ill patients: possible role of endothelin and atrial natriuretic hormone. *Journal of Clinical Endocrinology and Metabolism* **80**, 1238–1242.

Hypothalamic-Pituitary-Adrenal Axis

M F Dallman, S Bhatnagar and V Viau
University of California, San Francisco, San Francisco,
CA, USA

This article is reproduced from the previous edition
article by M F Dallman, S Bhatnagar and V Viau, volume 2,
pp 468–476, © 2000, Elsevier Inc.

The Hypothalamic-Pituitary-Adrenal Axis Is One
  Neuroendocrine Arm of the Central Corticotropin
  Releasing Hormone Stress System
Characteristics of the Hypothalamic-Pituitary-Adrenal
  Axis
Target Sequelae of Corticosteroid Responses to Stress

Glossary

Adrenocorti-cotropic hormone (ACTH)	A proopiomelanocortin-derived peptide of 39 amino acids that is released from the corticotroph and acts on MC-3 receptors on adrenocortical cells to stimulate the synthesis and secretion of adrenal corticosteroids.
Arginine vasopressin (AVP)	A peptide that, in addition to its behavioral and antidiuretic roles, potentiates the action of corticotropin-releasing factor to cause ACTH secretion from the corticotroph.
Corticotropin releasing hormone (CRH)	A 41-amino-acid peptide that acts centrally as a neurotransmitter and releasing factor for ACTH.
Cortico-sterone (B)	The major corticosteroid synthesized and secreted by rat adrenals; also called Kendall's compound B.
Cortisol (F)	The major corticosteroid synthesized and secreted by human adrenals; also called Kendall's compound.
Glucocorticoid receptor (GR)	A receptor found in cells throughout the body that mediates most of the systemic effects of corticosteroids secreted by the adrenal.
Heterotypic stress	The application of a novel stimulus to animals that have been previously or chronically stimulated by another stressor.
Homotypic stress	The reapplication of the same stressor that has been applied to animals previously.
Paraventricular nucleus (PVN)	The hypothalamic site of CRH and AVP neurons, which subserve both neuroendocrine and autonomic functions.
Proopiomela-nocortin (POMC)	The 13-kDa precursor protein of ACTH that is synthesized in the anterior pituitary corticotrophs in response to CRH.

The hypothalamic-pituitary-adrenal (HPA) axis,
which ultimately controls the secretion of glucocorticoids from the adrenal cortex, is simply one arm of a
central CRH system that appears to be responsible for
coordinated behavioral, neuroendocrine, autonomic,
and immune responses to alterations in homeostasis. There are marked circadian rhythms in the HPA
axis, well integrated with other circadian activity to
optimize the daily release of CRH and AVP, and
its primary function is to stimulate steroidogenesis
by the adrenal cortex. In addition, the HPA axis is
responsive to stimuli (stressors) that threaten homeostasis, either psychological or physically. Responses
to acute stressors are essential for life, and they turn
on and off rapidly. Chronic stressors appear to change
the response characteristics in the HPA axis, possibly
through recruiting central neural pathways that normally contribute in only a minor fashion to the acute
stress response. During chronic stress, both the CRH-
and the glucocorticoid-regulatory components of the
HPA axis serve to inhibit activity in other, energy-
expending hormonal systems of the body, thus conserving energy stores for immediate use.

The Hypothalamic-Pituitary-Adrenal Axis Is One Neuroendocrine Arm of the Central Corticotropin Releasing Hormone Stress System

CRH in the PVN is the essential driver of the anterior
pituitary corticotroph, causing the synthesis and secretion of ACTH, which then activates adrenocortical synthesis and the secretion of the corticosteroids:
cortisol (F) in humans and corticosterone (B) in rats.
ACTH appears to be a slave to hypothalamic release
of CRH and AVP, and its primary function is to stimulate steroidogenesis by the adrenal cortex. Both F and
B have important effects on central CRH synthesis,
behavior, the immune system, and energy balance.

Neuroendocrine Corticotropin Releasing Hormone Neurons

CRH neurons, primarily in the medial parvocellular
portion of the PVN, are known as neuroendocrine
neurons. Their axons end at the hypothalamic median eminence, and CRH secreted from these diffuses
into the hypophysial-portal blood supply to excite,
through its action on CRH receptor 1 (CRH-R1), the
synthesis of POMC and secretion of ACTH into the
general circulation. ACTH secreted from the pituitary

appears to have the single peripheral function of exciting adrenocortical MC-3 receptors to cause the synthesis and secretion of aldosterone from the zona glomerulosa and F (in humans) or B (in rats), or combinations of the two in other species from the zona fasciculata. The neuroendocrine CRH-synthesizing neurons in PVN also cosynthesize and secrete AVP, which greatly potentiates the effect of CRH on corticotroph ACTH secretion. The amount of AVP synthesized varies with the state of the organism. After adrenalectomy and the removal of F or B negative feedback or after some chronic stressors, AVP synthesis increases markedly in CRH cells. The increase in CRH neuronal AVP allows persistent responsivity in the HPA axis under conditions when a high corticosteroid feedback signal would otherwise damp the system.

Autonomic Corticotropin Releasing Hormone Neurons in the Paraventricular Nucleus

There are also CRH cells in the dorsal, lateral, and medial parvocellular regions of PVN that innervate the dorsal vagal complex and interomedial lateral portions of the spinal cord, suggesting that they affect neural outflow to the peripheral autonomic nervous system.

Other Corticotropin Releasing Hormone Neuronal Groups

Within the brain, there are clusters of other CRH-synthesizing neurons, in addition to those in the PVN, that also appear to play key roles in behavior, autonomic activity, and energy balance. Some of these CRH-expressing cell groups are located in the central nucleus of the amygdala (CeA), bed nucleus of the stria terminalis (BNST), lateral hypothalamic area, parabrachial nuclei, and dorsal motor nucleus of the vagus. Evidence from lesion studies and central injections of CRH and its antagonists suggests strongly that the central CRH system regulates not only the neuroendocrine and autonomic but also behavioral and possibly the neural recruitment responses to applied stressors.

Several studies have shown that CRH expression in the PVN is decreased by corticosteroid treatment, whereas CRH in the CeA and BNST is increased, suggesting that the corticosteroids exert opposite effects on CRH at different sites in brain. However, recent evidence suggests strongly that neurons in the PVN inhibit neuronal expression of CRH in the amygdala; that is, it is not a direct effect of glucocorticoids on extra-PVN cells that causes increased CRH expression but rather neural signals from the PVN to the amygdala that are altered by decreased or increased corticosteroids. Thus, it appears that at least some

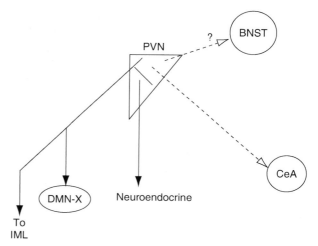

Figure 1 The PVN is central to the stress responsive systems of brain. CRH neurons in the PVN regulate activity in the HPA axis. Neurons in the PVN also regulate autonomic nervous system activity through the innervation of the dorsal motor nucleus of the vagus (DMN-X) and the interomedial lateral cell column of the spinal cord (IML) containing sympathetic preganglionic neurons. Recent results from Palkovits et al. show that pathways from the PVN also regulate CRH expression in the central nucleus of the amygdala (CeA). Although not documented, a similar pathway may exist for CRH neurons in the bed nucleus of the stria terminalis (BNST). Solid and dashed arrows indicate stimulatory and inhibitory connections, respectively.

central CRH pathways are also affected by activity in the PVN (**Figure 1**). It now seems possible that signals from the PVN serve to orchestrate the activity of the rest of the central CRH system.

Characteristics of the Hypothalamic-Pituitary-Adrenal Axis

The HPA axis exhibits three prominent characteristics that interact to alter the regulation of ACTH and corticosteroid secretion: a circadian rhythm in basal activity, sensitivity to corticosteroid (F and B) feedback, and responsivity to stressors. The response to a single stress differs considerably from responses to either homotypic or heterotypic stressors on the background of chronic stress, suggesting major regulatory changes occur in the central neural pathways that activate the HPA axis.

Circadian Rhythm of Glucocorticoid Secretion

Vertebrates exhibit peak circulating corticosteroid levels at the onset of their daily activity cycle and trough levels during the early period of inactivity. The circadian rhythm is driven by the biological clock in the suprachiasmatic nuclei in mammals and fish and in the pineal in birds. In humans and rodents, F and B levels change over a wide range between the peak and trough of the rhythm, and both peak and trough values are regulated by negative feedback effects of F or B on hypothalamic secretion of CRH. During the trough of the rhythm in rats, it appears that there is no CRH/AVP drive from the hypothalamus because neither lesions nor passive immunization with CRH antisera changes ACTH or B secretion; by contrast, CRH(AVP) secretion is essential to drive the circadian increase in B, as shown in the same experiments. Similarly, either adrenalectomy or reduction in normal B levels by use of adrenal B synthesis inhibitors elevates ACTH at both times of day. Both ACTH and direct neural regulation appear to account for the marked circadian rhythm in the amplitude of adrenal corticosteroid production.

Corticosteroid Feedback

Feedback regulation of stress-induced ACTH secretion is markedly affected by the circadian rhythm in HPA activity. There is high feedback sensitivity at trough times and relatively low sensitivity during peak times. In rats with fixed B levels, this is independent of the corticosteroid levels at the time of stressor application, but appears to correlate with the circadian drive to the CRH neurons.

Stressors

Acute signals that alter the balance in the organism stimulate acute HPA responses. These stimuli are most often termed stressors; however, there are also HPA responses associated with stimuli to hypothalamically regulated functions, such as feeding and copulation.

Acute stressors Acute, punctate stressors such as a 30-min psychological stress in humans or a similar period of restraint in rats provoke acute HPA responses that are usually completed within 2 h (**Figure 2**). The intensity and duration of the acute stimulus are related directly to the magnitude of the HPA response. These acute HPA responses are also modified to an extent by glucocorticoid feedback acting in the fast and intermediate time domains on mineralocorticoid receptors (MRs) and GRs. In rats, there is a clear behavioral role of the acute rise in B acting at GR-containing cells in the amygdala to consolidate memory of aversive events.

Persistent or chronic stressors markedly alter regulation in the hypothalamic-pituitary-adrenal axis Under conditions of chronic stress, there are changes in the amplitude of circadian rhythms, with increasing intensity of stress resulting in decreases in the amplitude of the rhythm through the elevation of trough values. Moreover, the magnitude and duration of acute stress responses under conditions of chronic stress depend on familiarity with the stressor. Chronic

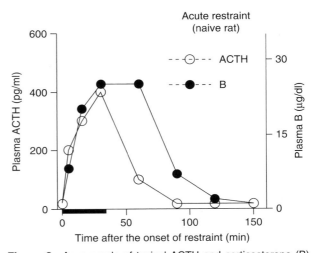

Figure 2 An example of typical ACTH and corticosterone (B) responses to acute restraint in naïve rats not previously exposed to stressors. The duration of restraint was 30 min; thereafter rats were returned to their home cages. The ACTH response ceases at the end of restraint; because ACTH levels are high, the B response is prolonged for 30 min beyond the period of restraint.

or prior stress appears to recruit neural pathways that alter regulation of acute HPA responses.

Circadian rhythm Under resting conditions, without additional acute stress, the signs of mild chronic stress are increased trough corticosteroid levels, suggesting strongly that under chronically stressful conditions there is hypothalamic stimulation of ACTH secretion at all times of day. With increasing intensity of chronic stressors, ACTH and corticosteroid secretion is elevated above normal around the clock (**Figure 3**). The elevation of the trough corticosteroid values is biologically significant and has been shown to enhance glucocorticoid-dependent target responses.

Altered responses to homotypic and heterotypic stressors When acute stress is presented to chronically stressed rats, it becomes clear that marked stress-induced alterations in control of the HPA axis have occurred. In rats, it has been shown that if the acutely applied stimulus is a repetition of the chronic stimulus (homotypic stress), the duration and magnitudes of ACTH and B responses are markedly inhibited compared to the responses of the naïve rat (**Figure 4a**; cf. **Figure 2**). By contrast, if the acutely applied stimulus is novel and different from the chronic stimulus (heterotypic stress), the duration and magnitudes of ACTH and B responses may be markedly facilitated compared to the responses of the naïve rat (**Figure 4b**; cf. **Figure 2**). These results described for restraint as a final stimulus appear to be generalizable to other types of chronic stress followed by either homotypic stress or heterotypic stress.

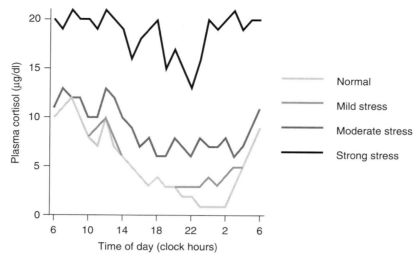

Figure 3 Examples of the effects of chronic stress of differing intensity on basal cortisol concentrations in humans. These examples are collected from a number of clinical papers and show stressors ranging from aging (which some may not perceive as a stress but which bears the hallmarks of chronic stress) or brief fasting at the low end to anorexia nervosa or coronary infarction at the high end. Note that under conditions of mild stress, only the trough levels of the basal rhythm are affected; as the stimulus intensity increases, mean F levels increase until, at highest intensity, the normal circadian rhythm disappears.

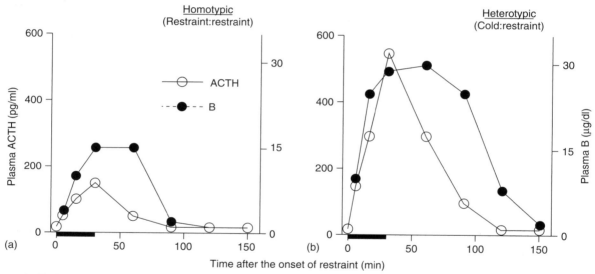

Figure 4 Typical HPA responses to restraint. a, As a homotypic stressor (restraint : restraint); b, As a heterotypic stressor (cold : restraint). Clearly, homotypic HPA responses are diminished (adaptation) and heterotypic responses are exaggerated (facilitation) in chronically stressed rats compared to naïve rats exposed only to the acute stress or restraint (see **Figure 2**). These are representative results (relative to results in concurrently run naïve rats) from separate sets of experiments of (a) Viau and (b) Bhatnagar.

If we were dealing only with repetitions of the same stimulus, it would be appealing to suppose that the final ACTH and B responses were reduced because of the prior and repeated stress-induced increases in B and its feedback effects on brain; however, because heterotypic stimuli elicit either normal or larger than normal responses, it is clear that prior stress-induced increases in B cannot explain the effect of chronic stress on regulation of the HPA axis.

Neural pathways mediating acute hypothalamic-pituitary-adrenal responses in chronically stressed animals There must be, as well, alterations in the neural pathways that respond to homotypic and heterotypic stimuli in chronically stressed rats.

In recent years, either *in situ* hybridization or immunocytochemical techniques have been used to measure changes in immediate early gene (most usually Fos) expression with time after stressors applied to stress-naïve rats in order to determine which neural structures are excited by specific stimuli. These studies have shown that most stimuli activate a common set of structures; among these are the nucleus of the tractus solitarius (NTS), ventrolateral medullary and pontine catecholaminergic cell groups, lateral parabrachial nuclei, raphe nuclei, locus coeruleus (LC), PVN, thalamic paraventricular nuclei (PVTh), amygdala, BNST, lateral septum, and prefrontal cortex. Recently, these techniques have been used in chronically stressed rats exposed to either a homotypic or heterotypic stressor. In both sets of experiments, the numbers of Fos immunoreactivity (Fos-ir) cells in a given structure were compared in naïve and chronically stressed rats after a final stress (foot shock : foot shock and cold : restraint). In both reports, more neurons in PVTh stained with Fos in the chronically stressed rats. In marked contrast to the increased number of Fos-staining cells in the PVTh, after homotypic stress the numbers of Fos-expressing cells in the amygdala, PVN, raphe nuclei, and LC were decreased compared to naïve rats experiencing the stressor for the first time; the reduction in Fos-ir cells in the PVN probably reflected a reduction in ACTH that generally occurs after the nth application of a homotypic stressor. After heterotypic stress, the opposite was observed; the numbers of Fos-positive cells in the amygdala, PVN, raphe nuclei, and LC were increased in the chronically stressed rats compared to naïve rats experiencing restraint. In this case, the increase in PVN Fos-ir cells was shown to reflect elevated ACTH responses that occurred after the heterotypic stressor.

The role of the PVTh on acute restraint-induced ACTH secretion was studied in naïve and chronically cold-stressed rats by lesions of the structure. Lesions of the PVTh augmented restraint-induced ACTH secretion in chronically stressed rats, although they had no effect on the amplitude of the ACTH response to restraint in stress-naïve rats. Thus, it appears that the PVTh normally acts to inhibit HPA activity in chronically stressed, but not naïve, rats; perhaps, therefore, the increased number of activated cells in this structure represents a memory of prior stress. Because the number of Fos-positive cells in the PVTh increases after both homo- and heterotypic stressors, it does not seem likely that this structure exhibits opposite functional effects after the two types of stressors; it is more likely that the output of the PVTh on the HPA response to acute stress in chronically stressed rats is generally inhibitory and independent of the type of acute stress.

The output of the posterior PVTh, where increased numbers of Fos-ir neurons were found after heterotypic restraint stress, is quite discrete; this portion of the nucleus innervates the basolateral nucleus of the

amygdala (BLA), basomedial nucleus of the amygdala (BMA), and CeA – also sites where decreased numbers of Fos-ir cells were found after homotypic shock stress and where increased numbers of Fos-ir cells were found after heterotypic restraint stress in cold-exposed rats. Based on Fos staining in rats after the application of homotypic and heterotypic stressors and some functional results, the diagrammatic circuit in **Figure 5** shows that some pathways to the activation of the HPA axis may be recruited in the chronically stressed individual.

Figure 5 clearly emphasizes the major role played by the amygdala in responding to acute stress under conditions of chronic or prior stress. Only a small amount of the known anatomic connectivity is shown in the figure. For instance, both the NTS and lateral parabrachial nucleus directly innervate all the other cell groups as well as the PVTh; the LC and raphe nuclei also innervate all the other cell groups shown in the diagram; and the PVN also innervates the amygdala, LC, raphe nuclei, lateral parabrachial nucleus, and NTS. Thus, the proposed circuit is massively parallel in nature. Afferent input probably ascends primarily through parallel inputs from the NTS (and ventral medullary aminergic pathways) and the parabrachial nuclei to more anterior brain sites. It is assumed that, under conditions of both homo- and heterotypic stress, the PVTh inhibits activity in the amygdala that leads to the activation of the HPA axis as well as behavioral and autonomic activity. The raphe nuclei, through secretion of serotonin at the lateral nucleus of the amygdala, may inhibit amygdalar activity, possibly mediating HPA adaptation to homotypic stress.

Although the circuit in **Figure 5** is based primarily on changes in the number of Fos-positive neurons after a final application of the same or a novel stress in chronically or repeatedly stressed rats, to date there has been no attempt to identify the phenotype of the increased Fos-positive cells after the application of novel stimuli. Validation of the model shown in **Figure 5** will require this identification and will also require the identification of the terminal fields of the neurons whose activity is altered specifically under conditions of novel stress on a background of chronic stress.

It is clear from this discussion that chronic stress alters the central regulation of stress-induced HPA function. In addition, the altered neural emphasis also effects changes in behavioral and autonomic outputs. The altered amygdalar output that proceeds through the CeA is compatible with changes in the activity of the amygdalar CRH system, which innervates all the indicated output structures. Thus, the major central stress mediator, CRH, may be in large part responsible

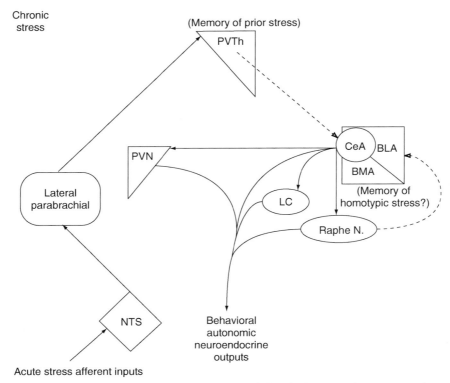

Figure 5 Model of pathways that are emphasized in HPA responses of chronically stressed rats to acute homotypic or heterotypic stressors. We assume that afferent inputs excited by stress excite the brain through activating neurons in the nucleus of the tractus solitarius (NTS) and, in turn, the lateral parabrachial nucleus. Based on results of Fos immunoreactivity (Fos-ir), the number of excited neurons in the thalamic paraventricular nuclei (PVTh) is increased after both types of chronic stressors. By contrast, compared to controls, the number of Fos-ir neurons is decreased after homotypic stress and increased after heterotypic stress in amygdala (CeA, BMA, and BLA), the PVN, the locus ceruleus (LC), and the raphe nuclei. Solid and dashed arrows indicate stimulatory and inhibitory connections, respectively. Only a selected portion of the interconnectivity is shown; both NTS and the parabrachial nucleus innervate all the other structures shown and, in turn, are innervated by the other structures. Moreover, the LC and raphe nuclei innervate all other structures. Thus, this is a massively parallel system.

for the changes in HPA responsivity observed after chronic stress.

Target Sequelae of Corticosteroid Responses to Stress

Because all cell types contain GRs, corticosteroid secretion above normal levels affects function in most tissues of the body. The alterations include changes in behavior and in endocrine and immune responses as well as in intrinsic activity of individual organs. Acute HPA responses to a single application of a stressor probably have considerable utility in that the elevated corticosteroid levels ensure an adequate substrate for increased metabolic need and help to sustain blood pressure and to depress immune function. However, chronic elevations in glucocorticoid levels induced by chronic stress can be deleterious to the organism. In addition to altering the expression of many gene products in the central nervous system, the elevation of glucocorticoid levels inhibits central catecholaminergic systems and stimulates the expression of neuropeptide Y (NPY). The diminution of enzymatic activity in catecholaminergic systems has been correlated with reduced systemic catecholaminergic function. The stimulation of NPY in the hypothalamic arcuate nucleus has been correlated with increased food intake. In addition, glucocorticoids have been shown to be required at the amygdala for the consolidation of the memory of conditioned stimuli as well as for the inhibitory action of serotonin on glutamate-induced stimulation of lateral amygdalar cell activity. Slight elevations of glucocorticoid secretion above normal inhibit activity in the thyroid, growth hormone, and gonadal axes through actions both at the central nervous system and at the pituitary and peripheral endocrine targets.

At the tissue level, glucocorticoids inhibit immune responses and protect the organism through a sequenced feedback effect from the consequences of overactivity in this potent system. However, because the glucocorticoids also, through central nervous system effects, alter peripheral catecholaminergic activity, the effect of stress on immune system function depends markedly on when the stress, or glucocorticoid treatment, is provided in temporal relationship to the immune challenge. Thus, the literature on this subject is confusing, showing that stress, or glucocorticoids, can enhance or inhibit immune system activity. The effects of glucocorticoids on immune cells are legion. The direct effects of glucocorticoids on target tissue activity may seem somewhat simpler. By themselves, glucocorticoids are catabolic hormones; they mobilize free fatty acids and amino acids from adipocytes and muscle and cause hyperglycemia through increasing hepatic gluconeogenesis. However, glucocorticoids also enhance insulin secretion. Normally, stress decreases food intake and insulin secretion so that the catabolic effects of the glucocorticoids predominate under stressful conditions; nonetheless, the stimulation of insulin by stress-induced glucocorticoid secretion occurs. This effect is perhaps through antagonizing the hepatic effects of insulin, and it tends to remodel energy stores so that more fat and less muscle are stored under conditions of high glucocorticoid levels.

Bone loss has become a hallmark of chronic stress, depression, anorexia nervosa, or glucocorticoid treatment. Again, these effects of the glucocorticoids are dual. They act directly on bone to decrease matrix deposition and osteoblast activity and at the hypothalamic-pituitary-gonadal axis to decrease gonadal steroid production. The gonadal steroids have positive effects on bone formation, and excess glucocorticoids provide a double hit on bone by their dual actions.

In summary, the HPA axis is one arm of the central stress system defined by CRH. Chronic stressors alter the regulation of the HPA axis, possibly by increasing the emphasis on activity in CRH pathways. Although acute glucocorticoid responses to stressors can be taken as important for the maintenance of homeostasis, chronic elevations in glucocorticoid secretion appear, on the whole, to be deleterious for the organism.

See Also the Following Articles

Adrenocorticotropic Hormone (ACTH); Corticotropin Releasing Factor (CRF); Glucocorticoids, Role in Stress; Paraventricular Nucleus; Vasopressin.

Further Reading

Antoni, F. A. (1986). Hypothalamic control of adrenocorticotropin secretion: advances since the discovery of 41-residue corticotropin-releasing factor. *Endocrine Review* 7, 351–378.

Bhatnagar, S. and Dallman, M. F. (1998). Neuroanatomical basis for facilitation of hypothalamic-pituitary-adrenal responses to a novel stressor after chronic stress. *Neuroscience* 84, 1025–1039.

Buijs, R. M., Wortel, J., Van Heerikhulze, J. J., et al. (1997). Novel environment induced inhibition of corticosterone secretion: physiological evidence for a suprachiasmatic nucleus mediated neuronal hypothalamic-adrenal cortex pathway. *Brain Research* 758, 229–236.

Cullinan, W. E., Herman, J. P., Battaglia, D. F., et al. (1995). Pattern and time course of immediate early gene expression in rat brain following acute stress. *Neuroscience* 64, 477–505.

Dallman, M. F., Akana, S. F., Scribner, K. A., et al. (1992). Stress, feedback and facilitation in the hypothalamo-pituitary-adrenal axis. *Journal of Neuroendocrinology* 5, 517–526.

Dallman, M. F. and Bhatnagar, S. (1999). Chronic stress and energy balance: role of the hypothalamo-pituitary-adrenal axis. In: McEwen, B. S. (ed.) *Handbook of physiology: environmental physiology* (vol. 7), chap. 10. Washington, DC: American Physiology Society.

Dunn, A. J. and Berridge, C. W. (1990). Physiological and behavioral responses to corticotropin-releasing factor: is CRF a mediator of anxiety or stress responses? *Brain Research Reviews* 15, 71–100.

Herman, J. P., Prewitt, C. M.-F. and Cullinan, W. E. (1996). Neuronal circuit regulation of the hypothalamo-pituitary-adrenocortical stress axis. *Critical Reviews in Neurobiology* 10, 371–394.

Li, H.-Y. and Sawchenko, P. E. (1998). Hypothalamic effector neurons and extended circuitries activated in "neurogenic" stress: a comparison of footshock effects exerted acutely, chronically, and in animals with controlled glucocorticoid levels. *Journal of Comparative Neurology* 393, 244–266.

McGaugh, J. L., Cahill, L. and Roozendaal, B. (1996). Involvement of the amygdala in memory storage: interaction with other brain systems. *Proceedings of the National Academy of Sciences USA* 93, 13508–13514.

Munck, A., Guyre, P. M. and Holbrook, N. J. (1984). Physiological functions of glucocorticoids in stress and their relations to pharmacological actions. *Endocrine Review* 5, 25–52.

Owens, M. J. and Nemeroff, C. B. (1991). Physiology and pharmacology of corticotropin-releasing factor. *Pharmacological Reviews* 43, 425–473.

Palkovits, M., Young, W. S., III, Kovacs, K., et al. (1998). Alterations in corticotropin-releasing hormone gene expression of central amygdaloid neurons following long-term paraventricular lesions and adrenalectomy. *Neuroscience* 85, 135–147.

Stutzmann, G. E., McEwen, B. S. and LeDoux, J. E. (1998). Serotonin modulation of sensory input to the lateral amygdala: dependency on corticosterone. *Journal of Neuroscience* 18, 9529–9538.

Swanson, L. W., Sawchenko, P. E., Rivier, J., et al. (1983). Organization of ovine corticotropin-releasing factor immunoreactive cells and fibers in the rat brain: an immunohistochemical study. *Neuroendocrinology* **36**, 165–186.

Taché, Y., Martinez, V., Million, M., et al. (1999). Corticotropin-releasing factor and the brain-gut motor response to stress. *Canadian Journal of Gastroenterology* **13**(supplement A), 18A–25A.

Hypothalamus *See:* Hypothalamic-Pituitary-Adrenal; Neuroendocrine Systems.

Hypothermia

M J Taylor
Organ Recovery Systems, Inc., Charleston, SC, and Drexel University and Carnegie Mellon University, Pittsburgh, PA, USA

This article is a revision of the previous edition article by M J Taylor, volume 2, pp 484–495, © 2000, Elsevier Inc.

Definitions
Background to Hypothermia as a Stress
The Extent of the Problem of Death due to Hypothermia
Pathophysiology of Hypothermia

Glossary

Cold-induced fibrillation	Very rapid, irregular contractions of the muscle fibers of the heart resulting in a lack of synchronization between heartbeat and pulse, with a resultant lack of cardiac output.
Cold narcosis	A state of stupor, unconsciousness, or arrested activity produced by cooling.
Homeotherm	A warm-blooded animal such as humans that regulates its core temperature at a constant temperature (usually 37°C, or 98.6°C) irrespective of environmental temperature.
Ischemia	Localized deprivation of oxygen (hypoxia) and nutrients to a tissue due to interruption of blood supply.
Lipid phase transition	A temperature-induced change of state of the lipid component of biological membranes involving a change from a gel phase to a liquid crystal phase. These physical changes of membrane fluidity often result in functional alterations of membrane properties.
Thermogenesis	The production of heat in the body, usually by metabolic oxidation of food substrates.

Definitions

The prefix hypo means below or under, and therm means temperature, so hypothermia literally means below normal temperature. In humans and most other mammals, normal temperature is regarded as 37°C (98.6°F), but this single value belies the fact that normal temperature in healthy individuals varies within a degree or so, depending on factors such as the site of measurement (core or exterior) and time of day (circadian rhythm). Body temperature can be measured in a variety of ways. Exterior temperatures include sublingual (under the tongue), skin, or axillary (under the armpit) measurements. Core or interior temperatures reflect the mean temperatures of the vital organs and are approximated by esophageal, rectal, tympanic membranes, and pulmonary artery measurements. In humans, normal body temperature has traditionally been set at 37°C based upon 1 million axilliary measurements from 25 000 individuals carried out by the nineteenth century investigator Carl Wunderlich in 1868. Modern-day corroboration of these data has been provided by a study of 148 healthy men and women that showed a mean oral temperature of 36.8°C, with 37.7°C as the upper limit of normal.

Humans are homeothermic mammals (warm-blooded animals), which means that the core body temperature is precisely regulated and kept constant at about 37°C, irrespective of the ambient temperature. Even though core temperature is well maintained, the temperature of the peripheral shell (skin, fat, and muscle) ranges from 31°C to 35°C, with skin temperature at 28°C to 32°C. Thermoregulation impairment, prolonged exposure to an extreme environment, or both may lead to a decrease in core temperature and the onset of a pathological state. Nevertheless, under controlled conditions in a hospital setting, hypothermia can actually be used for therapeutic advantage in a variety of medical applications since cold can also be a protective modality. Hypothermia is defined in homeotherms as the reduction of core body temperature below 35°C (95°F), and clinically has been arbitrarily graded for convenience into degrees of hypothermia, as shown in **Table 1**.

Background to Hypothermia as a Stress

Hypothermia is a double-edged sword in that cold has been both a friend and a foe to humanity. Historically, we know that cold can be a devastating stress, as illustrated by the nineteenth century records that Napoleon watched helplessly as his army was annihilated by the bitter Russian winter. Hypothermia remains a modern-day problem, and much of what we know has been gleaned from data collected from victims of accidental hypothermia. These include victims from outdoor recreational activities in which otherwise healthy individuals succumb to injury, and even death, as a result of overexposure to the cold weather conditions, as well as victims of urban problems such as old people living in substandard accommodations without adequate heating in the winter or homeless people sleeping on the street. The latter cases introduce some complications to the interpretation of hypothermic exposure due to confounding issues such as disease, drug or alcohol abuse, or age. In sharp contrast, deep hypothermia has saved some individuals from inevitable death due to prolonged hypoxic ischemia. There are remarkable accounts of children who have been rescued and have made complete recoveries after lengthy submersion in icy water that reduced their core body temperature to below 25°C (77°F) and caused them to stop breathing for periods as long as 40 min.

Under controlled conditions, deliberate hypothermia, while still a stress, can be used as a highly effective therapeutic modality to control, or counteract, the effects of hypoxia or ischemia associated with various medical and surgical treatments. From the very earliest medical manuscripts in the third to fifth centuries BC, we know that cold was recommended as a treatment for wounds, infections, sprains, fractures, and gouty swellings and to suppress hemorrhage (uncontrolled bleeding) and head injuries. Even total body hypothermia was recommended for tetanus and convulsions. Since the 1950s, a vast literature has emerged describing the value of hypothermia in widely varying diseases, including head injury, cerebral hemorrhage, cardiac arrest, carbon monoxide poisoning, neonatal asphyxia, and eclampsia. Today, the elective use of moderate and deep hypothermia has found numerous clinical applications centered principally upon protection of the heart and brain to facilitate techniques in cardiothoracic surgery and neurosurgery. Moreover, the robust cerebroprotective effect of mild hypothermia demonstrated in animals is currently undergoing clinical trials in the management of traumatic brain injury and may in the future be applied as an adjunctive technique in other critical situations such as victims of stroke and hemorrhagic shock.

The Extent of the Problem of Death due to Hypothermia

Accidental hypothermia is regarded as an escalating problem, but accurate statistics are not readily available. This is largely due to the fact that records often do not recognize or specify hypothermia as the primary cause of morbidity or mortality in victims of accidental hypothermia. Official health statistics based on death certificates tend to underestimate the actual incidence of hypothermia. This is partly due to the use of a single-cause coding system; for example, if a death is recorded as bronchopneumonia due to hypothermia, the cause of death is recorded as pneumonia and no statistical record of hypothermia is made. The issue is further complicated by the fact that hypothermia is often not diagnosed or recognized by physicians. Nevertheless, predictions have been made that significant numbers of people die from hypothermia-related causes. For example, based upon the research of Taylor and Fox in Britain, it has been predicted that 20 000 hypothermia-related deaths occur per year, predominantly in the elderly. Similar estimates in North America predicted 25 000 hypothermia-related fatalities per year in the United States and 8 000 in Canada. There is a growing awareness of exposure hypothermia associated with

Table 1 Classification of hypothermia

Classification	Temperature range (°C)	Temperature range (°F)
Mild	32–35	90–95
Moderate	27–32	81–90
Deep or profound	10–27	50–81
Ultraprofound	<10	<50

recreation, cold water immersion, and to some extent socioeconomic problems among people with predisposing factors such as drugs, alcohol intoxication, and age. However, attention also needs to be given to secondary hypothermia, such as that induced during shock resulting from trauma.

Pathophysiology of Hypothermia

Systemic Effects of Hypothermia

Surviving hypothermic exposure in humans is generally associated with core temperatures above 25°C (77°F); however, surviving deeper exposure is possible if appropriate treatment is employed. Physiological responses to cooling and warming depend on how heat exchange is mediated and whether the patient is conscious or anesthetized. Heat exchange may be either by surface phenomena (conduction, convection, and radiation) or in the clinical setting by core perfusion techniques. The pathophysiology and treatment of accidental hypothermia victims are complex issues often compounded by the nonhomogeneity of the patient population. For example, a drowning person may become seriously cooled in a matter of minutes, while elderly people living in substandard accommodations may undergo an insidious cooling process that develops over several weeks. Under these circumstances it has proved difficult to compare different methods of treatments. However, in the comparatively controlled environment of the hospital operating room, the physiological responses to hypothermia are well characterized and documented.

Effect of hypothermia on thermoregulation   Hypothermia triggers an ordered progression of autonomic thermoregulatory responses. Initially, cutaneous vasoconstriction is initiated in the arteriovenous shunts of the extremities, mediated by noradrenergic sympathetic nerves. With moderate cooling, this reflex vasoconstriction of the skin is assisted by direct constrictor action of cold on the arterioles. Aided by reflex noradrenergic drive to the heart, the vasoconstriction can result in large increases in arterial pressure. So, the body tightly controls its core temperature, using its peripheral shell as a thermal buffer with the environment. As heat is lost from the periphery, the temperature gradient from the core to the periphery increases, and heat flows out of the core tissues into the peripheral shell. Eventually vasoconstriction can no longer compensate for the continuing heat loss of the periphery by sacrificing peripheral temperature, and shivering is necessary to maintain core temperature. With progressive cold exposure, reflex increases in muscle tone and shivering are brought about by somatic motor nerves, and this can increase heat production by as much as fivefold for many hours at a time. Interestingly, newborn infants do not shiver, but utilize a nonshivering thermogenesis that relies upon metabolic heat production from the oxidation of brown fat. In general, when hypothermia reaches moderate degrees (<33°C), shivering gradually decreases and is followed by stiffness of muscles and joints.

Effect of hypothermia on the heart and brain   Hypothermia has significant effects on nearly every organ system, but disturbances of cerebral and cardiac function as the temperature of the brain and heart fall below 35°C (95°F) are of most concern. One of the earliest signs of hypothermia is a change in personality. The individual may become uncooperative and show signs of listlessness, incoordination, and confusion, often with subsequent amnesia for events at the time of low body temperature. Loss of consciousness is highly variable and may occur at any point within the range 26–33°C. After an initial rise in cardiac output associated with shivering, cardiac function declines with slowed heart rate due principally to the direct effects of cold on the cardiac muscle. At temperatures between 17 and 26°C (63 and 79°F), the cardiac output is not sufficient to supply even the reduced oxygen requirements of the cold tissues. At 25°C (77°F), cardiac function is reduced to about 30% of normothermic levels. The most important and life-threatening complication of hypothermia is the associated cardiac irritability. Progressive cooling eventually causes cardiac arrhythmias, with atrial fibrillation occurring earlier (~30°C [~86°F]) than ventricular fibrillation (threshold at 28°C [82°F]). However, the latter is highly variable and is influenced by several factors, including acid–base balance. Rapid cooling of large, aged, or diseased hearts can predispose to early fibrillation, while small, immature hearts may not fibrillate at all during cooling but pass directly from bradycardia (slow heart rate) to diastolic arrest. Ventricular fibrillation may occur in the temperature range 20–27°C (68–81°F) and is the most dangerous and feared aspect of hypothermia, since death invariably ensues unless rewarming and defibrillation procedures are initiated.

The brain is a highly metabolic tissue requiring a constant supply of oxygen and, like the heart, is exquisitely sensitive to hypoxia and ischemic insult. Metabolism is markedly suppressed by a fall in temperature, and in general metabolic rate is decreased by 5–7% per degree Celsius. Oxygen consumption is a reasonable measure of metabolic activity, since for practical purposes, tissue and cellular stores of oxygen do not exist, and cells rely upon the circulation to deliver oxygen in quantities determined by the rate of O_2 consumption. Cerebral blood flow (CBF) and cerebral metabolic rate of oxygen consumption also decrease by about 50% for every 10-degree drop in temperature. This correlates with declining electrical activity (EEG) as the brain cools with electrocerebral silence (no measurable electrical activity) at $\sim$20°C. This profound effect of hypothermia on diminished oxygen demand is actually one of the most important protective aspects of clinical hypothermia. However, despite the unequivocal fact that hypothermia protects the brain from the effects of hypoxia, prolonged survival in hypothermia almost totally depends on having sufficient cardiovascular function for adequate perfusion of important organ systems for supply of substrates in addition to oxygen. Hypothermia also causes a shift of the oxygen-hemoglobin dissociation curve to the left, thus reducing tissue oxygen availability. This may contribute to the uncompensated metabolic acidosis that is commonly observed with hypothermia due to reduced tissue perfusion with accumulation of lactate and other acid metabolites.

Effect of hypothermia on respiration The rate of respiration decreases progressively during cooling to 30°C, but the partial pressure of oxygen remains essentially normal. CO_2 production is significantly elevated initially due to intense shivering, but as the core temperature falls, CO_2 production is diminished. Coupled with increased solubility of CO_2 in plasma at lower temperatures, this tends to decrease the partial pressure of CO_2 despite diminished respiratory rate. The net effect of these changes is a mild respiratory alkalosis in the early phase of acute hypothermia. This alkalosis is, however, gradually replaced by metabolic acidosis as cooling progresses, due to poor tissue perfusion and oxygenation, as discussed earlier. So, in general, respiration is depressed during hypothermia, but the rate is almost in proportion to metabolic needs until respiration becomes shallow and erratic and eventually stops in the region of 25–30°C.

Effect of hypothermia on the blood Hypothermia also results in marked hematological perturbations such as increased viscosity, leukopenia (abnormally low number of circulating leukocytes), and thrombocytopenia (reduced numbers of platelets leading to bleeding tendencies). Increasing blood viscosity, which changes by as much as 5% per degree Celsius, also contributes to an apparent rise in vascular resistance (decreased efficiency of vascular perfusion). Deep hypothermia also hinders clotting by slowing the enzyme-mediated coagulation cascade and by promoting fibrinolysis. Abnormalities in clotting mechanisms occur in 68–100% of patients subjected to clinical hypothermia, making bleeding tendencies a major concern in people subjected to prolonged hypothermia.

Physiological signs and symptoms of cold exposure Hypothermia is now recognized as the number one killer of outdoor recreationalists, and along with this has come the need for increasing awareness of the problem. As a consequence, many outdoor organizations are taking active measures to educate their members about hypothermia as an environmental hazard and are teaching emergency care for hypothermia. A critical part of this process is the ability to recognize the signs and symptoms of hypothermic exposure. **Table 2** illustrates some of the characteristic signs and symptoms at various stages of hypothermia.

Because survival after cold exposure is critically dependent on early intervention to reverse the effects of hypothermia, emergency personnel have become increasingly skilled over the past several years at managing and treating victims of hypothermia. It is beyond the scope of this article to describe the recommended treatments for victims of accidental hypothermia, but **Figure 1** illustrates an algorithm of recommended actions. It is noteworthy that some early interventions can be initiated in the field, while more aggressive treatments can not be considered until the patient is transferred to an adequately equipped emergency vehicle or hospital.

Enhancing tolerance to cold exposure The risk of accidental hypothermia is ever present for people who live at high altitudes, and efforts to protect against cold exposure have focused on methods of decreasing heat loss by improving insulation. Nevertheless, some research has been devoted to finding ways of improving cold tolerance by modifying the thermoregulatory response to cold. The principal strategies employed have been thermal acclimation, physical exercise, dietary enhancement of thermogenesis, pharmacological enhancement of thermogenesis, and manipulation of the thermoregulatory set point. While none of these approaches have been accepted routinely to improve cold tolerance, it can be concluded from some studies that the pharmacological enhancement of cold thermogenesis using ephedrine in combination with methylxanthine represents the most promising method for delaying the onset of hypothermia in humans.

Contrasting outcome between victims of accidental hypothermia and patients experiencing clinical hypothermia In considering the chances of survival after the stress of hypothermia, an important

Table 2 Characteristics of hypothermic stress at different stages of cooling

Stage	Core temperature	Signs and symptoms
Mild hypothermia	37–35°C (98–95°F)	Normal, shivering can begin, cold sensation, goose bumps, unable to perform complex tasks with hands, shiver can be mild to severe, hands numb
Mild–moderate hypothermia	35–33°C (95–93°F)	Shivering/intense, muscle incoordination becomes apparent, movements slow and labored, stumbling pace, mild confusion, may appear alert. Use sobriety test; if unable to walk a 30-foot straight line, the person is hypothermic
	33–32°C (93–90°F)	Violent shivering persists, difficulty speaking, sluggish thinking, amnesia starts to appear, gross muscle movements sluggish, unable to use hands, stumbles frequently, difficulty speaking, signs of depression, withdrawn
Moderate hypothermia	32–30°C (90–86°F)	Shivering stops, exposed skin blue or puffy, muscle coordination very poor, inability to walk, confusion, incoherent/irrational behavior, but may be able to maintain posture and appearance of awareness
	30–27°C (86–82°F)	Muscle rigidity, semiconscious, stupor, loss of awareness of others, pulse and respiration rate decrease, possible heart fibrillation
Deep hypothermia	27–25°C (82–78°F)	Unconscious, heart beat and respiration erratic, pulse may not be palpable
	<25°C (<77°F)	Pulmonary edema, cardiac and respiratory failure, death (death may occur before this temperature is reached)

Adapted from the Princeton University Outdoor Action Guide, with permission.

distinction has to be made between accidental hypothermia and clinical hypothermia. Even though the final core temperature of the individual may drop to the same level, the survival rate from clinically induced hypothermia is much higher than that of accidental hypothermia. In the latter case, homeotherms respond to hypothermic stress with immediate activation of heat production as well as inhibition of heat loss. The timing and intensity of the thermogenic response, as well as the duration over which the process can be maintained, depend on factors such as sex, age, and health of the individual. Hypothermia ensues when maximum thermogenesis fails to balance minimum heat loss and heat deficit results. As hypothermia progresses, cold narcosis of the central nervous system supervenes and respiratory support declines. Heart rate also slows with decreasing temperature, but the heart may continue to beat for some time depending upon the cooling rate. Eventually, when the core temperature drops to a specific level (in the range 15–25°C [60–77°F]), the heart either goes into ventricular fibrillation or arrests. In the battle to maintain core temperature, the subject has exhausted itself.

In contrast to the preceding scenario, clinically induced hypothermia is a sedate, relatively nonstressful, and intensively monitored condition. The patient is initially anesthetized and rapidly cooled, often with the aid of cardiopulmonary bypass support, with little or no metabolic resistance. Moreover, the patient is monitored continuously throughout so that presenting complications can be corrected expeditiously or rewarming employed before they become lethal. It is important to explain why hypothermia is sometimes induced electively in patients for clinical

benefit. As described in the next section, it has long been known that hypothermia is a highly effective modality for protecting cells against the deleterious effects of hypoxia and ischemia. In general, the extent of protection is directly related to the degree of hypothermia, with colder temperatures offering greater protection. This is based on the fundamental effect of cooling on biophysical and biochemical processes as molecular activity and mobility is slowed. In the fields of cardiovascular surgery, neurosurgery, and more recently in trauma medicine, there is often a need in complicated cases for the surgeon to implement a temporary cessation of blood flow to the heart or the brain. Adjunctive hypothermia is often used to protect the organs against hypoxia and ischemia. In recent years, there has been a renewed interest in the application of mild to moderate hypothermia as a potent neuroprotective modality, and consideration is being given to a potential therapeutic benefit of hypothermia to avert the complications of traumatic brain injury and stroke.

Cellular Responses to Hypothermic Stress

A complete understanding of the effects of hypothermia on the body calls for examination of the events at the cellular level, since this is where the pathophysiology of hypothermic stress is ultimately mediated. A great deal is known about the effects of cold on cells, since cooling has proved to be the foundation of nearly all effective methods of protecting and preserving cells and tissues for applications such as transplantation. Transplantation science calls for effective methods of preservation since donor cells, tissues, and organs are required to withstand a period of ischemia and hypoxia as part of any transplantation

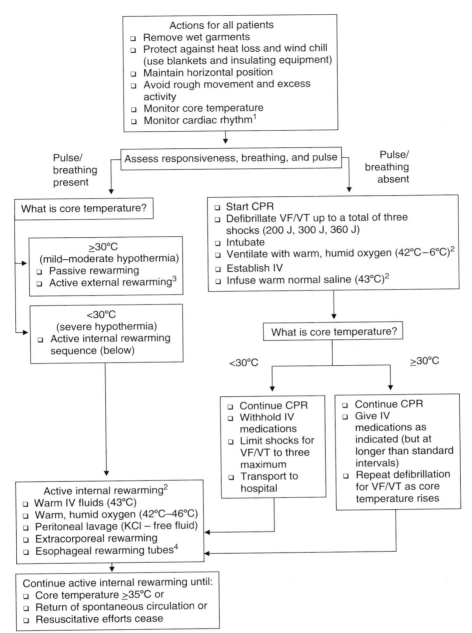

Figure 1 Algorithm for treatment of hypothermia. Notes: (1) This may require needle electrodes through the skin. (2) Many experts think that these interventions should be done only in hospital, though practices vary. (3) Methods include electric or charcoal warming devices, hot water bottles, heating pads, radiant heat sources, and warming beds. (4) Esophageal rewarming tubes are widely used internationally and should become available in the United States. Abbreviations: VF, ventricular fibrillation; VT, ventricular tachycardia; CPR, cardiopulmonary resuscitation; IV, intravenous. This algorithm is based on the Guidelines for Cardiopulmonary Resuscitation and Emergency Cardiac Care published by the American Medical Association (*JAMA*, **268**, 2171, Copyright 1992, American Medical Association, all rights reserved) and is adapted from the article 'JAMA protocol for hypothermia' at http://hypothermia.org/jama.htm

procedure when the blood supply is temporarily interrupted. The basis of this hypothermic protection is that cooling can help to combat the deleterious effects of ischemia, but the consequences of cooling are not exclusively beneficial, such that hypothermic storage is a compromise between the benefits and detriments of cooling. In the following, the detrimental effects only of hypothermic stress on cells is outlined.

General suppression of reaction rates The fundamental basis of all biological and chemical processes is molecular activity and mobility, which are governed by thermal energy such that as temperature is lowered, molecular motion is slowed. The removal of heat from a system slows down both physical and chemical processes in proportion to the loss of heat and therefore to the fall in temperature. Since the processes of deterioration associated with ischemia and anoxia are mediated by chemical reactions, it has proved well founded to attempt to prevent or attenuate these changes by cooling. Biochemical processes involve molecular interactions that are invariably catalyzed by enzymes in reactions that require energy input from cellular stores such as ATP or creatine phosphate. Cooling can affect all components of these reactions, including the energy status of the substrate molecules, the stability of the enzyme protein, and the capacity of the cell to supply biological energy. The rate of biophysical processes such as diffusion of ions and osmosis declines linearly with temperature by approximately 3% per 10°C. It is apparent, therefore, that biophysical events are relatively little affected by the comparatively modest temperature changes imposed during hypothermic storage of tissues for transplantation. It is only at much lower temperatures that the rates of biophysical processes become significantly important, especially at sub-zero temperatures, when phase changes lead to both ice formation and solute concentration changes.

By comparison, the rate of chemical reactions, including the biochemical processes that constitute metabolic activity, is slowed significantly more by a given degree of hypothermic exposure. It is well established that within the temperature range 0–42°C, oxygen consumption in tissues decreases by at least 50% for each 10°C fall in temperature. The quantitative relationship between energy requirements for biochemical processes and temperature changes has been expressed mathematically in different ways:

1. The Arrhenius relationship: Biochemical processes, in common with all chemical reactions, occur only between activated molecules, the proportion of which in a given system is given by the Boltzmann expression, $\exp(-E/RT)$, where E is the activation energy, R is the gas constant, and T is the absolute temperature. According to the Arrhenius relationship, the logarithm of the reaction rate, k, is inversely proportional to the reciprocal of the absolute temperature:

$$-\log k = A(-E/2.3RT).$$

A graphical plot of $\log k$ against $1/T$ will yield a straight line with a slope of $E/2.3R$ if the relationship represents a single rate-limiting step.

2. The Van't Hoff rule relates the logarithm of a chemical reaction rate directly to temperature and is commonly expressed in the form of the respiratory quotient or temperature coefficient, Q_{10}, where Q_{10} is the ratio of reaction rates at two temperatures separated by 10°C. Accordingly,

$$Q_{10} = (K_2/K_1)10^{(T2-T1)}$$

For most reactions of biological interest, Q_{10} has a value between 2 and 3, but some complex, energy-dependent reactions have a Q_{10} between 4 and 6 and are more likely to stop completely at low temperatures. Both Q_{10} and Arrhenius plots have been used to quantitate changes in metabolic processes occurring in biological systems, whether they are enzyme reactions in single cells or the oxygen consumption of the entire human body. The Q_{10} for whole-body oxygen consumption is approximately 2, indicating that, in general, metabolic rate is halved for each 10°C drop in temperature.

Metabolic uncoupling While it is clear that cooling has a profound effect on biochemical reaction rates and that this in turn can slow degradative processes and reduce the rate of substrate and energy depletion, it is important to realize that not all reaction rates are affected to the same degree, or even in the same manner, by cooling. One hypothesis of chilling injury states that at a certain critical temperature within the chilling injury range, the membrane lipids undergo a transition from a liquid-crystalline to a solid gel state. The two main consequences of the transition thought to eventually result in cell injury are an increase in membrane permeability and an increase in the activation energy of membrane-bound enzymes such as those controlling respiration in mitochondria. Thus, the result would be the accumulation or depletion of metabolites at the point of entry into mitochondria. Hence, the membrane phase transitions in subcellular membranes could cause metabolic imbalance and provide one component of injury sustained by homeothermic cells during cold exposure.

Figure 2 shows schematically the large number of different, integrated chemical reactions that constitute common metabolic pathways within a cell. Each of these reactions will be affected by cooling in a different manner and to a different degree such that the possibility exists for uncoupling reaction pathways and producing harmful consequences. In preservation, cooling prolongs *in vitro* survival because it slows metabolism, reduces the demand for oxygen and other metabolites, and conserves chemical

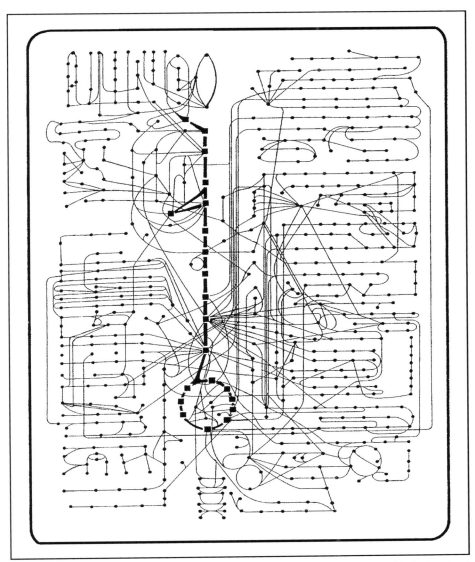

Figure 2 Schematic diagram illustrating the complexity of integrated biochemical pathways responsible for the structural and functional integrity of a typical cell. A healthy cell depends upon the synthesis and degradation of a wide variety of molecules. These processes are controlled by a complex series of biochemical reactions that produce and consume energy in a highly regulated manner. The diagram portrays schematically the complex integrated pathways that constitute the biochemical machinery of a typical cell. About 500 common metabolic reactions are shown by the connecting lines, with each metabolite represented as a filled circle. The centrally placed reactions of the main energy-producing pathways (glycolysis and tricarboxylic acid cycle) are shown as bold. A typical mammalian cell synthesizes more than 10 000 different proteins, a major proportion of which is enzymes. Each of these pathways can be affected differently by reduced temperatures such that the possibility exists for disruption of the normal metabolic processes, with harmful consequences as described in the text. Adapted from Alberts et al. (1994). *Molecular biology of the cell* (3rd edn.), Garland Publishing, with permission.

energy. However, it does not affect all reactions to the same extent, and the net result of cooling on an integrated, metabolizing system is complex, not entirely predictable, and not completely understood.

Studies of the effects of pure hypothermia on cell viability in the absence of any prior hypoxia have shown that the inactivation (killing) rates of cells exposed to reduced temperatures change slope at approximately 7–8°C, implying that there are distinct

mechanisms of hypothermic inactivation above and below this transition temperature. These values have been interpreted as suggesting that unbalanced metabolism is probably the rate-limiting step for hypothermic inactivation in the higher temperature range (8–25°C), and membrane lipid phase transition or cold denaturation of a critical protein is likely to be responsible for the strong temperature dependence in the lower range (<8°C).

Effect upon energy metabolism Under normal circumstances the supply of energy-rich compounds to fuel a cell's requirement for homeostatic control is continuously replenished by oxidative phosphorylation in the mitochondria. During cooling, however, there is a progressive exhaustion of chemical energy reserves in a cell despite the general suppressive effect of cooling on metabolism. The effect of cooling on metabolism is complex and should not be regarded as causing a simple uniform retardation of all biochemical reactions. For example, the complexity of low temperature effects on mitochondrial respiration is not limited to the impairment of translocase enzymes. It has been shown that other enzymes that control reactions of the tricarboxylic acid (TCA) cycle and the electron transport chain are affected differently by cold storage.

Effect upon ion transport and cell swelling Intracellular ionic composition and volume regulation of a cell are maintained by a pump-leak mechanism in which membrane-bound enzymes transport various ions and solutes to counter the passive diffusion driven by chemical potential gradients. These active pumps are inhibited by hypothermia both by its direct effect on enzyme activity and by the depletion of high-energy reserves as mitochondrial energy transduction fails. Nevertheless, the resultant passive redistribution of ions and water across the cell membrane and the concomitant change in the membrane potential have been demonstrated to be rapidly and fully reversible in the short term and may not be a source of permanent injury. Cells are known to have interrelated cation transport systems depending on energy supply and are thereby affected by reduced temperatures. Moreover, it is recognized that changes in the distribution of divalent cations (Ca^{2+}, Mg^{2+}) as a consequence of ischemia, hypoxia, and even cooling are especially important in cellular injury. The belief that calcium, in particular, is a mediator of cell death is based upon evidence accumulated over several decades from observations in a wide variety of tissues and pertains to cell death from a variety of causes. Cytosolic calcium concentration is 10 000-fold lower than extracellular concentrations, and it is now postulated that enhanced or unbalanced calcium influx across the plasma membrane represents a final common pathway in cell death mediated by various conditions that share the tendency to induce an abnormal membrane permeability for calcium. In recent years, the recognition of the central role of calcium-mediated effects in the death of cells of ischemically sensitive tissues such as heart and brain has led to intense scrutiny of the effects of perturbations in divalent cation homeostasis. Calcium functions as a second messenger in the regulation of numerous biochemical and physiological processes, often by activating regulatory proteins, which, in turn, can activate many intracellular enzymes, including protein kinases. It has recently been proposed that the significant protective effect of mild hypothermia against ischemic brain injury might be mediated in part by inhibition of calcium-induced effects and the prevention of inactivation of important Ca-dependent enzyme systems such as the kinases. However, it is generally recognized that cooling has no beneficial effect in preventing, and may even accentuate, inhibition of the (Ca^{2+}, Mg^{2+})-ATPase pump mechanism, which in general is the most important factor in controlling intracellular Ca^{2+} concentrations. The effects of cooling on calcium homeostasis result not only from the inhibition of transmembrane pumping, but also from the inhibition of calcium sequestration by intracellular organelles, particularly the endoplasmic reticulum and mitochondria.

Proton activity changes The principal events of the ischemic cascade show that elevation of the concentration of protons, i.e., increasing acidity, is regarded as a contributory central event in the process of cellular injury ensuing from O_2 deprivation and energy depletion. Moreover, reduced temperatures are also known to influence pH regulation, which is another important homeostatic mechanism for cell survival. It has frequently been reported that hydrogen ion concentration increases in a variety of mammalian cells during hypothermic storage such that tissue pH has been recorded to fall to 6.5–6.8 within a few hours of cold. Acidity is widely recognized as a hazard for cells, with the accumulation of protons contributing to a variety of deleterious processes, including metabolic block of glycolysis and structural damage. Destabilization of lysozomes releasing harmful proteases and catalysis of oxidative stress by mobilization of free heavy metals have been implicated as mechanisms of cellular tissue injury during acidosis.

Effect of hypothermia on the generation of oxygen free radicals The emerging role of oxygen-derived free radicals (ODFRs) in tissue injury and their participation in reperfusion injury is well established. In essence, it is recognized that cooling increases the susceptibility of cells to produce free radicals and attenuates the natural defense mechanisms by which cells normally deal with the low-level free radical production in metabolism. Due to a lower activation energy, free radical reactions are depressed less by temperature reduction than the enzymatic processes used to scavenge them. It is the balance between production and removal of free radicals that is crucial to the cell such that a combination of excessive radical generation and hindrance of normal defense mechanisms can redirect the processes in favor of injury. There is evidence that some of the natural defense mechanisms against free radicals become depleted during cold storage and that the addition of natural pharmacological scavengers including superoxide dismutase (SOD), catalase, or mannitol to cold storage media may improve the viability of hypothermically stored organs. It is clear, therefore, that in tissues exposed to cold there is potential for unbalanced free radical reactivity and elevated intracellular free calcium levels, and subsequent warming and reperfusion is likely to greatly potentiate these adverse events.

Structural changes The interrelationship between structure and function is fundamentally important for cellular homeostasis, which is governed by an intricate array of biochemical, physiological, and biophysical processes. Moreover, these processes are compartmentalized within the cell such that the structure of biological membranes and the cytoskeleton are integral components of cell viability and vitality.

The sensitivity of biological structures to temperature change is well known, and the thermal denaturation of proteins in particular is well documented. Thus, most proteins, as well as nucleic acids and many polysaccharides, are able to exist in their biologically active states only within a limited temperature range that is characteristic of the macromolecule and its environmental conditions such as ionic strength and pH. While a great deal more is known about heat denaturation of proteins at elevated temperatures, there are well-described examples of cold denaturation involving spontaneously unfolding of proteins or dissociation of the multisubunit structure into biologically inactive species that may or may not reassemble on rewarming to normal temperatures.

It has been postulated on the basis of measurements in both model systems and intact cells that a phase separation occurs within the plane of the membrane as cooling proceeds. Such cold-induced changes in the degree of membrane fluidity render it thermodynamically unfavorable for membrane proteins to remain in the gel phase such that they may be redistributed laterally into regions of low melting point lipids that remain in the liquid crystalline phase. This process is thought to result in packing faults due to the development of lipid-rich and protein-rich microdomains in a membrane undergoing phase transitions. One consequence of this could be a change in membrane permeability and alteration in the solute barrier function of the membrane. Phase separation of mammalian membranes has been demonstrated at temperatures

in the region of 10°C and below, and this correlates with the trend toward increased permeabilities to both ions and even large molecules such as proteins during cooling. In addition to phase separations, other forms of cold-induced membrane damage include the actual loss of membrane phospholipids, which is intuitively more deleterious than phase changes, which may in large part be reversible.

Cold-induced changes of cellular structural proteins that constitute cytoskeletal components such as microtubules have been known since the mid 1970s. This cold sensitivity appears to be mediated by depolymerization of component polypeptide units and in general is readily reversible upon rewarming. Nevertheless, the possibility exists for reassembly of the microtubules in a way that results in cellular abnormalities.

Thermal shock It has been discovered in some cells that the rate of cooling is also a determinant of injury; the phenomenon, which is not well understood, is referred to as thermal shock (cold shock) or chilling injury. The effects are thought to be related to the thermotropic properties of cell membranes involving phase transitions, as discussed briefly earlier. It has been proposed that rapid cooling in the absence of freezing can cause mechanical stresses on membranes induced by differential thermal contraction.

Cold shock proteins Changes in the structure of proteins are a common response to stress such that cells accumulate incorrectly folded proteins as a consequence of stresses such as hypoxia or temperature change. Proteins that experience unfolding or conformational changes do not remain soluble and are transformed into denatured proteins. It is now well established that one of the defense mechanisms adopted by cells to counteract such effects of stress is to synthesize new proteins commonly referred to as stress proteins or heat shock proteins (HSPs) because of their increased synthesis by many cell types after exposure to elevated temperatures. The general role of this group of highly conserved stress proteins is believed to be homeostatic in that they protect the cell against the harmful consequences of traumas and help promote a quick return to normal cellular activities once the shock has terminated.

The induction of stress proteins in response to cold (cold shock proteins) has been identified in invertebrate species such as bacteria and yeast, but it was not known until recently that similar families of cold shock proteins are also induced in mammalian cells.

Apoptosis vs. necrosis in cold-induced cell death It is now known that there are two distinct ways in which cells may die. Necrosis is caused by a general failure of cellular homeostatic regulation following injury induced by a variety of deleterious stimuli, including hypoxia, toxins, radiation, and temperature changes. Apoptosis (programmed cell death) by contrast, is a regulated process that has been distinguished from necrosis by numerous morphological, biochemical and physiological differences. While many of the diverse stresses known to cause necrotic cell death have also been reported to induce apoptosis in a variety of cells, the role of low temperatures as a possible stimulus of programmed cell death has yet to be investigated in depth. Nevertheless, it has been shown that cultured mammalian fibroblast cells at the transition from logarithmic to stationary growth were killed by brief exposures to 0°C and rewarming at 37°C. Moreover, the kinetics of cell death served to distinguish cold-induced apoptosis from the lethal effects of longer-term cold storage (hours or days), and also showed characteristics inconsistent with direct chilling injury (cold shock). It is possible, therefore, that apoptosis may represent another manifestation of cold injury. Susceptibility to cold-induced apoptosis seems to depend critically upon cell growth cycle and the temperature of exposure. Recent studies in cultured hepatocytes and liver endothelial cells have indicated that reactive oxygen species (free radicals) might play a key role in mediating cold-induced apoptosis.

Finally, it is important to emphasize that both the severity and the reversibility of the catalog of effects outlined here are highly dependent upon both the duration and the extent of hypothermic exposure. Many of the consequences of hypothermic stress manifest in cells subjected to prolonged exposure during cold storage do not develop during brief exposure to mild or moderate hypothermia.

See Also the Following Articles

Heat Resistance; Heat Shock Proteins: HSP60 Family Genes; Hyperthermia.

Further Reading

Bristow, G. K. (1985). Clinical aspects of accidental hypothermia. In: Heller, H. C., Musacchia, X. J. & Wang, L. C. H. (eds.) *Living in the cold: physiological and biochemical adaptations*, pp. 513. New York: Elsevier.

Collins, K. J. (1983). *Hypothermia: the facts*. New York: Oxford University Press.

Fuller, B. J. and Grout, B. W. W. (eds.) (1991). *Clinical applications of cryobiology*. London: CRC Press.

Kruuv, J. (1997). Survival of mammalian cells exposed to pure hypothermia in culture. In: Willis, J. (ed.) *Advances in molecular and cell biology* (vol. 19), pp. 143–192. Greenwich, CT: JAI Press.

Lee-Chiong, T. L., Jr. and Stitt, J. T. (1996). Accidental hypothermia: when thermoregulation is overwhelmed. *Postgraduate Medicine* 99(1), 77–80, 83–84, 87–88.

Lloyd, E. L. (1996). Accidental hypothermia. *Resuscitation* 32(2), 111–124.

Lønning, P. E., Skulberg, A. and Åbyholm, F. (1986). Accidental hypothermia: review of the literature. *Acta Anaesthesiologica Scandinavica* 30, 601–613.

Maher, J. and Hachinski, V. (1993). Hypothermia as a potential treatment for cerebral ischemia. *Cerebrovascular and Brain Metabolism Reviews* 5, 277–300.

Maier, C. M. and Steinberg, G. K. (2003). *Hypothermia and cerebral ischemia: mechanisms and clinical applications*. Totowa, NJ: The Humana Press.

Mercer, J. B. (1995). Enhancing tolerance to cold exposure – how successful have we been? *Arctic Medical Research* 54 (Supplement 2), 70–75.

Pozos, R. and Born, D. (1982). *Hypothermia: causes, effects, and prevention*. Piscataway, NJ: New Century Publisher.

Swan, H. (1973). Clinical hypothermia: a lady with a past and some promise for the future. *Surgery* 73, 736–758.

Taylor, M. J. (1987). Physico-chemical principles of low temperature biology. In: Grout, B. W. W. & Morris, G. J. (eds.) *The effects of low temperatures on biological systems*, pp. 3–71. London: Edward Arnold.

Taylor, M. J. (2006). Biology of cell survival in the cold: the basis for biopreservation of tissues and organs. In: Baust, J. G. & Baust, J. M. (eds.) *Advances in biopreservation* (chap. 2), pp. 15–62. Boca Raton, FL: CRC Press.

Taylor, M. J., Elrifai, A. M. and Bailes, J. E. (1996). Hypothermia in relation to the acceptable limits of ischemia for bloodless surgery. In: Steponkus, P. K. (ed.) *Advances in low temperature biology* (vol. 3), pp. 1–64. London: JAI Press.

Wilkerson, J. A., Bangs, C. C. and Hayward, J. S. (eds.) (1993). *Hypothermia, frostbite, and other cold injuries: prevention, recognition and pre-hospital treatment*. Seattle, Washington: Mountaineers Books.

Hypothyroidism

R T Joffe
McMaster University, Hamilton, Canada

This article is a revision of the previous edition article by R T Joffe, volume 2, pp 496–499, © 2000, Elsevier Inc.

Introduction
Thyroid and Psychiatric Symptoms
Types of Hypothyroidism
Clinical Hypothyroidism
Subclinical Hypothyroidism
Thyroid in Psychiatric Illness

Glossary

Clinical hypo-thyroidism	A disorder characterized by decreased production of thyroxine and triiodothyronine by the thyroid gland. It leads to a well-recognized clinical syndrome, of which psychiatric symptomatology is a prominent component.
Depressive symptoms	A group of mood, cognitive, and physical symptoms that commonly occur, but the number of symptoms are insufficient to qualify for the diagnosis of major depression.
Major depression	A characteristic syndrome that consists of mood, physical, and cognitive symptoms. This is one of the commonest psychiatric illnesses and is amenable to treatment with antidepressants and specific psychotherapies.
Subclinical hypothyroidism	A condition characterized by normal levels of circulating thyroxine and triiodothyronine but elevated levels of thyrotropin (TSH). There is also an enhanced TSH response to thyrotropin-releasing hormone (TRH). A well-described clinical syndrome is usually not evident.
Thyrotropin (TSH)	A hormone secreted by the pituitary that acts on thyroid cells to stimulate the production of thyroxine and triiodothyronine; also called thyroid-stimulating hormone.
Thyrotropin-releasing hormone (TRH)	A tripeptide hormone released by the hypothalamus that stimulates the release of TSH from the pituitary. TRH and TSH play an important role in the regulation of thyroid hormone secretion, both through a stimulatory effect on the thyroid and by negative feedback regulation of circulating thyroid hormone
	levels on the hypothalamus and pituitary. In this manner, appropriate thyroid hormone levels are maintained in the circulation.
Thyroxine (T_4)	One of two main circulating thyroid hormones produced by the thyroid gland. Although it is the major secretory product of the thyroid gland, this hormone is thought to exert its physiological action by conversion to triiodothyronine.
TRH test	A diagnostic test that involves the intravenous administration of TRH and the measurement of TSH at 15-min intervals for 90 min. In hypothyroidism, the TSH response to TRH is exaggerated, consistent with the high output of both TRH by the hypothalamus and TSH by the pituitary in response to a failing thyroid and decreased circulating T_4 and triiodothyronine levels. With the advent of new highly sensitive tests for the measurement of TSH, the TRH test is becoming obsolete.
Triiodothyronine (T_3)	One of two main circulating thyroid hormones produced by the thyroid gland. Only approximately 15–20% of circulating T_3 is secreted directly by the thyroid; the remainder comes from conversion from T_4. T_3 is approximately four times more metabolically active than T_4.

Introduction

Thyroid diseases, both hyperthyroidism and hypothyroidism, are among the commonest endocrine disorders seen in clinical practice. Excess or diminished production of thyroid hormone leads to the clinical syndromes of hyperthyroidism and hypothyroidism, respectively. A systematic evaluation of thyroid function tests helps verify the role of thyroid disease in the production of this symptomatology. This article reviews the clinical and biochemical features of hypothyroidism and, in particular, its relationship to psychiatric symptomatology.

Thyroid and Psychiatric Symptoms

It has long been known that there is an association between alterations of thyroid function and psychiatric symptomatology. Clinical thyroid diseases are commonly associated with psychiatric symptomatology, particularly alterations of mood and cognition. In particular, the association between hypothyroidism and depression has been documented consistently in the medical literature for more than 100 years.

Both hyperthyroidism and hypothyroidism may present with psychiatric symptomatology. In hyperthyroidism, a broad range of psychiatric symptomatology may present, but in hypothyroidism, depression and alterations of cognition are observed most commonly. Symptoms of anxiety and even psychosis are much less frequent. The observation of this very strong relationship between thyroid dysfunction and psychiatric symptomatology has led to the conclusion that thyroid hormones or the thyroid axis may be important in the pathophysiology of primary psychiatric disorders, especially major depression and the dementia disorders. As a result, it is common clinical practice to do a routine thyroid screening in patients who present with psychiatric symptoms, particularly disorders of mood or cognition. The best evidence is that most patients with depressive or dementia illnesses are euthyroid, and it has even been questioned whether routine thyroid screening of psychiatric patients is cost effective. However, this practice prevails because it does present an important opportunity, however uncommon, to identify an easily reversible major psychiatric disorder associated with hyper- or hypothyroidism.

Types of Hypothyroidism

Hypothyroidism is categorized according to the degree of thyroid failure. Since the mid-1970s, the definition of various degrees of hypothyroidism has become standardized. Grade I, or clinical, hypothyroidism is characterized by clinical symptoms of thyroid underactivity and is associated with abnormally decreased levels of thyroxine (T_4) and triiodothyronine (T_3), elevated basal thyrotropin (TSH) levels, and an enhanced TSH response to thyrotropin-releasing hormone (TRH). In grade I hypothyroidism, clinical symptoms of thyroid hormone deficiency are clearly evident. In grade II hypothyroidism, peripheral T_4 and T_3 levels are within normal limits, but both basal and TRH-stimulated TSH levels, using the TRH test, are elevated abnormally. Patients with this type of hypothyroidism do not have the classic symptoms of clinical hypothyroidism. Grade III hypothyroidism is characterized by no clinical features of hypothyroidism, normal circulating levels of T_4, T_3, and basal TSH, but an abnormally elevated TSH response to TRH. Each of these subtypes of hypothyroidism is considered separately here.

Clinical Hypothyroidism

Clinical hypothyroidism is a relatively uncommon disorder affecting approximately 1% of the population. However, its prevalence is influenced strongly by both gender and age; it is substantially more common in women and also increases in prevalence with advancing age. Therefore, the prevalence of clinical hypothyroidism in women over the age of 60 is approximately 4%. The features of clinical hypothyroidism are often vague and nonspecific. They include symptoms such as facial puffiness, dry skin, hair loss, myalgia, parasthesias, reduced tendon reflexes, cold intolerance, constipation, and fatigue. However, psychiatric symptoms occur in the majority of patients and are reasonably consistent for diagnosis. They include depressive symptoms or even a major depressive syndrome and, less commonly, evidence of cognitive deterioration. Anxiety and psychotic symptoms are much less common. The consistency of the psychiatric presentation in clinical hyperthyroidism is remarkable and highlights a need to exclude clinical hypothyroidism as a primary diagnosis in all patients presenting with depression or dementia, particularly in the elderly. These psychiatric syndromes associated with clinical hypothyroidism are generally not amenable to treatment with psychotropic drugs such as antidepressants and require correction of the underlying thyroid disease. However, in a minority of patients, psychiatric symptoms may persist even with correction of the underlying endocrine disorder, and further intervention with psychotropics may be necessary.

The diagnosis of clinical hypothyroidism is established on the basis of the clinical history as well as the measurement of T_4, T_3, and TSH. The specific treatment is dependent on the underlying pathology. However, thyroid replacement therapy is necessary to restore normal thyroid function.

Subclinical Hypothyroidism

This refers to both grade II and grade III hypothyroidism, as defined earlier. These abnormalities of thyroid function are usually detected on routine thyroid screening and are not associated with any particular clinical syndrome. Approximately 5–15% of depressed patients have evidence of subclinical hypothyroidism. These cases of subclinical hypothyroidism may be associated with a variety of causes, particularly iodine deficiency, autoimmune thyroid disease, and, less commonly, ablation treatment of clinical hyperthyroidism. The medical consequences of subclinical hypothyroidism are uncertain. Most studies have focused on grade II hypothyroidism, and these suggest that patients may have alterations in some physiological parameters such as myocardial contractility that may be reversed by thyroid hormone replacement therapy. Other studies have suggested that grade II hypothyroidism may be a risk factor for coronary artery disease due to alterations in serum lipoproteins. Although the clinical implications of grade II hypothyroidism require further clarification, it is known that between 5 and 10% per year of patients with subclinical hypothyroidism progress to clinical hypothyroidism.

The psychiatric consequences of subclinical hypothyroidism also remain to be clarified. As noted previously, approximately 5–15% of depressed patients have grade II or III subclinical hypothyroidism, although it is unclear whether this differs from the prevalence in the general population. Regardless, there is increasing evidence that subclinical hypothyroidism represents an increase in the vulnerability to depression and may also make patients more refractory to standard antidepressant therapies. Furthermore, if subclinical hypothyroidism is identified in a patient with depression, it is still a matter of controversy whether the depression in fact represents a clinical manifestation of the endocrine abnormality and, therefore, necessitates replacement therapy with thyroid hormone. Although the use of thyroid replacement therapy in subclinical hypothyroidism requires further study, the presence of treatment refractoriness may justify the use of thyroid hormones in order to enhance the response to antidepressants and, therefore, reduce the risk of chronicity and/or recurrence that are commonly associated with a major depressive illness.

Thyroid in Psychiatric Illness

As noted previously, the vast majority of patients with depression are euthyroid and have no evidence of thyroid dysfunction. Clinical hypothyroidism is extremely rare in major depressive illness, although 5–10% of patients with major depression have evidence of subclinical hypothyroidism. In fact, in the majority of patients with primary major depression, there is evidence of slight thyroid axis overactivity. It is suggested that primary major depression may be associated with a simulation of TRH, which in turn leads to increased release of TSH and, therefore, stimulates the thyroid gland to produce more T_4 and T_3. The most common alterations of thyroid function seen in primary major depression are slight elevations in measures of T_4, normal circulating levels of T_3, and blunted TSH responses to TRH. These alterations of thyroid function tests are suggestive of TRH stimulation. Although these alterations of thyroid function

tests are seen when groups of depressed patients are compared to either psychiatric or healthy controls, thyroid hormone levels in depressed patients are usually within normal limits.

Despite the fact that thyroid function is rarely decreased in depressed patients and in fact may be relatively increased, there is a long-standing practice of using thyroid hormones to treat depressive illness. Thyroid hormones used alone have not shown particular efficacy in treating depressive disorders, but T_3 in particular has been shown to augment therapeutic response when added to the antidepressant regimen in patients who have had no or only a partial response to treatment. The limited evidence to date suggests that T_3 may be more effective than T_4 in this regard. Although this remains to be clarified in future studies, the convention has been to use T_3 instead of T_4 in such cases, in contrast to thyroid replacement therapy for clinical hypothyroidism in which T_4 instead of T_3 is the usual treatment. There is insufficient evidence for the efficacy of either TRH or TSH in the treatment of depression. Although T_3 is gaining increasingly widespread acceptance as a treatment for resistant depression, its mechanism of action is unknown. However, it appears clear that it is not used to correct either clinical or subclinical hypothyroidism in the majority of cases.

See Also the Following Articles

Hyperthyroidism; Major Depressive Disorder; Thyroid Hormones.

Further Reading

Barzel, U. S. (1995). Hypothyroidism: diagnosis and management. *Clinical Geriatric Medicine* 11, 239–249.
Bilezikian, J. P. and Loeb, J. N. (1983). The influence of hyperthyroidism and hypothyroidism on alpha- and beta-adrenergic receptor systems and adrenergic responsiveness. *Endocrine Review* 4, 378–388.
Bunevicius, R., Kazanavicius, G., Zalinkevicius, R., et al. (1999). Effects of thyroxine as compared with thyroxine plus triiodothyronine in patients with hypothyroidism. *New England Journal of Medicine* 340, 424–429.
Gold, M. S., Pottash, A. L. C. and Extin, I. (1981). Hypothyroidism and depression: evidence from complete thyroid function evaluation. *Journal of the American Medical Association* 245, 1919–1922.
Haggerty, J. J., Jr. and Prange, A. J., Jr. (1995). Borderline hypothyroidism and depression. *Annual Review of Medicine* 46, 37–46.
Jackson, I. (1998). The thyroid axis and depression. *Thyroid* 8, 951–959.
Joffe, R. T. and Levitt, A. J. (1993). *The thyroid axis and psychiatric illness*. Washington, DC: American Psychiatric Press.

Hypoxia, Role in Stress *See:* Pressures, Effects of Extreme High and Low.

Hysteria

K Pajer
The Ohio State University, Columbus, OH, USA

This article is a revision of the previous edition article by K Pajer, volume 2, pp 500–502, © 2000, Elsevier Inc.

Definition and Historical Background
Treatment of Hysteria-Related Syndromes

Glossary

Conversion disorder	A psychiatric syndrome characterized by disturbances of bodily functions that do not correspond to known pathophysiological mechanisms.
Dissociation	The splitting of consciousness in an effort to repress painful memories; may result in either physical symptoms (somatization or conversion disorder), unconscious creation of alternative identities (multiple personality disorder), or inability to remain focused on present reality (borderline personality disorder).
Free association	A technique designed to uncover unconscious feelings. The patient lies down or sits comfortably and says anything that comes into his or her mind. Neither the patient nor the therapist makes any attempt to censor the thoughts, but the therapist listens and then interprets the associations.
Repression	Forgetting painful or frightening experiences. Repression is not a conscious process but, rather, an unconscious one; that is, the patient does not know that he or she has forgotten an event.
Somatization disorder	A psychiatric disorder in which the patient has many somatic complaints, but no underlying medical problem can be identified.

Definition and Historical Background

Clinical Vignettes

Patient 1 S.M. was 21 years old and in good health until she was out with her fiancé and he was hit by a swerving cab as he tried to push S.M. to safety. He died 3 days later. S.M. awakened on the day of the funeral to discover that she could not walk. She reported that she was paralyzed and could not walk or sit up. Her family tried to help her out of bed, and she simply collapsed. Her parents were quite upset, but she seemed relatively calm and told them it did not matter. She urged them to go to the funeral for her because she could not move. They consulted a prominent neurologist who could not find any abnormalities.

Patient 2 G.H. was 27 years old and sought treatment from a urologist for pain on urination and difficulty initiating urination. The urologist examined her and noted a urethral stricture that he treated with good success. Six weeks later, however, the patient called and said she was having pain in her pelvic area. He reexamined her, but could find nothing. The urologist suggested she consult her gynecologist, which she did. The gynecologist could not find any problem, but gave the patient some exercises to do to strengthen her pelvic muscles. The pain gradually subsided. However, the patient called 3 months later because of difficulties with her "bowels and stomach." The gynecologist referred her to a gastroenterologist who did a complete workup, but could not find any abnormalities. During the evaluation, G.H. did tell the gastroenterologist that she had recently begun her first sexual relationship and was having a great deal of difficulty with this. The gastroenterologist referred her to a psychiatrist, who worked with G.H. for several months before she finally elicited a history of severe and repeated sexual abuse that had occurred during childhood. This abuse had produced the urethral stricture and was now causing sexual and psychological difficulties for the patient as she tried to function in a normal adult romantic relationship.

Historical Changes in the Meaning of Hysteria

The word hysteria is familiar to most clinicians and lay people, but is elusive in definition. It is no longer used in psychiatric or psychological nomenclature, but, surprisingly, it was once the cornerstone of modern psychiatry. Several scholars of the history of psychiatry have proposed that the epidemic of hysteria afflicting American and British women in the late nineteenth and early twentieth centuries spawned the field of psychoanalysis. However, the disorder has now virtually disappeared. Furthermore, the term hysteria, once the focus of intensive treatment efforts and research, can scarcely be found in modern mainstream psychiatric literature.

The symptoms of hysteria can be found as early as 1900 BC in the Egyptian papyri (the actual word hysteria is derived from hystera, Greek for uterus). In both Egyptian and Greek writings, this multisymptom complex described in women was thought to be caused by a wandering uterus. Treatments were directed at coaxing the uterus to return to the pelvis and keeping it there once it returned. Assuming that sexual intercourse and childbirth would keep the uterus from moving, the most common prescription was for marriage and coitus.

Subsequent centuries brought changes in the definition and hypothesized etiology of hysteria. The definition became quite broad, referring to nearly any symptom of disease that was found more often in women than in men. Etiological explanations continued to focus on uterine pathology but also included causes such as satanic possession.

The nineteenth century brought a dramatic increase in the incidence of hysteria, although it is not clear why this happened. Treatments continued to focus on the uterus and newly discovered ovaries. The cauterization of the cervix, leeches applied to the cervix and vagina, and the removal of the ovaries were all common treatments that were only moderately successful. In the late nineteenth century, however, hypnosis was discovered to be useful for curing some symptoms of hysteria, such as the paralysis described earlier in S.M. Janet, Freud, and others believed that the mechanism of this cure was that hypnosis allowed the therapist, and then later the patient, to gain access to repressed feelings. In exploring these hidden feelings, buried conflicts could be resolved and the symptoms would disappear. The use of hypnosis diminished as Freud developed the technique of free association with interpretation by the analyst. This technique became the hallmark of psychoanalysis and was eventually used for many psychiatric disorders.

The *Diagnostic and Statistical Manual* 4th edn. (DSM-IV) has reclassified hysteria into two other disorders in the somatoform disorders category: conversion disorder (CD) and somatization disorder (SD). CD is a psychiatric syndrome characterized by disturbances of bodily functions (e.g., blindness, hearing loss, paralysis, and lack of sensation) that do not correspond to known pathophysiological mechanisms. SD is a psychiatric disorder in which the patient has many different somatic complaints but no underlying medical problem can be identified.

As with hysteria, these disorders are more common in women. However, we now know from clinical and research data on combat and natural disasters that men may also present with unusual physical symptoms that do not have medical explanations. The primary risk factor for both disorders in men and women is trauma or extremely stressful events over which the patient has no control. The trauma may be acute, as in the case of S.M. or exposure to battle, or chronic and repressed, as in the case of G.H., who had been the victim of repeated sexual abuse. She had remained asymptomatic until her first sexual relationship reawakened bodily sensations associated with a time of great stress earlier in her life.

Overwhelming stress in the context of helplessness seems to be the key feature of situations that produce SD or CD. However, studies of the function of either the sympathoadrenal or hypothalamic-pituitary-adrenal (HPA) axis components of the stress-response system have not demonstrated consistent abnormalities. It does appear that patient with SD are more subjectively sensitive to pain, with greater stress-response system reactivity. The multiple illnesses in SD may be due to a sensitization of the brain cytokine system by past adverse experiences such that it responds with a sickness pattern to a lower threshold of stress than is usually required in other people.

Treatment of Hysteria-Related Syndromes

Conversion Disorder

A complete medical and psychiatric workup is essential to rule out any medical pathology that merits treatment. In some cases, even an acute trauma is not known to the physician or psychologist (e.g., rape or an abortion of a hidden pregnancy). In this case, repressed trauma can sometimes be discovered with an interview that takes place when the patient is under the influence of amobarbital or lorazepam. On occasion, hypnosis is still used. The symptoms of a CD remit spontaneously in the majority of cases. The establishment of a nonjudgmental therapeutic relationship seems crucial for the treatment of patients whose symptoms do not subside quickly. With this type of a relationship, the exploration of latent trauma can be accomplished and healthier ways to cope with stress can be taught.

Somatization Disorder

As with CD, patients with suspected SD should receive complete medical workups. The primary danger in treating this disorder is that the patient can receive many invasive evaluations that are both expensive and disruptive to her life before someone notices the pattern of multiple, changing somatic complaints. There are three strategies for treating this disorder. The first is to control the frequent doctor shopping. This is accomplished most often by establishing a single physician to manage all aspects of care. This person keeps track of all medical care and schedules frequent contact with the patient. Second, some patients have had a positive response to antidepressant medication. The final treatment strategy is psychotherapy, focusing on any early trauma and the effect it may have on the patient's current ability to cope with stress. The prognosis for SD is not good unless the patient responds to an antidepressant or is motivated to embark on a course of psychotherapy.

See Also the Follwing Articles

Autonomic Nervous System; Combat Reaction, Chronic; Combat, Acute Reactions to; Corticosteroids and Stress; Posttraumatic Stress Disorder, Neurobiology of; Psychosomatic Medicine; Somatic Disorders; Trauma and Memory.

Further Reading

Dantzer, R. (2005). Somatization: a psychoneuroimmune perspective. *Psychoneuroendocrinology* **30**, 947–952.

Janet, P. (1920). *The major symptoms of hysteria.* New York: Macmillen.

Micale, M. (1989). Hysteria and historiography: a review of past and present writings, I–II. *History of Science* **27**, 223–261, 319–351.

Rief, W. and Barsky, A. J. (2005). Psychobiological perspectives on somatoform disorders. *Psychoneuroendocrinology* **30**, 996–1002.

Rief, W., Shaw, R. and Fichter, M. M. (1998). Elevated levels of psychophysiological arousal and cortisol in patients with somatization syndrome. *Psychosomatic Medicine* **60**, 198–203.

Scaer, R. C. (2001). The neurophysiology of dissociation and chronic disease. *Applied Psychophysiology and Biofeedback* **26**, 73–91.

Stone, J., Smyth, R., Carson, A., et al. (2005). Systematic review of misdiagnosis of conversion symptoms and "hysteria." *British Medical Journal* **331**(7523), 989–995.

Immobilization Stress

R Kvetnansky
Slovak Academy of Sciences, Slovak Republic
R McCarty
Vanderbilt University, Nashville, TN, USA

This article is a revision of the previous edition article by R Kvetňanský and R McCarty, volume 2, pp 503–506, © 2000, Elsevier Inc.

Variations in Immobilization
Advantages and Disadvantages
Acute versus Chronic Immobilization
Immobilization-Induced Gene Expression
Inventory of Neurohumoral and Genetic Responses to Acute Immobilization
Summary and Conclusion

Glossary

Immobilization	A model of stress that has been employed in studies of laboratory rats and mice. The procedure involves taping the four limbs of a rat or mouse to mounts secured to a metal frame using hypoallergenic tape. A pair of metal loops attached to the frame limits the range of motion of the animal's head. The frame, loops, and mounts are fabricated of stainless steel. The duration of a single episode of immobilization usually varies from 5 to 120 min or more. In addition, animals in chronic stress protocols may be immobilized each day for many weeks even months.
Restraint	A model of stress whereby laboratory rats or mice are restricted in their range of movement. Each animal is secured in a plastic tube or a wire-mesh container that is small enough to prevent the animal from moving about or turning. The frequency and duration of restraint stress vary depending on the questions being addressed by a given study, but a permanent restraint could last for many weeks.

Immobilization was introduced as a model of stress in animal experimentation in the mid-1960s. Since that time, Kvetnansky and colleagues have developed a standard protocol for immobilizing laboratory rats that involves securing the four limbs of a rat to mounts on a metal frame with hypoallergenic tape. The range of motion of an animal's head is limited by rings that are fixed to the metal frame. An acute episode of immobilization typically lasts from 5 to 120 min. In addition, animals can be immobilized daily (usually for 120 min) for many weeks to study the biological effects of adaptation to repeated immobilization stress.

During the first exposure to immobilization stress, laboratory rats or mice typically struggle vigorously to free themselves for 20–30 min. After that time, they will often cease struggling and remain motionless until a disturbance occurs. When one animal begins to struggle or if there is a sudden loud noise or some other form of sensory stimulation, many of the animals in the group that is being immobilized will begin to struggle again. Animals that have been immobilized daily for many days display signs of habituation to the stressor and calm down much sooner than naïve animals being immobilized for the first time.

Immobilization is a complex stressor and includes physical as well as psychological dimensions. The struggling and associated muscular exertion that occur during immobilization represent an intense form of physical exercise. After the first immobilization exposure, animals are so exhausted that they hardly move. In addition, the limited range of movement and exposure in an open area are significant sources of psychological stress to laboratory animals. It is also quite common for repeatedly immobilized adult rats to lose a significant amount of body weight over a 1- to 4-week period as a result of an increase in physical training and a decrease in food intake. After that period, repeatedly immobilized animals begin to gain weight at a rate that is similar to unstressed controls. However, the absolute body weights of stressed rats remain below those of control rats.

Variations in Immobilization

Since its introduction as a laboratory stressor, immobilization has been modified and adapted for the unique needs of different laboratories. Unfortunately, it is all too easy to assume that all models of stress involving immobilization are the same. In fact, it is very difficult to compare studies unless the technique for immobilization is comparable. For example, many investigators have used restraint as a model of stress. Restraint may involve placing the test animal into a plastic tube or a wire-mesh container that is well ventilated. Although the animal's range of movement is severely limited, the limbs are not secured and the animal remains within an enclosed area. Many have argued that restraint stress is less intense a stressor than immobilization, and comparative studies using neural and endocrine measures have supported this assertion.

Immobilization may also be combined with other stressors, such as cold temperatures or even placing the immobilization board in shallow water such that the animal is partially submerged. Caution should be exercised in comparing such studies with others because the addition of a second stressor affects an animal's physiological and behavioral responses.

Immobilization has also been employed in the development of an animal model of long-term weight-lessness. This model involves the continuous restriction of movement of laboratory rats for as long as 60 days to simulate some of the physiological changes that attend long-term space flight. The hypokinesia apparatus is modified such that the animal can gain access to food and water. It bears some similarity to studies with humans that have included long-term bed rest as a model of weightlessness associated with space flight.

Advantages and Disadvantages

Without doubt, immobilization has evolved into one of the most frequently employed models of stress in studies with laboratory rats and, recently, mice. There are several reasons for this. No special equipment is required other than the immobilization boards, which can be fabricated of stainless steel in a departmental or institute shop and used for many years (the authors have used the same boards for more than 30 years). Once the animals have been immobilized, the investigator is free to do other things in the laboratory until the end of the stress session for that day. In addition, the stressor is sufficiently intense such that most stress-responsive biological systems are altered and their regulatory processes may be studied (**Tables 1** and **2**). Immobilization is well tolerated by laboratory rats and mice and can be used in studies of chronic intermittent stress over weeks or even months. Finally, there is extensive literature on biological responses to immobilization that may be consulted when an investigator is planning an experiment that involves using an acute or a repeated stressor.

The immobilization model of stress does have its limitations, however. The intensity of the stressor cannot be altered, as we can do with foot-shock stress or cold stress, for example. In addition, measures of behavioral responses to immobilization stress are not usually an element of the experimental protocols. This limits the use of this model of stress when investigators have a specific interest in relating physiological and behavioral responses to the same stressful stimulus.

Acute versus Chronic Immobilization

Immobilization stress has provided an especially useful model for exploring the molecular and physiological adaptations that occur when animals are exposed to a regimen of chronic daily stress. Although immobilization is an intense stressor, considerable evidence shows that many neural and endocrine systems do exhibit decreases in the magnitude of their responses following repeated daily bouts of immobilization stress. These habituated responses are also characteristic of other laboratory stressors (e.g., restraint, foot shock, swim stress, handling, and open field testing) that are less intense than immobilization.

In laboratory rats that are exposed to repeated daily episodes of immobilization stress, there is an enhanced response of many neural and endocrine systems if the same animals are exposed to a novel stressor. The proper control group to demonstrate this sensitization effect is a group of naïve control rats with no prior history of experimenter-controlled stress that is exposed to the novel stressor for the first time.

Immobilization-Induced Gene Expression

In studies of transcriptional regulation of genes involved in neurotransmitter and hormone biosynthesis, immobilization has served as a valuable stress

Table 1 Selected neurochemical and neurohumoral responses of laboratory rats to acute immobilization stress[a]

Variable	Baseline	Stress	Peak time (min)
Norepinephrine			
Adrenal content (μg/adrenal)	3.2 ± 0.2	2.0 ± 0.3	120
Urine levels (μg/kg/24 h)	1.8 ± 0.2	4.9 ± 0.3	30
Plasma levels (pmol/ml)	1.25 ± 0.3	7.3 ± 1.2	20
Epinephrine			
Adrenal content (μg/adrenal)	17.5 ± 0.6	14.6 ± 0.4	120
Urine levels (μg/kg/24 h)	0.8 ± 0.06	2.6 ± 0.4	120
Plasma levels (pmol/ml)	0.20 ± 0.03	15.5 ± 2.7	5
Plasma levels of:			
DOPA (pmol/ml)	3.3 ± 0.2	3.9 ± 0.4	5
Dopamine (pmol/ml)	0.8 ± 0.09	1.25 ± 0.4	20
Dihydroxyphenylglycol (pmol/ml)	3.2 ± 0.3	9.3 ± 1.0	20
Methoxyhydroxyphenylglycol (pmol/ml)	15 ± 2.0	62 ± 15	60
Dihydroxyphenylacetic acid (pmol/ml)	5.2 ± 0.6	13.5 ± 0.2	20
Homovanillic acid (pmol/ml)	22 ± 4	55 ± 6	20
Plasma acetylcholinesterase (nmol/min/ml)	71 ± 5	112 ± 8	120
Plasma renin activity (ng/min/h)	4.4 ± 0.9	29.3 ± 4.7	10
Plasma aldosterone (pg/ml)	970 ± 90	3190 ± 460	120
Vasopressin (fmol/ml)	1.9 ± 0.2	6.1 ± 2.3	2
ACTH (pg/ml)	44 ± 4	790 ± 225	30
Corticosterone (μg/100 ml)	3.9 ± 0.2	24.5 ± 2.7	120
Prolactin (ng/ml)	7.2 ± 0.5	71 ± 17	20
Microdialysate norepinephrine (pg/ml)			
Paraventricular nucleus	178 ± 17	475 ± 37	30
Bed nucleus of the stria terminalis	92 ± 12	360 ± 38	30
Central nucleus of the amygdala	151 ± 8	425 ± 53	30

[a]Values are means ± SEM. All data on plasma levels of various substances were obtained from chronically catheterized animals. All data on microdialysate norepinephrine levels were obtained from animals that were surgically prepared with chronic microdialysis probes. All values are estimates of data presented in figures of published papers that employed immobilization stress in studies using laboratory rats.

Table 2 Quantitative changes in gene expression of catecholamine biosynthetic enzymes during acute immobilization stress[a]

Variable	Baseline	Stress	Peak time (h)
Adrenal medulla			
TH mRNA (amol/ng RNA)	0.46 ± 0.06	3.10 ± 0.56	3 after IMMO
DBH mRNA (amol/ng RNA)	6.00 ± 0.84	15.20 ± 1.57	3 after IMMO
PNMT mRNA (amol/ng RNA)	28.00 ± 2.36	141.0 ± 20.8	3 after IMMO
Stellate ganglia			
TH mRNA (amol/ng RNA)	0.017 ± 0.002	0.038 ± 0.005	24 after IMMO
DBH mRNA (amol/ng RNA)	2.60 ± 0.20	6.45 ± 0.61	24 after IMMO
PNMT mRNA	Present; not enough for quantification		
Brain stem			
TH mRNA (amol/μgRNA)			
Locus coeruleus	75.0 ± 8.7	268.0 ± 34.0	24 after IMMO
NTS (A2)	4.6 ± 1.0	9.6 ± 1.1	24 after IMMO
A1 area	17.0 ± 2.0	109.0 ± 11.0	3 after IMMO
Hypothalamus			
TH mRNA (amol/μg RNA)			
Paraventricular n.	5.2 ± 0.6	14.0 ± 1.8	3 after IMMO
Supraoptic n.	3.1 ± 0.9	10.4 ± 2.0	24 after IMMO
Dorsomedial n.	0.8 ± 0.1	5.5 ± 1.3	24 after IMMO
Arcuate n., lateral	8.0 ± 1.4	12.0 ± 0.6	24 after IMMO
Arcuate n., medial	11.0 ± 2.3	18.0 ± 2.5	3 after IMMO

[a]Values are means ±SEM. Values are from data presented in figures of published papers that employed immobilization stress in rats. DBH, dopamine-B-hydroxylase; IMMO, immobilization; n., nucleus; PNMT, phenylethanolamine N-methyltransferase; TH, tyrosine hydroxylase.

model. Kvetnansky, Sabban, Wong, and co-workers have examined changes in the transcription rates of genes for enzymes involved in catecholamine biosynthesis in central and peripheral tissues. These include genes for tyrosine hydroxylase (TH), dopamine-β-hydroxylase (DBH), and phenylethanolamine-N-methyltransferase (PNMT) (**Table 2**). For example, their work has shown that adrenal medullary TH mRNA concentration (expressed in amol ng^{-1} total RNA) increase approximately sixfold above control levels following a single 2-h period of immobilization. This increase is transient and levels of TH mRNA return to control levels within 24 h. However, if rats are immobilized for 2 h per day for 2–7 consecutive days, TH mRNA levels increase as much as sixfold above basal levels and these elevated levels are maintained up to 24 h later. The concentrations of DBH and PNMT mRNA in the adrenal medulla are 15–70 times higher, but are further elevated during immobilization stress. These increases are transient and within 24 h return to control levels. TH and DBH mRNA concentrations in the sympathetic ganglia show lower levels than those in the adrenal medulla. During immobilization, the ganglionic mRNA levels are significantly elevated; however, they stay increased even 24 h after the end of immobilization.

PNMT mRNA is also present in sympathetic ganglia in a very low concentration. PNMT gene expression has also been detected in other peripheral tissues such as the heart atria and ventricles, spleen, and thymus, and immobilization stress induced a many-fold increase of PNMT mRNA levels in these tissues.

TH mRNA levels also increase significantly within catecholaminergic cell bodies of the brain-stem areas, for example, the nucleus locus coeruleus, nucleus tractus solitarii, and A1 area, and in some hypothalamic nuclei following immobilization stress (**Table 2**). In these hypothalamic areas, catecholaminergic cells were not originally described.

The expression of genes that encode catecholamine biosynthetic enzymes is mediated by transcriptional mechanisms. Recent work identified various transcription factors that are associated with the brief or intermediate duration of a single or repeated immobilization stress exposure. It has been shown that the genes coding for the catecholamine biosynthetic enzymes contain several regulatory genomic elements in their promoters, for example, the cAMP response element (CRE), glucocorticoid response element (GRE), activating enhancer binding protein (AP)-1, AP-2, POU/Oct, and SP1 sites. The signaling molecules that may influence the transcription rates of the genes for TH, DBH, and PNMT, include P-cAMP response element binding protein (CREB), Jun N-terminal kinase (JNK), c-fos, Egr-l, Fra-1, and Fra-2.

With repeated daily stress exposure, Fra-2 was a major AP-1 factor induced in the adrenal medulla, but Egr-1 levels were also markedly elevated.

For PNMT gene expression, two transcription factors are important especially: glucocorticoid receptor and Egr-1. The crucial role of glucocorticoids in PNMT gene regulation has also been confirmed in corticotropin releasing hormone (CRH) (corticoliberine) knockout mice exposed to immobilization.

The signaling pathways triggered by immobilization differ in different tissues. In the adrenal medulla, immobilization triggered activation of the mitogen-activated protein kinase (MAPK), JNK, and induction of AP-1 factors, Egr-1 and phosphorylation of CREB. In contrast, in the sympathetic ganglia of immobilized animals were not observed changes in JNK and only little binding to the AP-1 motif of the TH promoter. However, there was an increase in CREB binding to the CRE site of the TH promoter. A single episode of immobilization also triggered the elevation of c-fos in the brain areas, especially in the locus coeruleus. In this area, increased phosphorylation of CREB was also observed after both single and repeated immobilization; however, the levels of Fra-2 and Egr-1 were not changed (in the adrenal medulla these transcription factors were highly activated). These results reveal differential mechanisms of regulation of gene expression of catecholamine biosynthetic enzymes by immobilization stress in two components of the sympathoadrenal system (adrenal medulla and sympathetic ganglia) as well as in the brain areas.

These findings related to the gene expression of catecholamine biosynthetic enzymes provide an excellent example of how immobilization has been useful in tracking the regulation of gene transcription during acute and chronic stress. In addition, these findings on gene expression may be compared with similar studies relating to the regulation of other genes because immobilization stress has been adopted as a model in a host of different laboratories.

Inventory of Neurohumoral and Genetic Responses to Acute Immobilization

Tables 1 and 2 present an abbreviated summary of biological responses of laboratory rats to a single 2-h period of immobilization stress. **Table 1** emphasizes the responses of the sympathetic nervous system, the adrenal medulla, and the hypothalamic-pituitary-adrenocortical system because of the importance of these systems in contemporary stress research. **Table 2** emphasizes changes in gene expression of catecholamine biosynthetic enzymes during the exposure of rats to an acute immobilization stress. This archival information was obtained from many journal articles (see Further Reading for secondary reference sources). This information provides a useful inventory with which we may compare the responses of the same biological systems to other types of laboratory stressors.

Summary and Conclusion

Since the mid-1960s, immobilization has become one of the most frequently employed laboratory models of stress. The protocols for acute and chronic immobilization have been described clearly, and many laboratories have incorporated this procedure into their studies of stress. A rich and varied literature is available on biological responses to immobilization, and these findings have provided important insights into the molecular, genetic, endocrine, and neural adaptations that occur in laboratory rats following acute versus chronic stress.

See Also the Following Articles

Adrenal Medulla; Adrenocorticotropic Hormone (ACTH); Animal Models (Nonprimate) for Human Stress; Corticosteroids and Stress; Genetic Factors and Stress; Hypothalamic-Pituitary-Adrenal.

Further Reading

Chrousos, G. P., McCarty, R., Pacak, K., et al. (eds.) (1995). Special issue on stress: basic mechanisms and clinical implications. Annals of the New York Academy of Sciences (771).

Kvetnansky, R., McCarty, R. and Axelrod, J. (eds.) (1992). Stress: neuroendocrine and molecular approaches. New York: Gordon and Breach.

Kvetnansky, R. and Mikulaj, L. (1970). Adrenal and urinary catecholamines in rats during adaptation to repeated immobilization stress. Endocrinology 87, 738–743.

McCarty, R., Aguilera, G., Sabban, E. L. and Kvetnansky, R. (eds.) (1996). Stress: molecular genetic and neurobiological advances. Amsterdam: Harwood Academic.

McCarty, R., Aguilera, G., Sabban, E. L. and Kvetnansky, R. (eds.) (2002). Stress: neural, endocrine and molecular studies. London: Taylor and Francis.

Pacak, K., Aguilera, G., Sabban, E. L. and Kvetnansky, R. (eds.) (2004). Special issue on stress: current neuroendocrine and genetic approaches. Annals of the New York Academy of Sciences (1018).

Sabban, E. L. and Kvetnansky, R. (2001). Stress-triggered activation of gene expression in catecholaminergic systems: dynamics of transcriptional events. Trends in Neurosciences 24, 91–98.

Usdin, E., Kvetnansky, R. and Axelrod, J. (eds.) (1984). Stress: the role of catecholamines and other neurotransmitters. New York: Gordon and Breach.

Usdin, E., Kvetnansky, R. and Kopin, I. J. (eds.) (1976). Catecholamines and stress. Oxford: Pergamon Press.

Usdin, E., Kvetnansky, R. and Kopin, I. J. (eds.) (1980). Catecholamines and stress: recent advances. New York: Elsevier North Holland.

Van Loon, G. R., Kvetnansky, R., McCarty, R. and Axelrod, J. (eds.) (1989). Stress: neurochemical and humoral mechanisms. New York: Gordon and Breach.

Yehuda, R. and McEwen, B. (eds.) (2004). Special issue on biobehavioral stress response: protective and damaging effects. Annals of the New York Academy of Sciences (1032).

Immune Cell Distribution, Effects of Stress on

F S Dhabhar
Stanford University School of Medicine, Stanford, CA, USA

This article is a revision of the previous edition article by F S Dhabhar, volume 2, pp 507–514, © 2000, Elsevier Inc.

Introduction
Stress
The Immune System
Stress-Induced Changes in Blood Leukocytes
Hormones Mediating a Stress-Induced Decrease in Blood Leukocytes
A Stress-Induced Decrease in Blood Leukocyte Numbers Represents a Redistribution Rather than a Destruction or Net Loss of Blood Leukocytes
Target Organs of a Stress-Induced Redistribution of Blood Leukocytes
Stress-Induced Redistribution of Blood Leukocytes
Conclusion

Glossary

B lymphocytes   The antibody-producing cells of the body, originating in the bone marrow. B lymphocytes are also identified by the surface expression of specific molecules such as CD19.

Fluorescence-activated cell sorter (FACS)	An instrument used to rapidly quantify the relative percentages of different cell types in a cell suspension. The identification of different cells is achieved based on the size, granularity, and fluorescence properties of the cell. Fluorescence is derived from fluorescently conjugated antibodies that bind specific markers on the cell surface.
Immune response	A reaction mounted by various components of the immune system, which consists of leukocytes, antibodies, cytokines and chemokines (messenger molecules), prostaglandins (inflammatory mediators), and accessory cells.
Leukocytes	Cells that constitute the immune system. These include T and B lymphocytes, natural killer (NK) cells, monocytes/macrophages, and granulocytes.
Lymphocytes	Leukocytes that specifically recognize and respond to foreign antigen.
Monocytes/ macrophages	Cells that phagocytose foreign particles and self tissues that are injured (monocytes generally flow through the blood and mature into macrophages after they are activated and extravasate into tissues). They produce cytokines, which recruit other leukocytes to the site of an immune response, and they perform an important function known as antigen presentation, which is crucial to the initiation of specific immune responses by lymphocytes. Also known as mononuclear phagocytes.
Natural killer (NK) cells	Large granular lymphocytes that lyse virally infected cells and tumors in the absence of specific antigenic stimulation. They are identified by surface molecules such as CD16 and CD56.
Neutrophils	Cells that perform functions similar to mononuclear phagocytes and that form an important component of an acute inflammatory response; also known as polymorphonuclear leukocytes.
T lymphocytes	Leukocytes that are mediators of cellular immunity. Like all leukocytes, they are formed in the bone marrow but mature in the thymus. Helper T lymphocytes (Ths) orchestrate immune responses by secreting cytokines and recruiting other leukocytes to the site of an immune reaction and activating them at that site; most Th cells express a surface protein called CD4, which is used to identify them. Cytolytic T lymphocytes (CTLs) lyse cells that are infected by intracellular viruses or bacteria; most CTLs express a surface protein called CD8, which is used to identify them.

Introduction

Effective immunoprotection requires the rapid recruitment of leukocytes into sites of surgery, wounding, infection, or vaccination. Immune cells or leukocytes circulate continuously on surveillance pathways taking them from the blood, into various organs, and back into the blood. This circulation is essential for the maintenance of an effective immune defense network. The numbers and proportions of leukocytes in the blood provide an important representation of the state of distribution of leukocytes in the body and of the state of activation of the immune system. Numerous studies have shown that stress and stress hormones induce significant changes in absolute numbers and relative proportions of leukocytes in the blood.

Dhabhar et al. were the first to propose that a stress-induced decrease in blood leukocyte numbers may represent an adaptive response. These investigators suggested that acute stress-induced changes in blood leukocyte numbers represent a redistribution of leukocytes from the blood to other organs, such as the skin and lining of the gastrointestinal and urinary-genital tracts and their draining lymph nodes. They also suggested that such a leukocyte redistribution may enhance immune function in those compartments to which leukocytes traffic during stress. In agreement with this hypothesis, it has been demonstrated that a stress-induced redistribution of leukocytes from the blood to the skin is accompanied by a significant enhancement of a skin immune response. Here we discuss stress- and stress hormone-induced changes in blood leukocyte distribution and investigate the functional consequences of a stress-induced redistribution of blood leukocytes.

Stress

Although the word stress generally has negative connotations, stress is a familiar aspect of life, being a stimulant for some but a burden for others. Numerous definitions have been proposed for the word stress. Each definition focuses on aspects of an internal or external challenge, disturbance, or stimulus; on the perception of a stimulus by an organism; or on a physiological response of the organism to the stimulus. Physical stressors have been defined as external challenges to homeostasis, and psychological stressors have been defined as the "anticipation justified or not, that a challenge to homeostasis looms." (Sapolsky, 2005, p. 648). An integrated definition states that stress is a constellation of events, consisting of a stimulus (stressor) that precipitates a reaction in the brain (stress perception), which activates physiological fight-or-flight systems in the body (stress response). The physiological stress response results in the release of neurotransmitters and hormones that serve as the brain's messengers to the rest of the body. This article examines the role played by stress and stress hormones in enhancing different aspects of an immune response. It is often overlooked that a stress response has salubrious adaptive effects in the short run, although stress can be harmful when it lasts a long time. An important distinguishing characteristic of stress is its duration and intensity. Thus, we define acute stress as stress that lasts for a period of a few minutes to a few hours and chronic stress as stress that persists for several hours per day for weeks or months. The intensity of stress may be gauged by the peak levels of stress hormones, neurotransmitters, by other physiological changes such as increases in heart rate and blood pressure, and by the amount of time for which these changes persist during stress and following the cessation of stress.

The Immune System

Immune Cells and Organs

The immune system consists of organs (bone marrow, spleen, thymus, and lymph nodes), cells (T cells; B cells; natural killer, NK, cells; monocytes/macrophages; and neutrophils), and messenger molecules (cytokines, chemokines, and prostaglandins). These components of the immune system are spread throughout the body and are in constant communication with one another. The appropriate distribution of immune cells in the body is crucial to the performance of the different functions of the immune system.

Functions of the Immune System

The functions of the immune system may be classified into six major categories:

1. Constant surveillance of the body in preparation for potential immunological challenges (such as those described in the other five categories).
2. Detection and elimination of infectious agents such as bacteria, viruses, fungi, and other microorganisms and parasites from the body.
3. Detection and elimination of noninfectious foreign matter from the body.
4. Wound repair and healing.
5. Clearance of debris that may result from noninjurious events such as programmed cell death (apoptosis) in host tissues.
6. Detection and elimination of tumors and neoplastic tissue.

Thus, the immune system may be regarded as the body's army with soldiers (immune cells) moving from their barracks (bone marrow, lymph nodes, spleen, and thymus) through highways (blood vessels and lymphatic ducts) and patrolling almost all organs within the body, especially those organs (skin, lining of gastrointestinal and urinary-genital tracts, lung, liver, lymph nodes, and spleen) that may serve as potential battle stations should the body's defenses be breached. In order to perform their functions, immune cells communicate with one another and with the rest of the body through messenger molecules such as cytokines and chemokines.

Immune Cell Trafficking

The appropriate distribution of immune cells between different tissues in the body is crucial to the performance of the immune functions. Leukocyte trafficking is the process by which leukocytes circulate between immune and nonimmune organs as they patrol the body and discharge their functions. Leukocyte trafficking is accomplished through interactions between adhesion molecules on leukocytes and endothelial cells that ultimately determine the location of immune cells within the body. The three major families of adhesion molecules are the selectins, the immunoglobulin superfamily, and the integrins. Adhesion molecules mediate three important steps (rolling, anchoring, and extravasation) that are involved in capturing leukocytes from the circulation. For example, a T cell flowing through the bloodstream may be selectively retained within the vasculature of the skin if a particular adhesion molecule is expressed on the T cell and its corresponding ligand is expressed on skin endothelial cells. Thus, hormones, cytokines, and chemokines may influence the location of leukocytes in the body by regulating the conformation or expression of adhesion molecules and/or their ligands on leukocytes and endothelial cells.

The Immune Response

It is important to note that, although immune reactions are classified into different categories (e.g., innate, acquired, cell-mediated, or humoral reactions), an immune response is often a combination of different immune reactions. The immune response protects the body from infections, wounds, and tumors. Although mechanisms for self- and counterregulation exist between various immune components, mechanisms also exist by which immune responses may be modulated or influenced by mediators such as hormones and neurotransmitters. Stress, and its consequent release of hormones and neurotransmitters, has been shown to influence specific immune parameters such as leukocyte trafficking, NK cell activity, lymphocyte proliferation, antibody production, effector cell function, and cell-mediated immune reactions.

Stress-Induced Changes in Blood Leukocytes

The phenomenon of acute stress-induced changes in blood leukocyte numbers is well known. In fact, decreases in blood leukocyte numbers were used as an indirect measure for increases in plasma corticosterone before methods were available to directly assay the hormone. Stress-induced changes in blood leukocyte numbers have been reported in fish, mice, rats, rabbits, horses, nonhuman primates, and humans. This suggests that the phenomenon of stress-induced leukocyte distribution has a long evolutionary lineage and that perhaps it has functional significance.

Many of these studies have shown that stress-induced increases in plasma corticosterone are accompanied by a significant decrease in numbers and percentages of lymphocytes and by an increase in numbers and percentages of neutrophils. FACS analyses have revealed that absolute numbers of peripheral blood T cells, B cells, NK cells, and monocytes all show a rapid and significant decrease (40–70% lower than baseline) during stress. These stress-induced changes in leukocyte numbers are rapidly reversed on the cessation of stress.

Hormones Mediating a Stress-Induced Decrease in Blood Leukocytes

Several studies have examined stress hormone-induced changes in blood leukocyte numbers. It has been shown in rats that both adrenalectomy (which eliminates the corticosterone and epinephrine stress response) and cyanoketone treatment (which eliminates only the corticosterone stress response) virtually eliminate the stress-induced redistribution of blood leukocytes. Studies have also shown that adrenal steroid and catecholamine hormones mediate the stress-induced changes in blood leukocyte numbers and that glucocorticoid treatment induces changes in leukocyte distribution in mice, guinea pigs, rats, and humans. These studies clearly show that glucocorticoid hormones induce a significant decrease in blood lymphocyte numbers when administered under acute as well as chronic conditions. Similarly studies have delineated the importance of catecholamine hormones in mediating stress-induced changes in blood leukocyte distribution in rodents and humans.

A Stress-Induced Decrease in Blood Leukocyte Numbers Represents a Redistribution Rather than a Destruction or Net Loss of Blood Leukocytes

From the discussion so far, it is clear that stress and glucocorticoid hormones induce a rapid and significant decrease in blood lymphocyte, monocyte, and NK cell numbers. This decrease in blood leukocyte numbers may be interpreted in two possible ways. The decrease in cell numbers could reflect a large-scale destruction of circulating leukocytes. Alternatively, it could reflect a redistribution of leukocytes from the blood to other organs in the body. Experiments were conducted to test the hypothesis that acute stress induces a redistribution of leukocytes from the blood to other compartments in the body.

The first series of experiments examined the kinetics of recovery of the stress-induced reduction in blood leukocyte numbers. It was hypothesized that if the observed effects of stress represented a redistribution rather than a destruction of leukocytes, we would see a relatively rapid return of leukocyte numbers back to baseline on the cessation of stress. Results showed that all leukocyte subpopulations that showed a decrease in absolute numbers during stress showed a complete recovery, with their numbers reaching pre-stress baseline levels within 3 h after the cessation of stress. Plasma levels of lactate dehydrogenase (LDH), which is a marker for cell damage, were also monitored in the same experiment. If the stress-induced decrease in leukocyte numbers were the result of a destruction of leukocytes, we would expect to observe an increase in plasma levels of LDH during or following stress. However, no significant changes in plasma LDH were observed, further suggesting that a redistribution rather than a destruction of leukocytes was primarily responsible for the stress-induced decrease in blood leukocyte numbers.

It is important to bear in mind that, although glucocorticoids are known to induce leukocyte apoptosis under certain conditions, they have also been shown to induce changes in various immune parameters and in immune cell distribution in the absence of cell death. It has been suggested that some species may be steroid-resistant and that others may be steroid-sensitive and that glucocorticoid-induced changes in blood leukocyte numbers represent changes in leukocyte redistribution in steroid-resistant species (humans and guinea pigs) and leukocyte lysis in steroid-sensitive species (mouse and rat). However, it is now accepted that, even in species previously thought to be steroid-sensitive, changes in adrenal steroids similar to those described here produce changes in leukocyte distribution rather than an increase in leukocyte destruction.

Target Organs of a Stress-Induced Redistribution of Blood Leukocytes

Based on this discussion, the obvious question we might ask is: Where do blood leukocytes go during stress? Numerous studies using stress or stress hormone treatments have investigated this issue. Using gamma imaging to follow the distribution of adoptively transferred radiolabeled leukocytes in whole animals, experiments showed that stress induces a redistribution of leukocytes from the blood to the mesenteric lymph nodes. It has been reported that anesthesia stress, as well as the infusion of adrenocorticotropic hormone (ACTH) and prednisolone in rats results in decreased numbers of labeled lymphocytes in the thoracic duct, whereas the cessation of drug infusion results in the normal circulation of labeled lymphocytes. This suggests that ACTH and prednisolone (which produce hormonal changes similar to those observed during stress) may cause the retention of circulating lymphocytes in different body compartments, thus resulting in a decrease in lymphocyte numbers in the thoracic duct and a concomitant decrease in numbers in the peripheral blood. It has also been reported that a single injection of hydrocortisone, prednisolone, or ACTH results in increased numbers of lymphocytes in the bone marrow of mice, guinea pigs, and rats. Fauci et al. suggested that glucocorticoid-induced decreases in blood leukocyte numbers in humans may also reflect a redistribution of immune cells to other organs in the body. Finally, corticosteroids have been shown to induce the accumulation of lymphocytes in mucosal sites, and the skin has been identified as a target organ to which leukocytes traffic during stress. *In vitro* catecholamine treatment has also been shown to direct leukocyte traffic to the spleen and lymph nodes.

It is important to note that in these studies a return to basal glucocorticoid levels was followed by a return to basal blood lymphocyte numbers, further supporting the hypothesis that the decrease in blood leukocyte numbers is the result of a glucocorticoid-induced redistribution rather than a glucocorticoid-induced destruction of blood leukocytes. In view of this, Dhabhar et al. proposed that a transient stress-induced decrease in blood leukocyte numbers reflects a redistribution or redeployment of leukocytes from the blood to other organs (e.g., lymph nodes, bone marrow, and skin) in the body.

Stress-Induced Redistribution of Blood Leukocytes

Molecular Mechanisms

It is likely that the observed changes in leukocyte distribution are mediated by changes in either the expression or affinity of adhesion molecules on leukocytes and/or endothelial cells. It has been suggested that following stress or glucocorticoid-treatment specific leukocyte subpopulations (being transported by blood and lymph through various body compartments) may be selectively retained in those compartments in which they encounter a stress- or glucocorticoid-induced adhesion match. As a result of this selective retention, the proportion of some leukocyte subpopulations would decrease in the blood and increase in the organ in which they are retained (e.g., the skin).

Support for this hypothesis comes from studies that show that acute psychological stressors such as public speaking can induce significant changes in leukocyte adhesion molecules. Prednisolone has also been shown to induce the retention of circulating lymphocytes within the bone marrow, spleen, and some lymph nodes, thus resulting in a decrease in lymphocyte numbers in the thoracic duct and a concomitant decrease in numbers in the peripheral blood. Moreover, glucocorticoid hormones also influence the production of cytokines and lipocortins that, in turn, can affect the surface adhesion properties of leukocytes and endothelial cells. Further investigation of the effects of endogenous glucocorticoids (administered in physiological doses, and examined under physiological kinetic conditions) on changes in the expression/activity of cell surface adhesion molecules and on leukocyte-endothelial cell adhesion is necessary.

Functional Consequences

It had been proposed that a stress-induced decrease in blood leukocyte numbers may represent an adaptive response, that is, a redistribution of leukocytes from the blood to other organs such as the skin, lining of gastrointestinal and urinary-genital tracts, lung, liver, and lymph nodes that may serve as potential battle stations should the body's defenses be breached. It has been suggested that such a leukocyte redistribution may enhance the immune function in those compartments to which leukocytes traffic during stress.

Thus, an acute stress response may direct the body's soldiers (leukocytes) to exit their barracks (the spleen and bone marrow), travel the boulevards (blood vessels), and take up position at potential battle stations (the skin, lining of gastrointestinal and urinary-genital tracts, lung, liver, and lymph nodes) in preparation for an immune challenge. In addition to sending leukocytes to potential battle stations, stress hormones may also better equip them for battle by enhancing processes such as antigen presentation, phagocytosis, and antibody production. Thus, a hormonal alarm signal released by the brain on detecting a stressor, may prepare the immune system for potential challenges (wounding or infection) that may arise due to the actions of the stress-inducing agent (e.g., a predator or attacker).

When interpreting data showing stress-induced changes in functional assays such as lymphocyte proliferation or NK activity, it may be important to bear in mind the effects of stress on the leukocyte composition of the compartment in which an immune parameter is being measured. For example, it has been shown that acute stress induces a redistribution of leukocytes from the blood to the skin and that this redistribution is accompanied by a significant enhancement of a skin cell-mediated immune (CMI) response. In what might at first glance appear to be contradicting results, acute stress has been shown to suppress splenic and peripheral blood responses to T-cell mitogens and splenic IgM production. However, it is important to note that in contrast to the skin, which is enriched in leukocytes during acute stress, the peripheral blood and spleen are relatively depleted of leukocytes during acute stress. This stress-induced decrease in blood and spleen leukocyte numbers may contribute to the acute stress-induced suppression of immune function in these compartments.

Moreover, in contrast to acute stress, chronic stress has been shown to suppress skin CMI and a chronic stress-induced suppression of blood leukocyte redistribution is thought to be one of the factors mediating the immunosuppressive effect of chronic stress. Again, in what might appear to be contradicting results, chronic stress has been shown to enhance mitogen-induced proliferation of splenocytes and splenic IgM production. However, the spleen is relatively enriched with T cells during chronic glucocorticoid administration, suggesting that it may also be relatively enriched with T cells during chronic stress, and this increase in spleen leukocyte numbers may contribute to the chronic stress-induced enhancement of immune parameters measured in the spleen.

It is also important to bear in mind that the heterogeneity of the stress-induced changes in leukocyte distribution suggests that using equal numbers of leukocytes in a functional assay may not account for stress-induced changes in relative percentages of different leukocyte subpopulations in the cell suspension being assayed. For example, samples that have been equalized for absolute numbers of total blood leukocytes from control versus stressed animals may still contain different numbers of specific leukocyte subpopulations (e.g., T cells, B cells, or NK cells). Such changes in leukocyte composition may mediate the effects of stress even in functional assays using equalized numbers of leukocytes from different treatment groups. This possibility needs to be taken into account before concluding that a given treatment changes an immune parameter on a per-cell rather than a per-population basis.

Conclusion

An important function of endocrine mediators released under conditions of acute stress may be to ensure that appropriate leukocytes are present in the right place and at the right time to respond to an immune challenge that might be initiated by the stress-inducing agent (e.g., attack by a predator or invasion by a pathogen). The modulation of immune cell distribution by acute stress may be an adaptive response designed to enhance immune surveillance and increase the capacity of the immune system to respond to challenge in immune compartments (such as the skin, the epithelia of the lung, and the gastrointestinal and urinary-genital tracts) that serve as major defense barriers for the body. Thus, neurotransmitters and hormones released during stress may increase immune surveillance and help enhance immune preparedness for potential (or ongoing) immune challenge.

See Also the Following Articles

Immune Response; Immune Function, Stress-Induced Enhancement; Immunity.

Further Reading

Benschop, R. J., Rodriguez-Feuerhahn, M. and Schedlowski, M. (1996). Catecholamine-induced leukocytosis: early observations, current research, and future directions. *Brain, Behavior, & Immunity* 10, 77–91.

Cox, J. H. and Ford, W. L. (1982). The migration of lymphocytes across specialized vascular endothelium. IV: Prednisolone acts at several points on the recirculation pathway of lymphocytes. *Cellular Immunology* 66, 407–422.

Dhabhar, F. S. and McEwen, B. S. (1996). Stress-induced enhancement of antigen-specific cell-mediated immunity. *Journal of Immunology* 156, 2608–2615.

Dhabhar, F. S. and McEwen, B. S. (1999). Enhancing versus suppressive effects of stress hormones on skin immune function. *Proceedings of the National Academy of Sciences USA* 96, 1059–1064.

Dhabhar, F. S. and McEwen, B. S. (2001). Bidirectional effects of stress & glucocorticoid hormones on immune function: possible explanations for paradoxical observations. In: Ader, R., Felten, D. L. & Cohen, N. (eds.) *Psychoneuroimmunology* (3rd edn., pp. 301–338). San Diego, CA: Academic Press.

Dhabhar, F. S., Miller, A. H., McEwen, B. S., et al. (1995). Effects of stress on immune cell distribution – dynamics and hormonal mechanisms. *Journal of Immunology* **154**, 5511–5527.

Dhabhar, F. S., Miller, A. H., McEwen, B. S., et al. (1996). Stress-induced changes in blood leukocyte distribution – role of adrenal steroid hormones. *Journal of Immunology* **157**, 1638–1644.

Dhabhar, F. S. and Viswanathan, K. (2005). Short-term stress experienced at the time of immunization induces a long-lasting increase in immunological memory. *American Journal of Physiology: Regulatory, Integrative & Comparative Physiology* **289**, R738–R744.

Dougherty, R. F. and White, A. (1945). Functional alterations in lymphoid tissue induced by adrenal cortical secretion. *American Journal of Anatomy* **77**, 81–116.

Fauci, A. S. (1975). Mechanisms of corticosteroid action on lymphocyte subpopulations. I: Redistribution of circulating T and B lymphocytes to the bone marrow. *Immunology* **28**, 669–680.

Goebel, M. U. and Mills, P. J. (2000). Acute psychological stress and exercise and changes in peripheral leukocyte adhesion molecule expression and density. *Psychosomatic Medicine* **62**, 664–670.

Mills, P. J. and Dimsdale, J. E. (1996). The effects of acute psychologic stress on cellular adhesion molecules. *Journal of Psychosomatic Research* **41**, 49–53.

Sapolsky, R. M. (2005). The hierarchy on primate health. *Science* **308**, 648–652.

Stefanski, V., Solomon, G. F., Kling, A. S., et al. (1996). Impact of social confrontation on rat CD4 T cells bearing different CD45R isoforms. *Brain, Behavior & Immunity* **10**, 364–379.

Viswanathan, K. and Dhabhar, F. S. (2005). Stress-induced enhancement of leukocyte trafficking into sites of surgery or immune activation. *Proceedings of the National Academy of Sciences USA,* **102**, 5808–5812.

Zalcman, S. and Anisman, H. (1993). Acute and chronic stressor effects on the antibody response to sheep red blood cells. *Pharmacology, Biochemistry & Behavior* **46**, 445–452.

Immune Function *See:* Immune Response; Immune Function, Stress-Induced Enhancement; Immune Suppression; Immune System, Aging; Immunity; Immune Surveillance – Cancer, Effects of Stress on.

Immune Function, Stress-Induced Enhancement

F S Dhabhar
Stanford University School of Medicine, Stanford, CA, USA

This article is a revision of the previous edition article by F S Dhabhar, volume 2, pp 515–522, © 2000, Elsevier Inc.

Stress

The Immune System

General Assumption: Stress Suppresses Immune Function and is Detrimental to Health – Reasons for Modifying This General Assumption

Studies Showing Stress-Induced Enhancement of Immune Function

Functional Implications

The Stress Spectrum Hypothesis

Conclusion

Glossary

Antigen	A foreign substance that induces an immune response.
Cytokines	Protein hormones that mediate various functions of immune cells.
Immune response	A reaction mounted by various components of the immune system, which consists of leukocytes, antibodies, cytokines and chemokines (messenger molecules), prostaglandins (inflammatory mediators), and accessory cells.
Leukocytes	Cells that constitute the immune system. These include T and B lymphocytes, natural killer (NK) cells, monocytes/macrophages, and granulocytes.

Stress

Although the word stress generally has negative connotations, stress is a familiar aspect of life, being a stimulant for some but a burden for others. Numerous definitions have been proposed for the word stress. Each definition focuses on aspects of an internal or external challenge, disturbance, or stimulus; on the perception of a stimulus by an organism; or on a physiological response of the organism to the stimulus. Physical stressors have been defined as external challenges to homeostasis, and psychological stressors have been defined as the "anticipation justified or not, that a challenge to homeostasis looms." (Sapolsky, 2005, p. 648). An integrated definition states that stress is a constellation of events, consisting of a stimulus (stressor) that precipitates a reaction in the brain (stress perception), which activates physiological fight-or-flight systems in the body (stress response). The physiological stress response results in the release of neurotransmitters and hormones that serve as the brain's messengers to the rest of the body. This article examines the role played by stress and stress hormones in enhancing different aspects of the immune response. It is often overlooked that a stress response has salubrious adaptive effects in the short run, although stress can be harmful when it lasts a long time. An important distinguishing characteristic of stress is its duration and intensity. Thus, we define acute stress as stress that lasts for a period of a few minutes to a few hours and chronic stress as stress that persists for several hours per day for weeks or months. The intensity of stress may be gauged by the peak levels of stress hormones, neurotransmitters, by other physiological changes such as increases in heart rate and blood pressure, and by the amount of time for which these changes persist during stress and following the cessation of stress.

The Immune System

Immune Cells and Organs

The immune system consists of organs (bone marrow, spleen, thymus, and lymph nodes), cells (T cells; B cells; and natural killer, NK, cells; monocytes/macrophages; and granulocytes), and messenger molecules (cytokines, chemokines, and prostaglandins). These components of the immune system are spread throughout the body and are in constant communication with one another. The appropriate distribution of immune cells in the body is crucial to the performance of the different functions of the immune system.

Functions of the Immune System

The functions of the immune system may be classified into six major categories:

1. Constant surveillance of the body in preparation for potential immunological challenges (such as those described in the other five categories).
2. Detection and elimination of infectious agents such as bacteria, viruses, fungi, and other microorganisms and parasites from the body.
3. Detection and elimination of noninfectious foreign matter from the body.
4. Wound repair and healing.
5. Clearance of debris that may result from non-injurious events such as programmed cell death (apoptosis) in host tissues.
6. Detection and elimination of tumors and neoplastic tissue.

Thus, it has been suggested the immune system may be regarded as the body's army with soldiers (immune cells) moving from their barracks (bone marrow, lymph nodes, spleen, thymus) through highways (blood vessels and lymphatic ducts) and patrolling almost all organs within the body, especially those organs (the skin, lining of gastrointestinal and urinary-genital tracts, lung, liver, lymph nodes, and spleen) that may serve as potential battle stations should the body's defenses be breached. While performing their various functions, immune cells communicate with one another and with the rest of the body through messenger molecules such as the cytokines and chemokines.

Types of Immune Responses

Natural or innate immunity Natural or innate immune responses are initially mounted when an organism encounters an antigen or pathogen. These responses are rapidly activated and generally regarded as the first line of defense. Epithelial barriers, immune cells, the complement system, circulating proteins such as C-reactive protein, cytokines such as the α and β interferons (IFNs), tumor necrosis factor (TNF), interleukin (IL-)12, and IL-15 are involved in mediating innate immune reactions. Macrophages, neutrophils, and NK cells are the primary cellular mediators. Cells of the innate immune system recognize pathogens through surface receptors such as the toll-like receptors (TLRs), which recognize pathogen-associated molecular patterns (PAMPs). Innate immune responses are not enhanced by repeated exposure to antigens.

Acquired or specific immunity Acquired or specific immune responses are mounted following prior exposure to an antigen; they are mediated by lymphocytes (T and B cells) and antibodies and are primarily regulated by lymphocyte-derived cytokines such as IL-2, IL-4, and IFN-γ. Acquired immune responses are directed against specific antigens and are often enhanced following repeated exposure to antigens. Acquired immunity can be divided into two broad categories: cell-mediated immunity (CMI) and humoral immunity.

Cell-mediated immunity CMI can be adoptively transferred from an immunized organism to naïve organism by the transfer of T cells and primarily involves cell-mediated clearing mechanisms. Intracellular infectious agents such as certain bacteria (e.g., *Listeria monocytogenes* or *Mycobacterium tuberculosis*) and viruses require a CMI response for their elimination. This response involves T helper (Th) cells which recognize infected cells with the help of specialized antigen-presenting cells (APC). On antigen recognition, Th cells release cytokines and chemokines, and they orchestrate a series of reactions involving cytolytic T cells (CTL), macrophages, and NK cells. These cells move to the site of infection and lyse or phagocytose infected cells and destroy them. In addition to their protective effects, CMI responses are also involved in harmful reactions such as organ transplant rejection, graft versus host disease, and certain autoimmune diseases. Delayed type hypersensitivity (DTH) is a form of CMI in which the macrophage is the major effector cell. The tuberculin skin test is a classic example of a CMI response. A characteristic CMI response peaks at 24–48 h following exposure to the antigen. Depending on the nature of the antigen, CMI reactions mediate beneficial (resistance to viruses, bacteria, and fungi) or harmful (allergic dermatitis, autoimmunity) aspects of the immune function.

Humoral immunity A humoral immune response is adoptively transferred from an immunized organism to a naïve organism by the transfer of cell-free plasma or serum and primarily involves antibody-mediated clearing mechanisms. Extracellular infectious agents such as bacteria (e.g., *Staphylococcus*, *Streptococcus*, or *Escherichia coli*), protozoan, and helminthic parasites require antibody-mediated responses for their elimination. Antibodies are proteins produced by B cells that neutralize extracellular infectious agents, which are then destroyed by macrophages, neutrophils, or complement proteins.

The integrated immune response It is important to note that, although immune reactions are classified into different categories, an immune response is often a combination of innate as well as acquired immune reactions. *In vivo* immune responses necessarily involve intricate interactions between both the innate and adaptive arms of the immune system. Different components of the immune system work in synchrony to protect the body from infections, wounds, and tumors. Although mechanisms of self- and counter-regulation exist between various immune components, mechanisms also exist by which immune responses may be modulated or influenced by mediators such as hormones and neurotransmitters. Stress, and its consequent release of hormones and neurotransmitters, has been shown to influence specific immune parameters such as blood leukocyte numbers, NK cell activity, lymphocyte proliferation, antibody production, effector cell function, and CMI reactions. The immunoenhancing effects of stress are the focus of the rest of this article.

General Assumption: Stress Suppresses Immune Function and is Detrimental to Health – Reasons for Modifying This General Assumption

It is generally assumed that stress suppresses immune function and hence is detrimental to health. However, the suppression of immune function under all stress conditions should not be evolutionarily adaptive. It seems paradoxical that organisms should have evolved to suppress immune function at a time when an active immune response may be critical for survival, for example, under conditions of stress when an organism may be injured or infected by the actions of the stress-inducing agent (e.g., a predator). Stress is an intrinsic part of life for most organisms, and dealing successfully with stressors is what enables survival. Environmental challenges and most selection pressures, the chisels of evolution, are stressors that may be psychological (fear and anxiety), physical (wounding and infection), or physiological (food or water deprivation). One of the primary functions of the brain is to perceive stress and to warn and enable an organism to deal with its consequences. For example, when a gazelle sees a charging lion, the gazelle's brain detects a threat and orchestrates a physiological response that first prepares and then enables the gazelle to flee.

It has been suggested that under short-duration stress conditions, just as the stress response prepares the nervous, cardiovascular, musculoskeletal, and neuroendocrine systems for fight or flight, it may also prepare the immune system for challenges (e.g., wounding or infection) that may be imposed by the stressor. In contrast to this hypothesis, it had previously been suggested that a stress-induced suppression of immune function may be evolutionarily adaptive because immunosuppression may conserve energy that is required to deal with the immediate demands imposed by the stressor. However, immunosuppression does not necessarily conserve energy, and some of the proposed mechanisms for immunosuppression, such as apoptosis of leukocytes, may expend rather than conserve energy. Moreover, the immune system may often be critically needed to respond immediately to the actions of the stress-inducing agent (e.g., wounding by a predator). Thus, whereas ovulation, copulation, and digestion can wait for the cessation of stress, the immune response cannot be assumed to be dispensable in terms of meeting the immediate demands of stress. Moreover, the time course for many of the proposed mechanisms for stress-induced immunosuppression, such as inhibition of prostaglandin synthesis, cytokine production, or leukocyte proliferation, is significantly longer than that seen during acute stress conditions. Thus, although energy conservation may play a role in stress-induced immunosuppression under some conditions, it is not clear that it does so under all stress conditions.

Another well-known paradoxical observation is that, on the one hand, stress is thought to suppress immunity and increase susceptibility to infections and cancer and, on the other, it is thought to exacerbate inflammatory (e.g., cardiovascular disease and gingivitis) and autoimmune (e.g., psoriasis, arthritis, and multiple sclerosis) diseases that should be ameliorated by the suppression of immune function. If stress were solely immunosuppressive, we would expect stress to ameliorate, not exacerbate, these diseases. A stress-induced enhancement of immune function would help explain the stress-induced exacerbation of diseases mediated by immunopathological reactions.

Keeping these considerations in mind, and based on their initial observations of the effects of stress and of the circadian corticosterone rhythm on leukocyte redistribution in the body, Dhabhar and McEwen demonstrated that stress has bidirectional effects on immune function such that acute stress is immunoenhancing and chronic stress is immunosuppressive. This article focuses on the immunoenhancing aspects of stress.

Studies Showing Stress-Induced Enhancement of Immune Function

A majority of studies in the field of psychoneuroimmunology have focused on the immunosuppressive effects of stress, but several studies have also revealed that stress can be immunoenhancing. A stress-induced enhancement of immune function may be an important evolutionarily adaptive response that prepares an organism for potential immunological challenges for which stress perception by the brain, and subsequent stress hormone and neurotransmitter release, may serve as an early warning. Studies showing stress-induced enhancements in immune parameters *in vivo* and *in vitro* are briefly reviewed next.

Skin Cell-Mediated Immunity

There exist several mechanisms by which stress may enhance immune function. Studies showed that acute stress (2-h restraint) results in a significant redistribution of leukocytes from the blood to other organs (the skin, lymph nodes, and bone marrow) in the body and that adrenal stress hormones are the major mediators of this leukocyte redistribution. Because the skin was one of the targets to which leukocytes trafficked during stress, it was hypothesized that such a leukocyte redistribution may increase immune surveillance and consequently enhance immune function should the skin be exposed to an antigen following acute stress.

To test this hypothesis, researchers examined the effects of acute stress on skin immunity, using rodent models of CMI. In order to induce CMI, researcher initially sensitized animals to 2,4-dinitro-1-fluorobenzene (DNFB) by administering the chemical antigen to the skin of the dorsum. The sensitization phase of a CMI reaction is one in which the organism develops an immunological memory (through the generation of memory T cells) for the antigen with which it is immunized. Following sensitization, the ability of the animals to mount a CMI response against DNFB was examined by administering DNFB to the dorsal aspect of the right pinna. The CMI response was subsequently measured as an increase in pinna thickness that was proportional to the intensity of the ongoing immune reaction. This phase, also known as the challenge phase, involves the recruitment of memory T cells and effector cells such as macrophages, which mount an immune response against the antigen to which the animal was previously sensitized. Acute restraint stress administered immediately before the introduction of the antigen resulted in a large and long-lasting enhancement of skin CMI. Histological analysis identified significantly larger numbers of leukocytes in the skin of stressed animals both before and after exposure to antigen, and this suggested that a stress-induced redistribution of leukocytes was one of the factors mediating the stress-induced enhancement of skin immunity. Acute stress has similarly been shown to enhance skin CMI in mice and, under certain conditions, may also enhance the CMI response in human subjects.

It has also been shown that the acute stress-induced enhancement of skin CMI is mediated by adrenal hormones. Thus, adrenalectomy, which eliminates the glucocorticoid and epinephrine stress response, eliminated the stress-induced enhancement of skin CMI. Low-dose corticosterone or epinephrine administration significantly enhanced skin CMI and produced a significant increase in T-cell numbers in the lymph nodes draining the site of the CMI reaction. These results suggest a novel role for adrenal stress hormones as endogenous immunoenhancing agents. They also show that hormones released during an acute stress response may help prepare the immune system for potential challenges (e.g., wounding or infection) for which stress perception by the brain may serve as an early warning signal.

Humoral Immunity

Wood et al. showed that exposure to foot shock stress enhanced humoral as well as CMI to keyhole limpet hemocyanin (KLH). These investigators administered a single acute foot shock session on days −1, 0, 1, and 3, relative to sensitization (day 0). They observed that, compared to nonstressed controls, animals stressed on days 0 or 1 showed enhanced immune responses with respect to serum anti-KLH IgG levels, splenocyte proliferation, and skin CMI to the KLH antigen. Similar results were almost simultaneously reported by researchers who found that the timing of stressor exposure was critical for determining its immunoenhancing effects. Several other studies have reported stress-induced enhancement of humoral immune responses. For example, stress has been shown to accelerate antigen removal in mice, rats, and pigs. It has also been proposed that glucocorticoids may shift the balance of an ongoing immune response in favor of humoral immunity, and physiological doses of glucocorticoids have been shown to enhance immunoglobulin production by mitogen- and IL-4-stimulated human lymphocytes in culture.

Cytokine Function

Several lines of evidence indicate that glucocorticoid stress hormones may act synergistically with cytokines to enhance specific immune reactions. Thus, although glucocorticoids inhibit the synthesis of cytokines under some conditions, they have also been shown to induce the release and potentiate the actions of cytokines under other conditions. For example, stress has been shown to induce increases in plasma levels of IL-1, IL-6, and glucocorticoids to induce the production of migration inhibitory factor (MIF), which is, in turn, proposed to counter the actions of glucocorticoids. Moreover, glucocorticoids synergistically enhance the induction of acute phase proteins by IL-1 and IL-6. Glucocorticoids similarly enhance the biological responses of other cytokines such as IL-2, IFN-γ, granulocyte colony-stimulating factor (G-CSF), granulocyte macrophage colony-stimulating factor (GM-CSF), and oncostatin M. It has been suggested that synergistic interactions between glucocorticoids and cytokines may be mediated by the glucocorticoid-induced upregulation of cytokine receptors on target cells.

Proliferative Responses and Phagocytosis

Acute stressors such as handling and foot shock have been shown to enhance the mitogen-induced proliferation of blood lymphocytes. Acute stress has also been shown to enhance macrophage phagocytic function and blood NK cell activity. Several studies have shown that the *in vitro* administration of stress hormones to immune cells can enhance different aspects of the immune function. Low physiological concentrations of corticosterone have been shown to stimulate mitogen- and anti-T-cell receptor-induced proliferation of splenocytes. Similarly, glucocorticoid hormones have been shown enhance nitric oxide and IL-1β secretion by macrophages.

Functional Implications

The studies described here show that, under certain conditions, stress can enhance immune responses. These studies may help reconcile the apparent contradiction between reports showing that, on the one hand, stress suppresses immunity and increases susceptibility to infections and cancer but, on the other, exacerbates autoimmune diseases that should be ameliorated by the suppression of immune function. For example, under natural conditions, acute stress may serve a protective role by enhancing an immune response directed toward a wound or infection. However, a stress-induced enhancement of immune function could also be detrimental if the immune response is directed against an innocuous (poison ivy, nickel in jewelry, latex, etc.) or autoimmunogenic antigen, and this could explain the well-known stress-induced exacerbations of autoimmune diseases. It is also known that chronic stress suppresses immune function. This may explain stress-induced exacerbations of infections and cancer and the stress-induced suppression of wound healing. It has also been reported that high doses or prolonged administration of corticosterone or low doses of dexamethasone are potently immunosuppressive, in keeping with their clinically well-known antisuppressive effects.

It is important to note that humans as well as animals experience acute or chronic stress as an intrinsic part of life. They also experience stress in conjunction with many standard diagnostic, clinical, and experimental manipulations. Unintended stress may significantly affect diagnostic measures and overall health outcomes. Thus, it may be important to account for the effects of acute versus chronic stress when conducting clinical, diagnostic, or experimental manipulations.

The Stress Spectrum Hypothesis

In view of the data presented here, and in view of the widely demonstrated immunosuppressive effects of stress, Dhabhar and McEwen proposed that a stress response and its consequent effects on immune function may be viewed in the context of a stress spectrum. One region of this spectrum is characterized by acute stress or eustress (i.e., conditions of short-duration stress that may result in immunopreparatory or immunoenhancing physiological conditions). An important characteristic of acute stress is a rapid physiological stress response mounted in the presence of the stressor, followed by a rapid shut-down of the response on cessation of the stressor. The other region of the stress spectrum is characterized by chronic stress or distress (i.e., repeated or prolonged stress that may result in dysregulation or suppression of immune function). An important characteristic of chronic stress is that the physiological response either persists long after the stressor has ceased or is activated repeatedly, which results in an overall integrated increase in the exposure of the organism to stress hormones. The concept of allostatic load has been proposed to define the psychophysiological wear and tear that takes place while different biological systems work to stay within a range of equilibrium (allostasis) in response to the demands placed by internal or external chronic stressors. We suggest that conditions of high allostatic load result in the dysregulation or suppression of immune function. Significantly, a disruption of the circadian corticosterone/cortisol rhythm may be an indicator and/or mediator of distress or high allostatic load.

The stress spectrum also proposes that acute or chronic stress is generally superimposed on a psychophysiological health maintenance equilibrium. The extent and efficiency with which an organism returns to its health maintenance equilibrium after stress depends on resilience, which we define as the reserve capacity of psychophysiological systems to recover from challenging conditions. Factors such as coping mechanisms, sense of control, optimism, social support, early life experiences, learning, genetics, and sleep may be important mediators of psychological resilience. Factors such as neuroendocrine reactivity, genetics, environment, nutrition, and sleep may be important mediators of physiological resilience. The psychophysiological basis of resilience and reserve capacity are underinvestigated and provide an important opportunity for future research.

The stress spectrum, taken together with the preceding discussion, shows that the duration, intensity/concentration, and timing of exposure to stressor-induced physiological activation (neurotransmitters, hormones, and their molecular, cellular, organ-level, and systemic effects) are critical for determining whether stress enhances or suppresses/dysregulates immune function. The model shows that the stressor itself can be acute or chronic. Stress perception and processing by the brain and mechanisms mediating psychological and physiological resilience are critical for determining the duration and magnitude of the physiological stress response. Psychological resilience mechanisms are especially important in humans because they can limit the duration and magnitude of chronic stress responses. Psychogenic stressors are also very important in human subjects because they can generate stress responses long after stressor exposure (e.g., posttraumatic stress disorder following a severe traumatic experience or, in a milder form, lingering anger/mood disturbance following a social altercation) or even in the absence of a physical stressor or salient threat (e.g., worrying about whether one's romantic feelings will be reciprocated). Therefore, following stressor exposure and its processing by the brain, there ensues a physiological stress response. This response may consist of acute or chronic physiological activation (neurotransmitters; hormones; and their molecular, cellular, organ-level and systemic effects) that results in psychophysiological states that have different effects on overall health and immune function.

Conclusion

Stress has long been suspected to play a role in the etiology of many diseases, and numerous studies have shown that stress can be immunosuppressive and hence may be detrimental to health. Moreover, glucocorticoid stress hormones are widely regarded as being immunosuppressive and are used clinically as anti-inflammatory agents. Due to a host of psycho-sociopolitical factors, stress has unfortunately become an increasing and inevitable part of people's lives. Stress is also a major factor during the diagnosis, treatment, and follow-up of most diseases. However, as this discussion shows, some stress conditions (i.e., acute or short-duration stressors) produce immunoenhancement. A determination of the physiological mechanisms through which stress and stress hormones enhance or suppress immune responses may help our understanding and treatment of diseases thought to be affected by stress. Thus, future studies should aim at developing biomedical treatments that harness an individual's physiology to selectively enhance (during vaccination, wounding, infections, or cancer) or suppress (during autoimmune or inflammatory disorders) the immune response, depending on what is most beneficial for the patient.

Further Reading

Altemus, M., Cloitre, M. and Dhabhar, F. S. (2003). Cellular immune response in adult women with PTSD related to childhood abuse. *American Journal of Psychiatry* 160, 1705–1707.

Dhabhar, F. S. and McEwen, B. S. (1996). Stress-induced enhancement of antigen-specific cell-mediated immunity. *Journal of Immunology* 156, 2608–2615.

Dhabhar, F. S. and McEwen, B. S. (1997). Acute stress enhances while chronic stress suppresses immune function in vivo: a potential role for leukocyte trafficking. *Brain, Behavior & Immunity* 11, 286–306.

Dhabhar, F. S. and McEwen, B. S. (1999). Enhancing versus suppressive effects of stress hormones on skin immune function. *Proceedings of the National Academy of Sciences USA* 96, 1059–1064.

Dhabhar, F. S. and McEwen, B. S. (2001). Bidirectional effects of stress & glucocorticoid hormones on immune function: possible explanations for paradoxical observations. In: Ader, R., Felten, D. L. & Cohen, N. (eds.) *Psychoneuroimmunology* (3rd edn., pp. 301–338). San Diego, CA: Academic Press.

Dhabhar, F. S., Satoskar, A. R., Bluethmann, H., et al. (2000). Stress-induced enhancement of skin immune function: a role for IFNγ. *Proceedings of the National Academy of Sciences USA* 97, 2846–2851.

Dhabhar, F. S. and Viswanathan, K. (2005). Short-term stress experienced at the time of immunization induces a long-lasting increase in immunological memory. *American Journal of Physiology: Regulatory, Integrative & Comparative Physiology* 289, R738–R744.

Glaser, R. and Kiecolt-Glaser, J. K. (2005). Stress-induced immune dysfunction: implications for health. *Nature Reviews Immunology* 5, 243–251.

Pruett, S. B. and Fan, R. (2001). Quantitative modeling of suppression of IgG1, IgG2a, IL-2, and IL-4 responses to antigen in mice treated with exogenous corticosterone or restraint stress. *Journal of Toxicology and Environmental Health A* 62(3), 175–189.

Sapolsky, R. M. (2004). *Why zebras don't get ulcers* (3rd edn.). New York: W. H. Freeman.

Sapolsky, R. M. (2005). The influence of social hierarchy on primate health. *Science* 308, 648–652.

Saul, A. N., Oberyszyn, T. M., Daugherty, C., et al. (2005). Chronic stress and susceptibility to skin cancer. *Journal of the National Cancer Institute* 97, 1760–1767.

Sephton, S. and Spiegel, D. (2003). Circadian disruption in cancer: a neuroendocrine-immune pathway from stress to disease? *Brain, Behavior & Immunity* 17, 321–328.

Straub, R. H., Dhabhar, F. S., Bijlsma, J. W. J., et al. (2005). How psychological stress via hormones and nerve fibers may exacerbate rheumatoid arthritis. *Arthritis & Rheumatism* 52, 16–26.

Viswanathan, K. and Dhabhar, F. S. (2005). Stress-induced enhancement of leukocyte trafficking into sites of surgery or immune activation. *Proceedings of the National Academy of Sciences USA* 102, 5808–5813.

Wood, P. G., Karol, M. H., Kusnecov, A. W., et al. (1993). Enhancement of antigen-specific humoral and cell-mediated immunity by electric footshock stress in rats. *Brain, Behavior & Immunity* 7, 121–134.

Zalcman, S. and Anisman, H. (1993). Acute and chronic stressor effects on the antibody response to sheep red blood cells. *Pharmacology, Biochemistry & Behavior* 46, 445–452.

Immune Response

P J Delves
University College London, London, UK

Innate and Adaptive Immune Responses
Recognition of Pathogens and Other Antigens
Generation of the Immune Response
The Anatomy of the Immune Response
Protective Immune Response
Avoidance of Harmful Immune Responses
Neuroendocrine–Immune Interactions

Glossary

Adaptive (acquired) immune response	Immunity mediated by lymphocytes and characterized by antigen-specificity and memory.
Complement	A group of serum proteins, some of which act in an enzymatic cascade, producing effector molecules involved in inflammation (C3a, C5a), phagocytosis (C3b), and cell lysis (C5b–C9).
Cytokines	Low-molecular-weight proteins that stimulate or inhibit the differentiation, proliferation, or function of immune cells.
Dendritic cell	Refers to an interdigitating dendritic cell which is major histocompatibility complex (MHC) class II-positive, Fc receptor-negative, and presents processed antigens to T cells in the T cell areas of secondary lymphoid tissues.
Granulocyte	Myeloid cells containing cytoplasmic granules (i.e., neutrophils, eosinophils, and basophils).
Innate immune response	Immunity which is not intrinsically affected by prior contact with antigen, i.e., all aspects of immunity not directly mediated by lymphocytes.
Primary immune response	The relatively weak immune response which occurs upon the first encounter of naive lymphocytes with their specific antigen.
Secondary immune response	The much stronger immune response which occurs upon the second encounter of primed lymphocytes with their specific antigen.
Toll-like receptors (TLRs)	A family of pattern recognition receptors involved in the detection of structures associated with pathogens or damaged host tissues.

The immune system has evolved to protect the body from foreign pathogens. It does so using quite a number of different cell types, most of which arise from pluripotent hematopoietic stem cells in the bone marrow and are collectively referred to as leukocytes (white blood cells). These stem cells can enter one of two differentiation pathways, the myeloid pathway which gives rise to monocytes/macrophages, dendritic cells, granulocytes (neutrophils, eosinophils, basophils, and mast cells), erythrocytes, and platelets, and the lymphoid pathway which gives rise to lymphocytes and natural killer (NK) cells (**Figure 1**). The bone marrow is referred to as a primary lymphoid organ and is where many of these cell types, including the B lymphocytes (B cells), reach maturity. However, the precursors of the T lymphocytes (T cells) need to leave the bone marrow and travel to the thymus in order to become fully developed. Given that a thymus is obligatory for the generation of T cells it is also referred to as a primary lymphoid organ. Upon maturation the lymphocytes, together with specialized antigen-presenting dendritic cells, primarily locate to secondary lymphoid organs (mucosa-associated lymphoid tissue (MALT), lymph nodes, and spleen) where the local architecture permits optimal stimulation of the immune response.

In order to become activated, the cells of the immune system need to detect the presence of a pathogen. Structures that can potentially be recognized by the immune system are broadly referred to as antigens and comprise an almost unlimited variety of protein, carbohydrate, lipid, and small molecular moieties. Antigenic structures are therefore associated not only with foreign organisms (viruses, bacteria, fungi, and parasites) and molecules (ingested, inhaled, or absorbed substances) but also the body's own (self) molecules and cells. Despite this capacity of the immune system to recognize an almost infinite variety of antigens, it must avoid making potentially damaging responses against self-antigens and against beneficial commensal organisms, food antigens, and so on. Thus, the cells of the immune system normally respond when they detect structures associated with pathogenic organisms.

Innate and Adaptive Immune Responses

Most cells of the immune system react with similar vigor however many times they encounter the same pathogen. This type of response is referred to as innate immunity (**Figure 2**) and involves phagocytic cells and

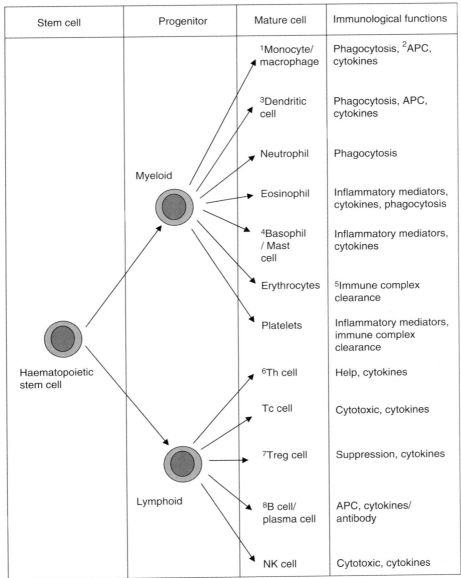

Stem cell	Progenitor	Mature cell	Immunological functions
		[1]Monocyte/ macrophage	Phagocytosis, [2]APC, cytokines
		[3]Dendritic cell	Phagocytosis, APC, cytokines
		Neutrophil	Phagocytosis
	Myeloid	Eosinophil	Inflammatory mediators, cytokines, phagocytosis
		[4]Basophil / Mast cell	Inflammatory mediators, cytokines
		Erythrocytes	[5]Immune complex clearance
		Platelets	Inflammatory mediators, immune complex clearance
Haematopoietic stem cell		[6]Th cell	Help, cytokines
		Tc cell	Cytotoxic, cytokines
	Lymphoid	[7]Treg cell	Suppression, cytokines
		[8]B cell/ plasma cell	APC, cytokines/ antibody
		NK cell	Cytotoxic, cytokines

Figure 1 The major players in the immune response derived from hematopoietic stem cells in the bone marrow. Myeloid and lymphoid progenitors differentiate into a number of different cell types that, upon activation, mediate various immunological functions (examples of which are indicated). [1]Monocytes in the blood have functions that generally become more pronounced when these cells enter the tissues and differentiate into macrophages. [2]APC, professional antigen-presenting cell that uses MHC class II molecules to present processed antigen to CD4 (usually helper) T cells. [3]Dendritic cells (DC) come in a variety of forms. In addition to the myeloid dendritic cells, lymphoid dendritic cells (not shown) arise from lymphoid progenitors and have similar immunological functions to those of myeloid DC. Note that DCs are the only cell type that can act as APCs for naive T cells (i.e., T cells that have not previously encountered an antigen). There is also an entirely separate population of cells with a dendritic morphology that are present in secondary lymphoid organs and are referred to as follicular dendritic cells (FDC). FDC are nonphagocytic and lack the MHC class II required of professional APC, but instead present nonprocessed antigen (held on their surface in the form of immune complexes) directly to B cells. [4]Blood basophils and tissue mast cells share functional properties but it is thought that they are independently derived rather than blood basophils giving rise to tissue mast cells. [5]Immune complexes are composed of antigen bound to antibody and also often including complement components. [6]Th cells assist other cells in the immune system partly by secreting immunostimulatory cytokines but also using cell-contact dependent mechanisms. [7]Treg cells are heterogeneous, some inhibit other cells in the immune system by secreting cytokines with immunosuppressive properties while others use cell-contact dependent mechanisms to suppress immune responses. [8]B cells can act as professional APCs for antigen-experienced Th cells, and when activated can themselves secrete cytokines. When B cells differentiate into plasma cells their role is to secrete large amounts of antibody.

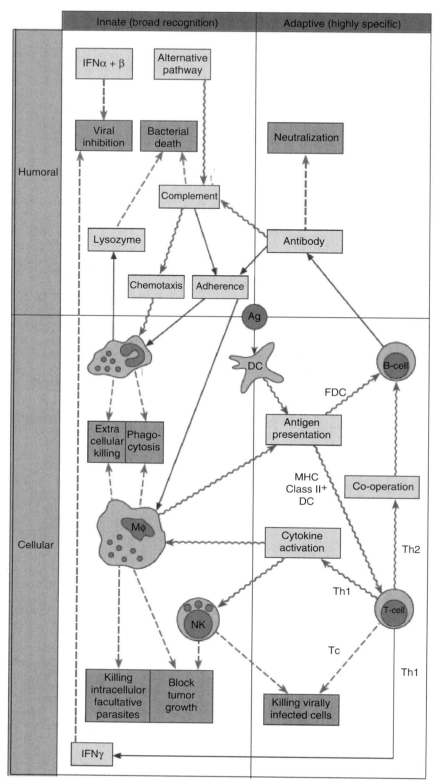

Figure 2   Some innate and adaptive immune responses. Humoral responses are those that are mediated by soluble molecules such as complement and cytokines in the innate response and antibody in the adaptive response. MHC class II⁺ dendritic cells act as professional APC to present processed antigen to T cells, while the entirely different follicular dendritic cells (FDC) can present native antigen to B cells. Ag, antigen; IFNγ, gamma interferon; Mφ, macrophage. Green wavy lines indicate processes that activate, whereas red dotted lines indicate processes that inhibit or kill. (Modified with permission from Delves PJ, Martin SJ, Burton, DR, and Roitt IM. (2006). *Roitt's essential immunology*, 11th edn. Oxford: Blackwell Publishers).

NK cells, as well as basophils and mast cells. The phagocytic cells comprise short-lived neutrophils present in both the circulation and in the tissues, blood monocytes which differentiate into the more actively phagocytic macrophage upon entering the tissues, and dendritic cells in the tissues. Eosinophils are also weakly phagocytic but they are more adept at killing organisms that are too large to be engulfed and onto which they release toxic molecules. Basophils in the blood, and the functionally related mast cell in the tissues, release inflammatory mediators such as histamine, prostaglandins, and leukotrienes. The NK cells, present in both the circulation and the tissues, kill infected or malignant cells. Thus, the innate immune response can call upon a number of fundamentally different cell types. In contrast, the adaptive (also referred to as acquired) immune response is mediated by lymphocytes. These cells are exquisitely specific for individual antigens and when they encounter 'their' antigen for the first time they mount a primary immune response that produces not only cells and molecules to deal with the threat at hand but also memory cells. The latter constitute a population of lymphocytes that are expanded in number and have the capacity to generate the qualitatively and quantitatively superior secondary immune response. Of the two main populations of lymphocytes, B lymphocytes (B cells) and T lymphocytes (T cells), it is the B cells that are responsible for producing antibody molecules. T cells can be divided into three main subpopulations. Helper T cells (Th) assist, and regulatory T cells (Treg) can suppress, other cells in the immune response. Cytotoxic T cells (Tc), also referred to as cytotoxic T lymphocytes (CTL), kill infected or foreign eukaryotic cells. Most Th and Treg express a molecule called CD4 on their cell surface, whereas most Tc express CD8 instead.

Recognition of Pathogens and Other Antigens

In order to mount an immune response the cells of the immune system need to detect the presence of a threat. They do this using cell surface receptors which can be grouped into two main types: broadly reactive receptors and antigen-specific receptors.

Broadly Reactive Receptors

The cells involved in innate immune responses have a large number of receptors which are each encoded by entirely separate genes and which recognize structures that are common to many different organisms. These types of receptors are referred to as pattern recognition receptors (PRR) and their ligands designated pathogen-associated molecular patterns (PAMPs). Recently PRRs have been found to also be present on the cells of the adaptive immune response (i.e., lymphocytes), and some PRRs have been shown to recognize certain endogenous (self) ligands as well as recognizing PAMPS. Although the receptors are highly specific for the structures they recognize, their ligands are molecules that are widely distributed amongst many different species of pathogen. Examples include the toll-like receptors (TLRs; such as TLR3 which recognizes viral double-stranded ribonucleic acid (RNA) and TLR5 which detects bacterial flagellin) and the mannose receptor. The latter binds to the terminal mannose structure characteristic of prokaryotes but which is always covered by other sugars in glycoproteins of eukaryotic origin.

Antigen-Specific Receptors

Lymphocytes possess highly antigen-specific receptors on their cell surface. The B-cell receptor for antigen is a transmembrane version of the antibody molecule, while the analogous receptor on T lymphocytes consists of an $\alpha\beta$ or $\gamma\delta$ T-cell receptor (TCR) heterodimer. These receptors contain variable regions which, as their name suggests, vary from one receptor to another and which confer antigen specificity. All the antigen receptors on an individual lymphocyte will possess the same variable region sequence, but those on a different lymphocyte will bear a different variable region and hence specificity for a different antigen. The receptors are generated by a unique gene recombination mechanism in which the nucleotide sequence encoding the variable region of the protein is constructed from more than one gene. Thus, one gene sequence is picked in a fairly random fashion from each of two (for immunoglobulin (Ig) light chains and for TCR α or γ chains) or three (for Ig heavy chains and for TCR β or δ chains) gene pools referred to as variable (V), diversity (D, if utilizing all three gene pools), and joining (J) gene segments and these sequences spliced next to each other (**Figure 3**). The Ig genes undergo recombination in the precursors of B lymphocytes while TCR genes undergo recombination in early T cells. In each lymphocyte a different recombination occurs and, together with a variety of additional molecular mechanisms which further increase diversity, leads to an almost infinite variety of antigen-specific receptors being generated. Therefore one lymphocyte will have antigen receptors that are specific for a particular component of streptococcus, another lymphocyte will be specific for an antigen from staphylococcus, another for a part of the influenza virus, and so on. There will only be a handful of lymphocytes specific for each antigen but collectively

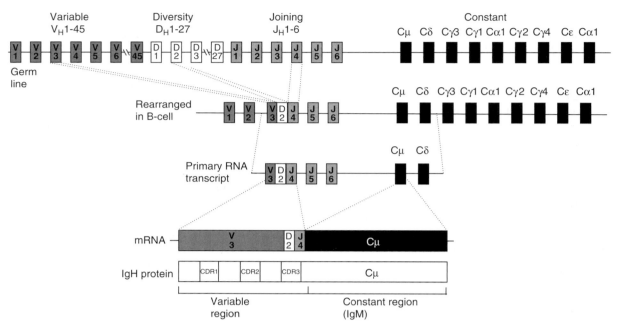

Figure 3 Antigen receptor gene recombination. In this example, immunoglobulin heavy chain (IgH) gene recombination is illustrated, but immunoglobulin light chain genes and the TCR genes undergo similar recombination processes in order to create a large number of different variable region sequences from a relatively small gene pool. Here the B cell has recombined the V3, D2, and J4 immunoglobulin heavy chain gene segments (not drawn to scale) and is utilizing the $C\mu$ constant region gene segment from a primary RNA transcript that also includes $C\delta$. Alternative splicing of the primary RNA transcript is used to also produce IgD with the same antigen specificity. A different B cell might recombine V42, D16, and J6, etc., and would therefore have a different heavy chain variable region sequence. Recombination to provide variability for the immunoglobulin light chain variable region (not shown) is brought about by similar mechanisms using separate gene loci containing only V, J, and C segments. The heavy chain constant region gene transcription can include transmembrane exons. The heavy and light chain proteins polymerize into the 4 chain (2H + 2L) immunoglobulin molecule, which then sits in the cell surface membrane to function as the antigen-specific B-cell receptor. In plasma cells the transmembrane exons are not utilized and a secreted version of the antibody, with identical antigen-specificity, is produced. In the case of IgM the antibody polymerizes into pentamers prior to secretion. Class switching occurs later in the immune response with $C\mu$ and $C\delta$ usage being replaced with, for example, $C\gamma1$ which specifies the IgG1 subclass of antibody but utilizing the same variable region and thus with the same antigen specificity. The areas of the variable region in both the heavy and the light chain which make contact with the antigen are referred to as complementarity determining regions (CDR).

all the lymphocytes will provide cover against virtually all antigens that might be encountered.

Generation of the Immune Response

Innate responses are initiated when the PRRs on the surface of phagocytic and other cells detect the presence of PAMPs. Additionally, foreign antigens will very often become coated with proteins that are generated by the complement system, a cascade of molecules activated during immune responses. Later on in the immune response the antigen will additionally be coated with antibody. Among the many different types of molecules on the surface membrane of immune system cells are receptors for complement molecules and for the nonantigen-binding end (Fc) of the antibody molecule. Microorganisms coated with antibody and/or complement are said to be opsonized for phagocytosis, the antibody and complement linking the organism to the phagocyte. Complement carries out other functions; it acts

as a chemotactic factor for phagocytes, it stimulates the release of inflammatory mediators from mast cells, and can mediate lysis of certain strains of bacteria.

The response of lymphocytes to an encounter with an antigen is somewhat different to that of the cells of the innate immune response. Whereas the latter go straight ahead with the task required, be it phagocytosis or the release of inflammatory mediators, the lymphocyte undergoes rapid cell division. The clone of lymphocytes with the appropriate antigen-specific receptor thus become greatly amplified in number during the adaptive immune response. T cells (at least the main population of T cells which bear an $\alpha\beta$ TCR) cannot recognize antigens directly, but instead see antigen that has been processed and presented. With respect to Th cells which have not previously encountered their specific antigen, i.e., naive T cells, this involves dendritic cells which phagocytose or endocytose antigen, then demolish its protein components using proteases which generate short peptides of around 15 amino acids in length within the endosomal compartment of the cell. While still inside the endosomes these antigenic peptide fragments are combined with major histocompatibility complex (MHC) molecules of the class II type, and the complex of antigen peptide plus MHC class II is transported to the cell surface of the dendritic cell. It is the combination of peptide–MHC that is recognized by the TCR on the T cell, with the dendritic cell also expressing other cell-surface molecules such as CD80 and CD86 which supply the potent co-stimulation obligatory for the activation of naive T cells. Both macrophages and B cells also express peptide-bearing MHC class II molecules on their cell surface but due to their less profound ability to provide high levels of co-stimulation they only activate antigen-experienced T cells. Dendritic cells, macrophages, and B cells are collectively referred to as professional antigen-presenting cells (APC), a euphemism for cells which present antigen to CD4 T cells using MHC class II molecules. However, virtually all cells in the body are able to present peptide antigens using MHC class I molecules. In this case the peptides are usually generated from antigens present within the cytosol of a cell, including foreign antigens such as viruses. Cytosolic proteolysis for subsequent antigen presentation utilizes a modified version of the proteasome enzyme complex that carries out the normal cellular degradative processes. Peptide–MHC class I complexes expressed on the surface of infected cells are recognized by CD8+ Tc cells. Thus CD4+ T cells use their αβ TCR to recognize peptides presented by MHC class II molecules on professional APC whereas CD8+ T cells use their αβ TCR to recognize peptides presented by MHC class I molecules on infected cells.

The MHC is given a different name in different species, in humans it is referred to as human leukocyte antigen (HLA; although present not only on leukocytes) while in mice it is called H-2. In humans there are three main MHC class I gene loci, HLA-A, HLA-B, and HLA-C, and three class II loci, HLA-DP, HLA-DQ, and HLA-DR. In mice the main class I loci are H-2K and H-2D while the class II loci are referred to as I-A and I-E. The MHC molecules are encoded by the most polymorphic of all of the genes in the genome, and thus can vary enormously from individual to individual. It is this MHC polymorphism that is largely responsible for the immune system recognizing and subsequently rejecting organs or tissues from other members of the same species (allografts). The MHC genes are co-dominantly expressed and therefore each individual expresses two polymorphic variants of HLA-A, two of HLA-B, and so on. Certain variants are more common in the population than others and with common variants such as HLA-A2

in Caucasians it is quite frequently the case that an individual will be homozygous at that particular genetic locus.

The Anatomy of the Immune Response

The cells of the innate response such as phagocytic cells can act individually at the site of an infection. They are attracted to such sites by chemotactic factors, and their passage from the circulation out into the tissues is facilitated by the upregulated expression of adhesion molecules on vascular endothelial cells, ligands for which are expressed on the leukocyte cell surface.

As discussed previously, the Th cells of the adaptive response need to interact with professional APC in order to be activated. This requires cell–cell contact as the TCR on the T cell must bind to the peptide–MHC on the APC. The Th cells are also required to be in close proximity with the cells that will receive their help, which is provided by a combination of soluble molecules such as cytokines and by interactions between cell surface molecules on the Th cell and on the cell being helped. There are different subsets of cytokine-producing Th cells (e.g., Th1 cells, Th2 cells) and depending upon which subset is involved, the cytokine-mediated help that is given may facilitate antibody production by B cells, activation of Tc to kill infected cells, or enhancement of macrophage function (**Figure 2**). Given that Th, Tc, and B cells are all antigen-specific, that there are only a handful of cells specific for a given antigen, and that T cells require antigen to be presented to them, there is a need for a meeting place where the relevant cells can get together. This is the role of the secondary lymphoid organs; the spleen, lymph nodes, and MALT. These are the locations in which adaptive immune responses are initiated. Because the majority of pathogens will enter the body by ingestion or inhalation the MALT collectively provides a critical first line of defense against infection and acts as a major effector site for protective immune responses.

Protective Immune Response

The immune response is aimed at destroying foreign pathogens. Engulfment of microorganisms by phagocytes leads to their elimination when a wide variety of microbicidal compounds including toxic metabolites of oxygen such as hydroxyl radicals and enzymes such as lysozyme kill the invader. Eosinophils release toxins to achieve extracellular killing. Mast cells and basophils produce a plethora of molecules which collectively facilitate an acute inflammatory response with recruitment of leukocytes to the site of the infection. Infected cells, and some tumor cells, are dealt with by Tc and NK cells which can both induce apoptotic cell death in the target cell. Many cells in the body are capable of releasing cytokines but Th cells are particularly adept at doing so. In addition to providing help for other cells in the immune system, some cytokines can be directly cytotoxic (e.g., tumor necrosis factor (TNF)). B cells produce antibody molecules which are collectively found in their secreted form at high levels (10–15 mg ml^{-1}) in the circulation and, with the exception of the physically large pentameric IgM, also readily diffuse into the tissues. Antibodies are able to directly neutralize bacterial toxins, prevent viruses binding to cells, agglutinate microorganisms and thereby immobilize them, activate complement, opsonize microorganisms for phagocytosis, and mediate antibody-dependent cellular cytotoxicity (ADCC) in which leukocytes of various types become linked by antibody to infected cells and then kill them.

Avoidance of Harmful Immune Responses

The immune system can potentially react against the body's own components, resulting in immunity to self (autoimmunity). This only becomes a problem if the autoimmune reactions cause pathology, in which case the individual develops an autoimmune disease. Approximately 3–5% of individuals develop autoimmune disease at some time in their life. There are an extremely large number of different diseases in which autoimmune responses are thought to play a role, with the most common including psoriasis, thyroid autoimmune diseases (primarily Hashimoto's thyroiditis and Graves' disease), rheumatoid arthritis, vitiligo, systemic lupus erythematosus, Sjögren's syndrome, celiac disease, Crohn's disease, pernicious anemia, ankylosing spondylitis, type I (insulin-dependent) diabetes, and multiple sclerosis. The fact that the vast majority of individuals do not develop pathogenic autoimmune responses is due to the phenomenon of immunological tolerance. Encounter with self-antigen early on in the development of a lymphocyte leads to its clonal deletion by apoptosis. This occurs in the thymus for T cells and in the bone marrow for B cells. The T cells undergo thymic education involving positive and negative selection events in the thymus. Cells are positively selected if the random rearrangement of their TCR genes generates a receptor capable of recognizing peptides presented by that individual's polymorphic variants of MHC (self-MHC). However, if the TCR recognizes peptides derived from self antigens then a subsequent negative selection step will induce apoptosis of the autoimmune T cell. Thus, the only T cells which leave

the thymus are ones that recognize foreign peptides presented by self-MHC. A somewhat similar process of negative selection occurs for B cells in the bone marrow, although their antigen receptor (the antibody molecule) recognizes antigen directly and therefore there is no requirement for positive selection for recognition of self-MHC molecules. The clonal deletion of T and B cells is not foolproof and some of the cells that leave the primary lymphoid organs are self-reactive. Therefore there are backup mechanisms to prevent harmful autoimmunity arising. Pathogenic foreign antigens are normally seen in the context of co-stimulatory activity whereas self-antigens do not provide co-stimulatory signals. When the lymphocyte receives a signal only through its antigen receptor in the absence of co-stimulation the result is not cell activation but rather cell inactivation, a process referred to as anergy. Unlike clonal deletion where the cell is eliminated, this leaves anergic cells which potentially can be re-activated. A further level of control rests with Treg cells that act to suppress any potentially harmful self-reactive cells. There are a number of different types of Treg cells, some of which arise naturally in the thymus and exert their effect via poorly understood cell contact-dependent mechanisms. Other Treg cells are induced to secrete cytokines that can mediate immunosuppressive activity, such as interleukin (IL)-10 and transforming-growth factor-β (TGFβ).

While the avoidance of harmful immune responses to self-antigens is something that operates with a fair degree of success, the capacity of the body to prevent allergic responses to what should be innocuous foreign antigens would appear to be rather less effective. A substantial minority of individuals (estimates vary, but perhaps even as many as 45% of children and 30% of adults) suffer from allergies to varying degrees. This frequently involves atopy, a capacity to produce raised levels of the IgE class of antibody against the allergen. The class of antibody is of paramount importance here because the IgE becomes bound to the surface of mast cells and basophils by virtue of the fact that these cells possess high-affinity receptors for the Fc region of IgE (FcεR). If the IgE has specificity for environmental antigens (allergens) these cross-link the IgE molecules. As a consequence, cross-linking of the FcεRs occurs leading to degranulation of the cells with the release of inflammatory mediators such as histamine.

Neuroendocrine–Immune Interactions

Although immune responses are driven by encounter with antigen and subject to regulation by a variety of cells and molecules which are clearly components of the immune system, it is also known that factors such as nutrition, hormones, and neuropeptides can modify the immune response. Stressors such as exam anxiety, restraint, and noise are known to influence various immune functions including lymphocyte proliferation, IgA secretion, phagocytosis, and the activity of NK cells. Receptors for endorphins, enkaphalins, acetylcholine, β-adrenoceptor agents, corticosteroids, insulin, growth hormone, estradiol, testosterone, and prolactin have all been described on various types of immune cell and their expression presumably infers some functional significance. To give an example, the cytokines IL-1, IL-6, and TNF act via the hypothalamic-pituitary-adrenal (HPA) axis to stimulate the release of glucocorticoids which are then capable of downregulating the activity of both Th1 cells and macrophages. Androgens and glucocorticoids generally suppress, while growth hormone, thyroxine, and insulin generally stimulate, immune responses. Lymphoid tissues, including the thymus, spleen, and lymph nodes, are richly innervated by norepinephrine-releasing sympathetic neurons. There is evidence from studies in knockout mice that in the absence of this neurotransmitter there is impaired production of the Th1-derived cytokines interferon (IFN)γ and TNF in response to challenge with antigen. Dendritic cells bear β-adrenoceptors and it has also been suggested that sympathetic nerves may be involved in controlling the migration of these APCs from the sites of inflammation to the local draining lymph nodes.

See Also the Following Articles

Apoptosis; Cytokines; Cytotoxic Lymphocytes; Glucocorticoids, Overview; Immune Cell Distribution, Effects of Stress on; Immune Function, Stress-Induced Enhancement; Immune Suppression; Immune System, Aging; Immunity; Infection; Lymph Nodes; Leukocyte Trafficking and Stress; Lymphocytes; Macrophages; Natural Killer (NK) Cells; Neuroendocrine Systems; Neuroimmunomodulation; Primate Models, Behavioral-Immunological Interactions; Prostaglandins; Serotonin; Thymus; Vasoactive Peptides; Inflammation; Organ Transplantation, Stress of; Vaccination.

Further Reading

Abbas, A. K. and Lichtman, A. H. (2006). *Basic immunology: functions and disorders of the immune system* (2nd edn.). Philadelphia, PA: Saunders.

Ader, R. (ed.) (2006). *Psychoneuroimmunology* (4th edn.). San Diego: Academic Press.

Daruna, J. H. (2004). *Introduction to psychoneuroimmunology*. San Diego: Academic Press.

Delves, P. J., Martin, S. J., Burton, D. R., et al. (2006). *Essential immunology* (11th edn.). Oxford: Blackwell Science.

Delves, P. J. (2006). Biology of the immune system. In: Beers, M. H., Porter, R. S., Jones, T. V., et al. (eds.) *The Merck manual* (18th edn, pp. 1320–1331). Whitehouse Station, NJ, USA: Merck.

Goldsby, R. A., Kindt, T. J., Osborne, B. A., et al. (2003). *Immunology* (5th edn.). New York: WH Freeman.

Padgett, D. A. and Glaser, R. (2003). How stress influences the immune response. *Trends in Immunology* **24**, 444–448.

Reiche, E. M., Nunes, S. O. and Morimoto, H. K. (2004). Stress, depression, the immune system, and cancer. *Lancet Oncology* **5**, 617–625.

Rhen, T. and Cidlowski, J. A. (2005). Mechanisms of disease: antiinflammatory action of glucocorticoids – new mechanisms for old drugs. *New England Journal of Medicine* **353**, 1711–1723.

Shepherd, A. J., Downing, J. E. and Miyan, J. A. (2005). Without nerves, immunology remains incomplete – *in vivo* veritas. *Immunology* **116**, 145–163.

Sternberg, E. M. (2006). Neural regulation of innate immunity: a coordinated nonspecific host response to pathogens. *Nature Reviews Immunology* **6**, 318–328.

Vedhara, K. and Irwin, M. (2005). *Human psychoneuroimmunology*. Oxford: Oxford University Press.

Immune Suppression

P Prolo and F Chiappelli
UCLA School of Dentistry, Los Angeles, CA, USA

This article is a revision of the previous edition article by F Chiappelli and D Hodgson, volume 2, pp 531–535, © 2000, Elsevier Inc.

Allostasis

Type I and Type II Allostatic Responses

The Allostatic Modulation of Immune Suppression

T Cell Anergy and Apoptosis

A New Strategy: Molecular Cartography

Glossary

Allostasis	Psychobiological process that brings about stability through change of state consequential to stress. The allostatic response encompasses a range of psychobiological outcomes that reflect physiologically important changes in the balance between the psychoneuroendocrine and the immune systems. Allostasis overload leads to statistically significant and clinically relevant damage to the organism due to excessive energy expenditure in the response to stress.
Anergy	A state of immune unresponsiveness, induced as soon as the antigen receptor of the T cell is stimulated, which stops T cell responses waiting for second signal from the antigen-presenting cell.
Apoptosis	The process of programed cell death needed to eliminate cells that represent a threat to the integrity of the organism.
Circadian	A term derived from the Latin *circa diem* meaning about a day, refers to biological rhythms that have a cycle of about 24 hours.
Molecular cartography	The science of recognizing and identifying multifaceted and intricate array of gene interaction and gene products that characterize the function of each individual cell in the context of cell–cell interaction, tissue, and organ function.

The renowned XIX century French physiologist, Claude Bernard (1813–78) first proposed that defense of the internal milieu (*le milieu intérieur*, 1856) is fundamental to physiological regulation, from when the phrase homeostasis originated. Walter Cannon (1871–1945) proposed that organisms engage in a dynamic process of adjustment of the physiological balance of the internal milieu in response to changing environmental conditions. Hans Selye (1907–82) established the cardinal points of the generalized stress response in his demonstration of concerted physiological responses to stressful challenges.

The immune response is finely regulated at the molecular, cellular, and physiological levels. Bacteriokines (i.e., bacterial cytokine inducers), produced by infectious pathogens, contribute to the control of the pathological inflammatory response. This article focuses on the homeostasis of the immune response from the perspective of the psychoneuroendocrine and cellular events that contribute to the suppression of immunity in response to stressors.

Allostasis

Allostasis refers to the psychobiological process that brings about stability through change of state consequential to stress. Psychoemotional stress can be defined as a perceived lack of fit of one's perceived abilities and the demands of the environment (i.e., person/environment fit). The perception of stress leads to anxiety, irritability and anger, tension, depressed moods, fatigue, a compendium of symptoms referred to as the sickness behavior (e.g., lethargy, nausea, and fever), and to a set of other bodily manifestations, including perspiration, blushing or blanching of the face, increased heart rate or decreased blood pressure, and intestinal cramps and discomfort, and suppressed immune resistance to antigenic challenges.

Sterling and Eyer (1988) defined allostasis as the set of mind–body systemic events aimed at regulating the recovery from stress. Heterostasis came to describe the situation where the demands upon the organism exceed its physiological capacity.

The process of allostatic regulation signifies the recovery and maintenance of internal balance and viability amidst changing circumstances consequential to stress. It encompasses a range of behavioral and physiological functions that direct the adaptive function of regulating homeostatic systems in response to challenges. The allostatic load refers to the set of physiological, psychological, and pathological side effects of the allostatic process, whereas allostatic overload signifies psychobiological collapse, and is associated with a variety of health outcomes systemically.

Type I and Type II Allostatic Responses

The allostatic response encompasses a range of psychobiological outcomes that reflect changes in the balance between the psychoneuroendocrine and the immune systems. Allostasis overload leads to statistically significant and clinically relevant damage to the organism due to excessive energy expenditure in the response to stress.

Type I

Type I allostasis utilizes stress responses as a mean of self-preservation by means of developing and establishing temporary or permanent adaptation skills. The organism aims at surviving the perturbation in the best condition possible, and at normalizing the normal lifecycle. An example of Type I allostatic response is recurrent aphthous stomatitis (RAS, canker sores), a stress-associated T cell-dependent pathology of the gingival mucosa. RAS lesions are characterized with increased Th1 patterns of cytokine *in situ* (e.g., interleukin (IL)-2). Ongoing work confirms a statistically significant correlation between the clinical incidence of RAS, based on stringent clinical and diagnostic criteria, and scores on a version of the short form-36 health survey questionnaire (SF-36) adapted for dentistry.

Other examples of Type I allostatic response manifested in the oral cavity include teeth grinding: tooth pain that cannot be attributed to carries, cracked tooth syndrome, pulpitis or other circumdental inflammatory process (e.g., gum disease), temporomandibular disorder and pain, and pain at palpation of the masticatory muscles, altered dental anatomy at the coronal surfaces. When the subjects are followed up prospectively, changes in vertical distance of occlusion and the angle of Spee that refers to the curved line that follows the occlusal surface of the posterior teeth of the mandible and is viewed from a sagittal plane are also noted.

Examples of systemic Type I allostatic response include the physiological responses to electromagnetic field. In a paired double-blind study, healthy young adults were exposed to electromagnetic field during controlled sleep. A sharp reduction in secreted melatonin was observed, which was transient and not correlated with any alterations of note in immune responses. The observed twofold increase in IL-2 serum levels failed to alter significantly natural killer cell activity.

Type II

In Type II allostatic load, the stressful challenge is excessive, sustained, or continued, and drives allostasis chronically. An escape response cannot be found. The psychobiological and pathological responses to stress become chronic (e.g., depression, anxiety, hypercortisolemia, and glucocorticoid resistance), with consequential erosion in health and immune surveillance mechanisms.

Oral Lichen Planus

Lichen planus of the oral mucosa (oral lichen planus; OLP) is one example of a Type II allostatic response with evident manifestations of immune suppression in the oral cavity. This form of oral lichenoid lymphocytic mucosal inflammation involves basal cell lysis, and lymphocyte transmigration into the epithelial compartment, and brings about a statistically significant increase in incidence of oral squamous cell carcinoma, which implicates OLP as a premalignant lesion. This chronic inflammatory disorder afflicts 2–3% of the population, and may be in part attributed to aging-associated decrease in the subject's ability to recover from the psychoneuroendocrine-immune changes consequential to stress since OLP is prevalent in individual over 50 years of age. Men are at risk at an earlier age than women (40–49 years with men versus 50–59 years with women). OLP lesions are exacerbated with nonsteroidal anti-inflammatory drugs, antirheumatic drugs, angiotensin-converting enzyme inhibitors, antihypertensive drugs, antibiotics, or β-blockers. These pharmacologic treatments share the commonality of suppressing one or another arm of cellular immunity, suggesting a pathological parallel between OLP lesions and mucositis. The nervous system may play an important role *in vivo* in regulating cellular immune responses in OLP lesions, as suggested by the suggestive alignment of autonomic innervation with lymphocytes (**Figure 1**). Immune suppression is modulated by sympathetic innervation, and by the cholinergic anti-inflammatory pathway, which inhibits proinflammatory cytokine production and secretion. The relationship between OLP and immune suppression is confirmed by the observation that it appears to result from an abnormal immune response to an unidentified causative agent. Over 75% of invading T cells express the memory phenotype (CD45RO+), the β1 integrin, CD29+, which renders them essentially sessile. A large proportion of the invading cells also appear phenotypically to be activated Treg (CD25+CD69+). Altered antigenicity of cell-surface epithelial cells causes them to be recognized as immunogenic, in a manner akin to an autoimmune disorder. Human hepatitis C virus (HCV) seems to be a predisposing factor for OLP, and comorbidity of HCV infection with OLP is noted in association with the HLA-Dr6 allele. The genetic propensity for OLP is emphasized by the observation that expression of HLA-Bw57 favors OLP, whereas HLA-Dql expression provides resistance against it.

Chronic Pain

A systemic example of Type II allostasis is chronic pain. Patients with fibromyalgia demonstrate altered

Control section   OLP section

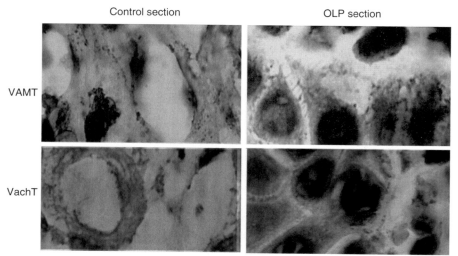

Figure 1 Double-label immunohistochemical staining of erosive OLP lesions with CD3 for T cells, and vesicles of acetylcholine transport (VachT; lower panels) and vesicles for monoamine transport (VAMT; upper panels) for autonomic innervation (magnification ×100, oil immersion).

function of β-adrenoceptors. Activation of G-protein coupled receptors, such as the adrenoceptors, leads to an increase in the intracellular level of cAMP. Levels of cAMP serve to assess, albeit indirectly, the functional state of these receptors in immune cells. Patients with fibromyalgia were compared to sex- and age-matched control subjects, and basal and stimulated intracellular cAMP levels were measured, using the β-agonist, isoproterenol (10^{-3} M–10^{-5} M, following a 5 min preincubation). Basal cAMP levels were shown to be elevated in patients with fibromyalgia (3.02 ± 0.44 pmol/10^6 cells, P = 0.124), compared to control subjects (2.26 ± 0.39 pmol/10^6 cells). Stimulation with isoproterenol at 10^{-3} M significantly increased intracellular cAMP in both groups; but isoproterenol at 10^{-5} M failed to produce this outcome in the patient group (P = 0.74), compared to the stimulation by isoproterenol obtained in the control group (P = 0.012). Taken together, these data show that patients with fibromyalgia harbor diminished adrenoceptor function in circulating immune cells.

Mucositis

Another example of Type 2 allostasis may be the clinical condition of mucositis. Oropharyngeal mucositis is a common and treatment-limiting side effect of cancer therapy. Oral and gastrointestinal mucositis can affect up to 100% of patients undergoing high-dose chemotherapy and hematopoietic stem cell transplantation, 80% of patients with malignancies of the head and neck receiving radiotherapy, and over 50% of patients receiving chemotherapy. Oral mucositis can be so severe as to lead to the need to

interrupt or discontinue the therapy protocol, and to hinder cure of the primary disease. Mucositis leads to immune suppression, and to an increased risk of local and systemic infection, opportunistic infections, and mortality due to sepsis. It is a critical condition since in 2004 alone, close to 1.5 million Americans were diagnosed with cancer and received some combination therapies for this disease, including surgery, radiation, chemotherapy, immunotherapy, and/or cell transplantation, and mucositis is the principal oral complication from cancer therapies.

The Allostatic Modulation of Immune Suppression

One important regulatory mechanism in allostasis is the interactive neuroendocrine-immune loop. Stress alters the regulation of both the sympathetic and the parasympathetic branches of the autonomic nervous system, and modulates immune suppression. Autonomic activation, and the elevation of hormones, including those produced by the hypothalamic-pituitary-adrenal axis, play a pivotal role in regulating cell-mediated immune surveillance mechanisms, including the production of cytokines that control inflammatory and healing events.

The experience of stress and of traumatic events leads to the release of glucocorticoids, which regulate cellular immune activity *in vivo* systemically and locally: they block the production of proinflammatory cytokines (e.g., IL-1β, IL-6) and of Th1 cytokines (e.g., IL-2) at the molecular level *in vitro* and *in vivo*, but have little effects upon Th2 cytokines (e.g., IL-4). The activity of the proinflammatory cytokine IL-1β is blocked by IL-1 receptor antagonists (IL-1Ra, sIL-1RII) in combination with the soluble IL-1 accessory protein (IL-1R AcP). This results in a long-term beneficial effect in chronic inflammatory diseases. The net effect of challenging immune cells with glucocorticoids is to suppress immune T cell activation and proliferation, while maintaining antibody production. The secretion of glucocorticoids by the adrenal cortex is under the control of the anterior pituitary adrenocorticotropin hormone (ACTH). Immune challenges release proinflammatory cytokines (e.g., IL-1β, IL-6), which induce hypothalamic secretion of the ACTH inducing corticotropin releasing hormone (CRH). It follows that the consequences of stress are not uniform. The immune-physiological impact of stress may be significantly greater in certain people, compared to others. The impact of stress is dynamic and multifaceted, and the same person may exhibit a variety of manifestations of immune suppression in response to stress with varying degrees of severity at different times. The outcome of stress can be multivalent, and individuals may position themselves along a spectrum of allostatic regulation, somewhere between Type I and Type II allostasis.

Several experimental protocols have been characterized for testing allostasis in animal and human research. Human subjects under stress (e.g., caregivers of elderly patients with dementia and spouses of military personnel in active combat duty) can be subjected to cognitive, sensory, or physiological challenges aimed at studying the allostatic process of immune-physiological adaptation to the challenge in addition to basal states of the stress response.

The Stroop Test

The Stroop color-word interference test is an example of a cognitive challenge that was originally developed in 1935 to examine patterns of cognitive decline. The Stroop challenge is measured as reaction time, and is high in patients with mild to moderate aging-related dementia of the Alzheimer's type (DAT). Patients with more severe dementia show less Stroop interference effect, when the reaction time is adjusted for color naming performance. These observations confirm the need and the importance of partitioning out underlying deficits for the understanding of complex cognitive processes in aging. Principal-components analyses show that disruption of semantic knowledge and speeded verbal processing in certain patients (e.g., patients with neuro-AIDS, patients with DAT) is a major contributor to the incongruent trial. The Stoop challenge is an effective modality for testing the glucocorticoids-cytokine response in healthy young men and women. Two groups of responders can be distinguished based on salivary and plasma glucocorticoids response to the challenge. The bottom 40% of the responders for cortisol responses to the challenge characteristically manifested significantly higher salivary and plasma levels of IL-6, but lower subjective experience of stress, compared to the high-glucocorticoids responders (top 40 percentile). This confirms that individual variations exist in the response of the glucocorticoids-cytokine axis to mild stress, and that these variations can have potentially adverse health outcomes.

An ongoing study is comparing patients with major depression (Diagnostic and Statistical Manuel of Mental Disorders, 4th edition (DSM-IV) criteria) with age-, sex-, and ethnicity-matched control subjects for the response on the Stroop test. Preliminary data indicate that the median Raw Color-Word score is 20% higher in the control, compared to the depressed subjects. The median predicted interference score based on Color-Word scores is indistinguishable among healthy and depressed subjects. These data confirm the literature in the substantial differences in percentile position of the median T scores: 66% percentile (depressed patients) versus 42% percentile (healthy control subjects). An important caveat of the Stroop challenge is that color confusion can be inconsistent in certain subgroups of subjects, especially as subjects advanced in age. The Stroop test should not to be used for clinical diagnostic purposes, but rather limited as an experimental tool.

The Cold Pressor Test

Another widely used stress paradigm for testing allostasis in human subjects is the cold pressor challenge. The physiological mechanism underlying the response to this challenge, which consists in the immersion of the nondominant hand in an ice bath, involves a response temperature as constriction to blood flow of both superficial and deep tissues of the hand, and associated strong perception of pain. This challenge test is an adequate model to study psychobiological responses to stressful discomfort because cold-induced vasospasms are frequently present in syndromes of chronic pain, but it may have adverse effects in subjects with cardiovascular dysfunctions. Pain latency (e.g., length of time of hand immersion) is significantly shorter in certain populations of patients, such as patients with fibromyalgia and secondary concomitant fibromyalgia, compared to healthy control subjects.

This challenge alters the glucocorticoids-cytokine axis responsivity in healthy young adult men and women, and leads to time-dependent patterns of change in the circadian patterns of salivary IL-6.

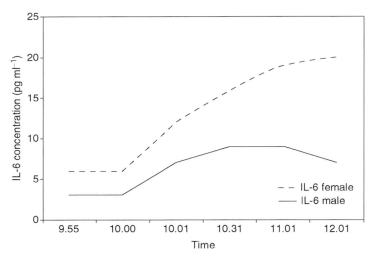

Figure 2 Salivary IL-6 response after cold pressor test applied at 10.00 a.m. on healthy volunteers. IL-6 response to stress was more pronounced in female (dashed line) compared to male subjects (solid line) ($P < 0.05$).

The cold pressor test significantly alters salivary IL-6 in control subjects. IL-6 levels were measured at times $t = -5$ min, $t = 0$ min (baseline levels), and $t = 1$, 31, 61, and 91 min postchallenge. Salivary IL-6 rose two- to threefold during the 90 min after cold pressor test. This effect was more pronounced in female compared to male subjects ($P < 0.05$; **Figure 2**).

The Dexamethasone-Suppression Test

The dexamethasone-suppression test (DST) is a widely used physiological challenge to study the functional response of the glucocorticoids-cytokine axis. Administration of 1–5 mg of dexamethasone (DEX) to healthy subjects in the evening (23.00 h) results in a flattened cortisol plasma level the following morning and day. The cortisol suppression response is an indication of DEX-sensitivity and normal hypothalamic-pituitary-adrenocortical (HPA) response. Significant changes in the migratory properties of circulating CD4+ T cells occur in DEX-sensitive control subjects. The use of the DST challenge is in monitoring the glucocorticoids-cytokine response in a variety of patient populations. In DEX-resistant (i.e., no cortisol suppression following DST) subjects, the migratory properties of circulating CD4+ T cells are not altered. An intimate relationship is evident between the physiological regulation of the neuroendocrine and cellular immune systems *in vivo* in healthy subjects, compared to patient populations. Stress states can lead to enhanced suppression of cortisol by DEX following the DST challenge, although discrepancies exist among reports. Neither low basal cortisol nor enhanced suppression of cortisol are consistent markers of a posttraumatic stress disorder, for instance, major depression, or DAT. The lack of reliability, validity, and specificity of the DST as a diagnostic instrument, however, has not reduced the usefulness of this challenge modality to better understand neuroendocrine-immune interactions and the physiological regulation of immune suppression. Another caveat of this paradigm is that it provides a static challenge to the neuroendocrine-immune system: it leads to a shut-off, albeit temporarily, of glucocorticoids flux by acting on its feedback system. In that respect it presents a reflection of the regulatory response, rather than of the glucocorticoid-cytokine axis potential *per se*, as, for example the CRH stimulation test does. Therefore, the DST challenge is a static challenge of glucocorticoids-cytokine responses.

Alcohol and Substance Abuse

Subjects who abuse alcohol or other substances (e.g., cocaine) characteristically exhibit a deregulated pituitary-adrenal axis, elevated cortisol levels, a blunted T cell activation, and consequential immune suppression. Associated is a deregulated distribution of CD4+CD62L+ cells, which upon withdrawal of alcohol or cocaine abuse, normalizes together with plasma cortisol. Indeed, nicotine and ethanol, at concentrations approximating those found in the plasma of smokers and alcohol abusers, decrease immune surveillance of oral carcinoma by interfering with immune cell-mediated clearance of the tumor target. Significant ($P < 0.05$) diminution of migration, binding, activation, and cytotoxic activity by nicotine when coupled with ethanol contributes to the observed immune suppression.

Experimental Findings

Circulating memory CD4+CD45R0+ cells in patients with OLP comprise 66% of the circulating leukocyte population, compared to 49% in healthy control subjects, suggesting an imbalance between naïve and memory T cells. Moreover, serum levels of tumor necrosis factor (TNF)-α and IL-6 are significantly elevated in patients with OLP. These patients also exhibit significant alterations in pituitary-adrenal/cellular immune regulation, as do close to 50% of patients with DAT. In these patients, whole saliva can be used for the reliable assessment of neuroendocrine products and cytokines.

Serum, saliva, and cervicular fluid samples were collected for the determination of IL-6 in healthy age-matched control subjects, in patients with DAT, and in their caregivers. Subjects were assessed by a multidimensional evaluation that included collection of demographic data, cognitive function, level of impairment, and assessment of mood states by means of the profile of moods states. Mean IL-6 levels in both plasma and saliva were higher in the group of patients with DAT, compared to the caregiver and control subjects. Crevicular fluid determinations were unreliable due to the small volume collected. Saliva and plasma IL-6 levels were well correlated. Profiles of moods states scores were significantly higher in the caregiver group (54.80 ± 65.45; -16–166), compared to the patient group with DAT (39.6 ± 50.5; 6–129), and the control subjects (9.4 ± 12.1; -26–2) (Wilcoxon, $P < 0.05$). Caregivers showed lower emotional well-being and more emotional stress than patients and healthy noncaregiver controls.

T Cell Anergy and Apoptosis

T cell activation can lead to the proliferative response. Alternative pathways can attenuate or prevent the response of T cells, and lead to anergy (i.e., absence of response) or apoptosis (i.e., spontaneous programed cell death), and consequential immune suppression.

T cell stimulation by triggering through the T cell receptor (TcR) in the absence of CD28-mediated costimulatory signals induces unresponsiveness to further stimulation in T cells, a phenomenon known as anergy. Anergic T cells do not produce IL-2 when challenged, and are defective in their ability to upregulate protein binding and transactivation at two critical IL-2 DNA enhancer elements: NF-AT (nuclear factor of activated T cells; a sequence that binds a heterotrimeric NFATp, fos, and jun protein complex), activator protein-1 (AP-1; that binds fos and jun heterodimers), the Janus tyrosine kinases (Jak), and the signal transducers and activators of transcription (Stat) act as key regulatory components. The impaired DNA-protein interactions in anergic T cells is related to poor expression of the inducible AP-1 family members c-fos, fosB, and junB, attributable, at least in part, to a selective block in the expression of the AP-1 Fos and Jun family members in anergic T cells. Ligation of CD28 results in its phosphorylation and subsequent recruitment and activation of phosphatidylinositol (PI)3-kinase. Pharmacological and mutational analysis data show that disruption of PI3-kinase association with CD28 is neither necessary nor sufficient for costimulation of IL-2 production. T cell anergy also involves transcription regulators.

Calmodulin

Calmodulin (CaM) is an intracellular Ca^{2+}-binding protein that mediates many of the effects of Ca^{2+}. CaM binds to Fas directly and identifies the CaM-binding site on the cytoplasmic death domain (DD) of Fas. Fas (APO-1/CD95) is a cell-surface receptor that initiates apoptotic pathways, and its cytoplasmic domain interacts with various molecules suggesting that Fas signaling is complex and regulated by multiple proteins. The processes of T cell anergy and apoptosis are intertwined and act together to play critical role in immune suppression.

The Apoptosis Process

The process of apoptosis is a complex network, with different nodes connected by physical interactions of critical domains, including the caspase recruitment domains (CARDs); death effector domains (DEDs); DDs; BIR (baculovirus inhibitor of apoptosis proteins (IAP) repeat) domains of IAPs; Bcl-2 family proteins; caspase protease domains; and endonuclease-associated CIDE (cell death-inducing DNA fragmentation factor (DFF)45like effector) domains. Apoptotic cell death is thus a multifaceted process, whose initial signal is triggered in part by members of the TNF receptor superfamily, including Fas. When Fas interacts with the Fas-ligand, transmembrane signals are initiated through the associated FADD/MORT-1 motif, which interacts with caspase-8. Up to 10 caspases have been identified to date, which have been numbered based upon the chronological order of publication of their respective cDNAs. Active caspases are released from cleavage from the pro-enzyme into a larger peptide (17–22 kD) and a smaller peptide (10–12 kD) that associate to form the active enzyme in cells undergoing apoptosis. Caspase-8 possesses two motifs near the 5′-terminal that associate with FADD, referred to as the death effector domain. Activated caspase-8 in turn activates other caspases, and acts directly on mitochondrial permeability and metabolism.

Mitochondria

Mitochondria are involved in apoptosis through release of soluble molecules, such as bcl-2 that is normally situated in the outer mitochondrial membrane near the inner–outer membrane contact sites where permeability pores form. The action of bcl-2 is to protect against apoptosis by preventing the opening of these pores and release of a 50-kD protease and cytochrome C. Additional events involve changes in the plasma membrane and translocation of phosphatidyl-serine from the inner to the outer aspect of the membrane, which can be reliably detected by its high affinity to the Ca^{2+}-dependent phospholipid-binding protein, Annexin-5 (35–36 kD). Signals reach the nucleus for activation of nucleases and degradation of chromosomes into nucleosomal subunits. These metabolites are detected either as fragments of increasing length on an agarose gel or as cytoplasmic content of nucleosomal proteins.

β-Amyloid

Case in point, the peptide found in the neural plaques that characterize Alzheimer's disease, β-amyloid, significantly modulates T cell-mediated immunity.

The 1–42 β-amyloid peptide leads to T cell anergy, and impairs the generation of CD4+CD25+ and CD8+CD25+ Treg by up to 25%. This effect is attributable to the 28–35 portion of the peptide, the same that is responsible for impairing the maturation of T cell *in vitro*. The peptide also induces apoptotic cell death of healthy human T cells, as monitored by augmentation of cytoplasmic oligonucleosomes following treatment with β-amyloid, and a over threefold induction of caspase 3 (**Figure 3**).

A New Strategy: Molecular Cartography

Molecular cartography is the science of recognizing and identifying the multifaceted and intricate array of interacting genes and gene products that characterize the function and specialization of each individual cell in the context of cell–cell interaction, tissue and organ function. The relevance of molecular cartography pertains to every domain of physiology, including immunity.

Molecular cartography provides the fundamental knowledge and understanding of the genomic, the proteomic, and interactomic processes that regulate the emergence, stability, and function of immune cell populations, and the mechanisms by which the psychoneuroendocrine system regulates immunity. It produces new fundamental knowledge with respect to the processes that regulate immune suppression.

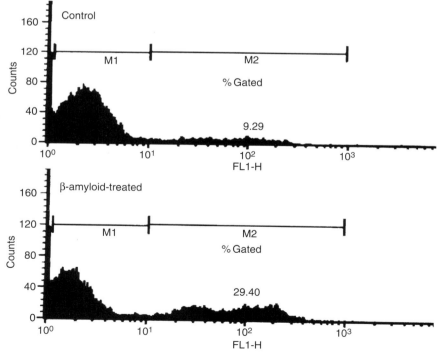

Figure 3   Caspase 3 induction in healthy human T cells exposed to β-amyloid peptide (1–42) for 48 h. Upper panel shows untreated (control) cultures. Lower panel shows β-amyloid-treated cultures. β-amyloid stimulated over threefold induction of caspase 3.

Further Reading

Carli, G., Suman, A. L., Biasi, G., et al. (2002). Reactivity to superficial and deep stimuli in patients with chronic musculoskeletal pain. *Pain* 100, 259–269.

Chiappelli, F., Kung, M. A., Nguyen, P., et al. (1997). Cellular immune correlates of clinical severity in oral lichen planus: preliminary association with mood states. *Oral Diseases* 3, 64–70.

Chiappelli, F. (2005). The molecular immunology of mucositis: implications for evidence-based research in alternative and complementary palliative treatments. *Evidence-Based Complementary and Alternative Medicine* 2, 489–494.

Chiappelli, F. and Cajulis, O. S. (2004). Psychobiological views on "stress-related oral ulcers" *Quintessence International* 35, 223–227.

Chiappelli, F. and Hodgson, D. (2000). Immune suppression. In: Fink, G. (ed.) *Encyclopedia of stress*, (vol. 2), pp. 531–536. San Diego: Academic Press.

Chiappelli, F., Prolo, P., Fiala, M., et al. (2005). Allostasis in HIV-1 infection and AIDS. In: Minagar, P. A. & Shapshak, P. (eds.) *Neuro-AIDS*. Hauppauge, NY: Nova Science Publisher (in press).

Chiappelli, F., Prolo, P., Iribarren, J., et al. (2006). Alzheimer's disease: new frontiers for the XXI century.

In: Welsh, E. M. (ed.) *Trends in Alzheimer's disease research*, pp. 233–258. Hauppauge, NY: Nova Science Publishers.

Czura, C. J., Friedman, S. G. and Tracey, K. J. (2003). Neural inhibition of inflammation: the cholinergic anti-inflammatory pathway. *Journal of Endotoxin Research* 9, 409–413.

Kunz-Ebrecht, S. R., Mohamed-Ali, V., Feldman, P. J., et al. (2003). Cortisol responses to mild psychological stress are inversely associated with proinflammatory cytokines. *Brain Behavior and Immunology* 17, 373–383.

Maekawa, K., Twu, C., Lotaif, A., et al. (2003). Function of β-adrenergic receptor on mononuclear cells in female fibromyalgia patient. *Journal of Rheumatology* 30, 364–368.

McEwen, B. and Wingfield, J. C. (2003). The concept of allostasis in biology and biomedicine. *Hormones and Behavior* 43, 2–15.

Sterling, P. and Eyer, J. (1988). Allostasis: a new paradigm to explain arousal pathology. In: Fisher, S. & Reason, J. (eds.) *Handbook of life stress, cognition, and health*, pp. 629–645. New York: Wiley.

van der PouwKraan, T. C., Kasperkovitz, P. V., Verbeet, N., et al. (2004). Genomics in the immune system. *Clinical Immunology* 111, 175–185.

Immune Surveillance – Cancer, Effects of Stress on

D Spiegel and F S Dhabhar
Stanford University School of Medicine, Stanford, CA, USA

Stress Reactivity and Disease Progression
Stress Hormones and Cancer Progression
Stress and Tumor Immunosurveillance
Psychosocial-Biobehavioral Intervention and Cancer

Glossary

B cells	Class of white blood cells that mount the humoral immune response, attacking foreign antigens such as those found on bacteria.
Chemokines	Proteins that attract the activity of various white blood cells.
Cytokines	Proteins that regulate immune activity and also affect the functioning of the central nervous system.
DNA ploidy	The relative disorganization of DNA replication in tumor cells.
Helper and cytolytic T cells	Class of white blood cells that kill virally infected or tumor cells.
Hypothalamic-pituitary-adrenal (HPA) axis	A major hormonal stress response system in the body that regulates the secretion of cortisol, which mobilizes glucose into the bloodstream.
Immuno-suppression	The reduction of the activity of components of the immune system.
Natural Killer (NK) cells	A class of white blood cells that attacks transformed or dying cells, such as tumor cells.
Neuroimmune effects	Interacting effects of the central nervous system on immune function.
Proopiomelano-cortin (POMC)	A precursor protein that is the source of adrenocorticotropic hormone, which triggers cortisol release, and of endogenous opiates

Cancer can be understood as, among other things, a series of stressors: the diagnosis, arduous treatments, fears of death, and changes in social and physical environment. For example, as many as 80% of breast cancer patients report significant distress during initial treatment. Estimates of the prevalence of psychiatric disorders among newly diagnosed cancer patients has ranged from 30–44%, and 20–45% exhibit emotional morbidity 1–2 years later. Although the majority of cancer patients do not have a psychiatric diagnosis, for those who do depression is the most common one, and the vast majority experience the diagnosis of cancer as a major stressor. Up to 10% have severe maladjustment as long as 6 years later. Thus, cancer is a disease that causes considerable psychological stress.

Cancer is largely a disease of aging; it is rare below the age of 50 and increasingly common with advancing age. To the extent that abnormalities of the endocrine stress response system, the hypothalamic-pituitary-adrenal axis (HPA), increase with age and affect cancer progression, their impact should increase with advancing age due to a greater likelihood of abnormality and a higher prevalence of disease. The bulk of cancer research has productively focused on the pathophysiology of the disease, emphasizing tumor biology, especially tumor characteristics such as DNA ploidy and estrogen/progesterone receptor status as predictors of disease outcome at the expense of studying the body's psychophysiological reactions to tumor invasion. These reactions are mediated by brain–body mechanisms, including the endocrine, neuroimmune, and autonomic nervous systems. Although a large portion of the variance in any disease outcome is accounted for by the specific local pathophysiology of that disease, some variability must also be explained by host resistance factors, which include the manner of response to the stress of the illness. For example, in a series of classic experiments in animals, Riley showed that crowding accelerated the rate of tumor growth and mortality. In a recent authoritative review of human stress literature, McEwen documented the adverse health effects of cumulative stressors and the body's failure to adapt the stress response to them. The activation of the HPA axis is an adaptive response to acute stress, but over time, in response to cumulative stress, the system's signal-to-noise ratio can be degraded so that it is partially on all the time, leading to adverse physiological consequences, including abnormalities of glucose metabolism, hippocampal damage, accumulation of abdominal fat, and depression. Abnormalities of HPA axis function, including glucocorticoid receptor hypersensitivity, have also been found to be associated with posttraumatic stress disorder. Thus, adverse emotional events, ranging from traumatic stressors to cumulative minor ones, are associated with HPA axis dysregulation. Persistently elevated or relatively invariant levels of cortisol may, in turn, stimulate tumor proliferation via differential gluconeogenesis in normal and tumor tissue, the activation of hormone receptors in tumor,

or immunosuppression. Glucocorticoid dysregulation may be associated with other stress-related endocrine and immune dysfunction that could have consequences for host resistance to cancer progression.

Stress Reactivity and Disease Progression

Reactivity to stressors involves not only the initial response but the system's ability to reset itself after stress. Older organisms seem to reset themselves after a stressor less readily, leaving stress-responsive systems more tonically upregulated for longer periods of time after the cessation of the stressor. Cancer affects older people particularly, and chronic disease-related stressors are perhaps likely to further decrease the flexibility of stress response mechanisms. Sapolsky and colleagues found that stressed older animals had not only persistently elevated cortisol levels after the stress was over but also much more rapid growth of implanted tumors. This finding was confirmed in a study that also identified the suppressive effects of stress hormones on natural killer (NK) cells as one potential mediator of the effect. It may not be so much the magnitude of stress-induced elevation of corticosteroids that is important in cancer outcomes as the duration or persistence of the elevation. These findings are particularly relevant because there is evidence that persistent elevations of cortisol, as measured by slower rates of cortisol decline throughout the day, have been associated with both shorter cancer survival and the suppression of NK cells. These lymphocytes, identified with CD56 cell surface markers, do not attack specific antigens but rather destroy transformed or dying cells, such as cancer cells. The number and killing activity of these NK cells have been found to be associated with the progression of breast cancer. As the disease progresses, NK activity declines and, conversely, declining NK activity and counts predicts breast cancer progression.

Stress Hormones and Cancer Progression

Mechanisms have been proposed whereby the neuroendocrine correlates of stress may promote neoplastic growth. Stress hormones may suppress immune resistance to tumors or act via differential effects on gluconeogenesis in healthy versus tumor cells. Tumor cells may become resistant to the catabolic action of cortisol, which inhibits the uptake of glucose in numerous cell types. In such cases, energy would be preferentially shunted to the tumor and away from normal cells by cortisol. Several studies have found an association between the stress-related elevation of glucocorticoids and more rapid tumor growth in animals. Another hypothesis suggests that HPA axis hormones may promote the expression of breast cancer oncogenes due to activation of proopiomelanocortin (POMC) genes by corticotropin releasing hormone (CRH). The POMC promoter has homology with POMC transcription factors that bind to human MAT-1 breast cancer oncogenes. Also, fasting insulin levels have been found to predict subsequent mortality from breast cancer, whereas levels of insulin-like growth factor binding proteins predict recurrence but not mortality. Thus, there are a variety of means by which depression-related abnormalities in HPA axis function could affect the rate of cancer progression. One leading hypothesis is an association between HPA axis and immune dysfunction because glucocorticoids are potently immunosuppressive.

Stress and Tumor Immunosurveillance

Although some aspects of antitumor immune responses are still controversial, there is now ample evidence to show that under certain conditions the immune system plays a crucial and protective role by detecting and eliminating tumors. Recently, Dunn et al. introduced the concept of tumor immunoediting, which hypothesizes that the immune system plays a critical role not only in detecting and eliminating tumors but also in shaping the extent of immunogenicity or nonimmunogenicity of tumors that ultimately escape immunosurveillance and result in clinically observable malignant disease. Evidence for the immunosurveillance hypothesis comes from (1) studies that show an increased incidence of virally induced cancers, such as Kaposi's sarcoma and non-Hodgkin's lymphoma, in patients undergoing immunosuppressive treatments; (2) studies of patients with immunodeficiency diseases; and (3) studies using selective cytokine- or leukocyte-deficient mice. However, immunosurveillance is also thought to play an important role in the elimination of cancers that do not have a viral etiology (e.g., malignant melanoma, non-Kaposi's sarcoma, and lung tumors), and higher incidence ratios for these cancers are observed in immunocompromised hosts.

All major leukocyte subtypes, including macrophages, granulocytes, NK cells, helper and cytolytic T cells, and B cells, are thought to play a role in immune surveillance. However, under certain conditions, regulatory/suppressor leukocytes such as subsets of CD25+ and CD4+ T cells and natural killer T (NKT) cells, may inhibit antitumor immune responses. Specific cytokines and chemokines are thought to exert direct and indirect protective (suppression of tumor development and progression)

as well as harmful (promotion of tumor growth and metastasis) effects. Moreover, in contrast to protective, regulated, antitumor immune responses, dysregulated or chronic immune responses directed against pathogens or self-antigens can induce or exacerbate tumorigenesis through chronic tissue damage and activation.

Prolonged or chronic stress has been shown to affect most immune parameters thought to be important for tumor surveillance. Therefore, stress may affect immune function and susceptibility to cancer in several different ways. First, in general, chronic stress and stress hormone exposure have been associated with the suppression of NK activity, T-cell responses, and cell-mediated immune reactions; decreased telomere length and telomerase activity in circulating leukocytes; increased tumor metastases; enhanced growth of transplanted tumors; and increased tumor number, size, and density of skin cancer (squamous cell carcinoma). Second, stress may also suppress antiviral immune responses. The suppression of immunity to transforming viruses could significantly enhance the risk of tumor formation and progression. Third, chronic stress may contribute to immune dysregulation and promote or sustain chronic pro-inflammatory states that, in turn, induce or exacerbate cancer. Fourth, glucocorticoids are potently immunosuppressive, so the effects stress and hypercortisolemia may include functional immunosuppression as well, as has been shown extensively in animals and for which there is a growing body of evidence in humans. This, in turn, could influence the rate of cancer progression.

Psychosocial-Biobehavioral Intervention and Cancer

Understanding how psychosocial factors such as stress can suppress protective immune function may help in the design of psychosocial-biobehavioral interventions that may buffer against stress- and depression-induced effects, thereby improving patient quality of life and potential survival. Five of eleven published randomized trials demonstrate such an effect. The principles of such stress management techniques include helping cancer patients construct a new network of social support; encouraging the expression and management of the range of emotions typical of such stress-inducing illness, including anger, fear, and sadness; helping people face their fears of dying and death; and reordering life priorities. Other helpful components include improving social relationships; enhancing doctor–patient communication; educating the patient about coping skills, the disease, and its treatment; and teaching anxiety and pain management techniques. Such interventions clearly improve patient quality of life and may have a positive effect on survival time via effects on endocrine, circadian, and immune physiology.

Further Reading

Andersen, B. L., Farrar, W. B., Golden-Kreutz, D., et al. (1998). Stress and immune responses after surgical treatment for regional breast cancer. *Journal of the National Cancer Institute* **90**(1), 30–36.

Ben-Eliyahu, S. (2003). The promotion of tumor metastasis by surgery and stress: immunological basis and implications for psychoneuroimmunology. *Brain, Behavior & Immunity* 7(supplement 1), S27–S36.

Ben-Eliyahu, S., Yirmiya, R., Liebeskind, J. C., et al. (1991). Stress increases metastatic spread of a mammary tumor in rats: evidence for mediation by the immune system. *Brain, Behavior & Immunity* **5**(2), 193–205.

Derogatis, L. R., Morrow, G. R., Fetting, J., et al. (1983). The prevalence of psychiatric disorders among cancer patients. *Journal of the American Medical Association* **249**(6), 751–757.

Dhabhar, F. S. and Mcewen, B. S. (1997). Acute stress enhances while chronic stress suppresses cell-mediated immunity in vivo: a potential role for leukocyte trafficking. *Brain, Behavior & Immunity* **11**, 286–306.

Dunn, G. P., Bruce, A. T., Ikeda, H., et al. (2002). Cancer immunoediting: from immunosurveillance to tumor escape. *Nature Reviews Immunology* 3(11), 991–998.

Epel, E. S., Blackburn, E. H., Lin, J., et al. (2004). Accelerated telomere shortening in response to life stress. *Proceedings of the National Academy of Sciences USA* **101**(49), 17312–17315.

Epel, E. S., McEwen, B., Seeman, T., et al. (1999). Psychological stress and lack of cortisol habituation among women with abdominal fat distribution. *Psychosomatic Medicine* **61**, 107.

Glaser, R. and Kiecolt-Glaser, J. K. (2005). Stress-induced immune dysfunction: implications for health. *Nature Reviews Immunology* **5**(3), 243–251.

Glaser, R., Kiecolt-Glaser, J. K., Malarkey, W. B., et al. (1998). The influence of psychological stress on the immune response to vaccines. *Annals of the New York Academy of Sciences* **840**, 649–655.

Goodwin, P. J., Ennis, M., Pritchard, K. I., et al. (2002). Fasting insulin and outcome in early-stage breast cancer: results of a prospective cohort study. *Journal of Clinical Oncology* 20(1), 42–51.

Irvine, D., Brown, B., Crooks, D., et al. (1991). Psychosocial adjustment in women with breast cancer. *Cancer* 67(4), 1097–1117.

Kiecolt-Glaser, J. K. and Glaser, R. (1999). Psychoneuroimmunology and cancer: fact or fiction? *European Journal of Cancer* 35(11), 1603–1607.

Kissane, D. W., Grabsch, B., Love, A., et al. (2004). Psychiatric disorder in women with early stage and advanced breast cancer: a comparative analysis. *Australian and New Zealand Journal of Psychiatry* 38(5), 320–326.

Klein, G. and Klein, E. (1998). Immunology. Sinking surveillance's flagship. *Nature* 395(6701), 34–41.

Licinio, J., Gold, P. W. and Wong, M. L. (1995). A molecular mechanism for stress-induced alterations in susceptibility to disease. *Lancet* 346(8967), 104–106.

McEwen, B. S. (1998). Protective and damaging effects of stress mediators. *New England Journal of Medicine* 338(3), 171–179.

Omne-Ponten, M., Holmberg, L. and Sjoden, P. O. (1994). Psychosocial adjustment among women with breast cancer stages I and II: six-year follow-up of consecutive patients. *Journal of Clinical Oncology* **12**(9), 1778–1782.

Posener, J. A., Schildkraut, J. J., Samson, J. A., et al. (1981). Diurnal variation of plasma cortisol and homovanillic acid in healthy subjects. *Psychoneuroendocrinology* **21**(1), 33–38.

Riley, V. (1981). Psychoneuroendocrine influences on immunocompetence and neoplasia. *Science* 212(4499), 1100–1109.

Romero, L., Raley-Susman, K., Redish, D., et al. (1992). A possible mechanism by which stress accelerates growth of virally-derived tumors. *Proceedings of the National Academy of Sciences USA* **89**, 11084.

Sapolsky, R. M. and Donnelly, T. M. (1985). Vulnerability to stress-induced tumor growth increases with age in rats: role of glucocorticoids. *Endocrinology* **117**(2), 662–666.

Sapolsky, R., Krey, L. and McEwen, B. S. (1985). Prolonged glucocorticoid exposure reduces hippocampal neuron number: implication for aging. *Journal of Neuroscience* 5, 1222–1227.

Sephton, S. E., Sapolsky, R. M., Kraemer, H. C., et al. (2000). Early mortality in metastatic breast cancer patients with absent or abnormal diurnal cortisol rhythms. *Journal of the National Cancer Institute* 92(12), 994–1000.

Spiegel, D. (1999). A 43-year-old woman coping with cancer [clinical conference]. *Journal of the American Medical Association* 1282(4), 371–378.

Spiegel, D. (2002). Effects of psychotherapy on cancer survival. *Nature Reviews Cancer* 2(5), 383–389.

Immune System, Aging

M A Horan
University of Manchester Medical School, Salford, UK

This article is reproduced from the previous edition, volume 2, pp 536–540, © 2000, Elsevier Inc.

Immune Systems
Pattern of Immune Aging
Causes of Immune Aging
Aging and Infections

Glossary

Autoantibody	Immunoglobulin whose specificity is directed at self.
C-reactive protein	A small protein of the pentraxin family, secreted and catabolized only by the hepatocytes (liver parenchymal cells). It was named for its ability to bind with pneumococcal C-polysaccharide. Its synthesis is under transcriptional control, regulated by pro-inflammatory cytokines (especially interleukin 6), and it is one of the proteins that characterize the acute phase response.
Cytokine	A small protein or glycoprotein that generally acts locally to alter cell behavior or function. Cytokines may be considered locally acting hormones. The major classes of cytokines are interleukins, interferons, and tumor necrosis factors.
Endotoxin	Lipopolysaccharides from the walls of gram-negative bacteria that can activate lymphocytes and mononuclear phagocytes.
Epstein–Barr virus	A herpesvirus that, after a primary infection, remains latent in B lymphocytes and may be reactivated at some later time.
Lymphocyte	A small cell derived from the bone marrow that, after appropriate processing and maturation, can participate in specific immune responses. B lymphocytes (B cells) further differentiate into plasma cells, which secrete immunoglobulin (antibody).
Monoclonal antibody	An immunoglobulin of a single specificity produced by an expanded clone of plasma cells.
Mononuclear phagocyte	A cell of bone marrow origin, larger than a lymphocyte, that can phagocytose foreign material and present it to lymphocytes to bring about an immune response. Examples are monocytes, macrophages, and Kupffer cells.

Immune Systems

Two interactive immune systems are recognized: innate (natural) immunity and acquired (adoptive or specific) immunity. Innate immunity comprises polymorphonuclear leukocytes (neutrophils, eosinophils, and basophils), natural killer (NK) cells, and mononuclear phagocytes, and it uses the complement cascade as its main soluble protein effector mechanism. It also uses numerous recognition molecules, including C-reactive protein (CRP), serum amyloid protein (SAP), and mannose-binding protein (MBP). These molecules have been selected during evolution to bind carbohydrate structures that do not occur on eukaryotic cells and so differentiate potentially harmful invaders from innocuous self.

Acquired immunity employs several subtypes of lymphocytes and uses antibody as its effector protein. Antibody and the T-cell receptor (TCR) are the recognition structures. B lymphocytes can recognize protein, carbohydrate, and simple chemical structures, whereas T lymphocytes seem to recognize only peptides. Clones of lymphocytes with receptors of sufficient affinity are triggered by antigen to proliferate and differentiate into the various effector cells: T-helper (Th) cells, cytotoxic T cells, suppressor T cells, and plasma cells (which secrete antibody).

After an immune response subsides, specific antibody often persists in the blood for many years and even decades. This implies that humoral effector cells (plasma cells) persist and continue to secrete antibody. In contrast, the antibody response at mucosal surfaces is generally short-lived (a few months to a year). Effector T cells do not persist for very long, but antigen-specific clones remain expanded as memory lymphocytes, which can differentiate quickly into effector cells if the antigen is encountered again. In general, memory responses are most effective in protecting against systemic infections (e.g., measles, mumps, poliomyelitis, and smallpox). Localized infections at mucosal surfaces (e.g., rotavirus, respiratory syncytial virus, and rhinovirus) can recur before memory lymphocytes can differentiate into effector cells, although the subsequent episodes of disease are usually less severe.

The flexible nature of specific immunity poses the problem of differentiating innocuous (self) antigens from harmful ones, a problem that innate immunity does not have. One way of overcoming this is to delete potentially self-reactive clones during maturation in the thymus (for T cells) and at a yet unknown site for B cells. Further specificity is assured by interactions with innate immunity. For T cells, antigen presentation is the critical step. The uptake of antigen into antigen-presenting cells (e.g., mononuclear phagocytes and dendritic cells) is determined by the presence of carbohydrate moieties that are recognized by innate immunity. For B cells, the interaction with innate immunity seems to be their membrane receptors for the C3d component of complement, which is found in association with CD19. CD19 is needed for antibody production for T-cell-dependent antigens and amplifies signaling after the antigen binds membrane immunoglobulin. Covalent binding of C3d to microbial carbohydrate structures facilitates this process. Different pathogens require different types of response for their elimination: type 1 responses (characterized by dependence on macrophages for phagocytosis and intracellular killing) and type 2 responses (macrophage independent, relying on non-cytotoxic antibodies, mast cells, and eosinophils). Th cells are required for both types of response, but these exist as two subtypes, called Th1 and Th2. Th1 cells produce interleukin (IL)-2, IL-3, tumor necrosis factor (TNF)-α, and interferon (IFN)-γ, and this pattern of cytokines promotes type 1 responses. Macrophages are activated and B cells are switched to IgG1 production (in humans), which binds macrophage Fc receptors and activates complement, both of which promote phagocytosis. Activated macrophages produce IL-12, TNF-α, and IFN-γ. This pattern of cytokines (especially IL-12) induces the activation and proliferation of NK cells, the differentiation of naïve T cells into Th cells, and the expression of the Th1 phenotype.

Th2 cells promote type 2 responses. Th2 cells require IL-4 to prime naïve cells. Once activated, they produce IL-3, IL-4, IL-5, IL-6, IL-10, and IL-13. This pattern of cytokines leads to the growth and activation of mast cells and eosinophils. It also switches B lymphocytes to produce IgG4 (and IgE) and inhibits macrophage activation. This pattern of response is typical of helminth infections, and it may also be important for the downregulation of type 1 responses.

Pattern of Immune Aging

Of all body systems, the immune system is probably the best understood, and studies of it can be traced to the early part of this century (and even earlier). Perhaps the first publication was by Peter Ludwig Panum, a Danish physician best remembered for the discovery of endotoxins. He reported an outbreak of measles in the Faroe Islands in 1846. The islands had been free of measles since the previous epidemic in 1781. The reported outbreak affected 75–95% of the population, although "of the many aged people still living on the Faroes who had had measles in 1781, not one was attacked a second time."

The classic view of immune aging (immunosenescence) is of an immunodeficiency state that predisposes the host to infectious diseases and possibly also neoplasms. The state is often attributed to the involution of the thymus gland and is thought to be characterized by the decreased proliferation of T lymphocytes and impaired Th activity, which lead to impaired cell-mediated and humoral responses to T-cell-dependent antigens. B-lymphocyte numbers and function (antibody production) seem to change little, although in the intact organism antibody titers to a variety of vaccine antigens are generally reduced. Paradoxically, there is an increased incidence of autoantibodies (inevitably of low titer) and benign monoclonal B-lymphocyte proliferations with monoclonal antibody production. Interestingly, older people in Japan have a very low incidence of these benign monoclonal proliferations, suggesting the importance of genetic factors in outbred populations such as humans.

With the discovery of cytokines and their regulatory importance for many cell types (including the cells of the immune system), new insights have emerged concerning the mechanisms underlying immunosenescence. The patterns of cytokine secretion by T lymphocytes from young and old mice clearly differ. In the young, IL-2 and IL-4 predominate, whereas in the old it is IL-10 and INF-γ. The young pattern also characterizes Th1 responses and the old pattern the Th2 responses. It is also known that naïve T cells (which have never encountered antigen) exhibit Th1 responses and that memory T cells (which persist after antigen exposure) exhibit Th2 responses. Memory T cells are known to accumulate during aging. Furthermore, the change in the balance of Th1-to-Th2 responses can be partially reversed by thymic hormones and the steroid dehydroepiandrosterone. However, the altered Th1–Th2 balance is not explained simply by the accumulation of memory T cells. Th1 function clearly declines during aging. For example, old mice are unable to develop tolerance to Staphylococcal enterotoxin B and die from shock, whereas young mice develop a tolerance and do not die. Thus, thinking has changed from the classic view of immunosenescence toward a view based on immune dysregulation, predominantly the disturbed balance of Th1–Th2 responses, a change that also appears to occur in humans. Increased Th1 and reduced Th2 responses would be expected to predispose to infections, but what causes this change?

Causes of Immune Aging

Clearly, the accumulation of memory T cells could explain some of the change, but it cannot account for it entirely. In outbred populations such as humans, there are genetic polymorphisms in the promoter regions of many (if not all) cytokine genes and the selective survival of particular genotypes could play a part but cannot explain the change in an inbred strain. One intriguing suggestion is that inflammation could be a significant cause.

Inflammation

Of all inflammatory cells, macrophages have been given the closest scrutiny. When stimulated, they secrete a variety of inflammatory mediators, including the pro-inflammatory cytokines IL-1, IL-6, and TNF-α. *In vivo* administration of endotoxin to mice induces the production of TNF-α, IL-1, IL-6, and INF-γ, and the response is much exaggerated in old animals. IL-6 is produced constitutively, and circulating levels are higher in the older (mice and humans) subjects than in the young. Treating old mice with antibodies to IL-6 reduces the magnitude of the Th2 pattern. IL-6 is known to orchestrate the so-called acute phase response, including the production of CRP in the liver. CRP is familiar to most readers as a clinical marker for inflammation and may itself exacerbate tissue damage, but why is the constitutive production of IL-6 higher in the old? What signals might be present in them that may not be present in the young?

Aging as a Pro-inflammatory State

The evidence presented in this article argues strongly for an exaggeration of the macrophage component of inflammation. Is there evidence that other inflammatory cells are similarly affected? The cell type that arrives earliest at a site of infection or tissue damage is the neutrophil. The effects of aging on neutrophil function are controversial – some *in vitro* studies show impaired function, whereas others show no impairment. In contrast, *in vivo* studies are unambiguous in showing that the neutrophil influx is greater in the old. One interesting study in mice with experimental pneumonia revealed a greater neutrophil influx in the old, associated with a higher death rate. This finding is entirely consistent with the author's studies of endotoxin administration to aged rats. Older humans also seem to experience such exaggerated inflammatory responses. For example, the adult respiratory distress syndrome and the systemic inflammatory response syndrome are both largely conditions of the old, and both are characterized by unrestrained inflammation. More controlled studies of experimental cutaneous wound healing in humans also show more rapid and more marked neutrophil influx into the site of injury in older subjects. This leads to high collagen turnover and probably slower wound healing but a restoration of dermal architecture (unlike the disorganized collagen deposition in the young) and a cosmetically more appealing end result. Interestingly, this effect can be reversed by prior treatment with estrogen, at least in older women.

Replicative Senescence

Studies on aging murine and human T-cell clones have shown that a population remains with normal responses in the midst of a much larger population with reduced responses, including reduced proliferation. It has been suggested that this might be an *in vivo* manifestation of replicative senescence (Hayflick limit), thought to occur in other types of aging cells *in vitro*. *In vitro*, such senescent cells fail to express CD28, have shortened telomeres, and are clearly memory cells (and express CD45RO). *In vivo*, there is known to be a decline in CD28+, with telomere shortening as well as a minimal proliferative capacity. The majority of these CD28$^+$ are CD8$^+$. Almost identical changes have been documented in acquired immunodeficiency syndrome (AIDS), in which they may be due to prolonged or repeated episodes of human immunodeficiency virus (HIV)-induced T-cell proliferation.

Reactivation of latent viruses It has been proposed that the accumulation of T cells showing the characteristics of replicative senescence of aging occurs by a similar mechanism to that in AIDS, that is, periodic or chronic restimulation of memory T cells. The idea that immune aging might result from the presence of immune activators is not new. Because such episodes of antigenic stimulation might also induce nonspecific T-cell replication (bystander replication), their effect on the integrity of the aging immune system may have been underestimated. Candidates for such chronic restimulation may include latent viruses such as the Epstein–Barr virus (EBV) or pathogens with epitopes that are cross-reactive with self-antigens present on T cells (e.g., influenza A). The consequence of bystander lymphocyte senescence may be that fewer functional $CD8^+$ T cells may be available to combat infections and cancer. EBV is acquired asymptomatically in childhood, as a symptomatic disease in adolescence (glandular fever and infectious mononucleosis), or as a new infection in old age. Of the seven EBV seroepidemiological studies that include older people, all have shown the highest titers of antibodies in the old. Although this suggests that reactivation does indeed occur in old age, the symptoms of glandular fever are absent. EBV can also be detected in saliva. Twenty percent of people over the age of 50 excrete the virus, but the prevalence of viral shedding in a truly aged population is unknown. Immunosuppression is known to increase the prevalence of virus shedding to over 90%. Symptomatic reactivation has been associated with Hodgkin's disease, nasopharyngeal carcinoma, oral hairy leukoplakia, lymphocytic interstitial pneumonia, and B-cell lymphoproliferative disease. EBV reactivation syndromes have never been investigated in older people, and morbidity could arise from the inappropriate production of cytokines (particularly in people with certain promoter region polymorphisms) and the premature onset of replicative senescence.

Aging and Infections

When an organism arrives at a potential portal of entry into the host (usually an epithelial surface), three outcomes are possible: the organism is eliminated, the organism proliferates successfully but fails to invade tissues, or tissue invasion occurs. For most organisms, tissue invasion is a *sine qua non* for infection, although some induce changes in the host predominantly through the elaboration of toxins (e.g., cholera). When tissue invasion occurs, an acute inflammatory response is triggered, and it is usually by the recognition of the systemic consequences of this that we diagnose infections. The host feels unwell, anorexic, and somnolent (thought to be induced mainly by IL-6). The hypothalamic thermostat is reset to a higher level and the host feels cold and attempts to raise the core temperature to this new level (fever). This is achieved by reducing heat loss by vasoconstriction and behavioral means (e.g., extra clothes) and by shivering. The metabolic rate is increased, although this is a much more important mechanism for small mammals than for large ones. Uncontrolled studies suggest that the old often fail to produce a fever response, but more careful studies suggest that this may not be the case. First, care must be taken with the measurement of body temperature. Using inadequate instruments at sites of heat loss (e.g., mouth or axilla) almost guarantees the failure to detect fever. The rectum and the tympanic membranes are more reliable sites, and electronic and infrared thermometers equilibrate much faster than mercury-in-glass ones. Second, the ambient temperature may be too low for the host to overcome, and the core temperature may rise into the febrile range only in a warm environment. Finally, experimental studies with several pyrogenic cytokines suggest that the hypothalamic thermostat of the old may be desensitized (dose–response curve shifts to the right) but that the maximal response is unaffected by aging. Another important sign of infection is the detection of an elevation in the circulating white blood cell count (mainly neutrophils), and there is no evidence that aging impairs this response. Likewise, older people also increase the levels of CRP in a pattern indistinguishable from similarly infected young people.

Comorbid factors such as malnutrition, glucocorticoid administration, and so forth can certainly impair host responses and do so in both young and old. Further, diseases at other sites are common in the old and may obscure the characteristic findings of infections. Age-related changes in several body systems predispose to more general types of presentation, known as the giants of geriatrics: immobility, falls, delirium, and incontinence. Thus, it is important to consider infection as a possible diagnosis in any older person whose condition changes acutely, whether the characteristic features are present or not.

Are Older People Predisposed to Acquire Infections?

This question is very difficult to answer. Theoretically, age-related immune changes could well predispose to acquiring infections, but they are not the only factors involved. To acquire an infection requires exposure to a potential pathogen, and this exposure is greatly dependent on environmental and lifestyle factors. For example, people who do not practice unprotected sexual intercourse and who have never had a blood transfusion are highly unlikely to be exposed to HIV. To acquire a common cold or influenza requires contact with an infected person; those living a solitary lifestyle, not traveling on crowded public transport, and not visiting places where people congregate (school, work, football matches, and so forth) may have considerably reduced risks of exposure to potential pathogens. However, those living in relatively closed environments (e.g., nursing homes) may be at an extremely high risk if a potential pathogen is introduced (e.g., tuberculosis, methicillin-resistant *Staphylococcus aureus*, *Clostridium difficile*, or rotaviruses). Very few hard data exist that make any direct comparisons across age groups. Perhaps the most reliable data come from the American National Health Interview Surveys. These have shown the community-dwelling aged to be at a considerably lower risk of developing colds or influenza than any other age group and at only a modestly increased risk of developing pneumonia. What is not in doubt is that, once infected, the old will be sicker and more likely to die.

See Also the Following Articles

Aging and Stress, Biology of; Cytokines; Infection; Lymphocytes; Macrophages.

Further Reading

Ashcroft, G. S., Horan, M. A. and Ferguson, M. W. J. (1998). Aging and cutaneous wound healing. In: Horan, M. A. & Little, R. A. (eds.) *Injury in the aging*, pp. 147–153. Cambridge, UK: Cambridge University Press.

Effros, R. B. (1998). Human genetics '98: aging and senescence; replicative senescence in the immune system: impact of the Hayflick limit on T-cell function in the elderly. *American Journal of Human Genetics* 26, 165–181.

Horan, M. A. and Ashcroft, G. S. (1997). Ageing, defence mechanisms and the immune system. *Age and Ageing* 26 (supplement 4), 15–119.

Horan, M. A. and Parker, S. G. (1998). Infections, aging and the host response. In: Horan, M. A. & Little, R. A. (eds.) *Injury in the aging*, pp. 126–146. Cambridge, UK: Cambridge University Press.

Immune System   *See:* Immune Response.

Immunity

F Chiappelli
UCLA School of Dentistry, Los Angeles, CA, USA

This article is a revision of the previous edition article by F Chiappelli and Q N Liu, volume 2, pp 541–546, © 2000, Elsevier Inc.

T-Cell Proliferation
Migration
Regulation
Conclusion

Glossary

Immunological synapse	Complex assemblage of rafts that integrates the signaling cascades for the amplification and regulation of T cell activation.
Rafts	Microdomains determined by and anchored to the cytoskeleton of T cells, and important in coordinating the signaling response in T cell-mediated immunity.
Regulatory T cells (Treg)	Characterized phenotypically by the expression of the α chain of the interleukin (IL)-2 receptor, CD25, at the molecular level by the expression of FoxP3, the P3 member of the first forkhead-box (FOX) transcription factor, which functions as a transcriptional repressor at the nuclear factor for activation of T cell (NFAT)/ activating protein (AP)-1 sites in cytokine gene promoters, and functionally Treg act to impair proliferative and IL-2 production responses, thus blunting T cell-mediated immunity.
Suppressors of cytokine signaling (SOCS)	A family of seven known cytoplasmic proteins, the suppressor of cytokine signaling, which modulate cytokine-mediated regulation of immunity.

Immunity confers protection of the organism against pathogens. Innate immunity concerns humoral (e.g., complement) and cellular events (e.g., natural killer cells) that do not require priming by antigens. Antigen-specific immunity addresses that branch of cellular (e.g., cytotoxic T lymphocytes and plasma B cells) and humoral immune surveillance (e.g., cytokine patterns, immunoglobulins) that depends upon the phenotypic (e.g., memory CD4+ T cells, CD4+CD45R0+, and B cells) and functional stage maturation of lymphocytes following presentation of the antigen by the major histocompatibility complex (MHC).

Immunity comprises important innate and adaptive immune responses. Viruses, bacteria, or classical parasites all probe the limit of immunity, and of the three basic parameters of immunology – specificity, tolerance, and memory. The practical specificity repertoire of T and B cells is probably in the order of 10^4–10^7 specificities expressed by T cells or by neutralizing antibodies. Tolerance is best defined by rules of reactivity to eliminate infections while avoiding destruction of normal cells by complete elimination of T cells that are specific for antigens persisting in the blood and lymphohemopoietic system. Induction of a T-cell response is the result of antigens newly entering the lymph nodes or the spleen, initially in a local fashion and exhibiting an optimal distribution kinetics within the lymphohemopoietic system. Antigens that stay outside lymphatic tissues are generally immunologically ignored. Immunity is regulated by antigen dose, time, and relative distribution kinetics. Memory relates to the host's resistance following a second exposure to the same agent, and it correlates with antigen-dependent maintenance of circulating antibody titers, and with T-cell responses.

In a previous article, we discussed innate and antigen-dependent immunity in general. Recent research developments have established the central role of T cells in regulating immune surveillance. This article focuses on novel knowledge pertaining to T cell-mediated immunity. The vast domain of autoimmunity is not addressed in this article.

T-Cell Proliferation

T lymphocytes, 70–80% of the peripheral blood mononuclear cells, express the cluster of differentiation (CD)-3, but lack CD14 (i.e., monocyte-specific) and CD20/21 markers (i.e., B cell-specific). CD3 is proximal to the T-cell receptor (TcR), constituted by the α and β chains in circulating T cells, and by the γ and δ chains in the mucosal lymphoid tissue. T cells are stimulated *in vivo* via TcR, and *in vitro* by immobilized anti-CD3 antibody and the CD28 co-stimulus, lest the cells fail to proliferate and enter anergy, a state of stunted cell activation and proliferative capability.

Rafts

Lipids and proteolipids in the T-cell membrane are organized into rafts, microdomains determined by and anchored to the cytoskeleton. Rafts compose the immune synapse, a complex assemblage that integrates the signaling cascades. The synapse amplifies and regulates the activation of T cells. The assembly of the immune synapse at the antigen-presenting site depends on the interactions between rafts and the actin cytoskeleton, which controls the coalescence of smaller raft components into the larger immune synapse complex to integrate cellular responses to diverse signals. Phosphoinositide 1,5 bisphosphate (PIP2) regulates raft cytoskeletal structure by regulating proteins that control actin dynamics. Upon stimulation, PIP2 is converted to PIP3 and diacylglycerol. Ceramide mediates this clustering and insertion into the lipid bilayer by acetylation motifs.

Raft constituents change, define and determine the process of T cell activation, and maturation, as for instance the increase in raft-associated glycosphingolipid GM1. Compared to resting (CD69–CD25–) or naïve T cells (CD45RA+), activated (CD69+CD25+) or memory T cells (CD45R0+) have significantly higher GM1 levels. CD3/CD28 stimulation promotes recruitment into rafts of the Src family kinase lck, which co-localizes in rafts with glycosylphosphatidyl inositol (GPI)-anchored proteins, the adaptor protein LAT and Ras, but not with nonraft membrane proteins (e.g., protein tyrosine phosphatase, CD45). β-endorphin, which is released during stress and which significantly impairs PIP2 metabolism and associated kinase activity during T-cell activation, may alter rafts structure.

Membrane Markers of Cell Activation

T-cell activation results in change of morphology to blast cells with large cytoplasm-to-nucleus ratio, loss of CD62L, the peripheral lymph node homing receptor, expression of the integrin lymphocyte function-associated antigen (LFA)-1, and replacement of CD45RA with the maturation marker CD45R0. Activated T cells express CD69, the activation inducer molecule, a very early activation antigen (MLR-3, Leu-23), several hours before CD25 (**Figure 1**). CD69, a member of the natural killer cell family of signal-transducing receptors, is a type II transmembrane glycoprotein with a C-type lectin-binding domain in its extracellular domain. CD69 controls and regulates the expression of the interleukin (IL)-2 gene by its action downstream to the nuclear factor for activation of T cell (NFAT) and activating protein (AP)-1 transcription complexes.

Following expression of CD69, the IL-2 and CD25 genes are activated. CD25, the chain of the IL-2 receptor is expressed in high density on the cell membrane. Rafts regulate immune signaling in part by segregating cytokine receptors. The β chain of the IL-2 and the IL-15 receptors, for example, is enriched in rafts. This enrichment functionally ensures cytokine selectivity and specificity. Rafts thus assist in the

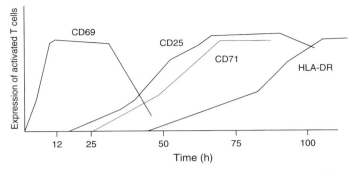

Figure 1 Comparative kinetics of expression of the membrane markers of activation, CD69, CD25, CD71, and human leukocyte antigen (HLA)-DR in activated healthy human adult T cells.

recruitment of CD25 to the vicinity of the signaling β chain, and promote formation of the (α,β,γ) high affinity IL-2 receptor complex. Activated T cells express the transferrin receptor, CD71, which is critical for the transport of iron from the extracellular environment into the cell during traversal of the DNA synthesis (S) phase. The expression of these and other membrane activation markers, including the exopeptidase CD26 (dipeptidyl peptidase IV) and CD137, the T cell co-stimulatory molecule (4–1BB) antigen, is transient, and exhibits finely controlled kinetics.

Traversal of the Cell Cycle

Successful traversal of the cell cycle depends on finely regulated biochemical pathways. At each critical juncture that signifies passage from one stage to the next, gatekeeper proteins allow or disallow the activated cell to progress. These molecular regulators are proteins, the cyclins, which associate with their respective kinase enzymes. Cyclin/cyclin-dependent kinase cdk phosphorylate key proteins that directly or indirectly modulate gene transcription and allow the activated T cell to move forward in the cycle. Cyclin D consists of a family whose members contribute to the regulation of G1/S transition. In T cells, cyclin D3 associates with either cdk4 or cdk6 late in Gap1 (G1). Cyclin D3-cdk4/6 kinase phosphorylates the retinoblastoma protein (Rb), which then releases the transcription factor E2F required for entry into the S phase and for DNA replication. For instance, at 10^{-9} M, Panax ginseng (Ginsenoside [20R]-Rg[3]Rc) blunts protein tyrosine kinase activity by 50%, impairs the phosphorylation of the retinoblastoma protein (Rb), and the expression of cyclin D3 (**Figure 2**), and leads to a threefold decrease in IL-2 production in response to CD3/CD28 stimulation. Expression of cyclin D3, and of the proliferating cell nuclear antigen (PCNA), and the phosphorylation of Rb are blunted in T cells by 0.1% ethanol, but enhanced by 12 ng ml^{-1} prolactin.

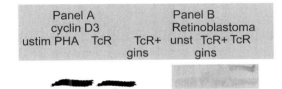

Figure 2 Modulation of cell cycle traversal by ginseng. Normal human T cells were stimulated *in vitro* with immobilized antiCD3/antiCD28 antibody, or the T-cell mitogen phytohemagglutinin, in the presence or the absence of 10^{-9} M ginsenoside Rc (Sigma) for 24 h. Cell extracts were obtained and used for assessment of cyclin D3 (panel A) or retinoblastoma (Rb) protein phosphorylation (panel B) by Western blotting with commercial monoclonal antibodies (Sta Cruz Biochemicals) to measure traversal of G₁. Note: Rb phosphorylation is measured as the ratio between the ratio of the upper, ppRb, and the lower pRb bands. TcR, T-cell receptor; PHA, phytohemagglutinin.

At 10^{-8}–10^{-7} M, the plasma levels of individuals taking ginseng herbal tea, ginseng significantly ($p < 0.05$) stimulates the expression of CD69, and induces a 60% increase in calcium/calmodulin-dependent kinase (CaM kinase) activity. Ion channels are indeed critical in the control of the membrane potential and calcium signaling, and modulate signal transduction pathways following stimulation.

The process and dynamics of cell cycle traversal is monitored by propidium iodine/bromodeoxy uridine (PI/BrdU) immunofluorescent flow cytometry analysis to obtain a timeline sequence monitoring of cells as they traverse G1, S, G2, and mitosis (M). At 10^{-6} M, ginseng has no effect on CD69 expression (4.04 ± 1.34-fold increase versus 4.30 ± 1.70-fold increase), on traversal of the cell cycle by PI/BrdU analysis (**Figure 3**), or on IL-2 production. By contrast, 10^{-6} M mercuric chloride (HgCl₂) blunts cell cycle traversal by accumulating activating T cell subpopulations in late S (% cells in S at 48 h, 76.0 ± 13.2 with control versus 91.0 ± 5.0 with HgCl₂, $p < 0.07$),

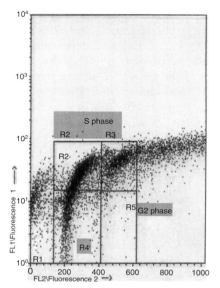

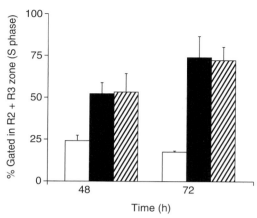

Modulation of cell cycle traversal by
10^{-6} M ginsenoside Rc

Figure 3 Modulation of cell cycle traversal by ginseng. Normal human T cells were stimulated in the presence or absence of 10^{-6} M ginseng, and the cultures were stained sequentially with propidium iodine (nuclear stain) and bromodeoxyuridine (DNA stain), followed by dual fluorescence flow cytometric analysis. Panel A shows the raw representation of the data from a representative culture, with highlighted the five regions (R1, R2, R3, R4, and R5) that constitute the population of cells traversing the phases of the cell cycle (G_1, S, G_2, and M). Panel B shows summary data of the effect of ginseng on cell cycle traversal as monitored by dual fluorescence propidium iodine/bromodeoxy uridine (PI/BrdU). Open bars, control unstimulated; closed bars, control stimulated; hatched bars, stimulated in the presence of 10^{-6} M ginsenoside.

which corresponds to a 50% drop in cell number traversing G_2 and M. However, 0.2% ethanol produces an accumulation of cells in late G1 (2.5-fold increase, compared to control).

T-Cell Memory – Cytokine Patterns

Monoclonal antibodies against CD45RA can serve to purify naïve T cells from memory T cells (93.94 ± 5.51% pure). Dual fluorescence flow cytometry is then used to monitor the maturation of T cells, i.e., the change in proportion from the naïve (CD45RA+) to the memory phenotype (CD45R0+) following CD3/CD28 stimulation. Kolmogorov-Smirnov analysis quantifies phenotypic T cell maturation. This approach has demonstrated that β-amyloid significantly ($p < 0.05$) blunts the ability of T cells to mature phenotypically.

Cytokines regulate immunity. One aspect of functional maturity of T cells, the variety of cytokines, depends on the initial antigen, and upon the physiological milieu (e.g., modulatory hormones and neuropeptides consequential to the stress response status of the organism). T helper (TH)1 and TH2 patterns of cytokine production are intertwined in terms of both their regulation and their relevance for the overall modulation of immune surveillance in health and disease.

Normal aging and aging-related dementia (e.g., dementia of the Alzheimer's type, DAT) are associated with significant changes in TH1 and TH2 cytokine production by circulating T cells. Intracellular cytokine staining, following stimulation of T cells in the presence of an inhibitor of protein transport thus retaining the cytokines inside the cell, and double-label immunofluorescence flow cytometry, reveals that normal subjects of 55–70 years of age have trace levels of cytoplasmic IL-10, interferon (IFN)γ, or IL-12 in T cells. Cohorts with DAT show significantly ($p < 0.05$) elevated levels of cytoplasmic IL-10 ($2.67 ± 1.15$ ng ml^{-1}), INFγ ($3.25 ± 2.25$ ng ml^{-1}), and IL-12 ($1.78 ± 19.00$ ng ml^{-1}) in T cells. In older (>70 years of age) patients with DAT, these levels drop to $1.99 ± 0.61$ ng ml^{-1}, $p < 0.06$; $1.25 ± 0.05$ ng ml^{-1}, $p < 0.09$; $1.04 ± 0.29$ ng ml^{-1}, $p < 0.01$ for cytoplasmic IL10, INFγ, and IL-12 in T cells, respectively. In addition, the process of immunological aging is evidently distinct in patients with DAT compared to normal subjects, and cytoplasmic levels of IL-10, IFNγ, and IL-12 in T cells rise to levels similar to their age-cohorts diagnosed with DAT in older normal subjects to $1.99 ± 0.70$ ng ml^{-1}, $2.75 ± 1.26$ ng ml^{-1}, and $1.33 ± 2.07$ ng ml^{-1}, respectively.

These changes can be attributed to a plethora of immunophysiological mechanisms within the context of stress and neuroendocrine immunity. The hypothesis has been put forward that age-associated alterations in immunity are associated with the reduction in hypothalamic dopaminergic tone with aging, related alterations in pituitary hormone, such as the anterior pituitary hormone, prolactin, and interference with the regulation of immunity. For example, 10–15 ng ml^{-1} prolactin increased IL-2 production by stimulated T cells *in vitro* close to twofold (8.15 ± 2.15 ng ml^{-1} versus 4.17 ± 1.22 ng ml^{-1}, respectively, p < 0.09). The prolactin effect is specific to Th1 cytokines, and is not obtained with the production of the TH2 cytokine, IL-4.

A third pattern of cytokines refers to the effect of certain growth factors (e.g., granulocyte macrophage colony stimulating factor; GM-CSF) in modulating the increase the production of bone marrow-derived antigen-presenting dendritic cells, and the production of IL-23 by these cells. IL-23 belongs to the IL-12 cytokine family, which shares p40, and binds to the IL12β1/IL-23R receptor complex to play a critical role in end-stage inflammation via signaling of the Janus tyrosine kinases (JAK) and signal transducers and activators of transcription (STAT) (JAK/STAT) pathway. Administration of IL-11 downregulates IL-12. IL-23 augments production of IL-17 by T cells, which becomes the significant cytokine in the involvement of T cells in inflammation. IL-17 leads to decreased neutrophilia in animal models, and *in vitro* administration of IL-17 synergizes the effects of tumor necrosis factor (TNF)-α for GM-CSF induction, for increased intercellular adhesion molecule (ICAM)-1 (CD54) expression by CD34+ progenitors, for increased neutrophil maturation, and for increased proinflammatory IL-6 and prostaglandin (PG)E2 and granulocyte-colony stimulating factor (G-CSF) growth factor production by keratinocytes and endothelial cells. IL-17 also favors increased secretion of the migration-inducing cytokine, IL-8. In human U937 cells, and probably in all lymphoid and myeloid cells, the JAK/STAT signaling pathway is responsible for transducing signals from the IL-17 receptor. Human vascular embryonic cells (HUVEC) express a homolog of IL-17R, as do ductal epithelial cells of human salivary glands, suggesting a significant role for IL-17 in immunity in the oral mucosa. In fact, in inflamed gingival tissue, IL-17 is the predominant cytokine in tissue proximal to 4–5 mm diseased periodontal pockets. IL-17 plays a critical role in immunity and mucosal inflammation, by modulating the effects of GM-CSF and other growth factors.

Migration

Cell migration is critical to immune surveillance. The migration of T cells is brought about by the concerted action of specialized factors and receptors, and is regulated by chemokines. Chemokines belong to three groups: C-X-C, C-C, and C depending on the number and position of cysteine. The first group (C-X-C) contains IL-8, growth-regulated oncogene (GRO)α, and GROβ and other chemokines with chemoattractant properties mainly, but not exclusively, towards neutrophils. The second (C-C) and third (C) groups comprise substances like monocyte chemoattractant protein (MCP)1, MCP2, MCP3, and macrophage inflammatory protein (MIP)1α and MIP1β, which mainly work on macrophages, lymphocytes, and eosinophils.

Recruitment of immune cells generally occurs by upregulating cell-surface adhesion molecule expression, such as endothelial leukocyte adhesion molecule (ELAM)-1 and increased ICAM-1, thereby enhancing cell adherence to the endothelial surface, and facilitating cell diapedesis through endothelial vessel walls. IL-8 mediates the recruitment and activation of immune cells in inflamed tissue, and increases endothelial permeability *in vitro*.

Plasma levels of IL-8 are raised in subjects with chronic alcoholism without liver disease and even more elevated in subjects with alcoholic hepatitis, who also show a rise in C-X-C chemokines. Alcohol abuse is a typical physiological stress that alters the distribution of monocytes and macrophages, and certain T-cell subsets, including a sharp decline in circulating CD4+CD62L+.

Regulation

Healthy human adult peripheral blood T cells express either CD4 or CD8. CD4 allows T cells to adhere by means of TcR to antigen-presenting cells (APC) that expose antigen in association with MHC-class 2. CD8 favors binding of the T cells to APC that present antigen via MHC-class 1. Most CD4+CD3+ cells act as TH cells, but a few CD4+ T cells are endowed with cytotoxic activity. CD8+ T cells are generally cytotoxic T lymphocytes, but they produce cytokines and growth factors that contribute to T cell-mediated immune regulation.

Membrane and Molecular Level

CD4 and CD8 are complexed lck, are members of the immunoglobulin gene superfamily, but are significantly divergent in their structure: CD4 is a monomer, while CD8 consists of two chains and occurs as a homodimer (α/α) or heterodimer (α/β). lck interacts with the CD4's 20 cytoplasmic relatively acidic residues (408–421), and with CD8α's 10 cytoplasmic residues (194–203) via ionic forces and by cysteine residues. The CD8β chain does not bind to lck. T cell stimulation leads to internalization of CD4:lck and its dissociation. The homodimeric form of CD8:lck may be internalized, but does not dissociate. The heterodimeric form of CD8:lck is not internalized, and does not dissociate. That is to say, active lck kinase is released in the cytoplasmic environment only following CD4+ cell activation.

A related src family member, fyn, associates primarily, but not exclusively with CD3, and other peptides generally implicated in the regulation of cell proliferation. The carboxyl domain of src family members exhibits a high degree of homology and contains the catalytic site. The N-terminal is unique to each peptide. The catalytic domain exhibits an adenosine triphosphate (ATP)-binding site at lysine 273, a site for autophosphorylation at tyrosine 394, and a site for tyrosine dephosphorylation mediated by CD45, or other phosphatases.

Related molecular events involved in the regulation of T cell stimulation include AkT (phosphoinositide 3-kinase, protein kinase B, PKB), the tumor suppressor, PTEN (phosphatase and tensin homolog deleted on chromosome 10, which removes phosphates primarily from lipids), Ras, mitogen-activated protein kinase (MAPK)/extracellular signal-regulated kinase (MEK), the dual threonine and tyrosine recognition kinase that phosphorylates and activates MAPK, and the novel tyrosine kinase inhibitor peptide, Tkip, a mimetic of SOCS-1 that binds to the autophosphorylation site of JAK2 and inhibits phosphorylation of STAT1α. Tkip could serve as a potentially important therapeutic target for both constitutive and IL-6-induced STAT3 activation.

Suppressors of cytokine signaling (SOCS) constitute a family of seven known cytoplasmic proteins that regulate the feedback attenuation of cytokine-mediated signal transduction. IL-2 stimulation of T cells induces signaling via JAK/STAT, and SOCS-3 inhibits the JAK/STAT cytokine signaling cascade by directly binding to it, and by preventing access to the signaling complex. IL-2 enhances SOCS-3 messenger ribonucleic acid (mRNA) and protein synthesis, and its phosphorylation on tyosine residues 204 and 221. SOCS-3 blocks the Ras/MEK activation pathway for c-fos and c-jun. Phosphorylation of SOCS-3 destabilizes its bond to proteosomes via elogin B and C, and leads to proteasomal destruction. In the 3T3 fibroblast model, activation of SOCS-1 and SOCS-3 inhibits focal adhesion kinase (FAK) activity *in vitro* and tyrosine phosphorylation of FAK. Activation of SOCS promotes polyubiquitination and degradation of FAK in a SOCS box-dependent manner. Together, these events lead to inhibited FAK-dependent signaling events, including cell motility on fibronectin.

Phosphorylation of FAK is an essential regulatory step in T-cell migration.

Another important pathway related to SOCS is the P3 member of the first forkhead-box (FOX) transcription factor (FoxP3). FoxP3 functions as a transcriptional repressor, targeting composite NFAT/AP-1 sites in cytokine gene promoters. The region responsible for NFAT inhibition has now been mapped to the N-terminus of FoxP3. Introduction of FoxP3 into conventional mouse T cells converts these cells to the regulatory T cell (Treg) phenotype (CD4+CD25+).

Cellular Level

Treg are defined phenotypically as CD4+CD25+ T cells. They constitute 7–10% of CD4+ T cells in peripheral blood from healthy donors, and can rise to up to 20% in patients with lymphoma. Depletion of CD4+CD25+ cells significantly ($p < 0.05$) enhances the proliferative response of the remaining CD4+CD25– population, but addition of sorted CD4+CD25+ cells to the CD4+CD25– T cell population blunts proliferative activity. Sorted CD4+CD25+ T cells are susceptible to apoptotic cell death, associated with low Bcl-2 expression, and prevented by IL-2 salvage.

Neuropilin-1 (Nrp1) is a plasma transmembrane receptor (120 kD) involved in axon guidance, angiogenesis, and the activation of T cells. It is a ligand to the class 3 semaphorin subfamily and the heparin-binding forms of vascular endothelial growth factor and placenta growth factor. It acts as another specific surface marker for CD4+CD25+ Treg cells. Nrp1 mediates contacts between the dendritic cells and T cells via homotypic interactions and is essential for the initiation of the primary immune response. It is constitutively expressed on the surface of CD4+CD25+ Treg cells independently of their activation status. Nrp1 is downregulated in naïve CD4+CD25– T cells following TcR stimulation.

Functionally, Treg are endowed with suppressing T-cell activation. Expression of FoxP3, the transcription factor for the scurfin protein product, is a master regulatory gene for the development and function of CD4+CD25+ subset. When transduced into T cells, FoxP3 recapitulates the hyporesponsiveness of naïve T cells, including impaired proliferation and production of cytokines including IL-2 and IL-10 upon TcR stimulation. FoxP3 is less efficient in reprogramming memory T cell subset into Treg cells, and is a reliable marker for functional Treg. Expression on the plasma membrane the glucocorticoid-induced TNF receptor (GITR) by Treg cells strongly suggests an important role for SOCS in neuroendocrine-immune regulation.

Different subsets of Treg cells have been identified. Naïve peripheral CD4+CD25− T cells can be induced *in vitro* into CD25+ anergic/suppressor cells through co-stimulation TcR and TGF-β, which induces Foxp3 gene expression. These TcR-challenged CD4+CD25− naïve can transit toward a regulatory T cell with Treg phenotype and potent immunosuppressive function. Treg are also divided into subsets according to cell-surface expression of CD62L. The suppressive function of the CD62L+ subset is far more potent on a per cell basis, can be expanded far more easily in culture, and is more responsive to chemokine-driven migration, compared to the CD62L− Treg population. Treg cells may be differentiated based on their expression of chemokine receptors, which may contribute to determine their migration properties: e.g., the traffic to and retention in bone marrow of certain Treg cells through CXCR4/CXCL12 signals.

Clinical Implications

Chemokine receptors serve as co-receptors for HIV-1 infection by binding to certain viral envelope proteins. For example, CXCR4 favors X4 HIV-1 strain tropism, and CCR5 favors tropism of R5 strain. Treg from healthy donors that express the HIV-co-receptor CCR5 are highly susceptible to HIV infection and replication. It is not surprising, therefore, that FoxP3-transduced T cells are markedly more susceptible to HIV infection, and that HIV-positive individuals with a low percentage of CD4+ and higher levels of activated T cells have greatly reduced levels of FoxP3+CD4+CD25+ T cells.

CD4+CD25+ T cells expand significantly in peripheral blood of HIV-seropositive patients receiving highly active antiretroviral therapy (HAART), and exhibit phenotypic (e.g., CD25), molecular (e.g., FoxP3), and functional characteristics (e.g., impaired proliferative and IL-2 production responses) of Treg cells. HIV-seropositive patients under HAART treatment supplemented with intermittent IL-2 show an increase of up to 79% (median, 61%) in CD4+CD25+CD69− cells, with a sharp increase in the proportion of cells expressing the CD45R0 memory phenotype, and Ki67 (proliferating cell antigen) expression.

Treg cells suppress Th1 cytokine responses, and ensure polarization of the Th2 pattern of cytokines during infection, such as schistosomiasis. A rat population of constitutive CD4+CD25+ T cells has been described that corresponds to Treg cells described in mice and humans, indicating that Treg phenomena are widespread among mammals.

Treg and T cells in general are critical to the regulation of immunity. We recall that T cells generally express either one of two major subtypes of the TcR. Most T cells in the peripheral blood and in lymphoid organs express the heterodimeric α/β chains TcR. The majority of T cells that express the TcR composed of γ/δ proteins are enriched in epithelial tissues. This distinction is evident to a lesser degree in humans, compared to other mammals (e.g., murine model). Human peripheral blood contains less than 5% of T cells that bear the γ/δ TcR subtype, and in the oro-pharyngo-gastrointestinal mucosa, γ/δ T cells predominate. T cells that express the α/β TcR contribute to the immune surveillance of mucosal tissues. For example, the demonstration that T-cell clones derived from peripheral lymph nodes, and expressing α/β TcR, preferentially home to gingival tissue following infection with the dental plaque micro-organism, *Actinobacillus actinomycetemcomitans*. This migration is blocked by anti-very late antigen (VLA)-4 antibodies. Constitutive Treg cells emerge in the peripheral blood from the thymus, and play a critical role in the control of intestinal inflammation. Lymph node-derived Treg cells can effectively counter established, severe, and progressive colitis. Syngeneic Treg cells obtained from spleens and administered to mice with colitis contribute to the resolution of the *lamina propria* inflammation, and to the reappearance of normal intestinal architecture. Treg cells proliferate in the mesenteric lymph nodes and the inflamed colon of mice under treatment. Another plaque-related organism, *Fusobacterium nucleatum*, induces a threefold increase in CD69 expression by CD4 T cells, and hence in the generation of inducible Treg, compared to a 4.15-fold activation in mitogen-stimulated control cultures. $HgCl_2$ at micromolar concentrations suppresses the *F. nucleatum*-mediated stimulation of CD69-expressing Treg by over 90%, and significantly ($p < 0.05$) blunts the production of IL-2. At supramicromolar concentrations (e.g., 10^{-5} M), $HgCl_2$ significantly ($p < 0.05$) increases the expression of CD25 by T cells by almost threefold. Taken together, these observations indicate that Treg from the peripheral and lymphoid system play an important role in the immune surveillance of inflammatory processes of mucosal immunity.

Conclusion

This article has discussed novel mechanisms of the regulation of T cell-mediated immunity. Future research in genomic, proteonomic, interactomic, and molecular cartography in general will elucidate the fundamental pathways in immunity and autoimmunity, and reveal new and improved modes of therapeutic intervention for immune-related diseases.

Acknowledgments

Support for our research efforts was obtained from the National Institutes of Health, the Alzheimer's Foundation, the MacArthur Foundation, the UCLA Psychoneuroimmunololgy program, and the UCLA Schools of Medicine and Dentistry.

Further Reading

Campos, M. and Godson, D. L. (2003). The effectiveness and limitations of immune memory: understanding protective immune responses. *International Journal of Parasitology* 33, 655–661.

Chen, W., Jin, W., Hardegen, N., et al. (2003). Conversion of peripheral CD4+CD25– naive T cells to CD4+CD25+ regulatory T cells by TGF-β induction of transcription factor Foxp3. *Journal of Experimental Medicine* 198, 1875–1886.

Chiappelli, F., Kavelaars, A. and Heijnen, C. J. (1992). β-endorphin effects on membrane transduction in human lymphocytes. *Annals of the New York Academy of Sciences* 650, 211–217.

Chiappelli, F. and Liu, N. Q. (2000). Immunity. In: Fink, G. (ed.) *Encyclopedia of stress* (vol. 2), pp. 541–547. New York: Academic Press.

Chiappelli, F., Kung, M. A., Stefanini, G. F., et al. (2000). Alcohol and immune function. In: Gershwin, M. E., German, J. B. & Keen, C. L. (eds.) *Nutrition and immunology: principles and practice*, Chap. 21, pp. 261–274. New Jersey: Humana Press.

Chiappelli, F., Prolo, P., Iribarren, J., et al. (2006). Alzheimer's disease: new frontiers for the XXI century. In: Welsh, E. M. (ed.) *Advances in psychology research*, pp. 233–258. New York: Nova Science Publisher.

Chiappelli, F., Prolo, P., Fiala, M., et al. (2006). Allostasis in HIV-1 infection and AIDS. In: Minagar, P. A. & Shapshak, P. (eds.) *Neuro-AIDS*. New York: Nova Science Publisher (in press).

Cogoli-Greuter, M., Lovis, P. and Vadrucci, S. (2004). Signal transduction in T cells: an overview. *Journal of Gravitational Physiology* 11, 53–56.

Crotty, S. and Ahmed, R. (2004). Immunological memory in humans. *Seminars in Immunology* 16, 197–203.

Eisenlohr, L. C. and Rothstein, J. L. (2005). Antigen processing and presentation. *Cancer Treatment Research* 123, 3–36.

Esche, C., Stellato, C. and Beck, L. A. (2005). Chemokines: key players in innate and adaptive immunity. *Journal of Investigative Dermatology* 125, 615–628.

Larsen, L. and Ropke, C. (2002). Suppressors of cytokine signalling: SOCS. *Acta Pathologica, Microbiologica, et Immunologica Scandinavica* 110, 833–844.

Liu, E., Cote, J. F. and Vuori, K. (2003). Negative regulation of FAK signaling by SOCS proteins. *EMBO Journal* 22, 5036–5046.

Maffei, A. and Harris, P. E. (1998). Peptides bound to major histocompatibility complex molecules. *Peptides* 19, 179–198.

Magee, T., Pirinen, N., Adler, J., et al. (2002). Lipid rafts: cell surface platforms for T cell signaling. *Biological Research* 35, 127–131.

Matsuzaki, J., Tsuji, T., Imazeki, I., et al. (2005). Immunosteroid as a regulator for Th1/Th2 balance: its possible role in autoimmune diseases. *Autoimmunity* 38, 369–375.

Meiri, K. F. (2004). Membrane/cytoskeleton communication. *Sub-Cellular Biochemistry* 37, 247–282.

Nishimura, M. I., Roszkowski, J. J., Moore, T. V., et al. (2005). Antigen recognition and T-cell biology. *Cancer Treatment Research* 123, 37–59.

Piccirillo, C. A. and Shevach, E. M. (2004). Naturally-occurring CD4+CD25+ immunoregulatory T cells: central players in the arena of peripheral tolerance. *Seminars in Immunology* 16, 81–88.

Reith, W., LeibundGut-Landmann, S. and Waldburger, J. M. (2005). Regulation of MHC class II gene expression by the class II transactivator. *Nature Reviews Immunology* 5, 793–806.

Romagnani, S. (1992). Human TH1 and TH2 subsets: Regulation of differentiation and role in protection and immunopathology. *International Archives of Allergy and Immunology* 98, 279–285.

Taams, L. S., Smith, J., Rustin, M. H., et al. (2001). Human anergic/suppressive CD4(+)CD25(+) T cells: a highly differentiated and apoptosis-prone population. *European Journal of Immunology* 31, 1122–1131.

Trowsdale, J. (2005). HLA genomics in the third millennium. *Current Opinions in Immunology* 17, 498–504.

van der Merwe, P. A. (2002). Formation and function of the immunological synapse. *Current Opinions in Immunology* 14, 293–298.

van Seventer, G. A., Salmen, H. J., Law, S. F., et al. (2001). Focal adhesion kinase regulates β1integrin-dependent T cell migration through an HEF1 effector pathway. *European Journal of Immunology* 31, 1417–1427.

Watford, W. T., Hissong, B. D., Bream, J. H., et al. (2004). Signaling by IL-12 and IL-23 and the immunoregulatory roles of STAT4. *Immunological Reviews* 202, 139–156.

Weiss, L., Donkova-Petrini, V., Caccavelli, L., et al. (2004). Human immunodeficiency virus-driven expansion of CD4+CD25+ regulatory T cells, which suppress HIV-specific CD4 T-cell responses in HIV-infected patients. *Blood* 104, 3249–3256.

Yagi, H., Nomura, T., Nakamura, K., et al. (2004). Crucial role of FOXP3 in the development and function of human CD25+CD4+ regulatory T cells. *International Immunology* 16, 1643–1656.

Zou, L., Barnett, B., Safah, H., et al. (2004). Bone marrow is a reservoir for CD4+CD25+ regulatory T cells that traffic through CXCL12/CXCR4 signals. *Cancer Research* 64, 8451–8455.

Immunomodulation *See:* Neuroimmunomodulation.

Impact of Terrorism on the Development of Mental Health Symptoms

R Yehuda
Bronx VA Medical Center, New York, NY, USA

Introduction
Relationship between Terrorism and Other Traumatic Experiences
Differentiating between Acute Mental Health Symptoms That Will Probably Abate and Those That Will Develop into Long-Term or Pathological Mental Health Consequences
Risk Factors for Chronic Posttraumatic Symptoms
The Role of Biological Studies in Helping to Identify Pathological Responses

Introduction

Because the broad goals of terrorism are ultimately psychological, it is imperative to understand the magnitude and scope of the psychological casualties in the wake of terrorism and their biological correlates so as to identify the appropriate means of immunizing people to these effects. Although the majority of people exposed to terrorism experience acute distress, the most important observation to emerge from longitudinal studies of people exposed to terrorism is that these symptoms are transient for the great majority. It therefore becomes important from a public health perspective to be able to predict those at greatest risk for long-term problems. Those at risk for long-term symptoms appear to have a more intense reaction at the time of the trauma (e.g., peritraumatic dissociation, panic, or related emotional distress), associated with a more negative appraisal of danger. It is not clear whether and to what extent pretraumatic risk factors (e.g., prior adversity, family history of psychopathology, cognitive risk factors, or preexisting personality traits) influence the intensity of the peritraumatic response to trauma, but presumably these risk factors are more relevant in situations in which exposure is less severe. Posttraumatic risk

factors, such as lack of social support, also seem to be important predictors of psychopathology, but the extent to which these reflect pre- or even peritraumatic risk factors is currently unknown.

In considering the strength of the information available regarding the psychological consequences of terrorism and their biological correlates, it is important to point to gaps in our knowledge with respect to these issues that currently preclude a thorough understanding of the psychological and biological consequences of terrorism. The first concerns whether psychological outcomes related to terrorism are comparable with those observed in the case of other traumatic events such as combat, interpersonal violence, and natural disasters, whose immediate and long-term consequences have been well established. The second concerns whether the immediate effects of terrorism are pathological, that is, requiring mental health intervention. In the absence of empirical data regarding these gaps in knowledge, governmental and privately sponsored interventions following terrorist attacks are modeled after those developed for responding to natural disasters. Thus, it is important to supply the missing information so that responses to terrorism can be tailored to the specific needs of survivors.

Relationship between Terrorism and Other Traumatic Experiences

Terrorism is a prototypic traumatic event (i.e., it meets the objective and subjective criteria as defined according to the *Diagnostic and Statistical Manual of Mental Disorders*, 4th edn., DSM-IV) for those who directly experience a threat to their life or physical integrity or who experience loss, most notably, the sudden loss of a loved one. However, terrorism is not only about life threat to single individuals, or even a small group of people; it is designed to instill fear in society at large. Thus, in addition to those who experience the effects of terrorism firsthand, there are collateral effects. People who were not in proximity to the target where the terrorist event occurred and people who were not directly affected by the loss of someone important to them can also be affected in terms of mental health outcomes, particularly because such events often receive repeated coverage on television and other media outlets. It is not known whether mental health consequences in people indirectly exposed to terrorism are qualitatively or quantitatively different from those who have been directly exposed. The additive effect of anticipatory anxiety is also not known, yet the real threat of imminent attack may be related to how quickly those exposed to terrorism can recover from its effects.

In applying knowledge from what has already been learned about the effects of other traumatic stressors, it is clear that a key variable in considering pathological outcomes is the passage of time. Although there are certainly immediate symptoms following any traumatic event, there is debate about whether and how to intervene in the acute aftermath of any trauma because, in most cases, such symptoms abate within weeks and months, and the consequences of interfering with the natural healing processes are unknown. One difference between terrorism and other traumatic events is that a single act of terrorism may represent the beginning or continuation of a situation or threat. In the context of an ongoing terrorist threat, identifying a persistent disorder may be more accurately defined only after the immediate threat of terrorism is substantially reduced in reality. This caveat does not suggest that people do not have mental health needs that should be met within this time frame; rather, it acknowledges that pathological responses that are defined by persistence and chronicity need to be considered in the context of actual ongoing threat.

Differentiating between Acute Mental Health Symptoms That Will Probably Abate and Those That Will Develop into Long-Term or Pathological Mental Health Consequences

The high rate of spontaneous recovery in the aftermath of terrorism raises an important question with respect to how initial symptoms should be understood and treated. If the initial symptoms are understood as transient reflections of distress, it is not clear that such symptoms require mental health intervention. Alternatively, it can be argued that treating early symptoms, even in those who will experience spontaneous recovery, might help prevent long-term responses in the 7–12% who generally remain symptomatic or deteriorate as the broad population begins to improve. Clarifying the causes of

high levels of immediate and long-term symptoms will no doubt lead to ideas about potential preventative treatments because it is now clear that the intensity of the exposure to trauma does not sufficiently predict who will develop or sustain symptoms.

In the absence of a linear relationship between acute stress reactions and longer-term adjustment, there are two theoretical models for pathological responses in the aftermath of a trauma. The first defines a pathological response to trauma by the persistence of the same symptoms that within a specified period of time immediately following the event would otherwise be considered normal. The second defines posttraumatic pathology by the presence of a fundamentally different initial response to stress, resulting in persistent symptoms of hyperarousal, recollection of intrusive events, and avoidance of reminders. Both models are consistent with the idea that posttraumatic mental health consequences are based on a failure to recover from the universal distress in the immediate aftermath of trauma. In the first case, the persistence of symptoms probably results from postexposure factors that prevent recovery, such as lack of social support or other coping resources. In contrast, the second model implies that the initial symptoms are fundamentally different at the outset and probably result from pre- or peritraumatic factors.

Supporting the idea that persistent responses are simply continuations of initial reactions are the findings that people who show high-magnitude posttraumatic stress disorder (PTSD) symptoms (i.e., intrusive, avoidance, and hyperarousal) in the first few days and from 1 to 2 weeks after the event are those at greatest risk for subsequent symptom severity. However, many researchers performing longitudinal studies of acute trauma survivors have not been able to identify specific symptoms that can convincingly predict pathological mental health outcomes. More promising clinical predictors appear to be the presence of a panic attack and/or intense dissociation during or immediately after a trauma, which suggests additional or fundamentally different immediate responses. Both panic attacks and dissociative responses reflect catastrophic or negative interpretations of the event. Such interpretations may further perpetuate arousal associated with stress responses and reduce the body's ability to achieve homeostasis following the trauma. The presence of catastrophic attributions (e.g., that posttraumatic symptoms signify a major problem and will not ultimately resolve) provides a way of drawing a distinction between being terrorized and being terrified. People exposed to a traumatic event are not traumatized unless they are deeply distraught at the time of the event and then make catastrophic interpretations that may result in fundamentally different biological stress responses.

Indeed, although trauma exposure certainly results in the release of stress hormones such as catecholamines and cortisol, it has been noted that dissociation and panic attacks are specifically associated with increased catecholamine levels. It may be that a peritraumatic panic attack or other intense distress during and immediately after the traumatic event leads to higher levels of stress hormones that might, in turn, strengthen traumatic memories and increase the probability of intrusive recollections. On the other hand, extreme reactions of panic and dissociation may be facilitated by relatively lower levels of stress hormones, such as cortisol, that play an important role in containing the catecholamine response to stress.

Risk Factors for Chronic Posttraumatic Symptoms

The finding that only a proportion of those exposed to trauma develop short- and long-term symptoms justifies an exploration of both the factors that increase the risk for and the factors that might serve to protect individuals from developing such symptoms following trauma exposure. Although there is not much known about the long-term consequences of terrorism specifically, there is information about factors that contribute to the development of chronic PTSD following exposure to other types of traumatic events. Putative risk factors for PTSD can describe the characteristics of the event or the response to the event or the characteristics of the people who experience those events. Indeed, a wide variety of risk factors, ranging from situational or environmental factors to familial or even genetic risk factors, for PTSD have now been identified. The identification of specific patterns of risk factors is relevant to an understanding of different types of acute reactions and for providing prophylaxis.

It appears on the basis of retrospective studies that those at greatest risk for developing chronic symptoms following a traumatic event are people with prior exposure to trauma, specific cognitive factors, and certain preexisting personality traits, such as proneness to experiencing negative emotions and having poor social supports. However, increasingly, family and genetic studies are pointing toward the role of genetic contributions to posttraumatic stress reactions. The adult children of Holocaust survivors with PTSD show a greater prevalence of PTSD to their own traumatic events than the adult children of Holocaust survivors without PTSD. It is difficult to know the extent to which increased vulnerability to PTSD in family members of trauma survivors with PTSD can be attributed to being raised by a parent with this disorder, to exposure of the fetus to the mother's stress hormones during pregnancy, or to genetic factors. Evidence that family resemblance with respect to PTSD may be at least partly explained by genes comes from twin studies in which concordance for PTSD was examined in monozygotic and dizygotic twins. However, identifying those at risk will depend on identifying how these genetic factors interact with patterns or risk factors such as childhood trauma, low educational attainment, personal or family history of anxiety or mood disorders, history of heavy alcohol use in the months prior to the incident, poor social supports in the posttraumatic period, and greater levels of exposure during the incident together with symptoms in the peritraumatic period.

The Role of Biological Studies in Helping to Identify Pathological Responses

There appears to be a distinct set of biological alterations in trauma survivors who develop chronic posttraumatic symptoms. Some of these reflect changes in stress-responsive systems that are qualitatively different than those predicted on the basis of the stress literature. Furthermore, the alterations in individuals with PTSD have been found to be distinct from those of similarly exposed individuals without PTSD and also different from those found in other psychiatric disorders, such as mood and other anxiety disorders. Together, these findings suggest that the biology of PTSD is not simply a reflection of a normative stress response but, rather, a pathological one.

For example, in contrast to the normal fear response, which is characterized by a series of biological reactions that help the body cope with, and gradually recover from, stress (e.g., high cortisol levels), some recent prospective biological studies have demonstrated that individuals who develop PTSD symptoms appear to have attenuated cortisol increases in the acute aftermath of a trauma compared to those who do not develop this disorder. Moreover, people who develop PTSD show higher heart rates in the emergency room and at 1 week posttrauma compared to those who ultimately recover, suggesting a greater degree of sympathetic nervous system activation. Thus, it may be that long-term symptoms following trauma are facilitated by a failure to contain the normal stress response at the time of the trauma, resulting in a cascade of biological alterations that lead to intrusive, avoidance, and hyperarousal symptoms.

This difficulty may occur because of pretraumatic biological risk factors.

Basic science research on both memory consolidation and fear conditioning have demonstrated that heightened adrenergic activation can promote the consolidation and retrieval of fear-provoking memories. Thus, extreme sympathetic arousal at the time of a traumatic event may result in the release of stress-related neurochemicals (including norepinephrine and epinephrine), mediating an overconsolidation of trauma memories. The enhanced elevation of catecholamines in the immediate aftermath of a traumatic event may increase the probability of intrusive recollections in the first few days and weeks posttrauma.

One of the major gaps in our knowledge concerns the interplay of biological responses at the time of a traumatic event and cognitive factors. Indeed, it is easy to see how an increased catecholaminergic response to trauma could be the proximal cause of intense panic. Furthermore, it seems plausible that people who find themselves in a more intense biological state of fear might be likely to appraise a situation as more immediately dangerous. On the other hand, it may be that preexisting cognitive factors mediate the catcholaminergic response to the trauma that leads to the panic. These preexisting cognitive factors, in turn, may or may not be the cause, result, or correlate of a preexisting biological alteration that sets the stage for an extreme response.

Clarifying the causes of high levels of immediate and long-term symptoms will no doubt lead to ideas about potential preventative treatments. For example, to the extent that panic reactions are associated with increased catecholamine responses at the time of trauma, aggressive intervention with adrenergic-blocking agents (such as propranolol) or cortisol or cognitive-behavioral stress management techniques emphasizing relaxation rather than any form of retelling (i.e., reexposure, as in debriefing) may be the most appropriate immediate interventions for people who panic in the hours immediately following a traumatic experience. For people who are not in a position to receive intervention within several hours or days posttrauma, it will be necessary to determine the impact of posttraumatic risk factors such as lack of social support on the longitudinal course of pathological responses to trauma.

Further Reading

Breslau, N., Chilcoat, H. D., Kessler, R. C., et al. (1999). Previous exposure to trauma and PTSD effects of subsequent trauma: results from the Detroit Area Survey of Trauma. *American Journal of Psychiatry* 156, 902–907.

Bryant, R. A. and Panasetis, P. (2001). Panic symptoms during trauma and acute stress disorder. *Behaviour Research Therapy* 39, 961–966.

Galea, S., Ahern, J., Resnick, H., et al. (2002). Psychological sequelae of the September 11 terrorist attacks. *New England Journal of Medicine* 346, 982–987.

Keane, T. M., Kaufman, M. L. and Kimble, M. O. (2001). Peritraumatic dissociative symptoms, acute stress disorder, and the development of posttraumatic stress disorder: causation, correlation or epiphenomena. In: Sanchez-Planell, L. & Diez-Quevedo, C. (eds.) *Dissociative states*, pp. 21–43. Barcelona: Springer-Verlag.

Schelling, G., Kilger, E., Roozendaal, B., et al. (2004). Stress doses of hydrocortisone, traumatic memories, and symptoms of posttraumatic stress disorder in patients after cardiac surgery: a randomized study. *Biological Psychiatry* 55, 627–633.

Yehuda, R. (1999). *Risk factors for posttraumatic stress disorder*. Washington, DC: American Psychiatric Press.

Yehuda, R. (2002). Post-traumatic stress disorder. *New England Journal of Medicine* 346, 108–114.

Yehuda, R., Engel, S. M., Brand, S. R., et al. (2005). Transgenerational effects of posttraumatic stress disorder in babies of mothers exposed to the World Trade Center attacks during pregnancy. *Journal of Clinical Endocrinology and Metabolism* 90, 4115–4118.

Impotence, Stress and

M R Gignac, G M Rooker and J K Cohen
Pittsburgh, PA, USA

This article is reproduced from the previous edition, volume 2, pp 547–550, © 2000, Elsevier Inc.

Overview
Physiology of Erection
Erectile Dysfunction
Evaluation and Treatment

Glossary

Erectile dysfunction (ED)	Failure to obtain sufficient erectile rigidity of the penis to allow vaginal penetration, also known as impotence.
Erection	Tumescence or engorgement of the corporal bodies leading to elongation, widening, and rigidity of the penis.
Intrinsic/ extrinsic stress	Psychological forces a person experiences. Intrinsic stress, for example, could result from guilt over marital infidelity; extrinsic stress, for example, could result from the death of one's parents.
Libido	The desire to have sex.
Nocturnal erection	Normal physiological erection of the penis that occurs subconsciously during the rapid eye movement sleep cycle and, when present, is thought to exclude organic disease as a cause of erectile dysfunction.

Overview

The inability to obtain sufficient penile rigidity to allow vaginal penetration, regardless of the cause, is termed impotence or is perhaps better described as erectile dysfunction (ED). ED is an exceedingly common problem. In fact, nearly half of all men over the age of 40 suffer from some degree of ED at various times. ED is also strongly associated with advancing age. ED is commonly related to medical conditions as well as psychological disorders, and most physicians agree that in many cases there is significant overlap. Stress in the medical literature has been defined as physical or psychological forces experienced by a person. An example of a physical force leading to ED is severe vascular disease; this leads to failure of the physical erectile mechanism. A typical psychological stress leading to ED is depression, which may not only be the cause but also the result of ED. The role stress plays in the development of ED is significant and often difficult to define.

Physiology of Erection

Neurological and Psychological Aspects

The events that lead to normal penile erection are complex and involve psychological and physiological mechanisms. Volitional erection usually begins with psychological arousal. This involves all of the senses (sight, touch, smell, taste, and hearing) as well as imagination. The sensory input arrives to special areas of the conscious brain via afferent neural pathways. In the case of positive input, the signals are used to create the sensations and fantasy associated with sexual arousal. This process can be modulated by stress and hormonal imbalance. Next are the descending pathways from the brain, leading to erection centers in the spinal cord. From the spinal cord, the pathway leads to the paired cavernosal nerves running alongside the prostate (neurovascular bundles), which are responsible for the induction of erection. This series of neural connections can collectively be termed the efferent pathway. Stimulation of the genital organs sends signals to the spinal erection center, some of which are transmitted up to the brain and others of which lead to the reflex stimulation of the cavernosal nerves. Thus, three types of penile erection are thought to exist. Psychogenic erection is the result of conscious sensory input and fantasy. Reflexogenic erection occurs by a reflex pathway in the spinal cord initiated by genital stimulation. Finally, nocturnal erections occur by an as yet unknown mechanism.

Mechanical Aspects: Penile Hemodynamics

The physiological mechanics of penile erection are fairly well understood. Essentially, the efferent neural activation leads to a change in the blood flow pattern to the penis whereby more blood is trapped in the paired erectile bodies (corpora cavernosum). Thus, there is greater inflow compared to outflow, and the penis elongates, increases in diameter, and develops sufficient rigidity for vaginal penetration. This requires normally functioning arterial, cavernosal, and venous systems. It is obvious on the basis of our current understanding of sexual function that a complex interaction must occur between the psychological and physical aspects of erection and there are many potential areas in which stress can affect the outcome.

Erectile Dysfunction

For treatment purposes, clinicians commonly classify patients as having either organic or nonorganic causes of ED. This division roughly corresponds to physical and psychological causes, respectively.

Organic and Nonorganic Erectile Dysfunction

Organic causes of ED relate to specific malfunctions in the physiological mechanisms of erection, in other words, any pathological process that affects the afferent input, efferent output, or mechanics of erection. For example, multiple sclerosis can disrupt the afferent and efferent pathways, vascular disease or antihypertensive medications can interfere with the erectile hemodynamics, and diabetes may affect multiple physiological mechanisms.

Nonorganic ED refers to problems that cannot be explained easily by the failure of physiological mechanisms; it is also commonly referred to as psychogenic impotence. This type of ED has defied universally accepted classification; however, it has been subdivided into five major categories: type 1, anxiety, fear of failure (e.g., performance anxiety); type 2, depression; type 3, marital conflict, strained relationship; type 4, ignorance and misinformation, religious scruples (e.g., about normal anatomy or sexual function); and type 5, obsessive-compulsive personality (e.g., anhedonia).

Stress and Erectile Dysfunction

The role stress plays in the causation of ED has been difficult to study and therefore information is lacking. Several commonsense inferences can be made. First, the presence of ED, regardless of the cause, leads to psychological stress such as fear of underlying disease and loss of self-image. Second, intrinsic and extrinsic causes of psychological stress can lead to physiological changes altering the afferent and efferent pathways as well as the mechanical function of erection. For example, anxiety states can be associated with higher circulating levels of catecholamines and these neurotransmitters can affect the hemodynamics of the penis, causing failure of the normal erectile mechanism. This may explain some cases of ED due to performance anxiety. Finally, emotional tone can have a strong influence on how the senses are interpreted, potentially turning positive signals into inhibition of erection; thus, stress can diminish libido profoundly.

Evaluation and Treatment

History and Physical Examination

The evaluation of patients with ED has generally been performed by either urologists or psychiatrists. With changing attitudes toward sexuality and the advancement in the science of ED, many different types of doctors now possess the appropriate evaluation and management skills. Still, however, sexual dysfunction often remains overlooked in the treatment of many patients. The initial evaluation begins with a thorough history and physical examination. In cases in which psychological factors seem to predominate, the careful elucidation of the history is especially important and often is the only means by which the psychological stress can be discovered. The encounter is best suited to a quiet, comfortable examining room and the history taken with the patient fully clothed, followed by the physical examination. This allows the interaction to occur in a minimally intimidating format. Elements of the history that are relevant include a specific description of the degree of dysfunction, duration, circumstances associated with the onset, coexisting medical problems, loss of libido, past surgeries, injuries, medications, psychiatric problems, and temporal relationship to major life events. On occasion, it is informative to interview the partner separately. The physical examination should focus on signs of systemic disease; thorough neurological evaluation; careful inspection of the genitalia, including rectal examination; and assessment for hormonal and vascular diseases.

Special Testing

On the basis of the initial interview, additional or second-line studies may be needed. These additional tests could include nocturnal penile tumescence (NPT) monitoring, injection cavernosometry and cavernosography, hormonal evaluation, and personality questionnaires.

Nocturnal penile tumescence monitoring The application of NPT monitoring is simple and can usually be performed at home by the patient. Either a one-time-use snap gauge device or an electronic monitor is applied to the penis at bedtime. The presence of normal nocturnal erections is considered proof that the mechanical aspects of penile erection are functioning appropriately. Both devices can measure the presence of an erection and, to some degree, the quality. The more sophisticated electronic monitor provides additional information, such as the number and duration of erections.

Injection cavernosometry and cavernosography Injection cavernosometry and cavernosography are invasive tests in which a vasoactive drug (e.g., prostaglandin) is injected directly into the body of the penis. The drugs work by stimulating the same hemodynamic changes as in normal erection. Before and after injection, pressures within the corporal bodies can be measured to determine an objective degree of tumescence, high-resolution ultrasound can be used to assess vascular changes, and intravenous contrast can be administered for the evaluation of venous leak.

These tests are used to detect arterial (inflow) and venous (outflow) diseases.

Both NPT and injection testing are intended to evaluate the physiological mechanism of erection. The use of these tests is directed not only by the suspected diagnosis but also, and perhaps more important, by potential therapeutic alternatives. Stated differently, extensive physiological testing affects the choice of treatment options infrequently and therefore is indicated only in select cases.

Hormonal evaluation Suspicion of a hormonal imbalance needs to be confirmed by blood tests assessing the function of the pituitary (prolactin), thyroid (thyroid hormones T_3 and T_4 and thyrotropin), and testicle (testosterone). Common abnormalities causing decreased libido include hypogonadism and hypothyroidism. It is important to note that psychological stress can decrease libido without lowering testosterone or thyroid hormone levels. If testosterone is found to be low, then prolactin should be measured; a significant elevation of prolactin can indicate a pituitary problem.

Personality questionnaires Another second line type of testing that is seldom used by urologists and occasionally used by psychiatrists is personality questionnaires. Many have been developed (e.g., the Minnesota Multiphasic Personality Inventory), and they are intended to elicit information similar to a sexual history. The use of this technique may offer advantages in assessing the degree of psychological stress. Many clinicians feel that a detailed personal interview is equally effective, if not more so, and requires less interpretation skills than these instruments. This explains their infrequent use.

Treatment

For the successful management of ED, it is necessary to understand the degree to which both psychological and physiological factors are contributing. For instance, the successful correction of anxiety disorder is helpful, but ignoring concomitant vascular disease will result in treatment failure. Likewise, the placement of a penile prosthesis can restore an adequate erection, but if the patient has a depressed mood he may not be interested in having sex. Treatment is therefore directed toward both the correction of physiological malfunctions and behavioral modification. Furthermore, managing the physiological and psychological factors must be considered in the context of available treatment options. A precise cause can often be determined, particularly when physiological disease predominates, but cannot be precisely corrected given the current limitations in treatment. Thus, in most cases of ED, treatment is directed at the symptoms and not the specific cause.

Physiological treatments There are several approaches to the physiological treatment of ED. These options, from least to most invasive, include an external vacuum erection device (VED); medications in oral pill, intraurethral pellet, and intracavernosal injection; and surgical prosthesis placement. The VED works by creating negative pressure around the penis, thereby causing blood engorgement and erection. It is useful in all types of ED and leaves no permanent changes. Various medications have been used and all affect penile hemodynamics. Oral medications leave no permanent change and effectiveness depends on the cause of ED. Typically, injection therapy is considered most reliable, but it can ultimately lead to corporal fibrosis. Penile prostheses are mechanical devices that are surgically implanted to replace the cavernosal tissue. Implants come in a variety of types, including semirigid and inflatable. In general, treatment is offered from the simplest to the most invasive, depending on the patient's wishes and therapeutic effectiveness.

A major breakthrough in ED medicament treatment was provided by the discovery that phosphodiesterase 5 (PDE5) inhibitors were effective in helping to induce penile erection. PDE5 inhibitors increase the concentration of cyclic guanosine monophosphate in the corpus cavernosum: this results in smooth muscle relaxation (vasodilation) with consequent increased inflow of blood into the corpus cavernosum and penile erection. In 1998, the FDA approved a potent PDE5 inhibitor, sildenafil ("Viagra"), as an oral treatment for ED. Since then several clinical trials, including three independent double blind controlled trials in patients with erectile dysfunction, have demonstrated that sildenafil was significantly more effective than placebo in producing sustained improvements in confidence, self-esteem, and almost normal erectile function. Other effective PDE5 inhibitors, tadalafil ("Cialis") and vardenafil ("Levitra"), are now also available and widely used for the treatment of ED.

Psychological treatment Incorporated into any ED treatment plan must be a provision for the psychological component. This is particularly relevant for ED associated with stress and is probably most useful in patients without significant organic disease. First, any discovered psychological diagnosis, such as depression, should be treated appropriately. Second, sex therapy counseling should be used, not only to uncover functional problems but also to direct intervention and alter negative patterns of behavior. Sex counseling is usually performed by therapists specially trained in sex therapy. The session or sessions will probably require both partners to participate and may involve assignments and exercises to be performed at home. The goals of this intervention are to identify and correct behavioral patterns and to develop coping skills for sources of internal and external stress. In many cases of stress-associated ED, a combination of both physiological and psychological therapies are used.

See Also the Following Article

Sexual Dysfunction.

Further Reading

Allen, J. R. (1987). Psychiatric treatment of erectile dysfunction. *Journal of the Oklahoma State Medical Association.* **80**, 19.

Althof, S. E., O'Leary, M. P., Cappelleri, J. C., Crowley, A. R., Tseng, L.-J. and Collins, S. (2006). Impact of erectile dysfunction on confidence, self-esteem and relationship satisfaction after 9 months of sildenafil citrate treatment. *The Journal of Urology* **175**, 2132–2137.

Blake, D. J. (1984). Issues in the psychiatric diagnosis and management of impotence. *Psychiatric Medicine* **2**, 109.

Hawton, K., Catalan, J. and Fagg, J. (1992). Sex therapy for erectile dysfunction: characteristics of couples, treatment outcome, and prognostic factors. *Archives of Sexual Behavior* **21**, 161.

Lue, T. F. (1998). Physiology of penile erection and pathophysiology of erectile dysfunction and priapism. In: Walsh, P. C., et al. (eds.) *Campbell's urology* (7th edn., pp. 1157–1179). Philadelphia: Saunders.

Tiefer, L. and Schuetz-Mueller, D. (1995). Psychological issues in diagnosis and treatment of erectile disorders. *Urologic Clinics of North America* **22**, 767.

Impulse Control

I-M Blackburn
Newcastle Cognitive and Behavioral Therapies Centre, Newcastle upon Tyne, UK

This article is reproduced from the previous edition, volume 2, pp 551–553, © 2000, Elsevier Inc.

Problems Associated with Uncontrolled Anger
Assessment of Anger
Methods of Anger Control
Conclusion

Glossary

Cognitive behavior therapy	A short-term psychotherapy for emotional disorders that aims at symptomatic, affective, and behavioral improvement through the evaluation and modification of an individual's dysfunctional way of processing information.
Idiographic measures	Measures that are not standardized but are devised to assess problems specific to an individual.
Nomothetic scales	Scales validated and standardized in normals and specific comparison groups, yielding norms for different client populations.

Impulse control can relate to several aspects of behavior, for example, anger, substance abuse, repeated self-harm, or suicidal attempts. Anger control is the primary concern of this article.

Problems Associated with Uncontrolled Anger

Anger can be seen as a normal emotional reaction experienced universally by adults and children, as well as by animals. As such, it serves a useful purpose in letting others know that their behavior is aversive so that they can alter their behavior if amicable or respectful relationships are to be maintained or restored. Anger directed at the self allows one to register unpleasant arousal, perhaps at transgressing one's own rules, again allowing for changes to occur. Anger or hostility can be seen as being composed of affective (irritability, full blown anger), physiological (increased arousal), cognitive ("you should not do that," "you are overstepping the mark"), and behavioral (sarcasm, verbal abuse, assault) components. It is when these interacting components reach the point at which anger and hostility are no longer controllable and are expressed in ways that entail negative social and interpersonal consequences that they become a problem. Thus, in the clinic, patients complain of their increased irritability, of anger being provoked by minor triggers, and of their fear of catastrophic consequences. In forensic settings, anger and impulse control are often the main treatment targets.

Anger and hostility have not been widely studied in the clinical literature, relative, say, to depression and anxiety. However, the rising rates of violent crime among adolescents, acts of uncontrolled anger as seen in road rage, violent familial discord, child abuse, and assaults have made uncontrolled anger and hostility a topical subject in the media. Moreover, poorly managed anger has been linked convincingly with a number of health problems, such as coronary artery disease and essential hypertension. Friedman and Rosenman postulated that type A behavior, characterized by striving for achievement, competitiveness, vigilance, impatience, and easily aroused hostility, predicted coronary heart disease (CHD). The wealth of research that followed has implicated anger and hostility as the component of the type A complex that best predicts CHD and mortality in general.

Several explanations have been put forward to explain the link between hostility/anger and health. The psychophysiological reactivity model proposes that hostile individuals react to stressors with extreme cardiovascular and neuroendocrine responses, which, over time, lead to the development of CHD and CHD symptoms such as myocardial infarction and angina. The psychosocial vulnerability model implicates increased interpersonal stressors and decreased social support, both at work and in daily life. The transactional model integrates the first two models – the hostile individual elicits negative reactions from others, which helps to confirm his or her views of others as antagonistic, increasing hostile tendencies further. Thus, there is a reciprocal relation between the cognitive and behavioral aspects of hostility, leading to increasingly exaggerated cardiovascular and endocrine reactions to intensifying interpersonal stressors. In a study of male patients with postmyocardial infarction and unstable angina, Hall and Davidson found that patients who had higher scores on a measure of hostile style, as rated during a standard interview, perceived the interviewer as more aggressive, although this perception was not corroborated by an independent rater.

Assessment of Anger

The assessment of anger in research studies is usually by standard interview or by nomothetic scales. Some studies have used physiological measures, such as systolic blood pressure in response to potentially anger-arousing stimuli; others have used observers' ratings of facial expressions or behavioral measures, such as hand dynamometer readings.

Interview methods are not validated easily, are time-consuming to administer, and are costly in terms of interviewer training and scoring. Self-rated questionnaires, tested psychometrically for their validity and reliability, have been most widely used. The Cook–Medley hostility scale relates more to cognitive than behavioral aspects of anger; in particular, high scores reflect a negative view of disparagement by others. The Buss–Durkee hostility inventory attempts to measure angry cognitions as well as the verbal and physical expression of anger. Anger, as a trait, can

be assessed by the trait anger scale, which measures cognitive and affective aspects of anger. Novaco developed the anger inventory to measure anger in response to a wide range of potential provocations. Deffenbacher and colleagues have devised a number of idiographic measures to assess anger in day-to-day living; the most intense, ongoing source of anger for the individual; and anger-related physiological arousal. These three idiographic measures are correlated positively with one another and with other indices.

More recently, Snyder and colleagues have developed a scale to measure hostile automatic thoughts (HAT). Automatic thoughts, as described by Beck, are the characteristic self-statements or images that flash into individuals' minds in reaction to external and internal triggers. They are not controlled, occur as reflexes, and are the products of assumptions, attitudes, and beliefs regarding ourselves and the world that derive from our past experiences. The HAT consists of 30 items, rated on five-point likert scales (1, not at all; 5, all the time), reflecting hostile thoughts that involve physical aggression, derogation, and revenge toward other people. It has been shown to be psychometrically valid and reliable.

Self-report measures are easy to administer and score, but they are not immune to faking if respondents desire to present themselves favorably. Hostility is generally considered to be socially undesirable, and low scores on hostility scales may be the result of faking good. This methodological issue may be resolved using a variety of scales that have been shown to be psychometrically sound, as well as using behavioral and observer ratings.

Methods of Anger Control

The majority of anger treatment outcome studies have used a cognitive-behavioral approach, involving methods aimed at reducing the occurrence of anger, regulating levels of arousal when angry, developing new skills in the face of provocation, and preventing conflictual situations from escalating. These treatment approaches have variously been labeled as stress inoculation training, based on Meichanbaum's methods for modifying self-statements in anxious patients; inductive social skills training, based on the principles of cognitive therapy; or cognitive relaxation coping skills. All these approaches have a lot in common, putting more or less emphasis on different aspects of cognitive-behavior therapy (CBT). Treatment can be applied individually or in groups.

Engaging the patient in treatment is of primary importance because patients with more anger are typically suspicious, avoidant, and provoking. Patients need to develop trust in the therapist, learn to differentiate between different types and levels of affect by self-observation and self-monitoring, recognize the costs of uncontrolled anger, and thus become motivated to change. Following this preparatory phase of treatment, various cognitive and behavioral methods are used. Cognitive restructuring aims to help patients modify their appraisals of threat and provocation, develop appropriate problem-solving thinking, adopt coping self-statements, and modify their basic attitudes regarding themselves and others.

To reduce arousal, methods such as controlled breathing, muscle relaxation, using relaxation imagery, and engaging in alternative tension-reducing activities are taught. Clients need to develop coping skills other than violent expressions of anger. These may include strategic withdrawal, negotiation, appropriate verbal and nonverbal communication, and respectful assertiveness.

In a recent meta-analytic study, Beck and Fernandez analyzed 50 studies incorporating 1640 subjects, published from 1970 to 1995, that used CBT. They reported a grand mean weighted effect size of 0.70, indicating that the average CBT client did better than 76% of untreated subjects in terms of anger reduction. This effect was statistically significant, robust, and relatively homogeneous across studies.

Conclusion

Anger, as other negative impulses, can be viewed as an affective stress reaction with cognitive and behavioral determinants. It can lead, when uncontrolled, to important catastrophic social, interpersonal, and physical health outcomes. Although ignored for a long time compared to other negative emotions such as depression and anxiety, it has been the subject of increasing interest in psychological and psychotherapeutic research.

See Also the Following Articles

Anger; Cognitive Behavioral Therapy; Hostility; Stress Management and Cardiovascular Disease; Type A Personality, Type B Personality.

Further Reading

Beck, R. and Fernandez, E. (1998). Cognitive behavioral therapy in the treatment of anger: a meta-analysis. *Cognitive Therapy and Research* **22**, 63–74.

Buss, A. H. (1961). *The psychology of aggression.* New York: John Wiley.

Cook, W. W. and Medley, D. M. (1954). Proposed hostility and pharisaic virtue scales for the MMPI. *Journal of Applied Psychology* **38**, 414–418.

Deffenbacher, J. L. and Stark, R. S. (1992). Relaxation and cognitive-relaxation treatments of general anger. *Journal of Counseling Psychology* **39**, 158–167.

Deffenbacher, J. L., Story, D. A., Brandon, A. D., et al. (1988). Cognitive and cognitive-relaxation treatments of anger. *Cognitive Therapy and Research* **12**, 167–184.

Deffenbacher, J. L., Thwaites, G. A., Wallace, T. L., et al. (1994). Social skills and cognitive-relaxation approaches to general anger reduction. *Journal of Counseling Psychology* **41**, 386–396.

Friedman, M. and Rosenman, R. H. (1974). *Type A behavior and your heart.* New York: Knopf.

Hall, P. and Davidson, K. (1996). The misperception of aggression in behaviorally hostile men. *Cognitive Therapy and Research* **20**, 377–389.

Novaco, R. W. (1975). *Anger control.* Lexington, MA: Heath.

Novaco, R. W. (1979). The cognitive regulation of anger and stress. In: Kendall, P. C. & Hollon, S. D. (eds.) *Cognitive behavioral interventions, theory, research, and procedures,* pp. 241–285. New York: Academic Press.

Snyder, C. R., Crowson, J. J., Houston, B. K., et al. (1997). Assessing hostile automatic thoughts: development and validation of the HAT scale. *Cognitive Therapy and Research* **21**, 477–492.

Spielberger, C. D. (1988). *State-trait anger expression inventory.* Orlando, FL: Psychological Assessment Resources.

Incest

A P Mannarino
Allegheny General Hospital, Pittsburgh, PA, USA

This article is a revision of the previous edition article by A P Mannarino, volume 2, pp 554–557, © 2000, Elsevier Inc.

Incest: Definition and Descriptive Characteristics
Diagnosis
The Psychological Impact of Incest
Treatment of Incest Victims

Glossary

Incest	A type of sexual abuse in which the abuser is a family member.
Nonoffending parent	The nonabusive parent, who typically has custody of the child.
Perpetrator	The family member who abuses the child.
Posttraumatic stress disorder (PTSD)	A stress disorder that includes three categories of psychiatric symptoms in response to a traumatic life event.
Sexual abuse	Sexual exploitation involving physical contact between a child and another person.

Incest: Definition and Descriptive Characteristics

Sexual abuse can be defined as sexual exploitation involving physical contact between a child and another person. Exploitation implies an inequality of power between the child and the abuser on the basis of age, physical size, and/or the nature of the emotional relationship. There can also be noncontact sexual abuse, which includes exposing a child to pornography, taking photographs or videotaping a child for sexual purposes, or sexual exploitation through the Internet.

Incest is a type of sexual abuse in which the abuser is a family member. The abuser may be a parent, stepparent, grandparent, older sibling, or other close relative. Sociological surveys by Finkelhor and others have suggested that 25–30% of all girls and 10–15% of all boys are sexually abused by the age of 18. The proportion of sexual abuse that is incestuous in nature is not absolutely known, but in clinical studies it seems to account for approximately one-half of all reported cases.

Incest is not limited to sexual intercourse. It also includes oral or anal intercourse, fondling of the breasts or genitals, and sexualized, inappropriate kissing. The empirical literature suggests that approximately 50% of incest cases involve oral, anal, or vaginal intercourse while the other half involve genital fondling. Violence is not typically perpetrated against a child victim as part of an act of incest, although threats of violence are common. A child may be coerced to participate in a sexual experience through the promise of rewards or the threat of punishment. In some families, children who are sexually abused may also be physically abused or witness domestic violence.

Children may be victimized by incest at any age. Despite the public misconception that only girls are victimized, boys may also be subjected to an incestuous relationship. The great majority of perpetrators of incest are male, with statistics suggesting that males account for 90% or more of reported cases. The severity of incest can vary from one episode of genital touching to hundreds of episodes of sexual abuse, including intercourse, which may extend over many years. Although incest is commonly reported across all socioeconomic classes, studies by Finkelhor have demonstrated that poor children are more vulnerable to this type of victimization.

Diagnosis

In the nomenclature of the American Psychiatric Association (*Diagnostic and Statistical Manual*, 4th edn.-TR), sexual abuse or incest is not usually considered to be a primary diagnosis (axis I) but is classified as a psychosocial stressor (axis IV) that may contribute to the primary diagnosis. (However, in situations in which the sexual abuse of the child is the primary focus of clinical attention, it can be coded on axis I.) Children who are victimized by incest do not manifest a unitary syndrome of traits, characteristics, or symptoms. Although, as a group, incest victims display more emotional and behavioral symptoms than normal children, these problems are typically diverse in nature. Moreover, approximately 30% of all incest victims are asymptomatic. Sexual preoccupation or sexualized behaviors are more common in incest victims than nonvictims, but the latter group may exhibit these problems as well. Overall, the general conclusion is that incest cannot be diagnosed based solely on the symptom presentation.

On medical examination, less than 20% of all incest victims display significant clinical findings. Even in cases in which the victim has been vaginally or anally penetrated, significant physical findings may not be present. Accordingly, the absence of significant physical findings does not mean that incest has not occurred.

Determining that incest has occurred is a complex legal and clinical problem. With very young children, they may engage in sexualized behaviors and only disclose alleged abuse after being questioned by the nonoffending parent. Older children may disclose the alleged victimization to a friend, relative, teacher, or other trusted adult. In the great majority of incest cases, the alleged perpetrator initially denies the victimization. In the absence of significant medical findings or a perpetrator confession, it is ultimately very difficult to prove that incest has occurred.

Interviewing the alleged victim is the most frequent method used to determine whether incest has been perpetrated. The nonoffending parent typically provides background data and information about what the child has previously disclosed. If the alleged perpetrator is a parent, he or she may also be interviewed; however, it is recommended that this be done at a separate time from the alleged victim. Most experts recommend that a comprehensive evaluation, including interviews with both parents, be conducted when incest is disclosed in the context of divorce or custody issues.

Over the past 15 years, many concerns have been generated regarding the procedures used to interview alleged sexual abuse and incest victims. Questions have been raised about children's memory and their ability to recall accurately what allegedly occurred. Laboratory research related to this issue has provided mixed results, with some studies suggesting that children do accurately recall the core features of significant events and other studies indicating that children can produce inaccurate information, particularly in response to repetitive or coercive-like questions. In this regard, criticism sometimes has been directed at child protective service workers, mental health consultants, and other investigative interviewers for allegedly pressuring children to make abuse disclosures or for using inappropriate interviewing techniques (i.e., leading questions). Unfortunately, with the exception of some highly publicized cases, it is impossible to know how often investigations of sexual abuse and incest have been contaminated by improper interview strategies.

In light of the significant issues related to interview methods, some professional guidelines have been promulgated to address this problem. For example, the American Professional Society on the Abuse of Children has developed guidelines for the evaluation of suspected sexual abuse in children, and the American Academy of Child and Adolescent Psychiatry has established practice parameters for the forensic evaluation of children and adolescents who may have been physically or sexually abused. Although it is impossible to know to what degree investigative interviewers are aware of and follow these guidelines, in the past few years there seem to be fewer concerns about inappropriate interviewing procedures.

The Psychological Impact of Incest

As mentioned earlier, children who have been victimized through an incestuous relationship may display a variety of emotional and/or behavioral difficulties subsequent to disclosure. Despite the diversity of the symptom presentation of this population, a number of studies have reported that 20–50% of sexual abuse and incest victims meet full or partial criteria for PTSD. The symptoms of PTSD fall into three categories: re-experiencing symptoms (i.e., intrusive thoughts, nightmares, and flashbacks), avoidance symptoms (i.e., avoid thoughts or feelings about the trauma, emotional detachment, and inability to recall important aspects of the trauma), and symptoms of increased arousal (i.e., sleep disturbance, hypervigilance, and difficulty concentrating). Other psychiatric sequelae of incest may include clinical depression, other anxiety disorders, low self-esteem, sexually reactive behaviors, and, for adolescents, substance abuse problems.

Recent studies have suggested that the frequency and severity of psychiatric symptoms in sexual abuse and incest victims may be mediated by their attributions and perceptions related to the victimization. Thus, victims who feel different from other children, who blame themselves for the abuse, who feel that others do not believe what they say, or have a decreased amount of interpersonal trust are at higher risk for

more serious symptomatology. In particular, children who feel that they are to blame for the victimization are more vulnerable to experiencing depressive disorders.

Legal proceedings may also have an impact on outcome. There is some evidence that when legal proceedings are delayed, emotional/behavioral symptoms in sexual abuse victims tend to increase. Also, when children have to testify in court and are subjected to a very hostile cross-examination or are required to testify multiple times, psychiatric symptomatology appears to worsen.

The psychological impact of being victimized by an incestuous relationship may be moderated by several factors. A number of major studies have demonstrated that emotional support of the victim from the nonoffending parent, which includes not blaming the child for the victimization, has a highly beneficial effect and is correlated with fewer psychiatric symptoms in the victim. Also, as we would anticipate, many nonoffending parents have highly intense emotional reactions to their child's disclosure of incest. These emotional reactions may include anxiety, guilt, anger, and shame. Recent empirical investigations have shown that, when nonoffending parents are able, over time, to resolve their emotional upset related to their child's victimization, this correlates with a reduction in the frequency and severity of the child's emotional and behavioral symptoms.

Treatment of Incest Victims

The treatment of incest may involve a variety of interventions, including individual and/or group therapy for the child victim, supportive therapy with the nonoffending parent, counseling for the perpetrator, and family therapy. Space does not permit a discussion of perpetrator treatment, except to say that most incest perpetrators initially deny victimizing the child and/or minimize its impact and typically require long-term therapy to address their difficulty in taking responsibility for the abuse, cognitive distortions, and issues related to potential relapse.

With the increased attention to and reporting of sexual abuse over the past two decades in the United States, a proliferation of clinical programs has occurred that focus on victim treatment. Unfortunately, the efficacy of the interventions offered in most of these programs has not been investigated. Nonetheless, there is now strong empirical evidence that Trauma-Focused Cognitive Behavioral Therapy (TF-CBT) is an efficacious treatment for sexual abuse and incest victims. Specifically, TF-CBT has been found to be superior to nondirective supportive therapy in reducing PTSD, depressive symptoms, shame, and general behavioral difficulties in the victimized child and parental distress and depressive symptoms in the nonoffending caretaker. This pattern of results has been replicated in a large multisite study of sexual abuse victims, most of whom had also been subjected to other traumatic events.

There are a number of core components of TF-CBT. These include psychoeducation, stress reduction strategies (e.g., relaxation training), creating a trauma narrative, cognitive processing to address inappropriate attributions (i.e, self-blame), and the development of safety and other coping skills.

Work with the nonoffending parent is an essential component of TF-CBT for sexual abuse and incest victims. Critical interventions with the nonoffending parents include addressing their attributions about the sexual abuse, enhancing their support of the victimized child, and behavioral management strategies.

In some treatment programs for incest families, family therapy is the intervention of choice. This is true even though family treatment has not been widely investigated empirically as a potentially effective therapeutic strategy for incestuous families. Family therapy for incest is based on the belief that family dynamics either contribute to the occurrence of the incestuous situation, help maintain the secrecy of the incestuous relationship, or can be changed to prevent future episodes of victimization. The perpetrator of the abuse may be included in family treatment, especially if there is a possibility of family reunification. However, the inclusion of the perpetrator in family sessions would typically occur only after the perpetrator has experienced extensive individual and/or group treatment and has been willing to accept total responsibility for the victimization.

See Also the Following Articles

Child Sexual Abuse; Familial Patterns of Stress; Sexual Assault.

Further Reading

American Academy of Child and Adolescent Psychiatry (1997). Practice parameters for the forensic evaluation of children and adolescents who may have been physically or sexually abused. *Journal of the American Academy of Child and Adolescent Psychiatry* 36, 432–442.

American Professional Society on the Abuse of Children (1990). *Guidelines for psychosocial evaluation of suspected sexual abuse in young children*. Chicago: Author.

American Psychiatric Association (2000). *Diagnostic and statistical manual* (4th edn.). Washington, DC: American Psychiatric Press.

Bruck, M. and Ceci, S. J. (1998). Reliability and credibility of young children's reports: From research to policy and practice. *American Psychologist* 53, 136–151.

Cohen, J. A., Deblinger, E. and Mannarino, A. P. (2005). Trauma-focused cognitive behavioral therapy for sexually abused children. In: Hibbs, E. & Jensen, P. (eds.) *Psychosocial treatments for child and adolescent disorders: empirically-based strategies for clinical practice.* (2nd edn., pp. 743–765). Washington, DC: American Psychological Association.

Cohen, J. A., Deblinger, E., Mannarino, et al. (2004). A multisite, randomized controlled trial for sexually abused children with PTSD symptoms. *Journal of the American Academy of Child and Adolescent Psychiatry* 43, 393–402.

Cohen, J. A. and Mannarino, A. P. (1996). A treatment outcome study for sexually abused preschool children: initial findings. *Journal of the American Academy of Child and Adolescent Psychiatry* 35, 42–50.

Deblinger, E., Lippman, J. and Steer, R. (1996). Sexually abused children suffering PTSD symptoms: initial treatment outcome findings. *Child Maltreatment* 1, 310–321.

Finkelhor, D. and Baron, L. (1986). Risk factors for child sexual abuse. *Journal of Interpersonal Violence* 1, 43–71.

Mannarino, A. P. and Cohen, J. A. (1996). Abuse-related attributions and perceptions, general attributions, and locus of control in sexually abused girls. *Journal of Interpersonal Violence* 11, 162–180.

Runyan, D. K., Hunter, W. M. and Everson, M. D. (1992). Impact of legal intervention on sexually abused children. *Journal of Pediatrics* 113, 647–653.

Saywitz, K. J., Goodman, G. S. and Lyon, T. D. (2002). Interviewing children in and out of court: current research and practice implications. In: Myers, J. E. B., Berliner, L., Briere, J., Hendrix, C. T., Tenny, C. & Reid, T. A. (eds.) *The APSAC handbook on child maltreatmen* (2nd edn., pp. 349–377). Thousand Oaks, CA: Sage.

Saywitz, K. J., Mannarino, A. P., Berliner, L., et al. (2000). Treatment for sexually abused children and adolescents. *American Psychologist* 55, 1040–1049.

Income Levels and Stress

S V Subramanian and I Kawachi
Harvard School of Public Health, Boston, MS, USA

Absolute Income and Health
Relative Income and Health
Income Inequality and Health
Income and Health: The Role of Social Comparisons

Glossary

Absolute income	The measure of the actual income of the individual; linked to the absolute income hypothesis.
Absolute income hypothesis	The idea that health of individuals depends on their own (and only their own) level of income.
Comparative group	The social group to which an individual compares him- or herself.
Income inequality	The measure of the extent of income dispersion in a society or a community; measures such as Gini coefficient are summary measures that quantify the extent of income dispersion in a society.
Membership group	The social group of which an individual feels a part.
Neomaterialist theory	A theory that emphasizes the importance of access to tangible material conditions, both elementary (e.g., food, shelter, and access to services and amenities) and nonelementary (e.g., car and home ownership and access to telephones and the Internet).
Normative group	The social group from which a person takes his or her standards or norms; this could be either the membership or the comparative group.
Pyschosocial effects	The direct or indirect effects of stress stemming from either being lower on the socioeconomic hierarchy or living in conditions of relative socioeconomic disadvantage, which facilitates constant social comparisons.
Relative deprivation	The condition in which individuals or groups subjectively perceive themselves to be unfairly disadvantaged compared to others who they perceive as having similar attributes and deserving similar rewards (typically their reference groups or groups to whom they typically compare themselves).
Relative income	The measure of the income of the individual in relation to the incomes of others in the society or group in which the individual resides. It is linked to the relative income hypothesis.
Relative income hypothesis	The idea that health depends not just on an individual's own level of income but also on the incomes of others in society.
Social comparison	The metric that results from an individual's self-comparison of some other individual or group of individuals on certain dimension, such as income, education, and material possessions.

Differential exposure to stressors is one of the links through which income is associated with health. Income can be conceptualized in absolute or relative terms, with each having distinct mechanisms through which income is hypothesized to influence stressful experiences, thereby affecting health.

Absolute Income and Health

The absolute income hypothesis posits that:

$$h_i = f(y_i), \quad f_i' > 0, \quad f_i'' < 0 \qquad (1)$$

where h_i is an individual's level of health, and y_i is that individual's own level of income. The relationship between individual income and individual health is concave; that is, every additional dollar is associated with diminishing returns to health. The relationship of individual income to health outcomes is often described as a gradient – at each level of income, individuals experience better health than those immediately below them. On the other hand, to describe the association between income and health as a gradient is possibly misleading because the relationship has been shown to be nonlinear; that is, there are diminishing returns to health improvement with additional rises in income. The concave relationship between income and health has been corroborated in numerous empirical demonstrations, in affluent countries as well as in poor countries. The absolute income hypothesis has been closely associated with the neomaterialist interpretation of the relationship between income and health, which posits that income matters for health because it confers on individuals the ability to purchase goods and services (e.g., health insurance, housing, and nutritious foods) that are necessary for maintaining health, even though the absolute income hypothesis could equally well have a psychosocial effect.

We can also posit a societal or community-level analog of the absolute income hypothesis, such that:

$$h_{ij} = f(Y_j, y_{ij}) \qquad (2)$$

where the health of individual i in community j is now hypothesized to be a function of not just his or her own income (y_{ij}) but also of the average income level of the community (Y_j) in which the individual resides. Indeed, a neomaterialist interpretation of the absolute income hypothesis need not be restricted to the availability of income at the individual level; it can also reflect the presence or absence of collective infrastructure at a population or community level. Deprived communities (i.e., communities with high levels of absolute poverty) are less likely to have services and amenities (e.g., health clinics and supermarkets) that are essential for protecting and promoting the health of their residents. Even if an individual resident is not poor, his or her health may be detrimentally affected by living in such a community. A growing number of multilevel studies have now demonstrated that community poverty is linked to higher mortality, higher morbidity, and a more adverse pattern of health behaviors, even after taking into account individual incomes.

Relative Income and Health

In contrast to the absolute income hypothesis, the relative income hypothesis posits that:

$$h_i = f(y_i - y_r) \qquad (3)$$

where health of an individual i is a function of the term $(y_i - y_r)$, which denotes the relative gap between an individual's income y_i and the income of some reference population y_r. The reference population could be the income of coworkers, neighbors, or the national population. The concept of relative deprivation was first rigorously formulated by Runciman. According to Runciman, "we can roughly say that A is relatively deprived of X when (i) he does not have X, (ii) he sees some other person or persons, which may include himself at some previous or expected time, as having X (whether or not this is or will be in fact the case), (iii) he wants X, and (iv) he sees it as feasible that he should have X" (Runciman, 1966: 10).

Runciman further conceptualizes the concept of relative deprivation in terms of magnitude, frequency and degree. "The magnitude of the relative deprivation is the extent of the difference between the desired situation and that of the person desiring it (as he sees it). The frequency of a relative deprivation is the proportion of a group who feel it. The degree of a

relative deprivation is the intensity with which it is felt" p.10.

Runciman went on to elaborate three types of reference groups. The first is the membership group, of which an individual feels a part; the second is the normative group, "the group from which a person takes his standards" (Runciman, 1966: 12); and the third is the comparative group, which is the group to which an individual compares him- or herself. Significantly, these different sources of relative comparisons may well coincide, as in Runciman's example of members of the middle class who aspire to be aristocracy and who try to emulate the behavior of the upper class (the normative reference) as well as to attain their status (the comparative reference). Building on these sources of relative comparisons, he further proposed two forms of relative deprivation, depending on the source: egoistic deprivation (relative deprivation of an individual with respect to his or her own group) and fraternalistic deprivation (relative deprivation of an individual's own group compared to other groups in society).

Note that relative deprivation theory, as the phrase suggests, presumes that individuals typically make relative comparisons of themselves to those who are better off than they are and not to those who are worse off. The latter comparison is referred to as relative gratification or relative satisfaction. Indeed, relative deprivation measures happen to be correlated with relative satisfaction.

Although the theory of relative deprivation is quite sophisticated, the empirical identification of reference groups has proved tricky. Empirically, the relative income hypothesis has been operationalized using variations of equation (3), with an important operationalization provided by Yitzhaki, following Runciman's theory. Thus, for a person i with income y_i who is part of a reference group with N people, Yitzhaki's index is given as:

$$RD_i = (1/N)\sum_j (y_j - y_i), \quad \forall y_j > y_i \qquad (4)$$

where the amount of relative deprivation (RD) for individual i is the sum of the incomes of j individuals who have incomes higher than that individual. The summation in equation (4), $\sum_j (y_j - y_i)$, is divided by the number of people in the reference group, N, making the measure invariant to size. If income is the object of relative comparison, then we can assess relative income deprivations by groups, based on, for instance, the state of residence, age group, race, educational attainment, gender, or occupation.

The British Whitehall Study of civil servants is frequently cited as evidence showing the health effects of relative deprivation (even though the study did not include any specific or explicit measures of relative deprivation). In that study, relatively lower-ranked civil servants were shown to have three times the mortality rate as the highest ranked civil servants, despite having access to the same National Health Service. Moreover, none of the subjects in the civil service cohort was deprived in an absolute sense; that is, they all had adequate nutrition, housing, and access to other material amenities. The mortality differential between civil service grades was thus attributed – at least in part – to the adverse psychosocial consequences of relative deprivation. Indeed, systematic tests suggest that people do take into account relative income position when making real-life decisions such as choosing between two earning schemes. For instance, Frank and Sunstein (2001) hypothesized two possible scenarios. In scenario A, the individual earns $110,000 per year and others earn $200,000; in scenario B, the individual earns $100,000 per year (less than in world A), but others earn only $85,000. Contrary to traditional economic perspective (wherein world A should be preferable because it offers higher absolute consumption), a substantial number of respondents opted for world B.

As we mentioned earlier, the absolute income hypothesis tends to be interpreted in materialist terms, whereas the relative income hypothesis tends to be interpreted in psychosocial terms. This dichotomy is unwarranted. For instance, the absolute income hypothesis is equally compatible with the psychosocial interpretation. That is, if lower income is associated with more stess (e.g., inability to pay the bills and to plan for the future), then an individual could end up with an income–health gradient even if no social comparison is taking place.

Analogously, the relative deprivation hypothesis could also be interpreted both ways (neomaterial as well as psychosocial). That is, an individual's social comparison to a reference group could be stressful (the psychosocial interpretation) or he or she may be unable to function in society because of limited access to material commodities (e.g., car ownership, Internet access, or air conditioning). For example, rising community living standards are often associated with an enlargement of the range of consumer goods that are necessary for an individual to function as a member of that community. Many consumer goods, such as central heating/air conditioning, telephone, and access to the Internet, have followed this trajectory, starting out as luxury goods and eventually ending up as necessities. Even if an individual is not deprived in any absolute sense (i.e., has adequate nutrition and housing), relative deprivation (compared to the standard basket of commodities that everyone else has access to) could adversely affect his or her health. In this sense, relative deprivation may affect health

because it reflects the ability of affected individuals to access material goods and services that in turn promote well-being. This underscores the futility of distinguishing material from psychosocial effects of income – any effect of income on health could be simultaneously operating through material as well as psychosocial pathways.

Income Inequality and Health

The community-level analog of relative deprivation leads us to the idea of income inequality, which can be stated as:

$$h_{ij} = f(I_j, y_{ij}) \qquad (5)$$

where I_j refers to summary measure of income distribution (e.g., the Gini coefficient) for community j in which the individual resides. Income inequality and relative deprivation are conceptually related because, as income inequality rises, those at the bottom end of the distribution become more relatively deprived. Various measures are available to quantify the extent of income inequality in a given community or society; of these, the Gini coefficient is frequently used. Algebraically, the Gini coefficient is defined as one-half of the arithmetic average of the absolute differences between all pairs of incomes in a population, the total then being normalized on the mean income. If incomes in a population are distributed completely equally, the Gini value is 0; and if one person has all the income (the condition of maximum inequality), the Gini is 1.0. The Gini coefficient can also be illustrated through the use of Lorenz curve (**Figure 1**). On the horizontal axis, the

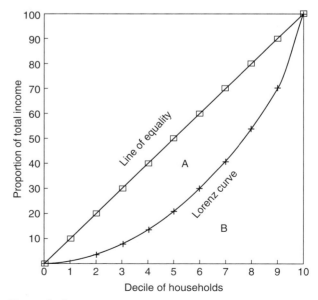

Figure 1 Lorenz curve.

population (in this case, households) is sorted and ranked according to deciles of income, from the lowest-decile group to the top-decile group. The vertical axis then plots the proportion of the aggregate income within that community accruing to each group. Under conditions of perfect equality in the distribution of income (Gini = 0), each decile group would account for exactly 10 percent of the aggregate income and the Lorenz curve would follow the 45° line of equality. In reality, the Lorenz curve falls below the 45° line of equality because the bottom groups in the income distribution earn considerably less than their equal shares. In **Figure 1**, for instance, the bottom one-half of households accounts for just 20% of the aggregate income. The degree to which the Lorenz curve departs from the 45° line of equality is a measure of income inequality. As it turns out, the Gini coefficient is the ratio of the area between the Lorenz curve and the 45° line of equality (A) and the area of the triangle below the 45° line of equality (A + B).

There is some debate as to whether income inequality is a valid community analog of relative deprivation at the individual level. Some argue that Gini coefficient is the measure of relative deprivation. For instance, the relative deprivation curve that represents the gaps between an individual's income and the incomes of all individuals richer than him or her (as a proportion of mean income) turns out to be the Gini coefficient. Others have presented a generalization of Gini, the s-Ginis, that can be interpreted as indices of relative deprivation. Indeed, it has been stated that "the Gini coefficient may be interpreted as a transformation of an index of 'envy' evaluated through the comparison of the income of an individual and that of all other individuals richer than him/her"(Atkinson and Bourguignon, 2000: 43).

As mentioned earlier, the relationship between individual income and health status is concave, such that each additional dollar of income raises individual health by a decreasing amount. The concave relationship between income and health has important implications for the aggregate-level relationship between income distribution and average health achievement, as noted by Rodgers. As illustrated in **Figure 2**, in a hypothetical society consisting of just two individuals – a rich one (with income x_4) and a poor one (with income x_1) – transferring a given amount of money (amount $x_4 - x_3$) from the rich person to the poor person will result in an improvement in average health (from y_1 to y_2) because the improvement in the health of the poor person more than offsets the loss in health of the rich person. Indeed, it is possible that, by transferring incomes from the relatively flat part of the

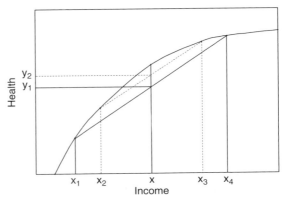

Figure 2 The individual-level relationship between income and health.

income–health curve, there may be no loss in health for the wealthy person.

Consequently, researchers have posited that an aggregate relationship between the average health status of a society and the level of income inequality in a society could be observed if the individual-level relationship between income and health (within the society) is concave. That is, the aggregate relationship between income inequality and health may be observed simply due to the underlying concave functional form of the individual income–health relationship and assuming an x amount of transfer of money from rich to the poor. Indeed, such a transfer also implies a reduction in the income inequality level in that particularly society, and as such, the society with the narrower distribution of income will have a better average health status, all other things being equal. It is worth emphasizing that, if the relationship between income and health at the individual level is linear (not concave), then a transfer of income from the rich to the poor will reduce the level of income inequality but will not lead to improvements in the average health status of that society.

Occasionally, this expected relationship between income distribution and the average health status of a population (which is a direct function of the concave relationship between individual income and health) has been described as a statistical artifact of the concave relationship between individual income and health. The use of the term artifact is misleading here because it suggests that the potential for improving the health of the poor through income redistribution is a statistical illusion. Indeed, there is nothing artifactual about improving the health of the poor (and hence, average population health) through income and wealth redistribution – indeed the success of much philanthropy (e.g., donating money to provide vaccines to the world's poor) rests on the validity of this assumption.

In addition to the concavity effect just described, researchers have posited an additional contextual effect of income inequality on health. This is the hypothesis that the distribution of income in society, over and above individual incomes as well as societal average income, matters for population health such that individuals (regardless of their individual incomes) tend to have worse health in societies that are more unequal. Thus, income inequality *per se* may be damaging to public's health by causing a *downward shift* in the income–health curve. Thus, the income inequality hypothesis is viewed as an independent contextual effect akin to a social pollution effect.

Income and Health: The Role of Social Comparisons

Wilkinson argued that income inequality is harmful to health because it leads to invidious social comparisons among individuals in society and that these comparisons, in turn, may act as a stressor in the form of feelings of shame, anxiety, and social exclusion and, as such, impact physiological systems. The economist Juliet Schor described how widening inequalities have given rise to a culture of upward social comparisons (and the attendant frustration of aspirations). Thus, a mechanism linking income inequality to health involves psychosocial pathways that have adverse physiological consequences. Models of the direct effects of stress on physiological systems include allostatic load, which describes the wear and tear on the organism caused by exposure to daily adverse life circumstances. Stress may also affect health indirectly by leading to a more adverse profile of behaviors, such as smoking and excess drinking. This line of explanation links the community income inequality and individual health through individual relative deprivation (including those related to income). Researchers interested in adult health and mortality have argued that inequality worsens adult health through social comparison. They have argued that income inequality affects health because ranking low in the social hierarchy produces negative emotions such as shame and distrust that lead to worse health via neuroendocrine mechanisms and stress-induced behaviors such as smoking, excessive drinking, and drug use. Although the human body is remarkable in adapting to occasional bouts of stress, they have argued that cumulative exposures to stressors (such as chronic poverty, low socioeconomic status, and constant social comparisons) eventually result in strain on regulatory systems.

Although we have discussed here the role of social comparisons as a source of stress, there are other mechanisms that link income and health that can also be explained through stress-based explanations. For instance, a chronic exposure to unpredictable social and economic circumstances (associated with low income) can also be a source of stress in addition to inhibiting access to important material goods necessary to sustain desirable levels of well-being. The challenge for researchers on income and health is to elucidate the specific pathways through which the different conceptualizations of income may impact on health through differential types of stressors.

Acknowledgments

S. V. Subramanian is also supported by a National Institutes of Health/National Heart, Lung, Blood Institute Career Development Award (1 K25 HL081275).

See Also the Following Articles

Economic Factors and Stress; Health and Socioeconomic Status; Social Status and Stress.

Further Reading

Atkinson, A. B. and Bourguignon, F. (2000). Introduction: income distribution and economics. In: Atkinson, A. B. & Bourguignon, F. (ed.) *Handbook of income distribution*, (vol. 1), pp. 1–58. Amsterdam: Elsevier Science.

Deaton, A. (2003). Health, inequality, and economic development. *Journal of Economic Literature* 41, 113–158.

Duclos, J.-Y. (2000). Gini indices and the redistribution of income. *International Tax and Public Finance* 7, 141–162.

Frank, R.H. and Sunstein, C.R. (2001). Cost-benefit analysis and relative position. *University of Chicago Law Review*, 68: 323–374.

Kakwani, N. (1984). The relative deprivation curve and its applications. *Journal of Business and Economic Statistics* 2, 384–394.

Kawachi, I. (2000). Income inequality and health. In: Berkman, L. F. & Kawachi, I. (ed.) *Social epidemiology*, pp. 76–94. New York: Oxford University Press.

Kawachi, I. and Kennedy, B. P. (2003). *The health of nations*. New York: The New Press.

Marmot, M. (2002). The influence of income on health: views of an epidemiologist. *Health Affairs* 21(2), 31–46.

McEwen, B. S. and Seeman, T. S. (1999). Protective and damaging effects of mediators of stress: elaborating and testing the concepts of allostatis and allostatic load. *Annals of the New York Academy of Sciences* 896, 30–47.

Rodgers, G. B. (1979). Income and inequality as determinants of mortality: an international cross-section analysis. *Population Studies* 33, 343–351.

Runciman, W. G. (1966). *Relative deprivation and social justice.* London: Routledge.

Schor, J.B. (1998). *The overspent American.* New York: Basic Books.

Subramanian, S.V., Belli, P., and Kawachi, I. (2002). The macroeconomic determinants of health. *Annual Review of Public Health* **23**: 287–302.

Subramanian, S.V., and Kawachi, I. (2004). Income inequality and health: what have we learned so far. *Epidemiologic Reviews* **26**: 78–91.

Subramanian, S.V., and Kawachi, I. (2006). Whose health is affected by income inequality? A multilevel interaction analysis of contemporaneous and lagged affects of state income inequality on individual self-rated health in the United States. *Health and Place* **12**: 141–156.

Subramanian, S.V., Kawachi I. (2006). Being well doing well: on the importance of income for health. *International Journal of Social Welfare* **15**, S1: S13–S22.

Wagstaff, A. and van Doorslaer, E. (2000). Income inequality and health: what does the literature tell us? *Annual Review of Public Health* **21**, 543–567.

Wilkinson, R. G. (1996). *Unhealthy societies – the afflictions of inequality.* London: Routledge.

Wilkinson, R.G. (2005). *The impact of inequality.* New York: New Press.

Yitzhaki, S. (1979). Relative deprivation and the Gini coefficient. *Quarterly Journal of Economics* **93**(2), 321–324.

Indigenous Societies

W W Dressler
University of Alabama, Tuscaloosa, AL, USA

This article is a revision of the previous edition article by W A Dessler, volume 2, pp 558–564, © 2000, Elsevier Inc.

Introduction
Stress in Unacculturated Indigenous Societies
Stress and Acculturation in Indigenous Societies
Stress and Migration
Conclusion

Glossary

Acculturation	The process by which a society is culturally influenced by another society.
Culture-bound syndromes	Local idioms for the expression of distress, consisting of socially recognized illness categories that have no acknowledged counterpart in Western biomedicine.
Cultural consonance	The degree to which an individual approximates in his or her own behavior the prototypes for behavior encoded in shared cultural models.
Extended kin support systems	Systems in which help or assistance is most appropriately sought from individuals who are related by common ancestry or marriage.
Indigenous societies	Societies that are native to a particular locale, in which people speak a distinctive language and have a distinctive social heritage and which are often technologically less complex. Usually, the way of life of the people is on the periphery of the major world industrial societies. Indigenous societies can also be referred to as traditional societies.
Modernization	A special case of acculturation in which an indigenous society is undergoing economic change or development.
Status incongruence	A discrepancy between an individual's aspirations for social status or prestige and his or her resources for actually achieving those aspirations.

Introduction

An indigenous or traditional society is characterized as native to a specific region, with a distinctive language and way of life. Also, the way of life of the people is peripheral to global capitalist market systems. This does not mean that such a society is unaffected by global market systems; in fact, one major source of stress in indigenous societies is the impact of economic change emanating from those larger systems. Nor does this mean that an indigenous society cannot be embedded within a modern, industrial society (e.g., Native Americans). Rather, in an indigenous society, culture and related systems of social organization are structured more in terms of local context and local systems of meaning, and less in terms of the middle-class values of industrial society. Understanding stress and its effects in indigenous societies requires an examination of both social arrangements that generate stresses within the indigenous social structure and the way in which traditional culture and social structure interact with outside influences to generate stresses.

Stress in Unacculturated Indigenous Societies

Anthropologists conventionally describe the relative degree of external influence on a society or community along a continuum of acculturation. A society that is relatively unacculturated or traditional has been minimally influenced by processes of modernization. Usually this means that households tend to practice a mix of economic pursuits for subsistence (i.e., raising food directly for consumption within the household) and for exchange in local markets. With respect to material lifestyles, although there is some access to imported consumer goods, these often are primarily related to subsistence activities (e.g., agricultural implements, outboard motors). Most goods consumed by a household are produced locally. What wage labor exists is usually within the community, and there is little formal education. Social relationships tend to be dominated by kinship. Systems of kinship can range from large groups formed around descent from a common ancestor (or unilineal descent groups) to somewhat more loosely structured kindreds that are like large ego-centered social networks. Finally, belief systems reflect local meanings and understandings, even when there have been modernizing influences (e.g., missionaries).

Patterns of morbidity and mortality within traditional societies provide one clue to patterns of stress in those societies. Generally speaking, rates of high blood pressure, coronary artery disease, stroke, and cancer tend to be very low. In traditional societies, patterns of morbidity and mortality tend to be dominated by infectious and parasitic disease, especially in childhood, and by trauma in adulthood. Although any generalizations must be tempered by reference to local ecological conditions, in many traditional societies life expectancy beyond 5 years of age is comparable to life expectancy in industrial societies, and in the aged in these societies there is little evidence of the kind of pathologies (e.g., atherosclerosis) associated with aging in industrial societies.

What has been most illuminating in the study of stress in unacculturated societies is the study of culture-bound syndromes. Culture-bound syndromes are local idioms of distress. They can be thought of as culturally appropriate ways of experiencing and expressing distress arising from stressful social relationships. Some attempts have been made to equate the culture-bound syndromes with Western psychiatric diagnoses, but recent evidence indicates that there is not a direct correspondence between culture-bound syndromes and biomedical psychiatric diagnoses; it is probably more useful to think of culture-bound syndromes and Western psychiatric diagnoses as comorbid.

A classic example of a culture-bound syndrome is *susto* in Latino societies of Central and South America. The individual suffering from *susto* experiences a loss of energy, difficulty in maintaining customary activities, frequent spells of crying, and diffuse somatic symptoms such as loss of appetite and sleep disturbance. As the name in Spanish implies, *susto* is attributed to a sudden fright (e.g., seeing a snake), at which time the soul of the individual leaves the body and wanders freely.

Research has shown that the distribution of *susto* is socially patterned. The prevalence is higher in females, tends to increase with age, and tends to be higher in relatively poorer communities. Furthermore, the greatest risk of *susto* has been found among persons experiencing difficulty in enacting common social role expectations. This usually arises from a lack of specific kinds of social resources (e.g., not having a large kinship network) that can be called on in carrying out expected role obligations (such as contributions to community work groups). Similar findings have been obtained in research on other culture-bound syndromes such as *ataques de nervios* in Puerto Rico, *debilidad* in the Andean highlands, heart illness in Iran, and *nervos* in Brazil. Culture-bound syndromes occur when individuals are low in cultural consonance; that is, they are unable to approximate in their own behaviors the prototypes for behaviors that are encoded in widely shared cultural models.

The experience of a culture-bound syndrome is important in two respects. First, it makes meaningful and intelligible the experience of social stress both to the person suffering the stress and to his or her social network. Second, in many societies, there are cultural practices, including healing rituals and participation in religious organizations, that deal directly with the syndrome and the underlying difficulties in social relationships. The aim is to mend the tear in the fabric of social relationships and hence end the individual's suffering.

The existence of these beliefs and practices that are helpful in ameliorating cultural stresses may in part account for patterns of morbidity and mortality in indigenous societies. As noted previously, the diseases conventionally associated with stress in industrial societies are relatively less important in indigenous societies. Also, in most cases an increase of blood pressure with age is not observed in indigenous societies. Other patterns of disease distribution that are taken for granted in industrial societies are not observed in traditional societies. One of the more striking of these is the association of blood pressure with African descent ethnicity. While it is assumed that persons of African descent have higher blood pressures, in fact this is true primarily for those of African descent in the Western hemisphere, and more specifically in societies in which Africans had formerly been enslaved. So, for example, when communities of African descent are compared, communities in Africa have the lowest average blood pressures, communities in the West Indies have intermediate average blood pressures, and African American and African Brazilian communities have the highest average blood pressures. Recent findings show also that *quilombo* or refugee communities descended from escaped slaves in isolated areas of Brazil have low average blood pressures and exhibit little increase of blood pressure with age.

These patterns suggest two things. First, there may be a relatively higher level of social integration in indigenous societies, along with practices that help to moderate the impact of social stressors, that account for the lower prevalence of conditions and diseases associated with stress in industrial societies. Second, the process of social change leading to the modern industrial state may itself generate profound social stresses that contribute to the distinctive pattern of morbidity and mortality in those societies.

At the same time, it is important not to romanticize life in indigenous societies, in the sense of overemphasizing social integration and cohesion, because stresses will be generated within any system of social relationships. What is important to specify across different cultural contexts is the process by which social stresses are generated and the ability of indigenous support systems to deal with those stresses.

Promising results in this regard are emerging from research on hormones and neurotransmitters associated with the stress process. Newer techniques of data collection under difficult field conditions, along with techniques for the analysis of those data, are beginning to show how variation in social behavior within traditional societies is associated with inter- and intra-individual variation in stress hormones, which in turn is associated with acute illness. For example, research in a peasant village in the West Indies has shown that men who are perceived by their peers to emulate the ideals of manhood in this community have lower circulating levels of cortisol. Similarly, children growing up in families that are closer to the cultural ideal of the family have lower circulating cortisol levels and experience fewer acute illnesses. This research, coupled with research on local idioms of distress, suggests that stresses in

unacculturated societies are deeply embedded in the system of social relationships that organizes everyday life.

Stress and Acculturation in Indigenous Societies

Societies that are undergoing acculturation are those that are being influenced by other social and cultural systems. In the study of stress and disease, the effect of modern industrial societies on local sociocultural systems has been of particular interest. There is considerable imbalance in this type of acculturation, because of the unequal power and influence that modern industrial states exert on traditional societies. The terms modernization and development have been used to describe this kind of influence.

Modernization in traditional societies was initiated by colonial expansion and has been particularly prominent since World War II and related processes of globalization. This influence has not been inadvertent. The aim has been to take advantage of both physical and social resources in developing societies.

These changes have had large effects on local social systems, including a transition from subsistence occupations to wage labor occupations, the replacement of indigenous languages by European languages, increased urbanization, increased emphasis on formal education, decreased emphasis on traditional social relationships, especially kinship, and substantial changes in indigenous belief systems. Everyday life can change at a rapid pace in modernizing contexts, the result being a stressful lack of consonance between traditional culture and the demands of modern life.

Specific and general aspects of this modernization process have been found to be associated with increasing rates of chronic diseases. Urbanization has been found to be associated with increasing rates of hypertension, independent of changes in diet and physical activity. Some investigators have used summary measures of acculturation both for individuals and for communities. When communities are ranked along a continuum of traditional, intermediate, and modern (depending on aggregate characteristics of the population by the variables noted previously), rates of hypertension, obesity, diabetes, and coronary artery disease consistently increase in communities with higher levels of acculturation or modernization. Also, daily circulating levels of hormones such as cortisol appear to increase in association with acculturative stress.

The results have been somewhat less consistent using measures of acculturation operationalized at the level of the individual. The pattern can still be observed in many studies, but the strength and the consistency of the associations are not as great. This has led some researchers to speculate that the linear model of stress and acculturation is not specified well enough to describe the process at the individual level.

Because the general model of stress and acculturation has not worked very well at the level of the individual, researchers have adapted the stress model, as it has been developed for European and American populations, and applied it to communities experiencing change and development. A major challenge in this research has been to identify factors that generalize across different cultural contexts and to distinguish those from factors that are culturally specific. There is emerging evidence to suggest that at least one set of social stressors generalizes across modernizing societies, primarily because these stressors are generated by the modernization process itself. In most societies undergoing modernization, there is an increased availability of Western consumer goods. Frequently the ownership of these goods becomes highly valued as symbols of status or prestige, often supplanting traditional indicators of higher status. This by itself contributes to the climate of change in a modernizing community. In addition, however, aspirations for the lifestyles of the Western middle class can quickly outstrip the ability of a developing economy to provide the kinds of jobs and salaries necessary to maintain such a lifestyle. Therefore, a kind of status incongruence can occur, in which the desire to attain and maintain a Western middle-class lifestyle exceeds an individual's economic resources for such a lifestyle. This kind of status incongruence has been found to be related to psychiatric symptoms, high blood pressure, elevated serum lipids, the risk of diabetes, and immunological status in developing societies in Latin America, the Caribbean, and Polynesia.

Resources for coping with stressors have been found to be more culturally variable. Social support systems are a good case in point. Social support can be defined as the emotional and practical assistance an individual believes is available to him or her during times of felt need; the social network in which this assistance is available is the social support system. In research in Europe and North America, generally speaking, emphasis has been placed on the nature of the assistance or social support transactions, rather than on who might provide that assistance. There is a growing body of cross-cultural research indicating that, in many societies, who provides the assistance is critical in determining the relationship between social support and health. This is probably a reflection of a continuing importance of kinship in defining who is and who is not an appropriate individual with whom to enter into a social relationship.

For example, in Latin American societies people have traditionally lived in large extended families organized around a father and his married sons (known as a patrilineal extended family). In addition to these extended family relationships, there is a social practice known as *compadrazgo*, through which individuals, especially men, establish formal, kinship-like relationships with unrelated persons (known as fictive kinship). The term *compadrazgo* literally means co-parenthood, and this carries the expectation of mutual support. These ties of fictive kinship are used to establish economically and politically important alliances. Research has shown that men who perceive greater amounts of support from both their extended and their fictive kin have lower blood pressures. Women are expected to restrict themselves to the household and domestic duties. Not surprisingly, with respect to health status, women benefit primarily from support available within the household. These studies show that the definition and effects of social supports are closely related to cultural and social structural factors and can only be understood within that context.

Other forms of stress resistance show similar differences cross-culturally, although the evidence is not quite as consistent as with social support. For example, in European and North American studies, a direct action coping style has been found to be helpful in moderating the effects of stressful events or circumstances. In this style of coping, attempting to directly confront and alter stressful circumstances contributes to better health status. In some research in traditional societies, this same relationship has been observed. In others, the opposite effect has been observed, i.e., a direct action coping style actually exacerbates distress and poor outcomes. In the specific case of this coping style, this probably has to do with the actual resources available to individuals and families in coping with stressors. When social and economic resources are meager at best, the belief that an individual can truly change the circumstances that are often thrust upon him- or herself may, in the long run, be deleterious.

A major source of stress in societies undergoing modernization is the increase in socioeconomic inequity that accompanies modernization. Generally speaking, the distribution of wealth becomes more unequal, resulting in marked social stratification, whereas previously such stratification was, if not absent, at least muted. Recent studies point to the effects of such stratification on cultural consonance as a potent source of stress. The capacity of an individual to achieve higher cultural consonance is severely compromised by lower socioeconomic status. Lower cultural consonance has been found to be associated with higher blood pressure and psychological distress and to mediate the effects of socioeconomic status in contexts of modernization. The inability to act on these widely shared cultural models is a potent source of stress in developing societies.

Stress and Migration

The other way in which social and cultural change can influence indigenous communities is through migration. This century has seen remarkable movements of people from traditional societies to North America and Western Europe, along with internal migration within developing societies that takes migrants into cosmopolitan urban centers in their own societies. Rarely can migration be considered an individual matter. Rather, it is much more common for entire communities of migrants to become established in their host country. This usually occurs because migration follows patterns established through social networks, especially kinship networks. Individuals and households take advantage of kin-based social support systems established in host countries in order to establish themselves there.

Research suggests that a similar pattern of stress and response develops in cases of migration like that observed in developing societies. That is, migrants come to the new setting with aspirations for a new life, aspirations that are reinforced in host countries through the depiction of middle-class lifestyles in advertising and other media forms. At the same time, migrants typically occupy the lowest levels of socioeconomic status in their host countries. Therefore, the ability of the migrant to amass the economic resources necessary to achieve a middle-class lifestyle is severely compromised. This status incongruence again has been found to be associated with chronic disease risk factors such as blood pressure and glucose levels.

Patterns of social support that can help an individual to cope with this kind of social stressor will often again be found in the kin support system. There are, however, several additional complications. First, kin support systems will often be fragmented. Only some people will migrate, not entire support systems. This can mean that some households and individuals are socially isolated, lacking even the most basic social supports. This can also mean that a large burden can be placed on a support system that is fragmented, and that the resulting demands for support are simply too

much for the system to bear. Second, the migrant, especially to North America, is entering a highly competitive and individualistic society. The kinds of mutual rights and obligations entailed by kinship have ceased to be recognized as strongly, for example, in the United States as in traditional societies in Latin America or Southeast Asia. Therefore, in some specific situations, the kin support system can come to be a source of stress and tension, as opposed to a resource for resisting stress.

The complications entailed here are illustrated by migrants from Samoa to northern California. Traditionally organized into large extended kin groups represented by chiefs, Samoans have transplanted their social organization to some U.S. urban centers. Traditionally, the chief (or *matai*) controls economic decision making for the entire extended family. In the American urban setting, however, the economic demands of daily life for an individual household can conflict with the decisions made for the extended family, causing this traditional form of social organization to become a source of stress. At the same time, within the larger extended family, core systems of kin-based social support have emerged, especially involving networks of adult siblings. Individuals and households with a strong support system of this kind have better health status in spite of social stressors such as status incongruence. This specific case illustrates the importance of understanding the adaptation of migrants in a host society in relation to their traditional cultural context, as well as the demands of the new social setting.

Some research on migrants from the developing world has shown the long-term effects of major life events experienced by families in the society of origin. This has been observed in immigrants from Latin America and Southeast Asia who have been exposed to protracted civil war and related conflicts. For example, it was found that persons who had had relatives kidnapped or murdered by nonmilitary death squads in Guatemala had continuing high levels of anxiety and depression years after the event. Similarly, anxiety and depression levels in migrants from Southeast Asia to the United States were associated with time spent in refugee camps, independently from other stressors and demographic control variables. These major crises associated with large-scale political events and circumstances can have effects that continue well after the initial, acute stages.

Conclusion

The study of stress and indigenous societies has helped to illuminate various aspects of the stress process. Perhaps the most important has been the clear demonstration of the link between the stress process and the social and cultural context in which individuals and families live. When stressors and resistance resources are examined only within a single cultural context, it can appear as if individual differences in exposure to stressors or in access to resistance resources are the only key to understanding the process. What is lost is the recognition that what counts as a stressor or a resistance resource is itself a function of the cultural context and related social influences. Furthermore, the relationship between stressors, resources, and outcomes can also be modified by social and cultural context. Comparing the stress process in different cultural contexts has been integral to revealing this aspect of the process.

Future research must be explicitly comparative in scope in order to expand on findings produced thus far. For example, research in developing societies suggests that the most important stressors in those societies are actually a function of the development process itself, such as status incongruence. Put differently, this aspect of the stress process is comparable across different settings. On the other hand, the most important resources for resisting stress appear to be specific to the local setting, as in the way in which systems of social support are structured by the existing systems of social organization. Continuing to refine these studies, including better measurements of the physiological dimensions of stress, will increase our understanding of human adaptation.

See Also the Following Articles

Cultural Factors in Stress; Cultural Transition; Economic Factors and Stress; Evolutionary Origins and Functions of the Stress Response; Familial Patterns of Stress; Health and Socioeconomic Status; Industrialized Societies; Minorities and Stress; Psychosocial Factors and Stress; Social Capital; Social Status and Stress; Social Support.

Further Reading

Decker, S., Flinn, M., England, B. G., et al. (2003). Cultural congruity and the cortisol stress response among Dominican men. In: Wilce, J. M., Jr. (ed.) *Social and cultural lives of immune systems*, pp. 147–169. London and New York: Routledge.

Dressler, W. W. (1994). Cross-cultural differences and social influences in social support and cardiovascular disease. In: Shumaker, S. A. & Czajkowski, S. M. (eds.) *Social support and cardiovascular disease*, pp. 167–192. New York: Plenum Publishing.

Dressler, W. W. (1999). Modernization, stress and blood pressure: new directions in research. *Human Biology* **71**, 583–605.

Dressler, W. W. (2004). Culture, stress and cardiovascular disease. In: Ember, C. R. & Ember, M. (eds.) *The encyclopedia of medical anthropology*, pp. 328–334. New York: Kluwer Academic/Plenum Publishers.

Dressler, W. W. and Bindon, J. R. (2000). The health consequences of cultural consonance. *American Anthropologist* **102**, 244–260.

Flinn, M. V. and England, B. G. (1997). Social economics of childhood glucocorticoid stress response and health. *American Journal of Physical Anthropology* **102**, 33–54.

Janes, C. R. (1990). *Migration, social change and health*. Stanford, CA: Stanford University Press.

McDade, T. W. (2001). Lifestyle incongruity, social integration, and immune function among Samoan adolescents. *Social Science and Medicine* **53**, 1351–1362.

Panter-Brick, C. and Worthman, C. W. (eds.) (1999). *Hormones, health, and behavior*. Cambridge: Cambridge University Press.

Rubel, A. J., O'Nell, C. W. and Ardon, R. C. (1984). *Susto: a folk illness*. Berkeley and Los Angeles, CA: University of California Press.

Indoleamines *See:* Serotonin; Serotonin in Stress; Serotonin Transporter Genetic Modifications.

Industrialized Societies

J Siegrist
University of Duesseldorf, Duesseldorf, Germany

This article is reproduced from the previous edition, volume 2, pp 565–569, © 2000, Elsevier Inc.

Process of Industrialization and Epidemiological Transition
Stressful Social Environments and Health
Concluding Remarks

Glossary

Epidemiological transition	The changing pattern of most prevalent diseases from infectious to chronic degenerative diseases.
Formal rationality	The purposeful calculation of the most efficient means to achieve a goal where rational choices are made to maximize individual benefit.
Gender roles	The cluster of social expectations and norms guiding typically male vs. typically female behavior.
Health-related lifestyle	A collective pattern of health-promoting or health-damaging behavior based on routinized choices people make about food, exercise, hygiene, safety, relaxation, and so on. This pattern is structured by specific needs, social norms, and constraints.
Social disintegration	A weakening of social ties and an absence of cooperative exchange resulting in a lack of social rules and trust and, ultimately, in a breakdown of a social order.

Process of Industrialization and Epidemiological Transition

The industrial revolution started in Great Britain during the second half of the eighteenth century and has subsequently spread across a number of economically advanced countries. This revolution, together with the political revolution initiated in France, must be considered one of the most radical changes in human history. Within a very short time period, fundamental ways of living and working were transformed from a basically agricultural society to a society that is driven increasingly by technology and market economy. With the invention of engines and machines, productivity was increased in an unprecedented way.

A large part of the workforce, employed formerly as peasants and craftsmen, moved to urban areas to engage in unskilled or semiskilled work. The rapid growth of cities and the formation of an industrial workforce contributed to two subsequent, most significant demographic trends: (1) a take-off period of population growth with declining infant mortality rates and (2) a decline in fertility with slow population growth in combination with increased life expectancy. At the same time, the social institutions of marriage and family underwent a marked transformation, and a new division of labor between the sexes started to develop.

After severe poverty and economic exploitation in the early stages of industrial capitalism, economic progress and the development of a welfare state were experienced by a growing proportion of industrial populations. This progress included the availability of healthier food, increased opportunities of energy consumption, better housing, transport, education, and general hygiene. In terms of population health, the process of industrialization was associated with a marked increase in life expectancy and a change in the pattern of prevailing diseases. Overall, 2 to 3 years are added to life expectancy at birth with each decade passing in advanced societies. This increase cannot be attributed to the fact that people, once becoming older, live substantially longer than in previous generations. Rather, increases in life expectancy were, and still are, mainly due to a reduction of death rates at earlier ages and, thus, to increased probabilities of survival. The most substantial decline has been in infant mortality, followed by reductions in childhood and midlife mortality. A dramatic reduction in mortality from infectious diseases played a major role in this process. The typical pattern of leading causes of disability and death in advanced societies is characterized by chronic conditions such as coronary heart disease, cancer, stroke, accidents, and metabolic and mental disorders. This change is referred to as the epidemiological transition.

While the development of modern medicine and related improvements of health care are a direct outflow of the broader processes of industrialization and modernization, it has been demonstrated that the impact of medicine on this major change in the pattern of morbidity and mortality has been limited. In fact, the bulk of the decline in mortality from infectious diseases came before medicine had developed effective forms of treatment and prevention. This means that public health measures and factors related to a general rise in living standards may have accounted for this change more significantly than medicine.

With this epidemiological transition from infectious to degenerative diseases, medicine and public health face new challenges. A substantial part of these challenges directly or indirectly concerns, the impact of stressful social environments on health. The following section discusses three different aspects of this impact in more detail.

Stressful Social Environments and Health

Stressful Experience and Health-Related Lifestyles

Many of the aforementioned degenerative diseases are considered diseases of affluence because they were prevalent to the extent that life became more comfortable. For instance, with technological advances and with the expansion of commercially available food and drugs, a number of behavioral health risks were programmed, e.g., access to a car reduced physical activity significantly, and, more importantly, it also increased the number of injuries and deaths from accidents. Frequent consumption of fat and meat, at first available to the wealthier groups, contributed to elevated blood lipids, overweight, and associated health risks. Spending money on drugs such as cigarettes or alcohol increased the risk of cancer and heart disease, among others. Consequently, during the first stage of the epidemiological transition, these behaviorally induced risks associated with a wealthier lifestyle were more prevalent among socially and economically privileged groups. At a later stage of the process of industrialization and modernization, however, this social pattern changed: diseases of affluence increasingly became the diseases of the poor. In contemporary societies, this is clearly the case in almost all northern, western, and central European countries, in the United States, and in Canada. The same pattern may be experienced in the near future in countries that are currently exposed to a process of rapid industrialization.

Hence, substantial social inequalities in health are observed, mainly due to higher rates of the former affluent diseases among lower socioeconomic groups.

To explain this shift in the social distribution of a broad range of degenerative diseases and their behavioral risk factors (e.g., smoking, alcohol consumption, overweight, hypertension, metabolic disorders, cardiovascular diseases, some manifestations of cancer, AIDS), the concept of health-related lifestyle needs to be described more precisely.

Health-related lifestyles are collective patterns of health-promoting or health-damaging behavior based on routinized choices people make about food, exercise, hygiene, safety, relaxation, and so on. In many cases, these choices form a coherent pattern that is structured by specific needs, attitudes, and social norms and by the constraints of a group's socioeconomic condition. Once established among a sociocultural group, such behavioral patterns may be transferred from one generation to the next through socialization processes or they may be adopted by model learning from peer groups during adolescence. Unfortunately, the latter is often the case with respect to health-damaging behaviors (smoking, alcohol and drug consumption, unsafe sex practices, etc.). As these behaviors are experienced as relief and reward in stressful psychosocial circumstances they may be reinforced easily and, thus, trigger careers of addiction later in life.

Alternatively, with higher levels of education and knowledge and with the availability of alternative means of coping with stressful psychosocial circumstances, health-damaging lifestyles may be abandoned more easily. This is most probably what happened to the wealthier populations in advanced societies in the recent past and what contributed, and still contributes, to the widening gap in life expectancy between socioeconomic groups.

To date, there are still powerful constraints toward maintaining health-damaging lifestyles among less privileged social groups. A major constraint concerns the exposure to adverse living and working environments. A large number of epidemiologic studies document associations between the amount of exposure to these unfavourable circumstances and the prevalence of unhealthy behavior. For instance, with respect to cigarette smoking, conditions such as heavy workload, shiftwork, social isolation at work, and job instability were identified. Moreover, people who suffer from unfavorable social comparison, e.g., regarding education, income, or general social standing, are at risk of exhibiting a health-damaging life-style. In all these cases, relief and reward experience in terms of some form of addictive behavior may be needed to mitigate a stressful experience.

Some of these processes operate in more subtle ways. It is well known that the processes of primary socialization vary considerably according to the parent's socioeconomic status. In particular, children born into families with a low educational level face more difficulties in deferring their gratifications and in pursuing long-lasting goals in future life. Their sense of self-efficacy and self-esteem is low, and they are more likely to experience their environment as uncontrollable and fateful. Thus, when facing frustrations, they may be less capable of coping in an active, effective way. Rather, they may seek relief in passive behavior, including drug consumption and related health risks.

This knowledge, derived from sociological and psychological research, has direct implications for health promotion activities and the design of preventive programs. It is evident that comprehensive approaches tackling structural and individual conditions are needed to change health lifestyles in a successful way.

Unfortunately, influential economic interests operate in almost all advanced societies to counteract these measures, most evidently the tobacco and alcohol industry. Advertising activities in mass medias and diffusion of new fashions through opinion leaders are effective means to maintain drug consumption. Efforts to equalize gender roles and to assimilate female attitudes and activities to behaviors that were typical attributes of the traditional male gender role resulted in an unprecedented increase in cigarette consumption among young women. Moreover, women in recent years, as compared to the 1950s, are more likely to work in occupations that were once almost exclusively male. As a consequence of these large-scale societal changes, some of the most advanced industrial societies, such as the United States, are moving toward greater equality in mortality between the sexes.

Impact of Social Disintegration on Health

Industrialized societies are characterized by a high level of mobility. A substantial part of this mobility is due to migration. Economic constraints and wars are the major causes of large migration waves that have shaped the life of many generations throughout the processes of industrialization and modernization. Social mobility is a second component of these secular trends. As mentioned briefly, the onset of early industrialization in Europe and the United States has been facilitated by a broader sociocultural development of modernization that promoted formal rationality and individualism as the dominant modes of thinking and behaving in western societies. Formal rationality is the purposeful calculation of the most efficient means to achieve a goal. Rational choices are made to maximize individual benefit. With the expansion of individual rights, duties, and life chances, traditional ways of maintaining group solidarity, social norms, and obligations lost their significance and attraction. Individual striving for an improved standard of living has become the dominant motivation

overriding traditional social constraints. Thus, a large proportion of people was, and currently is, subject to intragenerational social upward (and downward) mobility in occupational life.

For a long time, social mobility and increased individualism were considered the ultimate benefits of modernization, as legitimized by substantial gains in the quality of life. However, more recently, awareness of the limits, risks, and possible health adverse effects of this development has been growing. One line of thinking along these lines concerns the negative effects on health produced by social disintegration.

Social disintegration is an often reported consequence of enhanced social mobility and related gain in individual freedom. It becomes manifest through a weakening of close social ties (e.g., among family members) and a decrease in reciprocal social exchange or solidarity. Under these conditions, the stability of social relationships is threatened, and commitments held among affiliates may lose their significance. Social disintegration is often associated with a state of social anomie, i.e., a lack of rules and orientations guiding interpersonal exchange. In a society characterized by anomie, individual behavior cannot be predicted by social norms any longer as these norms have lost their validity.

A growing number of investigations conducted by social epidemiologists and medical sociologists document adverse health effects among people who experience social disintegration. Lack of social cohesion or social support, shrinking social networks, and elevated proportions of societal members suffering from social isolation, social exclusion, or individual struggle are different facets of this general trend. For instance, in a cross-cultural perspective analyzing data from 84 different societies, one study concluded that with greater involvement in a money economy a systematic increase in mean blood pressure was evident, even after adjusting for important confounders such as salt consumption and body mass index. With greater involvement in modern money economy, individual competition and striving for benefit became dominant at the expense of cooperative social relationships. In a review of more recent investigations it was concluded that at least eight community-based prospective studies in industrialized societies reveal an association between social disintegration and mortality rates, usually death from all causes. In particular, mortality risks are elevated among people who lack social ties to others. Even at a more distant, macrosocial level, current evidence suggests that a decline in overall mortality, now familiar in most advanced societies, is prevented in an economy that is maximizing shareholder profit at the expense of investments into community life, culture, and social security.

Although the precise mechanisms that transform stressful experience resulting from social disintegration into increased susceptibility to fatal or nonfatal bodily disease are far from clear, impressive evidence is available from social experiments in mammals. It illustrates the critical role of rewarding and securing experiences that social exchange, affiliation, and affection play in regulating the body's basic physiological processes. It may well be that the cultural canon of modern industrialized societies heavily weighted toward formal rationality, control, and individual striving substantially diminishes the health gain associated with progress in human evolution. This latter conclusion is supported further by a third line of investigation focusing on the impact of modern working life on health.

Stress at Work and Health

The most profound change evoked by the process of industrialization concerns the nature of human work. For a large part of the workforce, work and home become two different places and two different types of social organization. In all economically advanced societies, work and occupation in adult life are accorded primacy for the following reasons. First, having a job is a principal prerequisite for continuous income and, thus, for independence from traditional support systems (family, community welfare, etc.). Increasingly, the level of income determines a wide range of life chances. Second, training for a job and achievement of occupational status are important goals of socialization. It is through education, job training, and status acquisition that personal growth and development are realized, that a core social identity outside the family is acquired, and that goal-directed activity in human life is shaped. At the same time, occupational settings produce the most pervasive continuous demands during one's lifetime, and exposure to harmful job conditions is an important determinant of disability and premature death in midlife.

The nature of work has changed dramatically over the past hundred years. Industrial mass production no longer dominates the labor market. This is due, in part, to technological progress, in part to a growing number of jobs available in the service sector, and, most importantly, in person-based service occupations and professions. In this latter case, unlike in the industrial sector, the potential of rationalization and related cut down in personnel is limited. However, even within industrial work, major changes have taken place. With less focus on physically strenuous work, with improved safety measures against chemical and physical hazards at work, and with more demands for psychomentally stressful jobs (e.g., information processing, controlling, coordinating activities, often performed under time pressure) new health risks emerged. Meanwhile, there has been a recognition that the importance of work for health goes beyond traditional occupational diseases as there is growing evidence of adverse health effects produced by psychomentally and socioemotionally stressful jobs.

Before describing these health risks briefly, additional important changes in occupational life need to be mentioned. They are related to the structure of the labor market. There has been an increasing participation of women in the labor market, an increase in short term or part-time working and other forms of flexible job arrangements, and, most importantly, an increase in job instability and structural unemployment. This latter trend currently hits the economically most advanced societies as well as economies that lag behind. Overall, a substantial part of the economically active population is confined to insecure jobs, to premature retirement, or to job loss. Loss of job, as well as continued experience of job insecurity, was shown to be associated with an elevated risk of mortality in a number of prospective studies. In view of the rather high prevalence of these labor market conditions, the adverse effects on health produced by the economy are obvious.

Even within a continuously employed workforce, exposure to stressful psychosocial work environments carries the risk of ill health. Examples of this latter trend are shift work, irregular working hours and overwork, social isolation at work, conflicting demands, lack of control, and monotony. People working in jobs that are defined by a combination of at least some of these characteristics are at risk of developing chronic disease conditions such as hypertension, coronary heart disease, low back pain, or depression at least twice as often compared to people working in more favorable jobs. Additional evidence documents substantially elevated health risks among workers and employees who suffer from an imbalance between high efforts spent at work and low rewards received in terms of money, esteem, or promotion prospects. In many cases, such unfavorable job conditions are maintained, e.g., due to lack of alternatives in the labor market.

Concluding Remarks

In conclusion, despite substantial progress in life expectancy and the standard of living, the process of industrialization in technology, science, economy, and sociopolitical development has produced a substantial health burden that is attributable to an increasingly stressful social environment. Three aspects of this development were analyzed: (1) the impact of psychosocially adverse circumstances on health-damaging lifestyles; (2) health risks associated with social disintegration; and (3) afflictions of stressful working life and labor market conditions on well-being and health. It seems unlikely that these trends will be diminished in the near future as the process of economic and sociocultural globalization is progressing at a high pace. Moreover, pressures originating from population growth in rapidly developing parts of the world, new socioenvironmental risks, and man-made disasters may aggravate rather than moderate this burden. At the same time, with scientific progress in understanding the determinants and dynamics of stress-related health risks and with new worldwide public health efforts evolving, there is still hope that modernization and industrialization of human societies result in a sustainable humane and more healthy future.

See Also the Following Articles

Economic Factors and Stress; Gender and Stress; Health Behavior and Stress; Indigenous Societies; Social Support; Workplace Stress.

Further Reading

Blaxter, M. (1990). *Health and lifestyles*. London: Routledge.

Cockerham, W. C. (1998). *Medical sociology* (7th edn.). Upper Saddle River, NJ: Prentice Hall.

Henry, J. P. (1997). *Cultural change and high blood pressure*. LIT Publishing, Germany: Münster.

Henry, J. P. and Stephens, P. M. (1977). *Stress, health, and the social environment*. Berlin: Springer.

Hobfoll, S. E. (1998). *Stress, culture, and community*. New York: Plenum.

Karasek, R. A. and Theorell, T. (1990). *Healthy work: stress, productivity, and the reconstruction of working life*. New York: Basic Books.

Marmot, M. G. and Wilkinson, R. (1999). *Social determinants of health*. Oxford: Oxford University Press.

Weber, M. (1958). *The protestant ethic and the spirit of capitalism*. New York: Scribner.

Infection

H Friedman and S H Pross
University of South Florida College of Medicine, Tampa, FL, USA

This article is a revision of the previous edition article by H Friedman and S Specter, volume 2, pp 570–580, © 2000, Elsevier Inc.

Introduction
Central Nervous–Immune–Endocrine System Interactions
Stress Hormones and Infections
Bacterial Infections and Steroids
Virus Infections and Stress
Discussion and Conclusion

Glossary

Adrenocorticotropic hormone (ACTH)	A secreted serum factor from the adrenal glands that is considered a stress hormone.
Cytotines	Soluble proteins secreted by one type of cell that interacts and activates immune cells.
Legionella pneumophila	An opportunistic bacterium that causes Legionnaire's disease and primarily infects macrophages, a class of immune cells responsible for host resistance to infectious diseases.
Lentiviruses	A retrovirus, such as human immunodeficiency virus, that primarily infects immune cells and can induce acquired immunodeficiency syndrome.
Opportunistic infections	Infections caused by otherwise lowly pathogenic microbes in individuals who have some immunodeficiency.
Respiratory viruses	Small microorganisms that preferentially infect the cells of the respiratory system.

Introduction

Stress is a major factor in the progression of infectious diseases in humans as well as in experimental and domestic animals. In this regard, it is now known that the central nervous system (CNS), the endocrine system, and the immune system are complex systems that interact with one another. In particular, the brain and CNS exert a profound effect on the immune system, including mechanisms necessary for resistance to microbial infection. Stress dysregulates the immune response by affecting the interplay of these systems. New knowledge developed during the last few decades through experimental and clinical studies provide evidence that many immune alterations are due to stressful events that provoke health changes. Stressors, including specific stressful events, can stimulate the activities of the hypothalamic-pituitary-adrenal (HPA) axis as well as the sympathetic nervous system to enhance an individual's ability to adapt physiologically in response to a threat (**Figure 1**). Furthermore, psychological stress ensues when events or environmental demands exceed an individual's perceived ability to cope. Stress can increase susceptibility to infectious agents, influence the severity of infectious diseases, diminish an immune response to a vaccine, reactivate a latent herpesvirus, and in general depress resistance to opportunistic infectious organisms that otherwise should not cause overt disease. Moreover, stressful events and the stress they evoke also may substantially increase the production of pro-inflammatory cytokines associated with a wide range of diseases, especially chronic immune diseases.

Not only the CNS is complex; there is now much new knowledge about the complexity of the immune

system, which consists of both cellular and humoral elements. Many immune responses are mediated by soluble factors such as cytokines produced by lymphoid cells and by factors important for control of the CNS, including steroids and various neuropeptides and neurohormones produced by neuronal cells (**Figure 1**). Important mechanisms whereby stress influences susceptibility or the more rapid progression of infectious diseases are becoming clearer because of new experimental and clinical studies by investigators worldwide. Specifically, the current explosion of new knowledge concerning the nature and mechanism of the immune response system has focused attention on the important role of various lymphoid cells for resistance versus susceptibility to microbes, especially intracellular pathogens such as opportunistic bacteria, viruses, fungi, and even parasites. It is now known that the brain and CNS in general have profound effects on immunity. The interaction between the brain and immune system entails a complex series of activities involving responses of many cells to multiple stimuli.

Central Nervous–Immune–Endocrine System Interactions

The modulation of the immune response by the CNS is mediated by a complex network of bidirectional interactions between the nervous, endocrine, and immune systems. The HPA axis and autonomic nervous systems provide two key pathways for immune system dysregulation. For example, stress may activate the sympathetic adrenomedullary (SAM), as well as the HPA axis, and thereby result in the release of pituitary and adrenal hormones, including catecholamines (epinephrine and norepinephrine), ACTH, cortisol, growth hormone, and prolactin, which are influenced by stressful events, including negative emotions. Each of these soluble factors results in quantitative and qualitative changes in immune activity. For example, external factors, including stress, increase cortisol levels, which may induce adverse immunological alterations. Immune cells express receptors for one or more factors associated with the HPA and SAM axes, generally called hormones. Immunomodulation by hormones occurs through two pathways: directly, through binding to a specific cell receptor, or indirectly, by the induction of cytokines such as interferon (IFN-)γ, interleukins (ILs), and pro-inflammatory cytokines such as tumor necrosis factor (TNF-)α. Such cytokines interact with various target cells. Furthermore, the interaction between the CNS and the immune system is bidirectional. For example, immune cell-derived ILs such as IL-1 affect the production of corticotropin releasing hormone

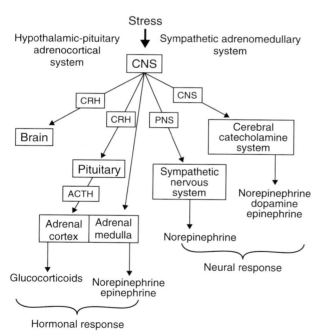

Figure 1 Arrangement of the hypothalamic-pituitary-adrenocortical and sympathetic adrenomedullary systems. The central noradrenergic system is activated in parallel with the peripheral sympathetic nervous system, and it is the central nervous system counterpart. The cerebral catecholamine system (i.e., dopamine and epinephrine) is activated under stress. ACTH, adrenocorticotropic hormone; CNS, central nervous system; CRH, corticotropin releasing hormone; PNS, peripheral nervous system.

(CRH) by the hypothalamus in the brain. An increase in stress hormone levels results in the further dysregulation of immune function. Similarly, lymphocytes produce many hormones such as ACTH, prolactin, and growth hormone.

Resistance to microbes, including bacteria, viruses, and parasites, depends on both innate and adaptive immune responses, consisting of a variety of cell types such as T and B lymphocytes; phagocytic monocytic cells, such as dendritic cells and macrophages; neutrophils; and polymorphonuclear cells. Soluble factors produced mainly by lymphoid cells, including ILs, IFNs, and other cytokines, are essential for host resistance. Immune resistance is based on primary and secondary antibody responses and cell-mediated immunity due to T lymphocytes such as Thl effector and Th2 helper cells, as well as Th3 regulatory cells. Such cells produce the many humoral factors important for immunoregulatory and protective pro-inflammatory activity, especially to intracellular opportunistic microbial pathogens.

Stress Hormones and Infections

As already indicated, many types of signals to the brain (e.g., visual, tactile, and emotional) cause the hypothalamus to release CRH, and, in turn, this stimulates the pituitary gland to release ACTH into the circulation, which then stimulates the adrenal cortex to produce glucocorticoids. ACTH inhibits the response of lymphocytes to antigenic or mitogenic stimulation, depresses cytokine responses by lymphocytes, and suppresses natural killer (NK) cell activity and antibody responses to a variety of antigens, including those associated with microorganisms. It is widely recognized that increased glucocorticoid production is by no means the only response to stress. The levels of several neuropeptides, including vasoactive intestinal peptides, substance P, prolactin, and growth hormones are increased, as are catecholamines such as epinephrine and norepinephrine. Localized increases in catecholamine levels probably account for the suppression of lymphocyte responses to mitogens or antigens. The immune system also returns signals to the CNS to close this circle. As previously stated, immune cells synthesize a number of neuropeptide hormones, including ACTH and β-endorphin. Moreover, cytokines produced by lymphocytes and macrophages have effects that are signals to the brain. Various ILs, including TNF-α, stimulate the hypothalamus, resulting in the induction of fever and release of corticosteroid hormones. Receptors for neuropeptides are present on lymphoid cells (**Table 1**), and neuropeptides derived from neural or immune cells stimulate leukocytes (**Tables 2–3**).

Table 1 Receptors for neuropeptide hormones on cells of the immune system[a]

Hormone	Receptor site
ACTH	Rat spleen T and B cells
β-Endorphin	Rat spleen T and B cells
Calcitonin gene-related peptide	Rat spleen T and B cells
CRH	Human PBL
Growth hormone	Rodent spleen, thymus, human PBL
Growth hormone-releasing hormone	Rodent spleen, human PBL
Luteinizing hormone-releasing hormone	Rat thymocytes
Prolactin	Human and mouse T and B cells
Somatostatin	Human PBL
Substance P	Mouse T and B cells
Thyrotropin	Human neutrophils, monocytes, B cells

[a]ACTH, adrenocorticotropic hormone; CRH, corticotropin releasing hormone; PBL, peripheral blood leukocytes.

Table 2 Stimuli for leukocyte-derived peptide hormones[a]

Hormone	Stimulator
Arginine vasopressin	Unknown
Corticotropin and endorphin	Newcastle disease virus
	Lymphotrophic viruses
	Bacterial lipopolysaccharide
	CRH
	Arginine vasopressin
	IL-1
Follicle-stimulating hormone	Con A
Growth hormone	Growth hormone-releasing hormone
	Growth hormone
Luteinizing hormone	Luteinizing hormone-releasing hormone
Metenkephalin	Con A
Neuropeptide Y	Unknown
Parathyroid hormone-related protein	Human T-cell lymphotrophic virus
Prolactin	Con A
Somatostatin	Hypersensitivity
Substance P	Unknown
Thyrotropin	Staphylococcal enterotoxin A
	Thyrotropin-releasing hormone
Vasoactive intestinal peptide	Histamine liberators
	Hypersensitivity

[a]Con A, concanavalin A; CRH, corticotropin releasing hormone; IL, interleukin.

Many studies have shown that increases in stress, especially those resulting in increased levels of stress hormones such as corticosteroids, alter the susceptibility of experimental animals to infectious diseases significantly (**Table 4**). The study of effects of

Table 3 Modulation of immune responses by neuropeptides[a]

Neuropeptide	Immune response
Arginine vasopressin	T-cell helper function
	Functions for IFN-γ production
Corticotropin	Antibody synthesis IFN-γ production
	B-lymphocyte stimulation
Endorphins	Antibody synthesis
	Mitogenesis
	NK-cell activity
Growth hormone	Cytotoxic T-cell activity
	Mitogenesis
Growth hormone-releasing hormone	Inhibit NK-cell activity
	Inhibit chemotactic response
Luteinizing hormone	Cytokine formation
Prolactin	IL-2 receptor production
Somatostatin	Reduces IFN-γ production
Substance P	Stimulate chemotaxis
	Stimulate proliferation
	Modulate cytokine levels
Thyrotropin	Antibody synthesis
	Co-mitogen
	Co-mitogenic with Con A

[a]Con A, concanavalin A; IFN, interferon; NK, natural killer.

Table 4 Effect of glucocorticoids on microbial immunity[a]

Organism	Glucocorticoid effect
Bordetella pertussis	Promotes initial protective effect, then promotes microbial survival
Candida albicans	Exacerbates infection
Escherichia coli	Decreases inflammation but not bacterial clearance
Legionella pneumophila	Exacerbates infection
Listeria monocytogenes	Increases susceptibility, impairs monocyte function
Mycobacterium avium	Impairs macrophage function
Mycobacterium leprae	Alters IFN-γ effects on monocytes
Mycobacterium tuberculosis	Increases cellular infiltration, increases bacterial growth
Neisseria gonorrhoeae	Increases infection rate
Plasmodium berghei	Decreases parasitemia
Pneumocystis carinii	Increases susceptibility
Propionibacterium acnes	Exacerbates infection
Pseudomonas aeruginosa	Increases susceptibility
Staphylococcus aureus	Ameliorates IP route infection
Streptococcus faecalis	Increases resistance
Trichinella spiralis	Decreases nematode clearance, cellular infiltration
Yersinia pestis (Pasteurella pestis)	Increases invasive infection, bacteremia

[a]IFN, interferon; IP, intraperitoneal.

neuroendocrine–immune interactions on microbial pathogenesis and immunity during the course of infectious disease is an important area of interdisciplinary research, and various studies showed that physiological stress and psychiatric illness can compromise immune function and alter susceptibility to infectious agents (**Table 5**). It is widely known that patients with psychiatric disorders, including schizophrenia and even depression, are more likely to have infectious diseases. This may be associated with altered HPA activity or physiological dysfunction related to immunomodulation associated with drugs that affect the brain. Unconventional life styles, eating disorders, poor hygiene, and other factors associated with severe mental health problems may contribute to altered immune function. In this regard, it is now recognized that the recreational use and abuse of illegal drugs such as marijuana, cocaine, heroin, and other opiates, as well as more widely used legal substances such as alcohol and tobacco, have marked effects on the CNS and the immune system. Individuals who use these drugs frequently are more susceptible to opportunistic microorganisms. The detrimental effects of such abused drugs on immunity in both humans and animals have now been extensively studied. These drugs are known to increase corticosteroid levels in both humans and experimental animals, either at the time of addiction or during withdrawal, and this effect has been related to altered immune resistance to microbial infection. Addiction to a psychoactive substance (as in the stimulation of the HPA axis) induces enhanced adrenal corticosteroid secretion, followed by consequential increases in serum glucocorticoids and the activation of the sympathetic nervous system. These responses result in immune dysregulation and increased susceptibility to microbial infections, especially to opportunistic pathogens.

Numerous early clinical observations reported that individuals often become more susceptible to infections following stressful situations. However, the concept of stress was not defined sharply. A stressor was often defined as any type of external or internal challenge, visual, tactile, or emotional, that disrupts the physiological equilibrium or homeostasis of an individual. For example, a number of studies showed that infection by mycobacteria, which cause tuberculosis, is increased by stress.

Alterations in the susceptibility to other opportunistic bacteria, as well as to viruses and parasites in general, have been studied extensively. Increases in infections due to stress occur not only in human populations but also in farm animals and experimental animals. There is now a large body of biomedical literature showing that stress alters susceptibility to infection. The mechanism of the stress includes effects on humoral function such as the production of glucocorticoids. The effects of stresses on two types

Table 5 Effects of stress on microbial immunity

Pathogen	Animal species	Stressor	Effect
Escherichia coli	Chicken	Cold	Increases resistance
	Chicken	Social	Increases resistance
Hymenolepis nana	Mouse	Predator	Increases reinfection rate
Mycobacterium avium	Mouse	Restraint	Increases susceptibility, impairs macrophage function
Mycobacterium tuberculosis	Rabbit	Tumbling	Increases susceptibility
Plasmodium berghei	Mouse	Electric	Increases survival
Salmonella enteritidis	Chicken	Fasting	Decreases antibody response
Salmonella typhimurium	Mouse	Crowding	Increases susceptibility

of infective diseases, bacterial and viral, are discussed next as examples.

Bacterial Infections and Steroids

Legionella pneumophila, an opportunistic ubiquitous bacterium, is the causative agent of Legionnaire's disease. Although almost all individuals are exposed to *Legionella*, only a small percentage of individuals exposed to these organisms are infected clinically. Indeed, when *Legionella* was first discovered in the outbreak of Legionnaire's disease in Philadelphia in the late 1970s, most of the 2500 conventioneers exposed to this organism from the air conditioning system in the Belleview Stratford Hotel developed significant titers to these bacteria. However, only approximately 200 individuals became clinically ill, and a significant number of these people died. These individuals had certain factors associated with their susceptibility, including increased alcohol consumption, cigarette smoking, (in general) being older, and being more immunocompromised. It is now well recognized that *L. pneumophila* causes clinical infection mainly in immunocompromised individuals, including patients who are treated with immunosuppressive drugs in hospitals for cancer chemotherapy or for organ transplantation.

Increases in susceptibility to infection by *Legionella* associated with steroid use have been studied in detail (Table 4). Although steroid therapy for various diseases has had revolutionary therapeutic effects and is widely recognized as constituting a major success for modern medicine, it is often associated with serious side effects; steroids have both beneficial and nonbeneficial features, and these may be inseparable. The anti-inflammatory and immunosuppressive activities of steroids are considered essential for the therapy of certain diseases, including autoimmune diseases, and to prevent organ rejection following transplantation. However, steroids may also result in an increased susceptibility to infections, especially by an opportunistic bacterium such as *L. pneumophila*. Although the spectrum of microbes causing infections in patients

during steroid therapy is not completely clear, experimental animal studies showed that steroid treatment is associated with increased infections caused by certain groups of opportunistic bacteria, including *Legionella*. The general consensus concerning the mechanism whereby steroids induce altered susceptibility to bacterial infection is that steroids suppress the immune response system.

The most important host defense mechanism against invading intracellular opportunistic bacteria is phagocytosis by macrophages, followed by intracellular killing and digestion of the microbes. It is now clear that steroids suppress the number and function of macrophages and neutrophils (**Figures 2–3**). For example, experimental studies have shown that peritoneal macrophages from hydrocortisone-treated mice are more susceptible to infection and killing by *L. pneumophila in vitro*. The steroid-involved impairment of antimicrobial activity by macrophages from mice infected with *Legionella* is generally similar to that reported for *Listeria monocytogenes*. For example, *in vivo* treatment of mice with hydrocortisone acetate affects the ability of peritoneal macrophages from the animals to kill *L. pneumophila in vitro*, as well as other microorganisms such as *Listeria monocytogenes, Streptococcus pyogenes, Staphylococcus aureus, Staphylococcus epidermidis, Escherichia coli*, and *Pseudomonas aeruginosa*.

The treatment of macrophages with steroids *in vitro* may affect antimicrobial immunity directly. For example, the ability of macrophages treated with steroids to kill *L. pneumophila* and organisms such as *Staphylococci in vitro* is markedly reduced. The specific mechanisms involved in the steroid impairment of macrophages, however, are unclear. In general, the intracellular killing of bacteria and other microbes by macrophages requires lysosomal migration to and fusion with the microbe-containing phagosome. It is probable that the mechanism of the steroid-induced impairment of antimicrobicidal activity of monocytes or macrophages is associated with the stabilization of lysosomes by steroids, which prevents their fusion with phagosomes. However, the possibility exists that

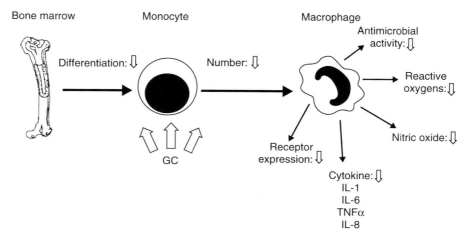

Figure 2 The effect of steroids on macrophages and monocytes. Glucocorticoids have a direct action on the number and function of phagocytic cells, including cytokine production and receptor expression. ⇓, decrease; GC, glucocorticoid; IL, interleukin; TNF, tumor necrosis factor.

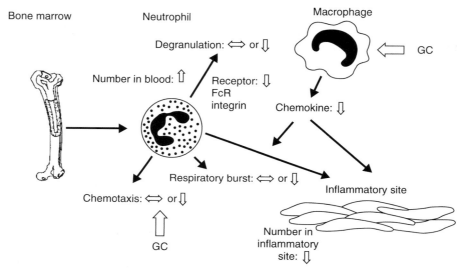

Figure 3 Prevention of neutrophil accumulation at local inflammatory site by steroid treatment. The chemotactic activity of neutrophils from steroid-treated animals or humans was enhanced, inhibited very weakly, or unaffected, except for neutrophils from inflammatory exudates, which showed reduced chemotactic activity. ⇓, decrease; ⇑, increase; ⇔, minimal or no change, FcR, Fc receptor; GC, glucocorticoid.

steroids induce the impairment of the antimicrobial activity of macrophages by suppressing the synthesis of one or several specific proteins of the killing system of the phagocytes. Nevertheless, several observations have indicated that macrophages treated with steroids ingest microorganisms at a normal rate and, after phagocytosis, secrete the usual reactive oxygen intermediates and exhibit normal fusion of lysosomes and phagosomes (i.e., the oxidative killing systems). Steroid-treated macrophages react to a cytokine such as IFN and are normally primed to secrete reactive oxygen intermediates on challenge. Thus, there have been reports negating the likelihood there is a direct

deleterious effect of steroids on the antimicrobial activity of macrophages.

Virus Infections and Stress

Virus infection can be exacerbated by stress hormones such as cortisone. For example, hydrocortisone-treated mice show an increased susceptibility to challenge with viruses such as influenza virus, Coxsackie virus, or even mouse hepatitis virus. Peritoneal macrophages from cortisone-treated mice are almost 1000 times more susceptible to challenge with the mouse hepatitis virus *in vitro* than are macrophages from untreated mice. Resistant macrophages from normal mice succumb to cytolysis by mouse hepatitis virus when cultured with spleen cells from cortisone-treated mice but not with spleen cells from normal mice, suggesting that a soluble product from lymphoid cells may be involved in increased susceptibility of the macrophages due to steroids.

Various studies have reported the association between naturally occurring stresses and individuals' susceptibility to upper respiratory tract viral infections. Although most of these studies provide some support for the hypothesis that stress is associated with an increased risk of upper respiratory viral infections, it is not yet clear how this occurs. Longitudinal studies performed with large populations of individuals suggest that stress is a significant factor in increasing the susceptibility to viral infection.

A number of studies have been performed testing the possibility that stress is involved in experimentally induced upper respiratory tract viral infections. Psychologically stressed, experimentally infected individuals had significantly higher levels of upper respiratory tract infections, but there were no differences in the incidence of infections or the amount of shed virus in nasal secretions between these and unstressed individuals. Several studies reported that stress precedes the onset of upper respiratory tract viral infection episodes, especially in children; for example, several studies reported a significant increase in minor stresses a few days before the onset of upper respiratory tract infection symptoms. The likelihood exists that the severity of the symptoms of upper respiratory tract infections rather than the incidence of infection may be affected by different types of psychological stress. So far, it is apparent that more clinical studies must be performed before we can fully understand the relationship between stress and upper respiratory tract viral infections in patient populations. In addition, little is known about how the timing of the stressor and viral exposure influences the development of these infections. There is some evidence suggesting that stress occurring after experimental viral exposure may increase susceptibility; however, there are differing published findings, some indicating an increased and some a decreased susceptibility even when stress precedes viral exposure.

Studies have been reported concerning stress and progression of acquired immunodeficiency syndrome (AIDS) in human immunodeficiency virus (HIV)-positive subjects. For example, a study published by investigators from the University of Miami School of Medicine, supported by the National Institute of Mental Health, showed that HIV-positive high-risk subjects had less evidence of progression to clinical AIDS when psychological intervention techniques,

such as stress reduction by counseling, music therapy, or exercise, were used. This study supported the view that psychological stress in HIV-positive individuals can result in a more rapid progression to clinical AIDS and that psychological stresses were often related to lack of an effective support system and with the notification of HIV-positive status. Such findings suggested that psychological stress and its intervention may be associated with the progression of chronic life-threatening viral infections, such as HIV.

There are also well-known studies concerning the effects of stress on herpesvirus exacerbation. A landmark study performed at the Ohio State University Medical School reported that medical students taking a routinely scheduled examination had increased psychological stress immediately preceding the examination and that this was associated with decreased immune function and the increased recurrence of herpesvirus titers, indicative of the reactivation of the herpesvirus. The study was particularly well controlled, consisting of medical students who were generally healthy and immunologically mature (i.e., approximately the second decade of life). All the students had normal immune functions, but at the time of the examination they were shown by psychological tests to have a significant stress level and increased serum glucocorticoids. Simultaneously, they showed a decrease in an immune function important in resistance to viral infection, NK cell activity and T-cell levels. Many of the students had an exacerbation of latent herpes shortly after the examination (with its associated stress).

Note that temporal relations often cannot be controlled readily in population studies. Furthermore, little is known about the differential effects of acute (short-term) versus chronic (long-term) or repetitive stressors. The clinical literature suggests that chronic stress may have particularly strong pernicious effects on health. But it is difficult to undertake true experimental studies of stress exposure in human populations because it is difficult to randomly assign subjects to defined stressor conditions. Although challenge viral exposure in experimental studies appears to be relatively controlled, it is often not because of independent variables and because stress is difficult to assess and manipulate. Furthermore, little is known about the biological pathways that may be responsible for the association between stress and increased viral infection in patient populations.

The effect of psychosocial interventions in ameliorating a number of infectious problems in patients with diseases as diverse as cardiovascular disease and cancer is currently being investigated. Many investigators believe that appropriate psychosocial intervention may result in reduced stress and thus reduced viral infections. Nevertheless, most studies to date with patient populations and viral infections suggest only that there is an association between stress and increased susceptibility to infection.

Discussion and Conclusion

It is now widely accepted that stress plays an important role in altering the susceptibility to infectious agents such as bacteria, viruses, and even parasites. Furthermore, stress is also acknowledged to be involved in increasing the susceptibility to the progression of autoimmune diseases and malignancies. Many studies have suggested that the stress hormones, especially cortisone and ACTH, are important in altering the immune mechanisms, especially in the lymphoid cells, which are important in the resistance to opportunistic microorganisms such as intracellular bacteria and viruses.

Various studies showed that a variety of stressors increase the susceptibility of experimental animals to bacterial infections. Some of the most defined studies to date were performed with mycobacteria, organisms that cause tuberculosis in humans and in domestic and experimental animals. Infection by mycobacteria is known to be increased by stress; for example, a number of widely known studies showed that mice that were normally resistant to mycobacterial infection showed increased susceptibility when given certain stressors. This has been related to increases in glucocorticoid levels, which are known to affect lymphoid cell function.

Glucocorticoids produced by the adrenal cortex under the influence of ACTH from the pituitary gland in the brain affect both humoral and cellular immune responses. Mice treated with glucocorticoids often show increased cellular infiltration following infection with mycobacteria and increased growth of the bacteria. Glucocorticoids have been shown to increase the susceptibility of experimental mice to infectious agents such *Listeria monocytogenes* and *Pneumocystis carinii*. However, glucocorticoids promote the survival of *Bordetella pertussis,* the causative agent of whooping cough in humans, although initially this hormone provides some protection against challenge infection. Furthermore, cortisone ameliorates infection by *Staphylococcus aureus* in experimental animals, but has been reported to increase the susceptibility to *Pseudomonas aeruginosa* in humans and animals and also to exacerbate infection by the ubiquitous fungus *Candida albicans*. Thus, there is a marked variability in the effects of corticoids on infection, depending on the organisms involved; the reasons for this remain unknown. For example, various studies showed that infection with

Propionibacterium acnes is exacerbated by corticosteroids but that infection with *Streptococcus faecalis* is decreased by them. Furthermore, animals infected with *Plasmodium,* the cause of malaria, showed decreased parasitemia due to corticosteroids.

It is clear that corticosteroids decrease the accumulation of neutrophils at a local inflammatory site. Such neutrophil accumulation is important in clearance of or resistance to bacterial infection. It has also been reported that the chemotactic activity of neutrophils from steroid-treated animals or humans can be enhanced, inhibited very weakly, or unaffected; however, most studies showed that neutrophils obtained from inflammatory exudates in steroid-treated mice showed reduced chemotactic activity. Such data indicate that the poor accumulation of neutrophils in inflammatory sites may be mediated by the inhibition of the release of local chemotactic factors rather than a direct effect on neutrophils. This possibility seems likely because steroid treatment does not inhibit neutrophil accumulation induced by the injection of a chemotactic complement component into human skin. It has been demonstrated that the treatment of purified human neutrophils with the synthetic steroid deoxymethasone does not inhibit neutrophil chemotaxis in response to a range of concentrations of known chemoattractants.

There are several mechanisms for gene regulation by the steroid–receptor complex. Glucocorticoid response elements regulate the rate of transcription initiated by promoters of the corresponding glucocorticoid response genes. Another possible regulation mechanism is the interaction with DNA-binding proteins associated with regulatory elements of DNA, such as the glucocorticoid modulatory element protein. Thus, it appears that steroids regulate the transcription of certain genes coding for proteins that augment steroid effects.

The infection of animals with the ubiquitous bacterium *L. pneumophila* is modulated markedly by steroids. Thus, steroid levels are an important factor in the increased susceptibility of organ-transplant patients, who are often immunosuppressed with steroids prior to the transplant and thus may become more susceptible to an opportunistic infection such as *Legionella* in hospitals. Viral infections have also been shown to be exacerbated by stress hormones, including cortisone. It is well known that hydrocortisone-treated mice show an increased susceptibility to challenge with a variety of viruses, including influenza virus, Coxsackie virus, and mouse hepatitis virus. It seems likely that, because stress is often associated with increased corticosteroid levels only, changes in the level of this hormone may be related to the apparent increased susceptibility of individuals to an upper respiratory tract viral infection following a stressful event. Results obtained using animal models show an increased susceptibility to challenge infection with bacteria or viruses, and studies of humans, infected either naturally or experimentally, strongly suggest a relationship between stress-induced immunomodulatory hormones and increased susceptibility to infection.

The complex interrelationship between the nervous and the immune system parallels the association of the susceptibility or resistance to infections by various microorganisms under conditions of stress. This is even more likely because it is known that the immune response is modulated markedly by a wide variety of neuropeptides associated with the CNS, not only corticotropin but also other hormones such as endorphins, prolactin, growth hormone, vasopressin, and somatotrophin. Neuropeptides affect a wide variety of immune responses, including antibody formation, mitogenic responses of lymphocytes, cytotoxicity by T cells, NK cell production and activity, and cytokine production. Thus, neuropeptides, hormones, and their receptors, present not only in the CNS but also on immune cells, are important factors in immunomodulation related to altering the susceptibility to infection by microorganisms, especially intracellular opportunistic bacteria and viruses. However, because of the complexity of both the CNS and the immune system, it is difficult to isolate the various pathways that are important in this altered susceptibility to infection associated with stress. Further studies in numerous laboratories, including those mainly concerned with the neurological system and those concerned with infectious diseases and immunity, will undoubtedly provide a greater understanding of the role of stress in infection.

See Also the Following Articles

Antibody Response; Desensitization; Disease, Stress Induced; Herpesviruses; HIV Infection/AIDS; Immunity; Leukocyte Trafficking and Stress; Natural Killer (NK) Cells.

Further Reading

Ader, R. and Cohen, N. (1993). Psychoneuroimmunology: conditioning and stress. *Annual Review of Psychology* **44**, 53–71.

Ader, R., Felten, D. and Cohen, N. (1991). *Psychoneuro-immunology* (2nd edn.). San Diego, CA: Academic Press.

Akira, S. and Kishimoto, T. (1992). IL-6 and NFκB in acute phase response and viral infection. *Immunological Reviews* **127**, 26–41.

Baue, A. F. (1989). Neuroendocrine response to severe trauma and sepsis. In: Faist, E., Ninnemann, J. & Green, D. (eds.) *Immune consequences of trauma, shyock and sepsis*, pp. 17. New York: Springer-Verlag.

Bayle, J. E., Guellati, M., Ibos, F., et al. (1991). *Brucella abortus* antigen stimulates the pituitary-adrenal axis through the extra-pituitary B-lymphoid system. *Progress in Neuroendocrinimmunology* **4**, 99–112.

Beisel, W. R. (1975). Metabolic response to infection. *Annual Review of Medicine* **26**, 9–29.

Blalock, I. E. (1992). Production of peptide hormones and neurotransmitters by the immune system. In: Blalock, J. E. (ed.) *Neuroimmunoendocrinology* (2nd edn.). Basel: Karger.

Friedman, H., Klein, T. W. and Friedman, A. L. (1996). *Psychoneuroimmunology, stress and infection*. Boca Raton, FL: CRC Press.

Friedman, H., Klein, T. W. and Specter, S. (1996). *Drugs of abuse, immunity and infections*. Boca Raton, FL: CRC Press.

Friedman, H., Newton, C. and Klein, T. W. (2003). Microbial infection, immunomodulation and drugs of abuse. *Clinical Microbial Reviews* **16**, 209–220.

Glaser, R. and Kiecolt-Glaser, J. K. (2005). Stress-induced immune dysfunction: implications for health. *Nature Reviews Immunology* **5**, 243–252.

Hart, B. L. (1988). Biological basis of the behavior of sick animals. *Neuroscience and Biobehavioral Reviews* **12**, 123–129.

Jefferies, W. M. (1991). Cortisol and immunity. *Medical Hypotheses* **34**, 198–215.

Kass, E. H. and Finland, M. (1958). Corticosteroids and infections. *Advances in Internal Medicine* **9**, 45–61.

Padgett, D. A. and Glaser, R. (2003). How stress influences the immune response. *Trends in Immunology* **24**, 444–453.

Rabin, B. S. (1999). *Stress, immune function, and health: the connection*. New York: Wiley-Liss & Sons.

Schattner, A. and Schaffner, T. (1987). Glucocorticoid-induced impairment of macrophage antimicrobial activity: mechanisms and dependence on the state of activation. *Review of Infectious Diseases* **9**, 5620.

Sheridan, J. F., Dobbs, C., Brown, D., et al. (1994). Psychoneuroimmunology: stress effects on pathogenesis and immunity during infection. *Clinical Microbial Reviews* **7**, 200.

Stone, A. and Bovbjerg, D. (1994). Stress and humoral immunity: a review of human studies. *Advances on Neuroimmunology* **4**, 49.

Stone, E. A. (1975). Stress and catecholamines. In: Friedhoff, A. J. (ed.) *Catecholamines and neuropsychopharmacology*, (vol. 2), p. 31. New York: Plenum Press.

Webster, J. I., Tonelli, L. and Sternberg, E. M. (2002). Neuroendocrine regulation of immunity. *Annual Review of Immunology* **20**, 126–163.

Inflammation

G Z Feuerstein, R R Ruffolo, C Coughlin, J Wang and D Miller
Wyeth Research, Collegeville, PA, USA

Glossary

Apoptosis	A process of cell death that results from the activation of specific signaling pathways that lead to the intracellular disruption of mitochondrial integrity, activation of cascade of proteases (e.g., caspases), and cell disintegration while maintaining the cell membrane intact.
Chemokines	A family of polypeptides that comprises about 50 members and 20 different receptors. This family of polypeptides is all involved in leukocyte traffic. Their diverse biological actions include interactions with viruses and cell receptors in numerous tissues.
Chemotaxis	The orientation and movement of a cell along a specific chemical concentration. Positive chemotaxis denotes movement of the cell toward the high-concentration site of the chemical; negative chemotaxis denotes movement of the cell away from the source of the chemical. Chemotactic properties are prevalent in all forms of leukocytes and in a wide variety of substances released in sites of tissue injury or activated cells.
Complement system	The entire functionality of approximately 20 distinct plasma proteins, their receptors, and ancillary/regulatory proteins that are responsible not only for immune cytolysis but also for reactions such as anaphylaxis, phagocytosis, opsonization, and hemolysis. Two major pathways for activation of the complement system are known: the classic pathway in which all components C1–C9 participate in the reaction and the alternative pathway in which only part of the plasma factors participate along with others that are not essential in the classic reaction.
Cytokines	Nonantibody peptides and polypeptides that are released by activated cells (e.g., T cells) and transfer signals to other cells. Lymphokines (cytokines produced by lymphocytes) and monokines (cytokines produces by monocytes) are cytokines.
Inflammation	A localized protective response elicited by injury or destruction of tissues, which serves to destroy, dilute, or wall off (sequester) both the injurious agent and the injured tissue. It is characterized in the acute form by the classic signs of pain, heat, redness, swelling, and loss of function. Histologically, it involves a complex series of events, including the dilation of the arterioles and capillaries, extravasation of fluids, and migration of plasma proteins and leukocytes into the injured area.
Interleukins (ILs)	A generic term for a group of multifunctional cytokines that are produced by a variety of lymphoid and nonlymphoid cells. Originally believed to play a role only in leukocyte biology, ILs are now recognized as the products of diverse nonlymphoid cells that also act on diverse receptors on multiple cells outside the lymphoid system. Over 20 ILs have been identified to date that act via different receptors with large divergent and cross-activation among the IL family members. ILs are involved in many disease processes and are targets for promising drug discovery.
Leukocytes	Colorless blood cells capable of ameboid movement; they are capable of moving directionally in response to chemical stimuli (chemotaxis). Leukocytes are divided morphologically into granular cells (basophils, eosinophils, and neutrophils) and nongranular cells (lymphocytes and monocytes). Leukocytes are the primary cells that launch immune and inflammatory reactions. Leukocytes are present in the systemic circulation and in special lymphoid tissue such as the lymph node, bone marrow, and thymus.
Lymphocytes	Mostly mononuclear, nonphagocytic leukocytes found in the blood and

lymphoid tissue that make up the primary body of immune competent cells. Lymphocytes belong to two primary classes – T cells (thymus dependent) and B cells (Bursa dependent) – but several other subclasses with various functional and biochemical markers are known. Lymphocytes function via direct cell–cell interaction (specialized receptors) and via humoral mediators such as cytokines, interleukins, and chemokines as well as antibodies (a primary B-cell function). T cells are primarily responsible for cell-mediated immunity.

Mast cells
A connective tissue cell that elaborates highly reactive mediators such as cytokines, histamine, and enzymes, which can modulate matrix proteins such as chymotrypsin and tryptase. Mast cells (or mastocytes) are believed to play an important role in allergic rhinitis and asthma and, via enzymes released, to contribute to inflammation and atherosclerosis.

Matrix metalloproteinases (MMPs)
Zinc-dependent endopeptidases known for their ability to cleave one or several constituents of the extracellular matrix. MMPs consist of a large family of proteases that share common structural and functional elements.

Metabolic syndrome
A clinical condition that manifests four or five risk factors for cardiovascular and metabolic disorders. These include obesity, high glucose levels, high blood pressure, and aberrant plasma lipid levels (high triglycerides and low high-density lipoproteins).

Monocytes
Mononuclear phagocytic leukocytes that originate in the bone marrow. Monocytes are the source of tissue macrophages, which are abundant in lung and liver.

Nonsteroidal anti-inflammatory drug (NSAID)
Small organic (synthetic) chemicals that have been developed to suppress inflammation of various mechanisms, locations, and durations. They are commonly compounds that do not act like the steroid hormones (e.g., glucocorticoids). This class of medicines contains primarily inhibitors of the cyclooxygenase enzymes (which produce pro-inflammatory metabolites of the fatty acid arachidonate) and displays various proportional inhibitory capacities toward the cyclooxygenase 1 or 2 enzymes. Many such agents are marketed for pain relief from conditions such as arthritis and other muscular-skeletal conditions.

Sepsis
A condition that results from a harmful or host response to infection. Sepsis is marked by endotoxemia (the presence of bacterial or other toxins in the blood) and the activation of multiple systems such as the immune, cardiovascular, respiratory, coagulation, and complement systems. Sepsis can lead to multiple organ failure and death.

Introduction

Inflammation is a fundamental reaction of the body to injury. It is a complex biological phenomenon that comprises diverse cellular, neural, hormonal, and humoral systems. Inflammation involves the vascular system as well as blood-borne components linked via a complicated network of mediators. Inflammation can be the result of endogenous or exogenous injurious events. Inflammation is fundamentally viewed as a purposeful reaction aimed to repair, salvage, and restore the structure, function. and integrity of the injured tissue, organ, and organism well-being at large.

However, inflammation may also become a destructive or pathological condition that underlies numerous diseases in humans. Such diseases include bone and cartilage diseases (rheumatoid arthritis and osteoarthritis), skin diseases (psoriasis), central nervous system (CNS) diseases (multiple sclerosis and Alzheimer's disease), vascular diseases (atherosclerosis), cardiac diseases (heart failure and myocardial infarction), respiratory diseases (asthma and chronic obstructive pulmonary disease, COPD), gastrointestinal diseases (inflammatory bowel disease and Crohn's disease), and chronic unresolved infectious diseases (e.g., tuberculosis). In recent years, inflammation is increasingly recognized as a fundamental contributing element in many human diseases that have not been traditionally associated with inflammation. Conditions such as obesity, diabetes, metabolic syndrome, stroke, and cancer are all recognized as harboring various immune and inflammatory cells and mediators.

Inflammation is invariably linked to general homeostasis systems (e.g., coagulation and fibrinolysis) as also to the immune, complement, and the nervous system. As such, intervention in or modulation of specific pro-inflammatory mediators might result in broader consequences than the intended anti-inflammatory objective. Moreover, many mediators of inflammation are actually part of the normal physiological repertoire of molecules and cells that secure essential function and health. Therefore, the modulation (blockade or enhancement) of many recognized pro-inflammatory mediators, although potentially to providing medical benefits, could also harm. Thus a fine balance needs to be preserved in many cases so as not to disrupt functionalities that require the same mediators to be at a level context and duration that, if not secured, could lead to pathological conditions on their own.

The advances made in understanding the cellular elements and mediators that initiate, propagate, and amplify various forms of inflammation have already yielded important therapeutics. Nonsteroidal anti-inflammatory drugs (NSAIDs), steroids, and, more recently, ant-cytokines and interleukin mimetics have an important role in the treatment of inflammation. It is, however, important to keep in mind that no anti-inflammatory therapeutic introduced into medical practice is free of adverse effect.

Immune and Inflammatory Cells in Acute Inflammation: Role of Endothelium and Adhesion Molecules

Acute injury to tissues, such as bruises, blunt-force trauma, or infectious agents, elicit a typical inflammatory reaction. The early response consists of local neurovascular reaction and release of preformed mediators that induced vasodilation, microvascular permeability, and extravasation of plasma components into the injured zone. This early stage is followed by the recruitment and migration of leukocytes from the systemic circulation with primary role of the polymorphonuclear (PMN) cells. The PMN cells are followed by monocytes, which together with the PMS cells and tissue macrophages provide the local tissue with the ability to conduct phagocytosis of invading pathogens, engulf cell debris (e.g., necrotic cells), and set the stage for tissue repair. The recruitment of leukocytes into the injury zone is governed by two key processes: chemotaxis and cell adhesion. The directional influx of leukocytes into the injured tissue is dependent on mediators such as chemokines or complement factors, which, along with cytokines and interleukins, also activate the leukocytes. In addition, the endothelium along the microvessels associated with the injury zone express adhesion molecules (in addition to constitutive ones) that enable the interaction with ligands that are expressed on the leukocytes. These cell adhesion molecules act as a cascade of events – from loose rolling, loose adhesion, committed adhesion, and final migration mostly through the endothelium junction. The key adhesion molecules are the. vascular cell adhesion molecule (VCAM-)1; intercellular adhesion molecule (ICAM-)1, selectins (E, P, and L), and platelet-endothelial cells adhesion molecules (PECAMs).

Inflammation, Artherosclerosis, and Cardiovascular Diseases

The major pathological process that underwrites heart attacks, strokes, and peripheral vascular diseases is arteriosclerosis. Although the role of lipids (cholesterol in particular) in initiation and propagation of the arteriosclerotic pathology is well documented, inflammation is considered to be a major pathological feature in the evolution of this vascular disease. Lipid-loaded cells are the hallmark in any vascular atheroma, or plaque, which are macrophages (derived from blood monocytes) that phagocytosed modified cholesterol within lipoproteins particles. This process leads to the activation of the macrophages and release of cytokines, chemokines, interleukins, and other pro-inflammatory mediators such as arachidonic acid metabolites (lipoxygenase and cyclooxygenase). Apoptosis of excessively loaded macrophages (also called foam cells) is believed to release numerous inflammatory mediators that exacerbate the inflammatory process and increase the likelihood of its rupture. Most significantly in this regards are matrix metalloproteinases (MMPs; especially MMP-2 and -9), which are believed to reduce the fibrous cap of the atheroma and enhance plaque rupture, leading to the initiation of thrombosis and vascular occlusion. The atheromatous plaque is also rich in other inflammatory cells such a mast cells and T cells. The vascular inflammation part of the atherosclerosis process is viewed as an important therapeutic target and a component of the efficacy of major anti-atheroslerosis drugs such as the statins.

Inflammation and Cancer

A causal link between cancer and chronic inflammation has been demonstrated in the more than 1 million cancer patients linked to viruses and bacteria. Infection with human papillomaviruses, HCV, HBV; *Helicobacter pylori*; and Epstein–Barr virus are major risk factors for the development of cervical, gastrointestinal (GI), and hepatocellular cancer and lymphoma, respectively. The link between inflammation and cancer is not limited to infectious agents; chronic inflammation from cigarette smoke, asbestos, inflammatory bowel disease, silica, and so on contributes to the development of malignancy in the lungs, bladder, and GI tract. The activation of innate inflammation has been shown to contribute to cancer progression, including tumor necrosis factor (TNF)-α, and nuclear factor (NF)-κB signaling. The disruption of the adaptive (or antigen-specific) immune response to tumors has been shown to be crucial to carcinogenesis. Many studies have documented the anergic antitumor immune responses contrasting with the favorable prognosis conferred by the infiltration of tumors with cytotoxic killer T cells in several malignancies. In contrast, infiltration with supportive immune elements, such as growth-promoting macrophages, confers a worse prognosis in some malignancies. Finally, the association between multiple inflammatory biomarkers, such as interleukin (IL-)8, macrophage inflammatory protein (MIP-)1a, and various chemokines, whose expression levels correlate directly with worse prognosis, underlies the intimate relationship between inflammation and cancer development and progression.

Inflammation and Metabolic Syndrome

Metabolic syndrome emerges as the twenty-first-century epidemic that threatens both developed and less developed nations. Although the original concept defining metabolic syndrome focused on insulin resistance, namely, the poor responsiveness of target cells to insulin's ability to advance glucose metabolism, it has been recently recognized that inflammatory mediators are likely to be causally associated with the state of insulin resistance and, hence, metabolic syndrome. Most notable in this regards are the cytokines TNF-α, and IL-6. These cytokines, and primarily TNF-α, reduce the efficacy of insulin to enhance glucose uptake into the cells, a situation that manifests itself as hyperglycemia, a hallmark of the insulin resistant condition. Obesity, a key feature of the metabolic syndrome, is considered a pro-inflammatory state. Obesity is associated with increased oxidative stress, a biochemical condition prone to activating NF-κB, NADPH, and other factors. Oxidative stress-induced inflammation increases endothelial leukocyte adhesion molecules that enhance leukocyte engagement with the endothelium, a primary step for their entry into the tissue, their activation, and the further release of inflammatory mediators. Excessive caloric intake, from carbohydrates or fats, is considered to significantly contribute to the inflammation state that drives key elements of metabolic syndrome.

Inflammation and Respiratory Diseases

Chronic obstructive pulmonary disease (COPD) is a chronic lung disorder that is mostly the result of smoking and other environmental toxic agents. The disorder is characterized by the accumulation of inflammatory cells such as macrophages and neutrophils, which are activated to release numerous mediators. The inflammation resides within the terminal bronchioles (small airways) and alveoli (small vesicular spaces where oxygen and CO_2 exchange takes place). The persistent inflammation ultimately leads to the destruction of these pulmonary structures and respiratory failure. Prominent in the COPD pathomechanism are the inflammatory products of arachidonic acid and MMPs released by the activated inflammatory cells. MMP-9 and, in particular, MMP-12 play a predominant role in COPD by degrading the matrix proteins such as elastin, a matrix protein that is vital to the recoil of the bronchioles (small airways) and to alveolar health. MMP-12-mediated elastin degradation is believed to lead to emphysema, a state of destruction of the normal architecture of the lung respiratory elements. MMP-12 also plays a role in macrophage recruitment. Promising data emanating from recent research suggest that selective inhibitors of MMP-12 might be useful drugs in the treatment and prevention of COPD.

Bronchial asthma, a disease of lung airway spasm that leads to severe respiratory distress and severe forms to death, has strong inflammatory components. Arachidonic acid metabolites of potent inflammatory properties figure prominently in this disease. Lipoxigenase products called leukotrienes, prostanoids (prostaglandins and thromboxane A2), and isoprostanes have been implicated in this disorder. Indeed, anti-inflammatory agents such as glucocorticosteroids have been a cornerstone of asthma-attack prevention, largely due to their inhibition of inflammatory eicosanoids. In addition, specific inhibitors of cysteinyl leukotriene have proven to serve additional therapeutic efficacy.

Inflammation and Joint Diseases

Several joint and bone diseases, such as rheumatoid arthritis and osteoarthritis, are probably the result of degenerative (the former) or immune and inflammatory (the latter) processes. Rheumatoid arthritis is a chronic systemic disease primarily affecting the joints in which severe chronic inflammation leads to the destruction of the joint structure and, ultimately, functional disability. Misdirected inflammation is the cardinal feature of rheumatological diseases. It involves both the initiation and maintenance phases of the disease, and the processes and players (cells and mediators) involved are similar to that in other diseases. Major cells in the immune system (i.e., neutrophils, macrophages, dendritic cells, B cells, and T cells) are the major culprits in the development and exacerbation of the disease. Although autoimmune mechanisms (including the generation of antibodies against joint tissue components) are believed to play a major causative role, the chronic condition is probably sustained by numerous inflammatory mediators, including cytokines, ILs, chemokines,

MMPs, prostanoids, and reactive oxygen radicals. Traditional anti-inflammatory agents such as the NSAIDs have been widely used to alleviate pain in and swelling of the joint, but their efficacy in mitigating the fundamental pathological process remained questionable. Likewise, the more recent class of antirheumatoid arthritis drugs, the COX-2 inhibitors, have a proven efficacy, yet at the cost of some increased risk for a cardiovascular adverse event. More recently, disease-modifying anti-arthritis drugs (DMARDs) have been successfully introduced into the medical management of rheumatoid arthritis. Such agents neutralize the cytokine TNF-α. Other cytokines and ILs (e.g., IL-6, IL-1, and IL-18) as well as interferon (IFN)-γ and endothelium leukocyte adhesion molecules (ICAM-1, VCAM-1, and selectins) are also targeted by therapeutic agents, as well as angiogenesis promoters such as vascular endothelium growth factor (VEGF).

The role of inflammation in osteoarthritis is less clear, although many of the cytokines already discussed are believed to play a key role in the destruction of bone and cartilage. Cartilage destruction probably involves cytokine activation of aggrecanase, an enzyme that destroys a major constituent of the normal cartilage.

Inflammation and Sepsis

Sepsis is a complex clinical syndrome that results from the harmful host response to infection; it results from the failure of the innate and acquired immune mechanisms to resolve the infectious condition and the damage induced by the toxins elaborated by the infectious agent. The bacterial toxins activate many of the inflammatory cells (in particular, neutrophils and monocytes/macrophages) but also other cells such as the endothelium. As a result of the toxins' action on the inflammatory cells, numerous preformed and newly elaborated mediators are produced, including oxygen radicals, bioactive lipid mediators, cytokines, chemokines, enzymes, and pro- and anticoagulation factors. Although many of the inflammatory cell products are helpful in confining and eliminating the infectious agent and its toxins, multiple tissues, organs, and system are also affected. Oxygen radical have bactericidal action, yet also affect the vasculature. Chemokines and cytokines modify the endothelium to support the fast recruitment of inflammation cells into the tissue to remove the invading agent while ILs activate and enhance the neutrophils, lymphocytes, and endothelium function. The inflammation cells also play a role in tissue repair and rehabilitation via the generation and release of growth factors that enhance

the regeneration of the damaged circulation, the matrix elements, and tissue integrity. The immune and inflammation cells and mediators are the most critical systems that secure defenses in sepsis. The failure of these defenses could lead to organ failure and death.

Summary

Inflammation plays a key role in acute injuries as well as chronic diseases. The immune and inflammatory reactions serve as the major defense mechanism against numerous external injurious events and pathological events that emerge as a result of endogenous aberrant genetic and biochemical imbalances. However, immune and inflammatory reactions can also evolve as a cause of diseases such as autoimmune diseases; granulomatous conditions; cancer; respiratory, joint, and bone diseases; and atherosclerosis. Thus, anti-inflammatory drugs emerge as an important source of novel therapeutics for diverse diseases such as cancer, metabolic syndrome, atherosclerosis, joint and bone diseases, and respiratory tract disorders.

Further Reading

Barish, G. D., Narkar, V. A. and Evans, R. M. (2006). PPARδ: a dagger in the heart of the metabolic syndrome. *Journal of Clinical Investigations* **116**, 590–597.

Bloomgarten, Z. T. (2005). Inflammation, atherosclerosis, and aspects of insulin action. *Diabetes Care* **28**, 2312–2319.

Cohen, J. (2002). The immunopathogenesis of sepsis. *Nature* **420**, 885–891.

Dandona, P., Aljada, A., Chaudhuri, A., et al. (2005). Metabolic syndrome: a comprehensive perspective based on interaction between obesity, diabetes and inflammation. *Circulation* **111**, 1448–1454.

Fontech, A. N. and Wykle, R. L. (2004). Arachidonate remodeling and inflammation. In: Parnham, M. J. (ed.) *Progress in Inflammation*, pp. 1–243. Basel: Birkhauser Verlag.

Lagente, V., Manoury, B., Nenan, S., et al. (2005). Role of matrix metalloproteinases in the development of airway inflammation and remodeling. *Brazilian Journal Medical Biological Research* **38**, 1521–1530.

Libby, P. and Theroux, P. (2005). Pathophysiology of coronary artery disease. *Circulation* **111**, 3481–3488.

Morgan, D. W., Forssmann, U. J. and Nakada, M. T. (2004). Cancer and inflammation. In: Parnham, M. J. (ed.) *Progress in inflammation*, pp. 1–201. Basel: Birkhauser Verlag.

Moser, B., Letts, G. and Neote, K. (2006). Chemokine biology – basic and clinical application. Vol. 1: Immunology of chemokines. In: Parnham, M. J. (ed.) *Progress in inflammation research*, pp. 1–205. Basel: Birkhauser Verlag.

Rolin, S., Masereel, B. and Dogne, J-M. (2006). Prostanoids as pharmacological targets in COPD and asthma. *European Journal of Pharmacology* **533**, 89–100.

Schottenfeld, D. and Beebe-Dimmer, J. (2006). Chronic inflammation: a common and important factor in the pathogenesis of neoplasia. *Journal of Clinical Investigations* **56**, 69–83.

Simmons, D. L. (2006). What makes a good anti-inflammatory drug target? *Drug Discovery Today* **11** (5–6), 210–219.

Van den Berg, W. B. and Miossec, P. (2004). Cytokines and joint injury. In: Parnham, M. J. (ed.) *Progress in inflammation*, pp. 1–291. Basel: Birkhauser Verlag.

Weizmann, M. N. and Pacifici, R. (2006). Estrogen deficiency and bone loss: an inflammatory tale. *Journal of Clinical Investigations* **116**, 1186–1193.

Zelcer, N. and Tontonoz, P. (2006). Liver X receptors as integrators of metabolic and inflammatory signaling. *Journal of Clinical Investigations* **116**, 607–614.

Inhibition   *See:* Emotional Inhibition.

Injuries   *See:* Acute Trauma Response.

Insomnia   *See:* Sleep, Sleep Disorders, and Stress.

Instinct Theory

R Gardner Jr
University of Wisconsin, Madison, WI, USA

This article is a revision of the previous edition article by R Gardner Jr., volume 2, pp 581–582, © 2000, Elsevier Inc.

The word instinct stems from a Latin root meaning impulse or instigation. Historically, the term differentiated innate from learned actions. Instincts were untaught, genetically preprogrammed, stereotypic, goal-directed behaviors and behavior chains shaped by natural selection. They exhibited more complexity than reflexes and occurred mostly in nonhuman animals. Nobel Prize-winning ethologist Konrad Lorenz described fixed motor patterns; releasers, the triggering stimuli of instinctive responses; and imprinting, wherein a newly hatched bird followed and attached itself to any moving object located before it, replacing its mother.

The concept of inherited behavior remains important. However, Nikos Tinbergen, who shared the 1972 Nobel Prize with Lorenz, pointed out that the popular use of the term instinct has three meanings: (1) behavior driven from within (e.g., the mating instinct emerges in the spring), (2) nonlearned behavior (e.g., the newborn knows instinctively how to suckle its mother's nipple), and (3) unpremeditated behavior (e.g., the driver instinctively puts his foot on the brake). The term instinct, therefore, is often omitted in works of present-day ethologists, sociophysiologists, behavioral ecologists, and other workers in animal and human behavior.

Prior to the ethologists, the theoretician–psychoanalyst Sigmund Freud used the word instinct (also libido and drive) to carry forward his machine metaphors of the mind (which had been popular in the nineteenth century), employing, for example, hydraulic and expended-fuel metaphors (as Lorenz also did for a time). Later John Bowlby, in contrast, defined instinct as behavioral-system actions that follow a recognizably similar pattern typical of the species, that have survival value, and that emerge even without the ordinary opportunities for learning.

Machine models hold little interest for modern theorists and researchers. Indeed, explosions of biological research on all fronts have rendered distinctions between learned and innate knowledge impossible. The capacity for learning is clearly inherited, a property that is expanded more in humans than in other animals. Moreover, research in molecular biology, notably in deciphering the genomes of many living forms, has demonstrated numerous conserved genes held in common by species, from bacteria to flies to fish to humans. Many influence behavior. Modern mammals exhibit reactions that ancestral vertebrates surely also had, for example, the flight-or-fight response.

Many anciently determined behaviors hinge on conspecific recognition and interaction (conspecifics are members of a same species), and these entail learning and behavioral modifications to varying extents. Certainly mating, social rank hierarchy, nurturance, eliciting nurturance, making in/out-group distinctions, and play behaviors must be included. These behaviors go awry in psychiatric disorders; examples include

1. Persecutory delusions, in which the patient has the conviction that he or she is targeted by hostile out-group members.
2. Mania, which involves the patient behaving in a commanding (dominant) fashion inappropriate for circumstances.
3. Depression, which involves the patient behaving like someone of low rank.
4. Paraphilias, which can be redefined as displaced mating urges.
5. Autism, in which children elicit nurturance poorly from parents and do not play spontaneously with other children.

Humans possess a brain three times heavier than their nearest relatives among the great apes, probably from greater sociality, which seems to enhance adaptation more than it costs in childbirth complications. However, 98.5% of primate genomes remain identical. Inherited neurons, altered to varying extents by experience, clearly determine all behaviors. Neuroscientist–psychiatrist Eric Kandel stressed that all learning reflects altered gene transcription and neuronal action. Learned behavior, once the antonym of instinct, now instead implies additional choices for the individual. Psychiatric leader Daniel X. Freedman noted that biological psychiatry is a redundancy; there is no unbiological psychology or sociology. All animal behavior, including human action, represents genetically programmed performances influenced by individual experience.

See Also the Following Articles

Evolutionary Origins and Functions of the Stress Response; Fight-or-Flight Response.

Further Reading

Allman, J. M. (1999). *Evolving brains.* New York: Scientific American Library.

Bowlby, J. (1969). *Attachment and loss* (vol. 1). New York: Basic Books.

Gardner, R. (1997). Sociophysiology as the basic science of psychiatry. *Theoretical Medicine* 18, 335–356.

Gardner, R. (2001). Affective neuroscience, psychiatry and sociophysiology. *Evolution & Cognition* 7, 25–30.

Kandel, E. R. (1998). A new intellectual framework for psychiatry. *American Journal of Psychiatry* 155, 457–469.

Lorenz, K. (1965). *Evolution and modification of behavior.* Chicago: University of Chicago Press.

Price, J. S., Gardner, R. and Erickson, M. (2004). Depression, anxiety and somatization as appeasement displays. *Journal of Affective Disorders* 79, 1–11.

Tinbergen, N. (1969). Instinct. In: *Encyclopedia Britannica,* (vol. 12), pp. 323–324. Chicago: William Benton.

Verhulst, J., Gardner, R., Sutton, B., et al. (2005). The social brain in clinical practice. *Psychiatric Annals* 35 (10), 803–815.

Integrative Medicine (Complementary and Alternative Medicine)

D Spiegel

This article is a revision of the previous edition article by D Spiegel, volume 1, pp 512–514, © 2000, Elsevier Inc.

Introduction
Acupuncture
Biofeedback
Nutritional and Herbal Treatments
Homeopathy
Hypnosis
Manipulative Therapies
Mindfulness-Based Stress Reduction
Relaxation Training
Conclusion

Glossary

Acupuncture	The insertion of thin needles at specific meridians or points in the body thought to affect the balance of the body's ability to manage pain and other medical illnesses, a practice originally developed in China.
Homeopathy	A treatment based on the idea that tiny amounts of substances can change the properties of water in a way that triggers the body's ability to respond to a disease.
Hypnosis	A state of highly focused attention, coupled with reduced awareness of experiences at the periphery of attention, and a heightened responsiveness to social cues.
Integrative medicine	The integration of many alternative or culturally sanctioned techniques into mainstream Western medical practice.

Introduction

While modern medical science has provided cures for many bacterial infections, life-extending treatments for viral infections such as HIV, and symptom-reducing interventions for heart disease, and has converted many kinds of cancer from a terminal to a chronic disease, it is especially striking that large numbers of Americans now turn to allied medical traditions and recently developed treatments for help with disease. More people than ever are living with serious illness, which is a chronic and severe stressor. Thus,

traditional medicine's very success has created a whole new set of problems. The acute disease model emphasizes diagnosis, definitive treatment, and cure. In some situations this works, but in many it does not. The leading killers of Americans, heart disease, stroke, and cancer, are by and large chronic and progressive rather than curable illnesses. The application of a curative model, in a setting in which disease management is often the most productive approach, leaves both doctors and patients frustrated. Rather than feeling satisfied when a disease is well managed, doctors and patients often feel disappointed that it has not been cured, and there is little emphasis on managing pain, anxiety, fatigue, and other debilitating aspects of illness and its treatment. The oldest adage of medicine is that our job is to "cure rarely, to relieve suffering often, and to comfort always." At the end of the twentieth century, it is as though that adage has been rewritten, that our job is now to "cure always, relieve suffering if one has the time, and leave the comforting to someone else."

Patients do indeed turn elsewhere for comfort. Complementary and alternative medicine professionals are one such place. They spend on average 30 min with their patients, compared with the typical 7 min allocated for physican–patient visits. Americans spend more out of pocket on complementary and alternative treatments than on visits to outpatient physicians or hospital care. An illness can be a lonely journey, and patients crave people who understand what the journey is like and who can stay with them during its course. Thus, the apparent appetite for complementary and alternative medicine is stimulated by the lack of help in coping with serious illness in modern medical care, which has become increasingly technological. This problem is being intensified by the business constraints in modern American medicine, which include frustration at obtaining appropriate reimbursement, increased paperwork burden, limited continuity of care, and second-guessing of treatment decisions. This can only further desiccate the doctor–patient relationship and limit the opportunities for medical compassion to enhance medical care.

Close to one-half of Americans utilize some form of alternative treatment, a substantial increase from the already sizeable figure of one-third in 1990. However, more than two-thirds of them utilize standard medical treatment as well, suggesting that as far as the patients are concerned, these interventions are complementary rather than alternative. A study in the

Kaiser health-care system indicated that the majority of complaints that lead to seeking alternative services are pain (52%) and anxiety (25%). Thus, patients seek complementary care for sensible reasons, bringing problems that are not life-threatening and that are often ignored or minimized in mainstream medical treatment. However, the relationship between complementary and standard medical care is complicated by the fact that three-quarters of those individuals who use alternative services do not tell their primary care physicians that they were obtaining these alternative or complementary services, so their use of them had the potential to undermine or at least complicate their medical care.

These data provide support for the use of the term integrative rather than complementary or alternative. The idea is to integrate the best of other treatment traditions into modern medical care. The NIH now has a National Center for Complementary and Alternative Medicine (NCCAM) that conducts studies and disseminates information on such treatments. Centers for integrative medicine have been opened at a number of prominent academic and proprietary medical centers. The modalities described briefly below have been shown to be helpful in stress management.

Acupuncture

This ancient Chinese technique is primarily employed in the United States for chronic pain, and to a lesser extent for habit problems or substance abuse. Given the interaction between pain and stress in chronic illness, the pain relief obtained through this technique can also reduce secondary stress and anxiety. Needles are inserted in locations thought to mediate pain perception and healing, usually alone, but sometimes with either mild electrical stimulation (electroacupuncture) or the combustion of a herbal preparation (moxibustion). Acupuncture analgesia has been found to be reversed by administration of naloxone, an opiate antagonist, so mediation of its effects via endogenous opiates is possible. Many patients find that they achieve a sense of well-being after acupuncture treatment that provides them with a respite from the stress of chronic illness.

Biofeedback

Biofeedback involves the use of telemetry recording peripheral muscle tension, skin temperature, or skin conductance (reflecting sweating) to inform people about their physiological responses and their ability to modulate them. This approach has been effective in treating tension and migraine headaches, managing stress, and treating psychophysiological disorders

such as Reynaud's disease, which involves vasoconstriction. Training with the equipment is utilized to teach patients how to enhance their ability to manage physiological responses to stress, tension, or other symptoms and thereby feel less secondary anxiety when a stressful situation arises.

Nutritional and Herbal Treatments

There are longstanding traditions of herbal treatments that contain a mixture of generally low-potency and complex combinations of substances that may have specific therapeutic benefit in some cases, or that may be ineffective or even harmful in others. Digitalis, a mainstay in the treatment of congestive heart failure and other cardiac disease, was originally the active component of foxglove, used as a herbal treatment for dropsy. Research supported by NCCAM has shown that omega-3 fatty acids, found in some fish oils, may be helpful in the management of autoimmune inflammatory diseases. Arthritis and other such diseases may be helped by a combination of interventions, including gentle movement such as *tai chi,* a Chinese technique of exercise designed to redirect energy flow in the body, and pain management including hypnosis and biofeedback. However a recent large study by NCCAM found that the herb hypericum, also known as St. John's Wort, did not appear effective in relieving the symptoms of depression, as had been found in previous studies. L-tryptophan, an amino acid precursor of serotonin, has been used in attempt to increase serotonin levels in the brain. Low serotonin has been linked to depression and impulsive behavior, and the most widely used antidepressants, selective serotonin reuptake inhibitors, increase the activity of serotonin in the synapses between neurons in the brain. However, one manufacturer of these dietary supplements produced batches with a small amount of a very harmful contaminant that produced inflammatory muscle pain in many and a number of deaths as well. While their product has been withdrawn from the market, it is an example of how apparently benign dietary supplements can be harmful. The use of some herbs may enhances peoples' sense of control over their disease, independent of specific effects, and thereby at least temporarily alleviate disease-related stress.

Homeopathy

This treatment regimen, developed in Germany and the United States, utilizes serial dilutions of substances thought to impart therapeutic properties in the water or alcohol that may initially mildly provoke and then help the body to heal symptoms of disease. Homeopathy and also other techniques such as traditional Chinese medicine emphasize a complex assessment of all bodily systems, treating imbalances in these systems and not just focusing on specific diseased parts of the body. Studies conducted through NCCAM and elsewhere have not proven specific effectiveness of homeopathic remedies beyond what might be expected from placebo response.

Hypnosis

There are a variety of well-established and thoroughly studied methods for teaching patients how to increase their control over mental distress and concomitant somatic discomfort. Hypnosis, for example, is a state of aroused, attentive focal concentration accompanied by a reduction in peripheral awareness. It has proven effectiveness in facilitating anxiety control and inducing analgesia. The techniques most often employed involve a combination of physical relaxation and imagery that provides a substitute focus of attention for the painful sensation. Hypnosis can be quickly induced in a matter of seconds, and patients can be taught self-hypnosis to provide ongoing anxiety and pain control. The ability of hypnotizable individuals to dissociate, or separate psychological from somatic response, can be used to maintain physical relaxation even in the face of emotional distress. This can also help patients to restructure their understanding of the situation that is making them anxious, in part because they are approaching it while in an unusually relaxed state. This is an important concept in many complementary treatments for anxiety such as meditation, massage, biofeedback, and hypnosis: the patient may not be able to alter the stressor itself, but can enhance his or her control over his or her psychological and somatic response to the stressor. This can, in turn, enhance the array of options available to the patient for dealing with that stressor, since he or she is more in control of somatic symptoms and less preoccupied with the effect of the stressor.

Self-hypnosis, for example, has been shown to be quite useful in helping medical patients suffering from procedure anxiety. A recent randomized trial employing hypnosis during interventional radiology procedures demonstrated that patients offered training in hypnosis had less pain, fewer procedural interruptions, less cardiovascular instability, and less anxiety while utilizing only 12% as much analgesic medication from a patient-controlled analgesia (PCA) device.

Manipulative Therapies

Approaches such as osteopathy, chiropractic, and therapeutic massage approach symptoms such as pain and limitation of movement, especially involving musculoskeletal disorders, through careful assessment of anatomical problems and physical manipulation of them. In chronic and severe but difficult-to-treat problems such as lower back pain, such approaches have shown effectiveness equivalent to more invasive surgical treatment in many cases. They may also help to reduce stress related to pain and disability. These treatment approaches are based upon the idea that one way that stress is experienced and can be treated is in the body. Psychological tension can manifest itself in physical tension and misalignment or dysfunction of parts of the body. The goal is to restore more normal structure–function connections in the body. Realigning physical movement is believed to reduce adverse effects of psychological as well physical stress.

Mindfulness-Based Stress Reduction

Similarly, other techniques involving breathing exercises, self-monitoring and regulation, and meditation, several based on adaptations of Buddhist meditation practices, have proven quite effective in stress management in the medical setting. Jon Kabat-Zinn has developed a model that involves teaching patients with pain, anxiety, and other illness-related problems a mindfulness meditation practice designed to help them

1. control their attentional processes
2. induce physical comfort and relaxation
3. maintain a present orientation
4. enhance empathic connection with others

This method helps patients learn to experience more choice in the management of their perceived stress and to reduce anxiety about the future by more richly immersing themselves in the range of their present experiences, both positive and negative. This helps them accept but put into perspective worries about the future by maintaining enjoyment of the present.

Research with this technique has produced promising results. Kabat-Zinn and colleagues demonstrated in a randomized trial that psoriasis patients who listen to an audiotape teaching mindfulness-based stress reduction had significantly more rapid healing of their skin lesions than control patients who listened to music. Thus, mindfulness training may influence the course of disease as well as reducing stress-related anxiety and pain.

Relaxation Training

Other techniques based upon meditative traditions have also been introduced for stress reduction. Benson and colleagues have popularized an approach that involves brief exercises designed to help patients manage daily stress and have termed the approach the relaxation response. Simple, brief relaxation exercises have been helpful in managing such problems as mild to moderate hypertension and are recommended in such situations prior to or in conjunction with antihypertensive medication treatment.

Conclusion

There is little doubt that Americans are voting with their pocketbooks and their feet for integrative approaches. Recent research has shown that some of these approaches produce specific therapeutic benefits, while others clearly do not. Even if relief of symptoms is a small but real effect, when the big picture is overwhelming, small amounts of mental and/or physical control can go a long way toward reassuring patients that they can more effectively manage the course of their life with disease. Stress is a normal part of life, and a natural if unwelcome part of the course of disease. The extent to which stress produces distress can be modified by a variety of treatments that engage patients as participants in their care. While results vary, these approaches should be viewed as an opportunity rather than a threat, a potentially useful addition to the management of stress in health care.

See Also the Following Articles

Disease, Stress Induced; Hypnosis; Meditation and Stress; Relaxation Techniques.

Further Reading

Doan, B. (1998). *Alternative and complementary therapies.* New York: Oxford University Press.

Eisenberg, D. M., Davis, R. B., et al. (1998). Trends in alternative medicine use in the United States, 1990–1997: results of a follow-up national survey. *Journal of the American Medical Association* **280**, 1569–1575.

Gore-Felton, C., Vosvick, M., et al. (2003). Alternative therapies: a common practice among men and women living with HIV. *Journal of the Association of Nurses in AIDS Care* **14**(3), 17–27.

Lang, E. V., Benotsch, E. G., et al. (2000). Adjunctive non-pharmacological analgesia for invasive medical procedures: a randomised trial. *The Lancet* **355**, 1486–1490.

Luskin, F. M., Newell, K. A., et al. (1998). A review of mind-body therapies in the treatment of cardiovascular disease. Part 1: implications for the elderly. *Alternative Therapies in Health and Medicine* **4**(3), 46–61.

Newell, S. A., Sanson-Fisher, R. W., et al. (2002). Systematic review of psychological therapies for cancer patients: overview and recommendations for future research. *Journal of the National Cancer Institute* **94**(8), 558–584.

Spiegel, H. and Spiegel, D. (2004). *Trance and treatment: clinical uses of hypnosis.* Washington, D.C.: American Psychiatric Publishing.

Vincent, C. and Furnham, A. (1996). Why do patients turn to complementary medicine? An empirical study. *British Journal of Clinical Psychology* **35**, 37–48.

Wetzel, M. S., Eisenberg, D. M., et al. (1998). Courses involving complementary and alternative medicine at US medical schools. *Journal of the American Medical Association* **280**(9), 784–787.

Zeltzer, L. K., Tsao, J. C., et al. (2002). A phase I study on the feasibility and acceptability of an acupuncture/hypnosis intervention for chronic pediatric pain. *Journal of Pain and Symptom Management* **24**(4), 437–446.

Interactions Between Stress and Drugs of Abuse

P V Piazza and M Le Moal
Université de Bordeaux, Bordeaux, France

This article is reproduced from the previous edition, volume 2, pp 586–594, © 2000, Elsevier Inc.

Introduction
Influence of Stressors on Drug Self-Administration
Factors Influencing Effects of Stressors
Mechanisms of Stress Action
Does Stress Induce a Drug-Prone Phenotype?
Conclusions

Glossary

Dopamine	A neurotransmitter that, with norepinephrine and serotonin, belongs to the class of monoamines. In the central nervous system there are two principal groups of dopaminergic neurons, one in the mesencephalon projecting to a large number of brain structures and the other in the hypothalamus, controlling hormonal function in the hypophysis. Mesencephalic dopaminergic neurons are divided into two major subgroups: (1) The nigrostriatal neurons (A9) that

Drug self-administration	Intravenous drug self-administration is one of the most used models for studying drug abuse in animals. This test measures the learning of an operant response, such as pressing a lever, which stimulates drug infusion, i.e., this test measures the capacity of pharmacological substances to act as positive reinforcers.
Gluco-corticoids	Consisting of cortisol in humans and corticosterone in rodents, this is the final step of the activation of the hypothalamo-pituitary-adrenal axis. These hormones have large effects in the periphery, where they modify energy metabolism and the activity of the immune system. Glucocorticoids also act at the level of the central nervous system. These hormones cross the blood–brain barrier easily and bind to two types of specific intracellular receptors, which are hormone-activated transcription factors. Glucocorticoids also seem to have direct membrane effects, although the mechanism of this action remains unclear.
Negative reinforcer	A stimulus that induces a subject to respond in a manner that interrupts the response. Foot shock is the most common negative reinforcer used in animals. Stressors are usually stimuli that can also act as negative reinforcers.
Positive reinforcer	A stimulus that increases the probability of a response. For example, positive reinforcers are food, a receptive sexual partner, and drugs of abuse.

have cell bodies in the substantia nigra-pars compacta (SNc) and that principally project to the dorsal striatum and the caudate nucleus and (2) the meso-limbic-cortical neurons (A10) with cell bodies in the ventral tegmental area (VTA) and that project to the ventral striatum, nucleus accumbens, and cortical and limbic structures, such as the amygdala and the hippocampus.

Introduction

This article analyzes the interactions between stress and the responses to drugs of abuse. In particular, it focuses on intravenous drug self-administration, one of the principal experimental models of drug abuse. Much of our information on the interaction between stress and drugs of abuse is based on experimental studies and in particular from research in rats. Although several authors have proposed that stress is related positively to abuse of both opioid and psychostimulant drugs, a firm causal link between

stress and drug abuse cannot be established on the basis of studies in humans. There are two main reasons for this. First, the variables under investigation, i.e., the history and the experiences of the subject, in humans cannot be manipulated directly under controlled experimental conditions, but only assessed indirectly on the basis of retrospective self-reports of stress. Second, a reliable measure of the outcome of stress on drug abuse implies that all individuals have equal access to drugs under identical environmental conditions. Again, this experimental setting is impossible to achieve in humans. As will be reviewed, this type of experimental investigation has revealed some of the biological factors that mediate stress-induced propensity to self-administer drugs of abuse.

Influence of Stressors on Drug Self-Administration

Definition of Stress

Stress is a very vague concept often used with different meanings that principally refer to a subjective state with a strong negative connotation. Because subjective states cannot be investigated directly in animals, experimental research on stress has focused principally on the behavioral and biological responses to the forced exposure to stimuli or situations that are normally avoided by the individual. This is why stimuli used as experimental stressors are very often identical to aversive stimuli used as negative reinforcers in learning tasks. Consequently, stress, as studied in animals, probably corresponds to "the internal status induced by the exposure to threatening and aversive stimuli." However, what is principally studied in stress research is a panoply of responses induced by aversive stimuli.

Model of Intravenous Drug Self-Administration

The experimental study of drug abuse has been made possible by the discovery that animals self-administer drugs intravenously. This behavior shares many similarities with drug use in humans. First, animals self-administer practically all the drugs that induce addiction in humans. Second, the patterns of self-administration of the different drugs in humans and animals are similar. Finally, the large individual differences in the response to drugs of abuse that characterize humans are also found in animals.

Self-administration measures positive reinforcing effect of drugs, i.e., the learning of an operant response, such as pressing a lever, that has as a consequence the delivery of a drug infusion. In general, changes in the rate of the response reinforced by the drug are considered to reflect changes in the sensitivity to its addictive properties.

Self-administration is usually studied using three different and complementary approaches: acquisition, retention, and reinstatement. The influence of different forms of stress on the three aspects of self-administration will be analyzed separately.

Influence of Stress on the Acquisition of Self-Administration

Acquisition studies evaluate the propensity of an individual to develop drug self-administration. For this purpose, the effects of first contact with low doses of the drug are studied, and parameters such as threshold or rate of acquisition are taken into account.

In adult animals, artificial and physical stressors, such as repeated tailpinch (**Figure 1**, top) and electric foot shock, facilitate the acquisition of the self-administration of psychostimulants, such as cocaine and amphetamine. Food restriction is another physical stressor that facilitates the acquisition of psychostimulant, opiate, and alcohol self-administration.

The acquisition of psychostimulant self-administration is also enhanced in male and female rats exposed to an aggressive biological 'congener' and in male rats raised in colonies in which there is a high level of social competition, i.e., colonies in which male rats fight to establish and maintain the social hierarchy that will determine access to females. Facilitation of the acquisition of morphine and alcohol oral self-administration, as well as of heroin intravenous self-administration is also induced by social isolation.

Early life events, such as prenatal stress, also increase the propensity to develop amphetamine self-administration. Such an effect has been observed in adult rats whose mothers had been submitted to a restraint procedure during the third and fourth weeks of gestation.

Influence of Stress on Retention

Retention studies are performed after prolonged training with high doses of drug and allow estimation of changes in (i) the sensitivity to the reinforcing effects of drugs and (ii) the motivation to self-administer drugs. The sensitivity to drugs is assessed by performing dose–response curves. In this case, the dose of the drug per infusion is varied, usually between sessions, and the rate of responding is recorded. Motivation for drugs is evaluated principally by means of progressive ratio schedules. In this case, the dose is maintained constant and the ratio requirement (number of responses necessary to obtain

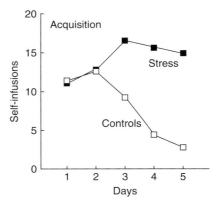

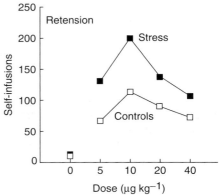

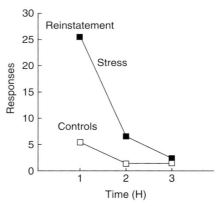

Figure 1 Examples of the effects of stress on intravenous self-administration. Top: effects of tail pinch on the acquisition of the self-administration of amphetamine (10 μg/infusion). Center: effects of food restriction on the dose–response curves of etonitazene self-administration. Bottom: influence of electric foot shock on the reinstatement of heroin self-administration. Stress facilitates the acquisition of self-administration, induces an upward shift of the dose–response function, and triggers the reinstatement of drug-seeking behavior. Redrawn with permission from, respectively, Piazza, P. V., Deminiere, J. M., Le Moal, M., et al. (1990). Stress- and pharmacologically-induced behavioral sensitization increases vulnerability to acquisition of amphetamine self-administration. *Brain Research* **514**, 22–26; Carrol, M. E. and Meich, R. A. (1984). Increased drug-reinforced behavior due to food deprivation. *Advances in Behavioral Pharmacology* **4**, 47–88; and Shaham, Y. and Stewart J. (1995). Stress reinstates heroin-seeking in drug-free animals: an effect mimicking heroin, not withdrawal. *Psychopharmacology* **111**, 334–341.

one infusion) is increased progressively. The highest ratio reached by the subjects (breaking point) is considered an index of its motivation to self-administer drugs.

Changes in dose–response functions for psychostimulant and/or opiate self-administration have been observed after social stress, social isolation, and food restriction (**Figure 1**, center). In all these cases, the stressors induce an increase in the rate of response over a large range of doses, resulting in a vertical upward shift of the dose–response function. This type of shift in dose–response curves suggests an increase in the reinforcing efficacy of drugs in stressed animals. This idea is confirmed by progressive ratio studies. Thus, over a large range of doses, the breaking point for heroin self-administration has been consistently higher for animals subjected to repeated electric foot shock than for control rats.

A large variability has been observed in the effect of social isolation. Indeed, higher, slightly higher, equal, or lower sensitivities to cocaine have all been described in socially isolated rats as compared to grouped rats. The conditions that were considered as controls could also contribute to such variability. In fact, the rate of self-administration of control animals, and not the one of isolated rats, is what really differentiates some of these reports. Not surprisingly, the effects of social isolation appeared weaker when other conditions that facilitate self-administration, such as priming injections of the drug and pretest periods of food restriction, were used concomitantly.

Influence of Stress on Reinstatement

Reinstatement studies are considered a measure of relapse in drug intake. In this case, the behavior is studied after the extinction of previously acquired self-administration. Extinction is usually obtained by substituting the drug with a vehicle solution. Following extinction, the administration of stimuli known to induce craving for the drug in abstinent human addicts, such as low doses of the drug, will reinstate responses to the stimulus that elicited the infusion of the drug during acquisition. The rate of response to this stimulus is the principal measure of reinstatement.

Stressors increase reinstatement of drug self-administration. In rats in which the response to heroin (**Figure 1**, bottom) or cocaine has been extinguished by substituting the drug with a saline solution, repetitive electric foot shock induces the reinstatement of response to the drug. Stress-induced reinstatement seems to be a very robust and well-documented phenomenon, and it is of comparable intensity to the one induced by other experimental manipulations known

to induce reinstatement, such as the infusion of low doses of the self-administered drugs.

Factors Influencing Effects of Stressors

Predictability and Intensity

Predictability and intensity seem important variables in mediating the effects of stress on drug self-administration. Unpredictable stressors have higher effects than predictable ones. Furthermore, stressors, especially when acute, need to be of a certain intensity in order to increase self-administration. The relationship between the intensity of the stressor and its outcome on drug seeking is also shown by reinstatement studies. Thus, the rate of reinstatement has been found to be a function of the duration of the shocks. However, in the case of prolonged exposure to stress, the duration of the stress seems less important. Similar facilitory effects on self-administration have been found for stressors that are continuous and for those that are of short duration and administered repeatedly.

Physical Versus Psychological Threats

Although 'physical' stressors involving a noxious stimulus such as electric foot shock and tail pinch increase self-administration, physical aggression per se does not seem to be a necessary condition for mediating stress effects. In fact, pure psychological stress is also able to increase drug self-administration. For example, it has been shown that witnessing another rat receiving foot shocks facilitates the acquisition of cocaine self-administration. Similarly, in social aggression experiments, the facilitation of self-administration is also found when the intruder is always protected by a screen grid and consequently never submitted to physical attacks.

Time Contingencies

Both acute and repeated exposure to stress can increase the propensity to develop drug self-administration. However, acute and chronic stress are influenced differently by temporal contingencies. In the case of acute stressors, a short interval between the stressful event and the exposure to the drug appears to be crucial. In contrast, after a prolonged exposure to stress, the interval between the termination of the stress and the exposure to the drug does not seem to be a relevant variable. In this case a facilitation of drug self-administration has also been found when the stress is terminated weeks before the start of the self-administration session. These observations are important from a pathophysiological point of view.

They indicate that repeated stress can induce long-lasting modifications that result in a drug-prone state that becomes independent from the actual presence of the stressor.

Mechanisms of Stress Action

Different mechanisms could mediate the effects of stress on drug self-administration and much remains to be done on this field of research. We will focus principally on the possibility that stressors sensitize the endogenous system of reward by an action on dopaminergic neurons and glucocorticoid hormones. Mesencephalic dopaminergic neurons, particularly their projection to the nucleus accumbens, are considered one of the principal substrates of drug-reinforcing effects. Glucocorticoid hormones are the final step of the activation of the hypothalamic-pituitary-adrenal axis. The secretion of glucocorticoids by the adrenal gland is considered one of the principal biological adaptations to external aggression.

Clearly, an interaction between glucocorticoids and dopamine should not be considered as the only possible mechanism mediating stress effects, but as the best studied of only one of the likely possibilities. **Figure 2** shows schematically the interactions among stress, glucocorticoids, and dopaminergic neurons.

Sensitization of the Reward System

One of the mechanisms by which stress could modify the sensitivity of an individual to drugs of abuse is by modifying the activity of those neurobiological systems that mediate the addictive properties of drugs.

Role of mesencephalic dopaminergic neurons Mesencephalic dopaminergic neurons seem to be a likely candidate for such a neurobiological system. The role of these neurons in drug abuse has been emphasized in several good reviews. In particular, the release of dopamine in the nucleus accumbens is considered one of the major mechanisms of the addictive properties of drugs. Practically all drugs of abuse increase

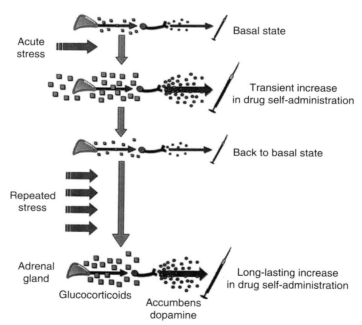

Figure 2 Possible pathophysiological mechanisms of the increase in drug self-administration induced by acute and repeated stress. The concentrations of glucocorticoids (large squares) determine the level of dopamine release in the nucleus accumbens (small squares). In basal conditions (basal state), glucocorticoid secretion and dopamine release are low, as is sensitivity to drugs of abuse. Acute stress increases glucocorticoid secretion, which, by enhancing the release of dopamine, results in an increase in the sensitivity to the reinforcing effects of drugs of abuse. However, activation of the negative feedback that controls the secretion of these hormones brings the system back to basal levels within 2 h. The increase in the concentrations of glucocorticoids induced by repeated exposure to stress will progressively result in a long-lasting increase in the secretion of these hormones and in the release of dopamine in the nucleus accumbens. These changes will, in turn, determine a long-lasting increase in the sensitivity to the reinforcing effects of drugs of abuse. The transient increase in glucocorticoids and dopamine observed after acute stress may explain why, in this case, an increase in drug self-administration is found only if the exposure to drugs closely follows the stressor. The long-lasting increase in the activity of these two biological factors could explain why, after repeated stress, an increase in the sensitivity to drugs is also found long (weeks) after the end of the stressor.

dopamine release in this brain area, and an increase or a decrease in dopaminergic activity in the nucleus accumbens corresponds, respectively, to an increase or a decrease in the reinforcing properties of drugs. Several types of acute stress transiently increase dopamine release in the nucleus accumbens. In parallel, repeated stress induces a long-lasting increase in the release of this neurotransmitter, particularly of drug-induced dopamine release.

Role of glucocorticoid hormones Glucocorticoid hormones seem to be the link between environmental experiences and mesencephalic dopaminergic neurons. In basal conditions, the administration of glucocorticoids at levels that are in the stress range can increase dopamine release in the nucleus accumbens, whereas the suppression of glucocorticoid secretion has the opposite effect. During stress, a selective blockade of stress-induced secretion of glucocorticoids reduces dopamine release by around 50%. Finally, the development of the long-lasting sensitization of the dopaminergic response to psychostimulants and opioids induced by stress is suppressed by the blockade of corticosterone secretion.

That glucocorticoids hormones, through their action on dopamine release, could increase the behavioral responses to drugs is supported by a supplementary set of data. First, administration of glucocorticoids, at levels that are in the stress range, increases the propensity to self-administer amphetamine. Second, the blockade of stress-induced corticosterone secretion induces a downward shift in the dose–response curve for cocaine self-administration, i.e., changes opposite to those observed after stress. Third, the blockade of corticosterone secretion can reverse the stress-induced sensitization of the dopaminergic and behavioral responses to cocaine.

Mechanisms of reinstatement The hypothalamic-pituitary-adrenal axis and dopaminergic neurons also seem to play a role in reinstatement, but in a way that differs from the one described for drug self-administration.

For example, a concomitant blockade of D1 and D2 dopaminergic receptors is needed to block stress-induced reinstatement, whereas selective antagonists of either receptor suffice to decrease the positive reinforcing effects of drugs. In parallel, although the injection of glucocorticoids alone can induce reinstatement, blockade of the secretion of these hormones does not prevent the stress-induced reinstatement of heroin self-administration. In contrast, the blockade of glucocorticoid secretion seems to block the stress-induced reinstatement of cocaine self-administration.

Stress-Induced Impulsivity

Changes in impulsivity could be an alternative mechanism by which stress modifies drug self-administration. A deficit in the inhibitory processes that normally operate to control the reward effect of a stimulus is considered an important dimension of impulsivity. This type of impairment could contribute to the increase in drug self-administration induced by stress. This idea is prompted by the effects of social aggression on the rate of responding during time-out periods, i.e., fixed time periods that follow each drug infusion and during which responses are not expected. During time-out, control animals learn quickly to reduce response rates and to wait for the next period of drug availability, whereas stressed rats maintain high rates of response during these time periods. The possibility that an inhibitory deficit is involved in excessive drug consumption is also backed by the finding that the inability to delay gratification predicts alcohol self-administration.

Although stress-induced impulsivity seems an interesting mechanism, further experiments should specifically test the actual occurrence of such a change in behavior. At the neurochemical level it will be important to correlate such potential changes in behaviors with neurobiological modifications involved in impulsivity, such as a decrease in serotoninergic activity.

Does Stress Induce a Drug-Prone Phenotype?

The Individual-Centered Vision of Addiction

It is a common observation that although a large number of people take drugs for variable periods of time, only few of them develop a true addiction, i.e., a compulsive drug use that becomes the main goal-directed activity of the subject. One of the theories that has been used to explain such individual differences in the development of addiction postulates the existence of a drug-prone phenotype, i.e., drug abuse is a pre-existing pathological condition revealed by the drug. Addiction would appear only in certain individuals because their biological phenotype will generate a 'pathological response' to drugs. This pathological response would make the addictive properties of drugs much greater in some subjects, increasing their likeliness to develop drug abuse.

Knowledge about Drug-Prone Phenotypes

Research in rodents has identified some of the biological factors that could determine a drug-prone phenotype. As indicated earlier, large individual differences in the propensity to develop drug self-administration have been described in laboratory rats, and the propensity of an individual animal to develop self-administration correlates with its behavior in other experimental situations. For example, animals that show the highest locomotor activity when exposed to a novel environment, a procedure that can be seen as a model of mild stress, also show the highest propensity to self-administer amphetamine.

Animals predisposed to drug addiction show a faster acquisition of drug self-administration, an upward shift of the dose–response function, and reach higher ratio requirements. They also show a higher release of dopamine into the nucleus accumbens in response to a drug challenge and a longer glucocorticoid secretion in response to stress. Finally, the higher dopaminergic activity of animals that are spontaneously drug prone seems to be glucocorticoid dependent. These rats are more sensitive to the dopaminergic effect of glucocorticoids, and blockade of glucocorticoid reduces their dopaminergic hyperactivity.

Stress-Induced Phenotype

Data presented in this article suggest that stressful experiences are one of the determinants of a drug-prone phenotype. Indeed, stressors can induce a long-lasting increase in drug self-administration, and such an effect occur place at an early stage of life, as exemplified by prenatal stress. Further support for this idea arises from the comparison of the characteristics of individuals who are spontaneously drug prone with those of subjects in which such a predisposition has been induced by stress. Indeed, dopaminergic hyperactivity and a dysregulation of glucocorticoid hormone activity, similar to that observed in subjects susceptible to drug addiction, have also been found in individuals made vulnerable by stress.

Conclusions

In conclusion, stress experiences increase the propensity of an individual to develop drug self-administration, inducing a drug-prone phenotype. Stress-induced increases in the secretion of glucocorticoids, which in turn enhance the drug-induced release of dopamine in the nucleus accumbens, seem to be an important substrate of such an effect of stress.

These observations highlight the importance of environmental experiences in the etiology of drug abuse. This confirms the hypothetical role of stress suggested by correlative studies in humans. Second, the observations support the idea that drug abuse is not simply induced by chronic drug intake, but that the phenotype of the individual plays an important role in determining the development of such a pathological behavior.

See Also the Following Article

Drug Use and Abuse.

Further Reading

Carrol, M. E. and Meich, R. A. (1984). Increased drug-reinforced behavior due to food deprivation. *Advances in Behavioral Pharmacology* **4**, 47–88.

de Kloet, E. R. (1992). Brain corticosteroid receptors balance and homeostatic control. *Frontiers of Neuroendocrinology* **12**, 95–164.

Kalivas, P. W. and Stewart, J. (1991). Dopamine transmission in the initiation and expression of drug- and stress-induced sensitization of motor activity. *Brain Research Reviews* **16**, 223–244.

Piazza, P. V. and Le Moal, M. (1996). Pathophysiological basis of vulnerability to drug abuse: Role of an interaction between stress, glucocorticoids and dopaminergic neurons. *Annual Review of Pharmacology and Toxicology* **36**, 359–378.

Piazza, P. V. and Le Moal, M. (1997). Glucocorticoids as an endogenous substrate of reward. *Brain Research Reviews* **25**, 359–372.

Piazza, P. V. and Le Moal, M. (1998). The role of stress in drug self-administration. *Trends in Pharmacological Sciences* **19**, 7–74.

Schuster, C. R. and Thompson, T. (1969). Self-administration and behavioral dependence on drugs. *Annual Review of Pharmacology* **9**, 483–502.

Shaham, Y. (1996). Effect of stress an opioid-seeking behavior: Evidences from studies with rats. *Annals of Behavioral Medicine* **18**, 255–263.

Wise, R. A. (1996). Neurobiology of addiction. *Current Opinion in Neurobiology* **6**, 243–251.

Interferons and Interleukins *See:* Cytokines; Immune Response; Multiple Sclerosis; Prostaglandins; Chronic Social Stress: GR Sensitivity in Leukocytes.

Intervention, Behavioral *See:* Stress Management and Cardiovascular Disease.

Ireland, Studies of Stress in *See:* Northern Ireland, Post Traumatic Stress Disorder in.

Ischemia *See:* Cardiovascular System and Stress.

IVF *See:* Stress Effect of Assisted Reproduction.

J

Job Insecurity: The Health Effects of a Psychosocial Work Stressor

J E Ferrie
University College London Medical School, London, UK
P Martikainen
University of Helsinki, Helsinki, Finland

Job Insecurity and the Labor Market
The Job Insecurity Concept
Mechanisms
Psychological Health
General Measures of Physical Health
Health Outcomes of Interest to the Organization
Effects beyond the Individual and the Workplace
Who Experiences Job Insecurity: The Public Health Impact
Summary

Glossary

Downsizing	The most common name given to the process whereby an organization reduces its workforce through natural wastage, early retirement, or redundancy.
Employment security	While job security represents the ability to remain in a particular job, employment security represents the likelihood of being able to remain in paid employment, even if this is a succession of jobs.
Job insecurity	In general terms, the discrepancy between the level of security a person experiences and the level he or she prefers. It can cover both the loss of any valued condition of employment and the threat of total job loss. The depth of the job insecurity experience is dependent on the perceived probability and perceived severity of the job loss. Job insecurity has a large subjective appraisal element that is highly context dependent, and the job insecurity experience may effect employees who do not lose their job as much as those who do. Job insecurity arising from the threat to a particular job may lead to loss of employment security if subsequent jobs prove hard to find. Job insecurity can be self-reported or externally attributed. The population in studies of self-reported job insecurity is composed of individuals who report their job as insecure. In studies of attributed job insecurity, the study population is deemed to be under threat of job loss by the researchers. Associations observed in studies of attributed job insecurity are likely to be underestimates, as the study population will contain respondents who do not perceive themselves to be under threat.
Primary labor market	The highly regulated section of the labor market in which employees have traditionally enjoyed long-term, secure employment with many benefits, such as occupational pensions, maternity cover, etc.
Psychological contract	Worker's beliefs regarding the terms and conditions of her or his employment. Fairness and good faith are implied in the psychological contract, and breaches have implications for the worker's trust in the organization, performance, and behavior.
Secondary labor market	That section of the labor market in which wages are low and employment rights are few. Such employment is often seasonal, part-time, or temporary and is frequently used to buffer short-term changes in labor requirements.
Sickness presenteeism	Describes the phenomenon that occurs when an employee, despite a level of ill health that should prompt rest and absence, still turns up at work.

Job Insecurity and the Labor Market

Over the past 25 years, large changes have taken place in the structure of the labor market in most industrialized countries. The major determinants of this restructuring have been deindustrialization, technological innovation, globalization, and a commitment to a free market economy, including the privatization of public services. There has been a marked shift from economies driven by manufacturing toward those dominated by employment in services. Technological innovation has allowed many routine functions largely to be replaced by electronic devices (such as cash dispensers), and global information systems have facilitated the rapid transfer of work to newly industrializing countries where labor is cheaper. This deindustrialization and technological change have generally been accompanied by the expansion and strengthening of the role of market forces. Many workers, who previously thought that they had a job for life, now feel much less secure, and job insecurity has become more widespread in all the countries belonging to the Organisation for Economic Co-operation and Development (OECD) since the mid-1980s. Like all social transformations, these changes have the potential to affect the health of individuals and populations.

The Job Insecurity Concept

Research during the major recessions of the 1930s and 1980s provided unequivocal evidence of the adverse effects of unemployment on health, particularly mental health. However, although it is a major determinant of unemployment, much less work has been done on job insecurity. This is partly because job insecurity did not excite attention until it affected white-collar workers in the 1990s and partly because it is less obvious that job insecurity could affect health, as, unlike unemployment, it involves no actual loss of income or status. However, some research has suggested that job insecurity may have detrimental consequences equal to those of job loss. This is consistent with the central proposition in stress research that anticipation of a stressful event provokes as much, if not more, anxiety than the event itself. For workers accustomed to long-term, secure employment, the threat of job loss involves a breach of the psychological contract and generates uncertainty, which, in addition to emotional reactions, can trigger changes in other psychosocial stressors, such as job involvement. The level of stress generated by job insecurity depends on the perceived probability and perceived severity of the threatened job loss. As job insecurity in the primary labor market has increased

and research on psychosocial stressors has gained credence and prominence, interest in the effects of job insecurity has also developed.

Job security is a vital concern for both employees and their organizations. The general concept has been defined by Jean Hartley and colleagues as the discrepancy between the level of job security a person experiences and the level he or she prefers. Job insecurity can also be generated by deteriorating employment conditions and career opportunities, so some investigators have extended the concept to include loss of any valued condition of employment. These definitions encompass large numbers of workers who have insecure jobs, often seasonal, part-time, or temporary. For workers in this secondary labor market, job security is not part of the psychological contract and insecurity is an integral part of their work experience. However, widespread downsizing, privatization, outsourcing, mergers, and closures have led to the suggestion that job insecurity, even for employees in the primary labor market, is no longer a temporary break in an otherwise predictable work life pattern, but is becoming a structural feature of the new labor market. This new employment insecurity brings employees in the primary labor market closer to those in the secondary labor market.

The difficulty in studying the health effects of job insecurity among workers in the secondary labor market is working out whether poor health outcomes can be attributed to job insecurity and unemployment, or whether it is those already in poorer health who are selected into the secondary labor market. For this reason much of the published research has concentrated on workers in the primary labor market.

Job insecurity can be self-reported or externally attributed. Studies of self-reported job insecurity examine workers who say their job is insecure, while studies of attributed job insecurity examine workers deemed to be under threat of job loss because downsizings or workplace closures are expected or are taking place. There is a strong association between self-reported and attributed job insecurity. However, as stress levels are determined by the perceived probability and perceived severity of the job loss, self-reported job insecurity is generally considered to be the more potent stressor.

Mechanisms

Work examining potential explanations of any association between job insecurity and health remains patchy. Studies to date have implicated at least the following: pre-existing ill health; personal characteristics, such as pessimism; material factors, such as financial hardship; non-work psychosocial stressors,

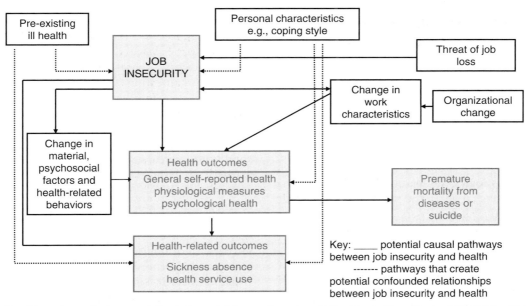

Figure 1 Possible pathways in the association between job insecurity and morbidity. Adapted from Ferrie, J. E., Shipley, M. S., Marmot, M. G., Martikainen, P., Stansfeld, S. and Davey Smith, G. (2001). Job insecurity in white-collar workers: towards an explanation of associations with health. *Journal of Occupational Health and Psychology* **6**, 26–42.

such as life events; other psychosocial and physical characteristics of the work environment, such as decreased job involvement; and health-related behavior (**Figure 1**).

The personal characteristics of pessimism, vigilance, neuroticism, mastery, and self-esteem have been found to explain part of the association between self-reported job insecurity and ill health and health-related outcomes. One of the main explanations of associations between unemployment and health is loss of income. Although job insecurity involves no loss of income, pre-existing deprivation and fear of financial insecurity have been shown to explain part of the association between self-reported job insecurity and self-reported psychological and physical health outcomes. Much has also been made of the potential for job insecurity to interact with other material and psychosocial stressors outside work and to precipitate increases in smoking and drinking.

It seems obvious that organizational change, which involves a reduction in the size of the workforce, in addition to generating job insecurity, is likely to result in changes to other characteristics of the work environment. This has been examined in a number of studies on changes in other psychosocial work characteristics, in particular, loss of job satisfaction, job control, and social support at work. Other work has shown a synergistic adverse effect on health in workers with both high job insecurity and high job strain. Despite this work, much of the association between job insecurity and ill health remains unexplained and

may be due either to direct effects of stress on the autoimmune system or to unobserved health-related selection.

Psychological Health

Most studies that have examined the effects of self-reported job insecurity on health have looked at psychological ill health as an outcome, often as the only outcome. Every study has documented consistent adverse effects on all measures of psychological health, although a combined analysis of the association between job insecurity and mental health outcomes in 37 study samples has estimated the effect size for self-reported psychological ill health to be medium rather than large, with a standardized effect of approximately 25%.

Good evidence for an association between job insecurity and poor psychological health has come from the observation of a dose–response relationship; that is, the higher the level of job insecurity, the greater the increase in psychological ill health. However, a dose–response relationship would be observed whether job insecurity increased psychological ill health or whether ill health increased the likelihood of reporting of job insecurity. In addition, self-reporting of both exposure (job insecurity) and outcome (psychological health) could contaminate the results if some participants have a tendency to report their situation, both work and health, in a negative light. Stronger evidence for the causal precedence of job insecurity comes from the study of change in job security. For example, it has been shown that, compared to employees whose jobs remain secure, psychological ill health increases among those who report a loss of job security. Studies that follow workers over time also show that self-reported job insecurity acts as a chronic stressor. This means that workers exposed to ongoing job insecurity experience the highest levels of psychological ill health.

Almost all studies of attributed job insecurity have documented an association between insecurity and psychological ill health. Findings from the most notable exception, an early factory closure study in the United States, surprised the investigators. "In the psychological sphere the personal anguish experienced by the men and their families does not seem adequately documented by the statistics" (Cobb, S and Kasl, S. V. (1977). Termination: the consequences of job loss. Cincinnati: DHEW-NIOSH Publication no. 77–224, National Institutes for Occupational Safety and Health, p. 180). The observation was attributed to imperfect measurement techniques, as numerous adverse psychological outcomes in individuals were documented in an eloquent narrative account of the closing. Another notable exception comes from a longitudinal study of white-collar civil servants, which took advantage of a natural experiment. In such experiments, a naturally exposed group is compared to an unexposed reference group. This means that there is no plausible selection process involved, and factors such as poor health or age are not influential in increasing the risk of job insecurity. Inferences about causality are strong under such conditions. In this particular natural experiment, well after the initial survey, one of the 20 departments in the study was unexpectedly sold to the private sector, a transfer of business in which most of the workforce lost their jobs. However, no effects on psychological health were seen in either sex in the run-up to the sale. A possible explanation of these seemingly contradictory findings recently emerged from a study that took advantage of a similar natural experiment in the Netherlands. One of the government agencies in the study was threatened with closure after the initial survey. Psychological ill health among employees in this agency was compared with that for employees in agencies unaffected by threat of closure, adjusting for ill health at baseline. Over the 13 months following the closure announcement, the number of new cases of psychological ill health in the closure group was significantly higher than in the nonclosure group. However, the increase in psychological distress among those working in the agency targeted, but who did not think they were at risk of job loss, was not significant; thus, self-reported rather than self-attributed job insecurity appeared to have been driving the association.

General Measures of Physical Health

Evidence is growing that self-reported job insecurity has adverse effects on self-reported general physical health measures, independent of effects on psychological health, although a combined analysis of the association in 19 study samples estimated the effect size for self-reported general physical health measures to be small, with a standardized effect of approximately 16%.

Reasonably consistent findings have been obtained for a number of health outcomes in both cross-sectional and longitudinal studies. Self-reported job insecurity has been shown to be associated with poor self-rated health, sleep disturbance, chronic insomnia, fatigue, migraine, colds and flu-like symptoms, longstanding illness, and musculoskeletal disorders. Evidence of a dose–response relationship and evidence from studies of change have provided more convincing evidence of a causal association, and there is evidence that self-reported job insecurity acts as a chronic stressor in relation to physical health. The small number of studies that have been able to examine associations between attributed job insecurity and self-reported measures of physical health have observed associations similar to those for self-reported job insecurity. However, there appears to be no evidence that attributed job insecurity acts as a chronic stressor, so it is possible that the finding for self-reported job insecurity may be due to a general tendency for negative reporting.

Very few studies have looked at the effect of either category of job insecurity on biomedical risk factors. There appears to be only two studies that have examined the association between self-reported job insecurity and blood pressure. Both studies found a significant increase in blood pressure compared with control workers who did not report job insecurity. Two studies of attributed job insecurity similarly found significant increases in blood pressure, but another two studies that examined a change in attributed security observed either no significant differences or effects in some groups but not others. Studies that have examined effects on body weight similarly report mixed findings, with no change as well as gain and loss in mean weight being observed. Resolution of these apparently divergent findings may lie in the observation that job insecurity has bidirectional effects on weight. A study of occupational factors and 5-year weight change among Danish men showed that job insecurity increased the likelihood of weight gain among obese men and weight loss among men who were lean.

Apart from two Scandinavian studies, there has been even less interest in biomedical risk factors other than blood pressure and body weight. Attributed job insecurity has been associated with nonsignificant increases in the stress hormone, cortisol, and in cholesterol in a mainly female blue-collar workforce, and levels of adrenal hormones have been shown to be raised among women at the bottom of the white-collar employment hierarchy. However, evidence on cholesterol from a longitudinal study of white-collar civil servants is mixed, and it remains uncertain what clinical relevance the observed changes in biomedical risk factors may have. Hardly any work has examined the effect of job insecurity on diagnosed diseases. Three studies have documented an association between self-reported job insecurity and various measures of coronary heart disease, and an association has been observed between attributed job insecurity and risk of ischemia (abnormal ECG or diagnosed angina) relative to unexposed employees. However, overall the evidence is limited. While the findings were indicative of adverse changes, these were modest and not significant after adjustment for major confounding somatic and behavioral coronary risk factors.

In part because job insecurity was rarely studied until the recession of the 1990s, there has been little research on the effect of job insecurity on mortality from diseases or suicide. Studies of self-reported job insecurity have not been documented, and there is no compelling evidence yet of an association between attributed job insecurity and premature death. Most work prior to the 1990s was a spin-off of studies of unemployment and health and found no significant differences between groups of workers exposed and unexposed to attributed job insecurity. More recently, a factory closure study in New Zealand examined mortality at the end of an 8-year follow-up as an outcome under the conditions of a natural experiment. The study found no statistically significant difference in the death rate for any cause between workers in the closing plant and in the control plant. This was by far the largest factory closure study to date, with nearly 2000 in both the study group and the control group. However, the number of deaths after 8 years was still relatively small, and instability in the sector, which led to the closing of the control plant by the end of the follow-up, may mean that these findings are minimum likely estimates of effects. Although temporary workers are generally considered to be part of the secondary labor market, recent work using Finnish data has looked at the effect on mortality of transfer from temporary to permanent employment. Moving from temporary to permanent employment is associated with a significantly lower risk of death, while remaining in temporary employment is associated with a significantly higher risk of death than being continuously in permanent employment. While moving the fittest temporary workers into permanent employment is likely to explain part of this effect, change in exposure to job insecurity may also contribute.

Consistent with the evidence of effects on psychological health, a review of eight studies of unemployment and suicide that used longitudinal data for individuals showed that in all but one there was greater job instability and occupational problems among suicides compared to nonsuicides. In the New Zealand factory closure study discussed previously, there was a significant, 2.5-fold increased risk of serious self-harm that led to hospitalization or death from suicide, and out of 46 men who lost their job during a U.S. factory closure, two committed suicide. Although this was 30 times the number expected, the number of people in the study population was too small to draw firm conclusions.

Health Outcomes of Interest to the Organization

A small number of studies have looked at the effect of self-reported job insecurity on safety at work. The main finding from this research is that job insecurity increases workplace injuries and accidents through detrimental effects on employee safety motivation and safety compliance. Both self-reported and attributed job insecurity have been associated with increases in short spells and medically certified spells of sickness absence from all causes, musculoskeletal disorders, and trauma. And a longitudinal study in Finland has shown that downsizing increases sickness absence more among low-income than high-income employees. In contrast to these findings, studies of British civil servants and Finnish workers on fixed-term contracts have shown that in some cases attributed job insecurity is associated with decreases in sickness absence, even when the workforce is known to have a higher level of ill health. This phenomenon is called sickness presenteeism and tends to occur when workers feel that being absent from work may increase their chance of redundancy. Unsurprisingly, sickness presenteeism appears to be more common among workers in the secondary labor market.

Job insecurity has also been widely studied in the organizational and managerial literature as a determinant of a number of outcomes that have adverse consequences for organizations, such as commitment, work effort, and productivity. Findings from the Netherlands have shown that not only is job insecurity a strong determinant of job change, but it is often the most valuable individuals that are most inclined to seek other job alternatives.

Effects beyond the Individual and the Workplace

A downstream effect of the stress caused by self-reported and attributed job insecurity is an increase in health service use: general practitioner (GP) consultations, hospital referrals, hospital attendance, and use of prescribed medicines, in particular, tranquilizers and antidepressants. However, as for sickness absence, effects can go either way, so there is also evidence that those with high levels of job insecurity may forgo a medical consultation or neglect care of themselves for fear of missing work. An in-depth study of effects on health service use also showed that these effects were not restricted to the workers themselves. GP consultations, hospital referrals, and attendance also increased significantly in the workers' families. Other effects on the family include increases in work–family conflict and tension in the home. Evidence of this spill-over confirms results from studies of both categories of job insecurity that have reported adverse effects on family members, family relationships and the behavior of children.

Who Experiences Job Insecurity: The Public Health Impact

Job insecurity is not evenly distributed throughout the working population. Along with unemployment, it falls more heavily on those with fewer skills, those with less education, and those at a disadvantage in the labor market such as immigrants and the disabled. Several studies have now demonstrated a strong inverse association between job insecurity and socioeconomic position, measured as occupational grade, social class, or education. This means that those at the top of the social hierarchy, however measured, are less likely to experience job insecurity than those at the bottom. Such inverse gradients have been demonstrated in specific occupational groups and in general population samples. There is also evidence that the effect of job insecurity on health is highest among those in the lowest socioeconomic group.

Studies of large companies or government employees – contexts in which most studies on the health effects of job insecurity have been carried out – may underestimate the extent of job insecurity in the general working population. A survey of a large sample of the working population in Taiwan found that job insecurity affected 50% of workers, and a study in Switzerland in 1997 showed that 10% of the working population reported a high level of job insecurity.

These may be two extreme examples, but an OECD study showed that in 1996 experience of job insecurity was very common, with on average 67% of workers unable to agree strongly with the statement "my job is secure." With the experience of job insecurity being this common, any detrimental effects of job insecurity on health can have major repercussion on the health of the working population as a whole.

Summary

Unequivocal evidence of a causal association between job insecurity and health would require longitudinal studies, with information from a period of secure employment for those subsequently exposed to job insecurity, in addition to a well-matched control group who remained in secure employment. Such prerequisites mean that opportunities for ideal studies are rare. Consequently, although research interest in the health consequences of job insecurity has increased, strong evidence of a causal link between job insecurity and many health outcomes remains limited. Despite this, there is now firm evidence of a causal association between both self-reported and attributed job insecurity and all measures of psychological ill health, and evidence of an association with a number of self-reported physical health outcomes.

Self-reported and attributed job insecurity are associated with adverse changes in most biomedical risk factors that have been examined, but effects are mostly nonsignificant. There is an indication that attributed job insecurity is associated with an increase in heart disease, but no evidence yet of an association between job insecurity and death from diseases or suicide. Job insecurity has been shown to increase workplace injuries and accidents through detrimental effects on employee safety motivation and safety compliance. Most studies show that attributed job insecurity is accompanied by an increase in self-certified and medically certified sickness absence. However, lower rates of sickness absence as well as sickness presenteeism among temporary workers and employees facing imminent threat have also been demonstrated. Both self-reported and attributed job insecurity result in increased use of health services and medications among both those directly affected and their families.

It has been proposed that the effect of job insecurity on health may be mediated via changes in health-related behaviors. However, there is little evidence to support or refute this hypothesis. Although some studies have found the effect of job insecurity on health to be partially explained by other work characteristics such as job satisfaction, social support at work, and job control, much of the association between job insecurity and ill health remains unexplained and may be due either to direct effects of stress on the autoimmune system or to unobserved health-related selection.

Recent work has demonstrated a synergistic adverse effect on health in workers exposed to both high job insecurity and high job strain. In a context of downsizing and reliance on outsourced labor, perceptions of insecurity are likely to be widespread and, as fewer people do more, occur alongside increasing demands and perceptions of low control. If current trends continue, the number of employees exposed to both job insecurity and job strain will probably increase. Despite its limitations, existing research on the stress of job insecurity has much to contribute to policies that will improve the health of workers and their families and prevent adverse effects on the organizations that employ them.

See Also the Following Articles

Demand–Control Model; Effort-Reward Imbalance Model; Unemployment, Stress and Health; Workplace Stress.

Further Reading

Bartley, M. and Ferrie, J. E. (2001). Unemployment, job insecurity and health – glossary. *Journal of Epidemiology and Community Health* 55, 776–781.

Burchell, B., Day, D., Hudson, M., Ladipo, D., Mankelow, R., Nolan, J., et al. (1999). *Job insecurity and work intensification*. York: Joseph Rowntree Foundation.

Ferrie, J. E., Marmot, M. G., Griffiths, J. and Ziglio, E. (eds.) (1999). *Labour market changes and job insecurity: a challenge for social welfare and health promotion*. European Series No. 81. Copenhagen: World Health Organisation.

Hartley, J., Jacobson, D., Klandermans, B. and Van Vuuren, T. (1991). *Job insecurity: coping with jobs at risk*. London: Sage Publications Ltd.

Quinlan, M., Mayhew, C. and Bohle, E. (2001). The global expansion of precarious employment, work disorganisation, and consequences for occupational health: a review of recent research. *International Journal of Health Services* 31, 335–414.

Platt, S., Pavis, S. and Akram, G. (1998). *Changing labour market conditions and health: a systematic literature review (1993–1998)*. Dublin: European Foundation for the Improvement of Living and Working Conditions.

Kidney Function

W J Welch
Georgetown University, Washington, D.C., USA

Introduction
Renal Vascular Resistance (RVR)
Sodium Reabsorption
Does Chronic Stress Cause Hypertension by a Renal Mechanism?
Summary

Glossary

Renal sympathetic nerve activity	Net activity (measured in Hz) of renal nerve bundles supplying the kidney.
Renal vascular resistance	Vascular resistance of blood flow through the kidney, calculated as systemic mean arterial blood pressure factored by renal blood flow.
Sodium retention	Excess reabsorption of Na^+ from various segments of the nephron, resulting in increased extracellular volume.

Introduction

The kidney's primary function is to maintain homeostasis by the efficient elimination of excess fluid and solute. This key function is regulated by both extrarenal and intrarenal mechanisms that control the kidney's ability to maintain proper fluid and electrolyte balance. The sympathetic nervous system (SNS) is an integral part of the homeostatic control system that maintains normal kidney function, with an extensive network of nerves identified in most renal tissues. The SNS modulates short-term regulation of renal function, and under normal conditions renal sympathetic nerve activity is low. During acute stress, however, elevated renal sympathetic activity depresses renal function. Chronic stress studies have been less conclusive and are difficult to design due to additional pathologies induced by stress, such as hypertension and cardiovascular complications. Major renal effects of mental stress include increased renal vasoconstriction, causing greater renal vascular resistance (RVR), and increased Na^+ transport, causing greater Na^+ retention. Both of these effects may contribute to the development of hypertension, and some investigators propose that this may be the primary mechanism of human essential hypertension. Therefore, most studies on the renal effects of stress have focused on its relationship to hypertension. Though the effects of stress are more pronounced in hypertensive humans and animals, stress increases renal vasoconstriction and Na^+ retention in normal subjects and animals, as well.

Renal Vascular Resistance (RVR)

The systemic blood pressure determines the renal perfusion pressure (RPP) and is a major determinant of RVR. The kidney has a unique ability to autoregulate its own blood flow that is efficient over a wide range of RPPs. Renal blood flow (RBF) changes very little over a large range of RPPs, therefore maintaining a stable RVR. This is due to the exquisite control of vascular tone in the primary renal resistance vessels, the preglomerular afferent arterioles and the postglomerular efferent arterioles. However, many hormonal and neural disturbances can alter autoregulation, often targeting these arterioles, leading to inappropriate increases in RVR. Increased sympathetic activity increases arteriolar resistance and RVR. Increased RVR exacerbates hypertension via its contribution to overall increased total peripheral resistance (since RBF is 20–25% of cardiac output) and its ability to promote Na^+ reabsorption. Stress can induce both neural and hormonal changes that affect RVR.

Renal Sympathetic Nerve Activity (RSNA) and RVR

Multiple studies using several types of acute stress in rats have shown that RBF is reduced and blood pressure (BP) and RVR over the period of stress are elevated. Renal sympathetic nerve activity (RSNA) when measured is increased and is now associated with the stress-induced changes in RVR. Renal sympathetic nerves act primarily by release of norepinephrine (NE), and nerve endings extend to most renal structures, including arterioles and tubules. In studies designed to test the effects of RSNA alone, higher RSNA frequencies within the range observed during stress increased RVR. The mechanism of RSNA stimulation on vascular tone is linked to increased release of NE and higher circulating epinephrine, acting on α- and β-adrenergic receptors, modulated by Ang II.

Experiments that stimulated RSNA show that there are at least three renal neuroeffector targets: renin-containing juxtaglomerular cells, the tubule, and the arterial vascular resistance. The sequence of RSNA input shows that renin is released at lower levels of RNSA, tubular reabsorption is increased at slightly higher intensities, and renal vasoconstriction occurs at even higher intensities. Each system appears to be regulated differently over a range of RSNA. Nonetheless, it appears that only moderate stress is sufficient to increase RSNA to levels that can alter major renal effectors. The role of RSNA on the renal contribution to hypertension is less clear. In studies in which periodic or prolonged periods of stress increased RSNA, there are only short-term effects on BP.

Many of the RSNA pacing studies have been limited to anesthetized rats, which may have altered basal RSNA. However, recent radiotelemetry techniques developed to measure RSNA in conscious rabbits exposed to stress have confirmed the role of renal nerves on increased RVR and have been used to explore the mechanisms. In response to air jet or white noise stress, RSNA was increased by 55 and 40%, respectively, within 1–2 min, and returned to normal by 9 min in conscious rabbits. Following treatment with rilmenidine, an imidazoline I (1) receptor agonist that reduces sympathetic-induced vascular tone, basal RSNA was reduced. However, the early response to air jet stress was reduced by 35%, whereas rilmenidine had no effect on white noise stress. Therefore, stress stimulates RSNA, but different stressor pathways may involve different central processing.

Increased RSNA impairs renal autoregulation, but the effects appear to be greater in hypertensive animals, suggesting a critical interaction with BP and RPP. However, stress also increases RSNA and BP in normotensive animals. WKY rats exposed to two different strategies of territorial stress (TS) developed higher BP over 5 months compared to control,

unstressed rats. There was no evidence that changes in renal function contributed to the hypertension. Indeed, renal function in spontaneously hypertensive rats (SHR) in which higher BP correlates to RSNA is not different from normotensive WKY. However, in this study TS rats had higher levels of serum corticosterone and catecholamines early in the study, but the values were similar to unstressed rats after 10–12 weeks. This suggested that early exposure to stress might have long-term effects. To test this idea, young normotensive rats were exposed to acute injection of the α-1 adrenoreceptor agonist phenylephrine, which transiently increased BP and decreased glomerular filtration rate (GFR). After recovery, the animals were normotensive, but developed hypertension with reduced GFR when exposed to a high-salt (HS) diet, 8–10 weeks later. Together, these studies suggest that stress-induced surges in catecholamines, rather than constant stress, may enhance the susceptibility to other environmental stimuli, such as HS intake, and lead to hypertension and renal injury.

Based on the results from rat denervation studies, chronic increases in RSNA impact renal function. Under normal conditions, RSNA is low and renal denervation does not lead to changes in RBF or RVR. However, when RSNA is high, such as in the SHR or in heart failure rats, renal denervation increases RBF and decreases RVR. This occurs despite the similar RBF measured in intact SHR and WKY rats. Denervation does not alter RBF in WKY. This shows that chronic stress/increased RSNA tends to suppress RBF and increase RVR in SHR. However, it is not clear whether this effect contributes to the development of hypertension in SHR.

The role of stress on RVR has also been studied in human models, where stress-induced renal vasoconstriction also increases RSNA. RSNA is determined by measuring plasma or renal outflow of NE. In healthy volunteers, a short period of mental stress was accompanied by increased renal release of NE and epinephrine (Epi) and renin release, which led to a 48% increase in RVR. Renal arteries also appear to be more sensitive than other visceral vessels to stress in humans. Renal artery (RA) and small mesenteric artery (SMA) resistance and blood velocity were measured by simultaneous pulse and echo Doppler ultrasound flowmetry in 16 young female volunteers for 3 min before and 3 min during a mental stress test. RA vascular resistance was increased and RA blood velocity was decreased during the first minute of stress. SMA resistance was modestly increased, but velocity was unaffected by stress. This suggests that renal blood flow is exquisitely sensitive to mental stress and the accompanying increase in RSNA.

Hormonal Modulators

In addition to direct actions of renal nerves and activation of α-adrenergic receptors, multiple vasoactive hormones may contribute to stress-induced RVR. Endothelin is a peptide hormone that acts on receptors in endothelial cells and on vascular smooth muscle cells, generating vasoconstriction. In a series of human trials in elderly and young women, acute mental stress (30 min) increased BP, heart rate (HR), plasma NE, effective renal plasma flow, and RVR, but its effect on RVR was more prolonged in the elderly group. Urinary excretion of endothelin-1 was elevated in both groups, whereas excretion of vasodilating prostaglandins and nitric oxide (NO) was high only during the mental stress period in elderly subjects but was sustained at a higher excretion levels in young subjects. The balance between these opposing vasoactive hormones may therefore determine the level of stress-induced RVR. These studies provide good evidence that the balance between renal vasoconstrictors and vasodilators is invoked in the kidney's ability to autoregulate blood flow during mental stress. However, studies that evaluate the direct effects of endothelin infusion do not support a major role for endothelin as a potent vasoconstrictor during stress.

Several studies have shown that renin is released into the renal circulation during various forms of stress. However, it is not clear whether the levels of renin and locally produced Ang II are sufficient to contribute to the increased vasoconstriction that accompanies increased sympathetic activity. One report suggests that Ang II modulates the effects of catecholamine activation of adrenergic receptors, but the interaction has not been carefully investigated.

The role of NO was examined in adult borderline hypertensive rats (offspring of SHR and Wistar rats) during 5 weeks of crowding stress. Compared to unstressed controls, BP, HR, and nitric oxide synthase (NOS) activity in the aorta were higher. However, NOS activity in the heart, adrenal gland, and kidney was not affected. Superoxide (O_2^-), which scavenges NO, may contribute to RSNA. The higher RSNA activity in SHR compared to WKY was normalized by tempol, a powerful antioxidant, which reduced BP and RSNA to a greater extent in SHR than in WKY. However, the effect of reactive oxygen species on other influences on renal function could not be ruled out in this study.

The renal levels of neuropeptide Y (NPY) and calcitonin gene-related peptide (CGRP) were measured following a period of mental stress (word conflict test) or after low-dose adrenalin infusion in 12 healthy volunteers. Mental stress caused a threefold increase in NE renal overflow but had no effect on NPY or CGRP, whereas Epi infusion increased levels of all neurotransmitters.

The pro-inflammatory transcription factor nuclear factor-κB (NF-κB) has been linked to psychosocial stress as a possible mediator of organ damage, specifically in the kidney. NF-κB activation in renal tissue was greater in tissue from patients with renal complications. NF-κB in peripheral blood mononuclear cells (PBMC), which can be easily measured, correlated with the degree of albuminuria in diabetic nephropathy patients and was reduced by antioxidant therapy. Similar levels of NF-κB activation in PBMC were observed in healthy volunteers during a 15-min psychosocial stress test. The activation of NF-κB in PBMC correlated with the stress-induced increases in catecholamines and cortisol. Though the long-term effects of stress on NF-κB have not been tested, these acute studies provide a possible mechanism of kidney damage caused by stress.

Sodium Reabsorption

A major hypothesis for the development of hypertension invokes the role of the kidney in the inappropriate retention of solute and fluid resulting in increased fluid volume. In order to maintain homeostatic control of body fluids during periods of hypertension, the kidney excretes greater levels of urine and solute, resetting a lower extracellular fluid volume. However, the increases in BP seen during periodic stress does not always generate this pressure-natriuresis response, partially due to the increased RSNA, which simultaneously increases Na^+ reabsorption. As some studies suggest, the inability to excrete more solute and fluid during periods of increased BP may predispose those individuals to hypertension. The observation that acute stress can cause Na^+ retention has led to the popular theory that human essential hypertension is primarily due to chronic stress mediating excess extracellular fluid volume via a renal mechanism. Acute stress clearly increases RSNA, and several animal models of hypertension show increased renal sympathetic activity. However, RSNA is determined by postganglionic fibers and is controlled by the arterial baroreceptor reflex, which is not associated with long-term BP control. Though recent evidence shows a stronger correlation of RSNA and long-term control, RSNA generated by stress provides primarily acute regulation of renal function-induced hypertension.

Animal studies show that acute stress consistently increases RSNA and decreases Na^+ excretion in normotensive rats and dogs and does so to an even greater extent in hypertensive rats. The neurohormonal regulation of these effects has been the focus of several studies. In conscious rats, a 10-min air jet stress increased BP and RSNA and reduced urine volume and Na^+ excretion by three- to fourfold (**Figure 2**). After denervation, urine volume and Na^+ excretion were not affected by stress, demonstrating the dependency of neural activity. Treatment with an AT1-R antagonist also prevented a decrease in urine flow or Na^+ excretion after stress, though RSNA was not affected. This suggests that Ang II mediates the antidiuresis and antinatriuresis induced by stress without affecting nerve activity. Previous studies showed that increases in RSNA led to greater Na^+ reabsorption, which was mediated by α-2 receptors. Inhibition of Ang II also decreased the RSNA effect, suggesting that Ang II interacts with α-2 receptors to regulate Na^+ reabsorption. Therefore, changes in RSNA induced by mental stress may have similar regulation by Ang II and α-2 receptors.

Results from human studies are less consistent but do show the effects of stress, and the associated increases in sympathetic activity on Na^+ retention are more closely associated with hypertension than in normotensive humans. In a well-controlled human subject trial, two 20-min periods of stress increased BP and decreased Na^+ excretion in 10 normotensive adult males, without altering GFR, measured by the clearance of inulin, or renal plasma flow (RPF), measured by the clearance of para-aminohippurate (PAH). Fractional Na^+ reabsorption was increased by stress and was primarily due to increases in reabsorption in the proximal tubule (PT), based on fractional lithium clearance measurements. Rilminedine, an imidazoline-I1 receptor antagonist, lowered basal BP but did not alter the effects of stress.

In a study that tested the interaction of hypertension and stress on renal function, three groups were evaluated: normotensive offspring of hypertensives (HP), hypertensive subjects (HT), and normotensive offspring of normotensives (NP). Basal BP, which differed between groups, was elevated by stress in all groups. However, the BP increased more in HP than in the other groups (**Figure 1**). Basal GFR and RBF were higher in HP than in the other groups. However, GFR was reduced by stress in HP and HT but not in NP, and RBF was reduced in HT and NP but not in HP. More interesting, however, were the responses to stress in normal subjects. Stress increased the filtration fraction, which suggests that efferent arteriolar resistance was elevated. There was also a paradoxical decrease in Na^+ excretion given that BP was higher. Again, the decrease in Na^+ reabsorption was attributed to increased PT reabsorption, based on the changes in lithium clearance.

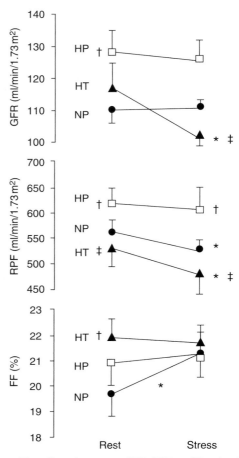

Figure 1　The effect of stress on GFR, RPF, and filtration fraction (FF) in normotensive (NP), normotensive with hypertensive parents (HP), and hypertensive (HT) subjects. From Ducher, M., et al. (2002). *American Journal of Hypertension* **15**, 346–350. © 2002 American Journal of Hypertension, Ltd.

However, Na^+ retention induced by stress is not always observed in normal subjects. In three groups designed to test the potential for the development of hypertension, the effects of mental stress on Na^+ excretion were evaluated in normotensive young males with and without a family of hypertension and compared to hypertensive males. Each subject was studied with or without 1 week of therapy with an angiotensin converting enzyme inhibitor (cilazapril). A 30-min period of mental stress led to increased BP, HR, and GFR and decreased RBF in all groups. However, Na^+ excretion was increased in both normotensive groups, eliciting the appropriate pressure-natriuresis response, whereas the hypertensive group failed to change. Angiotensin converting enzyme therapy restored the increased Na^+ excretion in the hypertensive group, suggesting that the failed natriuretic response is due to the observed elevation of Ang II in hypertensive subjects. Together, these studies suggest that individuals who respond to stress by decreasing

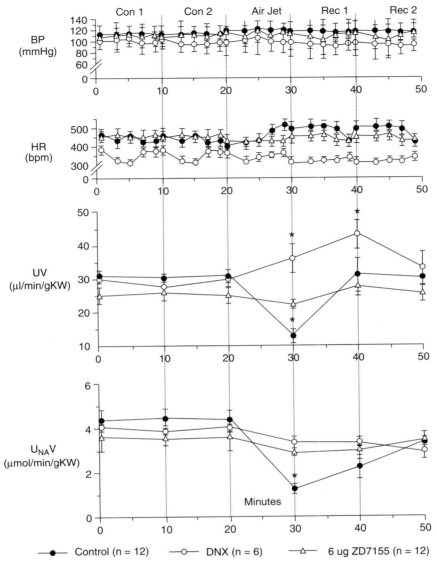

Figure 2 Effects of 10-min air-jet stress on BP, HR, urine flow rate (UV), and Na$^+$ excretion rate (U$_{NA}$V). UV and U$_{NA}$V are reduced during stress in conscious control rats. This effect is blocked by either denervation (DNX) or by Ang II, type 1 receptor blocker (ZD7155). From Veelken, R., et al. (1996). *Hypertension* **28**, 825–832.

Na$^+$ excretion are predisposed to Na$^+$ retention and hypertension, whereas normotensive humans with the appropriate natriuresis response to stress are less likely to progress to hypertension via stress.

Does Chronic Stress Cause Hypertension by a Renal Mechanism?

As discussed previously, most of the studies that have shown increased RSNA, RVR, and Na$^+$ reabsorption to stress were observed during acute stress. Under these acute conditions the increased RVR and renin release may contribute to the acute rise in BP. However, it is difficult to assign a role for Na$^+$ retention in

acute hypertension, which occurs almost immediately. Therefore, caution should be observed when using acute studies to interpret chronic stress-induced hypertension. Studies in normotensive rats and mice have shown that prolonged stress for as much as 4–5 months increases BP during this period. Mice have shown progressive arteriosclerosis, myocardial hypertrophy, increased catecholamine levels, and greater angiotensin sensitivity, since Ang II blockade prevented hypertension. However, there were no measurements of Na$^+$ balance during the development of hypertension to evaluate the kidney's role. In hypertensive models, such as SHR, renal function and volume status also rarely differ. The use of prehypertensive models has suggested a stronger role for the kidney in the development of hypertension but has not controlled adequately for the genetic backgrounds of these models. A more valuable set of data has been made in renal denervation studies, which have indicated that antinatriuresis and renal vasoconstriction may be due to the elevated RSNA in SHR.

Another issue of concern is that stress in rodents and humans may differ substantially. Human studies have not always found renal dysfunction in acute stress in normal subjects. This would be expected, since genetic predisposition appears to be necessary for the failure of the kidneys to adjust to high BP with appropriate natriuresis. It is possible that some normotensive subjects used in these studies had unknown genetic predisposition. Rodent studies have consistently shown the lack of renal compensation to acute stress, which is surprising but may not relate to the kidney's role, if any, in chronic stress. Indeed, chronic stress in rodents has been associated with cardiac and vascular remodeling.

The proper resolution of this question, at least in animals, will require a reproducible chronic stress model in rodents with noninvasive measurements of BP and renal function that can measure the critical components of renal influences on the development of hypertension over a chronic period. Lacking this type of information, the current evidence does not strongly support a role for changes in renal function contributing significantly to chronic stress-induced hypertension.

Summary

In summary, acute mental stress increases RSNA, BP, RVR, and Na^+ reabsorption in both animal and human studies. These effects are exaggerated in borderline hypertensive or hypertensive subjects, and many effects are blocked by Ang II inhibition, though multiple hormonal systems may be involved. The effects of chronic mental stress are more controversial, with few consistent observations. Though RSNA and general sympathetic activity is increased

in SHR, there are rarely any reports of renal dysfunction that would be expected if stress had permanent effects on renal function. The concept of mental stress altering renal function that leads to hypertension needs further experimental evidence.

See Also the Following Articles

Angiotensin; Blood Pressure; Hypertension; Regional Blood Flow, Stress Effects; Salt Appetite; Vasoactive Peptides.

Further Reading

Barrett, C. J., Ramchandra, R., Guild, S. J., et al. (2003). What sets the long-term level of renal sympathetic nerve activity: a role for angiotensin II and baroreflexes? *Circulation Research* **92**, 1330–1336.

Bierhaus, A., Wolf, J., Andrassy, M., et al. (2003). A mechanism converting psychosocial stress into mononuclear cell activation. *Proceedings of the National Academy of Science USA* **100**, 1920–1925.

Castellani, S., Ungar, A., Cantini, C., et al. (1999). Impaired renal adaptation to stress in the elderly with isolated systolic hypertension. *Hypertension* **34**, 1106–1111.

Di Bona, G. F. (2004). The sympathetic nervous system and hypertension: recent developments. *Hypertension* **43**, 147–150.

Di Bona, G. F. and Kopp, U. C. (1997). Neural control of renal function. *Physiological Reviews* **77**, 75–197.

Ducher, M., Bertram, D., Pozet, N., et al. (2002). Stress-induced renal alterations in normotensive offspring of hypertensives and in hypertensives. *American Journal of Hypertension* **15**, 346–350.

Schmeider, R. E., Veelken, R., Schobel, H., et al. (1997). Glomerular hypertension during sympathetic nervous system activation in early essential hypertension. *Journal of the American Society of Nephrologists* **8**, 893–900.

Schneider, M. P., Klingbeil, A. U., Schlaich, M. P., et al. (2001). Impaired sodium excretion during mental stress in mild essential hypertension. *Hypertension* **37**, 923–927.

Veelken, R., Hilgers, K. F., Stetter, A., et al. (1996). Nerve-mediated antidiuresis and antinatriuresis after air-jet stress is modulate by angiotensin II. *Hypertension* **28**, 825–832.

Korean Conflict, Stress Effects of

C A Goguen
National Center for PTSD, USA
M J Friedman
Dartmouth College, Hanover, NH, USA

This article is reproduced from the previous edition, volume 2, pp 595–598, © 2000, Elsevier Inc.

Critical Issues in Korean Conflict Trauma Research
Combat Exposure
Lasting Effects of Combat Exposure
Summary

Prior to the Korean conflict (1950–1953), combat-related posttraumatic stress reactions, variously termed battle fatigue, war neurosis, and combat exhaustion, were considered a temporary condition best treated close to the combat zone. Influential theoretical perspectives included Freudian concepts of defense mechanisms as adaptations to stress-induced intrapsychic conflicts and, later, Selye's general adaptation syndrome, stress reactions viewed as a three-stage physiological response. Psychiatry during World War II and the Korean conflict viewed traumatic war neurosis as a complex phenomenon resulting from "multiple physical and psychic forces struggling for emotional control . . . the stimuli of battle itself evoked a defensive process that sustained men in combat . . . the lonely, fearful battle environment forces individuals to join together for protection and emotional support" (Glass, 1954: 728). The military unit was seen as a key source of support and motivation for soldiers to return to active combat. Therefore, all but the most severe cases of psychiatric casualties were treated at the front lines.

Further reinforcing the belief that combat-related posttraumatic stress reactions were short-lived, the publication of the first edition of *Diagnostic and Statistical Manual of Mental Disorders* (DSM-I) in 1952 established responses to either combat or civilian catastrophe invoking overwhelming fear, "gross stress reaction," as a temporary condition. Any protracted course of symptoms was attributed to an unrelated neurosis. Subsequently, the 1968 edition, DSM-II, dropped "gross stress reaction," relegating combat-related posttraumatic stress reactions to an adult adjustment problem.

Critical Issues in Korean Conflict Trauma Research

Nevertheless, the most prevalent service-connected disability in a sample of former Korean prisoners of war (POWs) was anxiety neurosis (19.2%). Few researchers at the time examined the psychological impact of combat-related traumatic stress on Korean veterans. In fact, most clinical and empirical research on the possible long-term psychological sequelae of the Korean conflict did not begin in earnest until the 1980s, three decades later, and only after a substantial amount of research had been conducted on posttraumatic stress disorder (PTSD) among Vietnam veterans. These retrospective studies all suffer from sampling problems that make it difficult to generalize from their findings to all Korean conflict veterans. Some studies did not differentiate Korean veterans from World War II veterans, whereas all the remaining studies focused exclusively on treatment-seeking veterans or POWs, each a highly select group.

Combat Exposure

Despite limited data, certain trends can be seen. It is clear that some Korean combat veterans were exposed to high levels of war-zone stress. Indeed, Blake and colleagues found no significant differences for combat exposure or posttraumatic stress symptomatology between Korean combat veterans and either World War II or Vietnam combat veterans. In an early study, Korean veterans reported that their combat-related posttraumatic stress symptoms not only persisted but actually worsened over time.

One of the best-studied groups of Korean combat veterans are former POWs. Like non-POW Korean combat veterans, Korean POWs reported that they had continued to experience posttraumatic stress symptoms years, even decades, after the trauma. Consistent with studies demonstrating a dose–response relationship between traumatic exposure and posttraumatic stress symptoms, Korean POWs reported higher levels of posttraumatic symptoms than non-POW Korean combat veterans. Whereas Korean POWs experienced less combat exposure than non-POW Korean veterans, the combat they had experienced before their capture was fierce with heavy casualties. After capture, they were sent on death marches and were subjected to brainwashing techniques and long periods of physical deprivation, interrogation, and solitary confinement. Thirty-eight percent of Korean POWs died during captivity.

Lasting Effects of Combat Exposure

Despite the circumscribed number of empirical investigations, the existing database suggests that, in addition to PTSD, Korean POWs and combat veterans have experienced long-term consequences of traumatic exposure, including alcohol abuse, depression, and general psychiatric distress. Further, higher mortality rates, especially due to accidents, appear to occur among Korean POWs than are expected for U.S. males. With respect to their World War II counterparts, Korean veterans had a higher lifetime prevalence of suicide attempts, more frequent occurrences of drug abuse-related hospitalizations and outpatient treatment, and greater use of mental health outpatient treatment. However, fewer Korean veterans met diagnostic criteria for PTSD. Nevertheless, Korean POWs reported higher rates of posttraumatic stress symptomatology and depression than World War II POWs.

Compared to Vietnam counterparts, Korean veterans reported lower levels of alcohol or drug abuse and fewer occurrences of drug abuse-related hospitalizations and outpatient treatment. Korean veterans were more likely than Vietnam veterans to recognize, early in their disorder, the link between their symptoms and their combat exposure. However, less use of PTSD treatment programs was found among Korean veterans.

Summary

Relative to Vietnam and World War II veterans, few researchers have included Korean veterans in their studies. A caveat should be exercised when drawing conclusions from studies of highly selective samples of war-era groups that differ in important areas such as age, premilitary socioeconomic status, time since combat exposure, POW status, repatriation, and social attitudes. Nevertheless, it seems apparent that traumatized Korean veterans suffer chronic debilitating posttraumatic psychological consequences of their war-zone experiences.

See Also the Following Articles

Combat Stress Reaction; Persian Gulf War, Stress Effects of; Prisoners of War; Vietnam Veterans, Postwar Experiences and Health Outcomes; War-Related Posttraumatic Stress Disorder, Treatment of.

Further Reading

American Psychiatric Association (1952). *Diagnostic and statistical manual of mental disorders*. Washington, DC: American Psychiatric Association.

American Psychiatric Association (1968). *Diagnostic and statistical manual of mental disorders* (2nd edn.). Washington, DC: American Psychiatric Association.

Archibald, H. C. and Tuddenham, R. D. (1965). Persistent stress reaction after combat. *Archives of General Psychiatry* 12, 475–481.

Beebe, G. W. (1975). Follow-up studies of World War II and Korean conflict prisoners. II: Morbidity, disability, and maladjustments. *American Journal of Epidemiology* 101, 400–422.

Blake, D. D., Keane, T. M., Wine, P. R., et al. (1990). Prevalence of PTSD symptoms in combat veterans seeking medical treatment. *Journal of Traumatic Stress* 3, 15–27.

Druley, K. A. and Pashko, S. (1988). Posttraumatic stress disorder in World War II and Korean combat veterans with alcohol dependence. *Recent Developments in Alcoholism* 6, 89–101.

Engdahl, B. E., Harkness, A. R., Eberly, R. E., et al. (1993). Structural models of captivity trauma, resilience, and trauma response among former prisoners of war 20 to 40 years after release. *Social Psychiatry and Psychiatric Epidemiology* 28, 109–115.

Foy, D. W., Sipprelle, R. C., Rueger, D. B., et al. (1984). Etiology of posttraumatic stress disorder in Vietnam veterans: analysis of premilitary, military, and combat exposure influences. *Journal of Consulting and Clinical Psychology* 52, 79–87.

Glass, A. J. (1954). Psychotherapy in the combat zone. *American Journal of Psychiatry* 110, 725–731.

Goodwin, J. (1987). The etiology of combat-related posttraumatic stress disorders. In: Williams, T. (ed.) *Posttraumatic stress disorders: a handbook for clinicians*, pp. 1–18. Cincinnati, OH: Cincinnati Disabled American Veterans.

Keehn, R. J. (1980). Follow-up studies of World War II and Korean conflict prisoners. III: Mortality to January 1, 1976. *American Journal of Epidemiology* 111, 194–211.

Lee, K. A., Vaillant, G. E., Torrey, W. C., et al. (1995). A 50-year prospective study of the psychological sequelae of World War II combat. *American Journal of Psychiatry* 152, 516–522.

Mellman, T. A., Randolph, C. A., Brawman-Mintzer, O., et al. (1992). Phenomenology and course of psychiatric disorders associated with combat-related posttraumatic stress disorder. *American Journal of Psychiatry* 149, 1568–1574.

Page, W. F., Engdahl, B. E. and Eberly, R. E. (1991). Prevalence and correlates of depressive symptoms among former prisoners of war. *Journal of Nervous and Mental Disease* 179, 670–677.

Rosenheck, R. and Fontana, A. (1994). Long-term sequelae of combat in World War II, Korea and Vietnam: a comparative study. In: Ursano, R. J., McCaughey, B. G. & Fullerton, C. S. (eds.) *Individual and community responses to trauma and disaster*, pp. 359. New York: Cambridge University Press.

Selye, H. (1950). *The physiology and pathology of exposure to stress*. Montreal, Canada: Acta.

Sutker, P. B. and Allain, A. N. (1996). Assessment of PTSD and other mental disorders in World War II and Korean conflict POW survivors and combat veterans. *Psychological Assessment* **8**, 18–25.

Sutker, P. G., Winstead, D. K., Galina, Z. H., et al. (1991). Cognitive deficits and psychopathology among former prisoners of war and combat veterans of the Korean conflict. *American Journal of Psychiatry* **148**, 67–72.

U.S. Veterans Administration/Office of Planning and Program Evaluation (1980). *POW: study of former prisoners of war.* Washington, DC: U.S. Government Printing Office.

L

Learned Helplessness

D M Isaacowitz
Brandeis University, Waltham, MA, USA
M E P Seligman
University of Pennsylvania, Philadelphia, PA, USA

This article is a revision of the previous edition article by M E P Seligman and D M Isaacowitz, volume 2, pp 599–602, © 2000, Elsevier Inc.

Original Observations and Theory
Learned Helplessness and Psychopathology in Humans

Glossary

Explanatory style	A person's characteristic ways of explaining the causes of the events that happen in his or her life.
Shuttle box	Experimental apparatus for animals with two compartments separated by a barrier that can be adjusted by the experimenter.
Uncontrollable reinforcer	A reinforcer whose probability is the same whether an emitted response is present or absent. In this situation, the responding organism cannot control the reinforcer.

Original Observations and Theory

Learned helplessness refers to the motivational, cognitive, and emotional deficits that may follow from an organism's exposure to uncontrollable stressors. The theory arose from the observation that, after experiencing inescapable shock over which they had no control, dogs in the laboratory displayed a variety of behavioral deficits. In the original experiments on the learned helplessness phenomenon, the following design was typically used. The dogs were first given unpredictable and inescapable electric shocks in a Pavlovian hammock. Then, 24 h later, the dogs were placed in an experimental shuttle box. In this shuttle box, there were two compartments, and the dog was given 10 trials of escape/avoidance training. Shock was given in both compartments, but the termination of the shock took place when the dog jumped from one compartment to the other.

Approximately two-thirds of the dogs placed in the shuttle box after experiencing inescapable shock did not learn the escape/avoidance behavior; that is, they never learned that they could end the shock simply by jumping to the other compartment. Instead, they struggled at first and then stopped attempting to take action that might terminate the shock. The vast majority of dogs who had not experienced inescapable shock prior to entering the shuttle box had no trouble learning the escape/avoidance procedure to terminate the shock. The deficit in many of the previously shocked dogs was psychological rather than physical because these same dogs were able to run out of the shuttle box when the exit was opened.

This learned helplessness effect observed in the previously shocked dogs (i.e., they passively accepted later shock and did not learn to avoid it) was caused by the uncontrollability of the shocks experienced in the Pavlovian hammock. This was demonstrated by Seligman and Maier in 1967 using a yoked experimental design with three groups of dogs. The first group could press a panel in the hammock to terminate the shock. The second group received the same duration of shock as the first group, but could not control the onset or termination of its shock in the hammock. The third group received no shock prior to being placed in the shuttle box. The yoked group, which had received uncontrollable shock in the hammock, showed the strongest deficits in learning in the shuttle box. The dogs that had received the same amount of shock but could press to control the termination of the shock did not show these deficits.

The deficits observed in helpless dogs fall into three categories. First, motivational deficits exist because the dogs stop initiating voluntary behaviors, such as jumping from one compartment to the other. Cognitive deficits also appear in that the dogs do not learn that their responses have been effective even when they have indeed caused the desired effect. Finally, the dogs show transient helplessness effects that dissipate over time, suggesting that helplessness may be a passing emotional response. Interestingly, exposure to controllable shock in the shuttle box prior to experiencing uncontrollable shocks appears to immunize dogs against later helplessness deficits and forcibly exposing dogs to the appropriate response contingency (i.e., that jumping to the other compartment terminates the shock) can eliminate these deficits.

According to the researchers, the dogs who received uncontrollable, inescapable shock learned that outcomes were independent of their responses. When organisms experience uncontrollable outcomes, they may notice this contingency and learn that the outcomes are independent. They will then expect outcomes to be independent of their responses in the future. This expectation involves a cognitive representation of the contingency. The purpose of voluntary action is to cause certain outcomes, so a belief in response–outcome independence will reduce the organism's motivation to engage in voluntary responses. Because forming this expectation of independence is an act of learning, this cognitive representation will interfere proactively with future attempts to learn about response–outcome dependence. Finally, the fear that follows a traumatic event may be replaced with negative emotions when the organism realizes its lack of control in the situation. Thus, learned helplessness theory seeks to explain the three primary deficits observed through a cognitive pathway. In their 1976 review paper, Maier and Seligman reviewed alternative hypotheses for the observed deficits and argued that the helplessness account fits most parsimoniously with the available data.

Learned helplessness is not specific only to dogs in the shuttle box. Deficits have also been documented in cats, rats, and humans. These extensions of learned helplessness to animals other than dogs have been empirically and theoretically useful. One study found that helpless rats were less likely to reject cancerous tumors than nonhelpless rats, suggesting an important connection between helplessness and immune function. In humans, several studies used a yoked paradigm in which participants (college students) in the first group could turn off a loud noise by pressing a button. Students in the second group heard the same noise for the same duration of time as those in the first group, but the sound was not contingent on their pressing a button. A final control group did not hear any noise. In one study conducted by Hiroto, students then put their hand in a shuttle box; they were shocked but could escape by moving their hand to the other side. Just as in the dogs, the students in the uncontrollable group showed helplessness deficits; they did not learn the avoidance strategy and just took the shock. In another study by Miller and Seligman, students who heard the uncontrollable inescapable noise had more trouble solving difficult anagrams than did those who heard escapable noise and those who heard no noise at all.

Learned Helplessness and Psychopathology in Humans

Although these experiments demonstrate that learned helplessness deficits can be produced in humans, a large amount of research has investigated whether the learned helplessness model can be thought of as an analog for various psychological disorders in humans. The most work has been done on depression and posttraumatic stress disorder (PTSD), so we consider here how learned helplessness might be useful for the understanding and treatment of these two types of psychopathology. Although our focus in the remainder of this article is on links between learned helplessness and mental health, there is an additional, smaller body of work linking learned helplessness and physical health in humans.

Depression

In his 1975 book *Helplessness*, Seligman asserted that the learned helplessness phenomenon appeared to be very much like human depression. Specifically, the motivational, cognitive, and emotional deficits that appeared in helpless dogs seemed to mimic the symptoms of reactive depression, in which a human gets depressed after a major life stressor. Certainly the apparent emotional withdrawal and passivity shown by helpless dogs and college students paralleled depression; in addition, decreased motivation and increased cognitive difficulty, also parts of the helplessness experience, are major symptoms of depression. Based on these and other similarities, Seligman hypothesized that both learned helplessness and reactive depressions result from the expectancy that responses and outcomes are independent. Thus, gaining a sense of control would serve as an important part of treatment for depression.

Although the expectancy of future response–outcome independence served as a helpful stimulant for research on the cognitive predictors of depression in humans, there were several flaws with this original learned helplessness conceptualization of depression. First, just as not every dog became helpless after uncontrollable shock, not every human becomes depressed after experiencing stressful events with uncontrollable outcomes. Second, the theory could not distinguish between a depressed person feeling that he or she personally could not effect outcomes and the feeling that the response–outcome independence was true universally.

Abramson, Seligman, and Teasdale therefore offered a reformulated learned helplessness model of depression in their 1978 paper. This cognitively oriented reformulation centered on the notion that, when a life stressor takes place, people do not simply notice the contingencies involved. Rather, they ask themselves why the event happened. People tend to have usual ways of answering this question, and this is called their explanatory style. Causes for events generated by people tend to fall along three separate dimensions: (1) people may feel the cause is due to themselves or to other people or luck, (2) they will either attribute the cause to factors that are stable in time or temporary, and (3) the cause may affect many life domains or just the ones involved most specifically with the stressor. The theory follows a diathesis-stress model of depression onset – it claims that people who have a pessimistic explanatory style, in which negative events are explained with internal, stable, and global causes, will be especially vulnerable to depression when faced with uncontrollable life stressors.

There has been a large amount of empirical support for this model, using both questionnaires (primarily the Attributional Style Questionnaire) and content analysis of verbatim data and a wide range of experimental methodologies. A usual study followed a population prospectively over time to determine whether pessimists were more likely to get depressed after experiencing negative life events. In one series of studies, pessimistic college students experienced the most enduring depressive symptoms after doing poorly on a midterm. A meta-analysis supported the conclusion that a pessimistic explanatory style relates to depression, especially with regard to explanations for negative events. However, the vast majority of studies used either college students or adult psychiatric patients; there is some indication that the relationship between pessimism and depression may be slightly different in older adults. Nonetheless, prevention programs based on teaching pessimistic children and college students to dispute their automatic pessimistic thoughts and to become more realistically optimistic have produced lower rates of significant depressive symptoms in participants at high risk for depression. In addition, there is some evidence that successful cognitive-behavioral psychotherapy can cause a shift in explanatory style such that clients become more optimistic.

Post Traumatic Stress Disorder

Despite the reformulated learned helplessness model's prominence in research on cognitive approaches to human depression, it is the original learned helplessness model that has primarily (although not exclusively) influenced research on PTSD in humans. The behaviors that follow inescapable shock in animals appear to mimic many of the symptoms of PTSD in humans. As already noted, animals exposed to inescapable shock show cognitive, motivational, and emotional deficits. Similarly, humans exposed to traumatic stressors may show a variety of sequelae, including anxiety and hyperreactivity, isolation, and anhedonia, that are similar to the sequelae observed in helpless animals. After inescapable shock, animals experience a depletion of catecholamine in their central nervous system. Van der Kolk and his colleagues posit that catecholamine depletion, especially norepinephrine (NE) depletion, is also involved in the negative symptomatology of PTSD, such as lack of motivation. They also posit that an augmentation of locus coeruleus pathways causes intrusive PTSD symptoms, such as nightmares and flashbacks.

More important to van der Kolk and his colleagues' work is the analgesia response observed in helpless animals, such that they do not appear to experience pain in response to subsequent stressors presented within a short period of time after the administration of inescapable shock. This response is due to endogenous opioids in the body. Interestingly, there are many parallels between the symptoms of opiate withdrawal and PTSD, leading van der Kolk and colleagues (1985: 320) to hypothesize that "both are, at least in part, due to central noradrenergic hyperactivity associated with a relative decrease in brain opioid receptor binding." This hypothesis is supported by evidence that trauma survivors often put themselves in situations similar to the traumatic event, perhaps in an attempt to evoke endogenous opioid release and thus a sense of calm and control. However, this sense of calm is followed by symptoms of opiate withdrawal, such as hyperreactivity, thus immersing PTSD sufferers in a cycle of reexposure and withdrawal.

Other research on helpless animals finds that the NE depletion may be the outcome of a more immediate increase in NE when a helpless animal is exposed to a mild stressor. The hippocampus of the helpless animal appears to be conditioned by the inescapable, helplessness-inducing trauma to respond with increased NE to later lesser stressors. This increase in NE secretion immediately after later stressors could be part of the same general catecholamine dysregulation following traumatic stress as the NE depletion reported by van der Kolk.

In addition to the neurochemical and behavioral evidence for a learned helplessness approach to PTSD based on uncontrollable stress, evidence also exists supporting a relationship between helpless explanatory style and PSTD symptoms. McCormick and colleagues studied explanatory style among patients addicted to alcohol and/or gambling and found that patients with PTSD had a more pessimistic explanatory style than those who did not have PTSD. Although correlational, these results suggest that the cognitive reformulation of learned helplessness may also contribute to an understanding of the phenomenology of and potential treatments for PTSD. Moreover, recent work suggests that learning experiences can immunize animals against becoming helpless in the face of stress and that posttrauma therapeutic interventions centered on learning to predict and control stressors can be helpful in the treatment of PTSD in humans. This work suggests that the learned helplessness framework may be useful for both prevention and treatment of stress-related psychological disorders.

See Also the Following Articles

Cytokines, Stress, and Depression; Depression Models.

Further Reading

Abramson, L. Y., Seligman, M. E. P. and Teasdale, J. D. (1978). Learned helplessness: critique and reformulation. *Journal of Abnormal Psychology* **87**, 49–74.

Hiroto, D. S. (1974). Locus of control and learned helplessness. *Journal of Experimental Psychology* **102**, 187–193.

Isaacowitz, D. M. and Seligman, M. E. P. (2001). Is pessimistic explanatory style a risk factor for depressive mood among community-dwelling older adults? *Behaviour Research and Therapy* **39**, 255–272.

Maier, S. F. and Seligman, M. E. P. (1976). Learned helplessness: theory and evidence. *Journal of Experimental Psychology: General* **105**, 3–46.

Miller, W. R. and Seligman, M. E. P. (1975). Depression and learned helplessness in man. *Journal of Abnormal Psychology* **84**, 228–238.

Overmier, J. B. and Murison, R. (2005). Trauma and resulting sensitization effects are modulated by psychological factors. *Psychoneuroendocrinology* **30**, 965–973.

Peterson, C. and Bossio, L. M. (1991). *Health and optimism*. New York: Free Press.

Seligman, M. E. P. (1975). *Helplessness*. San Francisco: W. H. Freeman & Company.

Seligman, M. E. P. (1990). *Learned optimism*. New York: Pocket Books.

Seligman, M. E. P. and Maier, S. F. (1967). Failure to escape traumatic shock. *Journal of Experimental Psychology* **74**, 1–9.

Sweeney, P. D., Anderson, K. and Bailey, S. (1986). Attributional style in depression: a meta-analytic review. *Journal of Personality & Social Psychology* **50**, 974–991.

Van der Kolk, B., Greenberg, M., Boyd, H., et al. (1985). Inescapable shock, neurotransmitters, and addiction to trauma: toward a psychobiology of post-traumatic stress disorder. *Biological Psychiatry* **20**, 314–325.

Learning and Memory, Effects of Stress on

M Lindau
Uppsala University, Uppsala, Sweden
O Almkvist
Karolinska Institutet and University of Stockholm, Stockholm, Sweden
A H Mohammed
Karolinska Institutet, Stockholm, and Växjö University, Växjö, Sweden

This article is a revision of the previous edition article by M Lindau, O Almkvist, and A H Mohammed, volume 2, pp 603–609, © 2000, Elsevier Inc.

Introduction

Effects of Stress on Learning and Memory in Animals

Memory, Learning, and Their Anatomical Bases in Humans

Encoding in Stressful Situations

Effects of Anticipated Stress on Memory

Possible Mechanisms of the Relation between Stress and Memory

Summary

Glossary

Stressor	Stimuli that puts an extra demand on the organism.
Stress hormones	Hormones of the adrenal glands that serve to maintain bodily homeostatis in response to challenging external and emotional environment. These hormones are the glucocorticoids and epinephrine.
Corticosterone	A steroid hormone in many species including rodents produced by the adrenal cortex and involved in response to stress and immune reaction.
Cortisol	A steroid hormone in humans produced by adrenal cortex, involved in response to stress and has direct influence on the nervous system.
Hippocampus	A region of the cerebral cortex lying in the basal medial part of the temporal lobe thought to be important for learning and memory.
Amygdala	A group of nuclei involved in the medial anterior part of the temporal lobe regulating emotion and certain types of learning.
Emotion	Mental state of arousal.
Memory	Encoding of information, storage and recall.
Learning	A relatively permanent change in cognition as a consequence of the acquisition of new information and experience, directly influencing behaviour.

Introduction

Conceptually, the term stress describes a load on the organism. A stressful situation puts extra demands upon the system for cognitive or physical productivity. A stressor, which might be external or internal, can be anything that puts extra demands upon the system, such as a specific problem, issue, challenge, or personal conflict. A stress reaction is the individual's response to a given stressor on the physiological, cognitive, and/or emotional plane. Strain occurs when the organism is overloaded, exposed to prolonged stress, or placed in situations that the system can not cope with. The psychological consequence of strain is fatigue or exhaustion. Traumatic, salient memories that the individual would like to forget but can not may result in a neurotic fixation on the memories of the trauma, i.e., posttraumatic stress disorder (PTSD).

Physiologically, stress might be defined as a state of physiological and emotional arousal of the organism. It leads to the activation of the autonomic nervous system and the hypothalamic-pituitary-adrenal axis. The main signaling hormones of these systems are (nor)adrenaline, corticotropin-releasing hormone, and cortisol (corticosterone in most rodents).

It is generally accepted that stress affects learning and memory processes and that stress might improve as well as impair the acquirement of information. How is this possible? One answer to this question is that there are at least three types of stressors, physical, cognitive, and emotional, which affect different regions of the brain. Another answer lies in the progress that has been made in the knowledge of the effects of stress on the different stages of learning and memory processing.

Although the mnemonic system in animals is considerably more restricted than that in humans, much complementary knowledge about the effects of stress on learning and memory in humans has been gained through animal studies. The following section gives an account of some of the basic research about this topic in animals.

Effects of Stress on Learning and Memory in Animals

Animals learn about the relationship or association between two events. In classical conditioning, the animal learns to associate a stimulus such as a tone (conditioned stimulus) with food (unconditioned stimulus). In operant or instrumental conditioning, the animal learns to associate a response, for instance, pressing a lever (instrumental response), with food reward (reinforcement). It has been suggested by some researchers (e.g., Anthony Dickinson) that associative learning mechanisms have been shaped by evolution to enable animals to detect and store information about real causal relationships in their environment.

Stress Hormones and Learning

The impact of stress hormones in modulating associative learning and cognitive function in animals has been a subject of continued investigation. The studies that have documented the relationship of levels of the stress hormones with cognitive function, such as attention, perception, and memory, have been done mostly in rodents, in which investigators have examined the influence of stress hormones on acquisition, consolidation, and retrieval of information. Glucocorticoids are the stress hormones secreted by the adrenal glands in animals. In primates and dogs, the naturally occurring glucocorticoid is cortisol, whereas in rodents and birds it is corticosterone.

Fluctuations in corticosterone levels can be said to reflect emotional states related to stress. In experimental animals, changes in hormonal levels can be achieved by pharmacological means or environmental manipulations and their effects assessed. Several studies have shown that stress and glucocorticoids influence cognitive function.

The administration of low levels of corticosterone improves performance in learning tasks in animals. However, whereas short-term exposure to low levels of corticosterone can enhance cognitive function, it is known that short-term exposure to higher levels as well as long-term effects of high levels of corticosterone (e.g., through sustained exposure to restraint stress) have deleterious effects on learning, memory, and cognitive function. The biphasic effects of corticosterone on memory formation have been demonstrated in behavioral studies performed in chicks and rats.

Young chicks have a tendency to peck spontaneously at small salient objects in the environment. This natural behavior of chicks has been exploited to study learning. Chicks will peck spontaneously at bright beads, and if the bead is dipped in a distasteful substance, the chicks will peck once at the bead and show a strong disgust response. Subsequently, they will avoid pecking a similar but dry bead and learn this avoidance behavior. The strong emotional fear component involved in this passive avoidance response in chicks prompted Sandi and Rose to explore the role of stress hormones in learning in the chick. In tests of passive avoidance learning in the chick, they found that an inverted U-shaped curve emerged, in which low levels (0.1 μg) and higher levels (2 μg) of corticosterone were without effect, whereas an intermediate dose (1 μg) improved learning. Similarly, in rodents, an inverted U shape is seen between the dose of administration of corticosterone and performance in learning tasks. It has thus been seen that low doses of corticosterone can improve learning, whereas continuous exposure to glucocorticoids results in neuronal death in the hippocampus and in impaired learning ability. Aged rats that are impaired in cognitive function have elevated levels of corticosterone and increased hippocampal neuronal loss when they are compared with aged rats that are not impaired in cognitive function.

The effects of corticosterone on cognitive function are mediated through binding of the stress hormones to specific receptors in the brain. These receptors, known as glucocorticoid receptors, have been found to be abundant in the hippocampus, a brain region that is critically involved in modulating learning and memory. Another region in the brain that participates in cognitive function is the amygdala, which also has moderate amounts of receptors for corticosterone. The actions of corticosterone in the hippocampus and amygdala can be induced by the administration of selective drugs that interact with the glucocorticoid receptors. Drugs include those that enhance the effects of corticosterone (glucocorticoid agonists) or those that block or attenuate the effect of corticosterone (glucocorticoid antagonists). These drugs have provided powerful tools in dissecting the role of stress hormones in the hippocampus and amygdala in modulating cognitive functions in rodents. Pharmacological or environmental manipulation of the glucocorticoid receptors influences cognitive function in rats.

Hippocampus and Learning in Animals

Considerable evidence shows that the hippocampus mediates spatial learning in rodents. Spatial learning in rodents can be examined by the use of a water maze, known as the Morris maze. The procedure involves placing an experimental animal in a large pool of water of about 1.5 m in diameter. The animal has to use spatial cues in the experimental room to locate an invisible escape platform that is hidden 2 cm below the surface of the opaque water. After a few days of testing, the animals learn to locate the platform within seconds. It has been demonstrated that rats perform poorly in this test if hippocampal function is impaired. Thus, aged rats with pathological changes in the hippocampus show impaired spatial learning in the water maze compared to aged rats that do not show pathological hippocampal changes. Aged rats that had been exposed to repeated restraint stress have a reduction in glucocorticoid receptors in the hippocampus. This results in, among other things, an impaired spatial learning ability. In contrast, animals that have higher levels of glucocorticoid receptors in the hippocampus show an increased ability for spatial learning. Administration of a glucocorticoid receptor antagonist in the brain appears to impair information processing during spatial learning.

To sum up, spatial memory in animals is dependent on hippocampal function. Through their action in the hippocampus, stress hormones facilitate spatial information processing so that low levels of corticosterone improve learning, whereas higher levels impair performance.

Amygdala and Learning in Animals

Many studies have concentrated on the effects that stress hormones have on the hippocampus and its relationship to learning. Work by James McGaugh and colleagues has begun to explore the role of stress hormone receptors in the amygdala on learning. The amygdala is a region of the brain that plays a crucial role in acquisition and expression of fear responses. This brain region is thought to influence memory storage processes in other brain regions, such as the hippocampus and cortex. An interaction of stress hormones and amygdala nuclei appears to be important in modulating memory consolidation for emotional events. Binding of glucocorticoid receptors in the basolateral nucleus is known to affect memory storage. It was found that administration of the glucocorticoid receptor agonist in this area immediately after training enhanced retention of a passive avoidance response. Many studies have examined the effects of glucocorticoids on the acquisition of newly acquired information. In a test of memory retrieval of long-term spatial learning memory, it was found that stress caused impaired performance, and this impairment could be related to circulating levels of corticosterone. These findings point to a critical involvement of the amygdala in regulating stress hormone effects on learning and memory.

To conclude, the amygdala is a region of the brain known to be importantly involved in emotions. Stress hormones can affect the memory storage of emotional events by their actions on the amygdala. The impact of stress on the hippocampus and amygdala is highlighted by emerging evidence from animal studies that revealed that stress causes changes in hippocampal plasticity and can thus modify the information storage mechanism in the hippocampus and that the amygdala is involved in the emergence of stress-associated changes in the hippocampus.

Summary

Stress hormones have biphasic effects on learning and memory in animals. Low levels of stress hormones improve performance, whereas higher levels have a deleterious effect on learning. Two brain regions important in regulating learning and memory are the hippocampus and amygdala, which contain receptors for stress hormones. The effects of stress hormones on learning are mediated by these receptors in the hippocampus and amygdala. Research in rodents has revealed that emotional arousal regulates learning through the action of stress hormones, which activate receptors in the hippocampus and amygdala to affect memory formation.

Memory, Learning, and Their Anatomical Bases in Humans

Conceptualization of Learning and Memory

The contemporary conceptual frameworks of learning and memory emanate from experimental psychology. According to this model, human memory is not a unitary system, but is composed of a series of interdependent brain systems characterized by different features in terms of time for the registration of new information (immediate/extended in time), type of information (implicit/declarative or explicit), accessibility (immediate/search), amount of information stored (limited/unlimited), spontaneous duration of information in memory (limited/unlimited), and awareness of information (yes/no). These distinct memory systems appear to be subserved by separate neural networks, as shown by brain behavior studies and prior studies demonstrating specific effects on memory due to lesions in the brain.

One major division of memory is that between implicit or nondeclarative memory and declarative (explicit) memory. Nondeclarative memory includes procedural memory, classical conditioning, the perceptual representation system, and priming. In line with phylogenesis and ontogenesis, one early type is procedural memory, which is expressed as skilled behavior or motor procedures, which appear to be subserved by regions in the basal ganglia. One division of procedural memory is classical conditioning, which is the same as a stimulus–response connection. The hippocampus and certain parts of the cerebral cortex have been identified as important areas for this memory system. Another type of implicit memory is the perceptual representation system, which is concerned primarily with the acquisition and use of perceptual objects of the world. The predominantly responsible brain areas are the primary association cortices. Another branch of implicit memory is priming, which refers to an unconscious ability to process a stimulus due to prior exposure. Declarative memory can be described as the conscious recollection of facts and events (Krystal et al., 1995). To this memory system belongs short-term memory or working memory, semantic memory, and verbal as well as visuospatial episodic memory. Short-term or working memory processes and stores temporarily a very limited amount of information. Semantic memory covers acquisition and use of factual knowledge about the world and is mapped by association areas in the brain. Information unique in time, location, and person is involved in storage and recall of information from episodic memory, for which the medial temporal lobes are one crucial point of the subserving neural networks. Another important aspect of memory is learning. Some authors equate long-term storage with learning, for example, calling it the process by which information that may be needed again is stored for recall on demand (Peterson, 1967). A broader definition is that learning is the same as the modification of behavior according to earlier experiences.

The Anatomy of Human Memory

The hippocampus thus plays an important role in several of the subdivisions of the two main memory systems. In the hippocampus, stimuli from the external world are classified and stored, momentarily in short-term memory and for longer periods of time in long-term memory, and the spatial and temporal dimensions of the experiences are recorded. It is doubtful, however, that the hippocampus is responsible for the more permanent consolidation of memories. Adjacent to the hippocampal system is the amygdala, which plays an important role in the processing of emotional information in the brain. The amygdala consists of several distinct nuclei, whose functional properties vary. The basolateral amygdaloid complex appears to be the nucleus that is involved most crucially in memory performance. However, it is not critical for the consolidation of a memory trace per se. Instead, it has been suggested that the amygdala assigns emotional meaning to incoming free-floating feelings, integrates this emotionally meaningful information with associated emotional memories, and, through projections to the hypothalamus, hippocampus, and basal forebrain, directs emotional behavior. The amygdala also contributes to the enhancement of a memory trace that is related to emotional responses such as stress.

The frontotemporal area is the center for the executive function, short-term memory, and personality. This area of the brain has an elaborate network of connections to most other regions of the brain and a high concentration of stress hormone receptors, which has been found to assure the role of the frontal lobes in stress, learning and memory.

Vulnerability of Human Memory

The current conceptualization of human memory posits that the order of memory acquisition during ontogenesis, as described earlier, is reversed when the brain is exposed to various adverse influences such as aging, toxins, inflammatory agents, and stress. The meaning of this is that more sophisticated memory systems, such as declarative memory, are hit at an early stage, whereas more basic and ontogenetically earlier systems, such as procedural memory, are afflicted later on. Of course, the reversed order of degradation does not hold when there is a highly localized attack on the brain, as is the case for brain trauma. However, it is well known that episodic memory is highly sensitive for aging as well as for disease processes such as Alzheimer's disease. The next section describes changes that take place in relation to memory performance when humans are exposed to stress.

Encoding in Stressful Situations

Encoding is closely connected with attention and vigilance, which both influence the encoding of information into declarative as well as nondeclarative memory. Attention, like vigilance, is highly sensitive to stress. To be able to encode an all-embracing picture of an event, it is necessary that attention be unrestricted. During a stressful situation the attentional span tends to be narrowed to the most salient stimuli in the situation, whereas more peripheral stimuli are neglected. It has also been suggested that the hippocampus seems to shut down under severe stress, which may contribute to an incomplete encoding of the stressful situation. It has been demonstrated experimentally that people who have been exposed to pictures of a bloody car accident tend to remember central trauma-related items better than more peripheral details. This laboratory finding is related to a real-world phenomenon called weapon focusing. Witnesses to crimes committed with visible weapons have sharper memories of the weapon than of other aspects of the situation, including the face of the perpetrator, for which the memories are more diffuse. The explanation for this is that the gun is the carrier of the most emotionally salient information and therefore captures the attention at the expense of other aspects. This phenomenon has been found to be particularly pronounced in people reacting with anxiety at the sight of weapons.

Short-term memory, which demands that information be held in consciousness momentarily, has been found to be extra sensitive to stress because the situation demands a focus on stress-relevant stimuli and therefore attention tends to be biased. On the contrary, overlearned abilities, such as procedural memory, for which the memory traces are well consolidated, are found to be more stress resistant than recently acquired memories, which are destroyed more easily. In a laboratory test of declarative memory, spatial thinking, and procedural memory tested with a word stem priming task, high levels of cortisol impaired declarative memory and spatial thinking, whereas procedural memory was spared.

One reason why overlearned skills are more difficult to erase is that repetition contributes to a better memory. Thus, it appears that more recently registered material in long-term storage and short-term memory is more sensitive to stress.

Effects of Anticipated Stress on Memory

It is not always being in the stressful situation that causes emotional arousal; the anticipation of the incoming stressor may have the same effect. In an experiment by Lupien and colleagues, a group of 14 healthy elderly persons was given a nonstressful task and a stressful task. The nonstressful condition consisted of a computer task. The stressful condition consisted of a videotaped public-speaking task, for which the discourse was said to be evaluated by experts. Before and after each condition subjects were given a declarative memory task and a nondeclarative word completion task. Results showed that in the responders (individuals who react to stress with an increase in cortisol levels), high levels of cortisol were secreted long before the stressful condition, which was not the case in the nonresponders (no change in cortisol level due to stress). This signifies that the anticipation of the incoming stressor played a more important role in the secretion of cortisol than the actual stressor. The responders also

performed worse on the declarative memory task than the nonresponders, indicating that even the anticipation of stress has a detrimental effect on declarative memory. Nondeclarative memory was spared. The stress did not affect the nondeclarative memory significantly, either in the whole group or in the subgroups.

One concluding remark about the effects of stress on learning and memory is that stress seems to influence the modulation of memories through its effects on attention and vigilance during the encoding of information. This may be true both for being in a stressful situation and for anticipating of a fear-provoking event. Knowledge about the biological and psychological mechanisms behind the effects of stress on attention and memory storage may help individuals gain control over these processes in order to perhaps make use of the positive effects of stress on memory and learning and avoid the negative.

Possible Mechanisms of the Relation between Stress and Memory

It is possible to differentiate among physiological, cognitive, and emotional stress, which sometimes may partly overlap. These types of stress might be analyzed from two angles: context and time, and whether the stress is good or bad for learning and memory. Two types of learning that are enhanced by stress are classical fear and eyeblink conditioning, as well as processes related to learning about threatening stimuli. In the standard paradigm of eyeblink conditioning, the Pavlovian eyeblink conditioning, a human is exposed to an air puff to the eye, which evokes an involuntary eyeblink reflex as an unconditioned response (UR). When the air puff is directly preceded by a sound as the conditioned stimulus (CS), the human learns the association between the tone and the air puff and blinks in response to the tone, thus anticipating the air puff. The blink is the conditioned response (CR) and is an example of associative learning. Here we are dealing with a physiological stressful event that generates, not disturbs, new associative learning. Physical stressors are generally said to activate lower brain regions involved in, e.g., pain responses, whereas psychological stressors engage the limbic structures.

Concerning the effects of stress on cognition, particularly learning and memory, one of the greatest challenges for neuropsychological research today is to determine the effects of stress on the different stages of the memory process. It is suggested that stress has differential effects on distinct phases of the learning and memory processes. Consolidation of information is found to be enhanced by stress if the stress occurs concomitantly in time and in the same context as the thing to be remembered. The recall of information is impaired, however, if the system is exposed to stress shortly before the retrieval of information. One illustrative example of these conjunctions is given by Joëls et al. People passing a stressful examination may have difficulties in recalling the earlier learned, required information (impaired retrieval), but at the same time the traumatic experience of not remembering is burned deeply into their memories (enhanced consolidation). Retrieval difficulties have been interpreted as a negative consequence of the release of corticosteroid hormones. Inversely, the release of corticosteroid hormones facilitate new learning, which tends to compete with or overwrite the earlier acquired information. The competition between the access to earlier information and current challenges has been conceived as a kind of fruitful adaptation, since knowledge about new threats (i.e., risk of failure on the examination) may enhance the chances of future survival, in this context a better preparation for the next examination.

These findings are congruent with results showing that exposition for a psychological stressor preserves or enhances the memory for the emotional aspect of an event, while it simultaneously disrupts the memory for non-emotional or neutral aspects of the same event. This pattern may be explained by the fact that emotional and non-emotional memories are modulated by different structures of the brain. Encoding and retrieval of emotional memories are associated with the amygdala, whereas the encoding and retrieval of non-emotional memories are associated with the hippocampal formation. This pattern might also explain the gaps in memory and general memory impairment seen in patients suffering from traumatic memories.

Summary

Stress refers to an extra load on the organism. Neuroendocrinologically, stress reactions are characterized by the release of the stress hormones corticosterone in animals and cortisol in humans. Normally, increasing demands lead to increasing performance. However, this relationship holds up to a certain optimal level; thereafter, increasing demands lead to decreasing performance. This appears to be true for animal as well as human behavior in the domain of learning and memory. The mnemonic process in animals is characterized by associations between a few or several elements. Memory and learning in humans are more complex and may be

analyzed in two main systems: declarative and nondeclarative memory. In animals as well as in humans, the same cerebral structures have been identified as crucial in the mnemonic process: the hippocampus and the amygdala. The hippocampus is critical for learning and memory, whereas the amygdala is responsible for the transmission of emotional information during the mnemonic process. Stress hormone receptors in the hippocampus and amygdala make these cerebral structures responsive to stress. The frontal lobes are also involved in the memory process, through the region's accumulation of stress hormone receptors and rich connections to other parts of the brain. It is possible to differentiate among physiological, cognitive, and emotional stress, which might be analyzed from a time and context perspective and with respect to whether they are gold or bad for memory. Generally, declarative memory is more sensitive to stress than nondeclarative memory. Stress has different effects on the declarative memory depending on which phase in the memory process that it occurs.

See Also the Following Articles

Amygdala; Cognition and Stress; Hippocampus, Overview; Memory and Stress; Memory Impairment.

Further Reading

de Quervain, D. J., Roozendaal, B. and McGaugh, J. L. (1998). Stress and glucocorticoids impair retrieval of long-term spatial memory. *Nature* **394**, 787–790.

Joëls, M., et al. (2006). Learning under stress: how does it work? *Trends in Cognitive Science* **10**, 153–158.

Kim, J. J., Song, E. U. and Kosten, T. A. (2006). Stress effects in the hippocampus: synaptic plasticity and memory. *Stress* **9**, 1–11.

Krystal, J. H., et al. (1995). Toward a cognitive neuroscience of dissociation and altered memory functions in posttraumatic stress disorder. In: Friedman, M. J., Charney, D. S. & Deutch, A. Y. (eds.) *Neurobiological and clinical consequences of stress*, p. 249. Philadelphia, PA: Lippincott-Raven.

Lazarus, R. S. and Folkman, S. (1986). Cognitive theories of stress and the issue of circularity. In: Appley, M. H. & Trumbull, R. (eds.) *Dynamics of stress*, p. 63. New York: Plenum.

McEwen, B. S. and Sapolsky, R. M. (1995). Stress and cognitive function. *Current Opinion in Neurobiology* **5**, 205–216.

Payne, J. D., et al. (2006). The impact of stress on neutral and emotional aspects of episodic memory. *Memory* **14**, 1–16.

Peterson, L. R. (1967). Short-term memory. In: McGaugh, J. L., Weinberger, N. M. & Whalen, R. E. (eds.) *Psychobiology: readings from Scientific American*, pp. 141. San Francisco, CA: Freeman.

Pryce, C., Mohammed, A. H. and Feldon, J. (eds.) (2002). Environmental manipulations in rodents and primates: insights into pharmacology, biochemistry and behaviour. *Pharmacological and Biochemical Behavior* **73**, Special Issue.

Sandi, C. and Rose, S. P. (1994). Corticosterone enhances long-term retention in one-day-old chicks trained in a weak passive avoidance learning paradigm. *Brain Research* **647**, 106–112.

Shalev, A. Y. (1996). Stress versus traumatic stress. In: van der Kolh, B. A., McFarlane, A. C. & Weisaeth, L. (eds.) *Traumatic stress*, pp. 93. New York: Guildford Press.

Shors, T. J. (2006). Stressful experience and learning across the lifespan. *Annual Review of Psychology* **57**, 55–85.

Yerkes, R. M. and Dodson, J. D. (1908). The relation of strength of stimulus to rapidity of habit-formation. *Journal of Computational and Neurological Psychology* **18**, 459–482.

Lebanon, Studies of Stress in *See:* Combat, Acute Reactions to; Combat Reaction, Chronic; Korean Conflict, Stress Effects of; Posttraumatic Stress Disorder – Clinical; Posttraumatic Stress Disorder Overview; Traumatic Stress and Posttraumatic Stress Disorder, the Israeli Experience; War-Related Posttraumatic Stress Disorder, Treatment of.

Left Ventricular Mass

T G Pickering
New York Presbyterian Hospital, New York, USA

This article is reproduced from the previous edition, volume 2, pp 610–611, © 2000, Elsevier Inc.

Glossary

Echo-cardiography	A noninvasive technique for visualizing the structure and function of the heart using ultrasound. In its simplest form, a single beam (m mode) of ultrasound is aimed at the heart from a transducer placed on the chest wall, and reflections are detected from the cardiac structures hit by the beam. Two-dimensional echocardiography uses an array of beams that give a two-dimensional picture of the heart. Because traces can be recorded over several cardiac cycles, it is possible to gain information about the function of the heart as well as its structure.
Left ventricular hypertrophy	A left ventricular mass index that is above the upper limit of normal for the individual's gender and body size.
Left ventricular mass	Mass of the muscle of the left ventricle of the heart, calculated from echocardiographic measurements of the size of the chamber of the ventricle and the thickness of its walls. The size of the ventricle normally varies with the size of the

person, so for comparative purposes it is customary to normalize left ventricular mass to body surface area, as the left ventricular mass index.

Left ventricular (LV) mass is the weight of the left ventricle, typically estimated using echocardiography, and is thought to represent the cumulative effect of blood pressure on the heart. It is normally closely related to body size and is greater in men than in women. It also increases with age. It correlates more closely with blood pressure measured over prolonged periods of time (e.g., over several years in the Framingham heart study or by 24-h blood pressure monitoring) than with routine office measurements, but this correlation does not exceed 0.5, so that only 25% of the variance of LV mass can be explained by the blood pressure level. LV hypertrophy (defined as an LV mass that exceeds the normal range) is seen in about 30% of people with hypertension and is more common in older and more obese patients. The importance of LV mass also lies in the fact that it is an independent risk factor for cardiovascular morbidity; in fact, no other biological variable apart from age predicts cardiac risk better than LV hypertrophy. This may be partly because it represents a superior measure of the effects of increased blood pressure on the circulation, but it may also have direct pathological significance. Thus a high LV mass is associated with a decreased coronary flow reserve (i.e., the heart outgrows its blood supply) and it also makes the heart more susceptible to arrhythmias. Treatment of hypertension with either drugs or lifestyle measures (e.g., weight reduction) can reduce LV mass, and there is some evidence that the regression of LV hypertrophy is associated with an improved survival.

LV mass is usually measured by echocardiography, which is considered to be the gold standard. This is a noninvasive ultrasound test performed by holding an ultrasonic probe on the chest wall, which emits a single beam (m mode) or a two-dimensional array of beams, and detects the reflected beams from the tissues of the heart. Magnetic resonance imaging also enables visualization of the heart and may give an even more accurate assessment, but is also much more expensive.

While blood pressure is one of the major determinants of LV mass, there are others that may be of equal significance. Twin studies have shown that there is a genetic component, which may be linked closely to the genetic regulation of body weight. LV mass is related to salt intake, and the activity of the sympathetic nervous system and renin–angiotensin systems may also increase it; in healthy young adults, plasma angiotensin II is one of the determinants of LV mass. Like 24-h ambulatory blood pressure, measures of LV geometry, including LV mass and wall thickness, have provided important information about the significance of behavioral factors relating to heart disease due to hypertension. Studies have shown that occupational stress (measured as job strain) in men is associated not only with hypertension, but also with increased LV mass. The propensity to show exaggerated blood pressure responses to stress may also be associated with greater LV mass in African-American and white adolescents and adults. What remains uncertain is the causal relationship between these observations: (1) it could be that the increased LV mass is associated with structural changes in the arteries, which are responsible for the increased reactivity; (2) the left ventricle could produce an exaggerated response leading to the increased reactivity; or (3) the increased reactivity could be the cause of the increased LV mass. For the same level of clinic blood pressure, African-Americans have a greater LV mass than white people. The reason for this is unknown, but one contributory factor could be the comparatively higher nocturnal blood pressure in black people.

See Also the Following Articles

Blood Pressure; Cardiovascular System and Stress; Heart Disease/Attack.

Further Reading

Allen, M. T., Matthews, K. A. and Sherman, F. S. (1997). Cardiovascular reactivity to stress and left ventricular mass in youth. *Hypertension* **30**, 782–787.

de Simone, G., Ganau, A., Verdecchia, P., et al. (1994). Echocardiography in arterial hypertension: when, why and how? *Journal of Hypertension* **12**, 1129–1136.

Esler, M. (1996). The relation of human cardiac sympathetic nervous activity to left ventricular mass: commentary. *Journal of Hypertension* **14**, 1365–1367.

Harrap, S. B., Dominiczak, A. F., Fraser, R., et al. (1996). Plasma angiotensin II, predisposition to hypertension, and left ventricular size in healthy young adults. *Circulation* **93**, 1148–1154.

Koren, M. J., Devereux, R. B., Casale, P. N., et al. (1991). Relation of left ventricular mass and geometry to morbidity and mortality in uncomplicated essential hypertension. *Annals of Internal Medicine* **114**, 345–352.

Koren, M. J., Mensah, G. A., Blake, J., et al. (1993). Comparison of left ventricular mass and geometry in black and white patients with essential hypertension. *American Journal of Hypertension* **6**, 815–823.

Langenfeld, M. R. and Schmieder, R. E. (1995). Salt and left ventricular hypertrophy: what are the links? *Journal of Human Hypertension* **9**, 909–916.

Levy, D., Garrison, R. J., Savage, D. D., et al. (1990). Prognostic implications of echocardiographically determined left ventricular mass in the Framingham Heart Study. *New England Journal of Medicine* **322**, 1561–1566.

Schnall, P. L., Devereux, R. B., Pickering, T. G., et al. (1992). The relationship between "job strain," workplace diastolic blood pressure, and left ventricular mass index: a correction. *Journal of the American Medical Association* **267**, 1209.

Verhaaren, H. A., Schieken, R. M., Mosteller, M., et al. (1991). Bivariate genetic analysis of left ventricular mass and weight in pubertal twins (the Medical College of Virginia twin study). *American Journal of Cardiology* **68**, 661–668.

Leishmania, Stress Response in

M Shapira
The Ben Gurion University of the Negev,
Beer Sheva, Israel

This article is a revision of the previous edition article by
M Shapira, volume 2, pp 612–617, © 2000, Elsevier Inc.

Glossary

Amastigote	The life stage that resides within mammalian hosts, mostly in macrophages. An obligatory intracellular form.
Cutaneous leishmaniasis	A form of leishmaniasis that produces skin lesions, usually self-healing (*L. major*, *L. amazonensis*).
Leishmania	A protozoan parasite that belongs to the Kinetoplastida order. The parasites cycle between sand fly vectors and mammalian hosts, causing a wide range of clinical manifestations.
Metacyclic form	The infective life stage that resides in the sand fly vector, mainly in the proboscis.
Mucocutaneous leishmaniasis	A form of leishmaniasis in which the mucosal organs, primarily the nose and mouth, are attacked (*L. braziliensis*, *L. amazonensis*).
Promastigote	The parasite life stage that resides within the intestinal tract of the sandfly vector.
Visceral leishmaniasis	A systemic form of leishmaniasis in which visceral organs, mainly the liver and spleen, serve as targets for infection by parasites. Visceralization occurs in infections by certain species, such as *L. donovani*, *L. infantum*, and *L. ethiopica*. The disease is lethal if left untreated.

Leishmania: The Organism and Its Life Cycle

Leishmania parasites are flagellated diploid protists that belong to the order Kinetoplastida. This order is named after the kinetoplast, a unique organelle that harbors the mitochondrial DNA. Parasites of the genus *Leishmania* are the causative agents of a broad spectrum of human diseases. Different species of *Leishmania* vary in their clinical manifestations, ranging from lesions of the skin and mucosal organs to the lethal visceral form. Drug treatment is available, though toxic, and there is yet no safe vaccine available. *Leishmania* are distributed in large areas of the old and new world, causing both morbidity and mortality.

The parasites lead a digenetic life cycle, migrating between insect vectors and mammalian hosts. They exist as extracellular flagellated promastigotes in the alimentary tract of the sand fly vector. Promastigotes from the midgut of the sand fly are noninfective; however, upon proliferation they differentiate from procyclics into a virulent metacyclic form and migrate to the front part of the intestinal track. During the blood meal of female flies, the parasites are transmitted to the mammalian host, where they become obligatory intracellular amastigotes that reside within the phagolysosome vacuoles in macrophages. At all life stages *Leishmania* encounter hostile environments, which are characterized by high hydrolytic and proteolytic activities. Moreover, the parasites are exposed to growth conditions that differ significantly between vector and host in temperature, pH, nutrients, and serum components. Survival of *Leishmania* is facilitated by mechanisms that allow tolerance to pH and temperature shifts and resistance to complement lysis and to oxidative stress in the macrophage. Transformation includes morphogenesis and changes in metabolism and in enzymatic activities, as well as in the abundance of surface molecules. The adaptation necessary for parasite survival is acquired by alterations in gene expression, which can be modulated by the changing environment. The ability of *Leishmania* parasites to withstand the wide range of unfavorable conditions leads to their high virulence and therefore has been extensively studied.

Axenic Amastigotes: The Stress Response as a Differentiation Trigger

It has been well established that stage transformation of *Leishmania* parasites from promastigotes to amastigotes can be induced axenically upon exposure to elevated temperatures and reduced pH, conditions that mimic the environment in the mammalian host. Thus, in several *Leishmania* species, stage transformation may occur without a requirement for internalization within macrophages or other cells of the immune system. This has been shown for species of the new world, such as *L. amazonensis*, as well as for species that are distributed in the old world, such as *L. donovani*. Titration of the response to a gradual temperature elevation shows that axenic transformation is temperature restricted. It involves the increased synthesis of heat shock proteins; however, above a certain temperature threshold, translation of all other cellular proteins stops completely, preventing proper differentiation. Thus, axenic differentiation is restricted to a narrow range of temperatures, and above a certain threshold the parasites will die rather than transform. The temperature threshold varies for different species: the heat shock response in the visceralizing *L. donovani* parasites occurs at 39°C, whereas in *L. amazonensis*, a cutaneous disease agent, the stress response is induced at 33°C.

A host-free differentiation system for *L. donovani* was used to investigate the initial process of differentiation, by monitoring the induction of additional stage-specific genes. Within 1 h of exposing promastigotes to the differentiation signals that combine temperature elevation (37°C) and exposure to acidic pH (5.5), expression of the amastigote-specific A2 protein family was observed. At 5 h, morphological changes such as elimination of the flagellum and rounding up of the cells were observed, and the process was completed 7 h later. This morphological transformation occurred synchronously, while the cells were arrested at G1. Sequential exposure to elevated temperature (for 24 h) and acidic pH conditions indicated that heat was responsible for the growth arrest and the acidic pH was required for the actual completion of differentiation into amastigotes. Other inducers of the stress response such as ethanol and azetidine-2-carboxylic acid (a synthetic proline analog) were capable of replacing the heat treatment as a differentiation signal.

Expression of heat shock proteins is tightly associated with stage differentiation in *Leishmania*. Although members of the Hsp83 and Hsp70 proteins are abundantly expressed throughout the life cycle, the steady-state level of transcripts encoding these proteins increases in amastigotes, along with their preferential translation. Exposure of *Leishmania* parasites to geldanomycin, a drug that binds the ATPase site of Hsp90 and inactivates it, induces a stress response and triggers the differentiation process from the promastigote to amastigote life stage. In the presence of geldanomycin, expression of amastigote-specific genes such as A2 increases, and the cells transform into aflagellated and rounded amastigote-like cells. This effect of the drug is specific to *Leishmania* and is not observed with *Trypanosoma cruzi*,

for example, suggesting that the differentiation signals may vary between these two kinetoplastids.

As indicated, Hsp90 and Hsp70 are expressed in all life stages, although their regulatory pattern changes in response to the changing environment. However, it has been shown that thermotolerance is associated with Hsp100, which is expressed mainly in the amastigote stage of *Leishmania*. Knock-out mutants depleted from Hsp100 delay the development of skin lesions in infected mice, but did not have an apparent effect on growth of promastigotes. Virulence is partly recovered upon introduction of the missing gene into the knock-out parasite strain. The association of Hsp100 with thermotolerance has been shown for other organisms such as yeast, and it appears that this protein plays a similar role in *Leishmania*.

Gene Regulation in *Leishmania:* Studying Heat Shock Genes as Models

Genome sequencing projects of *L. major*, *T. cruzi* and *T. brucei* have been accomplished, and the sequencing of additional trypanosomatid genomes is currently under way (*L. infantum* and *L. braziliensis*). Protein-coding genes are arranged in huge unidirectional clusters that cover large portions of the chromosomes and are transcribed polycistronically. The mature, monocistronic transcripts are excised by *trans*-splicing and polyadenylation. *Trans*-splicing involves the addition of a short, capped leader to the 5′ end of the RNA, which is donated by an independent RNA molecule, denoted spliced leader RNA (SL RNA). Thus, capping of mRNAs is independent of the transcribing RNA polymerase, as in other eukaryotes.

Adaptation of trypanosomatids to different environments requires a tight control of gene expression. However, as a consequence of polycistronic transcription of protein coding genes, developmental regulation occurs posttranscriptionally by RNA processing, RNA stability, and translation efficiency. This has been established using heat shock genes as a model system, and unlike in most eukaryotes, transcriptional activation of these genes has been completely ruled out in *Leishmania*. The absence of transcriptional activation of protein coding genes fits well with the genomic organization of protein coding genes in *Leishmania* and their polycistronic transcription.

Splicing during Heat Shock

In higher eukaryotes, RNA splicing is disturbed by heat shock. Thus, heat shock genes often lack introns, except for Hsp83 in *Drosophila*. As a result, splicing of the hsp83 RNA is improved if a mild heat shock precedes a more drastic temperature stress.

In *Leishmania*, temperature elevation also affects *trans*-splicing in a stage-specific manner. For example, tubulin expression is altered during the life cycle. In the amastigote stage, the flagellum is adsorbed and the subpellicular microtubules do not reach the tip of the cells, causing them to round up. In accordance, processing intermediates of α-tubulin mRNAs accumulate at elevated temperatures. Counterwise, processing intermediates of Hsp70 can be seen only at 26°C, and not at mammalian like temperatures. This is in agreement with the increased steady-state levels of Hsp70 mRNAs that are observed in amastigotes.

RNA Stability during Heat Shock

Expression of stage-specific genes can be achieved by their differential stability at altered temperatures. Thus, transcripts of promastigote-specific genes are rapidly degraded at elevated temperatures, whereas transcripts encoding for heat shock genes, such as Hsp70 and Hsp90, are differentially stabilized at elevated temperatures. The stability determinants of these transcripts are found in their 3′ untranslated regions (UTRs), although they could not be associated with a specific sequence element. Almost any deletion in the 3′ UTR eliminated the preferential stability of the Hsp83 mRNA at elevated temperatures, suggesting that stabilization was acquired due to a specific RNA structure, which was sensitive to any change in the sequence of the 3′ UTR. Temperature control over RNA stability was observed for other genes that are differentially expressed throughout the life cycle, such as the gene encoding for a promastigote-specific protein kinase A (PKA). The PKA transcript has a much shorter $T_{1/2}$ at mammalian-like temperatures as compared to 26°C, the temperature at which promastigotes are grown. Thus, it is abundant in promastigotes but can hardly be detected in amastigotes. Control of transcript abundance during the life cycle of *Leishmania* by temperature and pH shifts was reported for the amastigote-specific A2 gene and the promastigote-specific surface protease gp63.

Preferential Translation at Elevated Temperatures

Similar to higher eukaryotes, *de novo* synthesis of heat shock genes in *Leishmania* increases dramatically at elevated temperatures, as observed in metabolic labeling experiments that measure directly the nascent incorporation of amino acids into polypeptide chains. This pattern of regulation can be transferred onto a transfected reporter gene, which is flanked by genomic sequences that include the UTRs on both sides of the coding gene, along with adjacent processing signals. Using a series of reporter constructs, it was shown that unlike in other eukaryotes, preferential translation in *Leishmania* is controlled mainly by the 3′ UTR of the Hsp83 gene, whereas the 5′ UTR alone can improve the effect of the 3′ UTR but cannot function alone in directing preferential translation. A similar observation was made for preferential translation of the Hsp70 gene, which is also controlled by the 3′ UTR. Furthermore, two types of 3′ UTR were found for Hsp70 genes, which differ in their ability to promote differential accumulation and translation at elevated temperatures, enabling expression at a broad range of conditions.

Translation regulation that is based on the 3′ UTR varies from what we know for Hsp70 in higher eukaryotes, where preferential translation is directed by the 5′ UTR. Great efforts were invested in understanding the mechanism that promotes and increases translation of heat shock genes at elevated temperatures in higher eukaryotes. Preferential translation cannot be assigned to binding of a specific protein factor to the 5′ UTR, and different reports have suggested potential mechanisms for directing preferential translation. For example, the 5′ UTR of heat shock genes is rich in adenosines and thus has minimal secondary RNA structures. Since heat shock impairs the ability to unwind RNA structures, which are common in 5′ UTRs of non-heat shock genes, only mRNAs with minimal structures can be efficiently translated. Another report showed that the 5′ UTR of Hsp70 contains boxes of sequence complementarity with the 18S rRNA, which may facilitate ribosome shunting, a mechanism by which the 40S ribosomal subunit binds the cap and bypasses large segments of the mRNA to reach the initiation codon. Preferential translation of *Drosophila* Hsp90 is also controlled by the 5′ UTR, but nucleotides close to the first AUG were implicated as essential for preferential translation at elevated temperatures.

In *Leishmania*, the 3′ UTR of the Hsp83 transcript appears to confer preferential translation at elevated temperatures. Deletion analysis mapped the regulatory region that controls translation of Hsp83 in *Leishmania* to sequences 201–472 of the 886-nt-long 3′ UTR. This element is required for preferential translation of a fused reporter gene at elevated temperatures. Interestingly, it functions irrespective of transcript stability. However, the minimal fragment that can induce preferential translation of a reporter gene is larger and requires the presence of the proximal half of the 3′ UTR (nts 1–472). Furthermore, mutations in the 3′ UTR that eliminate the increased stability of the mRNA do not affect their preferential translation at elevated temperatures, as long as the regulatory region is present in the 3′ UTR. The requirement for a relatively large regulatory region supports the possibility that a discrete RNA structure is required for promoting preferential translation during heat shock. However, to date, no specific proteins that bind to this region have been identified, and it is not clear how this 3′ UTR element functions.

Another 3′ UTR control element sized 450 nts directs preferential translation of amastigote-specific genes and appears to be conserved between the 3′ UTR of amastin and Hsp100 of *Leishmania*. The large size of this control region may also support a potential involvement of a specific RNA structure in regulating translation of amastigote-specific genes at elevated temperatures and acidic pH. RNA structure is known to be temperature sensitive and can even serve as a thermosensor molecule in prokaryotes, as well as in eukaryote organisms.

Heat Shock and Cell Death in *Leishmania*

Environmental stress conditions may cause multiple cell damages that include protein misfolding. Heat shock proteins can function as dedicated molecular chaperones in assisting the unfolding of damaged proteins and their proper refolding during recovery from stress. However, when repair is beyond reach, cells must be eliminated. Thus, events that are triggered by cell stress are closely associated with the decision process that targets a cell for its death. Programmed cell death (PCD) is a process that prevails in multicellular organisms, but an increasing number of reports indicate that single-celled organisms can die following a process that partly resembles PCD. Several apoptotic-like processes have been described in *Leishmania*; however, the issue of apoptotic death in this parasite is still controversial. Apparently, exposure of *Leishmania* to extreme conditions triggers stage differentiation rather than cell death. Despite their resistance to a broad range of environmental conditions, it is possible that upon passing a certain threshold, a PCD-like process will be induced. Preliminary reports indicate that stationary phase parasites of *L. donovani* present some of the basic features typical of PCD in response to treatment with antileishmanial drugs such as amphotericin B. These include nuclear condensation, nicked DNA in the nucleus, DNA ladder formation, increase in plasma membrane permeability, decrease in the mitochondrial membrane potential, and induction of a specific cysteine proteinase activity. Exposure to extreme temperatures also resulted in cell death, which could be rescued in part by overexpression of Bcl-X(L). Despite these results, major differences are observed between the apoptotic death in higher eukaryotes and the death process in *Leishmania*, trypanosomes, and other unicellular protists, such as *Tetrahymena* and *Dictiostelium*. It appears that lower eukaryotes possess the basic machinery that can drive cell death; however, the pathway of this process in these organisms is different from that found in multicellular organisms. Further studies are required to understand whether these PCD features are associated with the life cycle of *Leishmania* parasites.

Redox Control, Oxidative Stress, and *Leishmania*

Another type of stress faced by *Leishmania* parasites is oxidative stress. *Leishmania* parasites reside within macrophages, and cells of the immune system can inhibit the oxidative burst of their host cells. However, despite this feature, a strong system for detoxification of oxyradicals is also required. Thiol metabolism varies between *Leishmania* and their invertebrate vector or mammalian host cells. Redox control in kinetoplastid parasites is mediated by trypanothione, a compound that substitutes glutathione in defending the cell against chemical and oxidative stress. Trypanothione, the major reducing thiol molecule in *Leishmania* and other trypanosomatids, consists of a spermidine moiety that is linked with two glutathione molecules. It is of major importance for parasite survival, since the parasites reside within mammalian macrophages, which specialize in generating oxyradicals. It is also interesting to note that trypanothione and its metabolic pathway serve as a target for the popular antimony-based drugs. Moreover, trypanosomes lacking trypanothione reductase are avirulent and show increased sensitivity to trivalent arsenicals and oxidative stress.

Kinetoplastids, including *Leishmania*, do not encode for the glutathione S-transferase gene, and they also lack the enzyme catalase. Instead, they express the trypanothione S-transferase, which in *L. major* is associated with the eukaryotic translation elongation factor 1B (eEF1B). This association could have implications for translational control by sensing the redox state of thiol groups on proteins in the cell.

Summary

Leishmania is a parasitic protozoan that cycles between an invertebrate vector and a mammalian host and thus experiences a broad range of environmental conditions as part of its natural life cycle. Environmental stresses serve as a trigger for the parasite to differentiate from one life form to another, and as an obvious outcome, heat shock genes are abundantly expressed. Due to their conserved mode of regulation among eukaryotes, heat shock genes serve as an ideal system to study the unique molecular features of *Leishmania*, a very early and interesting eukaryote.

See Also the Following Articles

Apoptosis; Heat Shock Response, Overview; Oxidative Stress.

Further Reading

Ahmed, R. and Duncan, R. F. (2004). Translational regulation of Hsp90 mRNA. AUG-proximal 5'-untranslated region elements essential for preferential heat shock translation. *Journal of Biological Chemistry* **279**, 49919–49930.

Alzate, J. F., Barrientos, A. A., Gonzalez, V. M. and Jimenez-Ruiz, A. (2006). Heat-induced programmed cell death in *Leishmania infantum* is reverted by Bcl-X(L) expression. *Apoptosis* **11**, 161–171.

Argaman, M., Aly, R. and Shapira, M. (1994). Expression of the heat shock protein 83 in *Leishmania* is regulated post transcriptionally. *Molecular and Biochemical Parasitology* **64**, 95–110.

Barak, E., Amin-Spector, S., Gerliak, E., Goyard, S., Holland, N. and Zilberstein, D. (2005). Differentiation of *Leishmania donovani* in host-free system: analysis of signal perception and response. *Molecular and Biochemical Parasitology* **141**, 99–108.

Bates, P. (1993). Axenic culture of *Leishmania* amastigotes. *Parasitology Today* **9**, 143–146.

Charest, H., Zhang, W. W. and Matlashewski, G. (1996). The developmental expression of *Leishmania donovani* A2 amastigote-specific genes is post-transcriptionally mediated and involves elements located in the 3'-untranslated region. *Journal of Biological Chemistry* **271**, 17081–17090.

Davis, M. C., Ward, J. G., Herrick, G. and Allis, C. D. (1992). Programmed nuclear death: apoptotic-like degradation of specific nuclei in conjugating *Tetrahymena*. *Developmental Biology* **154**, 419–432.

Debrabant, A. and Nakhasi, H. (2003). Programmed cell death in trypanosomatids: is it an altruistic mechanism for survival of the fittest? *Kinetoplastid Biology and Disease* **2**, 7.

Fairlamb, A. H., Blackburn, P., Ulrich, P., Chait, B. T. and Cerami, A. (1985). Trypanothione: a novel bis(glutathionyl)spermidine cofactor for glutathione reductase in trypanosomatids. *Science* **227**, 1485–1487.

Folgueira, C., Quijada, L., Soto, M., Abanades, D. R., Alonso, C. and Requena, J. M. (2005). The translational efficiencies of the two *Leishmania infantum* HSP70 mRNAs, differing in their 3'-untranslated regions, are affected by shifts in the temperature of growth through different mechanisms. *Journal of Biological Chemistry* **280**, 35172–35183.

Garlapati, S., Dahan, E. and Shapira, M. (1999). Effect of acidic pH on heat shock gene expression in *Leishmania*. *Molecular and Biochemical Parasitology* **100**, 95–101.

Hess, M. A. and Duncan, R. F. (1996). Sequence and structure determinants of *Drosophila* Hsp70 mRNA translation: 5'-UTR secondary structure specifically inhibits heat shock protein mRNA translation. *Nucleic Acids Research* **24**, 2441–2449.

Ivens, A. C., et al. (2005). The genome of the kinetoplastid parasite *Leishmania major*. *Science* **309**, 436–442.

Johansson, J., Mandin, P., Renzoni, A., Chiaruttini, C., Springer, M. and Cossart, P. (2002). An RNA thermosensor controls expression of virulence genes in *Listeria monocytogenes*. *Cell* **110**, 551–561.

Jolly, C. and Morimoto, R. I. (2000). Role of the heat shock response and molecular chaperones in oncogenesis and cell death. *Journal of the National Cancer Institute* **92**, 1564–1572.

Krobitsch, S., Brandau, S., Hoyer, C., Schmetz, C., Hubel, A. and Clos, J. (1998). *Leishmania donovani* heat shock protein (100). Characterization and function in amastigote stage differentiation. *Journal of Biological Chemistry* **273**, 6488–6494.

Lee, N., Bertholet, S., Debrabant, A., Muller, J., Duncan, R. and Nakhasi, H. L. (2002). Programmed cell death in the unicellular protozoan parasite *Leishmania*. *Cell Death and Differentiation* **9**, 53–64.

Liang, X. H., Haritan, A., Uliel, S. and Michaeli, S. (2003). Trans and cis splicing in trypanosomatids: mechanism, factors, and regulation. *Eukaryotic Cell* **2**, 830–840.

Martinez-Calvillo, S., Yan, S., Nguyen, D., Fox, M., Stuart, K. D. and Myler, P. J. (2003). Transcription of *Leishmania major Friedlin* chromosome 1 initiates in both directions within a single region. *Molecular Cell* **11**, 1291–1299.

McGarry, T. J. and Lindquist, S. (1985). The preferential translation of *Drosophila* hsp70 mRNA requires sequences in the untranslated leader. *Cell* **42**, 903–911.

McNicoll, F., Muller, M., Cloutier, S., et al. (2005). Distinct 3'-untranslated region elements regulate stage-specific mRNA accumulation and translation in *Leishmania*. *Journal of Biological Chemistry* **280**, 35238–35246.

Morita, M. T., Tanaka, Y., Kodama, T. S., Kyogoku, Y., Yanagi, H. and Yura, T. (1999). Translational induction of heat shock transcription factor sigma32, evidence for a built-in RNA thermosensor. *Genes and Development* **13**, 655–665.

Purdy, J. E., Donelson, J. E. and Wilson, M. E. (2005). Regulation of genes encoding the major surface protease of Leishmania chagasi via mRNA stability. *Molecular and Biochemical Parasitology* **142**, 88–97.

Quijada, L., Soto, M., Alonso, C. and Requena, J. M. (2000). Identification of a putative regulatory element in the 3'-untranslated region that controls expression of HSP70 in *Leishmania infantum*. *Molecular and Biochemical Parasitology* **110**, 79–91.

Shapira, M., McEwen, J. G. and Jaffe, C. L. (1988). Temperature effects on molecular processes which lead to stage differentiation in *Leishmania*. *EMBO Journal* **7**, 2895–2901.

Siman-Tov, M. M., Aly, R., Shapira, M. and Jaffe, C. J. (1996). Cloning from *Leishmania major* of a developmentally regulated gene, *c-lpk2*, for the catalytic subunit of the cAMP-dependent protein kinase. *Molecular and Biochemical Parasitology* 77, 201–207.

Vickers, T. J. and Fairlamb, A. H. (2004). Trypanothione S-transferase activity in a trypanosomatid ribosomal elongation factor 1B. *Journal of Biological Chemistry* 279, 27246–27256.

Wiesgigl, M. and Clos, J. (2001). Heat shock protein 90 homeostasis controls stage differentiation in *Leishmania donovani*. *Molecular and Biological Cell* 12, 3307–3316.

Wyllie, S., Cunningham, M. L. and Fairlamb, A. H. (2004). Dual action of antimonial drugs on thiol redox metabolism in the human pathogen *Leishmania donovani*. *Journal of Biological Chemistry* 279, 39925–39932.

Yueh, A. and Schneider, R. J. (1996). Selective translation initiation by ribosome jumping in adenovirus-infected and heat-shocked cells. *Genes and Development* 10, 1557–1567.

Zilka, A., Garlapati, S., Dahan, E., Yaolsky, V. and Shapira, M. (2001). Developmental regulation of heat shock protein 83 in *Leishmania*. 3′ processing and mRNA stability control transcript abundance, and translation is directed by a determinant in the 3′-untranslated region. *Journal of Biological Chemistry* 276, 47922–47929.

Leptin, Adiponectin, Resistin, Ghrelin

A Gavrila, D Barb and C S Mantzoros
Beth Israel Deaconess Medical Center, Boston, MA, USA

Introduction
Adipose Tissue
Gastrointestinal Tract: Ghrelin
Conclusion

Glossary

Adipocytokine	Cytokines secreted by adipose tissue (i.e., leptin, adiponectin, and resistin).
Adiponectin	Hormone secreted by fat cells that modulates several physiological processes, such as glucose and fatty acid metabolism. Decreased plasma adiponectin levels are associated with obesity, insulin resistance, type 2 diabetes mellitus, and atherosclerosis.
Adipose tissue	Specialized connective tissue composed of fat cells (adipocytes), which store droplets of fat in the form of triglycerides and have many other important metabolic roles.
Adipostatic peptide	An agent that prevents adipocyte/fat cell accumulation.
Anorexia nervosa	An eating disorder that occurs most frequently in adolescent females and is characterized by the lack or loss of appetite, known as anorexia. Other features include excessive fear of becoming overweight, body image disturbance, significant weight loss, refusal to maintain minimal normal weight, and amenorrhea.
Anorexigenic peptide	An agent that transiently depresses food intake.
Cachexia	Extreme weight loss, usually associated with chronic disease.
Cytokine	A protein secreted by inflammatory leukocytes but also by nonleukocytic cells; cytokines act as intercellular mediators and differ from classic hormones in that they are produced by a number of tissues or cell types rather than by specialized glands.
Ghrelin	A peptide produced and secreted from stomach that stimulates growth hormone release and, in addition, increases appetite and food intake.
Insulin	A protein hormone secreted by the pancreas that plays a major role in the regulation of glucose metabolism, promoting the cellular use of glucose; also an important regulator of protein and lipid metabolism.
Leptin	A hormone secreted by fat cells and implicated in the regulation of food intake and energy balance, depressing appetite and increasing energy expenditure.
Orexigenic peptide	An agent that stimulates food intake.
Resistin	A hormone secreted by fat cells that may play a role in insulin resistance and inflammation associated with obesity.

Introduction

Obesity has become a public health problem due to its increasing prevalence and associated morbidity and mortality, mainly from cardiovascular disease, type 2 diabetes, and certain malignancies. In addition to a genetic predisposition, environmental factors, physical inactivity, a high-energy high-fat diet, smoking, and stress (which results in dysregulation of endogenous hormones) strongly contribute to the development of this multifcatorial disorder.

Obesity is known to be associated with insulin resistance and development of the metabolic syndrome. However, not all obese patients are insulin-resistant and total fat mass *per se* is not the most important factor contributing to insulin resistance but, rather, the presence of central or visceral obesity. Central obesity has been associated with the dysregulation of the hypothalamic-pituitary-adrenal (HPA) axis and the sympathetic nervous system. The stress hormones of the HPA axis (i.e., cortisol) and the sympathetic system (catecholamines) oppose the effects of insulin, and this may promote insulin resistance. A chronically stressed HPA axis leads to decreased circadian variations in circulating cortisol levels, and chronic glucocorticoid exposure may lead to increased food intake and obesity.

In parallel with the increasing prevalence of obesity, there has been a tremendous increase in research activity in a global effort to better understand energy balance and the regulation of metabolism and body weight. Although a biological basis for body fat regulation was first proposed more than 50 years ago, the hypothesis of an endocrine feedback loop regulating body weight remained elusive until the discovery of the adipocyte-secreted hormone leptin in 1994. This discovery has dramatically changed our understanding of adipose tissue from an inert depot of energy storage to an active organ producing and secreting various molecules that regulate metabolism and energy homeostasis, such as leptin, adiponectin, and resistin (see **Table 1**). In addition, it has recently been recognized that other peripheral organs, such as the gastrointestinal tract, secrete molecules that also convey information on energy intake and balance. For example, ghrelin, a novel gastrointestinal tract-secreted peptide, not only stimulates the secretion of growth hormone (GH) from the pituitary but also plays an important role in energy homeostasis, causing a positive energy balance by stimulating food intake.

The currently accepted model of energy homeostasis proposes that peripheral signals, such as molecules secreted into the circulation from the gut and the adipose tissue, are received and integrated by the central nervous system together with other signals/modulators of food intake and energy homeostasis, such as visual stimuli, smell, the presence of food, social habits or social behavior, and stress, with the final purpose to match food intake with energy expenditure. Signals from both adipose tissue and other peripheral organs not only are processed centrally in the brain to control body metabolism and energy but may also influence other physiological functions, such as the neuroendocrine and reproductive systems.

Various central and peripheral factors involved in energy homeostasis are being continuously discovered, and it is expected that a better understanding of these mechanisms will lead to effective treatments for the control of metabolism and obesity. This review discusses the potential role of four recently discovered molecules involved in metabolism and energy homeostasis: leptin, adiponectin, resistin, and ghrelin.

Adipose Tissue

The adipose tissue is considered today to be a very active and complex endocrine organ. Adipocytes produce and secrete a variety of bioactive molecules, including adipokines, which act at both the local (paracrine/autocrine) and systemic (endocrine) levels to exert diverse metabolic functions. These adipokines include leptin, tumor necrosis factor (TNF)-α, and interleukin (IL)-6, which have already been intensively studied, as well as newer molecules, such as adiponectin and resistin, which may prove to have important roles in controlling metabolism and energy homeostasis.

Leptin

Leptin (from Greek *leptos*, thin) is a 167-amino-acid protein discovered in 1994 as the product of the obese (*ob*) gene. Although known to have numerous other physiological functions in mice and humans, leptin is primarily involved in the control of the neuroendocrine and immune response to energy deprivation. Leptin is produced predominantly by adipose tissue and is secreted into the circulation at levels that are directly proportional to fat mass. Leptin is also expressed at low levels in the hypothalamus, pituitary, placenta, skeletal muscle, and gastric and mammary epithelia. Leptin is found in the peripheral circulation in both a free and a bound form; the free form crosses the blood–brain barrier, binds to the long isoform of a specific leptin class 1 cytokine receptor (also known as ObRb) and activates mainly the janus kinase (JAK)–signal transducer and activator of transcription (STAT) and phosphatidylinositol 3 (PI3)–AKT pathways to convey information to the central nervous system regarding the amount of energy stored in adipose tissue and acute changes in caloric intake. Leptin receptors are predominantly found in the hypothalamus, mainly in the arcuate nucleus but also in the brain stem and other regions of the central nervous system. The activation of hypothalamic receptors stimulates the production of anorectic

Table 1 Adipocytokines and ghrelin: effects on energy homeostasis[a]

Molecule	Site of production	Circulating levels	Target organ/tissue	Effect on insulin sensitivity	Effect on energy expenditure	Stress interaction	Other effects
Adiponectin	Adipose tissue (primary) Cardiomyocytes[b] Placenta[b]	Decreased in obesity, type 2 DM, CVD, malignancies	Muscle Liver Hypothalamus (PVN nucleus)	Increases insulin sensitivity Stimulates glucose uptake Stimulates fatty acid oxidation Decreases gluconeogenesis	Increases energy expenditure Decreases body weight without affecting food intake (ICV administration)	Exo- or endogenous glucocorticoids inhibit adiponectin secretion	Anti-inflammatory Anti-atherogenic Anti-carcinogenic
Ghrelin	GI tract: stomach (enterochromaffin cells) (primary) Hypothalamus (ARC nucleus)	Increased acutely before each meal Decreased in obesity Elevated in anorexia nervosa or cachexia	Pituitary (GH-releasing cells) Hypothalamus (NPY and AgRP neurons)	May reduce insulin sensitivity Decreased glucose disposal rate during ghrelin infusion Increases GH release Enhances the use of carbohydrates and reduces fat use	Decreases energy expenditure Increases appetite and stimulates food intake Reduces thermogenesis	Ghrelin stimulates ACTH release and activates HPA Acute psychological stress raises plasma ghrelin in rodents Activation of gut sympathetic nerves stimulate ghrelin secretion	Increases gastric motility and acid secretion Reduces locomotor activity
Leptin	Adipose tissue (primary) Hypothalamus[b] Pituitary[b] Placenta[b] Skeletal muscle[b] Gastric and mammary epithelia[b]	Increased in proportion to body fat	Hypothalamus (ARC) Brain stem	Increases insulin sensitivity Stimulates glucose uptake Stimulates free fatty acid oxidation	Increases energy expenditure Decreases appetite, food intake, and body weight Increases sympathetic activity Stimulates thermogenesis	Suppresses the activity of the HPA axis (CRH, ACTH, cortisol) Glucocorticoids stimulate leptin secretion, but excess may contribute to leptin resistance	Stimulates reproductive and thyroid functions Stimulates immunity Inhibits bone formation
Resistin	Adipose tissue Mononuclear leukocytes Macrophages	Variable in obesity	Liver ? Muscle ? Hypothalamus ?	Decreases insulin sensitivity in rodents (impairs insulin action on hepatic glucose production and may decrease fatty acid oxidation) Controversial in humans	May decrease energy expenditure in rodents Controversial in humans	Unknown	Inhibits adipocyte differentiation in rodents May have pro-inflammatory effects

[a]ACTH, adrenocorticotropic hormone; AgRP, agouti-related protein; ARC, arcuate nucleus; CRH, corticotropin releasing hormone; CVD, cardiovascular disease; DM, diabetes mellitus; GH, growth hormone; GI, gastrointestinal; HPA, hypothalamic-pituitary-adrenal; ICV, intracerebroventricular; NPY, neuropeptide Y; PVN, paraventricular nucleus.
[b]At low levels.

peptides, such as α-melanin-stimulating hormone (α-MSH) and cocaine and amphetamine-regulated transcript (CART), and inhibits the production of orexigenic peptides, such as neuropeptide Y (NPY) and agouti-related peptide (AgRP), resulting in the inhibition of appetite. In addition, leptin binding to hypothalamic receptors results in increased sympathetic activity, which stimulates free fatty acid oxidation and thermogenesis in brown adipose tissue, thus favoring energy expenditure in mice.

Leptin expression is mainly controlled by the amount of body fat mass; caloric restriction and weight loss results in decreased circulating leptin levels, whereas overfeeding and increasing adipose tissue mass results in increased leptin levels. Leptin production and secretion is also increased by insulin, glucocorticoids, TNF-α, and estrogens; it is decreased by β3-adrenergic activity, androgens, free fatty acids, growth hormone, and peroxisome proliferator activated receptor (PPAR)-γ agonists.

The direct involvement of leptin in the regulation of energy intake and expenditure (by signaling the adequacy of energy stores to the brain) was initially demonstrated in studies in mice. Mutations in the obese (*ob*) gene (leptin gene) and the diabetes (*db*) gene (leptin receptor gene) result in morbid obesity and diabetes, whereas the administration of leptin to leptin deficient (*ob/ob*) and normal rodents results in significant weight loss. However, diet-induced obese mice, the mouse model of obesity that most closely corresponds to garden-variety obesity in humans, are not able to lose weight significantly after leptin administration, indicating that these hyperleptinemic mice are leptin resistant, probably due to receptor or postreceptor defects.

Similarly, only a distinct minority of morbidly obese human subjects have congenital leptin deficiency due to mutations of the *ob* gene, which result in hyperphagia and early-onset, rapid weight gain. The administration of exogenous leptin to these patients results in the normalization of their hyperphagia, decreased caloric intake, and a significant loss of fat mass. Rare inactivating mutations of the leptin receptor gene have also been reported, which, similar to leptin gene defects, manifest clinically with hyperphagia and extreme obesity, as well as hypogonadotropic hypogonadism, but they are also associated with growth delay and secondary hypothyroidism. Our studies have shown that increasing leptin levels precede the onset of puberty, suggesting that leptin may be a permissive factor for the onset of puberty in humans.

Although exogenous leptin administration is an effective treatment, resulting in significant weight loss in obese leptin-deficient subjects, the majority of the cases of human obesity do not respond to leptin therapy. It is now known that most obese individuals have increased leptin production and secretion from adipocytes as well as high circulating leptin levels, features that are consistent with a state of leptin resistance. Several mechanisms are involved in the leptin resistance of obese individuals, including defective transport of leptin across the blood–brain barrier into the brain and/or reduced hypothalamic leptin signaling, in part due to the upregulation of specific inhibitors of leptin signaling. A complete understanding of the pathogenesis of leptin resistance in humans may open new pathways for the treatment of obesity.

Interestingly, a small study reported that exogenous leptin administration to replace leptin levels to preweight-loss levels, prevented the regaining of weight, and promoted the loss of fat mass in a small group of subjects participating in a weight loss program. These findings need to be confirmed by larger studies.

There is accumulating evidence that leptin has complex neuroendocrine functions, regulating the activity of the HPA and also the hypothalamic-pituitary-gonadal and -thyroid axes. It has been reported that leptin suppresses the activity of the HPA; that is, decreased leptin levels during fasting/starvation are associated with increased activation of the HPA and cortisol secretion. In accordance with this, in critically ill patients the nocturnal fall in leptin levels is associated with a paradoxical increase of nocturnal adrenocorticotropic hormone (ACTH) and cortisol levels. Leptin-deficient mice and humans fail to go through puberty, and leptin administration reverses this abnormality. We have shown that the decreased leptin levels found in food deprivation are responsible for the starvation-induced suppression of the hypothalamic-pituitary-gonadal axis as well as changes in the function of other neuroendocrine axes in humans. In addition, extremely thin women with hypothalamic amenorrhea have low leptin levels and exogenous leptin administration normalizes their neuroendocrine and reproductive functions. Thus, it seems that leptin may act as the critical link between adipose tissue and not only hypothalamic centers regulating energy homeostasis but also the reproductive system, indicating whether adequate energy reserves are present for normal reproductive function. Further larger trials are needed to conclusively prove whether leptin replacement treatment can ameliorate or treat the neuroendocrine dysfunction and also the immune abnormalities, osteoporosis, and infertility in women with hypothalamic amenorrhea.

In addition to signaling in the central nervous system, leptin also acts in the periphery and has important roles in regulating insulin action and lipid metabolism. Other peripheral endocrine effects include the direct regulation of immune function, hematopoesis, angiogenesis, and direct and indirect effects on bone metabolism.

Taken together, these findings suggest that leptin plays a significant role in the central regulation of energy balance and that leptin is a critical signal for neuroendocrine function in humans; this raises the possibility that leptin is indeed not only an adipostatic hormone but also a stress-related hormone crucial for survival.

Adiponectin

Adiponectin (Acrp30, apM1 protein, adipoQ, or GBP28) is a 247-amino-acid protein discovered simultaneously by four different research groups in the mid-1990s. Adiponectin is produced and secreted exclusively by differentiated adipocytes and represents one of the most abundant serum proteins that circulates in tightly associated trimers and higher-order oligomers. Eight adiponectin isoforms with variable potency have been isolated, which bind and activate at least two adiponectin receptors. Adiponectin receptor 1 (AdipoR1) is expressed ubiquitously but most abundantly in skeletal muscle and has a high affinity for globular adiponectin and a very low affinity for full-length adiponectin; adiponectin receptor 2 (AdipoR2) is found predominantly in the liver and has an intermediate affinity for both forms.

Adiponectin decreases with increasing overall and central adiposity and increases with prolonged weight reduction. In humans, although short-term fasting does not influence circulating levels of adiponectin, prolonged caloric restriction results in weight loss and increased adiponectin levels. In addition, daily caloric intake, macronutrient intake, and high fat intake do not correlate with and do not affect circulating adiponectin levels in humans, except possibly in obese individuals, but a Mediterranean-type diet, which has beneficial effects on morbidity and mortality, increases adiponectin levels. Interestingly, studies in rodents have revealed that central and peripheral adiponectin administration increases energy expenditure by stimulating free fatty acid oxidation and glucose uptake, thus reducing body weight and visceral adiposity without affecting energy intake.

Although its role has not been definitively established, there is accumulating evidence that adiponectin regulates insulin sensitivity and is also involved in inflammation and atherosclerosis. Initial animal studies showed that adiponectin-knockout mice develop insulin resistance either independently of diet or only after high-fat and high-sucrose diet, whereas adiponectin treatment improves their insulin resistance. In addition, lipoatrophic and obese mice have low adiponectin levels and insulin resistance, which improve partially after exogenous adiponectin administration. Moreover, the decrease in circulating adiponectin levels parallels the development of insulin resistance and type 2 diabetes in a longitudinal study of rhesus monkeys.

Studies in humans showed that there is a negative correlation of adiponectin levels with fasting glucose, insulin, and insulin resistance and a positive correlation with insulin sensitivity, independent of body–mass index (BMI). We also know that the adiponectin gene has the same location as one of the diabetes susceptibility genes on chromosome 3q27, and several longitudinal studies showed that human subjects with lower baseline adiponectin levels are more likely to develop type 2 diabetes, independent of adiposity. In contrast, type 1 diabetic patients may have elevated adiponectin levels compared to nondiabetic individuals, whereas chronically administered insulin does not have an effect on adiponectin levels.

Taken together, all these findings show that adiponectin levels are low in states of insulin resistance, such as obesity and type 2 diabetes, and adiponectin levels increase with improved insulin sensitivity after weight reduction or treatment with insulin-sensitizing drugs (thiazolidindiones). It is currently thought that adiponectin represents a link among obesity, insulin resistance, and various other metabolic abnormalities associated with obesity.

Adiponectin improves insulin sensitivity through multiple cellular and molecular mechanisms that are not entirely known at present. An important enzyme stimulated by adiponectin is AMP-activated protein kinase (AMPK), which, in turn, phosphorylates several intracellular proteins to alter various cellular functions, including the enhancement of insulin-stimulated glucose uptake into fat and skeletal muscle as well as the suppression of hepatic glucose production and stimulation of fatty acid oxidation. By increasing fatty acid oxidation through AMPK activation, adiponectin decreases circulating free fatty acids, resulting thus in improved insulin action. Adiponectin may also improve insulin sensitivity by inducing the activation of the insulin signaling system. Moreover, by stimulating nitric oxide (NO) formation, adiponectin may augment vascular blood flow to promote glucose uptake.

In addition to its insulin-sensitizing effects, adiponectin is also related to the lipid profile, another independent risk factor for cardiovascular disease. Previous studies reported a strong positive association between adiponectin and high-density lipoprotein (HDL) cholesterol and a negative association with serum triglyceride levels. However, there is no independent relationship between adiponectin and low-density lipoprotein (LDL) or total cholesterol. Adiponectin may lead to a favorable lipid profile by stimulating fatty acid oxidation, an effect probably mediated by AMPK. However, one study reported increased fatty acid oxidation in muscle cells in adiponectin-knockout mice, and a cross-sectional study of humans found that plasma adiponectin levels did not correlate with lipid oxidation, as measured by energy expenditure and respiratory quotient. Thus, further studies are needed to understand adiponectin's effects on fatty acid oxidation.

Adiponectin may also exert important anti-inflammatory and atheroprotective effects. It inhibits the production and action of several inflammatory factors involved in atherosclerosis, including TNF-α, and also suppresses monocyte adhesion and macrophage transformation to foam cells within the vascular wall. In addition, adiponectin inhibits smooth muscle cell proliferation in the vascular wall by inhibiting growth factors that promote hyperplasia and promotes vasodilation and angiogenesis by increasing NO production in endothelial cells through AMPK activation. In conclusion, adiponectin's involvement in cardiovascular disease is probably multifactorial, including its effects on risk factors such as insulin resistance and dyslipidemia but also a direct effect on the vascular system.

Furthermore, there is emerging mechanistic and epidemiological evidence supporting a protective role of adiponectin in malignancies. *In vitro* treatment of acute myelomonocytic leukemia cell lines with adiponectin suppressed the growth of myelomonocyte cells, induced apoptosis, and downregulated *Bcl-2* gene expression. More recently, adiponectin has been shown to be a direct inhibitor of angiogenesis *in vivo* and *in vitro* through the activation of caspases in endothelial cells. Consistent with the *in vitro* studies, which suggest that adiponectin is an important negative regulator of hematopoesis and the immune system, *in vivo* intratumoral administration of murine adiponectin resulted in significant suppression of T241 fibrosarcoma tumor growth. Adiponectin receptors are expressed by prostate, hepatocellular carcinoma, and various other cancer cell types (breast, endometrial, colon, and neuroblastoma cell lines). Recent experiments suggest that adiponectin may act on tumor cells directly through the activation of c-jun NH_2-terminal kinase, a mammalian MAPK family involved in the regulation of cell proliferation and apoptosis, and also through the suppression of the transcription factor signal transducer and activator of transcription (STAT)3, which also regulates cell proliferation, differentiation, survival, and apoptosis. Therefore, given its antiangiogenesis properties and the inactivation of STAT3 reported in obesity and

associated malignancies, adiponectin may prove to be an effective novel anticancer agent.

Epidemiological evidence also suggests that adiponectin plays an important role in the insulin-related pathways of carcinogenesis, independently of other known risk factors for cancers. We and others have recently reported that circulating adiponectin levels are inversely associated with risk for endometrial, breast, prostate, gastric, and colorectal cancer. In two recent case–control studies, we reported that women with high BMI and low plasma adiponectin had a 6.5-fold increased risk of endometrial cancer, independent of the possible effects of insulin-like growth factor (IGF-)1, IGF-2, IGF binding protein (IGFBP-)3, leptin, BMI, and other known risk factors of the disease. We also found in a prospective study in men that individuals in the highest quintile of adiponectin levels had an approximately 60% reduced risk for colorectal cancer compared to the lowest quintile. Significantly, these associations were also independent of body size and physical activity.

In addition, adiponectin levels may also correlate inversely with tumor size, histological grade, and disease stage in gastric and prostate cancer. Large association and prospective studies to prove adiponectin's role in the development of malignancies as well as mechanistic studies to address potential roles of adiponectin in cancer pathogenesis are needed.

Resistin

Resistin (adipose-tissue-specific secretory factor or FIZZ3) is a 94-amino-acid polypeptide with 11 cysteine residues. Resistin is almost entirely expressed and excreted from white adipose tissue in mice and circulates as a dimer. A single dicysteine residue is required for dimerization, whereas the remaining 10 cysteine residues are involved in determining the structure of the resistin monomeric unit.

Similar to adiponectin, resistin has been postulated to link obesity with insulin resistance, but these two molecules probably have opposite functions. In 2001, Steppan and colleagues reported that resistin secretion is decreased by the antidiabetic drug rosiglitazone and is increased in diet-induced and genetic mouse models of obesity. Moreover, the administration of antiresistin antibody improves blood sugar and insulin action in obese mice, and the administration of recombinant resistin impairs glucose tolerance and insulin action in normal mice. More recent studies have shown that resistin may increase hepatic insulin resistance by inhibiting AMPK and may also increase hepatic glucose production, thus controlling glucose and lipid metabolism. In addition, resistin has been postulated to regulate adipose tissue mass by inhibiting adipocyte differentiation and thus limit adipose tissue formation in response to increased energy intake. These observations have not been confirmed by other studies, however; thus, the role of resistin in mice remains controversial.

Human data are even more conflicting. Although resistin is expressed at very low levels in human adipose cells, high levels are expressed in circulating mononuclear leukocytes and macrophages. Similar to its distribution in rodents, resistin is found in human sera, and several studies (but not all) reported increased levels in obese and diabetic patients and a positive association with insulin resistance. One study showed that human resistin expression, but not serum levels, is proportional to insulin resistance, and several studies failed to show an association with insulin resistance. Resistin may have pro-inflammatory effects because recent *in vitro* studies found that resistin induces the expression of adhesion molecules such as vascular cell adhesion molecule (VCAM)-1 and intercellular adhesion molecule (ICAM)-1 in human endothelial cells.

Further studies are required to determine whether stress influences resistin levels and to elucidate the role of resistin in regulating insulin sensitivity. In addition, whether resistin influences obesity either directly or indirectly by altering glucose and insulin levels and whether resistin plays a role in inflammation associated with obesity warrant further investigation.

Gastrointestinal Tract: Ghrelin

Ghrelin, a 28-amino-acid lipophilic peptide with a labile octanoyl fatty acid side chain at the serine residue 3, was originally discovered by Kojima and coworkers during their search for an endogenous growth hormone secretagogue. This hormone is expressed primarily in specialized enterochromaffin cells (called X/A-like cells), which are located mainly in the mucosa of the fundus of the stomach. In addition, ghrelin-immunoreactive cells are also found in the intestine, with their concentration gradually decreasing from duodenum to colon; they are also found in the pancreatic islets, brain, and kidney. Ghrelin-producing neurons are located in the hypothalamus, more specifically in the hypothalamic arcuate nucleus, an important region controlling appetite, but also in previously uncharacterized neurons adjacent to the third ventricle, which send efferent fibers to NPY and AgRP neurons, stimulating the release of these orexigenic peptides.

Ghrelin binds to the growth hormone secretagogue receptor (GHS-R), a typical G-protein-coupled receptor, the activation of which by ghrelin results in increased intracellular calcium via the activation of the phospholipase C pathway. GHS-Rs are expressed in various regions of the brain, predominantly in the growth hormone-releasing somatotroph cells of the pituitary gland. Ghrelin stimulates the release of growth hormone from the pituitary in a dose-dependent manner and acts synergistically with growth hormone-releasing hormone (GHRH). In addition, ghrelin has a weak prolactin (PRL) and ACTH-releasing activity, but more important ghrelin can modulate gonadotropin-releasing hormone (GnRH) pulses, possibly being one of the signals that turns off the gonadal axis during starvation. The expression of ghrelin in the pituitary is high after birth and declines with puberty.

In addition to being a potent growth hormone secretagogue, ghrelin is a potent appetite stimulant. Ghrelin administration by intracerebroventricular, intravenous, or subcutaneous injection increases food intake and body weight, decreases fat use, and increases gastric acid output in a dose-dependent manner. Administered to rats by intracerebroventricular injections, ghrelin induces Fos protein expression, a marker of neuronal activation, in regions of primary importance in the regulation of feeding, including NPY neurons and AgRP neurons, but also in the neurons of the solitary tract nucleus and the dorsomotor nucleus of vagus. The latter may sustain a role for ghrelin in the central regulation of gastric acid secretion and gastric motility via vagal cholinergic pathways.

Ghrelin circulates in the bloodstream in two forms, acylated and desacyl ghrelin, with the acylated form being the biologically active form of ghrelin. Serum levels of ghrelin depend on the state of nutrition and are negatively correlated with the BMI. Accordingly, circulating ghrelin levels are decreased in obesity but elevated during fasting and in anorexia nervosa and cachexia, a finding that may reflect a compensatory mechanism. Acute psychological stress raises plasma ghrelin in the rat, and the activation of gut sympathetic nerves directly stimulate ghrelin secretion. Also, an increase in plasma ghrelin leads to the release of ACTH and the activation of the HPA axis. Recent human data demonstrated an inverse correlation between ghrelin and leptin that is independent of adiposity, but there is no regulation of ghrelin by leptin administration over the short term (a few hours to a few days).

In normal humans, plasma ghrelin levels rise immediately before each meal and in response to diet-induced weight loss and fall to minimum levels 1 h after feeding. This fall in ghrelin levels after a meal is correlated with insulin peak, suggesting that insulin may be a negative regulator of ghrelin secretion in the postprandial state. This fall in ghrelin levels after a meal is absent or blunted in obese humans, a fact that, researchers propose, may contribute to the development of their obesity. Significantly, obese patients who undergo gastric bypass surgery have significantly lowered ghrelin levels after surgery, which, on the basis of observational studies, has been proposed to contribute to maintaining decreased weight after bypass surgery.

Finally, what are potential clinical applications of ghrelin? It has been suggested that blocking or neutralizing ghrelin action may prove to be a reasonable pharmacological approach to reverse a chronically positive energy balance, such as in obesity. However, in contrast to predictions made from the pharmacology of ghrelin, studies in ghrelin-null mice showed that the deletion of ghrelin impairs neither growth nor appetite. In fact, ghrelin-null mice are neither anorexic nor dwarfs and display normal responses to starvation and diet-induced obesity, strongly suggesting that ghrelin is not critically required for viability, fertility, growth, appetite, or fat deposition. Thus, antagonists of ghrelin may not prove to be very successful antiobesity agents. In contrast, exploring its orexigenic activity for the treatment of eating disorders such as anorexia nervosa or the replacement of ghrelin in ghrelin-deficient states such as cachexia or other catabolic states seems to be a more reasonable approach.

Conclusion

This brief review has covered recent advances in the area of molecules regulating energy homeostasis and metabolism – leptin, adiponectin, resistin, and ghrelin. Most probably, we can expect other related hormones to be added to this list in the near future. In addition, synthetic analogs, agonists, or antagonists are expected to be developed by the pharmaceutical industry for the management of states of energy excess, such as obesity and type 2 diabetes, and states of energy deficiency, such as anorexia nervosa and hypothalamic amenorrhea.

See Also the Following Articles

Feeding Circuitry (and Neurochemistry); Food Intake and Stress, Non-Human; Ghrelin and Stress Protection; Glucocorticoid Negative Feedback; Metabolic Syndrome and Stress; Nutrition; Obesity, Stress and; Orexin.

Further Reading

Ahima, R. S. (2005). Central actions of adipocyte hormones. *Trends in Endocrinology and Metabolism* **16**, 307–313.

Barb, D., Pazaitou-Panayiotou, K. and Mantzoros, C. S. (2006). Adiponectin: a link between obesity and cancer. *Expert Opinions on Investigational Drugs* **15**, 917–931.

Bjorbaek, C. and Kahn, B. B. (2004). Leptin signaling in the central nervous system and the periphery. *Recent Progress in Hormone Research* **59**, 305–331.

Bluher, S. and Mantzoros, C. S. (2004). The role of leptin in regulating neuroendocrine function in humans. *Journal of Nutrition* **134**, 2469S–2474S.

Brennan, A. M. and Mantzoros, C. S. (2006). Drug insight: the role of leptin in human physiology and pathophysiology-emerging clinical applications. *Nature Clinical Practice: Endocrinology & Metabolism* **2**(6), 318–324.

Buren, J. and Eriksson, J. W. (2005). Is insulin resistance caused by defects in insulin's target cells or by a stressed mind? *Diabetes/Metabolism Research and Reviews* **21**(6), 487–494.

Chan, J. L. and Mantzoros, C. S. (2005). Role of leptin in energy-deprivation states: normal human physiology and clinical implications for hypothalamic amenorrhoea and anorexia nervosa. *Lancet* **366**, 74–85.

Gale, S. M., Castracane, V. D. and Mantzoros, C. S. (2004). Energy homeostasis, obesity and eating disorders: recent advances in endocrinology. *Journal of Nutrition* **134**, 295–298.

Haslam, D. W. and James, W. P. (2005). Obesity. *Lancet* **366**, 1197–1209.

Havel, P. J. (2004). Update on adipocyte hormones: regulation of energy balance and carbohydrate/lipid metabolism. *Diabetes* **53**(supplement 1), S143–S151.

Kadowaki, T. and Yamauchi, T. (2005). Adiponectin and adiponectin receptors. *Endocrine Review* **26**, 439–451.

Kojima, M. and Kangawa, K. (2005). Ghrelin: structure and function. *Physiological Reviews* **85**, 495–522.

Munzberg, H., Bjornholm, M., Bates, S. H., et al. (2005). Leptin receptor action and mechanisms of leptin resistance. *Cellular and Molecular Life Sciences* **62**, 642–652.

Shetty, G. K., Barb, D. and Mantzoros, C. S. (2006). Nutrients and peripherally secreted molecules in regulation of energy homeostasis. In: Mantzoros, C. S. (ed.) *Obesity and diabetes*, pp. 69–86. Totowa, NJ: Humana Press.

Steppan, C. M. and Lazar, M. A. (2004). The current biology of resistin. *Journal of Internal Medicine* **255**, 439–447.

Leukocyte Trafficking and Stress

S Hong
University of California, San Diego, La Jolla,
CA, USA
M U Goebel
University of Duisburg-Essen, Essen, Germany
P J Mills
University of California, San Diego, La Jolla,
CA, USA

Introduction

What Is Leukocyte Trafficking?

Acute Stress Paradigms

Chronic Stress Paradigms

Underlying Mechanisms and Mediators

Potential Clinical Implications

Summary

Glossary

Cellular adhesion molecules (CAMs)	Cell surface molecules that mediate leukocyte migration, homing, and cell-to-cell interaction. Types of adhesion molecules are the integrins, selectins, cadherins, and proteins of the immunoglobulin superfamily.
Cluster of differentiation (CD)	A uniform nomenclature system developed for distinguishing lineage or differentiation stage of leukocytes by identifying surface proteins that are recognized by a group of monoclonal antibodies.
Cytokines	Soluble proteins produced costly by activated immune cells during effector phases. They regulate and mediate immune and inflammatory responses.
Enzyme-linked immunosorbent assay (ELISA)	A serological assay that detects the concentration of bound antigen or antibody through a photometer.
Flow cytometry	A cellular research tool to characterize individual cells or other microparticles by size, granularity, and surface or intracellular markers using fluorescent-labeled antibodies.
Granulocytes	A subset of leukocytes that originate in the bone marrow and include neutrophils, eosinophils, basophils, and mast cells that possess abundant cytoplasmic granules. About 90% of the peripheral blood cells are granulocytes.
Inflammation	Process that begins with cytokines produced by activated immune cells upon recognition of the antigen presence.
Leukocytosis	An increase of leukocyte (white blood cells) numbers in the peripheral circulation.
Lymphocytes	A subset of leukocytes, including natural killer (NK), T, and B cells, that are major mediators of adaptive (specific) immunity in mammals. They originate in the bone marrow.
Monocytes	A subset of leukocytes that mature to become macrophages and that are phagocytic and produce cytokines.

Introduction

The immune system is the body's defense against disease-causing agents. It is complex yet well orchestrated and nearly self-regulatory. It provides surveillance throughout the body via circulation of white blood cells. The circulation of immune cells is an ongoing process under normal conditions (e.g., no infection), but the trafficking pattern changes under pathogenic conditions to accommodate the mounting of an immune response.

It is of great interest to researchers that there are other stimuli (that are not immunogenic) that lead to changes in trafficking of immune cells; one of these stimuli is stress. Stressors are acute immune system activators that lead not only to modulation in immune functions but also to leukocyte influx into the circulation. The effects of acute stress on leukocyte trafficking are mostly transient and fairly well understood, but the possible lasting effects of chronic stress on leukocyte mobilization are still largely unknown. While decades of research has helped delineated the effects of stress on leukocyte populations, it is only recently that the mechanisms underlying the phenomenon are being revealed, including various neurohormones and their respective receptors and cellular adhesion molecules.

This article reviews what is currently known about the effects of acute and chronic stressors on leukocyte trafficking, including discussion of mechanisms and potential clinical implications. It focuses on the evidence of changes in circulating leukocytes rather than in other tissues or lymphoid organs. The terms trafficking, demargination, leukocytosis, and mobilization are used interchangeably.

What Is Leukocyte Trafficking?

Surveillance and Inflammation

Even though only 2% of total leukocytes are in the peripheral circulation at any given time, they provide a diagnostic account of the functional status of the immune system. The majority are homed in lymphoid organs and the rest are diffusely distributed in other organs. During infection or injury migration of immune cells to different sites of antigen localization within the body is critical to host defense. Recognition of antigen leads to cytokine production, causing inflammation in the area that facilitates recruitment of circulating leukocytes to the infected site. Many of the mechanisms responsible for regulating these types of fundamental responses of the immune system, including cellular adhesion molecules (CAMs), are also central to the regulation of the immune response to stressors.

Major Players: Cellular Adhesion Molecules

Initial trafficking, rolling, and firm adhesion of leukocytes to sites of inflammation are mediated by cytokines and CAMs (e.g., L-selectin, LFA-1, VLA-4, and CD44), which are homing receptors on the immune cells, and their ligands on endothelial cells (molecules that binds to a macromolecule, such as a receptor, e.g., E-selectin, GlyCAM-1, ICAM-1, and VCAM-1). Inflammatory stimuli (e.g., cytokines

tumor necrosis factor-α [TNF-α] and interleukin-1 [IL-1] and chemokines [chemotactic cytokines]) and antigen recognition by immune cells lead to the expression of these molecules on both immune cells and endothelial cells. Leukocytes then attach to endothelial cells lining the infected areas (firm adhesion) and penetrate into the tissue (transmigration).

Adhesion of leukocytes to the endothelium involves multiple processes. First, the initial contact of leukocytes to the endothelium is mediated by L-selectin (CD62L), tethering them loosely to carbohydrate ligands like GlyCAM-1 as they roll along the surface, as shown in **Figure 1**. Until the leukocyte gets activated, this rolling process is reversible. Second, during activation, chemokines are released by the endothelium and trigger integrin LFA-1 (CD11a) expression on the leukocyte surface to bind tightly to the intercellular adhesion molecule ICAM-1 (CD54) on the endothelium. This event leads to an eventual transendothelial migration (extravasation). CAMs, such as L-selectin and ICAMs, are shed in a soluble form during the process and can further participate in biological processes. As mentioned previously, cytokines play a crucial role in trafficking and homing of leukocytes: inflammatory conditions, which activate macrophages and monocytes to release cytokines such as TNF-α, further activate the endothelium. This leads to upregulation of endothelial adhesion

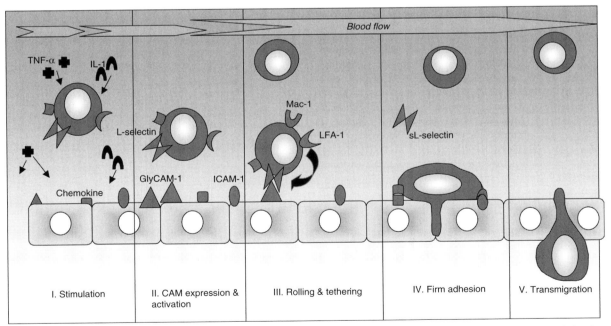

Figure 1 Schematic diagram of stages in migration and adhesion of leukocytes and cell adhesion molecules. (I, II) Stimulating factors including pro-inflammatory cytokines result in activation of leukocytes and endothelial cells and lead to increased expression and activation of adhesion molecules on both endothelial and immune cells. (III) Selectins (e.g., L-selectin) bind to ligands on the endothelium (e.g., GlyCam-1), causing leukocytes to be captured, roll, and tether. (IV) Activation and binding of integrins (e.g., LFA-1) to ligands (e.g., ICAM-1) leads to attachment and further activation of leukocytes. (V) Leukocytes transmigrate through the endothelial wall.

molecules, such as ICAM-1 and the vascular VCAM-1, which further attract leukocytes. Other cytokines, such as IL-2, IL-4, and IL-10, are suggested to have inhibitory effects through reduction of CAMs. The expression of CAMs is assessed by quantifying adhesion molecules on the surface of circulating leukocytes (using flow cytometry) and by determining the levels of their circulating soluble form (typically by enzyme-linked immunosorbent assay [ELISA]).

Acute Stress Paradigms

Numerous studies demonstrate that the immune system is responsive to acute psychological events. One example of immune reactivity to stress is the increased numbers of leukocytes in circulation. Evidence for this dates back to the 1930s, when Farris described the relationship among emotional stress, academic exams, and increases in the number of circulating leukocytes. A relatively parallel phenomenon in response to acute physical stress has also been documented. During the past two decades, with the more sophisticated research tools and techniques available, investigators have been actively examining the nuances of these phenomena, as well as researching the mechanisms that regulate them.

Psychological Stress

Researchers have used a wide variety of naturalistic and standardized stressors to investigate the phenomenon of acute psychological stress-induced leukocytosis. These stress paradigms include mental and emotional stressors such as uncontrollable stimuli (e.g., shock and noise), laboratory stressors (e.g., the color–word Stroop test and mental arithmetic test), and real-life stressors (e.g., academic examinations, piloting airplanes, giving a public speech, and parachute jumping). Regardless of the stress model used, psychological stress leads to leukocytosis at varying degrees depending on the type and duration of the stressor. The literature, for example, shows marked increases in the circulation of natural killer (NK) and $CD8^+$ T cell subsets, a decrease in the $CD4^+/CD8^+$ ratio, and small increases in helper T and B cells. Bosch and colleagues recently reported that a subset of NK cells is more responsive to a speech stressor such that the number of NK cells expressing low levels of CD56 (cytotoxic) tripled but the number of NK cells expressing high levels of CD56 (regulatory) did not change following a stressor. Together, such findings have raised several questions, including why selected subsets of leukocytes are more responsive to stress, and from which sites the leukocytes are being released? Regarding the first question, studies suggest that it is in part attributable to a different degree or

profile of CAM expression and receptors for neurotransmitters and stress hormones on different cell types. Regarding the second question, immune cells are released from the so-called marginal pools as well as from the spleen, which is a primary reservoir of circulating leukocytes, especially following sympathetic nervous system activation.

Psychological stress also leads to changes in CAM expression on peripheral (demarginated) leukocytes. It is consistently shown that the phenomenon of leukocyte redistribution in response to acute stress can be differentiated according to L-selectin (CD62L) expression. As seen in **Figure 1**, L-selectin serves a crucial role in a leukocyte's initial rolling on the endothelium. Findings suggest that it is primarily lymphocytes not expressing L-selectin ($CD62L^-$) that markedly increase in the circulation following acute stress (either psychological or physical). $CD8^+CD62L^-$ T cells, for example, show a two- to threefold increase in the circulation following acute stress as compared to $CD8^+CD62L^+$ T cells, which show either no change or a more moderate increase. A similar $CD62L^{-/+}$ response differentiation is shown for both $CD4^+$ and NK lymphocytes. This phenomenon most likely results from a combination of events, including a preferential release of $CD62L^-$ lymphocytes from the spleen and marginal pools, an increased rate of adhesion of $CD62L^+$ lymphocytes, and a downregulation or shedding of CD62L from the leukocyte's surface upon further activation.

Physical Stress

In addition to the phenomenon of psychological stress-induced leukocytosis, researchers report dramatic increases of immune cells in the circulation after a bout of exercise. It should be made clear here that a bout of exercise should be distinguished from longitudinal exercise training (see Physical Stress Models and Adaptation below). And, in this article, acute exercise is discussed as a physiological stressor, given the cardiopulmonary, metabolic, and hemodynamic demands of exercise on the individual. In addition, a large body of literature on the effects of exercise on the neuroendocrine system supports the notion that exercise is a biologically plausible paradigm to investigate stress-induced modulation of the immune system.

Changes in circulating cell numbers in response to exercise vary among subpopulations of leukocytes and are dependent upon the intensity and duration of the exercise challenge. There is a dose response in exercise-induced leukocytosis such that mild exercise results in smaller changes in cell numbers. Marked increases in numbers of most lymphocyte subsets, monocytes, and granulocytes are consistently observed. Similar to psychological stress, small or no changes are typically seen in numbers of B lymphocytes, even after exercise of a moderate to high intensity. Changes in NK cell and neutrophil numbers after exercise are most dramatic; the number of NK cells can increase two- to fourfold above resting levels. Interestingly, a small subset of monocytes that also expresses CD16 ($CD14^+CD16^+$) (CD16 is largely expressed on NK cells) is shown to be mobilized to the circulation during exercise at a larger degree than regular monocytes ($CD14^+CD16^-$). Not only cardiovascular exercise but also resistance exercise using relatively small muscle groups can significantly affect circulating immune cells.

In spite of the consistent findings on associations between exercise intensity and leukocytosis, exhaustive and prolonged exercise (e.g., a marathon or triathlon) results in decreased immune cell numbers (leukocytopenia; especially T and NK cells) in the circulation. Although the reason for this trafficking pattern after prolonged exercise is unclear, there are several possible explanations. It may well be that the initial leukocytosis for the first 20–30 min of a marathon may be followed by a gradual decline, resulting in leukocytopenia as the high-intensity exercise continues. As is discussed later, sustained activation of the hypothalamic-pituitary-adrenocortical (HPA) axis, resulting in high cortisol levels, may be a mediating factor for decreased immune cell numbers after a marathon. In addition, muscular tissue injury during a marathon or triathlon may also be a contributing factor, although whether the leukocytopenia seen after a marathon reflects the redistribution of the cells to the fatigued or damaged muscle tissue is not known.

During exercise, leukocytes may demarginate to the peripheral blood compartment in part by increased hemodynamic forces that detach cells that normally loosely adhere to the vessel walls at rest. Cells that are mobilized into the circulation during exercise appear to be from the secondary lymphoid organs (the spleen and lymph nodes) rather than the primary lymphoid organs (the thymus and bone marrow), given findings that a greater percentage of activated $CD62L^-$ memory T cells demarginate as compared to naive cells. Thus, exercise-induced leukocytosis appears to be a redistribution of cells from the spleen and lymph nodes rather than proliferation or differentiation of them from primary sources.

As with the psychological stress responses, $CD62L^-$ lymphocytes appear highly responsive to an acute exercise challenge. Granulocytes and lymphocytes show a significant decrease in the surface density of CD62L following exercise. A similar shedding process may also occur with the adhesion molecule ICAM-1. Such a shedding of ICAM-1 might lead to a further demargination of $CD62L^-$ leukocytes back into the circulation. Studies demonstrate an increase in levels of soluble ICAM-1 following exercise, supporting such a conjecture.

Pharmacological Stress

In order to test the hypothesis that leukocytosis following psychological or physical stressors may be mediated by sympathetic nervous system activation, investigators have examined leukocyte trafficking by administering sympathetic (adrenergic) agonists. Pharmacological infusion studies of such agonists provide direct mechanistic evidence for the stress–leukocytosis phenomenon. Infusion of the nonspecific β-adrenergic agonist isoproterenol (a pharmacological agent that leads to similar physiological effects as norepinephrine), for example, leads to increases in $CD8^+$ T and NK cell numbers in blood. Isoproterenol also leads to increased numbers of $CD62L^-$ but not $CD62L^+$ $CD8^+$ cells as well as a decrease of CD62L density and increased CD11a density. Activated/memory T cells appear more responsive to the infusion as compared to naive T lymphocytes. Studies using β-adrenergic antagonists such as propranolol to block sympathetic agonist effects in combination with stressors provide further evidence of adrenergic regulation of leukocytosis. Ingestion of propranolol for 5 days leads to a blunted stress-induced lymphocytosis to psychological and exercise stressors. For example, the $CD8^+CD62L^-$ T cell response to exercise is dramatically attenuated by treatment with propranolol. Together, these findings indicate that acute stress-induced leukocyte trafficking is mediated in part by β-adrenergic receptor activation.

Chronic Stress Paradigms

Psychological Stress

It is widely believed that more enduring stressors lead to downregulation of immune function and increased disease susceptibility. Studies report immune suppression under such chronic stressors as marital strife, bereavement, long-term caregiving, living in an unfavorable environment such as near a nuclear power plant, and environmental disasters such as floods and hurricanes. Immunosuppressive effects of chronic stress include a decrease in circulating leukocyte NK cell number and activity at rest, a lower cytokine release rate, and enhanced antibody titer for latent viruses such as herpes simplex virus type 1 and Epstein–Barr virus. Kiecolt-Glaser et al. reported that medical students who experience high stress levels and poorer social support during academic examination exhibit very low NK cell activity.

As with acute stress studies, CAMs appear to have an important role in mediating the effects of chronic stress on leukocytes. For example, one study was conducted on CD62L expression on T lymphocytes among elderly (average age of 75 years) spousal caregivers of Alzheimer patients experiencing high stress levels due to increased caregiving burden, who were compared to a group of caregivers with a relatively low stress burden from caregiving. The highly stressed caregivers showed significantly lower numbers of circulating $CD8^+CD62L^-$ and $CD4^+CD62L^-$ T cells at rest and during acute psychological stress but no differences in $CD62L^+$ T cells as compared to the control group. Lower numbers of $CD62L^-$ T cells in the circulation indicate that there is decreased availability of activated/memory T cells. In addition, this deficit in activated/memory T lymphocytes, cells that are critical in mounting immune responses, may imply a stress-associated accelerated decline of immunity in these older individuals, which, in turn, might have adverse consequences for health.

Physical Stress Models and Adaptation

It is of great interest to many researchers to determine if chronic exercise training or regular physical activity leads to a favorable modulation of the immune system. Contrary to findings of immunosuppression and potential increased disease susceptibility following chronic psychological stress, long-term regular exercise typically leads to improvements in health. It is unclear, though, whether regular exercise leads to enhanced immunity or changes in immune cell distribution that would support observations of improved health. In general, findings on the effects of chronic exercise (training) or physical fitness on resting peripheral blood leukocyte numbers and adhesion molecule expression are inconclusive, with no consistent effects shown for $CD4^+$, $CD8^+$, or B lymphocyte numbers among studies.

However, physical fitness might affect leukocyte trafficking in response to acute stressors. It has been shown that physically fit individuals exhibit attenuated lymphocytosis in response to a speech stressor and to a moderate exercise challenge (**Figure 2**). This blunted response to a stressor is not derived from the differences in cell numbers at rest and is only observed among T lymphocytes, not in monocytes, granulocytes, or NK cells. In addition, a significant attenuation of demargination is found for $CD4^+$ memory T cells that do not express the activation marker HLA-DR after exercise in fit individuals. Such findings imply that the effects of fitness on leukocytosis is cell type and activation stage specific.

Underlying Mechanisms and Mediators

How do stress-induced changes in leukocyte trafficking occur? How is selective and cell type-dependent mobilization explained? What factors influence CAM expression during leukocyte trafficking? There are two main underlying physiological pathways that address these questions.

Sympathetic Nervous System Activation

There is widespread direct communication between the sympathetic nervous system (SNS) and the immune system. Adrenergic projections and sympathetic nerve terminals are found in many organs of the immune system, including the spleen. Sympathetic agonists (catecholamines) are rapidly released from nerve endings following acute SNS activation and act directly on α- and β-adrenergic receptors. β_2-adrenergic receptors are found on all white blood cells, including lymphocytes, neutrophils, and monocytes. Activation of these receptors leads to lymphocytosis. Adherence of NK cells to endothelial cells is decreased in a dose-dependent manner after adding β_2-adrenergic agonists *in vitro*. As described previously, infusing the β-adrenergic agonist isoproterenol leads to demargination and trafficking of leukocyte subsets similar to those seen following a stressor. Catecholamines lead to increased recirculation of lymphocytes into the blood by decreasing the affinity of the lymphocyte to the vessel wall, and possibly through a shedding of adhesion molecules such as CD62L and ICAM-1 from the cell surface.

The HPA Axis

Neuroendocrine responses to stressors include increased levels of glucocorticoids in circulation as a result of HPA activation. Glucocorticoids are known for their immunosuppressive effects. Their pharmacological administration has wide-ranging effects, including the modulation of metabolic processes and immunosuppression. Glucocorticoids are widely used in the treatment of many inflammatory conditions, influencing the migration of immune cells to infected tissues. Studies demonstrate that glucocorticoids reduce the number of circulating leukocytes and downregulate cytokine production and chemotaxis, as well as downregulate adhesion molecules such as E-selectin and ICAM-1. *In vivo* studies demonstrate time-related effects of dexamethasone on ICAM-I expression, in which prolonged treatment (but not single acute doses) significantly reduces ICAM-1 expression on monocytes.

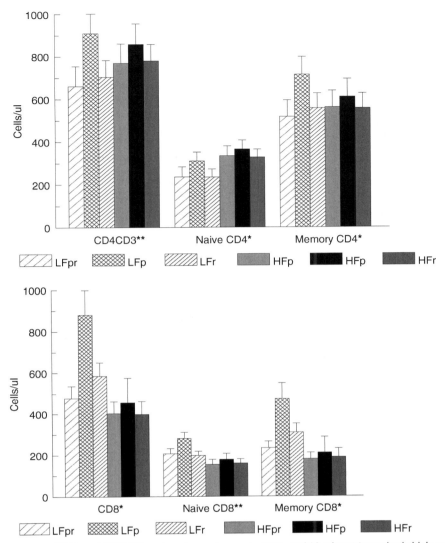

Figure 2 Naive and memory CD4⁺ and CD8⁺ T lymphocyte numbers pre-, post-, and 10-min postexercise in high- vs. low-fitness groups. Physically fit subjects showed reduced CD4⁺ and memory CD4⁺ T cell responses (indicated by *) but not in naive CD4 T cell responses. Fit subjects showed smaller CD8⁺ naive and memory cell responses. LF, low fitness; HF, high fitness; pr, pre-exercise; p, postexercise; r, recovery; * and ** denote significant ($p < 0.05$ and $p < 0.01$, respectively) time by group interactions (mean ± standard error).

Mediators

As with many other physiological processes, interindividual factors such as age, diet, gender, ethnicity, and psychosocial characteristics can affect leukocyte trafficking in response to stressors. Depression, lack of social support, or hostile personality, for example, can all lead to altered immune cell responses to acute stress. Although studies examining the effects of gender as a possible mediator of leukocyte trafficking during stressors have been inconsistent, studies examining the effects of reproductive hormones do indicate an effect. A low- versus a high-carbohydrate meal leads to attenuated leukocyte and neutrophil trafficking in response to exercise. Although aging appears to

be associated with a general decline in immune function, including a loss of naive T lymphocytes, few studies have systematically investigated whether age influences stress-induced leukocyte trafficking. As discussed earlier, physical fitness is a very important mediator of leukocyte responses to both exercise and psychological stressors.

Potential Clinical Implications

Are there potential clinical implications associated with exaggerated or perhaps diminished leukocyte trafficking responses to stressors? A few studies have endeavored to address this issue by studying clinical populations. For example, hypertension, or high blood pressure, is a well-established risk factor for atherosclerosis, which is an inflammatory disease. Patients with hypertension have elevated endothelial expression of the adhesion molecules ICAM-1, VCAM-1, E-selectin, and P-selectin. This enhanced CAM activation attracts leukocytes and monocytes to adhere to the endothelial surface, supporting inflammation. As previously discussed, the SNS plays a prominent role in leukocyte trafficking and CAM expression. Elevated sympathetic nerve activity and circulating catecholamines levels are common in hypertension. It is reasonable, therefore, to hypothesize that the sympathetic mediation of leukocyte trafficking and cell adhesion may be accentuated in hypertension. Incidentally, in addition to direct SNS activation effects, greater hemodynamic forces found in hypertension also contribute to the phenomenon of endothelial activation and increased expression of endothelial CAMs.

Findings show a greater expression of LFA-1 (CD11a) on circulating lymphocytes at rest and in response to stressors in hypertensive patients. In addition, the adhesion of lymphocytes to endothelial cells in hypertensives is enhanced in response to the stressor of exercise but reduced in people with normal blood pressure (**Figure** 3). Such differences in the adhesion characteristics of lymphocytes in hypertensives following stress might have clinical

relevance, as adherent mononuclear cells mediate endothelial injury associated with atherosclerosis as well as with ischemic disorders. However, whether such stressor-related effects on leukocytes are related to the etiology and/or progression of vessel disease in hypertension has yet to be demonstrated. More research is needed on the possible clinical relevance of stress-induced changes of immune cell adhesion before the significance of such observations can be fully understood. Stress-induced leukocyte trafficking also merits further investigation of its clinical implications in other clinical populations, including patients with cancer, multiple sclerosis, and rheumatoid arthritis.

Summary

Circulation of immune cells throughout the body is a critical immunosurveillance process for host defense. Many studies demonstrate mobilization of immune cells in response to acute and chronic psychological and physical stressors. Stress-induced leukocytosis is cell subset specific and there is a dose response based on the intensity of the stressor. CAMs, including CD62L, CD11a, and ICAM-1, play a crucial role in the phenomenon. Both the SNS and the HPA axis help regulate immune cell responses to a variety of stressors. Numerous important questions still need to be answered, including the identity of interindividual factors that significantly mediate immune cell responses to stressors, as well as the potential clinical implications of this interesting effect of stressors on the trafficking of immune cells in the blood.

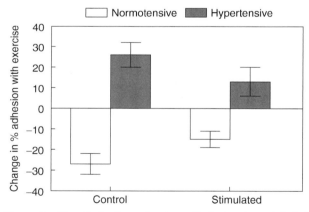

Figure 3 The effects of hypertension on the leukocyte-endothelial adhesion response to exercise. Percentage change of peripheral blood mononuclear cell (PBMC) adhesion to human umbilical venous endothelial cells (HUVEC) under control and cytokine-stimulated conditions at rest and in response to acute exercise in hypertensive patients and normotensive subjects. In response to exercise, PBMC adhesion to HUVECs was increased in hypertensives but decreased in normotensives under control and stimulated conditions ($p < 0.03$). Reprinted from Mills PJ, Maisel AS, Ziegler MG, et al. 2000. Peripheral blood mononuclear cell-endothelial adhesion in human hypertension following exercise, *Journal of Hypertension*. 18(12), 1804 with permission from the publisher.

See Also the Following Articles

Desensitization; Infection; Lymphocytes; Natural Killer (NK) Cells.

Further Reading

Bosch, J. A., Berntson, G. G., Cacioppo, J. T. and Marucha, P. T. (2005). Differential mobilization of functionally distinct natural killer subsets during acute psychological stress. *Psychosomatic Medicine* 67(3), 366–375.

Goebel, M. U. and Mills, P. J. (2000). Acute psychological stress and exercise and changes in peripheral leukocyte adhesion molecule expression and density. *Psychosomatic Medicine* 62(5), 664–670.

Hong, S., Johnson, T. A., Farag, N., Guy, H., Matthews, S. and Mills, P. J. (2005). Attenuation of T lymphocyte demargination and adhesion molecule expression in response to moderate exercise in physically fit individuals. *Journal of Applied Physiology* 98(3), 1057–1063.

Kiecolt-Glaser, J. K., McGuire, L., Robles, T. F. and Glaser, R. (2002). Psychoneuroimmunology and psychosomatic medicine: back to the future. *Psychosomatic Medicine* **64**, 15–28.

Mills, P. J., Farag, N. H., Hong, S., Kennedy, B. P., Berry, C. C. and Ziegler, M. G. (2003). Immune cell CD62L and CD11a expression in response to a psychological stressor in human hypertension. *Brain Behavior & Immunity* **17**(4), 260–267.

Sackstein, R. (2005). The lymphocyte homing receptors: gatekeepers of the multistep paradigm. *Current Opinion in Hematology* **12**(6), 444–450.

Leukocytes   *See:* Leukocyte Trafficking and Stress.

Life Events and Health

P Surtees and N Wainwright
Strangeways Research Laboratory and University of Cambridge, Cambridge, UK

Measurement
Health Associations
Individual Differences

Glossary

Annual prevalence	The proportion of people identified with a disease or other characteristic at any time during the period of a year.
Life event	A discrete incident or circumstance that may disrupt life, may require adaptation, and may be associated with, or result in, physical and/or emotional health change.
Major depressive disorder	A health state characterized by sustained feelings of sadness, hopelessness, helplessness, and worthlessness that is often also accompanied by suicidal thoughts, an inability to concentrate or to take pleasure in activities that were once enjoyable, and sleep, appetite, and memory problems.
Prospective cohort study	A study population defined according to risk factor exposure and prospectively followed up, for example, to ascertain incident disease endpoints.
Record linkage study	A study that brings together information included in two or more records based upon a unique identifying system.

On January 17, 1995, at 5:46:52 a.m., the southern part of Hyogo Prefecture in Japan was struck, without warning, by the Hanshin-Awaji earthquake, which measured 7.2 on the Richter scale and lasted for around 20 s. During the 3 months following this unexpected catastrophic natural disaster, in the districts of Awaji Island near the earthquake epicenter, heart attack rates increased by 50% and stroke rates by 90% in comparison with the same observation period during the previous year. Survivors in areas with the greatest loss and destruction of housing experienced the highest subsequent heart attack rates. While the occurrence of a profoundly stressful life event, such as the Hanshin-Awaji earthquake, provides a clear and dramatic incident from which to assess subsequent health, the attribution of health change to life events experienced more commonly across a lifetime is less straightforward.

Measurement

Life event assessment techniques have evolved to include the use of checklists and interview methods and have been used in a wide variety of research designs to aid understanding of the risk of life events to health.

Checklists

During the late 1940s, Thomas Holmes and colleagues at the University of Washington started to investigate the relationship between adjustment to social stress and illness onset using a self-administered instrument, the Schedule of Recent Experience (SRE). The SRE included a list of 43 life change events intended to represent most circumstances experienced by the patient groups studied, and to which differing degrees of readjustment were required. A subsequent scaling study was designed to take account of both the intensity and the relative time judged to be needed to adjust to each life event on the list. This Social Readjustment Rating Scale (SRRS) included the life events ranked according to these degrees of readjustment – subsequently termed life change units (LCUs). The event of highest rank was death of spouse (with a mean value score of 100), relative to marriage, with a mean value score of 50, and, for example, death of close friend, which scored 37. Typically the LCUs for all events reported on the checklist to have been experienced during a given time period (e.g., the past year) were summed to give a measure of the cumulative social stress experienced. With varying degrees of modification, the SRRS has served as a model of a questionnaire format for assessing life event experience in relation to health. For example, in psychiatry, scaling studies focused on the capacity of life events to induce distress and were scaled in terms of their associated upset or undesirability. While the checklist approach provided a powerful impetus to study the association between life events and illness, these techniques attracted criticism. This stemmed from suggestions that the circumstances to be rated were defined vaguely, resulting in variability in item interpretation, that symptoms were included in the event lists, and that the assumption of additivity of event effects was untested. Despite these criticisms, the list techniques can provide a reliable assessment of the occurrence of specified adverse experiences, although they may be limited in their capacity to provide details of the context surrounding their occurrence.

Interviews

The Life Events and Difficulties Schedule (LEDS), an interview method for the assessment of stressful life events, was developed in the late 1960s and over the subsequent 30 years by George Brown and colleagues at London University. In contrast to the early respondent-based checklist assessment techniques, this approach was based on using the interviewer as the measuring instrument. Through the LEDS, ratings of adverse experience followed from consideration of both the context and meaning of the immediate circumstances associated with a stressful situation. Use of the LEDS was designed to provide measures of the long-term threat of life events experienced, to attempt to date their occurrence accurately, and

to rate ongoing long-term difficulties. In addition, LEDS-based research drew attention to the importance of distinguishing the extent to which life events and long-term difficulties could be illness-related in order to help clarify their etiological significance for illness onset.

However, Bruce Dohrenwend and colleagues, at Columbia University, New York, raised fundamental criticisms of the LEDS core ratings of contextual threat. These criticisms were based upon their view that the contextual ratings represented a nonexplicit distillation of the event, the social circumstances surrounding its occurrence, and the personal history of the person who experienced the event, into one measure. Dohrenwend and colleagues argued that these situational and personal variables may themselves be important risk factors for illness, therefore creating ambiguity in understanding precisely which aspects of the stress process were associated with the illness outcomes of interest. They attempted to address these perceived problems with the LEDS approach through developing their own theoretical framework and measurement approach, using the Structured Event Probe and Narrative Rating method (SEPRATE) of life events measurement. The SEPRATE semistructured interview method was designed to provide measures that distinguished between the life event, the ongoing social situation present before event occurrence (for example, employment circumstances), and the personal dispositions and characteristics of the person who had experienced the life event. While the LEDS and SEPRATE share similarities in methodological approach, they differ markedly in their representation and rating of life event experience.

Health Associations

Efforts to synthesize research findings relating life events to health outcomes have been limited by the rarity of studies that meet stringent research design requirements. A commonly used set of criteria to help establish causality was proposed by the epidemiologist and statistician Sir Austin Bradford Hill. These criteria include consideration of the strength of the association, whether it is consistent (i.e., repeatedly demonstrated in different populations), whether there is evidence of temporality (i.e., the presence of the risk factor precedes onset of disease), and whether a dose–response relationship exists (i.e., disease risk increases monotonically with increasing exposure). These criteria have not yet been fully met for any health outcome following from stressful life event experience. However, increasingly persuasive evidence is now accumulating in relation to the onset, and subsequent prognosis, of some health outcomes.

Life Events and Psychological Health

Evidence from both prospective cohort and record linkage studies has consistently shown an association between the experience of stressful life events and the subsequent onset of episodes of major depressive disorder. The strength of this association has been shown to vary according to the way in which life events were assessed: generally stronger associations were reported when events were assessed using the LEDS approach, rather than through use of the list techniques such as the SRE. These studies have also suggested evidence of a dose–response relationship, with the risk of depressive disorder onset increasing broadly in step with the severity of the events experienced. A dose–response association between the number of recently reported stressful life events and the annual prevalence of depressive disorder is illustrated in **Figure 1**.

Record linkage studies, through their use of very large populations, provide a potentially powerful research design with which to investigate the relationship between severely stressful events and psychiatric health. For example, one study linked records from the Danish Civil Registration System with the Danish Psychiatric Central Register to investigate the association between death of a child and subsequent

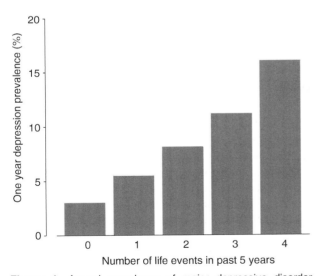

Figure 1 Annual prevalence of major depressive disorder according to the number of moderately or extremely upsetting (non-health-related) life events reported during the previous 5 years. Based upon 20 921 participants in the European Prospective Investigation into Cancer (EPIC)-Norfolk study in the United Kingdom.

parental admission to psychiatric hospital. Based on over a million persons identified in the registers and almost 12 000 deaths of children aged under 18 years, the study revealed a 67% increased risk of hospital admission for any psychiatric condition among the parents who had lost a child, with the risk being greatest for mothers and most pronounced for admission with a depressive condition.

The relationship between chronic enduring or progressively deteriorating stressful circumstances and psychiatric health is complex and difficult to study. For example, changes in the Japanese economy during the late 1980s, subsequently associated with escalating bankruptcy rates, has been interpreted as a significant contributory cause of increases in the male suicide rate, stemming from the high proportion of suicide notes in which economic circumstances were the stated reason for suicide. The Japanese male suicide rate increased from around 25 per 100 000 during the mid 1990s to over 35 per 100 000 at the beginning of the twenty-first century, when over 30 000 Japanese per year committed suicide, by then around twice the rate observed in the United States.

Life Events and Physical Health

Clinicians have long suspected stressful life events to be associated with the onset of physical disease (for example, this was noted by Sir James Paget, the surgeon and pathologist, in his *Clinical Lectures and Essays* in 1875). The assessment of stressful life event experience within chronic disease epidemiological study settings presents substantial methodological challenges related to cost, the need to limit participant burden, and the requirement of asking perhaps tens of thousands of study participants, ideally when they are all healthy, to recall their experience of stressful events over a particular time period. In consequence, within large-scale prospective cohort studies, the assessment of stressful life events has been largely restricted either to the use of short event lists or to specific events (e.g., bereavement). Record linkage research designs have investigated the risk of chronic disease and mortality associated with specific stressful events; for example, following the death or serious illness of a child or loss of a partner or twin. Both prospective cohort and record linkage studies have now provided evidence that under some circumstances such events may increase risk for congenital malformations, heart disease, and perhaps some cancers, just a few among many physical health outcomes studied.

Heart disease   Sudden and particularly catastrophic life events, such as the 1995 Hanshin-Awaji earthquake in Japan, the 1999 Ji-Ji earthquake in Taiwan, and the terrorist attacks on the World Trade Center in New York on September 11, 2001, have been associated with transient increases in blood pressure, increases in ventricular arrhythmias among patients with cardioverter defibrillators, and increases in the incidence of fatal and nonfatal cardiovascular events. Further, use of national registers in Denmark has shown that experiencing the unexpected death of a child (under 18 years) is associated with an increased subsequent risk of a heart attack (myocardial infarction) in the bereaved parents. The association between chronic stressful circumstances and cardiovascular events is less certain, but there is an increasing international consensus that a combination of high work demands and low job control is associated with cardiovascular events in certain occupational groups and that caregiving responsibilities for a disabled or ill partner for 9 or more h per week is associated with an increased risk of incident heart disease events in women.

Cancer Studies meeting stringent research design criteria that have been devoted to evaluating life events as possible determinants of cancer incidence and progression are rare. Evidence for the association between life events and cancer incidence is often contradictory, based on studies that often rely on imprecise case ascertainment methods, may be prone to recall bias in their assessment of life event histories, are able to include relatively few participants that develop cancer, and may be unable to include adjustment for factors known to be associated with cancer outcomes. Some of these limitations were overcome in a prospective study of a twin cohort of 10 808 women in Finland. During 15 years of follow-up, 180 incident breast cancers were diagnosed, and the results suggested that life events experienced during the 5 years before entry into the study were associated with an increased risk of breast cancer during follow-up. Three specific life events were found to be associated with an increase in breast cancer risk: divorce or separation, death of a husband, and death of a close relative or friend. The association between widowhood and divorce and subsequent cancer risk compared to married people has been investigated in a large Swedish study. A relatively consistent pattern of cancer risk was found in the divorced compared to the widowed (both with increases and decreases in risk, according to cancer site) that collectively may reflect changes in lifestyle following partner loss. Similar conclusions have been suggested to account for the evidence from record linkage studies that have found a slightly elevated overall cancer risk in mothers following death of a child.

Individual Differences

There are profound individual differences in the health consequences of stressful life events and difficult circumstances. These differences are most evident through studies of the health outcomes of people subsequent to their exposure to very stressful circumstances, including shipwreck, concentration camp experience, and terrorist attacks. Some people adapt to stressful circumstances more successfully than others. Not all people exposed to adverse or even traumatic circumstance experience health change. Identification of what distinguishes people in the way they are able to manage stressful life events can aid understanding of disease susceptibility and inform the design and delivery of effective care to reduce the long-term health impact of events. For example, a brief questionnaire designed to distinguish the extent to which people are optimistic about their lives and future expectations has shown that optimists have a reduced risk from dying due to cardiovascular causes over a 15-year period and after consideration of traditional risk factors. More direct evidence of individual differences in the capacity to adapt to stressful life events has followed from work originally inspired by Aaron Antonovsky's study of survivors of the Holocaust. This work has revealed how, despite their horrific experiences, some Holocaust survivors had subsequently been able to rebuild their lives successfully. Antonovsky defined sense of coherence (SOC), a theoretical construct based upon these observations, as a flexible and adaptive dispositional orientation enabling successful coping with adverse

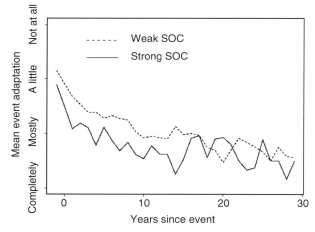

Figure 2 Mean reported adaptation to death of spouse or partner according to the elapsed time since the event occurred and according to sense of coherence (SOC). Based upon 20 921 participants in the European Prospective Investigation into Cancer (EPIC)-Norfolk study in the United Kingdom. Mean adaptation score was calculated from responses to the question "Do you feel that you have got over this now?" (1 = completely, 2 = mostly, 3 = a little, 4 = not at all).

experience. **Figure 2** shows that individuals with a weak SOC report that they take longer to get over the adverse effects of the death of their spouse or partner than those with a strong SOC and illustrates work that has provided support for the idea that SOC distinguishes adaptive capacity to adverse life event experience.

See Also the Following Articles

Cancer; Concentration Camp Survivors; Earthquakes, Stress Effects of; Heart Disease/Attack; Life Events Scale; Major Depressive Disorder; Terrorism.

Further Reading

Antonovsky, A. (1987). *Unraveling the mystery of health.* San Francisco, CA: Jossey-Bass.

Cooper, C. L. (ed.) (2005). *Handbook of stress medicine and health* (2nd edn.) Boca Raton, FL: CRC Press.

Dohrenwend, B. P. (1998). *Adversity, stress and psychopathology.* New York: Oxford University Press.

Giltay, E. J., Kamphuis, M. J., Kalmijn, S., Zitman, F. G. and Kromhout, D. (2006). Dispositional optimism and the risk of cardiovascular death. The Zutphen Elderly Study. *Archives of Internal Medicine* **166**, 431–436.

Hansen, D., Lou, H. C. and Olsen, J. (2000). Serious life events and congenital malformations: a national study with complete follow-up. *Lancet* **356**, 875–880.

Harris, T. (2000). *Where inner and outer worlds meet. Psychosocial research in the tradition of George W. Brown.* London: Routledge.

Holmes, T. H. and Rahe, R. H. (1967). The social readjustment rating scale. *Journal of Psychosomatic Research* **11**, 213–218.

Kessler, R. C. (1997). The effects of stressful life events on depression. *Annual Review of Psychology* **48**, 191–214.

Li, J., Laursen, T. M., Precht, D. H., Olsen, J. and Mortensen, P. B. (2005). Hospitalization for mental illness among parents after the death of a child. *New England Journal of Medicine* **352**, 1190–1196.

Lillberg, K., Verkasalo, P. K., Kaprio, J., Teppo, L., Helenius, H. and Koskenvuo, M. (2003). Stressful life events and risk of breast cancer in 10,808 women: a cohort study. *American Journal of Epidemiology* **157**, 415–423.

Stansfeld, S. and Marmot, M. (2002). *Stress and the heart: psychosocial pathways to coronary heart disease.* London: BMJ Books.

Surtees, P. G., Wainwright, N. W. J. and Khaw, K.-T. (2006). Resilience, misfortune and mortality: evidence that sense of coherence is a marker of social stress adaptive capacity. *Journal of Psychosomatic Research* **61**, 221–227.

Life Events Scale

E Wethington
Cornell University, Ithaca, NY, USA

This article is a revision of the previous edition article by E Wethington, volume 2, pp 618–622, Elsevier Inc.

General Assessment Issues
Major Life Events
Stress Appraisal
Chronic Stressors
Hassles or Daily Events

Glossary

Chronic stressor	An ongoing set of consistent, persistent physically or emotionally arousing demands on an organism; also referred to as a long-term difficulty.
Daily event	See hassle.
Distal stressors	Major events and stressors that occur earlier in life, usually in childhood or adolescence.
Event rating, contextual	An estimate of the severity of a stressor based on the objective demands posed for a particular individual who undergoes a more or less demanding stressor of that type.
Event rating, normative	A population-based estimate of the relative severity of a particular class of stressors.
Hassle	Minor life event whose effects disperse within a day or two; also referred to as a daily event.
Life event	A discrete occurrence believed to arouse a need for adjustment or to create negative emotions and physical reactions.
Proximal stressors	Recent events or stressors (e.g., within the past year).
Risk factor	A condition, such as stressor exposure, predisposing an individual to develop illness.

Stress appraisal	The individual evaluation of a stressor for its impact on well-being.
Stressor exposure	Exposure to life events, chronic stressors, or hassles in the environment.
Threat, contextual	The degree or type of demand posed by a life event or stressor.

A life events scale is a comprehensive list of external events and situations (stressors) that are hypothesized to place demands that tend to exceed the capacity of the average person to adapt. The difficulty in adaptation leads to physical and psychological changes or dysfunction, creating risk for psychological disorder or physical disease.

General Assessment Issues

It is now generally recognized that exposure to stressors in daily life, or over the course of life, is one of the most critical components of health and well-being. However, there remains ambiguity about the dimensions of stressor exposure that are involved in this process, specifically the types of stressors that have the more deleterious effects on health and that are risk factors for the development of physical and psychological illness. Variations in stressor assessment reflect different theories of how and why stressor exposure poses a risk to health.

Life events scales are the most commonly used means of naturalistic assessment of exposure to stressors, in distinction to the manipulation of stressor exposure in experimental research. Assessment of stressor exposure has been dependent on well-established research traditions in stress assessment. The first is the environmental perspective, which focuses on characteristics of events as risks for developing disease. The second is the psychological perspective, which focuses on perceptions and appraisals of threats. A third, and increasingly influential, is the life course perspective, which considers (1) the accumulation of stressors across the life span of individuals, (2) whether exposure to stressors early in life has long-term impact on health and well-being into adulthood, and (3) whether group differences in exposure to stressors (poor versus middle class; minority versus majority ethnic/racial status) are implicated in group-level differences in morbidity and mortality.

Four types of naturalistic stressor assessment predominate in the research literature: exposure to out-of-the-ordinary, demanding events, such as divorce, that have the capacity to change the patterns of life or arouse very unpleasant feelings (life events); self-reports of perceived stressfulness and appraisals of threat posed by events (stress appraisals); enduring or recurrent difficulties and strains in an area of life (chronic stressors); and exposure to smaller, relatively minor, and normally less emotionally arousing events whose effects disperse within hours or within a day or two (daily events or hassles). Although conceived of primarily as comprehensive lists of exposure to discrete events outside the organism, life events scales often combine two or more of these approaches, sometimes including appraisals of stressors, measuring dimensions such as severity, frequency, controllability, and expectedness of events.

A frequent goal of research on stressor exposure is to establish the relationship between exposure to stressors and some health outcome in order to evaluate stress as a risk factor for disease. If the research question is to estimate the size of the association between stressor exposure and distressed mood, then the usual procedure is to use a retrospective, simple count of likely stressful life events occurring in the months prior to the measurement of mood. However, if the researcher is interested primarily in the relationship between stressor exposure and the onset, timing of onset, or recurrence of onset of a major clinical disorder, then the stressor exposure measure shifts to a determination of the type, severity, and timing of events and preexisting chronic stressors that preceded the onset of disorder. Studies of daily variation in mood or of the onset of more transient physical disorders such as colds or body aches use measures of short-term exposure to relatively minor stressors, daily events or hassles, sometimes in combination with measures of preexisting chronic stressors. Studies focusing on diseases that develop over long periods of time, such as heart disease, tend to use measures of exposure to long-term, recurrent, and persistent chronic stressors in major life roles. In practice, these methods are increasingly combined as more investigators apply the life course perspective to research on health and disease. There is considerable interest in combining the measurement of more recent (or proximal) stressors with retrospective measurement of more distal stressors, particularly severely threatening stressor exposures occurring in childhood and adolescence.

Major Life Events

Two contrasting methods of life event measurement have developed: checklist measures and personal interview measures. The latter uses qualitative probes in order to specify more precisely the characteristics of life events believed to produce the actual risk of illness and the timing of life events in relation to the outcome studies. Because of their ease of administration and the amount of exploratory health research conducted, checklist measures predominate in studies of stressor exposure.

Checklist measures were derived from an environmental perspective on stress proposing that the basis of experienced stress is an event that brings about a demand for social, physical, or psychological readjustment. The earliest of these perspectives was the life change-readjustment paradigm, developed by Holmes and Rahe in1967. Other theoretical perspectives on stress, such as those developed by Lazarus, Dohrenwend, and Brown, have augmented their approach in significant ways.

A typical checklist measure consists of a series of yes/no questions, asking participants to report whether any event of situation like the one described has occurred over a past period of time (from a few months to a year or more). The typical checklist measure is self-administered, although there are exceptions. Many checklist measures have been elaborated to assess more detailed information about the time of occurrence and severity. For example, some ask respondents to report the date of occurrence. Others ask for a brief written description of the situation or who else was involved in the situation. Still others ask respondents to rate the relative stressfulness of the event (from "not at all" to "very"). Self-report descriptive questions are used to estimate the severity of the event and its likely relationship to an outcome. However, the typical checklist measure does not rely on descriptive information. A typical measure sums the absolute number of event reports or sums investigator-assigned severity ratings for the events reported. The investigator-assigned ratings, termed normative, are survey-established estimates of the relative severity of stressors such as deaths, job losses, marital problems, and moves. Checklist methods yield a summary score of the estimated, normatively derived stressfulness of changes experienced over a period of time. Related to the latter point, checklist measures tend to be used in studies that use continuous symptom or mood measures as outcomes, although they are also sometimes used in exploratory studies of the onset of illness.

The ancestor of most current measures is the Holmes and Rahe social readjustment rating scale. This measure included both positive and negative events because Holmes and Rahe theorized that change per se was associated with changes in health status. Over time, checklist (and other) life events measures have moved away from the change-readjustment paradigm to an emphasis on negative or undesirable events. This trend was based on much replicated findings that undesirable events are more predictive of health problems than positive events are. Life event scales intended for use in the general population have become more comprehensive and inclusive of events occurring to women, minorities, and other populations. Concomitantly, researchers have developed comprehensive events lists for age groups and special populations, including children, adolescents, and the elderly.

Despite their popularity, checklist measures have also been much criticized, most of these criticisms casting doubt on their reliability and validity as measures of stressor exposure. Criticisms include the vagueness and generality of the questions, which may lead respondents to misreport or overreport the occurrence of events or to report minor events as major. Life event scales have also been criticized for including events that are confounded with feeling states or psychiatric illness. There is also considerable evidence that life events scales suffer from recency bias: respondents are more likely to recall events that occur in the last month or two than those that occurred a year ago. Recall of events, moreover, is affected by mood at the time of recall.

The early development of personal interview methods for assessing life events used a theoretical perspective distinct from the change-readjustment paradigm, which informed the life events checklists. The major developer of interview methods, George W. Brown, proposed that social and environmental changes (and anticipations of those changes) that threaten the most strongly held emotional commitments are the basis for experienced severe stress. This perspective also holds that severe, rather than minor, stressors threaten health, distinguishing it from both change-readjustment and hassles paradigms.

Interview measures are not used commonly, primarily because of their greater expense and complexity. Investigators tend to use them under the following circumstances: (1) when more precise severity ratings are required; (2) where the relative timing of stress exposure and illness onset is critical to the study; (3) when the occurrence of an event, or series of events, may be related to respondent's preexisting illness or behavior (formally termed, independence from disorder); and (4) when there is interest in the specific effects of different types and severities of stressors on specific disease outcomes. Promoters of interview measures also claim that they are more comprehensive, reliable, and valid than checklist measures, although the debate is unresolved on this point. The complexity of interview methods precludes their use in lower-budget, very-large-sample (2000+), or more exploratory studies.

The Life Events and Difficulties Schedule (LEDS), developed by Brown and Harris, is the most widely used personal interview method. There are also several other personal interview methods, some based on different rating systems (e.g., Paykel's Interview for Recent Life Events and Dohrenwend's Structured Event Probe and Narrative Rating Method). All are semistructured survey instruments assessing a wide variety of stressors, many including more distal stressors that may have occurred in childhood or adolescence. The interviews consist of a series of questions asking whether certain types of stressors have occurred over the past 12 months (or longer) and a set of guidelines or optional probes for determining more objective features of those events. The probes are used by investigators to rate the long-term contextual threat of events; contextual-threat rating is the key component of these methods because the occurrence of a severely threatening event is believed to pose a risk for the onset of illness. Contextual ratings for different types of events are documented in dictionaries and available to those who complete training in the interview methods.

Stress Appraisal

Appraisal plays an important part in life event scales, as well as theories of the stress process, most notably the transactional model of stress developed and refined by Lazarus and Folkman. The appraisal of stressors is believed to underlie the emotional experience of stress. Measures of appraisal focus on the degree to which an event threatens well-being or threatens to overwhelm a person's resources to cope.

Life event scales differ in whether they explicitly include appraisal as a component or explicitly exclude appraisal. Several measures of stressor exposure consist of assessments of how well an individual coped with stressors (although these measures are not predominant in health research). Checklist and interview measures of life events, for the most part, aim to exclude appraisal from stressor exposure assessment, although some explicitly do not. Those that exclude appraisal do so because of concerns that stress appraisal is confounded with the health and psychological outcomes that stressor exposure is supposed to predict. Indeed, researchers have speculated that some stress appraisals are caused by underlying, persistent mood disturbance or ill health, rather than vice versa. The transactional model of stress posits that appraisals can be measured separately.

Chronic Stressors

Recent research on stress and illness has turned toward emphasizing the role of persistent, continuous, or regular exposure to stressors as an important risk factor for the development of disease. There are four main methods by which researchers measure chronic stress: (1) multi-item self-report interviews and questionnaires covering ranges of situations believed to produce chronic stressor exposure in a given setting, such as work-role demands, conflicts, and ambiguity; (2) intensive longitudinal surveys, such as daily-diary or experience-sampling methods, primarily using structured questions at regular (diary) or random (experience-sampling) intervals; (3) personal interview (contextual) measurement in life event interview instruments such as the LEDS; and (4) third-party observations of those believed to be at risk for stress exposure. The self-report interview or questionnaire is the most widely used method. Multi-item measures of chronic-stressors are an important class of life events scales.

A typical measure of chronic stressors is a set of questions designed to assess either the frequency or the severity of commonly occurring stressors in important life roles, such as work, marriage, and parenting. The strength of the multi-item approach is its grounding in the detailed, multidimensional assessment of environmental factors known to produce chronic stress, such as work and family. A weakness of the approach for some investigations is that the questions may be confounded with stress appraisal, particularly those scales assessing stressor severity.

Hassles or Daily Events

The research perspective in which measures of hassles were developed, the transactional model of stress (Lazarus), differs significantly from the research perspective in which major life event scales were developed. The hassles paradigm focuses attention on the potentially deleterious ways in which minor stressors, even those whose effects are relatively fleeting, can have negative impacts on health. Measures of hassles are life events scales, but assess exposure to minor hassles such as traffic jams, missed appointments, and quarrels with children. Although such events might in fact be major events for some people, the assumption of the hassles paradigm is that they are made more or less severe by the ways in which a person appraises and copes with the event.

Methods assessing daily events or hassles rely on diary methods of collection. These methods require participants to keep records of small events occurring over a given period of time, usually 1 day or a 24-h period, although weekly diaries have also been used. There are multiple styles of measurement: (1) open-ended approaches, which ask respondents to describe bothersome events of the day (not unlike personal interview measures, but usually self-administered rather than conducted in person); (2) structured question approaches, which are simple yes/no response questions modeled on life events checklists; and (3) combinations of checklists with open-ended questions. Hassles scales are almost always administered in tandem with measures of stress appraisal.

Current hassles scales share the strengths and weaknesses of related approaches to the measurement of more major life events. Because diary methods of data collection rely on written and self-report, there is concern that they may confound objective event occurrence with unmeasured appraisal process. Almeida's Daily Inventory of Stressful Events uses telephone interviews and investigator ratings of narrative event descriptions to reduce some types of appraisal bias. Experience sampling methods, which involve beeping a respondent at random times during the day and asking questions about the current situation, have emerged as an alternative method for measuring daily stressor exposure.

See Also the Following Articles

Environmental Factors; Life Events and Health.

Further Reading

Almeida, D. M., Wethington, E. and Kessler, R. C. (2002). The Daily Inventory of Stressful Events (DISE): an investigator-based approach for measuring daily stressors. *Assessment* 9, 41–55.

Brown, G. W. and Harris, T. O. (1978). *Social origins of depression: a study of depressive disorder in women.* New York: Free Press.

Brown, G. W. and Harris, T. O. (eds.) (1989). *Life events and illness.* New York: Guildford.

Cohen, S., Kessler, R. C. and Gordon, L. U. (eds.) (1995). *Measuring stress: a guide for health and social scientists.* New York: Oxford University Press.

Dohrenwend, B. S., Krashnoff, L., Ashkenasy, A. R., et al. (1978). Exemplification of a method for scaling life events: The PERI life events scale. *Journal of Health and Social Behavior* 19, 205–229.

Dohrenwend, B. P., Raphael, K. G., Schwartz, S., Stueve, A. and Skodol, A. (1993). The structured event probe and narrative rating method for measuring stressful life events. In: Goldberger, L. & Breznitz, S. (eds.) *Handbook of stress: theoretical and clinical aspects*, pp. 174–199 New York: Free Press.

Elder, G. H., George, L. K. and Shanahan, M. (1996). Psychosocial stress over the life course. In: Kaplan, H. B. (ed.) *Psychosocial stress: perspectives on structure, theory, life course, and methods*, pp. 247–292, San Diego, CA: Academic Press.

Holmes, T. H. and Rahe, R. H. (1967). The social readjustment rating scale. *Journal of Psychosomatic Research* 11, 213–218.

Kanner, A. D., Coyne, J. C., Schaefer, C., et al. (1981). Comparison of two methods of stress measurement: daily hassles and uplifts versus major life events. *Journal of Behavioral Medicine* 4, 1–39.

Lazarus, R. S. (1999). *Stress and emotion.* New York: Springer.

Lazarus, R. S. and Folkman, S. (1984). *Stress, appraisal and coping.* New York: Springer.

Paykel, E. S. (1997). The interview for recent life events. *Psychological Medicine* 27, 301–310.

Stone, A. A. and Shiffman, S. (2000). Capturing momentary self-report data: A proposal for reporting guidelines. *Annals of Behavioral Medicine* 24, 236–243.

Lifestyle Changes *See:* Life Events and Health; Life Events Scale.

Lockerbie Air Crash, Stress Effects of

H Livingston
Dykebar Hospital, Paisley, UK
M Livingston
Southern General Hospital, Glasgow, UK

This article is a revision of the previous edition article
by H Livingston and M Livingston, volume 2, pp 629–633,
© 2000, Elsevier Inc.

Researching the Impact of Disasters on Elderly People –
  Some Methodological Issues
What Happened to the Elderly at Lockerbie
What Do We Know about the Response of Elderly People
  to Experiencing Disasters?
Future Research

Glossary

Depression	A disorder of lowered mood typically associated with the loss of some or all of the following: interest, energy, pleasure, appetite, weight, concentration, and self-esteem. Disturbance of sleep, feelings of guilt, and wishing for death are also typical of depression.
Posttraumatic stress disorder (PTSD)	An anxiety disorder triggered by a traumatic and threatening event or events. Symptoms of PTSD are characteristically related to reexperiencing the event, the avoidance of triggers associated with the event, and increased arousal.

Researching the Impact of Disasters on Elderly People – Some Methodological Issues

Pan-Am flight 103 exploded in mid-air on December 21, 1988, over the small Scottish town of Lockerbie. This disaster continues to provoke media interest, not least because of the controversy over who were the perpetrators. The fireball of burning aviation fuel not only caused the death of all on board the aircraft but also death and injury to the inhabitants of the town. Survivors often had the harrowing experience of witnessing the mutilated bodies of the victims scattered over a wide area of the locality. The town hall was turned into a temporary mortuary as an army of police, firefighters, and other rescue services descended on Lockerbie. Disasters such as Lockerbie, the Hillsborough football stadium tragedy in England, and Piper Alpha, in which an oil rig in the North Sea caught fire, provide unique opportunities to research mental disorder. The main factor in the etiology of the subsequent psychiatric problems – the traumatic stressor – is known in a disaster. This is an unusual occurrence, not only in mental health research but also in psychiatric clinical practice.

However, there are a number of special methodological problems in postdisaster research. Obviously disaster research must be retrospective, an assessment of an event that has occurred generally as a random act of nature or as the result of unforeseen human error. The presence of a large number of health-care professionals and other services brought to the site of the disaster may affect the research outcome in several ways. (In the case of Lockerbie the town's population increased from 3500 to 10,000 virtually overnight.) The health-care and support services may be effective and succeed in reducing the level of distress experienced by the disaster victims, for example through the effects of early psychological intervention programs, although these remain controversial. In addition, the psychological impact of the disaster on the rescue and recovery workers themselves is often considerable, contributes to the overall rate and level of psychological distress and psychopathology that results, and is often little acknowledged by the workers themselves until they become dysfunctional at work. This is often because of a culture in the rescue services such as the police and the armed forces that encourages a macho image and in which the acknowledgment of emotional problems is perceived by staff workers to have an adverse effect on careers. Many of the staff workers in these services are young and ill-prepared for tasks such as collecting and identifying human remains, having never previously witnessed death and dying. They are required to work at a disaster site that may be some distance from their own homes and usual family and friend support networks. The consequent media attention and the possibility of compensation for psychological damage as well as physical injury and material loss are additional factors that have to be considered in a disaster research design.

The method of assessment is important also in postdisaster studies. A desire for compensation may (in theory at least) lead to a desire on the part of respondents to fake bad, or generate higher than warranted scores of distress. This is a phenomenon that is of even greater concern in the Internet era because of the ready access to questionnaires listing, for example, the phenomena of PTSD. In our view, therefore, such research should include not only self-report rating-scale measures but also some more objective evaluations such as clinical diagnostic assessments.

PTSD may persist for many years. A large study of Vietnam veterans found that the prevalence of PTSD was 15% after 19 years. It seems reasonable to expect that a significant number of disaster victims will continue to experience the psychiatric consequences of trauma into old age. This was certainly our impression when we were invited to examine survivors of the so-called Clydebank Blitz, the heavy German bombing of a small Scottish industrial town, important for the manufacture of ships and armaments, in March 1941 during World War II. The survivors of this event were recently encouraged to appeal to the benefits authorities in the United Kingdom for a war pension to compensate for the psychiatric consequences of exposure to two nights of intensive bombing that flattened large areas of the town and led to many casualties. Although not a systematic research study, our clinical impression was that many of these elderly people continued to experience psychiatric symptoms associated with an experience of traumatically induced stress more than 50 years prior to the clinical assessment, including full-blown PTSD.

A review has also examined the differing impact of a range of traumatic occurrences, such as the Holocaust, World War II, and the Vietnam and Korean wars. Curiously, elderly survivors of the Holocaust appeared to function well in life, unlike the combat veterans. In both groups, vivid imagery of what took place persisted, as well as disruption of sleep and a lack of trust in relationships. Furthermore avoidance of potential stressors that carried actual or symbolic relevance to the original traumatizing experience took place because these were likely to provoke a relapse or exacerbation of symptoms.

When the Lockerbie disaster occurred in 1988, there were no published studies on how traumatic stress impacted on elderly people at the time of the stress or soon after. It is possible to speculate that older people, faced with more loss-making events in a longer life, would either be better able to cope as a result or less so because of being sensitized by prior trauma. Solicitors acting for those involved in the Lockerbie explosion sought psychiatric input to assist the insurers in handling claims arising from the psychiatric damage sustained by the victims of the events

of December 1988. We decided therefore to study the clinical impact of traumatic stress on elderly people in the context of this Scottish disaster.

What Happened to the Elderly at Lockerbie

The initial assessment took place approximately 1 year after the incident, but avoided the anniversary of that event; the review took place 2 years later. Subjects were selected from a larger sample of survivors who had claimed that they had been traumatized by the explosion on the basis of a General Health Questionnaire (GHQ) score above the case cut-off level. The 31 elderly people in this category were seen, and their assessments were compared with 24 GHQ-case-designated younger survivors. Nineteen (61%) of the elderly were available for review, 2 had died, 1 was in the hospital for unrelated health problems, 1 had moved, 3 refused to participate, and 5 did not reply. Diagnosis was assigned using the *Diagnostic and statistical manual of mental disorders* (3rd edn. rev.; DSM-III-R). This classification system has since been revised, and DSM-IV is now in use. The psychological impact was measured by the Leeds scales, which assess anxiety and depression; the GHQ28, a measure of global psychological functioning; and the Revised Impact of Events scale (RIE), which quantifies posttraumatic symptoms.

The older survivors did not differ significantly from the younger in GHQ, Leeds, and RIE responses. Average GHQ28 scores were well above case level (score 4/5) 1 year after the disaster in both groups (younger 9.83 [SD, 8.20]; older 11.76 [SD 8.74]; not significant). Anxiety rather than depression tended to predominate on the GHQ and the Leeds scales. The younger and older survivors recorded high scores on the RIE intrusion (younger 15.09 [SD 9.44]; older 18.71 [SD 12.84]; not significant) and avoidance (younger 15.08 [SD 9.99]; older 17.71 [SD 11.76]; not significant) subscales. Clinically, all but five elderly survivors fulfilled DSM-III criteria for PTSD, as did all the younger subjects (Fisher test, not significant).

At the follow-up 2 years later, the proportion of GHQ cases among the elderly survivors had declined from 71 to 47%, but this was not statistically significant. The mean Leeds depression (initially 7.40 [SD 4.40]; at follow-up 3.76 [SD 2.59]; $p < 0.004$) and anxiety (initially 15.47 [SD 10.60]; at follow-up 4.87 [SD 4.87]; $p < 0.001$) ratings had declined significantly (see **Figure 1**). Both avoidance behavior and the level of intrusive thoughts (RIE) had also declined significantly (paired $t = 2.05$, $p = 0.07$; paired $t = 3.69$, $p = 0.003$, respectively) (see **Figure 2**). The proportion

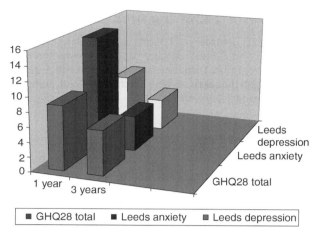

Figure 1 Emotional distress in elderly Lockerbie survivors, Leeds scales and General Health Questionnaire.

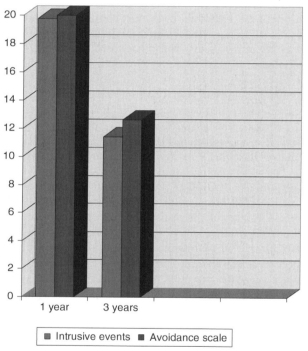

Figure 2 Impact of the disaster on elderly survivors, Revised Impact of Events scale.

of PTSD cases had declined significantly from 14/19 (74%) to 3/19 (16%) (χ^2 10.64, df = 1; not significant). Significantly, no new cases of PTSD had developed during the follow-up period. Persistent PTSD was associated with high Leeds anxiety and GHQ anxiety scores (anxiety and insomnia subscale and social dysfunction subscale). Furthermore, there was a positive correlation between persistent PTSD and a diagnosis of depression on DSM-III criteria, although none between a PTSD diagnosis and individual RIE items.

What Do We Know about the Response of Elderly People to Experiencing Disasters?

At the time we undertook our studies of elderly survivors following the Lockerbie disaster we were unaware of any other work on elderly people in such situations apart from occasional single case studies. Subsequently, reports on elderly victims of two other disasters appeared: the 1988 earthquake in Armenia and the 1995 Hanshin-Awaji earthquake in Japan.

The Armenian earthquake study was undertaken approximately 18 months after that event and involved the assessment of a total of 179 elderly and younger subjects. In young and old, as might be expected, the most traumatized were those who were closest to the earthquake epicenter. Age did not affect the level of distress suffered, regardless of the location of the victim relative to the epicenter, but elderly people tended to experience more symptoms indicative of emotional hyperarousal than did the young and to have less evidence of intrusive symptoms.

Following the Japanese Hanshin-Awaji earthquake, a study of the early psychological impact of the disaster on its victims was carried out that divided the subjects into two groups using an age cut-off of 60 years. Sixty-seven younger subjects and 75 older subjects were seen 3 weeks after the disaster. Fifty younger subjects and 73 older subjects were subsequently reviewed at 8 weeks after the disaster. The older people showed a significant decrease in symptoms in contrast with those under 60. The authors attribute this to the presence of more extensive social networks and some previous disaster experience among the older group of subjects, although it could also be argued on strong clinical grounds that previous experience of severe stress sensitizes rather than protects the sufferer from future stress related reactions.

A subsequent review looked at the effects of PTSD in groups of elderly people who were World War II veterans, were Holocaust survivors, and had experienced a natural disaster in later life. This review suggested that PTSD symptoms in the elderly can be persistent or intermittent. The severity of the trauma and premorbid psychiatric illness predisposed this group to the development of PTSD, and good psychosocial support seemed to protect against it. Older adults did not seem any more predisposed to developing PTSD than younger adults, and the symptoms appeared to be similar across the age groups.

Sadly, several other large-scale natural disasters have occurred recently – in 2004–2005 alone, the Asian tsunami, Hurricane Katrina, and the South Asian earthquake. To date, no studies of the responses of elderly people to these events have been published.

Obviously, the nature of disasters is such that they do not permit prospective study. Our sample of elderly victims was small, but remains the only long-term prospective follow-up of elderly people after a natural disaster. The multiple standardized assessment techniques used, including the application of diagnostic criteria in all cases, showed a remarkable degree of internal consistency. The major methodological flaw is that all our subjects were engaged in the process of claiming compensation from the airline on whose aircraft the explosion took place. We found that the elderly subjects had an initial emotional response to the disaster that was similar to the younger subjects, meeting the psychological case criteria in high numbers and recording high levels of anxiety and diagnosed PTSD. The level of distress diminished significantly over the 3-year time period of the studies, although one in six of the elderly subjects still had PTSD at follow-up, comparable to the findings in a study of the survivors (of all ages) of an Australian brush fire. No links between a PTSD diagnosis and specific aspects of the disaster were found at Lockerbie, although the disaster had a number of unique aspects, including a delay in recognizing that it was a terrorist act and in bringing the suspects to justice, which might be expected to adversely impact survivors' coming to terms with the event (analogous to mourning).

Future Research

Future work should attempt to assess a complete population of elderly survivors following a disaster early on and to review them over the long-term to obtain a clear idea of how traumatic stress in such situations affects older people. This work, just like the disaster-recovery effort, may require international organization, involving the creation of a disaster assessment team that can be mobilized at short notice. Such a team would be preequipped with a research design and appropriate measures. To maintain objectivity, the team needs to avoid being part of the therapeutic input or, indeed, the assessment process if a medical-legal issue is involved, such as a compensation claim. At the same time, the researchers have to strive to avoid artificially creating more stress by prolonging unnecessarily the process of assessment for an already bewildered and traumatized group of people.

See Also the Following Articles

Acute Stress Disorder and Posttraumatic Stress Disorder; Aging and Stress, Biology of; Community Studies; Disaster Syndrome; Disasters and Mass Violence, Public, Effects of; Earthquakes, Stress Effects of; Posttraumatic Stress Disorder, Delayed.

Further Reading

American Psychiatric Association (1987). *Diagnostic and statistical manual of mental disorders* (3rd edn.). Washington, DC: American Psychiatric Association.

Goenjian, A. K., Najarian, L. M., Pynoos, R. S., et al. (1994). Post-traumatic stress disorder in elderly and younger adults after the 1988 earthquake in Armenia. *American Journal of Psychiatry* 151(6), 895–901.

Goldberg, D. (1978). *The manual of the General Health Questionnaire*. Windsor, UK: National Foundation for Educational Research.

Hilton, C. (1997). Media triggers of post-traumatic stress disorder after the second world war. *International Journal of Geriatric Psychiatry* 12(8), 862–867.

Horowitz, M., Wilner, N. and Alvarez, W. (1979). Impact of events scale: a measure of subjective stress. *Psychosomatic Medicine* 41, 209–218.

Kato, H., Asukai, N., Miyake, Y., et al. (1996). Post-traumatic symptoms among younger and elderly evacuees in the early stages following the 1995 Hanshin-Awaji earthquake in Japan. *Acta Psychiatrica Scandinavica* 93(6), 477–481.

Kulka, R. A., Sclenger, W. E. and Fairbank, J. A. (1990). *Trauma and the Vietnam War generation*. New York: Brunner/Mazel.

Livingston, H. M., Livingston, M. G., Brooks, D. N., et al. (1992). Elderly survivors of the Lockerbie air disaster. *International Journal of Geriatric Psychiatry* 7, 725–729.

Livingston, H. M., Livingston, M. G. and Fell, S. (1994). The Lockerbie disaster: a 3 year follow-up of elderly victims. *International Journal of Geriatric Psychiatry* 9, 989–994.

McFarlane, A. C. (1989). The aetiology of post traumatic morbidity, predisposing, precipitating and perpetuating factors. *British Journal of Psychiatry* 154, 221–228.

Sadavoy, J. (1997). Survivors: a review of the late-life effects of prior psychological trauma. *American Journal of Geriatric Psychiatry* 5(4), 287–301.

Snaith, R. P., Bridge, G. W. K. and Hamilton, M. (1976). The Leeds scales for the self assessment of anxiety and depression. *British Journal of Psychiatry* 128, 156–165.

Weintraub, D. and Ruskin, P. E. (1999). Posttraumatic stress disorder in the elderly: a review. *Harvard Review of Psychiatry* 17(3), 144–152.

Loss Trauma

A Bifulco
Royal Holloway, University of London, London, UK

Glossary

Complicated bereavement	A pathological response to loss in which the usual bereavement process is impeded leading to psychopathology.
Eye movement desensitization and reprocessing (EMDR)	A treatment for trauma responses involving desensitization and rapid eye movements.
Loss	Death or long-term separation from a close other, but also experiences with loss of self-identity, security, or trust in others.
Loss trauma	A type of event combined with a pathological response, which involves characteristics of both trauma and loss.
Posttraumatic stress disorder (PTSD)	A classified anxiety disorder, with distinctive symptoms, specifically in response to a traumatic event.
Traumatic event	A type of severe life event, often involving horror, which has fundamental implications for one's safety and place in the world. Can be single or multiple.
Traumatic grief	A pathological response to death of a close other with symptoms similar to PTSD.

Introduction

The investigation of loss trauma is a relatively new psychological subdiscipline, based on the specification of a particular type of traumatic event (that of the death of a close person), with the identification of specific pathological responses, which, although similar to those identified in relation to other traumatic events, have identifiable symptoms associated with a grief response. Its identification as a new focus of study is marked by a new journal (*Journal of Loss and Trauma*) and by organizations such as the National Institute for Trauma and Loss in Children. It is also marked by variants of treatment protocols, which attend specifically to elements of the loss in trauma. However, there is as yet no widely recognized classification of traumatic grief as a disorder. The word trauma has a dual meaning, referring both to an event or circumstance and to the psychological impact of that event on an individual's well-being. In this article these meanings will be differentiated by traumatic event and trauma response.

Loss Trauma Events

A traumatic event is a type of life event, that is, an external circumstance that happens at a defined time. However, as trauma, it constitutes an event with a particularly high level of threat and unpleasantness, which has implications for a person's sense of safety and place in the world. Thus, it is usually sudden and unpredicted and is often accompanied by circumstances that involve horror or intense shock. Trauma events are usually public (e.g., witnessing a suicide, being involved in a terrorist bomb attack, being in the line of a major flood or tsunami) and are common in combat and war situations with both soldiers and civilians. However, trauma can also be private, for example, physical or sexual assault, which involves threat to life or personal integrity. Trauma events can be single or multiple, with different pathological responses associated with them. Loss trauma events are often single when deaths of others are involved. However, a context of severe illness, caring responsibility, or enforced separation may constitute a multiple or chronic course to the traumatic experience.

Loss trauma identifies traumatic circumstances specifically with loss events, usually the death of a close person. This usually involves a parent, partner, child, or close relative or friend, and usually under unexpected or horrific circumstances. Thus, suicides, accidents involving physical mutilation, or circumstances with a random aspect such as freak accidents would all be encompassed in loss trauma events. Loss trauma can also include losses of children or babies, for example, birth of a stillborn child or a child with multiple handicaps or deformities. As a category of event, loss events not only can involve deaths of close others and separations from a close other (e.g., parent, partner, child), but also can involve psychological losses such as loss of security (e.g., loss of job or home), sense of self (e.g., loss of reputation or physical losses such as limbs), or a meaningful relationship (e.g., revelation or betrayal). However, there has been less investigation of these wider losses in terms of loss trauma.

Responses to Loss Trauma

Any traumatic and major loss event will have some immediate psychological consequences such as shock, distress, denial, or numbing and possibly flashbacks to the event. However, in a small proportion of cases, posttraumatic stress disorder (PTSD) will ensue, a classified psychological anxiety disorder. Complicated bereavement responses may set in whereby the bereavement process is incomplete, the loss is unresolved, and traumatic grief may occur. Traumatic grief is seen as a variant of other disorders such as depression and PTSD and does not have a distinct classification in standard psychiatric manuals. However, there is ongoing debate about whether traumatic grief should constitute a disorder in its own right.

Posttraumatic Stress Disorder (PTSD)

PTSD involves response to a traumatic event described as actual or threatened death or serious injury, or a threat to the physical integrity of self or others. PTSD is one of several anxiety disorders. It was originally used for explaining combat reactions in terms of shell shock but is now linked with a range of traumatic events. PTSD symptoms exist for at least 1 month and include preoccupation with the horror of incident, hypervigilant scanning of the environment for potential threat or danger, avoidance of situations, futility about the future, shattered world view, excessive anger, cognitive dysfunction, and prolonged impaired social or occupational functioning. PTSD is often typed by whether the trauma provoking it is acute or chronic, that is, single exposure or multiple incidents and exposure. The latter is considered the most damaging in terms of functioning, particularly when occurring in childhood. In terms of prevalence, while it is estimated that most people (90%) experience at least one traumatic event in a lifetime, only 10% develop a history of PTSD. This is more likely after certain events. For example, prevalence ranges from as high as 50% in response to rape to less than 1% after hearing of serious injury to close relative or friend.

Complicated or Pathological Bereavement

When the response to loss (usually the death of a close person) does not follow the usual progression through the stages of grief work leading to acceptance, it is considered a pathological bereavement response. It impedes the development of new ties and inhibits adaptation to the loss both personally and socially. When this occurs in childhood, it is argued, it impedes adult functioning and leads to long-term problems. However, not all researchers accept the inevitability of grief work and claim that adaptive responses can occur without evidence of following particular stages in the process. Grief work thus may be required only following more severe losses or for individuals with high levels of distress or vulnerability to loss.

Traumatic Grief

Traumatic grief is a relatively new term that combines trauma with bereavement or grief responses. It is provoked by the death of a significant other and includes symptoms similar to PTSD but specifically focused on the lost person, including intrusive, distressing preoccupation with the deceased, hypervigilant scanning of the environment for cues of the deceased, the wish to be reunited with the deceased, separation anxiety features, futility about the future, difficulty acknowledging the death, shattered world view, and anger together with impaired social functioning.

Studies have examined traumatic loss among groups such as elderly caregivers of terminally ill spouses, young adults who lost a friend to suicide, and parents who lost a child in a traffic accident. These have shown ensuing symptoms in two categories: (1) separation distress, involving preoccupation with thoughts of the deceased, longing, searching, loneliness, and impaired functioning, and (2) traumatic distress, feeling disbelief, anger, mistrust, and detachment from others.

Peritraumatic Dissociation

Peritraumatic dissociation is a dissociated response to loss with expression of psychological shock, as indicated by a sense of reality having been abruptly altered. Thus, being in a daze, feeling disoriented, numb, or on automatic pilot, and experiencing the surroundings as unreal are typical, together with staring into space or feeling like a spectator. This response is usually associated with traumatic grief. The greater the experience of shock and overwhelming emotion, the more likely the dissociation, with PTSD following afterward. This is similar to the symptoms described in complicated bereavement or traumatic grief.

Childhood Loss Trauma

Loss trauma including loss of parents, loss of partners, and loss of close friends may be expected to occur at any life stage. However, when such losses occur off-time (i.e., nonnormatively), this may be a contribution to their traumatic nature and impact. Thus, losses of parents in childhood, losses of children, and widowhood in early- or mid-adulthood are all candidates for traumatic loss.

Psychoanalytic approaches to depression emphasize its relationship to loss experience, particularly in childhood. As a result there has been much investigation of childhood loss of a parent and vulnerability to adult disorders such as depression. Detailed investigation of childhood deaths of parents has shown that these have marked long-term impact only when neglectful or abusive parenting follows, or when the loss is considered aberrant in terms of abandonment. When death of a parent in childhood occurs in otherwise caring and supported circumstances, no long-term dysfunction occurs.

Childhood trauma has been extensively studied by Leonie Terr, who identified different symptoms following from single-blow or multiple-blow trauma. Type I trauma, that following a sudden single shock, was found to evince symptoms such as full repeated memories, strangely visualized or repeated, repetitive behaviors, trauma-specific fears, omens, and misperceptions. In contrast, type II trauma, following multiple or chronic shock, evinced denial and numbing, dissociation, and rage. In both instances childhood trauma led to changed attitudes about people, aspects of life, and the future.

Adult Loss Trauma

The most typical adult losses concern loss of a child or pregnancy and loss of a partner. These events can occur at any age, but death of a partner is clearly more common (and more normative) in later life. Again, the traumatic nature of the losses include suddenness and horror. PTSD is observed after pregnancy loss, and given that most losses of pregnancy are sudden and unexpected, these can constitute trauma, although those pregnancies that are lost in later weeks (or taken to term and ending in stillbirth) or those in which the fetal loss involves pain and bloodshed are more likely to constitute loss trauma. However, even with miscarriage in earlier weeks, a small proportion (7%) develops PTSD symptoms. However, more common responses are depression (30–50%) or anxiety (32%) occurring within 6 months of miscarriage. Research into widowhood (e.g., by Colin Murray-Parkes in the 1970s) showed individual variation in responses, but showed complicated bereavement with aspects such as intrusive thoughts, avoidant behaviors, yearning, loneliness, and loss of interest. Further work with elderly widows following an extensive caring role showed distinct traumatic grief responses.

Treatment for Loss Trauma

The core of treatment for trauma involves being able to talk about the traumatic experience within a therapeutic trusting relationship. The dilemma for the therapist is that reminders of trauma can trigger symptoms of PTSD, so symptoms can in the short term be worsened. Thus, trauma treatment must balance the degree of processing (of negative information) with containment (by the therapeutic relationship) in a secure setting. There are various approaches to treating trauma, which are not necessarily specific to loss trauma.

Critical Incident Stress Debriefing

Debriefing was originally developed for limited use as a brief group intervention to help mitigate psychological distress among emergency response personnel. This was then developed to be used on an individual rather than a group basis. However, global application of debriefing has been shown to be relatively ineffective and may at times impede recovery. This may be because it has been removed from its original purpose as a group bonding exercise for emergency workers, but also because it may impede the natural support that individuals can receive from those close at times of emergency. It has been argued that formalized debriefing can pathologize normal reactions and thus neutralize normal coping responses.

Cognitive-Behavioral Treatment (CBT)

CBT treatments used for affective disorder can help individuals to understand and manage anxiety associated with the trauma-related stimuli. Exposure treatment involving repeated confrontations with memories of the traumatic stressor in therapeutic settings has shown successful outcomes, although not specifically adapted for trauma responses. CBT can be helpful in conjunction with other techniques such as eye movement desensitization and reprocessing.

Eye Movement Desensitization and Reprocessing (EMDR)

EMDR was discovered by Francine Shapiro; it is a desensitization process that involves bringing the traumatic memory to mind while the patient simultaneously moves the eyes from side to side, following the movement of the therapist's finger back and forth in front of the face. After a series of eye movements the patient is instructed to let go of the traumatic images and say what comes to mind. Over the course of successful treatment, the emotional distress abates, traumatic images become less intrusive, and beliefs about the self become more positive. There is general agreement that the technique is successful in conjunction with other therapeutic techniques, but the precise mechanism for its action is not well understood, although it may directly work on brain mechanisms.

Dialectic Behavior Therapy (DBT)

DBT was invented by Marcia Linehan and although originally used mainly for borderline personality disorder in which self-harm is involved, it was found to also be effective for trauma. The therapy requires learning skills for coping with painful emotional states that lead to self-destructive behavior. Behavioral skills and emotional control are enhanced through emphasis on actively teaching and reinforcing adaptive behavior. It can be conducted both on an individual psychotherapy basis and in group meetings. Again, it is not specifically designed for loss trauma but has elements required to deal with some traumatic grief responses.

Resilience to Loss Trauma

Experience of traumatic events is common, but experience of trauma psychopathology is fairly rare. Therefore, it is argued, resilience must exist in the face of encountering trauma or, conversely, some individuals are vulnerable or sensitized to loss trauma. As with other psychological disorders, factors influencing vulnerability to PTSD include lack of social support, lack of education, family background, prior psychiatric history, and aspects of trauma response such as dissociative states.

It has been argued that resilience to loss trauma has been underestimated because of research focus on individuals developing disorders, which biases the field toward vulnerable individuals. For example, absence of grief, usually pathologized among patients, may in fact indicate resilience in hardier individuals. It is argued that there is little empirical support for the notion of delayed grief and that some individuals may adapt quickly to loss without going through grieving stages. Similarly, PTSD-type symptoms are common in the first few weeks after a traumatic event, but in most people these disappear and the full syndrome does not occur, thus indicating some process of resilience. Resilient and recovering individuals are often put into same category, since chronicity of symptoms is a key marker for pathological reactions and more resilient individuals adapt more quickly and may be perceived to have been treated rather than have drawn on personal resilience factors.

See Also the Following Articles

Childhood Stress; Childbirth and Stress; Dissociation; Familial Patterns of Stress; Grieving; Posttraumatic Stress Disorder in Children; Posttraumatic Stress Disorder, Delayed; Posttraumatic Therapy; Trauma and Memory; Trauma Group Therapy.

Further Reading

Allen, J. (2005). *Coping with trauma: hope through understanding* (2nd edn.). Washington, D.C: American Psychiatric Publishing.

Bifulco, A., Harris, T. and Brown, G. W. (1992). Mourning or early inadequate care? Reexamining the relationship of maternal loss in childhood with adult depression and anxiety. *Development and Psychopathology* 4, 433–449.

Bonnano, G. A. (2004). Loss, trauma and human resilience. *American Psychologist* 59, 20–28.

Bowlby, J. (1980). *Loss sadness and depression: vol. 3: Attachment and loss.* London: Hogarth Press and Institute of Psychoanalysis.

Figley, C. R., Bride, B. E. and Mazza, N. (eds.) (1997). *Death and trauma: the traumatology of grieving.* Washington, D.C: Taylor Francis.

Herman, J. L. (1992). *Trauma and recovery.* London: Pandora.

Horowitz, M. J. (1986). *Stress response and syndromes: PTSD, grief and adjustment disorders* (3rd edn.). Northvale, NJ: Jason Aronson.

Parkes, C. M. (1986). *Bereavement studies of grief in adult life.* Harmondsworth, UK: Penguin.

Prigerson, H. G., Shear, M. K., Frank, E., Silberman, R. and Reynolds, C. F. (1997). Traumatic grief: a case of loss-induced trauma. *American Journal of Psychiatry* 154, 1003–1009.

Terr, L. C. (1990). *Too scared to cry.* New York: Harper & Row.

Van der Kolk, B. A., McFarlane, A. C. and Weisaieth, L. (eds.) (1996). *Traumatic stress: the effects of overwhelming experience over mind, body and society.* New York: Guilford.

Lymph Nodes

T L Whiteside
University of Pittsburgh Cancer Institute,
Pittsburgh, PA, USA

This article is a revision of the previous edition article by
T L Whiteside, volume 2, pp 634–640, © 2000, Elsevier Inc.

Architecture of Lymph Nodes
Lymphocyte Migration within the Lymph Node
Antigen-Driven Interactions in the Lymph Node
Significance of Lymph Nodes
Interactions between the Central Nervous System
    and Lymph Nodes

Glossary

B cell-dependent area	Primary and secondary follicles located in the superficial cortex, underneath the subcapsular sinus. B cells migrate to and are organized into follicles.
Cortex	A major area of the lymph node consisting of a superficial cortex and a deeper region, the paracortex.
Fibroblast reticular cell (FRC) network	Network composed of collagen-containing reticular fibers that are produced by FRCs. It forms the infrastructure of the lymph node.
Lymph node (LN)	A key organ of the peripheral immune system.
Medulla	The second major area of the lymph node located beneath the paracortex, closest to the hilum, and subdivided into medullary cords and medullary sinus, which drains into the efferent lymphatic vessel.
Paracortical cords	The paracortex is made up of multiple cords. Each is a functional repeating unit of the cortex, which stretches from a medullary cord to the base of a B cell follicle. It consists of the central high endothelial venule (HEV) surrounded by a perivenular channel, a corridor, and a cortical sinus. HEVs are specialized segments of vessels localized deep in the paracortex, whose luminal surface is lined by high cuboidal endothelial cells serving as transmigration points for lymphocytes emigrating from the bloodstream to the lymph node. Perivenular channels are narrow spaces along the HEVs into which lymphocytes arrive, having crossed the endothelium, and where they seem to accumulate. To reach the corridor, they must next cross the barrier of overlapping fibroblast reticular cells, which form the perivenular sleeve. In the corridor, lymphocytes are able to migrate more freely and interact with antigen-presenting cells lining the corridor walls. The cortical sinus is a fluid-filled compartment that bounds the outer surface of the paracortical cords and connects the subcapsular sinus with the medullary sinuses.
T cell-dependent area	The interfollicular regions and the paracortex of the lymph node. T cells migrate preferentially to these anatomical locations.

Lymph nodes (LNs) are fundamental functional units of the immune system. They are the organs in which immune cells transact their business. Distributed strategically throughout the body, they are localized close to major junctions of the lymphatic channels. Naive lymphocytes recirculate continuously through the peripheral lymphoid organs, including LNs, passaging from blood to lymph and then back to blood via the thoracic duct. LNs play a key role in collecting information necessary for entering lymphocytes to make a decision about whether to respond to an antigen or to become tolerant and/or die, thus avoiding autoimmunity. Lymph draining the extracellular spaces of the body carries antigens from tissue sites to the nearest LN, where afferent lymphatic vessels converge. Antigens thus delivered to the LN are trapped, screened, and presented to those rare immune cells in the pool of T and B lymphocytes migrating through the node that are capable of antigen recognition. The process of recognition involves Ig receptor (e.g., 1 in 100 000 cells) on B cells and T cell receptor (TCR) on T lymphocytes and initiates a series of events orchestrated within the milieu of the LN, culminating in generation of an antigen-specific immune response. Virtually all primary immune responses take place in LNs and other secondary lymphoid organs, such as spleen or gut-associated lymphoid tissue. Hence, LNs are extraordinarily important sites of interactions between immune cells and antigens and are especially adapted to facilitate these interactions.

Architecture of Lymph Nodes

LNs are small, oval structures (about 0.5 cm or less in diameter) with complex architecture, which differs between species. The basic structural elements of lymph nodes are the cortex and the medulla (**Figure 1**). A section through a LN shows the outermost capsule; the subcapsular sinus draining afferent lymphatic vessels; the cortex, consisting of an outer region made up of B lymphocytes organized into lymphoid follicles and of deeper paracortical cords made up mainly of T lymphocytes; the medulla, organized into medullary cords, consisting of strings of macrophages and antibody-secreting plasma cells; and medullary sinus connected with efferent lymphatic vessels. This basic architecture of LNs undergoes dramatic changes during an antigenic challenge or in response to neural or inflammatory stimuli, and it is this remarkable plasticity of the critical architectural elements of a lymph node that facilitates immune cell interactions.

The cortex of a lymph node in larger animals and humans is subdivided into 10 or more lobules separated by fibrous bands called trabeculae (**Figure 1**). Each lobule has the follicle with a germinal center, the B lymphocyte-dependent area, and the paracortex corresponding to the T cell-dependent area. This area accommodates paracortical cords, which form the fundamental structural unit of the lymph node paracortex. **Figure 2a** provides a lateral view of paracortical cords, each with a central postcapillary high endothelial venule (HEV) bordered by the cortical sinus. Paracortical cords begin at the base of follicles and run parallel to each other to the corticomedullary junction, where they coalesce into medullary cords. In cross-section, a paracortical cord is a cylinder composed of sinus-lining cells at its periphery, concentric rings of barrier-type cells called fibroblastic reticular cells (FRCs), and a central HEV (**Figure 2b**). The concentric arrangement of FRCs creates a perivenular channel. The spaces between the rings are filled with lymphocytes and other cells and FRCs from an outermost layer of the channel, enclosing it like a sleeve.

Outside of the sleeve is a fluid-filled corridor bounded and supported by a network of FRCs. The corridors are 10–25 μm in diameter, and they join with and split from each other, creating no barriers and allowing for efficient cell migration. The boundary of flat sinus-lining cells separates the corridors from the surrounding paracortical sinus. A representative radius of a cord is 50–100 μm or roughly 10 lymphocyte diameters. However, paracortical cords are pliable structures, capable of stretching to easily accommodate masses of migrating lymphocytes.

The outermost aspect of a lobule, situated underneath the subcapsular sinus, is the B-dependent area of a LN. It is composed of tightly packed B lymphocyte formations referred to as primary follicles. Germinal centers are formed within follicles on antigenic stimulation of B cells and represent areas of extensive B cell proliferation. Occasional T cells are also present. An important cell resides in the follicular area, the so-called follicular dendritic cell (FDC), which is responsible for trapping and presenting antigens to B cells. The FDC is a highly specialized type of DC that binds immune complexes via Fc and complement receptors, internalizes them, and holds them for long periods of time. This function of FDC is crucial for memory B cell development. The germinal centers are surrounded by dense formations of small memory B cells. Interfollicular areas are populated by T cells and represent T-dependent regions of the LN. Follicles provide the microenvironment for the exposure of B cells to trapped antigens and for their proliferation. They are the anatomic site for somatic mutations. Although B cell differentiation to plasma cells occurs mostly in the deep paracortex and medullary cords, follicles are the site of B cell affinity maturation and memory development.

The medulla of a LN is a loose network of medullary cords and sinuses situated in the hilar area and

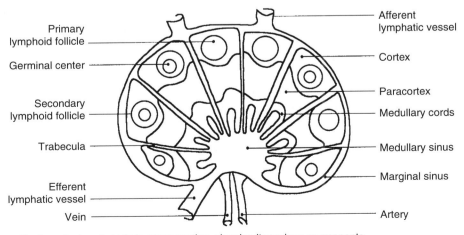

Figure 1 A schematic view of a lymph node in cross-section, showing its various components.

Primary lymphoid follicle

Germinal center

Secondary lymphoid follicle

Trabecula

Efferent lymphatic vessel

Vein

Afferent lymphatic vessel

Cortex

Paracortex

Medullary cords

Medullary sinus

Marginal sinus

Artery

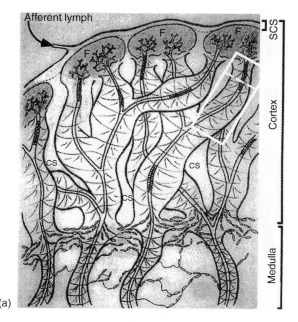

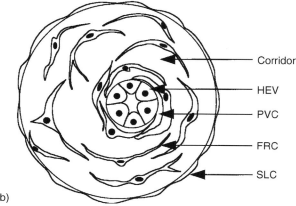

(b)

Figure 2 Functional units of a lymph node. (a) Paracortical cords in a longitudinal view. A white box indicates a representative cord. Note an extensive network of reticular fibers surrounding each postcapillary venule and high endothelial venules (HEV) shown as darker regions of the venules. Paracortical cords begin at the base of follicles (F), run the length of the cortex, and coalesce into medullary cords at the corticomedullary junction. Spaces around paracortical cords are cortical sinuses (CS). SCS, subcapsular sinus at the margin of the LN. Reproduced with permission from Kelly (1975). (b) A cross-section of a paracortical cord, indicating a control HEV surrounded by perivenular channels (PVC) and corridors supported by a framework of fibroblastic reticular cells (FRC) and bounded by sinus-lining cells (SLC).

separated loosely from the paracortex by a network of connective tissue fibers. Medullary cords contain both T and B cells and most of the plasma cells in the LN. B cells complete their maturation into antibody-producing plasma cells in the medulla, and lymph exiting via the efferent lymphatics is enriched in antibodies. In addition, scavenger macrophages line the medullary sinuses and are responsible for the removal of particulate antigens found in the lymph.

Lymph vessels carrying interstitial fluid deliver antigens to the LN. The lymph enters from afferent lymph vessels into the subcapsular sinus and is channeled around and through trabecular sinuses, across the LN parenchyma toward a medullary network of sinuses. From there, it can leave the LN via efferent lymph vessels and travel to the next LN in the chain. The intranodal lymph channels are enclosed by FDCs, sinus-lining endothelial cells, and macrophages, which sample the lymph and transport antigenic material for presentation to B and T cells. Antigens in the lymph do not have free access to the lymphocyte compartment, and FDCs serve to select and transport lymph-borne molecules to be presented to T and B cells that home to LNs from the blood.

Overall, the architecture of a LN is characterized by a high degree of compartmentalization, which appears to be necessary in order to maintain the constant and directed flow of lymphocytes from one compartment to another and to allow for cellular interactions to occur at the time and place best suited for optimal immune responses.

Lymphocyte Migration within the Lymph Node

Figure 3 is a diagrammatic representative of trafficking of lymphocytes in, within, and out of the LN. Lymphocyte migration is a continuous process. Naive lymphocytes enter the node from the bloodstream via specialized structures called HEVs in the paracortical cords. Adhesion molecules on the surface of lymphocytes are instrumental in their binding to and the subsequent transmigration through the high cuboidal endothelium. Antigens enter the LN through the afferent lymphatics and are trapped by specialized cells (dendritic cells [DCs]) for presentation to lymphocytes. Only the rare lymphocytes recognizing the antigen via the TCR or BCR are activated and stop recirculating. Lymphocytes that do not recognize antigen continue migrating through the LN and leave it via the efferent lymphatic vessel (**Figure 3c**).

Lymphocytes entering the paracortex cords from blood via HEV move outward through perivenular channels made up of concentric rings of FRCs. Lymphocytes spend 10–100 min moving through these channels, which are rich in extracellular matrix (ECM) components and provide an excellent substrate for lymphocyte migration. To reach the cord, lymphocytes must once again transmigrate, this time through tightly overlapping FRCs enclosing the perivascular channels like a sleeve. Once within the next compartment, called the corridor, the route of lymphocytes depends on whether they are T or B cells. T cells migrate to the T-dependent areas, whereas

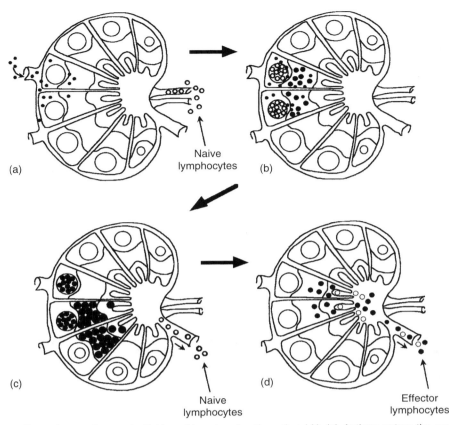

Figure 3 A diagram illustrating continuous trafficking of lymphocytes through a LN. (a) Antigen enters the nodes through afferent lymphatics, and small naive lymphocytes enter via the blood vessels from the bloodstream. In the cortex, lymphocytes enter through HEV (not shown). (b) Once in the node, T cells migrate to T cell-dependent areas, whereas B cells migrate to follicles. Antigen is taken up and processed by dendritic cells (not shown). (c) Lymphocytes that recognize the antigen stop recirculating, enlarge or blast and begin to proliferate. Masses of blasting T cell are seen filling the paracortex. Lymphocytes that do not recognize antigen continue migrating and leave the LN via the efferent lymphatic vessel. (d) After about a week, plasma cells appear in the medulla, and effector lymphocytes and antibodies leave the LN via the efferent lymphatic vessel.

B cells migrate to the follicles. It is not known how the cells select their route or how their traffic is directed. Lymphocytes end their journey through the cord by migrating between the sinus-lining cells into the cortical sinus.

The migration of lymphocytes through the cortex proceeds radially outward, from the HEV lumen to the outer sinuses. It is remarkable that during this journey lymphocytes manage to traverse across three cellular boundaries: the HEV endothelium, the FRC boundary in perivenular channels, and the sinus-lining cell. In addition, lymphocytes migrate more or less up and down within the cortex. They do so by crawling along the corridor walk or sinus boundaries, both richly expressing the ECM components. This oriented migration within the cortex is crucial for lymphocyte interactions with antigen-presenting cells (APCs) and for the connection between the follicular areas and the medulla. Also, the ability of differentiated effector T cells or plasma cells to leave the LNs

via efferent lymphatics depends on the open routes of migration within the cord.

Antigen-Driven Interactions in the Lymph Node

The presence of an antigen dramatically alters the appearance and size of the LN. Upon entering the node environment through afferent lymphatics, antigens are taken up by sessile APCs referred to as interdigitating dendritic cells (IDCs) and found in the cortex. These cells migrate via lymph from tissues to the corridor, where they attach to FRCs, providing an optimal milieu for lymphocyte–APC interactions. Aside from enlarging the surface available for these interactions, IDCs are rich in costimulatory molecules and cytokines. Lymphocytes typically spend 3–6 h in the corridor space. Thus, migrating T lymphocytes have the opportunity to screen IDCs immobilized on the corridor walls for antigens (peptides) presented by the major histocompatibility complex (MHC). When the TCR on the T cell encounters the peptide it recognizes, activation of the T cell occurs. This process can occur anywhere in the corridor space, allowing migrating T cells an opportunity for screening multiple IDCs along the way. Thus, corridors of the paracortex are the ideal sites for interactions of IDCs, T cells, and B cells, where the generation of the immune response is facilitated by efficient cell-to-cell contact. They also provide a suitable environment for the proliferation of activated T cells.

When a T cell traversing the paracortex meets its cognate antigen, the TCR transmits activation signals to the nucleus, and T cell proliferation begins within the corridor. Simultaneously, B cells migrating through the paracortex or moving along the axis of the corridor are also likely to encounter antigen recognized by the Ig receptor and to initiate proliferation. In an environment rich in cytokines secreted by activated T cells, B cells undergo differentiation. The clonal expansion of antigen-specific T and B cells leads to their accumulation in the corridors and to marked distention of the cords. The size of a LN increases dramatically during an immune response. In addition to ballooning, paracortical cords undergo elongation in reactive LNs, and endothelial cells in HEV also proliferate. Thus, the entire size of the LN increases several-fold in a relatively short period of time. Conversely, when the depletion of lymphocytes occurs, e.g., during thoracic drainage, the diameter of the cord shrinks. Large differences in the size of the cortex due to changes in lymphocyte numbers are the basis for a common perception that reactive LNs are large and nonreactive LNs are small. The enormous plasticity of LNs depends on their infrastructure of collagen fibers and FRCs, forming a loose reticular network amenable to shrinking and extension. The LN also has a network of nerve endings that connects it to the central nervous system (CNS). In an enlarged reactive LN, changes in the migration rate of lymphocytes occur: the traffic along the long axis of the cords becomes prominent, with effector T cells and differentiating B cells moving toward the medulla and other B cells, those destined to become memory cells, moving toward the follicles. This is possible because extended cords allow for easy access and enhanced lymph flow to the interfollicular area at the base of follicles. Similarly, medullary cords and sinus are also extended in reactive LNs and are able to accommodate more lymphocytes now migrating toward the efferent lymphatic vessel in the hilum. Before lymphocytes exit the LN, they spend a period of time in the medulla. Here, in the environment rich in cytokines and in the presence of helper T cells, B cell maturation into antibody-secreting plasma cells takes place. Antigen-specific effector T cells and plasma cells leave the LN through the efferent lymphatic vessel to enter the bloodstream and eventually to reach the site of infection or repopulate sites of antibody production, respectively.

Significance of Lymph Nodes

Because lymph-borne antigens enter the LN continuously and immune responses are generated to a variety of antigens at all times, immune cells leaving the LN contain effector cells primed to deal with a variety of different antigens. The LN environment is structured and organized to facilitate entry and migration of naive lymphocytes to areas of antigen presentation, to promote antigen recognition, to allow for activation and proliferation of antigen-specific T and B cells, and, finally, to assure the availability of immune effector cells to sites of infection. This series of events is accomplished in 4 to 6 days in primary immune responses and in a much shorter period of time in a secondary response. The presence in the follicular compartment of memory B cells surrounded by interfollicular T cells assures that anamnestic responses are initiated promptly at the site of antigen entry. Migration of activated T and B cells from the follicular area along the length of extended paracortical cords to medulla proceeds rapidly during secondary immune responses and may be facilitated by chemokines, by cytokines produced by activated lymphocytes or accessory cells, and perhaps by the directional flow of fluids in the corridors. The regulation of directed migration of lymphocytes during primary or secondary immune responses is a subject of intense investigation. To home to the LN, lymphocytes must execute a series of adhesion and signaling events that involve a variety of molecules. First, tethering and rolling of lymphocytes entering HEV of LNs is mediated by L-selectin (CD62L) and its ligands, such as MECA-79. Next, arrest of rolling lymphocytes is mediated by the integrin leukocyte function-associated antigen 1 (LFA1), interacting with ICAM1 and ICAM2 expressed on HEV. Activation of integrins on lymphocytes is mediated by the CC chemokine ligand 21 (CCL21, SLC, 6Ckine) constitutively expressed by HEV cells. It binds to its receptor (CCR7) on lymphocytes. A second CCR7 ligand, CCL19 (ELC, MIP3β) is expressed by the lymphatic endothelial and interstitial cell but not by HEV. Other integrin-activating signals involving chemokines and their receptors exist, and it is thought that T cells and B cells respond to different signals in HEV. Activation-dependent adhesion steps allow lymphocytes to stick firmly to HEV and to emigrate through the vessel wall and enter the LN environment. The LN represents a series of distinct micro environments, each adapted to optimize the function of immune cells. The key element is migration of these cells from one compartment to another. It is important to note that the migration of lymphocytes within the node can proceed in either of two directions, from HEV outward to the sinus in the paracortical cord or from the follicular area to the medulary sinus at the hilum. Naive lymphocytes entering the node via HEV take the first route; once activated and/or proliferating, lymphocytes tend to take the second path. The regulated movement of fluids and cells within the LN compartments is a wonderful example of the efficiency of the immune system in executing primary and secondary antigen-specific responses.

Interactions between the Central Nervous System and Lymph Nodes

Recent advances in the field of neuroimmunology have shown that the CNS and the immune system are intimately linked. The CNS influences responses of the immune system through the release of humoral factors such as cortisol or epinephrine from the hypothalamic-pituitary-adrenocortical (HPA) axis. Glucocorticoids released as part of a systemic stress response influence (downregulate) immune responses profoundly. Communication between nervous and immune systems is also maintained by the efferent neuronal sympathetic nervous system in lymphoid organs. LNs are innervated so that a close association exists between autonomic nerve terminals and immune cells. Local synthesis and colocalization of norepinephrine, neuropeptides, such as neuropeptide Y, and opioids have been documented in the nerve terminals of nerve fibers located in LNs. Immune cells present in this microenvironment have specific surface receptors for neurotransmitters and neuropeptides and are responsive to signals transmitted via the receptors. In addition to efferent nerve terminals, LNs contain afferent nerve fibers characterized by the expression of receptors for cytokines or other factors produced by immune cells. Thus, bidirectional traffic of biochemical mediators between the CNS and immune cells regulates their interactions.

An example of chemically mediated signal transmission in response to stress is shown in **Figure 4**. In this schema, stress or infectious agents induce the release of glucocorticoids from the HPA axis. Glucocorticoids have potent anti-inflammatory and immunosuppressive effects, including the downregulation of lymphocyte functions and of their migration into the LN. In the presence of cortisol, immune cells begin to produce a cytokine, migration inhibitory factor (MIF), which counteracts inhibitory effects of

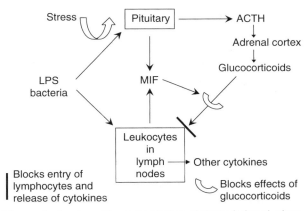

Figure 4 A schematic representation of stress-induced, glucocorticoid-mediated effects on lymphocyte entry into LN and on cytokine production by lymphocytes present in LN. ACTH, adrenocorticotropic hormone; MIF, migration inhibitory factor, LPS, lipopolysaccharide.

glucocorticoids at the local level. The pituitary also produces and releases MIF into the systemic circulation. MIF suppresses glucocorticoid production and restores the immune balance.

Trafficking of lymphocytes is fundamental to the generation of immune responses. Glucocorticoids inhibit lymphocyte migration into LNs and disrupt lymphocyte recirculation.

Lymphopenia observed in the presence of steroids is not due to death of lymphocytes but to redistribution of the circulating lymphocyte pool. Lymphocytes that normally enter LNs now migrate away from them, with the net result being the downregulation of lymphocyte entry into the LNs. The molecular mechanism responsible for this effect is a glucocorticoid-induced decrease in expression of L-selectin (CD62L), also known as a lymph node homing receptor, and of CD44 Hermes protein on the surface of lymphocytes. Because these adhesion molecules are involved in lymphocyte–HEV interactions and are necessary for lymphocyte entry into LNs, dysregulation of their expression naturally interferes with homing. It is probable that these interactions are not direct but are mediated via cytokines, whose local production is inhibited by glucocorticoids (see **Figure 4**). The profound effects of stress on the immune system are partly mediated via neurotransmission in LNs. Thus, the understanding of LN architecture and of lymphocyte migration patterns in LNs is necessary for the appreciation of stress-induced alterations in immune responses. The various aspects of the CNS–immune system communication and, especially, the role of cytokines in orchestrating these interactions are being intensely investigated today.

See Also the Following Articles

Cytokines; Immune Cell Distribution, Effects of Stress on; Immune Response; Lymphocytes.

Further Reading

Anderson, A. O. and Shaw, S. (1995). Lymphocyte trafficking. In: Rich, R. R., Fleischer, T. A., Schwanz, B. D., Shearer, W. T. & Strober, W. (eds.) *Clincal immunology*, pp. 39–49. St. Louis, MO: Mosby.

Calandra, T. and Bucala, R. (1997). Macrophage migration inhibition factors (MIF): a glucocorticoid counter-regulator within the immune system. *Critical Reviews in Immunology* **17**, 77–88.

Cyster, J. G. (1999). Chemokines and cell migration in secondary lymphoid organs. *Science* **286**, 2098–2102.

Eskandari, F. and Sternberg, E. M. (2002). Neural-immune interactions in health and disease. *Annals of the New York Academy of Science* **966**, 20–27.

Friedman, E. M. and Lawrence, D. A. (2002). Environmental stress mediates changes in neuroimmunological interactions. *Toxicological Science* **67**, 4–10.

Gretz, J. E., Anderson, A. O. and Shaw, S. (1997). Cords, channels, corridors and conduits: Critical architectural elements facilitating cell interactions in the lymph node cortex. *Immunology Reviews* **156**, 11–24.

Kelly, R. H. (1975). Functional anatomy of lymph nodes. I. The paracortical cords. *International Archives of Allergy and Applied Immunology* **48**, 836–849.

Straub, R. H., Westermann, J., Scholmerich, J. and Falk, W. (1998). Dialogue between the CNS and the immune system in lymphoid organs. *Immunology Today* **19**, 409–413.

Von Andrian, U. H. and Mempel, T. R. (2003). Homing and cellular traffic in lymph nodes. *Nature Reviews Immunology* **3**, 867–878.

Warnock, R. A., Askari, S., Butcher, E. C. and von Andrian, U. H. (1998). Molecular mechanisms of lymphocyte homing to peripheral lymph nodes. *Journal of Experimental Medicine* **187**, 205–216.

Wrona, D. (2005). Neural-immune interactions: an integrative view of the bidirectional relationship between the brain and immune systems. *Journal of Neuroimmunology* **172**, 38–58.

Lymphocyte Trafficking and Cell Adhesion Molecules (CAM) *See:* Leukocyte Trafficking and Stress; Lymph Nodes.

Lymphocytes

N R Rose
Johns Hopkins University School of Medicine, Baltimore, MD, USA

This article is a revision of the previous edition article by N R Rose, volume 2, pp 641–645, © 2000, Elsevier Inc.

Introduction
Origin and Development
B Lymphocytes
T Lymphocytes
Natural Killer (NK) Cells

Glossary

Anamnestic response	An accelerated secondary immune response.
B cell lymphoblasts	Large, metabolically active B cells.
Class I major histocompatibility complex (MHC)	The MHC expressed on all nucleated cells.
Class II major histocompatibility complex (MHC)	The MHC expressed mainly on antigen-presenting cells.
Cytokines	A diverse group of multifunctional proteins that play a key role in a variety of biological processes, including cell growth and activation, inflammation, immunity, hematopoiesis, tumorigenesis, tissue repair, fibrosis, and morphogenesis. Chemokines are a subgroup involved in chemotaxis. Cytokines are synthesized in a variety of cell types, including lymphocytes and cells of the mononuclear phagocyte system.
Endocytosis	Ingestion of molecules by the cell.
Epitope	Antigenic determinant.
Erythropoietin	The growth factor required for the generation of erythrocytes from the pluripotential stem cell.

Granulocyte/ monocyte- colony stimu- lating factor (GM-CSF)

The growth factor required for the generation of granulocytes and monocytes from the pluripotential cell.

Immuno- globulin

The antibody containing fraction of serum.

Stem cell

A self-renewing undifferentiated cell capable of developing into specialized cells.

Introduction

In vertebrates, the specialized function of acquired or adaptive immunity is assigned to the immune system. Like other specialized organs, the immune system comprises a number of differentiated cells that contribute to its special function; unlike most other organs, however, the immune system is distributed throughout the body (see **Immune Response**). This decentralized anatomical structure best serves its purpose of providing immunological surveillance and protection. The distinguishing features of the acquired immune response are its specificity (the ability to distinguish one antigenic molecule from another) and its memory. The immune system must recognize and respond to the vast universe of antigenic determinants and must learn to respond more vigorously at a second encounter. The cells specialized to serve these critical functions are the lymphocytes. This article focuses on the major population of lymphocytes: B lymphocytes, T lymphocytes, and natural killer (NK) cells.

Origin and Development

Figure 1 diagrams the early development of the hematopoietic system, of which the immune apparatus is a component. All of the blood cells develop from a single multipotential or pluripotential stem cell. Phylogenetically this cell arises in the yolk sac. In mammals, the pluripotential stem cell transfers to the liver during embryonic development, but later, during gestation and birth, it migrates to the bone marrow. Like all stem cells, it is capable of self-renewal but can differentiate into a number of specialized progenitor or precursor cells. These include the erythrocyte progenitor, which eventually develops into the erythrocytes; the megakaryocyte progenitor, which is the eventual source of platelets; and the myeloid progenitor of the granulocytes and monocytes, which is the source of all of the granulocytic leukocytes, such as polymorphonuclear neutrophils, eosinophils, and basophils and of the monocytes of the blood and the macrophages and dendritic cells of the tissues. Finally, the lymphocyte progenitor is the source of B lymphocytes, T lymphocytes, and NK cells. The production of these progenitor cells, as well as their continued differentiation into the mature functional cells of the lymphopoietic system, is driven by a family of peptide messengers, referred to collectively as colony-stimulating factors. At least two of them, erythropoietin, which promotes the production of erythrocytes, and granulocyte/monocyte-colony stimulating factor (GM-CSF), which fosters production

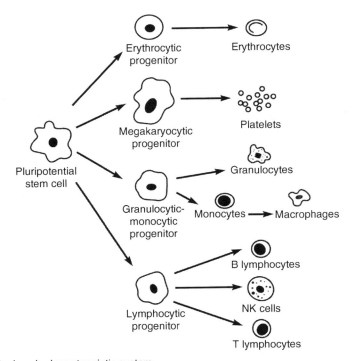

Figure 1 Development of the lympho-hematopoietic system.

of the granulocyte/monocyte lineage, have been isolated and used clinically to treat deficiencies of the respective cell populations.

B Lymphocytes

As indicated previously, B lymphocytes arise from the pluripotential stem cell in the fetal liver and later in the bone marrow. Directed by several stimulating factors, it matures into a functional B lymphocyte. These cells comprise approximately half of the approximately 10^{12} lymphocytes in the human body. They represent about 20% of the circulating lymphocytes but a majority of those found in the organized lymphoid tissues, such as the spleen and lymph nodes. The critical event in B cell maturation is the production of an antigen-specific receptor and its expression on the cell surface.

The B cell receptor (BCR) is a membrane-bound form of the immunoglobulin (Ig) molecule. The clonal selection theory of the immune response requires that there be an enormous diversity of these cell surface receptors, enough to bind any antigenic determinant or epitope that the B cell may encounter. The BCR is a heterodimeric molecule consisting of two heavy and two light chains, both of which have variable regions that contribute to the epitope-specific binding site. The required diversity of the receptors is produced by a specialized process of recombination, wherein one of a large set of variable (V) genes combines with one of a smaller number of diversity (D) genes (in the immunoglobulin heavy chain) and joining (J) genes to produce the variable regions of both the heavy and light chains. The pairing of a heavy and light immunoglobulin chain in a random manner further expands the diversity of BCR on different B cells. Another limited set of genes encodes the constant (C) region of the immunoglobulin molecule. Although initially apart on the chromosome, the V(D)J complex is joined with a C region gene to produce the immunoglobulin heavy chain or light chain. The assembly of immunoglobulin genes depends upon two recombination activator genes, RAG-1 and RAG-2. After completion of the immunoglobulin gene arrangement, the BCR is expressed on the cell surface with a μ heavy chain, representative of the IgM class of antibody. As the cell continues its maturation, a second class of immunoglobulins, IgD, composed of the same V(D)J segment but a δ constant region gene, is also expressed at the B cell surface. Finally, the mature B cell completes recombination by secreting immunoglobulin products with the δ constant region (i.e., IgG antibodies), the α constant region (IgA antibodies), or the ε constant region (IgE) antibodies. Circulatory antibodies of the IgG class are

mainly responsible for acquired protective immunity; IgA antibodies produced at mucosal surfaces serve immune functions in secretions; IgE antibodies are associated with allergic and hypersensitivity reactions.

A small population of B cells, termed B-1 cells, develops early during ontogeny and expresses the CD5 cell surface marker. The cells secrete low- to moderate-affinity IgM antibodies that are often broadly cross-reactive, including reactions to common pathogens and self-antigens. The antibodies are referred to as natural antibodies because their production does not appear to require the presence of a specific antigen. They may provide some initial protection against infectious agents.

The mature B cell is activated by binding an antigen that expresses the complementary (cognate) epitope recognized by its BCR. The activation process requires cross-linking of membrane BCR. The receptor is associated with a number of auxiliary molecules such as CD19, CD20, and CD21, which act in concert with the receptor and serve as distinguishing markers of B cells. These molecules transmit activation signals to the interior of the cell after receptor aggregation takes place on the cell surface.

This event sets in motion a series of metabolic steps, manifest mainly by the activation of tyrosine kinases, leading to tyrosine phosphorylation of a set of substrates that control intracellular signals. Early events of activation lead to development from a resting mature B lymphocyte into a metabolically active B lymphoblast with enlarged cytoplasm containing multiple mitochondria. The B cell blasts then divide repeatedly to produce a clone, each member of which bears the parental BCR and, therefore, expresses the same epitope specificity.

Upon binding to the BCR, antigen is endocytosed and processed for presentation to specialized T cells (see below). In addition to presenting antigens, B cells secrete a number of cytokines such as IL-10, IL-12, tumor necrosis factor-α (TNF-α), and lymphotoxin, which subsequently act to direct or regulate immune responses (see **Cytokines**).

Some of the activated B cells differentiate into plasma cells, which are the source of circulating antibody, whereas others differentiate into memory cells, which give rise to memory response upon rechallenge of the individual with the same antigen. The hallmarks of the immune response are both its specificity for the antigen that induced its formation and the enhanced immune response or anamnestic response on rechallenge.

Since a single B cell bears multiple BCRs with identical specificities, cross-linkage of the receptors requires that an antigenic molecule express more than one identical epitope. A number of microbial carbohydrates fulfill this requirement, and so B cells can be stimulated directly by the capsular polysaccharides of such microorganisms as pneumococci and meningococci. It is much less likely, however, that a globular protein will express more than one copy of an epitope. Under these circumstances, B cell activation requires help from a T cell capable of recognizing the same antigen. The endocytosed antigen is fragmented within the B cell, and the peptide fragments are loaded into the groove of a specialized cell surface glycoprotein, the class II major histocompatibility complex (MHC) molecule. The resultant class II/peptide fragment complexes are then inserted into the B cell surface. These complexes can be recognized by the antigen-specific receptors of the subset of T cells, referred to as CD4$^+$ or helper T cells.

The two-way interaction between T cells and B cells is critical for the development of a vigorous, adaptive immune response. On the one hand, B cells concentrate antigens and effectively present them to T cells that recognize the particular antigen. On the other hand, activated CD4$^+$ T helper cells produce cytokines that foster the activation and differentiation of B cells into plasma cells. When the T cell interacts with the MHC II/peptide fragment, it induces division of the B cell through the agency of costimulating surface molecules expressed by the T cell. CD154 of the T cell, for instance, engages CD40 of the B cell. In addition, T cell-derived cytokines, such as IL-4, IL-5, and IL-6, direct the B cell into an antibody-forming plasma cell. As the B cell progresses into the immunoglobulin-producing process, it undergoes a class switch; that is, the heavy chain C region, which originally expressed the specificities of the IgM and IgD classes, differentiates into cells that produce IgG, IgA, or IgE. This process allows the production of antibodies with differing biological functions while retaining the same antigen-combining site. At the same time, there is an increased affinity of the antibodies resulting from the extraordinarily high level of somatic mutation of the V genes, providing antibodies of high efficiency in combining with their antigenic targets.

T Lymphocytes

T lymphocytes constitute the second major class of lymphocytes, comprising approximately 70% of lymphocytes in the peripheral circulation and essentially all of the lymphocytes in the lymphatic circulation. They also derive from the hematopoietic stem cell through the lymphocyte progenitor, but undergo a process of differentiation in the thymus before they are seeded to peripheral lymphoid tissues and blood (see **Autotolerance**), (see **Thymus**). Like B cells,

mature T cells have a great diversity of antigen-specific cell surface receptors. T cell receptors (TCRs) are heterodimers made up of α and β chains or, rarely, γ and δ chains. Knowledge of the function of the latter subset of T cells is still limited.

Unlike the BCR, the TCR remains at the cell surface and is not shed into the medium. It is associated with a set of transmembrane proteins, referred to as the CD3 complex, which play a critical role in signal transduction. Through their agency, the T cell undergoes a process of activation similar to that described for the B cell. Like the BCR, the TCR is organized into a variable and constant portion. Furthermore, the same recombinational mechanisms are involved in the assembly of the V region genes in T cells and B cells. The process is controlled by RAG-1 and RAG-2, which together are required for T cell maturation. Antigen primed T cells may differentiate directly into effector or regulatory T cells. Following clonal expansion, a proportion of the antigen-stimulated T cells differentiates into long-lived memory cells. Memory T cells are responsible for the ability of the immune system to mount an anamnestic response when they encounter the same antigen. Thus, memory T cells play a central role in maintaining long-term protection against infection. In humans, memory T cells are usually CD45 RA$^-$ CD45 RO$^+$. Unlike effector T cells, they are not susceptible to programmed cell death following activation. Consequently, they survive for long periods of time in spleen and lymph nodes without undergoing division. Following a second encounter with their cognate antigen, memory T cells multiply rapidly and produce large amounts of cytokines so that even low levels of antigen can produce a vigorous secondary response. Memory B cells can be divided into central memory cells that inhabit secondary lymphoid organs and effector memory cells that migrate to inflamed areas.

T cells exert both regulatory and effector functions. The major regulatory T cells are the CD4$^+$ helper T cells, referred to previously. Their regulatory function depends on costimulatory molecules, such as CD154, as well as the production of particular cytokines. Some CD4$^+$ T cells develop into cells that primarily secrete the cytokines IL-4, IL-5, IL-6, and IL-13 (referred to as T$_h$2 cells) or into T cells that produce mainly IL-2, interferon-γ (IFN-γ), and lymphotoxin (referred to as T$_h$1 cells). The T$_h$2 cells help B cells to develop into antibody-producing cells, whereas T$_h$1 cells are primarily inducers of cell-mediated responses. Cell-mediated immunity is responsible for protection against intracellular microorganisms and involves the activation of macrophages as well as the generation of cytotoxic T cells. Cytotoxic T cells mediate the direct killer functions of cell-mediated immunity; they carry the CD8 marker in place of CD4 and are capable of lysing target cells that express the requisite antigen together with matched class I MHC. Virus-infected tissue cells, for example, may be eliminated from the host's cells by virus-specific CD8 T cells.

Under normal circumstances, the immune system is kept under strict control by a variety of regulatory mechanisms. Regulatory or suppressor T cells were recognized a number of years ago, but their identity remained elusive. Recently, several populations of T cells with regulatory capability have been identified. They include naturally occurring T regulatory cells (Tregs), which were first identified by their ability to prevent spontaneous autoimmune disease. They are characterized by the cell surface marker $CD4^+CD25^+$ and the transcription factor FoxP3. The critical role of the FoxP3 factor is attested by the demonstration that $CD4^+CD25^+$ T cells do not develop a regulatory function in FoxP3-deficient mice. In addition, retroviral transduction of FoxP3 into $CD4^+CD25^-$ cells converts them into functional regulatory T cells. $CD4^+CD25^+$ Tregs are anergic *in vitro*, failing to proliferate following nonspecific or antigen-specific stimulation. They can, however, mount an antigen-dependent proliferative response *in vivo*. The T cell growth factor IL-2 appears to play a critical role in their development, since mice genetically deficient in IL-2 have reduced numbers of Tregs. The distinguishing feature of Tregs is their ability to suppress a broad range of innate and adaptive immune responses; the suppression requires direct contact between the regulatory T cell and its target.

In addition to naturally occurring Tregs, naive T cells can be induced to differentiate into regulatory T cells following an encounter with their cognate antigen. These cells differ from the natural $CD4^+CD25^+$ Tregs in that they do not express FoxP3 and act primarily by the production of immunosuppressive cytokines such as IL-10 and transforming growth factor-β (TGF-β). They are referred to as Tr1 cells. These induced regulatory T cells are favored by antigen presentation through immature dendritic cells or by environments in which high levels of suppressive cytokines are present, such as at mucosal surfaces. Because induced Tr1 cells secrete these immunosuppressive cytokines, they can downregulate responses to other nearby antigens, a process called bystander suppression.

Recent studies have provided evidence of a number of other regulatory T cell populations. For example, $CD8^+$ T cells can mediate immune regulatory functions including allograft rejection. Although their mechanism of action is still unclear, they may induce suppression by cytolysis of helper $CD4^+$T cells.

NKT cells represent a distinct lineage of T cells that are characterized by an invariant TCR light chain as well as by the presence of characteristic NK cell markers. This invariant TCR does not recognize peptide presented in the usual fashion by class I or class II MHC molecules, but instead recognizes lipids and glycolipids presented by the nonclassical CD1 molecule. It appears that NKT cells are capable of both upregulating and downregulating immune responses.

Finally, a population of regulatory T cells bearing the $CD3^+$ marker but lacking $CD4^+$ or $CD8^+$ has been described. The cells are referred to as double-negative T cells, but their mode of action is still unknown.

T cell recognition differs from that of B cells. The BCRs recognize free antigens based on their complementary conformations. In contrast, T cells respond to antigens only on the surface of other cells, because they recognize the complex of a peptide fragment bound in the groove of a class II or class I MHC glycoprotein. $CD4^+$ T cells recognize peptides in class II MHC complexes, whereas $CD8^+$ T cells recognize peptides in class I complexes. In the case of class II recognition, the MHC/peptide fragment complex is generated within an antigen-presenting cell (APC). They may be B cells, as described previously, macrophages, interdigitating dendritic cells of the lymph nodes, circulating dendritic cells, or Langerhans cells of the skin (see **Lymph Nodes**). In all of these cells, endocytosed proteins are fragmented by proteolytic enzymes within the endosomal/lysosomal compartment, and the resulting short peptides are loaded into the class II MHC groove. The complexes are then expressed at the surface of the cell, where they can be recognized by those $CD4^+$ T cells that bear the requisite TCR. The recognition is based not on the conformation of the antigen, but rather on key amino acids.

$CD8^+$ T cells recognize antigens and peptides in conjunction with class I MHC molecules. Generally, these antigens are derived from internally synthesized proteins, including viral proteins (see **Herpesviruses**). The fragments are produced in cytoplasmic vesicles by proteolysis, translocated into the endoplasmic reticulum, and bound to the class I MHC molecules, which are then brought to the cell surface. There they can be recognized by $CD8^+$ T cells expressing the appropriate receptors. Generally, the antigenic epitopes loaded into class I MHC are approximately nine amino acids in length.

Two signals, specific and nonspecific, are required for T cell activation. Specificity is provided by the interaction of the TCR with an MHC/peptide fragment complex. A second, non-antigen-specific costimulating signal is given by membrane glycoprotein of the APC B7-1 (CD80) or B7-2 (CD86). Through their interaction with CD28 on resting T cells, these molecules trigger activation and clonal expansion of the T cell. Engagement of the TCR in the absence of B7 costimulation results in clonal anergy. Another receptor expressed on activated T cells, CTLA-4, binds B7 and may serve as a regulatory signal.

A number of other costimulatory receptors have recently been described, including inducible costimulator intracellular (ICOS) and programmed death-1 (PD1), which regulate the immune response.

Natural Killer (NK) Cells

NK cells are an important component of the innate as well as the adaptive immune system. In fact, in animals that lack the RAG-1 or RAG-2 genes, NK cells provide a substantial degree of protection against infection. They comprise about 10% of the circulating lymphocytes. Although closely related to T cells, they lack the conventional TCRs, but express two specialized receptors. One receptor allows them to recognize virally infected cells or tumor cells, permitting them to destroy such cells. They also express receptors for the host's class I MHC molecules, which inhibit lytic activity. Thus, the NK cell is disarmed in the presence of its corresponding MHC molecule. Often, tumor cells or virally infected cells diminish expression of class I MHC molecules, thus avoiding the attack of cytotoxic T cells. They may then become targets for killing by NK cells, which are no longer shut off by recognition of the host MHC class I molecules. In addition, some NK cells express receptors for the constant portion of the immunoglobulin molecule. Armed with an IgG, the NK cell then has acquired a specific receptor to direct its cytotoxic effects, lysing target cells that bear the appropriate antigen. This process is referred to as antibody-dependent, cell-mediated cytotoxicity (ADCC). Thus, the NK can mediate its cytotoxic actions through two different recognition mechanisms. NK cells also produce cytokines that regulate the development of acquired immunity, for example, IFN-γ, and stimulate macrophages to produce cytokines, such as TNF and IL-12, which enhance the development of cell-mediated immune responses.

See Also the Following Articles

Autotolerance; Cytokines; Herpesviruses; Immune Response; Lymph Nodes; Thymus.

Further Reading

Bendelac, A., Rivera, M. N., Park, S. H. and Roark, J. H. (1997). Mouse CD1-specific NK1 T cells: development, specificity and function. *Annual Review of Immunology* **15**, 535–535.

Bentley, G. A. and Mariuzza, R. A. (1996). The structure of the T cell antigen receptor. *Annual Review of Immunology* **14**, 563.

Jonuleit, H. and Schmitt, E. (2003). The regulatory T cell family: distinct subsets and their interrelations. *Journal of Immunology* **171**, 6323–6327.

Kisielow, P. and von Boehmer, H. (1995). Development and selection of T cells: facts and puzzles. *Advances in Immunology* **58**, 87–209.

Kronenberg, M. and Rudensky, A. (2005). Regulation of immunity by self-reactive T cells. *Nature Insight* **435**, 598–603.

Lanier, L. L., Corliss, B. and Phillips, J. H. (1997). Arousal and inhibition of human NK cells. *Immunological Reviews* **155**, 145–154.

Ohashi, P. S. (2002). T-cell signaling and autoimmunity: molecular mechanisms of disease. *Nature Reviews Immunology* **2**, 427–438.

O'Shea, J. J., Ma, A. and Lipsky, P. (2001). Cytokines and autoimmunity. *Nature Reviews Immunology* **21**, 37–45.

Pitkänen, J. and Peterson, P. (2003). Autoimmune regulator: from loss of function to autoimmunity. *Genes and Immunity* **4**, 12–21.

Reth, M. (1992). Antigen receptors on B lymphocytes. *Annual Review of Immunology* **10**, 97–121.

Sakaguchi, S. (2004). Naturally arising CD4+ regulatory T cells for immunologic self-tolerance and negative control of immune responses. *Annual Review of Immunology* **22**, 531–562.

Salomon, B. and Bluestone, J. A. (2001). Complexities of CD28/B7: CTLA-4 costimulatory pathways in autoimmunity and transplantation. *Annual Review of Immunology* **19**, 225–252.

Shevach, E. M. (2002). CD4+ CD25+ suppressor T cells: more questions then answers. *Nature Reviews Immunology* **21**, 389–400.

Lymphokine-Activated Killer Cells (LAKs) *See:* Cytotoxic Lymphocytes.

Macrophage Antimycobacterial Activity, Effects of Stress on

C S Boomershine and B S Zwilling
The Ohio State University, Columbus, OH, USA

This article is reproduced from the previous edition, volume 2, pp 657–662, © 2000, Elsevier Inc.

Introduction
Stress Influences Mycobacterial Infection
Summary

Glossary

Nramp   (*natural resistance associated macrophage protein*) A phagolysosomal membrane product encoded by the *Nramp1* gene that confers resistance to mycobacterial growth during the early nonimmune phase of infection. Susceptible mice differ from resistant mice in a nonconservative glycine-to-aspartic acid substitution within a predicted transmembrane domain of Nramp1.

Introduction

Tuberculosis, a worldwide public health problem, has also increased significantly in the United States. The increase in tuberculosis is partly due to depressed cellular immunity associated with HIV infection. However, tuberculosis has also increased independently of HIV infection. Only since 1997, following mobilization of the public health community, has the incidence of tuberculosis in the United States begun to resume its downward course. Tuberculosis is a highly complex disease with multiple determinants for disease progression and severity. The susceptibility of humans to mycobacterial disease is determined partly by genetic differences. One of the most important genetic factors determining resistance to mycobacterial infection is the ability of host macrophages to control the growth of the tubercle bacilli.

Innate Resistance against Mycobacteria

The innate resistance of macrophages to mycobacterial infection has been studied most thoroughly in mice. The ability of mice to control mycobacterial growth in the spleen, following intravenous injection of *Mycobacterium bovis* BCG, maps to a region on mouse chromosome 1. Mice resistant to mycobacterial growth are termed Bcg^r, whereas those strains in which mycobacteria grow exponentially are termed Bcg^s. The resistance of Bcg^r mice is mediated by the *Nramp1* gene, which has been cloned in both mice and humans. *Nramp1* codes for a phagolysosomal membrane product termed natural resistance associated macrophage protein. Susceptible mice differ from resistant mice in a nonconservative glycine-to-aspartic acid substitution within a predicted transmembrane domain of Nramp1. While the mechanism of Nramp-mediated resistance remains ill defined, work from the authors' laboratory suggests that Nramp1 acts as a transporter of iron into the macrophage phagolysosome.

Although the susceptibility of an individual to mycobacterial disease is influenced strongly by innate immunity, genetic differences alone cannot account for the recent rise in the incidence of tuberculosis. The vast majority (90–95%) of people exposed to pathogenic strains of mycobacteria are able to control the growth of the organism without any disease manifestations. While some macrophages are able to limit mycobacterial growth, they are not sufficient to resolve a primary mycobacterial infection. Fortunately, macrophages are the major antigen-presenting cells of the body. Enzymes in the macrophage phagolysosome digest microorganisms killed by the respiratory burst and some microbial peptides become associated with glycoproteins encoded by genes of the major histocompatibility complex (MHC). Peptides coupled to MHC class II glycoproteins are cycled to the cell surface where they serve as the sole basis for antigen recognition by CD4$^+$ T lymphocytes. These macrophages then travel to regional lymph nodes where they present this processed antigen to T cells.

Specific Immune Response to Mycobacterial Infection

T-cell activation results in the development of cell-mediated immunity and enhanced reactivity to the purified protein derivatives (PPD) of mycobacteria. Activated Th cells then travel to the area of the primary focus and release lymphokines that cause monocytes to migrate into the site and differentiate into specialized histiocytic cells termed epithelioid giant cells. The primary lesion becomes organized into a granuloma, with macrophages containing ingested mycobacteria located centrally surrounded by epithelioid giant cells and activated T cells. The production of interferon (IFN)-γ by activated T cells results in macrophage activation and enhanced antimicrobial activity resulting from the activation of IFN-γ responsive genes. Mycobacteria may persist within macrophages of the granuloma for decades, but in immunocompetent individuals, further multiplication and spread are usually confined. The relative strength of the cell-mediated immunity of the host ultimately determines if resumption in multiplication of the mycobacteria will occur. The consequence of a resumption in the multiplication of bacilli leads to tuberculosis with subsequent tissue destruction, systemic dissemination of disease, and, when left untreated, death. Reactivation of disease has been attributed to several environmental factors, including protein malnutrition associated with chronic alcoholism, immunosenescence associated with aging, and stress.

Stress Influences Mycobacterial Infection

One of the first observations that stressful life events can affect disease pathogenesis was made in studies of tuberculosis by Ishigami. Ishigami found decreased phagocytic cell activity during periods of emotional stress in chronically ill, tuberculous school children. He postulated that the stressful school environment led to the children's immunodepressed state and their increased susceptibility to tuberculosis. Contemporaneous studies have proven that physical and psychological stress can modulate susceptibility to tuberculosis as well as general immune function. Physiologic responses to stressors are mediated by both the hypothalamic–pituitary–adrenal (HPA) axis and the sympathetic nervous system (SNS).

HPA Axis Effects on Mycobacterial Infection

The HPA axis mediates the stress response by producing a cascade of hormones in response to a variety of stimuli, ultimately resulting in the enhanced production of glucocorticoids by the adrenal glands. Glucocorticoids then enter the circulation and exert their effects through binding to cytoplasmic receptors. Upon binding, the glucocorticoid–receptor complex is internalized and translocated to the nucleus where it binds to glucocorticoid response elements (GREs). The receptor-charged GREs enhance the transcription initiation of glucocorticoid-regulated genes influencing the amount of critical proteins within the cell. Glucocorticoids have been shown to suppress the immune response. Glucocorticoid hormones cause a species- and cell type-specific lysis of lymphocytes. They suppress the inflammatory response by decreasing the number of circulating leukocytes and the migration of tissue leukocytes, inhibiting fibroblast proliferation, and inducing lipocortins that blunt the production of prostaglandins and leukotrienes, which are potent anti-inflammatory molecules.

Mononuclear cells possess high-affinity (type II) glucocorticoid receptors and represent one of the best studied primary target cells for glucocorticoids. Studies have shown that the production of proinflammatory cytokines interleukin (IL)-1, IL-6, and tumor necrosis factor (TNF)-α by activated macrophages is blocked at the transcriptional and posttranscriptional level by glucocorticoids. The downregulation of these potent mediators of inflammation underlies some of the immunosuppressive and anti-inflammatory actions of glucocorticoids, but does not address the effect glucocorticoids have on macrophage–T-cell interactions. Due to the requirement for macrophage MHC class II expression in antigen presentation for the induction of an immune response, the authors began their work by evaluating the effect of restraint stress on the expression of MHC class II glycoprotein expression in murine macrophages.

MHC class II glycoprotein expression is induced in mice following the injection of antigen or microorganisms *in vivo* or by treatment of macrophages with recombinant IFN-γ *in vitro*. It was found that macrophages from resistant strains of mice are able to persistently express MHC class II following infection of the mice with *M. bovis* (strain BCG). It was shown subsequently that the treatment of macrophages from Bcg^r mice with rIFN-γ induced persistent MHC class II expression, whereas macrophages from

Bcg[s] mice expressed this glycoprotein only transiently. The regulation of MHC class II expression by macrophages from resistant and susceptible mice also differed. Glucocorticoid treatment of macrophages from susceptible mice resulted in decreased MHC class II expression, whereas MHC class II expression by macrophages from resistant mice was unaffected.

The regulation of MHC class II expression by glucocorticoids raised the possibility that stress could modulate class II expression following activation of the HPA axis. This hypothesis was confirmed by demonstrating that restraint stress suppressed MHC class II expression by murine peritoneal macrophages and that this suppression coincided with peak corticosterone levels in plasma. The authors' previous work that showed strain-specific differences in MHC class II glycoprotein expression was extended by showing that the stress-induced suppression of MHC class II expression was limited to certain strains of mice. Bcg[r] mice were resistant to the restraint stress-induced decrease in MHC class II glycoprotein expression observed in Bcg[s] mice. The resistance of Bcg[r] mice was not due to a decrease in HPA axis activation, as corticosterone suppressed the induction of MHC class II by macrophages from both resistant and susceptible mice.

Adrenalectomy ameliorated the suppressive effects of restraint stress on MHC class II expression in Bcg[s] mice by abrogating the increase in corticosterone that results from HPA axis activation. Later experiments showed that the difference in MHC class II expression by macrophages from resistant and susceptible mice was due to a difference in MHC class II mRNA stability (**Figure 1**). Cortisterone decreased the stability of MHC class II mRNA in macrophages from susceptible mice but not in macrophages from resistant mice. The stability of mRNA of other IFN-γ-induced genes was affected similarly. Thus, the increased mRNA stability of macrophages from Bcg[r] mice may account for the pleiotrophic effects that have been attributed to *Nramp1*.

The differential regulation of MHC class II glycoprotein expression by glucocorticoids could account for differences in tuberculosis susceptibility. The role of HPA axis activation in the control of the growth of mycobacteria in humans has been the subject of some discussion. Glucocorticoid treatment of human macrophages suppressed antimicrobial activity markedly. However, Rook and co-workers showed that dexamethasone increased the susceptibility of monocytes from some individuals to mycobacterial growth, but other donor monocytes were unaffected by glucocorticoid treatment.

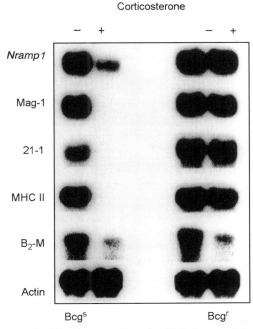

Figure 1 Stabilized expression of mRNA is associated with mycobacterial resistance controlled by *Nramp1*. Splenic macrophages from Bcg[r] and Bcg[s] mice were stimulated with rIFN-γ for 24 h followed by treatment with corticosterone. After 20 h, total RNA was extracted, and the effect of corticosterone on the expression of rIFN-γ-induced genes was determined by Northern analysis. Copyright 1997 by the American Society for Microbiology. Reprinted with permission from Brown *et al.* (1997).

These studies, together with previous work on MHC class II expression, led the authors to conduct a series of experiments to determine if mycobacterial growth, which is under *Nramp1* control, may also be affected differentially by HPA axis activation. It was found that activation of the HPA axis increased the growth of mycobacteria in susceptible mice but did not affect the ability of resistant mice to limit growth of the bacilli (**Figure 2**). The failure of restraint stress to increase the susceptibility of Bcg[r] mice was not due to unresponsiveness of this strain of mouse to HPA axis activation. HPA axis activation resulted in an increase in plasma corticosterone and ACTH levels in both strains of mice. The role of corticosterone in mediating the effects of HPA axis activation was demonstrated in three ways. First, adrenalectomy abolished the effect of HPA activation on mycobacterial growth. Second, treatment of Bcg[s] mice with the glucocorticoid receptor antagonist RU 486 abrogated the effects of restraint stress. Finally, the implantation of timed-release pellets that elevated plasma corticosterone levels to those attained by restraint increased the growth of mycobacteria in adrenalectomized susceptible mice. A subsequent *in vitro* study of macrophages

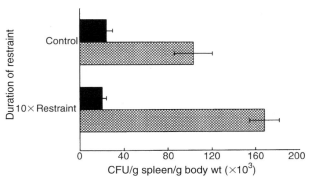

Figure 2 Regulation of mycobacterial growth by the hypothalamic–pituitary–adrenal axis: differential responses of *Mycobacterium bovis* (strain BCG)-resistant and -susceptible mice. Mice were restrained for ten 18-h cycles after infection with 5×10^4 CFU of *M. avium*. The numbers of CFU in the spleens were determined 12 days after infection. Data are the means ± SD for seven animals per group. The difference between growth of mycobacteria in the spleens of Bcg^r (■) mice versus growth in those of Bcg^s (■) mice was significant ($P < 0.001$). Copyright 1993 by the American Society for Microbiology. Reprinted with permission from Brown *et al.* (1993).

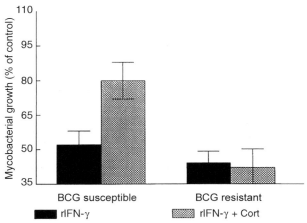

Figure 3 Cytokine-mediated activation of macrophages from *Mycobacterium bovis* (strain BCG)-resistant and -susceptible mice: differential effect of corticosterone on antimycobacterial activity and expression of the *Nramp1* gene. Splenic macrophages were treated with rIFN-γ for 24 h prior to infection with 4×10^5 CFU of *M. avium*. After 24 h to allow for phagocytosis and following removal of unphagocytized bacteria, the cultures were treated with 10^{-6} *M* corticosterone + rIFN-γ or just rIFN-γ for 5 days prior to lysis of the macrophages and pulsing of the bacteria with [^{3}H] uracil. Data are expressed as the percentage of the control value, which represents the amount of radioactivity incorporated by the bacteria after infection of cultures of macrophages treated with rIFN-γ divided by that of cultures not treated with rIFN-γ. The effect of corticosterone on the antimycobacterial activity of rIFN-γ-activated macrophages from Bcg^s mice was significant ($P \leq 0.03$). Copyright 1995 by the American Society for Microbiology. Reprinted with permission from Brown *et al.* (1995).

from Bcg^r and Bcg^s mice showed that corticosterone addition decreased the antimycobacterial activity of susceptible macrophages, whereas corticosterone had no effect on resistant macrophages (**Figure 3**).

Sympathetic Nervous System Effects on Mycobacterial Infection

Stress results in activation of the HPA axis as well as the SNS. The authors have also reported that epinephrine treatment of peritoneal macrophages suppressed MHC class II expression induced by rIFN-γ. Other observations found that restraint stress also increased epinephrine and norepinephrine levels in the spleen. Numerous other studies have reported that macrophage function can be suppressed or stimulated by catecholamines. It was found that catecholamine treatment of macrophages infected with mycobacteria inhibited intracellular growth of the bacilli. By using specific adrenoceptor agonists and antagonists, it was shown that this effect of catecholamines was mediated via the α_2-adrenergic receptor. The mechanism that accounts for this stimulation of macrophage functional capacity by catecholamines is under investigation. The use of macrophages harvested from Bcg^s mice in this study demonstrates that susceptible macrophages can be induced to control mycobacterial growth.

It has been reported that epinephrine treatment of *Mycobacterium avium*-infected macrophages increased IL-10 production. This effect was mediated by the β_r-adrenoceptor and could be mimicked by the addition of cAMP. IL-10 is a cytokine produced by a variety of immune cells that has a diverse array of actions. IL-10 production could play a role in tuberculosis by affecting the production of IFN-γ by T cells. IL-10 has been shown to inhibit MHC class II expression on monocytes and to inhibit T-cell proliferation directly. Preliminary studies in the authors' laboratory have also found that catecholamine treatment can inhibit macrophage activity. It has been shown that the addition of catecholamines during the infection of rIFN-γ-primed macrophages reduced reactive nitrogen intermediate production. Studies on the regulation of catecholamine-induced modulation of macrophage function are currently underway.

Summary

Differences in the resistance of certain mouse strains to mycobacterial growth have allowed us to study the effect activation of the HPA axis has on the innate mechanisms of mycobacterial resistance. It has been shown that macrophages from *M. bovis* BCG-resistant and-susceptible mice differ in their susceptibility to HPA axis-mediated effects. MHC class II glycoprotein expression by macrophages from Bcg^s mice decreased in response to increased plasma corticosterone levels induced by restraint. Restraint of Bcg[r] mice led to a similar rise in corticosterone levels, but MHC class II expression remained unaffected. Restraint stress also increased mycobacterial growth in susceptible mice but did not affect the ability of resistant mice to limit growth of the bacilli. These results suggest that activation of the HPA axis may account for the increase in susceptibility of Bcg[s] mice to mycobacterial growth. This suppression may be particularly apparent in individuals who express the mutation in *Nramp1* that results in susceptibility to mycobacterial disease and may account for the increase in the incidence of active tuberculosis among susceptible populations. Other work in the authors' laboratory has shown that catecholamine treatment of susceptible macrophages increased their ability to inhibit the intracellular growth of mycobacteria. The significance of these findings to mycobacterial disease is under investigation.

See Also the Following Articles

Cytotoxic Lymphocytes; Immune Response; Infection; Macrophages.

Further Reading

Ader, R., Felten, D. L. and Cohen, N. (eds.) (1991). *Psychoneuroimmunology* (2nd edn.). San Diego: Academic Press.

Beato, M. (1989). Gene regulation by steroid hormones. *Cell* **56**, 335.

Blackwell, J. M. (1996). Structure and function of the natural-resistance-associated macrophage protein (Nramp1), a candidate protein for infectious and autoimmune disease susceptibility. *Molecular Medicine Today* **2**, 205–211.

Bloom, B. R. (1992). Tuberculosis, back to the frightening future. *Science* **358**, 538–539.

Brown, D. H., Lafuse, W. P. and Zwilling, B. S. (1995). Cytokine-mediated activation of macrophages from *Mycobacterium bovis* BCG-resistant and -susceptible mice: Differential effects of corticosterone on antimycobacterial activity and expression of the *Bcg* gene (candidate *Nramp*). *Infection and Immunity* **63**, 2983–2988.

Brown, D. H., Lafuse, W. P. and Zwilling, B. S. (1997). Stabilized expression of mRNA is associated with mycobacterial resistance controlled by Nramp1. *Infection and Immunity* **65**, 597–603.

Brown, D. H., Sheridan, J., Pearl, D. and Zwilling, B. S. (1993). Regulation of mycobacterial growth by the hypothalamic-pituitary-adrenal axis: Differential responses of *Mycobacterium bovis* BCG-resistant and -susceptible mice. *Infection and Immunity* **61**, 4793–4800.

Centers for Disease Control and Prevention (1995). Tuberculosis morbidity—United States, 1994. *MMWR Morbidity and Mortality Weekly Report* **44**, 387–389, 395.

Chen, L., Boomershine, C. S., Wang, T., Lafuse, W. P. and Zwilling, B. S. (1999). Synergistic interaction of catecholamine hormones and *Mycobacterium avium* results in the induction of interleukin-10 mRNA expression by murine peritoneal macrophages. *Journal of Neuroimmunology* **93**, 149–155.

Collins, F. M. (1989). Mycobacterial disease: Immunosuppression and acquired immunodeficiency syndrome. *Clinical Microbiology Reviews* **2**, 360–377.

Dannenberg, A. M. (1993). Immunopathogenesis of pulmonary tuberculosis. *Hospital Practice* **1**, 51–58.

Fiorentino, D. F., Bond, M. W. and Mosmann, T. R. (1989). Two types of mouse T helper cells. IV. Th2 clones secrete a factor that inhibits cytokine production by Th1 clones. *Journal of Experimental Medicine* **170**, 2081–2095.

Ishigami, T. (1919). The influence of psychic acts on the progress of pulmonary tuberculosis. *American Review of Tuberculosis* **2**, 470–484.

Kuhn, D. E., Baker, B. D., Lafuse, W. P. and Zwilling, B. S. (1999). Differential iron transport into phagosomes isolated from the RAW264.7 macrophage cell lines transfected with Nramp1[Gly159] or Nramp1[Asp169]. *Journal of Leukocyte Biology* **66**, 113–119.

Lalani, I., Bhol, K. and Ahmed, R. (1997). Interleukin-10: Biology, role in inflammation, and autoimmunity. *Annals of Allergy Asthma and Immunology* **79**, 469–481.

Malefyt, R., Haanen, J., Spits, H., et al. (1991). IL-10 and viral IL-10 strongly reduced antigen specific T cell proliferation by diminishing the antigen presenting capacity of monocytes via down regulation of class II major histocompatibility complex expression. *Journal of Experimental Medicine* **174**, 915–924.

Malefyt, T., Yssel, H. and de Vries, J. E. (1993). Direct effects of IL-10 on subsets of human CD4+ T cell clones and resting T cells. *Journal of Immunology* **150**, 4754–4765.

Malo, D., Vogan, K., Vidal, S., et al. (1994). Haplotype mapping and sequence analysis of the mouse Nramp gene predict susceptibility to infection with intracellular parasites. *Genomics* **23**, 51–61.

Miles, B. A., Lafuse, W. P. and Zwilling, B. S. (1996). Binding of alpha-adrenergic receptors stimulates the anti-mycobacterial activity of murine peritoneal macrophages. *Journal of Neuroimmunology* **71**, 19–24.

Rook, G. A. W., Steele, J., Ainsworth, M. and Leveton, C. (1987). A direct effect of glucocorticoid hormones on the ability of human and murine macrophages to control the growth of *M. tuberculosis*. *European Journal of Respiratory Disease* **71**, 286–291.

Safley, S. A. and Ziegler, H. K. (1994). Antigen processing and presentation. In: Zwilling, B. S. & Eisenstein, T. K. (eds.) *Macrophage–Pathogen Interactions*, pp. 115–130. New York: Dekker.

Sheridan, J. F., Dobbs, C., Jung, J., et al. (1998). Stress-induced neuroendocrine modulation of viral pathogenesis and immunity. *Annals of the New York Academy of Sciences* **840**, 803–808.

Stead, W. W. (1992). Genetics and resistance to tuberculosis. *Annals of Internal Medicine* **116**, 937–941.

Vespa, L., Johnson, S. C., Aldrich, W. A. and Zwilling, B. S. (1987). Modulation of macrophage I-A expression: Lack of effect of prostaglandins and glucocorticoids on macrophages that continuously express I-A. *Journal of Leukocyte Biology* **41**, 47–54.

Wiegeshaus, E., Balasubramanian, V. and Smith, D. W. (1989). Immunity to tuberculosis from the perspective of pathogenesis. *Infection and Immunity* **57**, 3671–3676.

Zwilling, B. S. (1994). Neuroimmunomodulation of macrophage function. In: Glaser, R. & Kiecolt-Glaser, J. (eds.) *Handbook of Human Stress and Immunity*, pp. 53–76. New York: Academic Press.

Zwilling, B. S., Brown, D., Christner, R., et al. (1990). Differential effect of restraint stress on MHC class II expression by murine peritoneal macrophages. *Brain Behavior and Immunity* **4**, 330–338.

Zwilling, B. S., Brown, D., Feng, N., Sheridan, J. and Pearl, D. (1993). The effect of adrenalectomy on the restraint stressed induced suppression of MHC class II expression by murine peritoneal macrophages. *Brain Behavior and Immunity* **7**, 29–35.

Zwilling, B. S., Brown, D. and Pearl, D. (1992). Induction of major histocompatibility complex class II glyco-proteins by interferon-γ: attenuation of the effects of restraint stress. *Journal of Neuroimmunity* **37**, 115–122.

Zwilling, B. S., Kuhn, D. E., Wikoff, L., Brown, D. and Lafuse, W. (1999). Role of iron in *Nramp1*-mediated inhibition of mycobacterial growth. *Infection and Immunity* **67**, 1386–1392.

Zwilling, B. S., Vespa, L. and Massie, M. (1987). Regulation of I-A expression by murine peritoneal macrophages: differences linked to the Bcg gene. *Journal of Immunology* **138**, 1372–1376.

Macrophages

W P Fehder
New York University, New York, NY, USA
F Tuluc
Children's Hospital of Philadelphia, Philadelphia, PA, USA
W-Z Ho and S D Douglas
Children's Hospital of Philadelphia and University of Pennsylvania Medical School, Philadelphia, PA, USA

This article is a revision of the previous edition article by W P Fehder, W–z Ho and S D Douglas, volume 2, pp 663–668, © 2000, Elsevier Inc.

Origin and Function of Monocytes/Macrophages
Stress and Monocytes/Macrophages

Glossary

Activated macrophage	A macrophage that has been stimulated either biochemically or immunologically and exhibits an increase in one or more functional activities or the appearance of a new functional activity.
Cytokines	A class of low-molecular-weight soluble protein molecules released by immune cells during the course of immune response that serve to mediate and regulate the amplitude and duration of immune/inflammatory responses in the organism. Cytokines are produced during the effector phases of natural and specific immunity in a brief self-limited event. Many of the same cytokine substances are produced by different cells and may act on many different cell types. Cytokines exert their action by binding to target cell-surface receptors, which may be on the surface of the secreting cell (autocrine action), on the surface of a nearby cell (paracrine action), or on the surface of a cell in a remote location (endocrine action) reached through the bloodstream.
Interleukins (ILs)	Cytokines that are principally synthesized by leukocytes and act primarily on leukocytes.
Macrophages	Large, irregularly shaped white blood cells measuring 25–50 µm in diameter that are the major differentiated cells of the mononuclear phagocyte system.
Mononuclear phagocytes	A class of immune cells that have a common lineage that includes monoblasts, promonocytes, monocytes, and macrophages.
Neurokinin (NK-)1 receptor	A G-protein-coupled receptor that mediates the biological responses to substance P that has been demonstrated on T cells, B lymphocytes, neutrophils, mast cells, and monocytes/macrophages.
Substance P (SP)	An 11-amino-acid peptide present in the central nervous system that is involved in the pathogenesis of nausea/emesis, pain, mood disorders, stress, anxiety, reinforcement, neurotoxicity, and neurogenesis. It is a member of the tachykinin family of neuropeptides. Outside the central nervous system, SP regulates intestinal motility and secretion, causes vasodilation, and serves as a modulator of a number of important immunological functions. Circulating levels of SP become elevated in stressful situations; monocytes stimulated

Tissue macro-phages

by SP produce and release cytokines such as tumor necrosis factor α, interleukin-1, and interleukin-6.

Members of the monocyte/macrophage family that have migrated from the circulation into a body tissue, remaining adherent for several months and ultimately migrating to nearby draining lymph nodes for disposal at the end of their useful life. Some tissue macrophages may survive for the lifetime of the individual.

Macrophages are a diverse group of leukocytes (white blood cells) that share a common origin in the bone marrow and enter the circulation as incompletely differentiated monocytes. Macrophages are the major differentiated cells of the monocyte/macrophage system.

Origin and Function of Monocytes/Macrophages

The monocyte/macrophage system comprises bone marrow monoblasts and promonocytes, peripheral blood monocytes, and tissue macrophages. The peripheral blood monocytes differentiate into macrophages that are capable of phagocytosis of particles, cells, bacteria, and fungi; they also have major roles in antigen presentation and cytokine secretion. Monocytes remain in the circulatory system or migrate to different tissues where they increase in size, becoming tissue macrophages. Tissue macrophages become part of the architecture of specific tissues where they may remain, performing specific protective functions and functions unique to the organ. These tissue macrophages are given names according to their location (Table 1). Tissue macrophages may be stimulated by chemical messengers to break away from their attachment and migrate along with mobile macrophages and monocytes to areas of inflammation by a process known as chemotaxis. The term monocyte/macrophage system is virtually synonymous with, and has replaced in the nomenclature, the reticuloendothelial system.

Macrophages perform an essential function in the immune system by attacking and destroying invading bacteria, viruses, and other injurious substances, participating in a wide range of physiological and pathological processes. Although many micro-organisms are phagocytized and destroyed with ease by macrophages, certain pathogens such as listeria, salmonella, brucella, mycobacteria, chlamydia, rickettsia, leishmania, toxoplasma, trypanosoma, and legionella are able to parasitize nonactivated macrophages and replicate within them. Only when macrophages have been activated against these specific intracellular pathogens are they able to inhibit or destroy them. Monocytes and macrophages play an active role in the clearance and inactivation of most viral pathogens. Paradoxically, these same cells also represent a major target cell and infectious reservoir for many viruses. The human immunodeficiency virus (HIV-1) infects and replicates within monocytes and macrophages by binding to the CD4 and CCR5 receptors that are present on the macrophage cell membrane.

The macrophages in tissues and body cavities are a cell population that is regularly renewed by the influx of monocytes manufactured in the bone marrow and circulated via the blood. The control of monocyte production, release of monocytes into the blood, monocyte migration and extravasation into tissues, and finally differentiation into tissue macrophages are accomplished by means of soluble chemical factors. These soluble chemical factors are termed cytokines and are themselves influenced by stress-associated factors such as adrenocorticotropic hormone (ACTH), cortisol, adrenergic hormones, and neuropeptides such as substance P (SP), vasoactive intestinal peptide (VIP), and proopiomelanocortin (POMC). Macrophages secrete cytokines that produce effects on other immune cells, as well as receptors for cytokines produced by other immune cells, thereby promoting bidirectional communication. The major cytokines that produce effects on the monocyte/macrophage cells are: interferon (IFN-)γ, IFN-α, IFN-β, and interleukin (IL-)1. Monocyte/macrophages produce and secrete IL-1, IL-6, and tumor necrosis factor (TNF-)α.

Phagocytosis and Microbicidal Functions

The term macrophage was first used more than 100 years ago by Elie Metchnikoff to describe the large mononuclear phagocytic cells he observed in tissues. Through the process of phagocytosis, macrophages are

Table 1 Tissue-localized macrophage/monocyte cells

Location	Cell type
Bone marrow	Monoblasts, promonocytes, monocytes, macrophages
Peripheral blood	Monocytes
Skin	Langerhans cell and histiocyte
Lung	Alveolar macrophage
Bone	Osteoclast
Liver	Kupffer cell
Central nervous system	Microglia
Lymphoid organs	Tissue macrophages, dendritic cells
Spleen	Red-pulp macrophages
Gastrointestinal tract	Tissue macrophages
Serous cavities	Pleural and peritoneal macrophages

one of the most effective components of nonspecific immunity. Macrophages also play two essential roles in specific immunity, first as professional antigen presenting cells and then, with proper stimulation, as immune effector cells. Once activated by the immune system, macrophages become more powerful than neutrophils in their ability to phagocytize. Macrophages are able to engulf much larger particles such as whole red blood cells and malarial parasites or as many as 100 bacteria. Phagocytized particles are encapsulated and digested by intracellular proteolytic enzymes contained in lysosomes and other cytoplasmic granules. Macrophage lysosomes are unusual in that they contain lipases that aid in the digestion of the thick lipid bacterial membranes. Once the engulfed particles are digested, macrophages can extrude residual products. Macrophages perform many essential roles in the immune response such as the direct killing of damaged cells, bacteria, and viruses and antigen presentation. Macrophages produce and respond to cytokines and other chemicals central to both the inflammatory and the specific immune response. There are populations of macrophages that live throughout the life span of the organism.

Cytokine Mediation of Macrophage Response

Macrophages express major histocompatibility complex (MHC) class II on their surface and are important antigen-presenting cells for both B and T lymphocytes. Macrophages, when activated by cytokines produced by T helper (TH) cells, become effector cells of cell-mediated immunity. Macrophages are the first cells involved in an immune reaction and help orchestrate immune events both by the production of chemical signals (cytokines and SP) and by the processing and presentation of antigens to subsets of T lymphocytes that may either enhance or suppress specific immune responses. Activated macrophages also produce cytokines, such as IL-1, TNF-α, and IL-6, that augment T-cell function, as well as IL-8, macrophage colony-stimulating factor (M-CSF), granulocyte macrophage colony-stimulating factor (GM-CSF), and granulocyte colony-stimulating factor (G-CSF) that stimulate polymorphonuclear neutrophil (PMN) and monocyte activity. The ability of macrophages and lymphocytes to stimulate one another's functions provides an important amplification mechanism for specific immunity. Thus, macrophages play an important and central immunoregulatory role.

Toll-like Receptors

Toll-like receptors, identified in macrophages in mammals, are a relatively new family of membrane receptors able to recognize specific patterns of pathogen components, such as bacterial endotoxins and viral nucleic acids. Toll-like receptor (TLR)-4 is part of a molecular complex that recognizes and mediates intracellular responses to lipopolysaccharide (LPS). Pathogen recognition by TLRs activates the innate immune system through different signaling pathways, causing inflammatory responses such as cytokine production. Impaired adrenal stress response occurs in TLR-2-deficient mice, suggesting that TLR-2 and, possibly, TLR-4 may constitute an important link between the immune and endocrine stress systems at both the central and peripheral levels, particularly during inflammation and sepsis.

Stress and Monocytes/Macrophages

An examination of the role of macrophages in the modulation of immune function by stress is particularly compelling. A representation of the interactions among various stressors and the immune system is provided in **Figure 1**.

Macrophages play a pivotal role in immune responses, first as professional antigen-presenting cells stimulating the expansion of one of two sets of CD4$^+$ T-cell populations (TH1 or TH2) and finally, when activated themselves, functioning as major effector cells in cell-mediated immunity. The TH1 and TH2 responses are highly integrated and contraregulated, relying on two distinctly different profiles of cytokine production. Many of the cytokines produced by one or the other subpopulation have positive effector functions and, in addition, negatively regulate the activity of the alternate subgroup. The negative regulation may be at the level of either T-cell expansion or T-cell effector functions, including macrophage activation. Thus, an immune response in which TH1 cells are stimulated downregulates the co-stimulation of TH2 cells. Conversely, an immune response in which TH2 cells are stimulated downregulates both the co-stimulation of TH1 cells and their effector activity.

TH1 cells produce cytokines associated with aspects of classic cell-mediated immunity, producing IFN-γ, IL-2, IL-3, GM-CSF, TNF-α, and TNF-β, which activate macrophages. IFN-γ induces oxygen burst and nitric oxide production, which are essential for microbicidal reactions. IL-3 activates macrophages, causing increased antigen presentation. IFN-γ and IL-2 both stimulate macrophages to produce TNF-α, which in turn further stimulates macrophage activation in a cascade of events.

TH2 cells produce cytokines (IL-4, IL-5, and IL-6) that are associated with the B-cell responses of humoral immunity. IL-4 acts as a growth factor specific for TH2 cells, acts as an inhibitory factor for the

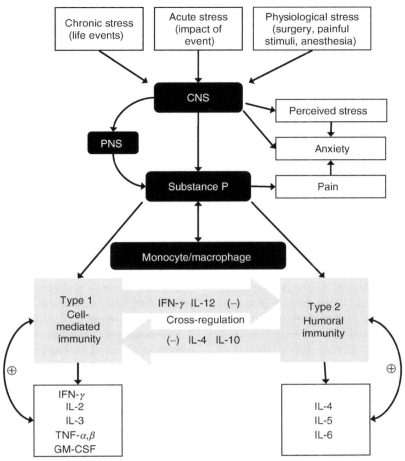

Figure 1 Stress effects on monocyte/macrophages. The effects of stress on the immune system are mediated by the neuropeptide substance P. The cells of the monocyte/macrophage system have receptors for and are able to synthesize and release substance P. Thus, they play a central role in mediating these effects. CNS, central nervous system; GM-CSF, granulocyte macrophage colony-stimulating factor; IFN, interferon; IL, interleukin; PNS, peripheral nervous system; TNF, tumor necrosis factor.

stimulation of TH1 cells by IL-2, and also effectively inhibits IFN-γ activation of macrophages. When appropriately stimulated by TH2 cytokines and antigen, B cells give rise to antibody-secreting plasma cells. The antigen–antibody complex serves as a powerful stimulator of the monocyte/macrophage phagocytosis of these circulating complexes.

In a mouse surgical-sponge model of inflammation, acute restraint-induced stress caused increase in leukocyte trafficking to the site of immune activation. Mice acutely stressed before sponge implantation presented 200–300% higher macrophage, neutrophil, natural killer cell, and T-cell infiltration than did nonstressed animals. Stress-induced increases in leukocyte trafficking may be responsible for immunoprotection during trauma, surgery, and infection, but it may also exacerbate immunopathological responses during inflammatory diseases, such as arthritis, cardiovascular disease, psoriasis, multiple sclerosis, and gingivitis.

Substance P as a Mediator of Stress Response

A major mediator of the effects of stress on monocyte/macrophage function is the neurotransmitter peptide SP, which is widely distributed in the central, peripheral, and enteric nervous systems. SP may have a major role in several inflammatory disease processes such as rheumatoid arthritis, bullous pemphigus, asthma, and inflammatory bowel diseases such as Crohn's disease and ulcerative colitis, as well as in the transmission of pain. SP may be the chemical messenger of a neurogenic alarm system that serves to communicate stress in a reciprocal manner among the central nervous system (CNS), endocrine system, and immune system. SP is associated with the sympathetic nervous system and is essential to the maintenance of adrenal catecholamine secretion from the adrenal medulla in times of stress.

Studies of surgical patients demonstrate that the stress of surgery shifts the TH1/TH2 cytokine balance toward TH2, suggesting that cell-mediated immunity was downregulated. Furthermore, the highest immune alteration was associated with the most stressful and invasive surgery. Several experimental animal studies indicate an association between stress and levels of SP. Two studies of SP in the brain tissue of rats that had been subjected to stressful stimuli found decreases in SP levels, which the authors attributed to tissue SP depletion following the increased release of SP. Experimental models of induced stress such as restraint stress and sequential removal of group-housed rats were found to be associated with increased levels of SP in the periaqueductal gray area of the brain. Insulin-induced hypoglycemia or mild electric foot shock were shown to increase the release of both catecholamines and SP from rat adrenomedullary cells. The intracerebroventricular administration of SP in conscious rats elicited an integrated cardiovascular, behavioral, and endocrine response in a pattern consistent with an integrated stress response in rodents. Experimental evidence in first-time parachutists and patients undergoing diagnostic procedures demonstrated increased levels of circulating SP associated with acute psychological stress. The high levels of circulating SP remained elevated long after the anxiety associated with the acute stressor diminished.

Macrophages, endothelial cells, eosinophils, and Leydig cells have also been identified as nonneuronal sources of SP. The presence of specific SP receptors on the surface of monocytes and the ability of macrophages to produce SP suggest its role in the autocrine regulation of SP gene expression.

The biological responses to SP are mediated by the NK-1 receptor, a 407-amino-acid G-protein-coupled glycosylated receptor that has been demonstrated on T cells, B lymphocytes, monocytes, macrophages, neutrophils, and mast cells. There is a connection between SP in the peripheral nervous system and the immune system. There is direct innervation of the spleen by SP-containing nerve fibers in splenic areas adjacent to lymphocytes, macrophages, and granulocytes, with evidence of its role in the traffic of lymphocytes from lymph nodes. SP modulates the effector phase of adaptive immunity and serves as a co-stimulator in the activation of monocytes, macrophages, T cells, and B cells, with the subsequent release of regulatory cytokines by these cells.

Effect of Stress on Monocytopoiesis

Macrophages synthesize and release two hematopoietic growth factors, M-CSF and GM-CSF, in response to external stimuli such as particles that are phagocytosed and endotoxin. Furthermore, macrophages release IL-1 and TNF, which in turn can induce fibroblasts and endothelial cells to produce M-CSF and GM-CSF, which stimulate the production of mononuclear phagocytes. The spiral of increased inflammatory response is further magnified by the synthesis of TNF-α by mononuclear phagocytes in response to GM-CSF simulation. Thus, macrophages play a pivotal role in regulating immune response. SP induces the production of hematopoietic growth factors IL-1, IL-6, and TNF-α from human monocytes. Bone marrow is innervated by nerve fibers that release SP in concentrations that induce tissue macrophages resident in bone marrow to release IL-1, IL-3, and GM-CSF.

Furthermore, macrophages express NK-1 receptors and serve as a nonneural source of SP. The release of SP by macrophages serves as a paracrine mechanism (by stimulating nearby macrophages) for amplifying the effect of stress on monocytopoiesis. Thus, stress acting through SP as a mediator may play a physiological role in regulating monocytopoiesis through two mechanisms: stimulation of the direct release of hematopoietic growth factors by monocytes and paracrine amplification.

Effect of Stress on Monocyte/Macrophage Function

The manner and extent to which stress influences immune response is, then, of vital concern. Stress may either enhance or inhibit macrophage function. Experimental evidence shows that SP plays a role in modulating immune response at each of the succeeding levels of response to foreign antigen. SP induces the release of stem cell factor and IL-1 in bone marrow stroma, thereby mediating hematopoesis. A summary of the effects of stress on the monocyte/macrophage system is provided in **Table 2**.

During acute inflammatory reactions, the number of circulating monocytes is increased with enhanced bone marrow production. This is mitigated by the decreased time that the monocytes are in the circulation due to efflux into inflammatory exudates. The SP-containing neurons have direct contact with immune and hematopoietic cells in the primary and secondary lymphoid organs. Thus, traffic of lymphocytes may be regulated by the secretion of neuroactive peptides such as SP from nerves.

Macrophages and monocytes increase phagocytosis and increase chemotaxis in response to SP. Increased levels of IL-6 are released by peritoneal macrophages in response to increased levels of SP produced by mice exposed to cold-water stress. Macrophages from humans and guinea pigs have receptors for and respond to SP-releasing cytokines

Table 2 Effects of stress on monocytes/macrophages

Source	Model	Effect
Animal (*in vitro*)	Macrophages exposed to salmonella	Increased SP receptors
Animal (*in vivo*)	Mice exposed to salmonella given SP antagonist	Increased mortality
	Mice exposed to cold-water stress	Increased SP; increased IL-6 release by macrophages
	Stressed rats (restraint and sequential removal)	Increased levels of SP in periaqueductal gray area of brain
Human (*in vitro*)	Bone marrow stroma cells exposed to SP	Increased stem cell factor, IL-1
	Monocytes/macrophages exposed to SP	Increased IL-1, IL-6, IL-7, IL-10, IL-12, TNF-α; chemotaxis, and phagocytosis
Human (*in vivo*)	Acute psychological stress in parachutists	Increased SP
	Acute psychological stress in medical diagnostic procedures	Increased SP, CD8$^+$
	Sickle cell patients in vaso-occlusive crisis	Increased SP correlated with pain; increased IL-8

IL, interleukin; SP, substance P; TNF, tumor necrosis factor.

IL-1, IL-6, and TNF-α. Macrophages in mice exposed to oral salmonella doses expressed higher levels of SP receptors and the administration of the SP antagonist spantide II resulted in higher mortality than in non-SP-antagonized mice. Treatment with spantide II was also associated with significantly reduced levels of IL-12 and IFN-γ. Thus, SP serves to amplify on-going immune reactions and serves as a mediator in stress-induced immune reactions.

See Also the Following Articles

Cytokines; Immune Response; Macrophage Antimycobacterial Activity, Effects of Stress on; Neuroimmunomodulation.

Further Reading

Bornstein, S. R., Zacharowski, P., Schumann, R. R., et al. (2004). Impaired adrenal stress response in toll-like receptor 2-deficient mice. *Proceedings of the National Academy of Sciences USA* **101**, 16695–16700.

Chancellor-Freeland, C., Zhu, G., Kage, R., et al. (1995). Substance P and stress-induced changes in macrophages. *Annals of the New York Academy of Sciences* **771**, 472–484.

Douglas, S. and Ho, W. (2006). Morphology of monocytes and macrophages. In: Lichtman, M. A. (ed.) *Williams hematology* (7th edn., pp. 960–970). New York: McGraw Hill.

Hassan, F. and Douglas, S. (1990). Stress-related neuro-immunomodulation of monocyte-macrophage functions in HIV-1 infection. *Clinical Immunology and Immunopathology* **54**, 220–227.

Lewis, C. and McGee, J. (1992). *The macrophage*. Oxford: Oxford University Press.

Ho, W. Z. and Douglas, S. D. (2004). Substance P and neurokinin-1 receptor modulation of HIV. *Journal of Neuroimmunology* **157**, 48–55.

Lai, J. P., Ho, W. Z., Kilpatrick, L. E., et al. (2006). Full-length and truncated neurokinin-1 receptor expression and function during monocyte/macrophage differentiation. *Proceedings of the National Academy of Sciences USA* **103**, 7771–7776.

McGillis, J., Mitsuhashi, M. and Payan, D. (1990). Immunomodulation by tachykinin neuropeptides. *Annals of the New York Academy of Sciences* **594**, 85–94.

Perry, V. (1994). *Macrophages and the nervous system*. Austin, TX: R. G. Landes.

Viswanathan, K. and Dhabhar, F. S. (2005). Stress-induced enhancement of leukocyte trafficking into sites of surgery or immune activation. *Proceedings of the National Academy of Sciences USA* **102**, 5808–5813.

Major Depressive Disorder

A B Negrão and P W Gold
National Institute of Mental Health, Bethesda, MD, USA

This article is reproduced from the previous edition, volume 2, pp 669–675, © 2000, Elsevier Inc.

Stress System
Syndromes of Major Depression

Glossary

Amygdala	Brain region involved in the expression and acquisition of conditioned fear.
Atypical depression	Major depressive disorder with a predominance of somatic features (increased appetite, sleep, and weight gain) that are the inverse of what is seen in melancholia.
Cushing's disease	A disorder characterized by the clinical effects of increased circulating glucocorticoids caused by a pituitary ACTH-producing microadenoma.
Major depression	A psychiatric disorder characterized by depressed mood, loss of pleasure in most activities, and symptoms that affect cognitive function, appetite, weight control, sleep patterns, and sexual function.
Melancholia	A historical term that designates the presence of decreased appetite, weight loss, complete lack of pleasure, insomnia, and early morning worsening of symptoms in a patient with major depression.

Stress System

The stress response consists of a simultaneous repertoire of behavioral and physiological adaptations that promote survival during threatening situations. The most apparent are fear-related behaviors that include anxiety, decreased exploration (or freezing), increased vigilance, and intense focus on the threatening stimulus. Concurrently, there is evidence of physiological activation of both the hypothalamic-pituitary-adrenal (HPA) axis and the sympathetic nervous system. Metabolically, a catabolic state ensues that mobilizes fuel for the stressed body site or the brain, and endocrine programs for growth and reproduction are inhibited. Finally, there is systematic inhibition of vegetative functions whose execution would impair the likelihood of survival during a life-threatening crisis (e.g., feeding, sexual behavior, and sleep).

This section focuses on the core stress systems, the corticotropin-releasing hormone (CRH) (including the HPA axis) and the locus ceruleus–norepinephrine (LC–NE) systems. We also discuss the importance of other relevant neural substrates to the stress response and major depression.

Corticotropin-Releasing Hormone

Several discrete CRH systems have been identified in the brain. CRH was first discovered as the hypothalamic hormone that plays the principal role in the regulation of the HPA axis. Intrahypothalamic CRH pathways contribute to the inhibition of feeding and sexual behavior and to the inhibition of endocrine programs for growth. Parvocellular CRH neurons in the paraventricular nucleus (PVN) of the hypothalamus send terminals to brain stem arousal and autonomic centers. An extrahypothalamic CRH system has been identified in the amygdala and is important in modulating aversively charged emotional memory. The administration of a CRH antagonist directly into the central nucleus of the amygdala (CEA) diminishes fear conditioning significantly. These CRH pathways represent the anatomical context for the observation that the intracerebroventricular administration of CRH recapitulates many of the metabolic, endocrine, autonomic, and behavioral features of the stress response. While it is well known that cortisol participates in a classic negative feedback loop to restrain the HPA axis, amygdala and descending hypothalamic CRH pathways are actually activated by cortisol. Cortisol also contributes significantly to the inhibition of programs for growth and reproduction seen during stress, as well as to feedback restraint on an activated immune system (**Figure 1**).

Locus Ceruleus–Norepinephrine System

The LC–NE system originates in the mid-pons and sends a dense network of terminals to many cortical and subcortical structures. The LC–NE system serves globally as a generalized warning system, inhibits vegetative functions such as grooming, eating, and sleeping, and contributes to accompanying increases in autonomic outflows. Ascending norepinephrine pathways project to the PVN CRH neurons and exert excitatory effects on the HPA axis. Brain stem norepinephrine, in turn, also influences other key structures that work together with the core stress system components, including the amygdala.

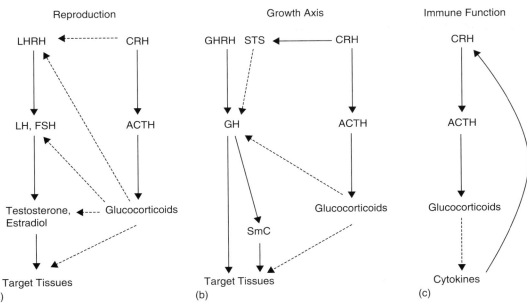

Figure 1 A representation of the interactions between the hypothalamic-pituitary-adrenal axis and other neuroendocrine systems: (a) reproductive axis, (b) the growth axis, (c) immune function. LHRH, luteinizing hormone-releasing hormone; CRH, corticotropin-releasing hormone; LH, luteinizing hormone; FSH, follicle-stimulating hormone; ACTH, corticotropin; GHRH, growth hormone-releasing hormone; STS, somatostatin; GH, growth hormone; SmC, somatomedin C. Dotted lines indicate inhibition and solid lines indicate stimulation.

CRH/LC–NE Systems and Interactions with Neural Substrates of Relevance to the Stress Response and Depression

Activation of the stress system sets into motion a range of fear-related behaviors and promotes the encoding of conditioned fear. The amygdala is the key structure involved in conditioned fear, and, as noted, CRH in the central nucleus of the amygdala in the rat plays an important role in this phenomenon. Activation of the amygdala is associated with activation of the HPA axis, most probably via direct projections from the CEA to the PVN. There is also evidence that the amygdala can activate the HPA axis indirectly via projections to brain stem catecholaminergic centers.

The classic effect of glucocorticoids on the CRH system is the negative feedback effect exerted on the HPA axis. Glucocorticoid receptors in the hippocampus play an important role in mediating this negative feedback restraint. However, not all glucocorticoid effects on the CRH system are inhibitory. Thus, glucocorticoids actually enhance the expression of CRH in the CEA and increase fear-related behaviors. This glucocorticoid effect provides the context for a feedforward loop between the amygdala and the HPA axis.

The core stress systems and the amygdala are also linked closely to the medial prefrontal cortex (MPC). This complex structure is important in promoting the extinction of conditioned fear encoded in the amygdala and, by doing so, exerts restraint on stress system activity. Pathways from the MPC to the brain stem

also inhibit brain stem autonomic centers. This structure also sends the only direct cortical connections to the hypothalamus, and the activation of glucocorticoid receptors located in the MPC inhibits the HPA axis. It has been shown that the chronic hypercortisolism of Cushing's disease is associated with a significant decrease in the size of the prefrontal cortex. This finding suggests the possibility of another feed-forward loop in the context of sustained hypercortisolism, a state in which the inhibitory actions of the MPC on the hypothalamus would be impaired due to cortisol-mediated atrophy.

The medial prefrontal cortex is also involved in a critical array of complex behaviors. This structure helps decide whether a particular situation is likely to result in reward or punishment and is involved in the shifting of affect from one state to another based on internal and external cues and in orchestrating sequences of sophisticated repertoires of motor activity and behavior. Activation of the amygdala takes the medial prefrontal cortex off line, thus inhibiting complex, innovative behaviors and promoting the kinds of autonomic, stereotyped repertoires that would be most adaptive in an immediately life-threatening situation.

Syndromes of Major Depression

Definition

Depression affects up to 15% of women and 8% of men worldwide. According to the World Health

Organization, depression is a greater source of morbidity for women than any other illness. The *Diagnostic and Statistical Manual of Mental Disorders*, 4th edition (DSM-IV), edited by the American Psychiatric Association, provides clinicians and researchers with criteria to diagnose someone who suffers from depression. Major depressive disorder, as the condition is named, is characterized by depressed mood or inability to experience pleasure and at least four of the following associated symptoms: feelings of worthlessness, suicidal thoughts, diminished concentration, and changes in weight, appetite, psychomotor activity, and sleep. The symptoms have to be severe enough to cause impairment in the patient's daily activities, and they have to last at least 2 weeks in order for the diagnosis to be firmed. The causes of the disorder are not known. Stressful life events play a role in the course of the disorder, and there are studies demonstrating the importance of heritable factors.

Phenotypic Subtypes of Major Depression

Major depression is a disorder that is clinically heterogeneous. Although the core symptoms (depressed mood and inability to experience pleasure) need to be present, there are many distinct clinical presentations of the disorder. Differences in the subtypes of major depression are determined by the combination of the associated features. Two subtypes of major depression, namely, major depression with melancholic features (melancholia) and major depression with atypical features (atypical depression), have received the greatest attention from investigators (**Table 1**).

Although the term depression implies a suppression of thought and feeling, melancholia is instead a state of hyperarousal and fear often stemming from a profound sense of personal unworthiness and pessimism about future prospects. Any loss in cognitive and emotional range is counterbalanced by the intensity of this anxiety, which coincides with, and is perhaps inseparable from, a loss of pleasure in everyday activities. Patients with severe melancholia seem to be in especially close contact with painfully charged memories of past losses and failures. The emotional intensity of melancholia is matched by indices of physiological hyperarousal (insomnia, early morning awakening, and hypercortisolemia). Patients also experience inhibition of vegetative functions: loss of appetite and libido, inhibition of growth, and sex steroid secretion.

In contrast to melancholia, patients with atypical depression often feel much less alive than usual and experience a profound inertia and fatigue that often isolates them and interferes with normal functioning. Characteristically, they sleep excessively, eat a lot,

Table 1 Characteristics of major depression with melancholic features (melancholia) and atypical features (atypical depression)

Characteristic	Melancholia	Atypical depression
Vegetative functions	Insomnia, anorexia, weight loss, diminished libido	Hypersomnia, increased appetite, weight gain
Behavior	Anxious, preoccupied with concerns about deficient self, preferential access to dysphorically charged memories	Partial reaction to positive stimuli, intense fatigue, diminished sense of connection to self
Stress system	Hyperactive	Hypoactive
Medical consequences	Osteoporosis, increased cardiovascular morbidity and mortality, prefrontal cortex abnormalities	Autoimmune disorders?
Response to treatment	Similar response to different classes of antidepressants	Preferentially to MAOIs[a]

[a]Monoamine oxidase inhibitors, an antidepressant medication that acts on the catabolic path of monoamines.

and usually gain weight. Like patients with melancholia, they have a diminished libido and a blunted capacity to experience everyday pleasure, although they may react temporarily to positive external and internal clues (mood reactivity).

Major Depression as a Disorder of Adaptation

As reviewed previously, the stress response system is a stereotyped, adaptive repertoire that ensures survival during threatened homeostasis. Major depression, by definition, is associated with relatively unshifting affect and simultaneous changes in fundamental biological processes that regulate sleep, food intake, metabolism, and reproduction. Similarities between the stress response and the phenomenology of melancholia prompted us to first postulate that the clinical and biochemical manifestations of this disorder reflect a dysregulation in stress system mediators. Changes seen during the stress response are under strict control by counterregulatory mechanisms that serve to limit the response in time and magnitude. Melancholia can be seen as a state of chronically and excessively activated stress response, possibly due to an escape of the usual regulatory influences. In that sense, melancholia would be a disorder of adaptation, more specifically, one in which the stress response required for survival becomes dysregulated and is the very source of the illness. In contrast, many symptoms found in atypical depression can reflect a pathological inactivation of stress system mediators. The remainder of this article reviews the lines of evidence indicating the convergence between a dysregulation of the stress response and the biochemical and neurobiological findings in both subtypes of major depression.

Major Depression with Melancholic Features

Hypercortisolemia and hypothalamic CRH secretion Sustained hypercortisolism has been demonstrated repeatedly in patients with major depression and is perhaps the best documented finding in the biology of psychiatric disorders. Many lines of evidence indicate that hypercortisolism of major depression is due to the hypersecretion of hypothalamic CRH neurons. Data obtained in brains taken from patients who had suffered with affective illness reveal overexpression of CRH in the hypothalamus.

Norepinephrine secretion Patients with melancholic depression show sustained and profoundly elevated levels of cerebrospinal fluid (CSF) NE when sampled through an indwelling lumbar drain for 30 h. Moreover, CSF NE levels were highly elevated during sleep, indicating that the hypersecretion of centrally directed norepinephrine was not an artifact of the conscious distress of the illness. Increased basal norepinephrine spillover into arterialized venous blood was noted in patients with major depression with melancholic features. We have subsequently replicated this finding in arterial plasma and have shown that patients with melancholic depression show significantly higher norepinephrine spillover than controls in response to psychological and pharmacological stimuli. Our patients also showed significantly higher basal heart rates and heart rate increases to psychological and pharmacological stressors.

Pathophysiology of melancholic depression The reciprocal connectivity of the structures that participate in the modulation of the core stress system suggests that similar phenotypes can be generated by primary defects in any of these structures, including the prefrontal cortex, the amygdala, or the CRH/LC–NE systems. For example, data showed a decrease in the volume and metabolic activity of the left subgenual prefrontal cortex in patients with major depression. Theoretically, an initial decrease in the function of the MPC could potentially enhance amygdala activation as well as the activation of the HPA axis and brain stem noradrenergic neurons. An activated amygdala and hypothalamic CRH centers would further activate brain stem arousal and autonomic centers.

An increased noradrenergic drive from the brain stem could potentiate the activity of the HPA axis. Hypercortisolism in major depression could be enhanced further by the capacity of glucocorticoids to damage or destroy hippocampal glucocorticoid receptor-containing neurons that mediate negative feedback on the HPA axis. In this regard, Sheline and colleagues found that patients with depressive episodes in the past had diminished bilateral hippocampal volumes compared to controls matched by age and medical conditions.

Taken together, a number of feed-forward loops among key components of the stress system could emerge that would intensify the stress system dysfunction in major depression, leading to a diminished activity of the medial prefrontal cortex and activation of the amygdala, HPA axis, and brain stem noradrenergic centers. The final result could be a syndrome associated with a relatively stereotyped affect, increased fear, and activation of the HPA axis and sympathetic nervous system. Such a syndrome would closely resemble the syndrome of melancholic depression.

Long-term medical consequences Patients with major depression exhibit a number of neuroendocrine and autonomic changes that could potentially predispose them to long-term medical consequences such as osteoporosis and premature ischemic heart disease. Hypercortisolism and suppression of the growth hormone and reproductive axes during depressive episodes would be expected to result in loss of bone mineral density. Unfortunately, bone mineral density, once lost, is not regained easily. In a study of premenopausal women (average age 41) with past or current major depression, almost 40% showed a loss of bone mineral density at the hip or spine that was at least 2 standard deviations below peak bone age, thus meeting American Osteoporosis Society criteria for osteoporosis. Because peak bone age is reached at around age 30, this means that these patients had lost more than an average of 1.5% of bone mineral density per year. Thus, by the time they enter menopause, these patients could have severe osteoporosis with losses as great as 35% below peak bone mass. Because each 10% decrease in bone mineral density is associated with a doubling of the fracture rate, the bone loss seen associated with depression represents an additional risk to fractures in aging women.

Patients with major depression show an overall increase in mortality regardless of age (independent of suicide). This relates, in part, to the fact that the relative risk for ischemic heart disease in patients with major depression is two or more and this increased risk is independent of traditional risk factors such as hypertension, dyslipidemia, and smoking. Many of the changes noted in depression could contribute to this enhanced susceptibility, including hypercortisolism and inhibition of the growth hormone and reproductive axes (leading to, among other things, increased visceral fat mass), with the resultant insulin resistance and its sequelae. Norepinephrine and epinephrine spillover studies showed that patients with depression had higher basal and stimulated heart rates and elevated norepinephrine spillover rates in the context of normal epinephrine secretion. These data strongly suggest increased cardiac sympathoneural activity in patients with major depression, another likely risk factor for ischemic heart disease. Thus, major depression with melancholic features is not only a disorder that affects fundamental parameters that define our humanity, such as self-regard, but also the product of sustained dysregulation in global neuroendocrine and autonomic functions acting on the myriad of peripheral substrates subjected to their influences.

Major Depression with Atypical Features

Biochemical manifestations and pathophysiology Relatively few studies have been conducted on the neurobiology of atypical depression; most have focused on HPA axis regulation. We studied patients with Cushing's disease, a rare illness characterized by severe hypercortisolism and a high incidence of depression. We demonstrated that depression in those patients was almost all of the atypical subtype. After having shown that the profound hypercortisolism of Cushing's disease was attributable entirely to a pituitary rather than central defect, we then focused on the function of hypothalamic CRH-containing neurons in Cushing's disease. In a series of studies, we showed that hypothalamic CRH-containing neurons in patients with Cushing's disease were suppressed by long-standing hypercortisolism. This confluence of atypical depression with a suppressed CRH system led us to hypothesize that some forms of atypical depression were associated with a pathological suppression rather than activation of arousal producing stress mediators.

In subsequent studies, we determined the pattern of plasma ACTH and cortisol responses to ovine CRH in patients with known hypothalamic CRH deficiency, secondary either to traumatic pituitary stalk section or to hypothalamic neoplasma. These patients often showed blunted and delayed plasma ACTH and cortisol responses, indicating that the adrenal cortex had been hypostimulated in these subjects. To test the hypothesis that patients with fatigue states and classic forms of atypical depression might show evidence of

hypothalamic CRH deficiency, patients with seasonal affective disorder and patients with chronic fatigue syndrome were studied. Seasonal affective disorder is characterized by the classical phenotype of atypical major depression. Both of these groups showed plasma ACTH and cortisol responses to CRH similar to those seen in patients with hypothalamic CRH deficiency. We have also shown this pattern in patients with atypical depression studied in the postpartum period.

In summary, these observations raise the question that the presentation of atypical symptoms (lethargy, fatigue, hypersomnia, and hyperphagia), as seen in Cushings' disease and in atypical depression, might be associated with hyposecretion of hypothalamic CRH. More studies will be needed to definitively document this important point.

Potential medical implications of HPA axis dysfunction in atypical depression If a centrally mediated hypoactivity of the HPA axis were documented in patients with atypical depression, this finding could have implications both for the clinical features of atypical depression, such as lethargy, fatigue, and hyperphagia, and for susceptibility to long-term medical consequences. Data show that peripheral inflammatory mediators such as interleukin-6 and tumor necrosis factor activate hypothalamic CRH neurons and the hypothalamic-pituitary axis. This circuit, during inflammatory stress, has been shown to promote HPA activation and glucocorticoid-mediated restraint of the immune response. The putative role of hypothalamic CRH and subsequent pituitary-adrenal activation is as a counterregulatory restraint on the immune response. Thus, it has been postulated that during the stress of a fight-or-flight situation, inflammatory mediators recruit the HPA axis to prevent the immune response from overshooting in the context of an anticipated injury and powerful inflammatory stimulus.

In *in vivo* studies, we and others have shown that adrenalectomized rats given an inflammatory stimulus show a profoundly exaggerated inflammatory response that, in some instances, resulted in death. In addition, we have shown that susceptibility to inflammatory disease in Lewis rats is associated with the hypoactivity of hypothalamic CRH in response to inflammatory mediators and other stimuli. Lewis rats also show significant attenuations in behavioral and other physiological responses to inflammatory mediators and other stressors. In the light of these data, we propose that patients with atypical depression could represent the tip of the iceberg of subjects who complain of lethargy, fatigue, and apathy, as well as an array of low-level but persistent complaints such as muscle pain, joint pain, and allergic phenomena. We are currently continuing to test this hypothesis utilizing new paradigms that will hopefully provide sufficient resolution to detect subtle hypoactivity of the HPA axis secondary to a change in CRH function.

See Also the Following Articles

Anxiety; Corticotropin Releasing Factor (CRF); Cushing's Syndrome, Medical Aspects; Cushing's Syndrome, Neuropsychiatric Aspects; Depression and Manic-Depressive Illness.

Further Reading

Chrousos, G. P. and Gold, P. W. (1992). The concepts of stress and stress system disorders: overview of physical and behavioral homeostasis. *Journal of the American Medical Association* **267**, 1244–1252.

Chrousos, G. P. and Gold, P. W. (1998). A healthy body in a healthy mind – and vice versa – the damaging power of "uncontrollable" stress. *Journal of Clinical Endocrinology and Metabolism* **83**, 1842–1845.

Gold, P. W., Goodwin, F. K. and Chrousos, G. P. (1988). Clinical and biochemical manifestations of depression: relation to the neurobiology of stress (1). *New England Journal of Medicine* **319**, 348–353.

Gold, P. W., Goodwin, F. K. and Chrousos, G. P. (1988). Clinical and biochemical manifestations of depression: relation to the neurobiology of stress (2). *New England Journal of Medicine* **319**, 413–420.

Herman, J. P. and Cullinan, W. E. (1997). Neurocircuitry of stress: central control of the hypothalamo–pituitary–adrenocortical axis. *Trends in Neuroscience* **20**, 78–84.

Michelson, D., Stratakis, C., Hill, L., Reynolds, J., Galliven, E., Chrousos, G. P. and Gold, P. W. (1996). Bone mineral density in women with depression. *New England Journal of Medicine* **335**, 1176–1181.

Sapolsky, R. M., Krey, L. C. and McEwen, B. S. (1986). The neuroendocrinology of stress and aging: the glucocorticoid cascade hypothesis. *Endocrine Reviews* **7**, 284–301.

Sternberg, E. M. and Gold, P. W. (1997). The mind-body interaction in disease. Special issue: Mysteries of the mind. *Scientific American* 8–15.

Sternberg, E. M., Hill, J. M., Chrousos, G. P., Kamilaris, T., Listwak, S. J., Gold, P. W. and Wilder, R. L. (1989). Inflammatory mediator-induced hypothalamic–pituitary–adrenal axis activation is defective in streptococcal cell wall arthritis-susceptible Lewis rats. *Proceedings of the National Academy of Sciences USA* **86**, 2374–2378.

Male Partner Violence

M Ingram, N P Yuan and M P Koss
University of Arizona, Tucson, AZ, USA

This article is a revision of the previous edition article by M P Koss and M Ingram, volume 2, pp 676–681, © 2000, Elsevier Inc.

Prevalence
Psychological Impact
Physical Impact
Prevention
Intervention
Conclusion

Glossary

Physical abuse	Physical violence directed toward an intimate partner including pushing, slapping, punching, kicking, choking, assault with a weapon, tying down, and restraining; threats of bodily harm and threats of violence directed at the woman's children; and behaviors liable to cause fear of physical safety such as leaving a woman in a dangerous place, driving fast and recklessly to frighten her, and refusing to help when she is sick or injured.
Psychological abuse	Abusive behaviors whose damage is primarily emotional including physical and social isolation, extreme jealousy, possessiveness, and removing access to communication or transportation; deprivation, degradation, and humiliation; emotional distress inflicted through threats to harm companion animals or livestock; and intimidation, intense criticizing, insulting, belittling, and ridiculing.
Sexual assault	Forced sexual acts or sexual degradation, such as coercing a woman to perform sexual acts against her will; hurting her during sex or assaulting her genitals, including using objects intravaginally, orally, or anally; pursuing sex when she is not fully conscious or otherwise un-

Stalking   able to consent; insisting on sex without protection against pregnancy or sexually transmitted diseases; and forcing her to have sex with others either privately or while being observed by the partner; often part of violent relationships.

Stalking   A pattern of repeated harassing or threatening behavior including following a woman, appearing at her home or place of business, making harassing phone calls, leaving written messages or objects, and vandalizing her property, even in the absence of threat of serious harm.

Male partner violence is broadly defined to be inclusive of the various types of behaviors that are used to coerce, control, and demean women. According to a report on intimate partner violence by the U.S. Department of Justice, 20% of all nonfatal violence against women in 2001 was committed by current or former spouses or boyfriends, whereas intimate partners committed 3% of nonfatal violence against men. Women are at a greater risk of assault, including rape and homicide, by a husband, ex-husband, boyfriend, or ex-boyfriend than they are by an acquaintance or stranger. Some methodologies generate data showing equal rates of intimate partner violence by men and by women; however, women are more likely to sustain minor or serious injuries. Violence within an abusive relationship is characterized as a recurrent experience when a woman is repeatedly placed in physical danger or controlled by the threat or use of force. Specifically included in these definitions, along with physical assault, are sexual assault, battering, threats, intimidation designed to obtain power and control by inducing fear in the victim, and stalking. The United Nations, the American Medical Association, and the American Psychological Association Presidential Task Force on Violence and the Family have established definitions of violence that recognize a pattern of physical, sexual, and/or psychological acts aimed at harming, intimidating, or coercing someone who is or was involved in an intimate relationship with the perpetrator.

Prevalence

Over the past 25 years, researchers have documented that violence by male intimates is one of the most prevalent and serious threats to the well-being of women in the United States and internationally. The landmark 1998 National Violence Against Women survey (NVAW), consisting of telephone interviews with 16,000 men and women, found that 25% of the women surveyed had been raped and/or physically assaulted in their lifetime by a current or former spouse, cohabiting partner, or date. The National Crime Victimization Survey (NCVS), an annual general survey of crime, indicated that the rate of intimate partner violence against women dropped by 49% between 1993 and 2001 but that the rate in 2001 was still high. There was an estimated 691,710 nonfatal incidents of violence committed by current or former spouses, boyfriends, or girlfriends, and the victims were primarily women (85%). These estimates, however, must be understood in the context of the limitations of the methods used to obtain them. National estimates based on telephone surveys are likely to be conservative due to the exclusion of the homeless, those too poor to own a telephone, people with limited English, recent immigrants who may be fearful of the government, and women whose partners control their ability to freely receive calls. Household-based samples mean that several living situations are missed in which women may be at high risk for violence including prisons, psychiatric hospitals, military settings, and colleges. These and other differences in methods contribute to substantial variation in estimate size across surveys.

Physical Assault

The NVAW documented that 22% of women were physically assaulted by current or former intimate partners during their lifetime. The majority of assaults were relatively minor, involving pushing, grabbing, and shoving. Few incidents involved more extreme forms of aggression, such as kicking or beating, threatening with a knife or gun, or using a weapon.

Sexual Assault

NVAW have shown that more than 7% of women report being raped by a current or former intimate partner in their lifetime. Those subjected to physical abuse are especially vulnerable to sexual abuse, with 26% to 52% of physically abused women reporting also being raped. Men who are both physically and sexually abusive are consistently found to perpetrate the most violent and severe assaults on their partners, with the majority of victims being repeatedly assaulted during the course of the relationship. Women who are victims of both physical and sexual violence are also at greater risk for abuse during pregnancy as well as at greater risk of homicide.

Psychological Abuse

Emotional abuse is generally concomitant with physical or sexual assault. In a recent study of primary-care patients, all women who were physically abused also reported emotional abuse in that relationship. The Canadian Centre for Justice Statistics National

Survey on Violence Against Women included questions on jealousy, limiting contact with family or friends, belittling and insulting female partners, preventing access to family income, and insisting on knowing a partner's whereabouts at all times. Approximately one-third of ever-married women in Canada reported that their current or previous partner was emotionally abusive in at least one of these five ways. In the majority of cases, emotional abuse was concomitant with physical or sexual abuse; only 18% of women who experienced emotional abuse reported no physical violence by a partner.

Stalking

Stalking by male partners also threatens the health of women. Based on a definition that includes experiencing fear, approximately 5% of women (compared to about 1% of men) have been stalked by a current or former intimate partner in their lifetime, according to the NVAW. Among women who were stalked by a former or current partner, 81% were also physically assaulted and 31% were sexually assaulted by the same man. Stalking frequently escalates among women who have left their abusive partners. The likelihood of being stalked by a male partner increases with the duration of time that the woman has been separated from the abusive relationship.

Risk Factors

Various factors increase the likelihood that a woman will be assaulted by a male partner. Research has identified several demographic risk factors. They include being younger in age; being single, divorced, or separated; having lower income; and having less education. In addition, ethnic minorities report higher rates of male partner violence compared to Whites. The NVAW indicated that American Indians/Alaska Native women had the highest rates, followed by African Americans. White and Hispanic women reported similar rates and Asian/Pacific Islanders reported the lowest rates of victimization by an intimate partner. These differences may reflect, in part, socioeconomic differences. However, researchers have found that differences in risk exist even after controlling for such variables. It is of note that studies consisting of only Native American samples have shown that some tribes have higher rates of partner violence, whereas others do not. Immigrant women experiencing partner violence are also a vulnerable population because they are often isolated in a foreign country, in constant fear of deportation, and feel at the mercy of their spouse to gain legal status. A history of childhood physical abuse, alcohol-related problems, drug use, and certain personality characteristics also increase the likelihood that women will be assaulted by a male partner. Certain characteristics of the male partner also increase the risk of victimization, including childhood exposure to intimate partner violence, partner alcohol-related problems, and emotionally abusive and controlling behaviors.

Psychological Impact

Victims of male partner violence are subject to physical, emotional, and perhaps sexual violence over an extended period of time. The impact on a woman's mental health is thus not derived solely from specific acts of violence but rather from the stress of living with recurrent, escalating, and unpredictable attacks. Not surprisingly, the severity and frequency of violence is associated with an increase in mental health symptoms, and symptoms have been shown to decrease when a woman is free from the abuse.

Posttraumatic Stress Disorder

Posttraumatic stress disorder (PTSD), as defined in the Diagnostic and Statistical Manual of Mental Disorders, fourth edition, has become the predominant diagnosis used to describe the various symptoms of psychological trauma exhibited by partner violence victims, with intensity of exposure being the primary etiological variable for PTSD. Rates of PTSD among abused women range from 31 to 84%. The occurrence of sexual assault in marriage is associated with greater trauma, more severe depression, and lower self-esteem than is found among victims of physical abuse alone. The most common symptoms of the disorder among abused women are nightmares, intrusive memories of abuse, avoidance of reminders of the abuse, and anxiety symptoms. Victims may also exhibit cognitive symptoms such as difficulty concentrating, problems with memory, and anger.

There is concern within the mental health profession and among victim advocates regarding the constructive use of PTSD as a diagnostic tool. PTSD pathologizes the victim's response to violence rather than focus the source of the trauma. In treating the symptoms of PTSD, the causal role of violence is neglected, placing victims at risk of misdiagnosis, inappropriate medication, and even possible further abuse. In addition, the victim may perceive the diagnosis as evidence of her own inadequacy rather than as condemnation of the violent behavior being perpetrated on her. Research has shown that access to both social support and victim advocacy services leads to a reduction in PTSD symptoms among abused women.

Depression

Prior to the introduction of PTSD, depression was the preferred diagnosis for victims of partner violence.

Today, depression continues to be prevalent among victims of intimate partner violence with rates varying between 39 and 83%. Women are more likely to be diagnosed with either depression or PTSD, and an investigation of the co-occurrence in physically abused women found that only 17% met the criteria of both. Depression is more likely among victims when psychological and sexual abuse occur within a physically violent relationship. Having low levels of social support has also been associated with depressive symptoms among victims.

Although it is imperative to investigate, document, and respond to the impact of trauma on the mental health of victims, the attempt to diagnose a woman trapped in a violent relationship with a mental disorder may be counterproductive.

Other Psychiatric Disorders

Victims of male partner violence are at greater risk of alcohol abuse and illicit drug use than nonabused women. Although partner violence may involve alcohol consumption by the female victim, or by the perpetrator and victim, increased alcohol use and illicit drug use by women frequently follows victimization. Compared to nonvictims, victims are also at higher risk for exhibiting eating disorders and more likely to report attempted suicide.

Physical Impact

Researchers and health-care providers worldwide single out partner violence as a major public health threat to women. The most severe physical outcome is death. Approximately 30% of murders of women that occurred between 1976 and 1996 were committed by male partners. The majority of these women were abused by a partner prior to being killed. Female victims also experience high rates of short-term and long-term health consequences. Children are also often affected because of prenatal or postnatal exposure to violence. Therefore, it is not surprising that women with a history of partner abuse demonstrate increased health-care use. Female victims of partner violence seek care for violence-related injuries, general health problems, and mental health problems.

Acute Injuries

Male partner violence is the largest single cause of injury to women requiring emergency medical treatment. Estimates of emergency department visits by women due to partner assault are between 13 and 25%. In a Bureau of Justice Statistics report on violence-related injuries treated in hospital emergency departments, only 14% of the injuries treated in

women were inflicted by strangers compared to 29% in men. Physically abused women experience injuries to multiple parts of the body, including injuries to the face, head, neck, throat, breast, chest, and abdomen. Battered women are more likely to have abrasions and contusions or pains for which no physiological cause can be discovered. Fractures, dislocations, and lacerations occur with about equal frequency in abused and nonabused women. One of the most troublesome aspects of male partner violence is the recurrent and often escalating nature of the abuse. Women who frequently present for medical treatment of trauma are likely to have been treated previously for injuries from abuse. Victims of partner violence have on average seven treatment episodes in the emergency service compared to two among nonbattered women. The pattern of escalation is also evident in homicide rates. In one study, 14% of the women who were killed had been in the health-care system for violence-related injuries. Approximately 47% had received health-care services for some type of problem during the year before they were killed.

Chronic Health Problems

Women of all ages with a history of past or current partner abuse are disproportionately represented among women receiving a variety of services in primary-care settings. The injuries, emotional stress, and fear associated with male partner violence can contribute to the development of chronic health problems. They include chronic pain (e.g., headaches and back pain) and central nervous system symptoms, such as fainting and seizures. Women who have been abused report higher rates of gastrointestinal symptoms and functional gastrointestinal disorders, such as irritable bowel syndrome and nonulcer dyspepsia, compared to other women. These disorders have no known pathogenesis or established treatment and are the most common chronic gastrointestinal conditions seen in primary care, as well as the most common reason for referral to gastroenterologists. In various clinical samples, between 44 and 67% of all female gastroenterology patients report a history of sexual violation, and between 32 and 48% of female patients had experienced severe physical trauma in childhood or adulthood. Gynecological problems are also long-lasting outcomes of male partner violence. Symptoms and conditions include HIV infection, other sexually-transmitted diseases, vaginal bleeding or infections, decreased sexual desire, genital irritation, painful intercourse, chronic pelvic pain, and urinary tract infections. The likelihood of having a gynecological problem is three times greater among women who are abused by spouses.

Birth Outcomes

Because young women in their most active childbearing years are at highest risk for abuse, abuse during pregnancy deserves special mention. Women who are abused and pregnant are more likely to engage in poor maternal health behavior. They frequently delay prenatal care. Compared to nonabused women, women who are abused are twice as likely to delay prenatal care until the third trimester. Pregnant women who are abused report higher levels of alcohol, tobacco, and drug use than other pregnant women. Pregnancy complications may include preterm labor, low birth weight, spontaneous abortion, anemia, and infections. It is also important to mention the effects of intimate partner violence on children. Children who observe violence against their mothers are at higher risk of emotional, behavioral, physiological, cognitive, and social problems.

Prevention

Primary Prevention

The aim of primary prevention, as applied in public health, is the reduction of the risk of obtaining a disease or health condition. Specific to male partner violence, primary prevention focuses on learning not to use violence. Primary prevention strategies include changing social norms promoting violence against women, changing male roles, promoting the status of women, and increasing the public's awareness of the problem of male partner violence. Other approaches focus on training to improve relationship, conflict resolution, and anger management skills.

Secondary Prevention

Secondary prevention occurs when an individual has a disease or health condition, but health consequences have not yet developed. One approach for partner violence is to conduct violence screening in health-care settings and non-health-care settings, such as workplaces, schools, and military bases. Intimate partner violence screening facilitates early identification and treatment referrals for female victims. Specific to perpetrators, secondary prevention efforts include training to deescalate aggression and counseling and hotlines for violent partners.

Intervention

The response to male partner violence must include effective interventions, not only in specific cases of victimization but in communities and from a societal perspective. Beyond providing victim services, communities need to develop a coordinated response across different types of agencies, and public policy needs to counter the systemic issues related to male partner violence.

Mental Health Services

Mental health clinicians have the potential to play a vital role in assisting the recovery process for survivors of partner violence. However, to avoid retraumatizing the survivors, clinical services must focus on providing specific interventions to counter the impact of trauma rather than on the mental disorders of the victim. For a woman living in a violent situation, mental health practitioners should prioritize her physical safety and assisting her to access victim services as a first step in addressing mental health concerns. Key to this process is assisting women to identify and develop formal and informal support networks that will help facilitate situational realities associated with both living in or leaving a violent relationship. For this to be feasible, strong linkages need to be fostered between clinical services and women's services, such as advocacy centers, domestic violence shelters, and rape crisis organizations. Additional resources are also needed to ensure that women who are using victim services, for example, those living in shelters, are able to access appropriate clinical services.

Coordinated Community Response

Mental health services should also be addressed within the framework of implementing a coordinated community response to partner violence. The development of coordinated community response is an outgrowth of the efforts of women's advocates to make reforms within the often-fragmented criminal justice system. The objective of the coordinated community response is to ensure that components of the system work together to form a consistent and systematic response that shifts responsibility away from victims and holds perpetrators of violence responsible for their behavior. Women's safety is considered of primary importance. Within this framework, emphasis is placed on batterer rehabilitation programs and support and advocacy for victims, but not specifically on the provision of clinical services for women suffering from trauma. Accessibility to immediate, appropriate clinical services could serve to avert the escalation of trauma symptoms.

Public Policy and Advocacy

Examples of proactive public policy are demonstrated in the Violence Against Women Act (VAWA) of 1994, which sponsored legislation to support increased police personnel, higher levels of prosecution, more severe penalties for perpetrators, and extended victim services. VAWA also recognized that immigration law placed abused women at risk and provided relief by giving abused immigrant women the means to establish lawful permanent residence without the help of a spouse. VAWA 2000 strengthened protections for battered immigrant women, sexual assault survivors, and victims of dating violence. Appropriate interpretation and enforcement of mandatory arrest laws is another area of public-policy intervention that should be pursued. Coupled with an advocacy agenda is the need for a public health response. This perspective, emphasizing the establishment of screening protocol, early interventions, and multiple approaches to prevention, offers hope of reducing the incidence of partner violence and minimizing its effects.

Conclusion

Women's Advocates Incorporated calculated in 2002 that intimate partner violence costs the U.S. economy $12.6 billion on an annual basis in legal services, direct medical care, policing, lost productivity, and victim services. Efforts have been made in the past decade to address this issue through initiatives such as mandatory arrest and sentencing laws within the criminal justice system and the development and implementation of screening protocols by health and social service organizations. However, the fact that thousands of women are injured or killed each year by an intimate partner indicates the need for social norms to be addressed. There is much to be done in terms of creating a comprehensive systematic response to male partner violence both in the United States and internationally, and the lack of such response contributes to the perception of societal support or even encouragement of violence. Although victims and perpetrators must both have access to appropriate intervention, the prevention of male partner violence is of paramount importance and requires action on a multiple levels.

See Also the Following Articles

Aggressive Behavior; Crime Victims; Familial Patterns of Stress; Marital Conflict; Posttraumatic Stress Disorder – Clinical; Pregnancy, Maternal and Perinatal Stress, Effects of; Sexual Assault; Violence.

Further Reading

Campbell, J. C. (2002). Health consequences of intimate partner violence. *Lancet* **359**, 1331–1336.

Coker, A. L. (2004). Primary prevention of intimate partner violence for women's health: a response to Plichta. *Journal of Interpersonal Violence* **19**, 1324–1334.

Crowell, N. A. and Burgess, A. W. (eds.) (1996). *Understanding violence against women, Panel on Research on Violence against Women, Committee on Law and Justice, Commission on Behavioral and Social Sciences and Education, National Research Council*, Washington, DC: National Academy Press.

Field, C. A. and Caetano, R. (2004). Ethnic differences in intimate partner violence in the U.S. general population: the role of alcohol use and socioeconomic status. *Trauma, Violence, & Abuse* **5**, 303–317.

Humphreys, C. and Stephens, J. (2004). Domestic violence and the politics of trauma. *Women's Studies International Forum* **27**(5–6), 449–570.

Koss, M. P., Goodman, L. A., Browne, A., Fitzgerald, L. F., Keita, G. P. and Russo, N. F. (1994). *No safe haven: violence against women at home, work, and in the community*. Washington, DC: American Psychological Association Press.

Koss, M. P., Bailey, J. A., Yuan, N. P., et al. (2003). Depression and PTSD in survivors of male violence: research and training initiatives to facilitate recovery. *Psychology of Women Quarterly* **27**, 130–142.

Max, W., Rice, D. P., Finkelstein, E., et al. (2004). The economic toll of intimate partner violence against women in the United States. *Violence & Victims* **19**, 259–272.

Plichta, S. B. (2004). Intimate partner violence and physical health consequences: policy and practice implications. *Journal of Interpersonal Violence* **19**, 1296–1323.

Rennison, C. M. (2003). *Intimate partner violence, 1993–2001*. Washington, DC: Bureau of Justice Statistics, Crime Data Brief, National Institute of Justice.

Tjaden, P. and Thoennes, N. (2000). *Extent, nature, and consequences of intimate partner violence*. Washington, DC: Office of Justice Programs, National Institute of Justice, U.S. Department of Justice.

Violence Against Women Act of 1994. (1994). Pub. L. No. 103–322, Title IV, 108 Sat. 1902. Washington, DC: Government Printing Office.

Waters, H., Hyder, A., Rajkotia, Y., Basu, S., Rehwinkel, J. and Butchart, A. (2004). *The economic dimensions of interpersonal violence*. Geneva: World Health Organization.

Manic Depression *See:* Depression and Manic-Depressive Illness.

Marital Conflict

P T McFarland and A Christensen
University of California, Los Angeles, Los Angeles,
CA, USA

This article is a revision of the previous edition article by
P T McFarland and A Christensen, volume 2, pp 682–684,
© 2000, Elsevier Inc.

What Is Conflict?
What Happens During Conflict?
What Are the Consequences of Conflict?

Glossary

Demand–withdraw interaction	A pattern of interaction in which one member of a couple attempts to engage in the discussion of relationship issues and pressures, nags, demands, or criticizes the other while the other member attempts to avoid such discussions and becomes silent, withdraws, or acts defensively.
Process of conflict	The interaction that takes place around a conflict of interest.
Psychoneuro-immunology	The study of the interactions among the psychological, neurological, and immunological systems.
Structure of conflict	The conflict of interest between spouses; the incompatibility of needs, desires, or preferences that characterize a couple's struggle.

What Is Conflict?

Conflict in marital relationships is normal and inevitable. Indeed, conflict occurs to a much greater extent in marriage than in any other long-term relationship. Although some theorists have suggested that conflict may serve constructive or functional purposes, such as allowing for the disclosure of feelings and the creative resolution of problems, the focus in the marital literature has generally been on the destructive or dysfunctional consequences of conflict.

An important distinction is made in the marital literature between the structure of conflict and the process of conflict. The structure of conflict refers to the conflict of interest between the spouses, that is, the incompatibility of needs, desires, or preferences that characterize the couple's struggle. The process of conflict refers to the actual interaction that occurs between the spouses regarding the conflict of interest.

It is important to note that a particular conflict of interest may give rise to a variety of conflictual processes. Couples may engage in overt conflict about the issue, or they may choose to avoid discussion about the issue altogether. Some theorists suggest that the decision to engage or to avoid is determined by spouses' beliefs about the likelihood that their efforts at resolving the conflict will be successful. Others have suggested that factors such as commitment to the relationship and negative feelings about the partner may also influence engagement or avoidance in conflict.

What Happens During Conflict?

Assuming that the management of conflict affects the quality and stability of the relationship, marital researchers have focused more of their attention on the process of conflict than on the structure of conflict. Researchers often study marital conflict by having couples discuss a conflict of interest in a laboratory setting for a predetermined amount of time (typically 10–15 min) while the resulting interaction is audiotaped or videotaped. Trained observers then code the problem-solving interaction for categories or dimensions of interest. Although the same type of discussion leads to more intense negative affect at home than it does in the laboratory, the observational research paradigm described does produce interactions that are similar to those experienced by couples in naturalistic settings.

One of the objectives of marital research has been to identify conflict behaviors that are associated with relationship satisfaction and thus differentiate between distressed and nondistressed couples. Although a number of differences have been identified, there are a few consistent findings across studies. First, distressed couples display higher rates of negative behaviors during conflictual interactions than nondistressed couples. These negative behaviors include criticism, complaints, hostility, defensiveness, denial of responsibility, and withdrawal. Second, compared to nondistressed spouses, distressed spouses exhibit greater reciprocity of negative behavior. That is, when a distressed spouse behaves in a negative manner, the other spouse tends to respond in kind, which escalates the conflict and leads to a cycle of negativity that is difficult to break. Third, nondistressed couples display higher rates of positive behaviors, such as approval and humor, during conflictual interactions than distressed couples. Similar to this cross-sectional research, longitudinal research has also demonstrated the deleterious effect of negative interactions on future satisfaction and stability.

A pattern of conflictual interaction that has received much empirical attention and has been found to be highly correlated with marital dissatisfaction is the demand–withdraw interaction pattern. In this pattern, one spouse (the demander) attempts to engage in the discussion of relationship issues and pressures, nags, demands, or criticizes the other while the other spouse (the withdrawer) attempts to avoid such discussions and becomes silent, withdraws, or acts defensively. Although both self-report and observational studies have demonstrated a gender linkage in roles in this pattern, with wives generally in the role of demander and husbands generally in the role of withdrawer, this gender effect is moderated by the specific issue that is being discussed. Specifically, the gender linkage in roles is apparent during discussions in which wives' issues are being addressed, but this linkage is not apparent during discussions in which husbands' issues are being addressed. Also, the pattern often occurs when a structural conflict of interest exists between partners whereby the partners have a differential investment in change on an issue. The spouse who desires a change that can only be achieved through the cooperation of the other (e.g., spending more time together) will generally take on a demanding role during discussion, whereas the spouse who seeks no change or change that can be achieved unilaterally (e.g., spending less time together) will generally take on the withdrawing role because discussion will only create an argument or undesired change.

In addition to studying overt behavior, marital researchers have also examined covert factors that may impact marital conflict and satisfaction, such as affective processes and perceptual differences between spouses. One area that has received much attention in the marital literature concerns the attributions that spouses make in accounting for events that occur in marriage. There is accumulating evidence indicating that attributions for negative events can promote conflict, such as when negative partner behavior is attributed to the selfish intent of the partner. Such attributions have been found to be related to less effective problem-solving behavior and to higher rates of negative behavior during problem-solving tasks. Moreover, research has demonstrated that attributions for negative partner behavior affect a spouse's own behavior toward the partner.

Recent years have seen a growing emphasis on the application of social psychological theories to the study of marital conflict. Attachment theory is one such theory that has been the focus of increased attention in marital conflict research. Attachment theory asserts that mental models of the self and other develop in the context of early parent–child interactions and that these models influence the communications and reactions of spouses to partner behaviors. Research findings generally suggest that spouses with secure attachment styles are more likely to compromise when dealing with conflict, whereas those with insecure attachment styles tend to employ less productive approaches to marital conflict.

What Are the Consequences of Conflict?

Conflict not only has an effect on the marital relationship itself, but it can also affect the health of individual partners. A growing body of research documents the association between marital conflict and the physical and mental well-being of spouses. Although married people tend to be healthier than those who are not married, marital conflict has been linked to an increase in physical illnesses such as rheumatoid arthritis and cardiac problems. Marital conflict also increases the risk for mental disorders. The association between marital conflict and depression is well established, as is the association between marital conflict and the physical and psychological abuse of spouses. Some of the most compelling data relating marital conflict to mental disorders are seen in the strong linkage between marital conflict and substance abuse.

The link between marital discord and poorer health outcomes has been systematically explored over the past decade. Negative and hostile behaviors during marital conflict are associated with various physiological effects in spouses, such as elevations in blood pressure and heart rate and changes in endocrine and immune functioning. Across studies, these negative physiological effects are more severe and persistent for wives than for husbands. Research in the field of psychoneuroimmunology suggests that there are negative long-term health consequences for spouses who are unable to physiologically recover from marital conflicts or cannot adapt physiologically to repeated conflicts.

In addition to its negative effects on spouses, marital conflict is related to problems in family functioning, including parenting and sibling relationships. Moreover, research has demonstrated the effects of marital conflict on the parent–child relationship, such as attachment difficulties and parent–child conflict, and to a wide range of adjustment problems in children, including internalizing problems such as depression and anxiety and externalizing problems such as aggression, delinquency, and conduct disorders. Exposure to frequent and severe marital conflict, such as physical aggression, seems to be particularly disturbing for children.

Not only is marital conflict itself a stressor, but other life stressors can affect marital conflict. For example, greater work demands among air traffic controllers and unemployment in blue-collar workers have been shown to be associated with more negative marital interactions. Stressful events may increase conflict by diminishing the capacity of spouses to provide support to one another, even as it increases their need for support. Such events may also affect marital interactions by giving rise to new conflicts of interest or by exacerbating old ones.

See Also the Following Articles

Marital Status and Health Problems; Marriage.

Further Reading

Aubry, T., Tefft, B. and Kingsbury, N. (1990). Behavioral and psychological consequences of unemployment in blue-collar couples. *Journal of Community Psychology* **18**, 99–109.

Beach, S. R. H., Fincham, F. D. and Katz, J. (1998). Marital therapy in the treatment of depression: toward a third generation of therapy and research. *Clinical Psychology Review* **18**, 635–661.

Bradbury, T. N. and Fincham, F. D. (1992). Attributions and behavior in marital interaction. *Journal of Personality and Social Psychology* **63**, 613–628.

Burman, B. and Margolin, G. (1992). Analysis of the association between marital relationships and health problems: an interactional perspective. *Psychological Bulletin* **112**, 39–63.

Christensen, A. and Heavey, C. L. (1990). Gender and social structure in the demand/withdraw pattern of marital conflict. *Journal of Personality and Social Psychology* **59**, 73–81.

Cummings, E. M. and Davies, P. T. (2002). Effects of marital conflict on children: recent advances and emerging themes in process-oriented research. *Journal of Child Psychology and Psychiatry* **43**, 31–63.

Ewart, C. K., Taylor, C. B., Kraemer, H. C., et al. (1991). High blood pressure and marital discord: not being nasty matters more than being nice. *Health Psychology* **10**, 155–163.

Gottman, J. M. (1979). *Marital interaction: experimental investigations.* New York: Academic Press.

Grych, J. H. and Fincham, F. D. (1990). Marital conflict and children's adjustment: a cognitive-contextual framework. *Psychological Bulletin* **108**, 267–290.

Halford, W. K. and Markman, H. J. (eds.) (1997). *Clinical handbook of marriage and couples intervention.* London: John Wiley.

Hazan, C. and Shaver, P. R. (1994). Attachment as an organizational framework for research on close relationships. *Psychological Inquiry* **5**, 1–22.

Kiecolt-Glaser, J. K., Malarkey, W. B., Chee, M. A., et al. (1993). Negative behavior during marital conflict is associated with immunological down-regulation. *Psychosomatic Medicine* **55**, 395–409.

Kiecolt-Glaser, J. K., Glaser, R., Cacioppo, J. T., et al. (1997). Marital conflict in older adults: endocrinological and immunological correlates. *Psychosomatic Medicine* **59**, 339–349.

Repetti, R. L. (1989). Effects of daily workload on subsequent behavior during marital interaction: the roles of social withdrawal and spouse support. *Journal of Personality and Social Psychology* **57**, 651–659.

Robles, T. F. and Kiecolt-Glaser, J. K. (2003). The physiology of marriage: pathways to health. *Physiology and Behavior* **79**, 409–416.

Marital Status and Health Problems

I M A Joung
Erasmus University, Rotterdam, Netherlands

This article is reproduced from the previous edition, volume 2, pp 685–691, © 2000, Elsevier Inc.

Health Differences among Marital Status Groups
Theories about the Explanation
Selection on Health and Determinants of Health
Social Causation, Intermediary Factors, and Biological
  Pathways

Glossary

Determinants of health	Factors associated with health and illness, such as socioeconomic status and alcohol consumption.
Intermediary factors	Determinants of health through which marital status affects health outcomes.
Unmarried	People who have never been married, are divorced, or are widowed.
Selection	The theory about health differences between marital status groups in which it is assumed that health affects marital status.
Social causation	The theory about health differences between marital status groups in which it is assumed that marital status affects health.

Marital status is associated with all kinds of health outcomes: both subjective health states (illness, e.g., self-perceived health) and objective health states (disease, e.g., clinically diagnosed conditions), both mental and physical health, and both morbidity and mortality. Health differences between marital status groups are generally assumed to result from both an effect of health on marital status (selection) and an effect of marital status on health (social causation). Marital status affects health through several intermediary factors; of these, psychosocial factors, especially psychosocial stress, occupy a central position.

Health Differences among Marital Status Groups

The general pattern for health differences among marital status groups is that married people have the fewest health problems, followed by never-married and widowed people, whereas divorced people have the most health problems. This ranking is found both among men and women; however, the differences among the marital status groups are generally larger among men than among women.

In most studies in which separated people are distinguished as a separate group, it is found that they have as many as or even more health problems than divorced people. However, in many studies on health differences among marital status groups, separated people have not been treated as a separate marital status category but have been grouped with either divorced or married people.

In many Western countries, nonmarital cohabitation is of increasing importance. The few studies that have addressed health differences between married people and people living in consensual unions have found either no health differences or that the health of people in consensual unions compared somewhat unfavorably with that of married people but favorably with that of the unmarried, noncohabiting people. The remainder of this article focuses on health differences among married, never-married, divorced, and widowed people.

Mortality

Mortality differences among marital status groups were described in the nineteenth century. For instance, in 1853 William Farr examined age-specific mortality rates for never-married, married, and widowed people living in France. He found that the mortality rates of married men and women compared favorably to those of never-married and widowed men and women. For example, at the ages 40–50 mortality rates were 17.7, 10.3, and 20.1 per 1000 for never-married, married, and widowed men, respectively.

Since then numerous researchers in many countries have looked at mortality differences among marital status groups. A considerable number of studies have been performed on this subject in the last decades. The results from these studies indicate very consistently that married people have lower mortality rates than unmarried people.

The sizes of the mortality differences between married and unmarried groups and the rankings of the mortality rates of the three unmarried groups have changed over time. For instance, in the Netherlands in the period of 1869–1872, the differences in total mortality between married and never-married women were rather small, and under the age of 40 never-married women actually had lower mortality rates than married women. This was mainly due to the high childbirth mortality rate among married women. In the following decades, the differences in total mortality between married and never = married women increased as, childbirth mortality rate, among others, decreased.

The relationship between marital status and mortality also shows some differences between countries. Hu and Goldman explored mortality differences between marital status groups in 16 industrialized countries for the period of 1950–1980. They found that, for the majority of countries, divorced men experienced the highest mortality rates among men and that, in about half of the countries, the same pattern existed for women. Generally, the mortality rates of divorced men and women were 2–2.5 and 1.5–2 times, respectively, those of their married counterparts. In Japan, however, the mortality rate of never-married men was as high as the rate of divorced men and never-married women had much higher mortality rates than divorced women. Also, mortality rate differences between the never married and married in Japan far exceeded the largest mortality rate differences by marital status in the other countries (being more than three times that of the married group).

The differences in total mortality rates among marital status groups are more or less mirrored in the differences in rates for specific causes of death. For the majority of causes of death, the largest differences are found between the rates for divorced and married people. In general, never-married and widowed people have higher rates of cause-specific mortality than married people, alternately occupying the position of the group with the second highest mortality rate. In comparison with the differences found for the total mortality rate, the relative size of the differences in the rates of mortality due to cardiovascular diseases and cancer is somewhat smaller, but it is considerably larger for the mortality rates due to external causes of death (e.g., accident and suicide). **Table 1** shows the age-adjusted relative risks of divorced men and women compared to married men and women for total mortality and mortality from a number of specific causes of death.

Morbidity

More recently, differences in morbidity, short-term disability, and health-care use among marital status groups have been studied. Morbidity differences largely have patterns similar to mortality rate differences: married people have the lowest rates, divorced people have the highest rates, and never-married and widowed people have rates in between. The size of the differences among marital status groups is generally larger for indicators of subjective health (e.g., self-perceived general health and subjective health complaints) than for indicators of objective health (e.g., chronic diseases) and is larger for mental than for physical health.

Morbidity differentials are by and large reflected in the patterns for health-care use and short-term

Table 1   Relative risks of divorced men and women compared to their married counterparts in the Netherlands, 1986–1990[a]

	Divorced men	Divorced women
Total mortality	1.6	1.5[b]
Cardiovascular diseases	1.5	1.4
Cancer	1.2	1.3
External causes	3.8	3.0
Infective diseases	2.2	2.1
Cirrhosis of the liver (with mention of alcohol)	9.1	6.0
Diabetes mellitus	2.2	1.4

[a]*Source*: Statistics Netherlands.
[b]For example, a relative risks of 1.5 means that the mortality rate of divorced women is 1.5 times that of married women.

disability. Widowed and divorced people have higher rates for physician contacts, hospital admissions, and use of medicines and report more bed days and days of restricted activity than married people. Never-married people, however, seem to have a lower health-care use and less bed disability days than married people, despite their higher morbidity rates.

Theories about the Explanation

Several explanations have been suggested for the association between marital status and health. First, it has been put forward that the association might be due to data errors and thus be an artifact. Although data errors might explain part of the association between marital status and health found in earlier studies, more recent studies have shown convincingly that there are genuine health differences among marital status groups. Other explanations that have been proposed can be grouped into two main theories: selection theory and social causation theory. According to selection theory, the relatively good health of married people is the result of the selection of healthy people into and unhealthy people out of the married state. According to social causation theory, marriage has a health-promoting or a health-protective effect, whereas the unmarried state has adverse health effects. Thus, in selection theory, health status precedes marital status; in social causation theory, marital status precedes health status. A graphic representation of these explanations is shown in **Figure 1**. In order to establish whether or to what extent health differences precede differences in marital status or vice versa, longitudinal data are required. Selection theory and social causation theory are not mutually exclusive, and it is generally accepted that a combination of

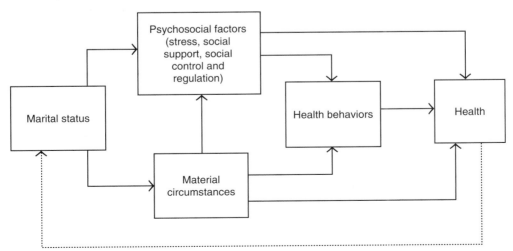

Figure 1   A representation of the explanations for health differences among marital status groups. →, social causation; ⤏, selection.

selective and causal factors are responsible for the observed health patterns in marital status groups.

Selection on Health and Determinants of Health

According to selection theory, the relatively good health of married people is the result of the selection of healthy people into and unhealthy people out of the married state, thus increasing the relative amount of unhealthy people in the unmarried states. A distinction can be made between direct selection and indirect selection. In direct selection, health itself is the selection criterion; in indirect selection, the determinants of health are the selection criteria.

The process of selection could occur with regard to first marriages as well as other marital transitions (divorce, bereavement, and remarriage) and could cause the health differences by marital status in several ways. Selection in partner choice is the most straightforward mechanism: unhealthy people may be less attractive marriage partners and thus may either not be chosen or, if illness develops during marriage, might be discarded as marriage partners. Selection may also operate through assortive mating, the fact that people generally tend to marry partners with traits that they themselves possess, such as physical attractiveness. Assortive mating could also includes health status and does not so much influence whether a person marries as whom the person marries. If, indeed, unhealthy people are more likely to marry unhealthy others, we could find that unhealthy married people are more likely to become widowed because their unhealthy partner is at greater risk of mortality. In addition, it is conceivable that relationships in which both partners are unhealthy are more stressful and therefore more prone to dissolution. Finally, with regard to the transition from the married to the widowed state, selection may also operate through processes independent of partner choice due to health considerations, for instance, through both spouses developing health problems after marriage for reasons such as a joint unfavorable environment (e.g., shared material deprivation or unhealthy behaviors). In this case, the health differences between married and widowed people are not caused by the conditions of widowhood itself (social causation) but are, instead, based in already existing health differences between those who will become widowed and those who will remain married (selection).

Direct Selection

It has been demonstrated in several longitudinal studies that direct selection is operative in marital transitions. However, the evidence is still partial and sometimes inconsistent. There are indications that the presence of disease decreases the marriage probabilities of never-married people and increases the divorce probabilities of married people. It has also been found that direct selection might be able to explain a considerable part of the health differences among marital status groups. However, other studies have been unable to demonstrate selection effects, and sometimes even evidence for adverse selection was found (i.e., that healthier people were less likely to marry).

Indirect Selection

As stated earlier, selection may operate not only through the exclusion of unhealthy people from marriage (direct selection) but also through selection on a wide range of determinants of health (indirect selection). The determinants of health that may operate in this way are, for instance, socioeconomic status, physical appearance (e.g., body length and obesity), and health-related habits (e.g., alcohol consumption). Research has demonstrated that indirect selection is indeed operative in marital transitions and that its direction is mostly, but not always, in accordance with the health differences observed among marital status groups. Adverse selection occurs, for instance, with regard to educational level among women – people with a higher educational level have more favorable health outcomes than those with a lower educational level, but women with a high educational level are overrepresented among never-married and divorced women.

Social Causation, Intermediary Factors, and Biological Pathways

According to social causation theory, health depends on marital status. Marital status may, on the one hand, affect the etiology of health problems: the married state may prevent people from becoming ill, whereas the unmarried state may be the cause of a decline in resistance to diseases. Marital status may, on the other hand, once health problems have developed, affect the course and outcome of the disease. Ample evidence from longitudinal studies shows that differences in marital status are associated with subsequent health differences; thus social causation mechanisms explain (part of the) health differences among marital status groups. The effect of marital status on health is not assumed to be a direct effect but to be intermediated by psychosocial factors (e.g., stress and social relationships), material circumstances (e.g., financial situation and housing conditions), and health behaviors (e.g., smoking and alcohol consumption).

Psychosocial Factors

Psychosocial stress is related causally to illness and mortality. Lazarus and Folkman defined psychosocial stress as "a particular relationship between the person and the environment that is appraised by the individual as taxing or exceeding his or her resources and endangering his or her well-being." Psychosocial stress varies among marital status groups. First, bereavement and divorce are stressful life events in themselves. On the social readjustment rating scale of Holmes and Rahe, a scale of 43 life events ordered on the basis of the assumed intensity and length of time necessary to accommodate to the life event, bereavement and divorce rank first and second, respectively. Understandingly, the loss of a beloved person is an important source of stress itself. Feelings of failure, lowered self-esteem, and sense of incompetence, which are often experienced by divorced people, also evoke stress. Furthermore, the many concurrent changes in the lives of bereaved or divorced people, such as lowered income, change in parental responsibilities, forced move to other housing, or the loss of familiar activities and habit systems, also contribute highly to the total amount of stress experienced.

Second, the differences in psychosocial stress among marital status groups are also caused by mechanisms other than the stressful character of the event of bereavement or divorce. Negative societal attitudes toward the marital status a person occupies can be a source of stress. Although societal attitudes toward alternatives to marriage have become more liberal in recent years, prejudices and stereotyped images of never-married people and divorced people still exist. Uncertainty about social roles is also a source of stress, and certainty about social roles differs according to marital status. Marriage provides people with clear and socially acceptable roles, whereas divorce lacks clearly defined norms.

Other psychosocial factors may also contribute to the effect of marital status on health. Several aspects of social relationships are associated with health status and differ among the marital status groups. First, social integration (the existence and quantity of social relationships) is related directly to health. Psychological and sociobiological theories suggest that the mere presence of, or sense of relatedness with, another organism may promote health through relatively direct motivational, emotional, or neuroendocrinal effects. Married people are, on average, more socially integrated for several reasons: they have at least one social tie in their spouse; their children constitute additional social ties, which most never-married people lack; and their social network is expanded with the social ties of their spouse. Consequently, the loss of a spouse also means a break in the social network.

Second, social support (the functional nature or quality of social relationships) has been found to be related directly and indirectly to health. With regard to the latter, social support is assumed to buffer the negative health effects of stress, thus modifying the relationship between stress and health. In this case, social support has no beneficial effect on the health of people who experience little stress, but the beneficial effects of social support increase with increasing stress. Social support is the aid that is transmitted between social network members. An distinction is often made between emotional and instrumental support. Emotional support includes expressions of affection, admiration, respect, or affirmation; instrumental support is the provision of advice, information, or more practical assistance. The availability and quality of social support differ by marital status. Partner relationships are, in general, more supportive than are other types of relationships. This also means that in cases of bereavement or divorce an important provider of social support is lost.

Finally, differences in social relationships among marital status groups result in differences in social regulation and control. Married people experience more social control; wives, in particular, try to influence their spouses' health behaviors. Furthermore, married people have a more regulated life, which facilitates health-promoting behaviors such as proper sleep, diet, and exercise; the moderate use of alcohol; the adherence to medical regiment; and seeking appropriate medical care.

Material Circumstances

Differences in material resources among marital status groups constitute another intermediary of the relationship between marital status and health. People who share a household profit from economies of scale in the purchasing and use of housing and other goods and services. In addition, changes in marital status are often associated with large changes in material resources. Bereavement and divorce are, especially among women, often accompanied by a decline of their financial situation and, consequently, a deterioration in other structural living circumstances (e.g., housing). This is most obvious in situations in which the husband is the sole wage earner. However, even in cases of double incomes the wife is likely to be worse off financially after divorce or bereavement. Women are generally married to men of a higher or equivalent educational level, and in many countries men earn on average more than women of an equivalent educational level earn. The fact that the material situation of women generally deteriorates after a divorce does not necessarily imply that men gain materially from divorce. In a divorce, possessions are divided between the former spouses, the ex-husband might be obliged to pay alimony, and economies of scale are lost. This might put divorced men in a materially disadvantaged position compared to married men. Widowed women are generally better off financially than divorced women, even with comparable levels of household income, because divorced women lose their house and must divide assets with their ex-husband, whereas widowed women more often keep the family home and other financial assets intact.

Health Behaviors

Differences in health behaviors among marital status groups are also seen as an intermediary of the association between marital status and health. Marriage often has a deterrent effect on negative health behaviors, such as smoking, excessive alcohol consumption, substance use, and other risk-taking behavior, and marriage promotes an orderly lifestyle. Differences in sexual and reproductive behavior among the marital status groups have been mentioned as explanations for differences in mortality rates from several malignant neoplasms – the excessive mortality rate among never-married women from breast cancer, uterine cancer, and ovarian cancer; the higher mortality rate among divorced women from cervical cancer; and the lower mortality rate among never-married men from prostate cancer.

Finally, differences in the use of health services among marital groups have been mentioned (e.g., married people are more inclined to use preventive health services) and in compliance with required prolonged treatment (married people are more willing to undertake the required treatments for diabetes mellitus and tuberculosis).

Interrelationships between Intermediary Factors

Psychosocial factors, material circumstances, and health behaviors have been mentioned as possible intermediary factors in the effects of marriage on health. However, the effects of marriage on health through intermediary factors cannot be viewed as three independent pathways. Several interrelationships could exist among the three intermediary factors. In the conceptual model of these interrelationships is shown in **Figure 1**, marital status is not assumed to have a direct effect on health behavior but to influence health behavior only indirectly through psychosocial factors and material conditions.

Psychosocial factors may have direct health effects or may operate through an effect on health behaviors.

Unmarried people experience higher levels of psychosocial stress. Cigarette smoking and alcohol consumption are palliative coping responses to psychosocial stress. In addition, social support is important in health behavior changes; partner support, for instance, is beneficial to smoking-cessation maintenance. Finally, the more regulated life of married people facilitates healthy behaviors, and married people attempt to influence the health behaviors of their spouses.

Also, the material circumstances associated with marital status may have direct health effects, increase psychosocial stress, or operate through changes in health behaviors. With regard to the latter, unhealthy eating habits and a lack of recreation possibilities could, in part, be determined by an individual's financial position.

Evidence from several studies shows that psychosocial factors, material circumstances, and health behaviors act separately as intermediary factors in the relationship between marital status and health. The relative importance of these three groups of intermediary factors has been addressed only recently. Tentative results suggest that psychosocial factors are the most important intermediary factor in health differences between marital status groups among men, whereas material circumstances constitute the major intermediary factor of health differences among women.

Pathways of Intermediary Factors to Health

The effects of health behaviors such as smoking, alcohol consumption, obesity, and lack of physical activity on health are relatively well known. For instance, smoking is, in the long term, associated with cardiovascular diseases, chronic obstructive lung diseases, and many malignant neoplasms such as cancer of the lung, bronchus, trachea, larynx, pancreas, and bladder. Excessive alcohol consumption is associated with diseases of the liver, stomach, and central nervous system and is related to external causes of death, such as traffic accidents and suicide. Obesity and lack of physical exercise are both associated with cardiovascular diseases and conditions of the locomotor system; obesity is also associated with the development of non-insulin-dependent diabetes mellitus.

There is also a considerable amount of research on the relationship between psychosocial stress and health. Stress may cause direct physiological changes in the endocrine, immune, and autonomic nervous systems. Evidence shows that these physiological changes increase susceptibility to infectious diseases, cancer, and cardiovascular diseases. It has also been suggested that marital status, mediated by psychosocial stress, enhances susceptibility to diseases in general rather than having specific etiological effects. This theory of generalized susceptibility might explain why marital status is associated with many apparently different causes of disease and death.

The direct links between social relationships and health are more speculative. Evidence suggests that biological and psychological mechanisms are involved. A variety of studies of animals and humans suggest that the mere presence of, and especially affectionate physical contact with, another similar or nonthreatening organism reduces cardiovascular and other forms of physiological reactivity. The psychological mechanisms are related to, but partially independent of, the biological mechanisms and might, for instance, be affective in nature (if there is a basic human need for relationships or attachments, people will feel better psychologically when that need is fulfilled, with physiological consequences).

The direct health effects of material circumstances (i.e., health effects not mediated by psychosocial stress or health behaviors) are also of a more speculative nature. In previous centuries, poverty might have been the cause of starvation, death from hypothermia, or increased susceptibility to infectious diseases because of undernourishment. However, the contribution of these causes of death to overall mortality are minimal in current Western societies. However, it is conceivable that unfavorable material circumstances still increase risks for respiratory infections or the transmission of infectious agents through effects on living conditions (damp houses, presence of fungal mold, and crowding). The results of studies on this subject are inconclusive, however. The health effects of material circumstances are presumably mediated mainly by changes in psychosocial stress and, to a lesser extent, by changes in health behaviors.

A final comment with regard to the social causation theory is that we should keep in mind that marital relationships are not always health enhancing. Marital relationships may also have negative health effects, whereas divorce may have positive health effects. Marital problems are a source of stress, and social control in an environment in which hazardous health behaviors are valued could have unfavorable consequences. With regard to the positive health effects of divorce, it has, for instance, been found that people improve their health after divorce, depending on the stress of the marriage. In addition, several studies have reported that unhappily married people are less healthy than divorced people and happy married people. On the average, however, marriage is associated favorably with intermediary factors and with health.

See Also the Following Articles

Bereavement; Economic Factors and Stress; Familial Patterns of Stress; Gender and Stress; Marital Conflict; Psychosocial Factors and Stress; Social Support.

Further Reading

Burman, B. and Margolin, G. (1992). Analysis of the association between marital relationships and health problems: an interactional perspective. *Psychological Bulletin* **112**, 39–63.

Joung, I. M. A. (1996). *Marital status and health: descriptive and explanatory studies.* Alblasserdam, Netherlands: Haveka.

Joung, J. M. A., van de Mheen, H., Stronks, K., et al. (1998). A longitudinal study of health selection in marital transitions. *Social Science & Medicine* **46**, 425–435.

Joung, I. M. A., Stronks, K., van de Mheen, H., et al. (1997). Contribution of psychosocial factors, material circumstances and health behaviours to marital status differences in self-reported health. *Journal of Marriage and the Family* **59**, 476–490.

Stroebe, W. and Stroebe, M. S. (1987). *Bereavement and health.* New York: Cambridge University Press.

Waldron, I., Weis, C. C. and Hughes, M. E. (1997). Marital status effects on health: are there differences between never married women and divorced and separated women? *Social Science & Medicine* **45**, 1387–1397.

Marriage

A C Yoneda and J Davila
State University of New York at Stony Brook,
Stony Brook, NY, USA

This article is a revision of the previous edition article
by J Davila, volume 2, pp 692–698, © 2000, Elsevier Inc.

Glossary

ABCX and double ABCX models	Models of family adaptation that suggest that successful adaptation is a function of the nature of the stressor, the family's resources for coping with the stressor, how they appraise the stressor, and the extent to which the family has experienced an accumulation of stress over time.
Adaptive strategies	Behaviors that spouses and couples use to negotiate and cope with problems or stressors; include skills in communication, problem solving, and provision of social support.
Infidelity	Sexual or emotional unfaithfulness to a spouse.
Infertility	Persistent inability to conceive a child for at least 1 year.
Marital functioning	A broad term that includes how spouses and couples think about, feel about, and behave in their marriage.
Marital stress generation model	A model, adapted from research on unipolar depression, that was designed to explain how marital stressors are created by troubled spouses and then negatively impact the subsequent individual well-being of spouses.
Marriage	The legal union of a man and woman as husband and wife.
Vulnerability stress adaptation (VSA) model	A model of marital outcomes that suggests that marital dissatisfaction results from the interplay among spouses' individual vulnerabilities, stressors the couple must face, and the skills the spouses and couples have for negotiating and coping with stressors.

This article is based on the definition of marriage in the United States as of February 2005. Because this definition may change in time to encompass more diverse sets of couples, the types of stressors faced by married couples may also change. Marriage is currently defined as the legal union of a man and woman as husband and wife. Recent U.S. census data indicate that approximately 80% of all Americans will marry at some point in their lives. However, more than 50% of all first marriages will end in divorce, and subsequent remarriages are even more likely to end in divorce. Relationship problems are one of the most common reasons why people in the United States seek counseling, and the development of prevention and intervention programs to combat marital distress and dissolution is proceeding rapidly.

The Relation between Stress and Marriage

Most people agree that stress plays a role in marital functioning, and there is clear evidence that stressful events and circumstances can have a negative impact on marriages. One of the difficulties in this field of study arises from problems inherent in defining the relations between stress and marriage. One distinction that must be drawn is whether the stressors are internal or external to the marriage. An external stressor is something that originates outside the marriage, such as unemployment or health problems. An internal stressor is something that originates inside the marriage, such as marital conflict or divergent needs and desires. A second distinction that must be drawn is between effects of stressors on marriage and effects of marriage on stressors. The effects of stressors on marriage are how stressors, either external or internal, influence marital functioning and the quality and stability of the marriage. The effects of marriage on stressors are how marital functioning affects the experience of stressors, again either external or internal. The experience of stressors, in this case, is how well an individual copes with stressors and the impact the stressor has on the individual in terms of his or her own well-being. The field is still expanding its understanding of the bidirectional relationship between stress and marriage, and advances in this domain are likely to follow in the coming years.

Major Models of Stress and Marital Functioning

There are presently three major models that were designed explicitly to explain the relations between stress and marriage.

The Vulnerability-Stress-Adaptation Model of Marital Outcomes

The VSA model was developed to understand precursors to marital dissatisfaction and marital dissolution. Prior to the development of this model, the study of marital outcomes was dominated by a behavioral and social-learning perspective on marriage, which maintains that marital dysfunction arises because couples do not have adequate skills to negotiate their problems. However, many felt that this perspective was limited, particularly because it failed to focus on the individual qualities of spouses and on stressful life experiences that might affect spouses' abilities to interact successfully with their partners. Hence, the VSA model was developed as an integrative perspective that incorporates three factors: enduring vulnerabilities (e.g., individual characteristics such as personality, psychological symptoms, and family of origin experiences) that spouses bring to the marriage, stressful events (e.g., external stressors) that individuals and couples encounter and experience, and adaptive processes (e.g., skills that couples have for communicating, problem solving, and providing support to one another) that may help the couple negotiate and cope with individual and marital difficulties and stressors.

The VSA model suggests that marital dissatisfaction results from the interplay of these three factors, and most directly from repeated experiences with poor adaptation (e.g., poor communication and social support). Once a couple is dissatisfied, it is then at risk for marital dissolution. Stressful life events in the VSA model are seen as factors that impact or interact with a couple's capacity for successful problem negotiation or social support in predicting marital dissatisfaction. For example, stressful life events will lead to dissatisfaction when a couple does not have the adaptive skills to successfully negotiate or cope with the stressor. Stressful life events might also erode a couple's capacity for successful coping (i.e., successful adaptation) if the events are severe enough. The VSA model also suggests that stressful life events can be created or exacerbated by spouses' enduring vulnerabilities and the inability to successfully negotiate problems. For example, people with certain personalities might be particularly prone to generating stress, and couples with poor communication skills may inadvertently contribute to the stressful events with which they then must contend. Hence, in this model, stressful life events play a very important role in marital dissatisfaction and dissolution.

Research largely supports the hypothesis that good adaptive processes moderate the impact of life stressors on marital functioning. This is particularly true for the moderating role of social support. Some research also indicates that problem-solving behaviors moderate the association between stressors and marital functioning. For example, Cohan and Bradbury found that levels of stressful life events were associated with emotions and behaviors displayed while couples were discussing marital problems. Furthermore, the association between life events and later marital satisfaction was moderated by problem-solving behavior. Higher levels of life events were associated with lower levels of marital satisfaction in couples when, for example, wives did not effectively express their anger about marital problems.

The ABCX and Double ABCX Models of Family Stress

Hill's 1949 ABCX model of family adaptation has largely guided family stress theory. His theory was based on his study of servicemen separated from their families during World War II, but the model is sufficiently general to be considered applicable to all families and marriages. Hill suggested that stressors have the potential to produce change in the family system and that family adaptation differs in response to stressors. He proposed that family adaption (X) was a function of the nature of the stressor (A), the family's resources (B), and the family's appraisal of the stressor (C). Regarding the nature of the stressor, the stressfulness of an event depends on exactly what the nature of the event is – some events are inherently more stressful than others. Family resources are similar to adaptive processes and enduring vulnerabilities in the VSA model. For example, family resources may be material, such as income; intrapersonal, such as education or family of origin experiences; or interpersonal, such as communication skills or family cohesion. More resources should minimize, and fewer resources should maximize, the negative consequences of stressful life events. The family's appraisal of the stressor determines how the family views the stressful life event. Families who view the event as a threat should fare worse than families who view the event as a challenge.

The Double ABCX model expands the ABCX model by including a mechanism to explain the development of family adaptation or distress over time. That is, whereas the ABCX model focuses on adaptation at one point in time in response to a concurrent stressor, the Double ABCX model includes the accumulation of stress over time as a predictor of longer-term adaptation. The notion is that family crises do not occur in isolation. They occur in conjunction with other preexisting stressful circumstances, and they initiate new stressful circumstances. Thus, the Double

ABCX model encompasses the accumulation of stressful circumstances (aA), existing resources and additional resources developed by responses to earlier stressors (bB), appraisals of the original stressor and the aftermath of the family's attempt to deal with it (cC), and longer-term family adaptation (xX). These two models have gained much empirical support in studies of families with diverse stressors, including families coping with wartime separations and families coping with children who have mental disorders. These models have also been used to inform the assessment and treatment of children and families facing severe life stressors. Although not explicitly designed to understand stress in marriage, these models have clear applications to marital outcomes in that when successful adaptation is not achieved, marital distress and dissolution may follow.

The Marital Stress Generation Model

The marital stress generation model was designed to explain how marital stressors (internal stressors) are created by spouses and how marital stressors impact the individual well-being of spouses. Hence, it differs from the other two models that focus on external stressors and how couples and families cope with them. The marital stress generation model proposes that symptomatic spouses (e.g., spouses with depressive symptoms) perceive their partners negatively and are deficient in their capacity to communicate with, negotiate with, or support their partners. These negative perceptions and deficiencies lead spouses to experience more stressors within their marriage, and these stressors subsequently maintain or exacerbate the symptomatic spouse's symptoms.

The marital stress generation model developed out of the stress generation model of unipolar depression, which stated that depressed people contribute to the occurrence of interpersonal stressors, which then contribute to further depression. Research has consistently supported this model and has suggested that a stress-generation process may not be specific to depression. Research on the marital stress generation model supports the model, at least for wives. For example, Davila et al. found that wives with depressive symptoms expect their husbands to be critical of them and then solicit and provide support in a negative manner when interacting with their husbands. This behavior leads to increases in marital stress, which in turn leads to increases in wives' depressive symptoms. Hence, the model describes how marital interactions (e.g., involving the provision and receipt of social support), marital stress and individual well-being can affect one another and keep spouses mired in a cycle of marital dysfunction and distress. In a

similar vein, some researchers hypothesize that in maritally discordant wives uncertainty about the future of the relationship and ongoing concerns about spousal disagreements may elicit and further perpetuate anxiety symptoms, and that reduced positive reinforcement from spousal interactions and helplessness about the ability to change the relationship may elicit and perpetuate depressive symptoms.

Summary

The three models described here address different types of stressors and different segments of the stress–marital functioning association. However, they have at least one significant commonality in that they all focus on the adaptive strategies used by couples to negotiate problems or to support one another. This highlights the fact that the manner in which couples cope with stressors is critical to their ultimate marital outcome.

Specific Types of Stressors Associated with Marital Functioning

A number of specific types of stressors and their association with marital functioning have been studied. Samplings of the major stressors are presented. Not all of these programs of study were conceived of as research on stress and marriage, but, by their nature, the variables they examine are stressful events and fit within the stress paradigms just described. Initial investigations of many of these stressors focused on direct associations between the stressor and marital functioning. Research has moved toward more integrated models, as described, particularly with respect to how the manner in which couples negotiate or cope with stressors affects associations between stress and marital functioning. Although such knowledge is expanding, further research on the mechanisms of the association between stress and marital functioning is still necessary.

Work-Related Stressors and Unemployment

Work-related stressors and unemployment (especially those ensuing financial hardship) are consistently shown to be associated with poorer marital and family functioning. Job loss and unemployment decrease the individual well-being of spouses, decrease marital satisfaction, and increase marital dissolution. Consistent with the models described earlier, research suggests that these negative effects can result from poor adaptation within the family (e.g., increased conflict and poor social support) and from increased depression among spouses. For example, financial strain can lead to increases in depressive symptoms, which lead to reductions in spousal support and increases in marital distress. Work-related stressors show similar associations. For example, couples have more negative marital interactions on workdays that are reported as more stressful and when daily workload is high. Different types of jobs may also be more or less stressful. For example, shift work or jobs involving separations may be more stressful for some couples than are other types of work. The negative impact of long working hours on marriage is receiving greater attention as the length of the typical work week increases. Related to this, a number of studies have examined differences between blue-collar and white-collar workers facing job stress, and they suggest that blue-collar marriages may be at greater risk than white-collar marriages, possibly because of the different strategies they use to cope with job stress. However, much variance exists within blue- and white-collar jobs. In summary, there is clear evidence that work-related stress, and the manner in which couples negotiate it, can have a serious negative impact on marriage.

Military Service

Military couples and families often deal with a unique set of stressors, such as frequent relocation, relationship maintenance during separation, reunion, and numerous other factors above and beyond those dealt with by nonmilitary couples. A number of studies, many deriving from early tests of the ABCX model of family stress, indicate an association between aspects of military service and marital functioning. For example, wives' perceptions of marital adjustment declined during husbands' military-related absences, and wives and children reported increased emotional distress during absences. In addition, higher levels of marital quality before husbands' military-related absences led to more successful family reintegration at the end of the absence. The higher levels of military life stress are also associated with lower levels of general well-being and global life satisfaction among military wives. Hence, being married to a man in the military and the stressors that come along with that may have negative outcomes for wives, although this is likely to be moderated by family adaptation. Newer lines of research are investigating the role of military women as well as couples in which both partners serve in the military. The implications of such roles for marital and familial relationships are still in an early stage of examination.

Health Problems

A relatively large literature has indicated that health problems are significant marital stressors and that marital quality has a significant impact on health outcomes. Longitudinal studies indicate that unhappy marriages are associated with morbidity and mortality. Although the relationship between poor marital quality and health problems is bidirectional and thus difficult to disentangle, examining the consequences is nonetheless of paramount importance. Numerous health problems have been studied, including chronic pain; cancer; cardiac disease; pulmonary disorders; renal, endocrine, and gastrointestinal disorders; and neurological disorders. In general, this research indicates that health problems both affect and are affected by marital functioning. Furthermore, social support may play an important stress-buffering role for individuals and couples. Coronary heart disease is one of the most well-researched stressors, and it provides a good example of how health problems and marital functioning can be related. For example, research has indicated that spouses of cardiac patients have higher levels of psychological distress and more marital tension postrecovery. Research has also indicated that spousal support (e.g., intimacy, and emotional and instrumental support) is associated with better outcomes for coronary heart disease patients, including lower mortality rates, whereas marital discord and conflict leads to worse outcomes. The association between coronary heart disease and marital functioning is considered so important that relationship-based interventions for cardiac patients and their partners are now emerging. Of course, different health problems may pose different challenges for individuals and couples. Hence, the associations between health stressors and marital functioning may be different depending on the health problem studied. Abrasive marital interactions appear to have negative consequences on endocrinological and immunological functioning. Studies examining negative behaviors during marital conflict have found that such activities are associated with increased levels of epinephrine, norepinephrine, growth hormone, and adrenocorticotropic hormone (ACTH), as well as greater immunological change over the following 24 h. Wives appear to be more reactive physiologically to marital conflict than husbands. Longitudinal studies have further supported such findings, with higher levels of stress hormones in newlyweds foreshadowing marital distress and dissolution 10 years later.

Infertility

Infertility is a significant stressor that affects approximately 10% of couples, according to recent estimates. Research suggests that infertility can have numerous negative effects for women and men, including lowered self-esteem, increased depression and anxiety, and feelings of guilt and shame. Some of these negative effects may be even more prominent among women. For example, studies have found that associations exist between infertile women who desire children (and have no social or biological children) and substantial and significant long-term psychological distress. Clinical and anecdotal evidence suggests that infertility also negatively affects marital satisfaction and marital functioning, particularly sexual satisfaction. The diagnosis, investigation, and/or management of infertility may interact with a couple's sexuality and sexual expression by exacerbating sexual problems, or the sexual problems themselves may be a contributory factor in childlessness. It is certain that couples dealing with infertility are faced with many issues that can strain a marriage beyond sexual difficulties alone, such as financial difficulties (from the high costs of fertility treatments) and reconceptualization of future plans and social roles. However, the empirical data indicate that couples with fertility problems are no more dissatisfied with their relationships than are other couples. In addition, there is evidence that infertility has positive effects on some couples. Successful coping with infertility can result in increased commitment and closeness. Hence, the effects of infertility on marital outcomes may depend on how couples adapt to or cope with the stressor. In line with this, data indicate that couples will fare worse when spouses have incompatible ways of coping with infertility.

Transition to Parenthood

Numerous studies have suggested that marriage suffers during the transition to parenthood. For example, marital satisfaction tends to decline and marital problems and conflict can increase, particularly in wives. However, research that contradicts these findings also exists. Methodological issues are problematic in prior studies showing decline; there are distortions such as the assessment of spouses during the third trimester of pregnancy and the failure to include comparison groups of couples at similar points in marriage who were not having children. Studies that include comparison groups and that assess spouses before, during, and after pregnancy have failed to find differences between the couples who were transitioning to parenthood and those who were not. There is some evidence, however, that marital factors affect which couples will fare better or worse during the transition to parenthood. For example, existing marital problems may lead spouses and couples to experience a more stressful transition, and, to the extent that spouses' child care and housekeeping

expectations for their partners are not met, couples may view their marriages more negatively. Hence, the transition to parenthood may not be equally stressful for all couples, but may instead depend on how couples negotiate the transition.

Psychopathology

Much research indicates that psychopathology is intrinsically linked with marital functioning. Although psychopathology is conceived of as an enduring vulnerability in the VSA model of marital outcomes and as a cause and an outcome of marital stress in the marital stress generation model, it may be reasonable to also consider psychopathology as a stressor, particularly when a spouse is in the active phase of a disorder. Various types of psychopathology, including depression, substance abuse, anxiety disorders, and schizophrenia, are associated with significant marital dysfunction and divorce. As such, they are stressors that have major implications for marital outcomes, largely because they interfere with important aspects of marital functioning. For example, skillful communication, adaptive emotion regulation, and the ability to be physically and emotionally available and supportive are important to good marital outcomes, but they are often impaired by psychopathology. Research consistently suggests that greater levels of psychopathology are associated with lower levels of marital satisfaction. It has also been found that depression in one spouse is significantly associated with lower marital satisfaction in both spouses. The association between psychopathology and poor marital functioning is so prominent that forms of marital and couple therapy are used to treat many disorders, highlighting the importance of examining the effects of psychopathology on both partners.

Infidelity

Infidelity is an important internal marital stressor that has recently garnered a great deal of attention. Although a paucity of empirical research on this stressor currently exists, both clinicians and scholars have recognized the significance of infidelity to couples. For example, Cano and O'Leary found the discovery of infidelity to be associated with increased levels of clinical depression in the noninvolved spouse. Given the significant negative role of psychopathology in marriages, as noted in a prior section, these findings highlight the importance of investigating infidelity as a marital stressor. Currently, researchers are investigating the differing effects of emotional versus sexual infidelity on wives and husbands. Findings are mixed as to whether gender differences exist in response to different types of infidelity. Present research has investigated differences in husbands and wives in terms of the amount of distress caused or the likelihood of forgiveness depending on the type of infidelity. It appears that men's distress is primarily predicted from the type of infidelity (greater distress from sexual infidelity than emotional), whereas women's distress is predicted from a number of factors (e.g., relationship commitment and whether the person the husband is having the affair with is a new person vs. an ex-partner). Relationship commitment appears to be highly associated with the likelihood to forgive for both husbands and wives. However, more research is needed on the interactions between gender differences and the type of infidelity.

Ethnic Differences in the Relations between Stress and Marriage

Research on ethnic differences in the association between stress and marriage is still in its early stages, but indicates that couples of varying ethnicities are likely to experience different types of stressors consistent with their ethnic/cultural backgrounds. These stressors may be altered or amplified in couples of differing ethnicities and cultural backgrounds. Ethnic minority couples also face different stressors at a societal level than do Caucasian couples (e.g., stereotyping and stigmatization), suggesting that couples of different ethnicities may face stressors that present unique challenges to the success of their marriages. Much of the existing research focuses on differences between Caucasian and African American couples and families; however, there is an increasing trend toward including Latino and Asian couples and families. In general, research indicates some similarities between couples of various ethnicities but also some potentially important differences. Stressors related to financial hardship and social networks may play a particularly important role in African American and Latino marriages. Because of these sorts of findings, some authors are now calling for a more comprehensive model of marital outcomes for various ethnic minority couples, similar to the models described earlier, that include the role of stressors and how couples adapt to them. A great deal of additional research is necessary before the ethnicity-specific associations between stressors and marital outcomes for all groups are more fully understood. Research on interracial marriages and their potentially unique stressors is also garnering an increasing amount of attention. Such research suggests higher levels of marital challenges due to lack of cultural understanding, racial pressure, and lack of familial support. However, much more research is needed in this area.

Methodological and Measurement Issues

The study of stress in general has been fraught with measurement and methodological problems, and many of these problems emerge in the study of stress and marriage. For example, both external and internal stressors typically have been assessed using self-report measures. People are asked to report whether a stressor has occurred and how much stress or negative impact was associated with the occurrence of the event. At issue here is the extent to which people are reliable reporters, particularly when assessing amount of stress or negative impact. These reports can be biased by mood. Hence, distressed or unhappy spouses may report higher levels of stress and negative impact than nondistressed spouses, and this may artificially inflate associations between stress and poor marital functioning. One solution to this problem draws on the contextual threat procedures developed by George Brown and colleagues. Participants are interviewed and interviewers or coders make ratings of objective stress, as opposed to spouses' subjective stress ratings. This procedure is used frequently in the study of stress and psychopathology, and it could easily be applied to studies of marriage and stress. However, it is a time-consuming procedure. Another option is the use of daily diaries. Although such methods rely on self-report data, if we are interested in data obtained through self-report, such as examining each partner's account of various life events, daily-diary information may prove very useful. Notably, in daily-diary studies there is a dramatic reduction in the likelihood of retrospection because the amount of time elapsed between an experience and the account of the experience is minimized. The recall of the frequency of various stressors and marital interactions, and the immediate response to such events, therefore, may be greatly improved. Another consideration for marital researchers is whether it is the number of stressors that spouses experience or the stressfulness of stressors (e.g., the nature of the stressor) that affects marriage. Similarly, there are numerous types of stressors, including discrete events, chronic strains, and daily hassles, which might affect marital functioning in different ways. Another issue in stress research that applies to marital research is the reliance on retrospective reports of stress. Current models of stress and marriage imply longitudinal associations between the two, which suggests that stressors should be examined prospectively over time. Finally, it may be important to study specific types of stressors individually rather than aggregating unrelated events. All stressors may not show similar associations with marital functioning.

Further Reading

Booth, A., Crouter, A. C. and Clements, M. (2001). *Couples in conflict*. Mahwah, NJ: Lawrence Erlbaum.

Bradbury, T. N. (1998). *The developmental course of marital dysfunction*. New York: Cambridge University Press.

Cann, A. and Baucom, T. R. (2004). Former partners and new rivals as threats to a relationship: infidelity type, gender, and commitment as factors related to distress and forgiveness. *Personal Relationships* 11, 305–318.

Cano, A. and O'Leary, K. D. (2000). Infidelity and separations precipitate major depressive episodes and symptoms of nonspecific depression and anxiety. *Journal of Consulting and Clinical Psychology* 68, 774–781.

Cano, A., O'Leary, K. D. and Heinz, W. (2004). Short-term consequences of severe marital stressors. *Journal of Social and Personal Relationship* 21(4), 419–430.

Cohan, C. L. and Bradbury, T. N. (1997). Negative life events, marital interaction, and the longitudinal course of newlywed marriage. *Journal of Personality and Social Psychology* 73(1), 114–128.

Cutrona, C. E. (1996). *Social support in couples: marriage as a resource in times of stress*. Thousand Oaks, CA: Sage.

Davila, J., Bradbury, T. N., Cohan, C. L., et al. (1997). Marital functioning and depressive symptoms: evidence for a stress generation model. *Journal of Personality and Social Psychology* 73, 849–861.

Demo, D. H. and Allen, K. R. (2000). *Handbook of family diversity*. London: Oxford University Press.

Dillaway, H. and Broman, C. (2001). Race, class and gender differences in marital satisfaction and divisions of household labor among dual-earner couples. *Journal of Family Issues* 22(3), 309–327.

Drummet, A. R., Coleman, M. and Cable, S. (2003). Military families under stress: implications for family life education. *Family Relations* 52(3), 279–287.

Fu, X., Tora, J. and Kendall, H. (2001). Marital happiness and inter-racial marriage: a study in a multi-ethnic community in Hawaii. *Journal of Comparative Family Studies* 32(1), 47–60.

Hammen, C. L. (1991). The generation of stress in the course of unipolar depression. *Journal of Abnormal Psychology* 100, 555–561.

Hetherington, E. M. (1999). *Coping with divorce, single parenting, and remarriage: a risk and resiliency perspective*. Mahwah, NJ: Lawrence Erlbaum.

Hill, R. (1949). *Families under stress*. Westport, CT: Greenwood Press.

Karney, B. R. and Bradbury, T. N. (1995). The longitudinal course of marital quality and stability: a review of theory, method, and research. *Psychological Bulletin* 118, 3–34.

Kreider, Rose M. (2005). Number, timing, and duration of marriages and divorces: 2001. In: *Current population reports*, pp. 70–97. Washington, DC: U.S. Census Bureau.

L'Abate, L. (1998). *Family psychopathology: the relational roots of dysfunctional behavior*. New York: Guilford.

Leiblum, S. R. (1997). *Infertility: psychological issues and counseling strategies*. New York: John Wiley & Sons.

Lundquist, J. H. and Smith, H. L. (2005). Family formation among women in the U.S. military: evidence from NLSY. *Journal of Marriage & Family* 67(1), 1–13.

McCubbin, H. I. and Patterson, J. M. (1983). The family stress process: the double ABCX model of adjustment and adaptation. *Marriage and Family Review* 6, 7–37.

McQuillan, J., Greil, A. L., White, L., et al. (2003). Frustrated fertility: infertility and psychological distress among women. *Journal of Marriage & the Family* 65(4), 1007–1018.

Revenson, T. A., Kayser, K. and Bodenmann, G. (2005). *Couples coping with stress: emerging perspectives on dyadic coping*. Washington, DC: American Psychological Association.

Robles, T. F. and Kiecolt-Glaser, J. K. (2003). The physiology of marriage: pathways to health. *Physiology & Behavior* 79, 409–416.

Root, M. P. (2001). *Love's revolution: interracial marriage*. Philadelphia: Temple University Press.

Schmaling, K. B. and Sher, T. G. (2000). *The psychology of couples and illness*. Washington, DC: American Psychological Association.

Story, L. B. and Bradbury, T. N. (2004). Understanding marriage and stress: essential questions and challenges. *Clinical Psychology Review* 23, 1139–1162.

Whisman, M. A., Uebelacker, L. A. and Weinstock, L. M. (2004). Psychopathology and marital satisfaction: the importance of evaluating both partners. *Journal of Consulting and Clinical Psychology* 72(5), 830–838.

Marriage, Same Sex   *See:* Homosexuality, Stress and.

Maternal Deprivation

R L Huot, C O Ladd and P M Plotsky
Emory University School of Medicine, Atlanta, GA, USA

This article is reproduced from the previous edition, volume 2, pp 699–707, © 2000, Elsevier Inc.

Introduction
Maternal Deprivation Models
Consequences of Maternal Deprivation
Biological Significance

Glossary

Corticotropin releasing hormone (CRH)	A 41-amino-acid peptide and the primary regulator of the pituitary-adrenal system that is activated in response to stressors. CRH also acts as a neuromodulator in corticolimbic and brain-stem areas and, thus, is believed to participate in the coordination of the mammalian neuroendocrine, behavioral, autonomic nervous system, and immune responses to a stressor.
Hypothalamic-pituitary-adrenal (HPA) axis	A system that transduces interoceptive and exteroceptive signals into an endocrine response, culminating in the synthesis and secretion of adrenal glucocorticoids that act throughout the body to mobilize energy substrates such as glucose for use by the individual in escape or fighting.
Maternal deprivation	A neonatal manipulation in which rat pups are briefly handled and separated from the dam for prolonged periods of time ranging from 3 to 24 h. This procedure is typically implemented between postnatal days 1 and 21, with either single or repeated exposures.
Stress hypo-responsive period (SHRP)	A period from postnatal days 3 to 14 when neonatal rat pups show attenuated pituitary-adrenal responses to stressful stimuli that would cause a response in the adult. This period is characterized by low levels of circulating glucocorticoids, although a majority of this steroid is in free form due to the low production of corticosteroid-binding globulin during this age period. It has been postulated that the maintenance of low glucocorticoid levels is necessary during this period for the normal development of the HPA axis and the central nervous system, especially the hippocampus.

Early experience is associated with long-term behavioral, neuroendocrinological, cognitive, and central nervous system (CNS) changes in rodents, guinea pigs, and primates. The specific effects of positive or negative stimuli during the neonatal period are believed to be dependent on the genetic background of the individual, developmental status of the CNS at the time of exposure, duration of the stimulus, type and severity of the experience, and other factors such as the availability of social support. A number of research laboratories have employed the paradigms of neonatal handling and neonatal maternal deprivation as probes of CNS plasticity during the postpartum period. In general, these paradigms exert opposite influences, with maternal deprivation being associated with long-term increases in anxietylike behavior, HPA axis responsiveness to stressors, and changes in the functional characteristics of the central neurocircuits involved in the perception of and response to environmental events. Due to the relative stability of the changes resulting from neonatal maternal deprivation, as well as the ability of antidepressant treatment to reverse these changes transiently, this paradigm has been explored as an animal model of affective disorders.

Introduction

Initial studies in the late 1950s and 1960s by Levine, Denenberg, Ader, and others showed that neonatal handling or infantile stimulation led to long-term adaptations in behavior and the stress response. Subsequently, numerous paradigms of prenatal stress, neonatal maternal deprivation, and isolation rearing have been developed by numerous laboratories to systematically study the effects of adverse early experience on the development of behavior, endocrine function, and the CNS. This review is primarily limited to the effects of neonatal maternal deprivation in the rat. Before introducing the neonatal deprivation models, we provide a brief review of the developmental status of the neonatal CNS, the HPA axis and stress response, and the role of maternal behavior in development.

Central Nervous System Plasticity in the Neonate

Genetic and environmental factors interact to guide CNS development throughout the life span. Although the basic structure and connectivity of the brain are specified by genetic factors, environmental factors play a key role in programming the patterns and density of connectivity that underlie the individual organism's perception of and responsiveness to its environment. These adaptations occur via a variety of processes, including activity-dependent plasticity and synaptic pruning. Frequently, this plasticity involves neurocircuits mediating the various aspects of the stress response, including the regulation of HPA axis activity.

Because many species spend their lifetimes within a narrow geographical range with respect to their birthplace, this interactive process may provide an adaptive advantage, serving as a mechanism by which an individual organism may optimize its neurocircuitry and develop behaviors appropriate for survival. As illustrated in **Figure 1** for the rat, many neurodevelopmental processes continue during and after the neonatal period. Furthermore, many of these processes are sensitive to circulating glucocorticoid hormone levels. Therefore, exposure to adverse conditions during the neonatal period can modulate the CNS developmental process through multiple mechanisms. This postpartum period of increased vulnerability to environmental factors varies among species, depending on the state of CNS developmental maturity at birth.

The Hypothalamic–Pituitary–Adrenal Axis and Regulation of the Stress Response

Internal and external stimuli (i.e., stressors) conveying actual or perceived threat, pain, metabolic imbalance, or failure of expectations are processed via widely distributed pathways and converge on the paraventricular nucleus (PVN) of the hypothalamus. Neurons in this structure produce the peptides corticotropin releasing hormone (CRH) and arginine vasopressin (AVP), which are transported to the median eminence nerve terminals and are released into the hypophysial-portal circulation, the functional link between the CNS and the endocrine system. At the anterior pituitary gland, these peptides stimulate the synthesis and release of adrenocorticotropic hormone (ACTH) into the systemic circulation. Circulating ACTH evokes the synthesis and secretion of glucocorticoids (cortisol in primates and corticosterone in rodents) from the adrenal cortex, which serve to mobilize energy substrates during stress. Plasma glucocorticoid levels are controlled tightly by glucocorticoid-mediated negative feedback on the secretion of CRH and ACTH by the activation of cytoplasmic mineralocorticoid receptors (MR) localized in the

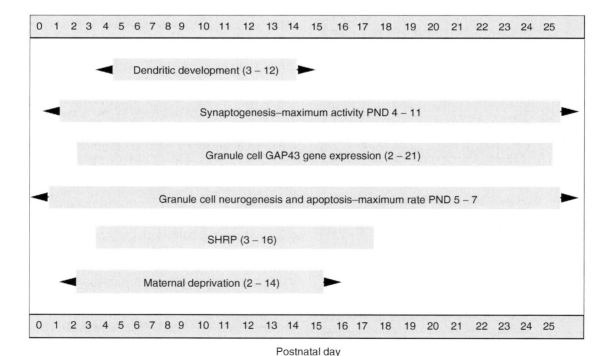

Figure 1 Developmental processes occurring during the neonatal period in rodents. Maternal deprivation paradigms overlap a significant portion of the stress hyporesponsive period (SHRP). Throughout the neonatal period, myelination, neurogenesis, and apoptosis, as well as synaptogenesis and synaptic pruning, are occurring. All these mechanisms represent targets for epigenetic and environmental modification of the basic genetic plan for CNS development.

hippocampus and septum and/or the activation of cytoplasmic glucocorticoid receptors (GR) located in the adenohypophysis and throughout the CNS.

HPA axis responses are adaptive and essential for survival in adulthood, but may be maladaptive in infancy while the brain is immature. In the normally developing rodent the brain is protected from catabolic and other effects of glucocorticoids due to a reduced sensitivity of the HPA axis to activation during the neonatal period, postnatal days (PND) 3–16, a developmental epoch known as the SHRP. This reduced responsiveness is not absolute and may be overcome by strong stressors, including maternal deprivation.

Role of Maternal Behavior in Postnatal Development

The early environment in many mammalian species is determined largely by the mother. In many primate species, including humans, early interactions between the mother and the infant serve as a template for all subsequent relationships. The neonatal rat is completely dependent on its mother for nutrition, temperature regulation, grooming, and regulation of micturition for the first 2 weeks of life. Alterations in the quality of maternal care have been shown to exert profound and long-lasting influences on the development of stress responsiveness and health in rodent offspring. This dependence and the subtle complexities of maternal behavior led Hofer to postulate the concept of the mother as a hidden regulator of physiological and behavioral development in the rat.

In many mammals, maternal care is quite stereotypic and involves a number of distinct behaviors. Maternal behavior in the rat consists of nest building, retrieval of the pups into the nest, nursing periods associated with an arched-back posture to encourage suckling, and anogenital licking to stimulate urination and defecation. Levine and colleagues showed that particular maternal behaviors modulate the development of the HPA axis at different levels and serve, in part, to reduce the responsivity of the HPA axis beginning a few days after birth and lasting until the pups are more independent.

Maternal Deprivation Models

Rodent Models of Maternal Deprivation

Numerous maternal deprivation models have been developed to study the effects of prolonged separations of infants from their mothers on behavioral and endocrine responsiveness. These deprivation manipulations vary greatly among research groups, ranging from a single 24-h deprivation to repeated maternal deprivation episodes lasting 12, 8, 6, or 3 h from PND

1–2 through PND 14–21. In addition, some paradigms require the isolation of pups from one another during the separation period, whereas in others the pups remain together as a litter during the period of separation.

In an open colony setting, the dam typically leaves her pups for periods of 5–15 min in order to forage for food and water; however, in some cases the dam may be away for periods of 60–180 min. Mimicking these observations, Plotsky and Meaney developed a maternal deprivation model in which Long Evans rat litters were standardized to eight male pups (or four male and four female pups) on PND 2 and then assigned randomly to one of four neonatal rearing conditions during PND 2–14, inclusive: (1) brief handling and 180 min per day of maternal separation (HMS180); (2) brief handling and 15 min per day of maternal separation (HMS15); (3) nonhandled (HMS0); and (4) animal facility rearing (AFR), in which litters were handled twice weekly beginning on PND 4 for cage changing. Bedding material in the home cages was replaced only partially (50%) with clean bedding once per week when the dams and pups were out of the cage (HMS15 and HMS180). In all deprivation studies, the dams were moved to an adjacent cage when they were off the nest in the morning and then the pups were placed in a transfer cage and moved to an incubator in another room. At the end of the daily separation, both HMS15 and HMS180 litters were returned to their home cage, rolled in the native bedding, and then reunited with their dam. All litters were weaned on PND 21–23 and group housed (two to three per cage) until adulthood (> PND 60).

Comparisons have been made between the maternally deprived animals (HMS180) and a control group consisting of nonhandled (HMS0), animal facility-reared (AFR), or handled (HMS15) rats. Despite the wide variations in the maternal deprivation protocols, adult animals that experienced neonatal maternal deprivation typically display high anxietylike behavior and HPA axis hyperresponsiveness, whereas adults that experienced neonatal handling exhibit reduced anxietylike behavior and conserved HPA axis responses to stressors. In this review, the control and experimental groups are presented as in the studies, but it should be kept in mind that the selection of the control group may have a profound effect on the conclusions drawn from the data.

Primate Models of Maternal Deprivation

The majority of nonhuman primate maternal deprivation studies have been performed in rhesus monkeys or squirrel monkeys. The specific nature of the maternal deprivation protocols varies widely in these studies from severe and prolonged maternal deprivation to less profound periods of deprivation. Maternal separation in primates is associated with increased oral behaviors and other stereotypic movements, anxietylike behavior, cognitive impairment, aggression, deficits in bonding, and exaggerated HPA axis function.

Consequences of Maternal Deprivation

Changes in Maternal Behavior

The dams of pups exposed to the HMS15 protocol exhibited increased maternal behavior, such as licking and grooming of the pups, as compared to the AFR group, whereas prolonged maternal deprivation (HMS180) was associated with reduced and deranged maternal behavior. Dams of the HMS180 group retrieved their pups with a longer latency on reunion and took longer to begin to nurse the pups as well as to lick and groom them. This decreased maternal behavior was largely responsible for the long-term resistance to stress as demonstrated in cross-fostering studies. In support of the role of maternal behavior, Meaney and colleagues demonstrated an inverse correlation between the amount of time the dam spent in licking, grooming, and arched-back nursing of her pups and subsequent adult stress responsiveness. Furthermore, the importance of anogenital licking for the development of the normal HPA axis stress response has been shown.

Hypothalamic-Pituitary-Adrenal Axis Adaptations

Handled, nonhandled, and maternally deprived rats show distinct and stable differences in their HPA response to stressors as adults, as summarized in **Table 1**. In adult rats, basal levels of ACTH and corticosterone typically do not differ among the rearing groups described earlier. However, in response to a psychological stressor (e.g., novel environment or air puff startle), exaggerated ACTH and corticosterone responses are apparent in maternally deprived and nonhandled rats as compared to handled or animal facility reared rats. Using a single 24-h period of neonatal maternal deprivation, van Oers and colleagues have shown that the age at which maternal deprivation occurred altered the outcome with respect to HPA axis function. Deprivation at PND 3 resulted in hyperresponsiveness of the pups at PND 20, whereas deprivation at PND 11 resulted in hyporesponsiveness. Similar experiments will be necessary to elucidate the neurocircuits and mechanisms mediating aspects of the overall neuroendocrine, behavioral, and cognitive effects of neonatal maternal deprivation.

Table 1 HPA axis effects of neonatal handling and maternal deprivation as compared to nonhandled rats

Variable	Neonatal handling[a]	Neonatal maternal deprivation[b]
HPA axis function		
Basal ACTH	⇔	⇔
Basal corticosterone	⇔	⇔
ACTH stress response	⇓	⇑
Corticosterone stress response	⇓	⇑
Dexamethasone resistance	⇔	⇑
CRH receptor binding		
Paraventricular nucleus	⇔	⇑
Pituitary	⇔	⇓
CRH content		
Paraventricular nucleus	⇔	⇑
Stalk median eminence	⇓	⇑
CRH mRNA		
Paraventricular nucleus	⇓	⇑
GR mRNA		
Hippocampus	⇑	⇓
Paraventricular nucleus	⇔	⇔
Pituitary	⇔	⇔
Prefrontal cortex	⇑	⇓

[a]HMS15 (brief handling and 15 min per day of maternal separation).
[b]HMS180 (brief handling and 180 min per day of maternal deprivation).

At the level of the hypothalamus, maternally deprived and nonhandled rats show significantly greater expression of CRH mRNA, specifically in the PVN, compared to handled rats. In addition, these rats have an elevated peptide content of CRH and AVP in the stalk median eminence as well as increased CRH and AVP concentrations in the hypophysial-portal circulation compared to handled rats. Also, maternally deprived and nonhandled rats show increased CRH receptor binding in the PVN compared to handled rats. This latter adaptation may reflect the increased expression of CRHR1-receptor mRNA in the PVN as a consequence of the stress of maternal deprivation. Thus, the brains of these animals exhibit increased CRH as well as potentially increased responsiveness to this CRH.

Impaired glucocorticoid-mediated negative feedback may contribute to the elevated expression of CRH as well as to the exaggerated secretion of ACTH and corticosterone seen in deprived rats, whereas an increased feedback tone may underlie the reduction in stress responsiveness observed in handled rats. The expression of the two types of glucocorticoid receptors is extremely vulnerable to neonatal experience. The type 1 or mineralocorticoid receptor (MR) is a high-affinity receptor that shows a high degree of saturation even under basal conditions. It is believed to be involved in the maintenance of basal HPA activity. In contrast, the type 2 or glucocorticoid receptor (GR) is a low-affinity receptor that becomes activated in the presence of elevated levels of glucocorticoids typical of stress. As adults, the density of hippocampal GR binding sites in the experimental groups is handled = AFR > nonhandled > maternally deprived; the levels of GR mRNA follow a similar pattern. An increased expression of GR in the hippocampus and prefrontal cortex may increase the negative feedback tone on the HPA axis, thus providing a mechanism by which handled rats dampen their stress response. Conversely, the reduction of hippocampal GR in maternally deprived rats may, in part, explain their HPA axis hyperresponsiveness to stressors. Reports also indicate that hippocampal MR mRNA levels are increased in HMS180 maternally deprived rats, perhaps accounting for the normal circadian trough and peak ACTH and corticosterone levels in these animals. These changes in GR and MR binding and expression are apparent from at least PND 21 in the HMS180 model.

However, in response to 24 h of maternal deprivation on PND 3, Levine's group found decreased binding for both MR and GR in the CA1 region of the hippocampus in males at PND 48. No changes were observed in binding of the MR in females at PND 48 or of mRNA for either MR or GR at PND 60. When deprivation was applied on PND 11 and the brains collected the next day, one study showed a decrease in both MR and GR mRNA in CA1, whereas another study showed a decrease only in the MR mRNA in CA1 and no changes in the GR mRNA. Thus, although these studies confirm the high degree of plasticity of the glucocorticoid receptors in the brain in response to early experience, the actual effects of maternal deprivation seem variable over time. Studies of the time sequence in glucocorticoid receptor expression changes in response to maternal deprivation are needed to sort these out among maternal deprivation paradigms.

Behavioral Consequences

Stress has long been associated with increased anxiety- or fearlike behavior. Using multiple tests of these behaviors (e.g., elevated plus maze, novel open-field locomotion, defensive withdrawal, and acoustic startle), many groups have shown that maternal deprivation is associated with increased anxiety- and fearlike behavior beginning in the neonatal period and persisting throughout adulthood.

When placed in a brightly lit, novel open field, rats initially spend more time near the walls and show reduced locomotor activity. HMS180 maternally deprived rats continue to display neophobia long after the AFR and HMS15 animals have habituated to the novel environment. Similar results were found in an open-field exploration test as well as in the latency to eating in a conflict test following overnight food deprivation, suggesting a heightened fearfulness in maternally deprived rats exposed to a novel arena.

In the defensive withdrawal test, HMS180 rats show an increased latency to exit from a safe compartment into the open-field arena and demonstrate an increased number of reentries into the cylinder as well as a greater total amount of time spent in the cylinder compared to AFR and HMS15 rats. Similarly, in the elevated plus maze, maternally deprived rats spent less time in the open arms compared to either handled or AFR rats. Nonhandled rats show a level of anxietylike intermediate between maternally deprived and handled rats in these tests. Thus, it appears that maternally deprived rats show greater anxiety and neophobia than do handled (HMS15), nonhandled (HMS0), or normally reared (AFR) rats.

Early experience can also affect an adult animal's cognitive performance. Infantile handling has been shown to prevent cognitive impairments as the animal ages. At 24 months, but not at 12 months, handled rats learn to find a hidden platform in the Morris water maze faster than nonhandled rats. This may be due to less exposure to glucocorticoids throughout the animals' life because elevated levels of these stress hormones are related to cognitive impairments. It has been hypothesized that maternally deprived rats should be impaired on tasks of learning and memory. Data from the authors' laboratory support this hypothesis; middle-age (120 days) maternally deprived rats show a slight, but significant, impairment on the learning of the Morris water maze.

Overall, these behavioral observations provide compelling support for the thesis that maternal deprivation during the neonatal period increases anxiety- or fearlike behavior that persists throughout adulthood. Thus, sensory experiences encountered during a critical window of development, particularly those associated with mother–infant interactions, significantly affect individual perception of the environment and responses to it throughout life. It is postulated that this process arises through a combination of stimulus-induced plasticity during postnatal development, activation of extrahypothalamic CRH neurocircuits, and glucocorticoid effects mediated through a cascade of transcriptional changes in critical sensory and limbic systems.

Extrahypothalamic Effects

Considering the effects of maternal deprivation on behavior and endocrine responses to psychological stressors, it would not be surprising to find a number of adaptations in the CNS, especially in systems involved in the regulation of stress and fear. Studies in the HMS180 maternal deprivation paradigm have shown that maternal deprivation and handling affect extrahypothalamic CRH systems, GABA and benzodiazepine pathways, and norepinephrine circuits as outlined in **Table 2**.

The involvement of extrahypothalamic CRH systems is particularly salient because these circuits appear to coordinate the neuroendocrine, behavioral, sympathetic nervous system, and cognitive responses to stressors. Furthermore, there are substantial interactions between these CRH-containing neurocircuits and brain-stem noradrenergic systems. CRH mRNA levels in the central nucleus of the amygdala and the bed nucleus of the stria terminalis were increased in HMS180 maternally deprived rats and decreased in HMS15 handled rats compared to nonhandled rats. The CRH mRNA levels in these brain regions of the HMS15 rats were equivalent to those of animal facility-reared animals.

Table 2 Extrahypothalamic effects of neonatal rearing paradigms

Variable	Neonatal paradigm[a]
CRH receptor binding	
Locus ceruleus	HMS180 > HMS0 > HMS15 = AFR
Raphe	HMS180 > HMS0 > HMS15 = AFR
CRF content	
Bed nucleus of the stria terminalis	HMS180 > HMS0 > HMS15 = AFR
Central nucleus of the amygdala	HMS180 > HMS0 > HMS15 = AFR
Hippocampus	HMS180 = HMS0 = HMS15 = AFR
Locus ceruleus	HMS180 = HMS0 = HMS15 = AFR
CRF mRNA	
Bed nucleus of the stria terminalis	HMS180 > HMS0 > HMS15 = AFR
Central nucleus of the amygdala	HMS180 > HMS0 > HMS15 = AFR
Hippocampus	HMS180 = HMS0 = HMS15 = AFR
GR mRNA	
Hippocampus	AFR = HMS15 > HMS0 > HMS180
Prefrontal cortex	AFR = HMS15 > HMS0 > HMS180
α_2-*Adrenergic receptor binding*	
Locus ceruleus	HMS15 > AFR > HMS0 > HMS180
Nucleus of the solitary tract	HMS15 > AFR > HMS0 > HMS180
GABA$_A$ receptor binding	
Amygdala	HMS180 = HMS0 = HMS15 = AFR
Locus coeruleus	AFR = HMS15 > HMS0 = HMS180
Nucleus of the solitary tract	AFR = HMS15 > HMS0 = HMS180

[a]AFR, animal facility-reared control; HMS0, nonhandled; HMS15, handled (brief handling and 15 min per day of maternal separation); HMS180, maternal deprivation (brief handling and 180 min per day of maternal deprivation).

These CRH-containing pathways project to brainstem areas such as the locus ceruleus, where CRH activates locus ceruleus noradrenergic neurons. This stress-induced activation may serve to increase autonomic nervous system information flow, enhance vigilance behavior, and provide additional drive to the HPA axis. In addition, the apparent reduction in α_2-adrenergic receptor binding in the locus ceruleus and nucleus of the solitary tract implies that, once activated, the firing rate of the locus ceruleus neurons may be difficult to shut off. Interestingly, HMS180 maternal deprivation was also associated with decreased central benzodiazepine (CBZ) receptor binding in the locus ceruleus and the nucleus of the solitary tract compared to handled rats. Thus, increased CRH and reduced CBZ, GABA$_A$, and α_2-adrenergic receptor binding all provide mechanisms for general hyperresponsiveness to psychological stressors as a result of maternal deprivation. It is not known whether these same changes result from other maternal deprivation paradigms.

Biological Significance

Accumulating evidence indicates that there are critical developmental windows during which the developing brain is very susceptible to environmental influences. It is postulated that cues related to the environment are transmitted primarily via the primary caregiver, which in most species is the mother. Transmission may be through factors transferred in the milk, aspects of maternal behavior, or both. Maternal–infant interactions and other sensory experiences during these sensitive periods sculpt the final form of the nervous system via multiple mechanisms. The processes of activity-dependent plasticity and hormonal programming act to fine-tune the genetically determined neurocircuitry by altering the strength of connections, changing the morphology of neurons, and altering the expression critical signaling molecules. These changes then lead to robust differences in how that individual decodes and responds to its environment.

Observations of rats exposed to the HMS180 maternal deprivation paradigm suggest a likely cascade initiated by adverse early experience. However, the sequence of this cascade is currently unknown. The initial events lead to impaired function of two primary inhibitory systems: the glucocorticoid-mediated negative feedback system and the GABAergic-CBZ system. Subsequent steps in the cascade involve the dysregulation of CRH and monoaminergic systems.

The relative loss of glucocorticoid tone, as well as of inhibitory GABAergic-CBZ tone in the amygdaloid complex and the locus coeruleus, appears to disinhibit ascending noradrenergic drive, thus further increasing CRH secretion and gene expression in hypothalamic and extrahypothalamic circuits. Overall, these processes underlie the complex neuroendocrine, behavioral, and cognitive changes observed in response to maternal deprivation in rodents.

Like young rats, both monkey and human babies exhibit elevated glucocorticoid responses during periods of brief maternal separation. Furthermore, early adverse experience in humans also leads to long-term changes in behavior and stress responsiveness. Childhood stressors, including the loss of a parent, neglect, or child abuse, have been associated with an increased vulnerability to mood and anxiety disorders. Models of neonatal maternal deprivation in rats may serve to elucidate the CNS changes occurring in response to adverse early experience in the human and may provide insights into effective prevention and treatment strategies. The mechanisms uncovered by these animal studies may provide a bridge between psychological and psychiatric constructs and their central systems and molecular neuroscience mechanisms.

See Also the Following Article

Childhood Stress.

Further Reading

Arling, G. L., Harlow, H. F., Sackett, G. P., et al. (1976). A 10-year perspective of motherless-mother monkey behavior. *Journal of Abnormal Psychology* **85**, 341–349.

Bhatnagar, S., Shanks, N., Plotsky, P. M. and Meaney, M. J. (1996). Hypothalamic-pituitary-adrenal responses to stress in neonatally handled and nonhandled rats: differences in facilitatory and inhibitory neural pathways. In: McCarty, R., Aguilera, G., Sabban, E. & Kvetnansky, R. (eds.) *Stress: molecular genetic and neurobiological advances.* New York: Gordonand Breach Science Publishers.

Caldji, C., Francis, D., Sharma, S., et al. (in press). The effects of early rearing environment on the development of GABA$_A$ and central benzodiazepine receptor levels and novelty-induced fearfulness in the rat. *Journal of Neuroscience.*

Caldji, C., Tannenbaum, B., Sharma, S., et al. (1998). Maternal care during infancy regulates the development of neural systems mediating the expression of fearfulness in the rat. *Proceedings of the National Academy of Sciences USA* **95**, 5335–5340.

Calhoun, J. B. (1962). *The ecology and sociology of the Norway rat.* Bethesda, MD: H. E. W. Public Health Service.

Cullinan, W. E., Herman, J. P., Helmreich, D. L. and Watson, S. J. (1995). A neuroanatomy of stress. In: Friedman, M. J., Charney, D. S. & Deutch, A. Y. (eds.) *Neurobiological and clinical consequences of stress: from normal adaptation to PTSD,* pp. 3–25. Philadelphia: Lippincott-Raven.

Dunn, A. J. and Berridge, C. W. (1990). Physiological and behavioral responses to corticotropin-releasing factor administration: is CRF a mediator of anxiety and of stress responses? *Brain Research Reviews* **15**, 71–100.

Francis, D., Diorio, J., LaPlante, P., et al. (1996). The role of early environmental events in regulating neuroendocrine development. *Annals of the New York Academy of Sciences* **794**, 136–152.

Francis, D. D. and Meaney, M. J. (1999). Maternal care and the development of stress responses. *Current Opinion in Neurobiology* **9**, 128–134.

Hall, F. S. (1998). Social deprivation of neonatal, adolescent, and adult rats has distinct neurochemical and behavioral consequences. *Critical Review of Neurobiology* **12**, 129–162.

Hennessy, M. B. (1997). Hypothalamic-pituitary-adrenal responses to brief social separation. *Neuroscience and Biobehavioral Reviews* **21**, 11–29.

Hofer, M. A. (1994). Early relationships as regulators of infant physiology and behavior. *Acta Paediatrica* (supplement) **397**, 9–18.

Jacobson, L. and Sapolsky, R. M. (1991). The role of the hippocampus in feedback regulation of the hypothalamic-pituitary-adrenal axis. *Endocrine Review* **12**, 118–134.

Kolb, B. and Whishaw, I. Q. (1998). Brain plasticity and behavior. *Annual Review of Psychology* **49**, 43–64.

Ladd, C. O., Huot, R. L., Thrivikraman, K. V., Nemeroff, C. B., Meaney, M. J. and Plotsky, P. M. (2000). Long term behavioral and neuroendocrine adaptations to adverse early experience. In: Mayer, E. & Saper, C. (eds.) *Progress in brain research: the biological basis for mind body interactions* (vol. 122), pp. 79–101. Amsterdam: Elsevier.

Levine, S. (1994). The ontogeny of the hypothalamic-pituitary-adrenal axis: the influence of maternal factors. *Annals of the New York Academy of Sciences* **746**, 275–288.

Levine, S., Wiener, S. G. and Coe, C. L. (1993). Temporal and social factors influencing behavioral and hormonal responses to separation in mother and infant squirrel monkeys. *Psychoneuroendocrinology* **18**, 297–306.

Liu, D., Tannenbaum, B., Caldji, C., et al. (1997). Maternal care, hippocampal glucocorticoid receptor gene expression and hypothalamic-pituitary-adrenal responses to stress. *Science* **277**, 1659–1662.

McEwen, B. S., de Leon, M. J., Lupien, S. J. and Meaney, M. J. (1999). Corticosteroids, the aging brain and cognition. *Trends in Endocrinology and Metabolism* **10**, 92–96.

Pellow, S., Chopin, P., File, S. E., et al. (1985). Validation of open:closed arm entries in an elevated plus maze as a measure of anxiety in the rat. *Journal of Neuroscience Methods* **14**, 149–167.

Plotsky, P. M. (1991). Pathways to the secretion of adrenocorticotropin: a view from the portal. *Journal of Neuroendocrinology* **3**, 1–9.

Plotsky, P. M. and Nemeroff, C. B. (1998). Molecular mechanisms regulating behavior. In: Jameson, J. L. (ed.) *Textbook of molecular medicine*, pp. 979–988. New Jersey: Humana Press.

Plotsky, P. M., Owens, M. J. and Nemeroff, C. B. (1998). Psychoneuroendocrinology of depression. *Psychoneuroendocrinology* **21**, 293–307.

Sapolsky, R. M. and Meaney, M. J. (1986). Maturation of the adreno-cortical stress response: neuroendocrine control mechanisms and the stress hyporesponsive period. *Brain Research Reviews* **11**, 65–76.

Spencer-Booth, Y. and Hinde, R. A. (1971). Effects of brief separations from mothers during infancy on behavior of rhesus monkeys 6–24 months later. *Journal of Child Psychology and Psychiatry* **12**, 157–172.

Takahashi, L. K., Kalin, N. H., Vandenburgt, J. A., et al. (1989). Corticotropin-releasing factor modulates defensive-withdrawal and exploratory behavior in rats. *Behavioral Neuroscience* **103**, 648–654.

Valentino, R. J., Curtis, A. L., Page, M. E., et al. (1998). Activation of the locus ceruleus brain noradrenergic system during stress: circuitry, consequences, and regulation. *Advances in Pharmacology* **42**, 781–784.

Van Oers, H. J., de Kloet, E. R. and Levine, S. (1998). Early vs. late maternal deprivation differentially alters the endocrine and hypothalamic responses to stress. *Developmental Brain Research* **111**, 245–252.

Weinstock, M. (1997). Does prenatal stress impair coping and regulation of hypothalamic-pituitary-adrenal axis? *Neuroscience and Biobehavioral Reviews* **21**, 1–10.

Wheal, H. V., Chen, Y., Mitchell, J., et al. (1998). Molecular mechanisms that underlie structural and functional changes at the postsynaptic membrane during synaptic plasticity. *Progress in Neurobiology* **55**, 611–640.

Medical Profession and Stress

K G Power and V Swanson
University of Stirling, Stirling, UK

This article is reproduced from the previous edition, volume 2, pp 708–712, © 2000, Elsevier Inc.

Sources of Occupational Stress for Medical Professionals
Mediators and Moderators of Occupational Stress
Stress Outcomes for Medical Professionals
Summary

Glossary

Consultant	A specialist medical practitioner providing secondary care, normally in a hospital setting.
General practitioner	A doctor working in primary care in the community; the first point of contact for medical cases of all kinds.
Mediators/ moderators	Intervening variables that alter (increase or decrease) the relationship between stressors and strains.
Strains	Physical, psychological, or behavioral outcomes of stressors.
Stressors	External demands or stimuli acting on an individual, perceived as taxing his or her resources.
Transactional models	Models that conceptualize stress as a dynamic interaction between the person and his or her environment.

Sources of Occupational Stress for Medical Professionals

Intrinsic Factors

Although medical work can be routine and repetitive, doctors have high levels of responsibility, necessitating intensive skill use. A wrong decision or diagnosis may put a life at risk or lead to litigation. Doctors must be familiar with a vast area of knowledge and increasingly complex technology, but often act and make decisions in isolation. The corollary of autonomy of decision making is therefore a heavy burden of responsibility and a high degree of accountability for errors. Many aspects of medical work are emotionally stressful, e.g., dealing with death, trauma, suffering, and serious illness and communicating difficult and emotional decisions to patients and relatives. There may be personal moral and ethical dilemmas involved in patient treatment, e.g., in dealing with abortion. Environmental factors may increase personal risk, including exposure to viral infections or contagious diseases such as hepatitis and HIV. There is risk of physical injury from abusive or violent patients, such as in emergency departments, from psychiatrically disturbed patients, or during home visits. Although clinical aspects of medical work can be a source of stress, intrinsic factors have been shown to contribute less to occupational stress than extrinsic or organizational factors. Rigorous training generally equips doctors to deal with clinical issues, facilitating the development of effective coping mechanisms to deal with clinical responsibilities. However, they may be less well equipped to cope with the hassles of day-to-day management and increased bureaucratization of health care. The repetitive or trivial nature of some patient consultations may be a source of irritation or hassle, and the expectations or demands of patients and their relatives may be perceived as unrealistic.

Workload

Doctors' workload and constant time pressure have been identified as major sources of occupational stress. Several factors may be considered, including overall volume of work, patient list sizes, number of consultations, home visits, unsocial hours and night work, time pressure, and time spent on call. Being on call is described as being in a state of heightened alert, during which it is difficult to relax. Dealing with night calls may result in disturbed sleep, leading to impaired physical and mental functioning. Howie and colleagues assessed the impact of workload in general practitioners (GPs) and found that larger than average list sizes, time pressures (e.g., appointments running late), and more patient-centered attitudes in doctors correlated positively with stress. Faster doctoring and poor time management were associated with less recognition of patients' psychosocial problems and higher rates of prescribing.

Organizational factors such as overbooked and late-running surgeries can lead to shortened consultations and reduced quality of care for patients, whereas improved time management leads to reduced stress for GPs. Agius and co-workers identified demands on time as a major stressor for consultants, including interruptions, meeting deadlines, finding time for research and teaching demands, having so much to do that everything cannot be done well, and conflicts between work and family time as main components. Compared with doctors in hospital settings, general practitioners working in the community may feel constantly visible and on call, leaving less time for self or family. In some countries, the development of GP cooperatives to manage on-call requirements addresses the issue of 24-h commitment to patient care, potentially reducing a major source of occupational stress.

Relationships at Work

Relationships with colleagues are a potential source of stress for doctors. In particular, relationships between medical students and consultants may be a source of stress. Furthermore, the previously competitive style of much medical training is at odds with recent emphasis on the health-care team in general practice. Team working may also introduce interprofessional role conflicts, uncertainties or ambiguities,

and a sense of a diminished role for doctors more accustomed to autocratic or autonomous working styles.

Gender Issues

Male and female doctors have different sources and levels of occupational stress. Despite intakes of women to some medical schools now standing at 50% or higher, women are underrepresented in some specialties (e.g., surgery) and hold fewer consultant grades overall. Patronage in some specialties and the old boys network are still considered to be important parts of the career system discriminating against women. The premise that an increased entry of females to the profession would lead to changes in the structural hierarchy of medical care has not been fulfilled. In India, where sex role segregation is commonplace, medical specialty choice is strongly associated with gender-based stereotypes, with female physicians dealing almost exclusively with women's and children's medical problems.

Role Conflicts: Home–Work Interface

Stress in the home–work interface is common for medical professionals. Stress between work and home is bidirectional and may affect male and female doctors differently depending on the complexity of domestic and occupational roles at different life stages. People-intensive and emotionally demanding medical work may leave the individual feeling drained and uncommunicative with spouse or family, and domestic relationship problems may adversely affect work performance. Female doctors fare less well than male colleagues in maintaining successful marriages, with approximately one-third of female doctors in the United Kingdom remaining single and divorce rates being higher for female than for male doctors.

Mediators and Moderators of Occupational Stress

Transactional psychological models emphasize the importance of individual differences in determining the link between stressors and stress outcomes or strains. Structural characteristics of both the job and the individual medical practitioner influence the stressor–strain relationship.

Structural Factors

The characteristics and type of medical practice (e.g., single-handed, group practice; government funded or profit based) or medical specialty may make them more or less demanding and threatening to doctors' general well-being. Some comparative studies have identified general practice as one of the most stressful areas of medicine. Anesthetics and psychiatry have also been singled out for being respectively more and less stressful than other specialties. However, evidence regarding the stressfulness of different types of medical specialty is not conclusive. Other studies comparing psychiatric morbidity in doctors in different specialties found no differences among gastroenterologists, surgeons, radiologists, and oncologists or among consultant physicians, surgeons, and radiologists.

Dispositional Factors

The psychological characteristics of individuals who chose a medical career may predispose them to experience work-related psychological distress. Cooper and colleagues suggested that a type A personality predicted reduced mental well-being in GPs, a finding confirmed in other studies, although only a small percentage of variance in strains tends to be explained by type A personality. An internal locus of control has been associated with reduced levels of stress in medical professionals, and neuroticism has been found to correlate highly with occupational stress, emotional exhaustion, depersonalization, and lowered job-related achievement in hospital consultants.

Coping

Doctors possess more resources for coping than most occupational groups due to their length of education and training, status, and financial security. However, few studies have considered coping in doctors. The association between neuroticism and emotion-focused coping strategies used by consultants was linked to a negative appraisal of job stressors by Deary and colleagues. Although maladaptive coping behaviors such as drug or alcohol abuse or work-related strategies such as increased prescribing have been examined, adaptive coping has been studied infrequently. Social support has been identified as an important intervening variable. Increased quality and quantity of social support are associated with a reduction in perceived stress, increased job satisfaction, and improved mental well-being in both male and female doctors, although female doctors utilize a wider range of social support and home- or work-based coping strategies than males.

Stress Outcomes for Medical Professionals

Job Satisfaction

Job dissatisfaction and lowered morale are commonly described outcomes of stress in medical professionals, with moderate negative correlations between job satisfaction and occupational stress being reported frequently. Job dissatisfaction is associated with poor work performance, mental ill health, and inappropriate prescribing. Female doctors have consistently been shown to report greater job satisfaction than males.

Physical Ill Health

Although medical knowledge is no guarantee of good health, doctors have improved rates of morbidity and mortality in comparison with the general population and other professionals. However, mortality for some causes (e.g., cirrhosis of the liver, road accidents) is substantially higher for doctors than for other comparable professional groups, and concerns have been expressed regarding the tendency of doctors to self-treat or neglect their own health. Because doctors have multiple sources of self-referral, the collection of accurate morbidity data may be more difficult for doctors than for other groups.

Mental Ill Health

Several studies have suggested that doctors have higher rates of mental distress, anxiety, and depression than norms. Because of long working hours, heavy workloads, and the emotional demands of medical practice, younger doctors and those in training may be more vulnerable to psychological distress than older colleagues. However, direct causal links between work stress and mental illness in doctors have not been established firmly. Many studies fail to take into account baseline gender differences in the prevalence of anxiety and depression. Some studies suggest that female doctors suffer from more mental health problems than male doctors or other female professionals, whereas others find no significant differences between female and male doctors or between female doctors and other professional women in stress-related mental distress.

Measures of burnout, encapsulating depersonalization and emotional exhaustion, may be particularly sensitive indicators of strain in medical professionals. One Australian study found that young male GPs were more likely to suffer burnout than young female GPs, suggesting that this may be due to a more empathetic and psychosocial approach to patient care in female doctors. However, other studies have found no gender differences in doctors' burnout. Furthermore, the concept of burnout may overlap a dispositional tendency toward negative affectivity and/or neuroticism, leading to confounding of dependent and independent variables in studies using burnout measures.

Behavioral Outcomes: Alcohol and Drug Use

Doctors generally exhibit a greater prevalence of alcohol and drug abuse than comparable social groups. A main source of drug misuse is via self-prescribing. Psychiatric admissions for alcoholism for male doctors in Scotland were 2.7 times greater than for a comparison group of social class 1 males, with 58% of psychiatric hospitalizations for male doctors in the 45 to 54 age group attributed to alcoholism. GPs in single-handed practices are also overrepresented in hospital admissions for doctors with drug and alcohol problems. General practitioners and some medical specialties, notably anesthetics, have higher rates of alcoholism and drug abuse than others. It has been argued that males in general are more likely to use alcohol as a means of coping with stress than females. This gender difference is reflected in studies of GPs. However, one longitudinal study of junior house officers, albeit in a mixed-gender sample, found no relationship between reported drinking habit and self-reported stress or depression.

Suicide

Suicide rates for doctors in the United States are twice that of the general population and three times that of other professions. Certain medical specialties may have an increased suicide risk, including anesthetics, pharmacy, and psychiatry, although a U.K. study confirmed the excess mortality of doctors from suicide in doctors under 40, but found no difference by medical specialty. Female doctors are also three to four times more likely to commit suicide than females in the general population. An explanation of the elevated suicide rate for doctors is necessarily speculative. The availability of means for suicide (e.g., access to drugs), technical skills, and knowledge ensuring the act is successful may be relevant. Personality characteristics of doctors, including obsessive–compulsive behavior and proneness to depression, may also be important, along with high rates of alcohol and drug abuse and the stress of the doctor's occupational role.

Impact on Patient Care

Although the media image of the overworked, sleep-deprived doctor persists, it has proved methodologically difficult to investigate the impact of stress on doctors' job performance and patient care. Long working hours and sleep deprivation affect work performance in junior hospital doctors, being linked to lowered arousal, attentional deficits, and poor information recall, with fatigued subjects giving less consideration to risks they take. Mechanic's classic studies of doctors related work frustration to short cuts in work performance, including inadequate examinations and prescribing. Prescribing behavior is one objective indicator of performance, and dysfunctional prescribing is related to job dissatisfaction in GPs. However, reaching agreement as to what constitutes efficient prescribing is difficult.

Summary

A review of studies investigating the extent and impact of occupational stress on doctors indicates that it is pervasive across specialties and cultures. It is therefore crucial for the future well-being of both doctor and patient to identify and manage stress in medical professionals. However, the measurement of stress and strain in this group, as in other occupational groups, has methodological problems. Measurement tools mainly comprise cross-sectional self-report questionnaire surveys and semistructured interview techniques. Response rates vary considerably, questioning representativeness, with some studies being small scale and parochial. The use of a wide range of measures and methods makes comparison among studies, specialties, and cultures difficult. Many studies employing standardized measures of mental ill health, such as the General Health Questionnaire, Maslach Burnout Inventory, and Hospital Anxiety and Depression Scale, report positive correlations between stress and psychological distress, particularly anxiety and depression.

However, few studies have addressed physical or behavioral aspects of the stress response or have considered individual differences as mediators/moderators of stressors/strains for medical professionals. This lack of methodological sophistication is an important omission. For example, where gender is taken into account, females, compared with male doctors, report greater job satisfaction, different behavioral outcomes (e.g., less alcohol and drug use), and a greater use of coping strategies. Similarly, dispositional factors such as neuroticism, which have been clearly associated with strain outcomes such as job dissatisfaction and mental ill health, are often not considered. A shift away from empirical/descriptive stimulus–response models toward more sophisticated transactional conceptualizations in the study of stress in medical professionals is required. This more sophisticated approach has implications for selection, training, and continued professional development of doctors, enabling doctors, managers, and educators to improve specific skills for coping with stress in those medical professionals who need them most. This has relevance for both medical professionals and the patients in their care.

See Also the Following Articles

Caregivers, Stress and; Workplace Stress.

Further Reading

Agius, R. M., Blenkin, H., Deary, I. J., Zealley, H. and Wood, R. A. (1996). Survey of perceived stress and work demands of consultant doctors. *Occupational and Environmental Medicine* 53, 217–224.

Cooper, C. L., Rout, U. and Faragher, B. (1989). Mental health, job satisfaction and job stress among general practitioners. *British Medical Journal* 298, 366–370.

Deary, I. J., Blenkin, H., Agius, R. M., Endler, N. S., Zealley, H. and Wood, R. (1996). Models of job-related stress and personal achievements among consultant doctors. *British Journal of Psychology* 87, 3–29.

Firth-Cozens, J. (1987). Emotional distress in junior house officers. *British Medical Journal* 295, 533–535.

Grol, R., Mokkink, H., Smits, A., et al. (1985). Work satisfaction of general practitioners and the quality of patient care. *Family Practice* 2, 128–135.

Howie, J. G. R., Hopton, J. L., Heaney, D. J. and Porter, A. M. D. (1992). Attitudes to medical care. The organization of work and stress among general practitioners. *British Journal of General Practice* 42, 181–185.

Mechanic, D. (1972). General medical practice: some comparisons between the work of primary care physicians in the United States and England and Wales. In: *Public expectations and health care*. New York: Wiley.

Richardsen, A. M. and Burke, R. J. (1991). Occupational stress and job satisfaction among physicians: sex differences. *Social Science and Medicine* 33, 1179–1187.

Riska, E. and Wegar, K. (1993). Women physicians: a new force in medicine? In: Riska, E. & Wegar, K. (eds.) *Gender, work and medicine*. London: Sage.

Sutherland, V. J. and Cooper, C. L. (1993). Identifying distress among general practitioners: predictors of psychological ill-health and job dissatisfaction. *Social Science and Medicine* 37, 575–581.

Swanson, V., Power, K. G. and Simpson, R. J. (1998). Occupational stress and family life: a comparison of male and female doctors. *Journal of Occupational and Organizational Psychology* 71, 237–260.

Winefield, H. R. and Anstey, T. J. (1991). Job stress in general practice: practitioner age, sex and attitudes as predictors. *Family Practice* 8, 140–144.

Meditation and Stress

J L Kristeller
Indiana State University, Terre Haute, IN, USA

Meditation: Overview and History

Types of Meditation

Theory and Mechanisms

Research Evidence and Clinical Application

Conclusions

Glossary

Loving kindness meditation	A group of guided meditative practices directed toward cultivating compassion toward oneself and others.
Mantra meditation	Also mantram. A widely practiced form of concentrative meditation in which a word or short phrase is repeated, usually silently, to oneself. In traditional usage, the mantra carries with it spiritual significance. Om, referring to the presence of the absolute within, is one of the most familiar mantras.
Shamatha	Sustained quieting or calming of the mind; meditative practices that are directed toward doing so.
Vedanta	Refers to the Vedas, part of the foundation of Hinduism, as interpreted in the mid-1800s by the Indian mystic Sri Ramakrishna, who promulgated an ecumenical world view of religion and meditative practice. The Vedanta Society was founded by Swami Vivekenanda, his chief disciple, in the United States in 1893, and maintains a number of centers today.
Vipassana	Insight or mindfulness meditation.
Yoga	To yoke or link the mind/spirit and body. Meditation is one traditional means by which this occurs. Hatha yoga, referring to practice of physical postures, is one branch of the traditional Yogic system.

Meditation: Overview and History

The therapeutic use of meditation may be unique within contemporary psychology, as it draws explicitly on non-Western traditions to inform both the practice and the conceptual understanding of meditation effects. Awareness of Hindu and Buddhist meditative and yogic traditions entered Europe and the United States from India, Japan, and China beginning in the 1800s, influencing the Theosophist movement, which adopted the term meditation to refer to a wide range of related practices. Interest was further sparked by the 1883 Parliament of the World's Religions; some Zen and Hindu-based practices in the United States can still be traced directly to this conference, through the influential writings of Alan Watts on Zen Buddhism and the Vedanta Society. The first documented secular adaptation of meditative practices to therapeutic use was Johannes Schultz's development of autogenic training in 1932, which used slow-paced breathing and mindful awareness of physical sensations to facilitate deep relaxation experiences. The writings of D. T. Suzuki on Zen practice stimulated interest in meditation in the 1950s by psychodynamic therapists, particularly Fromm and Horney, and fueled openness to more secular forms of meditation, such as transcendental meditation, a decade later. There is increasing recognition of similarities in meditative and contemplative practices across world religious traditions, including Christianity, Judaism, and Islam, in both process and purpose.

Types of Meditation

Meditative techniques are generally classified into two types: concentrative meditation and mindfulness meditation. Concentrative techniques involve sustained attentional focus on a specific object, such as a mantra (a repeated sound or word), with a goal of complete absorption, suspension of everyday preoccupations, and calming the mind, whereas mindfulness meditation cultivates sustained attentive awareness to whatever may emerge into conscious experience, without reaction or analysis. In addition, guided meditation, in which attention is directed to a particular type of experience (i.e., an emotion, such as anxiety, a physical feeling, such as pain, or a type of thought), can be considered a third category that may have particular value in regard to therapeutic effects. Tibetan Buddhist practices are particularly rich in complex guided meditations. However, these distinctions are a matter of degree: awareness cannot occur without sustained attention, and sustained attention or concentration cultivates awareness. Most traditional meditative approaches incorporate aspects of both concentrative and mindfulness practice. Focused concentration may be more powerful in inducing trancelike states. Yet, as active thinking and feeling processes are quieted, similar states of transcendent experience may be achieved through a

wide range of practices, as evident from phenomenological descriptions of meditative experience across traditions.

Concentrative Meditation

A wide variety of traditional concentrative techniques exist, but the most common involve focus on the breath (e.g., in Buddhist Shamatha meditation), focus on a word or phrase (e.g., the mantra), or visualization of an object (e.g., as in Tibetan mandala meditation). Transcendental meditation (TM), the most widely researched version of Hindu mantra or concentrative meditation that has been used therapeutically, was created in the 1960s for teaching in the West by the Maharishi Mahesh Yogi; other influential Hindu-based meditation groups in the United States include the Vedanta Society, founded in 1893, and the Himalayan Society, founded by Swami Rama in 1971. Recently, Catholic Centering Prayer, as being revived from early Christian practices by Father Thomas Keating, has garnered increasing attention, and is strikingly similar in many respects to other mantra meditations. In TM, the mantra is generally a Sanskrit word or phrase assigned by a TM teacher and is intended to have a spiritual, although not religious, meaning. TM practice involves sitting quietly in a relaxed posture for 20 min twice a day, with closed eyes. The mantra is repeated silently to oneself, with attention returned to it as thoughts wander to other experiences. Unlike some concentrative techniques, TM practitioners are instructed that attention is to be directed in an effortless manner.

Benson further secularized this practice in the 1970s for research and clinical applications, coining the term the relaxation response, and suggesting that practitioners use the word "one" as a mantra, but other words or phrases, whether of a secular or spiritual meaning, may be used. Eknath Easwaren, an Indian scholar and meditation teacher based in California, developed a transcultural approach that uses both mantra-based meditation and longer memorized textual passages; although he is deceased, his work is increasingly being utilized in treatment programs. These concentrative approaches have all been integrated into more comprehensive treatment programs.

Mindfulness Meditation

Mindfulness techniques have been introduced primarily through Vipassana or insight meditation drawn primarily from southeast Asian Theravadan practices (Thai, Vietnamese, and Burmese), Japanese Zen *shikantaza* ('just sitting'), and visualization and other techniques from the very rich Tibetan traditions.

Body-focused awareness is also cultivated in a number of traditions; the word yoga means to connect (or yoke) the mind and body. Influential venues by which these traditions entered the United States were a number of Zen monasteries founded beginning in the 1960s; the Naropa Institute in Boulder, CO, founded in 1974 by the Tibetan monk Chogyam Trungpa Rinpoche; and the Insight Meditation Society, founded in 1975 by Jack Kornfield, a psychologist who studied Buddhism in Thailand, and his associate Sharon Saltzburg, among others. The prolific writings of Thich Nhat Hanh, a Vietnamese Zen monk, have been particularly influential in regard to loving kindness meditation and walking meditation. A contemporary Asian mindfulness meditation retreat program, developed by S. N. Goenka in Burma and India, uses a traditional 10-day intensive practice format and has been explored for use in prison populations and with drug addicts in both India and the United States.

The Mindfulness-Based Stress Reduction (MBSR) program, developed by Jon Kabat-Zinn in 1981 at the University of Massachusetts Medical Center, is the most widely used and researched therapeutic approach drawing on mindfulness meditation techniques; it was influenced by both Vipassana and Korean Zen traditions, in combination with yoga and body-focused meditation. The MBSR program uses the breath as an attentional focus but also emphasizes cultivating detached, nonjudgmental awareness of whatever arises into consciousness. Practice is generally a single sitting meditation session per day of 40–45 min, though this may be shortened as appropriate for use with children or other groups. Maintaining an erect posture is emphasized, consistent with a goal of staying alert. Engaging a trancelike state is avoided. Variations on the MBSR program include Mindfulness-Based Cognitive Therapy (MBCT), developed by Teasdale, Segal, and Williams, and Mindfulness-Based Eating Awareness Therapy (MB-EAT), developed by Kristeller. MBCT incorporates cognitive therapy techniques designed to address depressive thinking; MB-EAT incorporates cognitive and self-regulation approaches to management of compulsive overeating and obesity. Linehan's Dialectical Behavior Therapy incorporates brief mindfulness meditation practices into an intensive group treatment program for borderline personality disorder.

Theory and Mechanisms

Meditation involves the intentional cultivation of moment-to-moment, nonjudgmental awareness of one's present experience, whether narrowly or more broadly focused. The goal of these practices is to develop an ability to bring stable and nonreactive awareness to one's internal (cognitive-affective-sensory) and external (social-environmental) experiences and thereby heighten the capacity to bring conscious control to responses and reactions. Within Buddhist psychology, meditation is identified as the most important means to bringing forth skillful action, speech, livelihood, effort, understanding, and thought. It is through meditation that higher wisdom in all areas of life is sought and achieved. These dimensions map fairly well onto the range of meditation effects that have been explored scientifically, including physical relaxation, emotional well-being, behavioral regulation, improvement in relation to self, growth in compassion toward others, and spiritual enlightenment or a sense of transcendence.

The psychology of meditation practice must therefore consider how it is that a group of relatively simple attentional and cognitive practices may bring about this range of effects. The means through which this is thought to occur within Buddhist psychology is again compatible with contemporary learning theory. Within contemporary Buddhist psychology, distress is viewed as a function of conditioning leading to cravings and aversions, which create *dukkha* (suffering or stress) and are incompatible with higher or wiser levels of functioning. The traditional goal of meditation practice is release from craving or conditioning. This is strikingly parallel to learning models of stress, as expressed in anxiety disorders, addictive behaviors, and depressed mood or cognitions.

Several fundamental mechanisms are likely to be involved in early and intermediate stages of practice. Advanced stages may engage more complex processes related to altered states of consciousness that are somewhat distinct, or that, as Austin posits, may be on a continuum with more fundamental shifts in neuropsychological functioning. First, focusing attention on a neutral repetitive object, whether it be the breath, a mantra, or a repeated chant, disengages attention from other targets that may be stress related. This process may produce stress-reducing effects similar to those of any distracter but is different in that the mind is not then caught up in an alternative source of attention. It is not uncommon with initial practice for individuals to note how profoundly relaxing they find the experience. The next step is cultivation of the ability to rest the attention on a neutral stimulus, such as the breath or the mantra, in a more sustained manner. This is intended to generalize to increased ability to sustain attention on other objects (sometimes referred to as bare attention). Linked to this process, and heightened in mindfulness meditation, is observing the occurrence of patterns of habitual or conditioned responding, a type of reflective self-monitoring. Initial practice often brings awareness of the chattering mind, the undisciplined pattern of racing thoughts. Sustained attention then leads to an active disengagement of usual reactivity, analysis, or letting the attention move unbidden to the next association, emotion, or response. Simply observing experiences such as pain sensations, anxiety, or cravings, without reacting, may share similarities with systematic desensitization, in that repeated exposure, without either withdrawal or reinforcement, interrupts the feedback loop of the conditioning process. Therapeutic value may be amplified by guided meditations that utilize specific objects as targets for mindfulness practice, such as the experience of pain, fear, anxiety, eating, or compassion. Another value in maintaining sustained attention is similar to what Marlatt describes in the addiction literature as urge surfing: coming to the realization that by observing an experience or impulse in a sustained way, one discovers that these experiences are not constant, but rise and then fall away.

One hallmark of highly conditioned reactive responses is that they occur so quickly or are so powerful that alternatives cannot emerge or are not experienced as sustainable. As automatic reactive patterns are disengaged, the potential emerges for alternative choices that may have been lying dormant. Meditators often report that they observe the

alternative choices that arise as fresh and in some way unexpected, yet emerging from their own capabilities, rather than being directed or prescribed from the outside. Even at early stages of practice, individuals will note that it becomes easier to introduce a moment of silence or space into daily choices and that making a healthier decision no longer feels like as much of a struggle as it once did.

Figure 1 illustrates several of these steps in regard to mindfulness practice. Awareness is heightened in regard to stress responses (1a), such as anger or overeating (Y), the trigger (X) for that response, and the connections between the trigger and the response (1b). Resting attention with this awareness then acts to disengage or disconnect the trigger from the response (2a) and the feedback/reinforcement value (2b) from the response to the trigger. When these links are disconnected, access to alternative choices (A, B, or C) becomes available (3); with further practice, a novel or wiser response (W) may emerge (4).

Cultivating bare attention also appears to disengage a sense of self-identification with the experience, i.e., being able to say "I feel the pain, but I am not my pain." This disidentification of self from experience is considered to play a primary mediational role within some meditative traditions; one counterpart in contemporary psychology is the recognition that the constructed self, along with critical self-judgment, is often central to distress and psychopathology. This

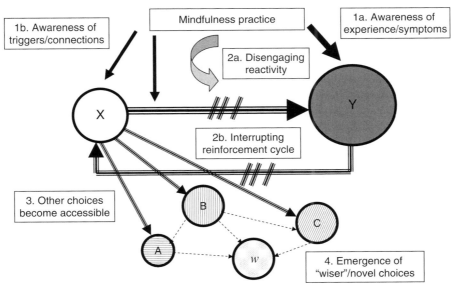

Figure 1 Illustration of several steps in regard to mindfulness practice. Awareness is heightened in regard to stress responses (1a), such as anger or overeating (Y), the trigger (X) for that response, and the connections between the trigger and the response (1b). Resting attention with this awareness then acts to disengage or disconnect the trigger from the response (2a) and the feedback/reinforcement value (2b) from the response to the trigger. When these links are disconnected, access to alternative choices (A, B, or C) becomes available (3); with further practice, a novel or wiser response (W) may emerge (4).

disidentification may be accompanied by a sense of liberation, a release from operating on automatic, whether from the usual chatter of the conscious mind or from more challenging patterns, such as anger, drinking, or compulsive eating.

Spiritual growth as a functional result of meditation practice may also occur due to disengagement of more immediate survival needs. Spiritual engagement is being increasingly recognized as a potent protective factor when individuals are under high stress conditions. While understanding the neuropsychological processes underlying spiritual or mystical experience is at an exploratory stage, meditative traditions universally aim to cultivate such experiences; disengagement of ordinary cognitive processing appears to be a necessary, if not sufficient, foundation for engaging spiritual or mystical experience.

Research Evidence and Clinical Application

Background

Contemporary research on meditation effects is generally dated from early studies in the 1950s on physiological effects in Indian yogis and Japanese Zen masters. Research on the clinical application of meditation is usually considered to date from the early work with TM or from the publication of Benson's *The Relaxation Response* in 1973. Murphy and Donovan's annotated 1996 bibliography summarizes more than 1000 studies on meditation.

It is useful to organize research evidence, both experimental and clinical, around the six domains noted earlier: cognitive/attentional, physiological/health, emotional, behavioral, relation to self/others, and spiritual. Clearly, these domains intersect and overlap, but such an approach helps in considering underlying mechanisms. For example, traditional perspectives on meditation practice have tended to focus on self-transformation and spiritual growth, yet it is apparent that substantial health and emotional effects in novice meditators can be obtained independently of such changes. The level of experience of research participants may vary from thousands of hours of meditation experience to individuals just being introduced to a given practice. Methodological quality varies greatly, and until recently, few studies met criteria for well-controlled randomized clinical trial research. Yet Grossman's meta-analytic review of 20 well-designed MBSR intervention trials found substantial effect size estimations of approximately 0.50, across various samples and problem areas. Neuroimaging techniques may prove particularly

valuable in identifying possible underlying processes, given the inherent introspective nature of the processes involved. Somewhat surprisingly, there are very few studies comparing concentrative and mindfulness meditation (or other meditation) techniques.

Individual differences have also been of interest; an early model suggested that individuals higher on cognitive anxiety might respond better to meditation techniques than to more body-centered relaxation interventions. However, several attempts to confirm this model either failed to do so or found that the variance accounted for was very small. Clinically, some individuals who drop out of meditation practice report that the experience is boring; conversely, others have difficulty with racing thoughts that they are unable to quiet. Beginning with shorter time periods, use of a mantra, or other techniques, such as breath counting, can help with these problems. Although the basics of meditation practice appear relatively simple, it is generally strongly emphasized that one should have a meaningful personal practice before using meditation therapeutically with others.

Efforts to use self-reporting to measure mindfulness have greatly accelerated in the past few years. Baer's factor analytic research has identified five facets of mindfulness that can be measured in both meditators and nonmeditators, including attending to experience, nonjudging, nonreactivity to inner experience, describing experience in words, and acting with awareness; this research is still in the formative stage. The revival of interest in spirituality as a psychological construct is also contributing to measurement of this aspect of meditation practice.

Cognitive and Attentional Effects

Most of the research on attentional and cognitive effects of meditation has investigated concentrative and TM approaches. Although evidence is not entirely consistent, there appears to be an improvement in field independence, reaction time, sustained attention, and ability to detect detail in rapidly presented material. Additional research is needed to investigate the role of meditation in affecting the cognitive processes hypothesized to mediate other effects.

To date, clinical application within this domain has been limited, but preliminary evidence suggests that there is value in using mindfulness meditation in treating attention-deficit disorder. Clinically, one of the notable cognitive effects is an experience of inner silence, of quieting the mind to the point that inner self-talk is not experienced. Beginning meditators often express frustration that they cannot silence their thoughts, not understanding that such silence is the result of practice and of the ability to disengage, and is difficult, if not impossible, to force. The occurrence of such silence may be an important marker of a shift in neuropsychological functioning and deserves further investigation.

Physiological and Health Effects

Within the domain of physiological effects, the most robust research findings are related to a shift in balance of less sympathetic to greater parasympathetic autonomic nervous system function, accompanied by feelings of relaxation, decreases in blood pressure, and lowered levels of stress hormones. This shift is essentially what Benson has referred to as the relaxation response. There are also primary physiological effects due to slowed breathing; respiration rates of two to four cycles per minute have been shown in separate studies by Benson and by Lehrer to lead to marked physiological changes, including increases in body temperature, in Tibetan and Rinzai Zen monks, two traditions in which such slow-paced breathing is cultivated. Central nervous system effects have primarily focused on changes in alpha and theta rhythm dominance during practice. The increase in theta activity is sometimes interpreted as indicating that meditators are simply falling asleep; while this may occur, a pattern of sustained (nondescending) theta suggests a distinct state of consciousness. More recent work is documenting increased synchronization of activity across regions of the brain and heightened gamma activity in advanced meditators.

Impact on health through lowering of cortisol levels, lowering of blood pressure in both adults and adolescents, and improved management of pain and immune functioning deserve further exploration. Chronic pain patients have been shown to respond remarkably well to the rigorous combination of sitting meditation, gentle hatha yoga, and body awareness practices, with decreases in pain experience and increases in pain tolerance. A randomized clinical trial documented improvement in fibromyalgia patients, but these effects were not replicated using an attentional-support control comparison group. Evidence is limited regarding improvement in immune functioning in cancer patients enrolled in an MBSR program, but research by Carlson and colleagues found improvement in several indicators of immune response in breast and prostate cancer patients, including interleukin (IL)-4. They also found improved diurnal profiles in salivary cortisol, which is associated with survival time. A notable use of guided mindfulness meditation practice has been in conjunction with standard treatment of psoriasis, leading to markedly faster clearing rates of this chronic skin disease.

Emotional Effects

Meditation can be considered one of the few tools for systematic cultivation of emotional equanimity, an advanced level of stress and affect tolerance. Improvement in emotional well-being has been documented in multiple studies with both concentrative and mindfulness meditation practice, and in both novice and more advanced meditators. Reduced anxiety, anger, and depression and heightened experience of well-being have been documented in a number of studies involving both clinical and non-clinical populations. The MBSR program has been used successfully to treat individuals with diagnosed anxiety disorders, producing long-term effects for those with panic attacks and agoraphobia. There is a growing literature showing the value of MBCT in preventing relapse in individuals with three or more previous episodes of major depressive illness. The MBCT program integrates cognitive-behavioral components into the structure of the MBSR program, in addition to using guided meditations in regard to depressive thoughts.

Meditation practice, however, may not uniformly result in a positive emotional experience. Because one of the mechanisms involved is interrupting dominant conditioned responses, emotionally painful experiences or even flooding with uncovered memories of traumatic events may emerge when constructed mechanisms for suppression are disengaged. In the general population, the incidence of these experiences is very low, but this may increase substantially in psychiatric populations, requiring tailoring of the meditation practice and guided support from the therapist. The value of mindfulness techniques, including brief meditation, with borderline personality disorder is now well supported in research on Linehan's Dialectic Behavior Therapy. There is a growing clinical literature by such individuals as Epstein, Rubin, and Germer and colleagues on the integration of meditation practice into psychodynamic psychotherapy.

Meditation and Behavior

Improved behavioral regulation may be the result of several factors: the interruption of chains of behavioral reactions as awareness is cultivated, improved emotional regulation, increasing receptivity to behavioral/lifestyle recommendations, or learning to tolerate and ride out waves of craving, rather than responding impulsively. Much of the research literature focused on behavior change has investigated the effects of TM on reductions of drug, smoking, and alcohol intake, with claims made of substantial improvement in long-term abstinence, depending on the amount and duration of practice. While suggestive, randomized clinical trials are needed to investigate the effects of both concentrative and mindfulness-based meditative interventions. The MB-EAT program has preliminary support of effectiveness in treating binge eating disorder, as does Dialectical Behavior Therapy.

Relation to Self and Others

Cultivating compassion toward oneself and toward others is central to Buddhism; cultivating the capacity to disengage from self-preoccupation is a central goal of meditative practice in all contemplative traditions. Overidentification of self with either positive or negative experience may contribute to stress and interfere with self-growth. Research evidence has supported the development of self-acceptance when under stress in more advanced meditators in both concentrative and mindfulness traditions. Such self-acceptance may come through disengaging from usual preoccupations and cultivation of insight, and may be heightened through use of loving kindness meditations. Increases in both self-growth and empathy have been observed in couples, therapists, and other health professionals enrolled in relatively brief (4- to 8-week) meditation programs.

Profound transformative experiences have been documented in incarcerated individuals enrolled in Goenka's week-long intensive meditation retreats in prisons in India and the United States. Evidence is accruing that advanced meditators practicing within Tibetan traditions that involve extensive guided meditation on cultivation of compassion exhibit strikingly higher left prefrontal cortex activity that underlies positive emotion. It is unclear whether such effects emerge inherently from intensive practice, are mediated through attentional and cognitive disengagement of self-preoccupation, or require domain-specific guided meditations, such as loving kindness practices.

Spiritual Well-Being

Recent research on spiritual well-being in medical populations suggests that it is a powerful factor in overall adjustment, despite high levels of stressors. Cultivation of spiritual growth and well-being is fundamental to virtually all meditative traditions, but different emphasis is placed on the centrality of achieving spiritual or transcendent experience across different traditions; furthermore, the degree to which this is viewed as a secular goal (as within TM or some schools of Buddhism and Hinduism) or as an inherently religious goal (as within Judeo-Christian contemplative traditions) varies substantially. Research with novice meditators using both concentrative and mindfulness practices is beginning to document modest shifts in spiritual well-being, using psychometrically sound self-report measures.

Concentrative meditative practices are recognized to more readily cultivate trance states even in novice meditators, and induction of mystical experience is being examined in neuroimaging studies in highly experienced meditators. D'Aquili and Newberg's research on advanced meditators has garnered substantial attention in positing a neurophysiological basis for suspending a sense of the self and engaging the experience of union with a higher being.

Conclusions

Meditation practice, as it is currently understood, engages mechanisms that promote effects far broader than basic physical or emotional relaxation. To summarize, meditation can affect the stress response in a number of ways: first, it serves as a neutral distractor; second, mindfulness meditation teaches the capacity for self-observation of patterns of experience; third, the capacity to sustain awareness without responding or reacting is heightened. With yet more practice, conditioned reactions and responses to inner experience gradually weaken; finally, in the course of this uncoupling, meditation appears to facilitate the emergence of more integrative responses. Specific therapeutic goals may be facilitated by directing meditative awareness toward the target of concern, such as anxiety symptoms or pain management. By understanding meditation practice as engaging these processes, it becomes clearer how a range of therapeutic effects may occur as a function of a relatively simple set of practices, much as other principles, such as cognitive restructuring, behavioral techniques, or insight-oriented psychotherapies, are applied to a wide range of therapeutic issues.

Both concentrative and mindfulness approaches have developed and gained acceptance over the past 30 years as valuable components of treatment programs for a wide range of disorders and presenting issues. The literature on meditation, as it can be incorporated into therapeutic modalities, continues to expand. Research also continues to explore underlying mechanisms, in ways that may inform a greater understanding of self-regulatory processes in general. As the theoretical framework for understanding meditation psychotherapeutically evolves, it becomes more evident that meditation cannot be dismissed either as an esoteric spiritual/religious practice or as only one of many relatively simple relaxation techniques.

See Also the Following Articles

Cognitive Behavioral Therapy; Relaxation Techniques; Stress Management, CAM Approach.

Further Reading

Austin, J. H. (1998). *Zen and the brain*. Cambridge, MA: MIT Press.

Baer, R. A., Smith, G. T., Hopkins, J., Krietemeyer, J. and Toney, L. (2006). Using self-report assessment methods to explore facets of mindfulness. *Assessment* **13**(1), 27–45.

Benson, H. (1975/2000). *The relaxation response*. New York: Harper Press.

Bodian, S. (1999). *Meditation for dummies*. Foster City, CA: IDG Books Worldwide, Inc.

Davidson, R. J., Kabat-Zinn, J., Schumacher, J., Rosenkranz, M., Muller, D., Santorelli, S. F., et al. (2003). Alterations in brain and immune function produced by mindfulness meditation. *Psychosomatic Medicine* **65**(4), 564–570.

Epstein, M. (1995). *Thoughts without a thinker: psychotherapy from a Buddhist perspective*. New York: Basic Books, Inc.

Germer, C. K., Siegel, R. D. and Fulton, P. R. (eds.) (2005). *Mindfulness and psychotherapy*. New York: Guilford Press.

Goleman, D. (1977/1996). *The meditative mind. Varieties of meditative experience*. Los Angeles, CA: Tarcher Books.

Grossman, P., Niemann, L., Schmidt, S. and Walach, H. (2004). Mindfulness-based stress reduction and health benefits. A meta-analysis. *Journal of Psychosomatic Research* **57**(1), 35–43.

Kabat-Zinn, J. (1990). *Full catastrophe living*. New York: Delacorte Press.

Murphy, M., Donovan, S. and Taylor, E. (1999). *The physical and psychological effects of meditation: a review of contemporary research with a comprehensive bibliography, 1981–1996*. Sausalito, CA: Institute of Noetic Science.

O'Connell, D. F. and Alexander, C. N. (eds.) (1994). Self-recovery: treating addictions using transcendental meditation and Maharishi Ayer-Veda. *Alcoholism Treatment Quarterly* **11**(1–4), Special Issue.

Segal, Z. V., Williams, J. M. G. and Teasdale, J. D. (2003). *Mindfulness-based cognitive therapy for depression. A new approach for preventing relapse*. New York: The Guilford Press.

Travis, F. T. (2001). Transcendental meditation technique. In: Craighead, W. E. & Nemeroff, C. B. (eds.) *The Corsini encyclopedia of psychology and behavioral science* (3rd edn., pp. 1705–1706). New York: John Wiley & Sons.

Walsh, R. and Shapiro, S. (2006). The meeting of meditative disciplines and Western psychology. *American Psychologist* **61**, 227–239.

Walton, K. G., Schneider, R. H., Nidich, S. I., et al. (2002). Psychosocial stress and cardiovascular disease. Part 2: Effectiveness of the Transcendental Meditation program in treatment and prevention. *Behavioral Medicine* **28**(4), 106–123.

Melanocortin Receptors *See:* Feeding Circuitry (and Neurochemistry).

Membrane Glucocorticoid Receptors

P J Gasser and M Orchinik
Arizona State University, Tempe, AZ, USA

This article is reproduced from the previous edition, volume 2, pp 713–720, © 2000, Elsevier Inc.

Glucocorticoid Receptors

Glucocorticoid Receptors in Liver

Glucocorticoid Receptors in Lymphocytes

Glucocorticoid Receptors in Adrenal Gland

Glucocorticoid Receptors in Pituitary

Glucocorticoid Receptors in Brain

Glucocorticoid Transport Proteins

Corticosteroid-Binding Globulins

Signal Transduction by Membrane Glucocorticoid Receptors

Glossary

Corticosteroid-binding globulin (CBG or transcortin)	A plasma protein that specifically binds corticosteroids.
Corticotropin releasing factor (CRF)	A 41 amino acid residue hypothalamic peptide that mediates the neural control of pituitary adrenocorticotropin secretion.
Dexamethasone	A synthetic glucocorticoid.
EC_{50}	The dose of a hormone or drug necessary to produce 50% of the maximal response.
GABA	γ-Aminobutyric acid, an inhibitory neurotransmitter.
$GABA_A$ receptor	A membrane protein complex that forms an agonist-gated chloride ion channel and mediates fast inhibitory synaptic transmission.
K_D	Equilibrium dissociation constant. The concentration of ligand at which 50% of the receptors are occupied.
Nongenomic	A mechanism of steroid hormone action that does not initially involve modulation of gene transcription.
RU38486 (Mifepristone)	A synthetic progesterone receptor antagonist that binds with high affinity to the cytosolic glucocorticoid receptor.
TBPS (t-Butylbicyclophosphorothionate)	A competitor for binding of GABA to the $GABA_A$ receptor.
Triamcinolone acetonide	A synthetic glucocorticoid.

Glucocorticoid Receptors

Cellular and organismal responses to glucocorticoid hormones are complex and integrative, involving immediate, short-term, and long-term components. Target cell responses to glucocorticoids are initiated by two main mechanisms. In the classical, genomic mechanism, glucocorticoids interact with intracellular receptors, which act as ligand-gated transcription factors. The ligand–receptor complex then regulates the transcription of specific genes by interaction with hormone response elements and/or AP-1 transcriptional regulatory sites. This mechanism produces responses that are usually apparent in hours or days.

In the other, nongenomic, mechanism, glucocorticoids initiate immediate or very short latency responses in target cells. These short latencies preclude the genomic mechanism of transcriptional activation/ inhibition and altered translation, although genomic responses may follow rapid responses. It is believed that these responses are mediated by glucocorticoid receptors that are integral to or associated with target cell plasma membranes. Membranal glucocorticoid receptors have not been cloned, but several membrane-associated glucocorticoid-binding proteins have been purified, and there are numerous reports of nongenomic physiological and behavioral responses to the hormones (**Table 1**). Receptor binding studies have characterized glucocorticoid binding to plasma membranes in various tissues from several species (**Table 2**), and some of the cellular signaling mechanisms activated by the hormones have been elucidated. Multiple classes of glucocorticoid-binding sites have been revealed in plasma membranes: (1) membranal glucocorticoid receptors distinct from intracellular glucocorticoid receptors, (2) membrane-associated forms of intracellular glucocorticoid receptors, (3) membrane receptors for corticosteroid-binding globulins (CBG), (4) membrane glucocorticoid-transporting proteins, and (5) other membrane proteins that also bind glucocorticoids. These proteins have been distinguished pharmacologically, based on binding specificity profiles for various natural and synthetic ligands, and immunologically, based on cross-reactivity with antibodies for intracellular glucocorticoid receptors. This article reviews the membrane glucocorticoid receptors and describes what is known of the mechanisms by which they initiate rapid cellular/organismal responses.

Glucocorticoid Receptors in Liver

The liver, a major target organ for glucocorticoid hormones during stress, shows both immediate and long latency physiological responses to glucocorticoid hormones and has both cytosolic and membrane glucocorticoid receptors. Radioligand binding and photo-affinity labeling reveal high-affinity ($K_D = 7\text{--}12$ nM) and low-affinity ($K_D = 90\text{--}344$ nM) membrane-binding sites for both dexamethasone and cortisol (see **Table 2**) in rat and chicken hepatocytes. The sites appear to be integral membrane proteins, as they can be extracted by detergent, but not by high salt. The sites for the two glucocorticoids also appear to be distinct from each other. Low-affinity dexamethasone binding is attributed to a 45-kDa protein, whereas two membrane proteins, 52 and 57 kDa, are responsible for cortisol binding. Glucocorticoid-binding sites have also been demonstrated visually in rat hepatocyte membranes. Gold-conjugated corticosterone–bovine serum albumin (BSA) specifically labels the apical, but not the lateral, membranes of hepatocytes (see **Table 2**).

During stress, glucose stores in the liver are mobilized rapidly by the activation of glycogen-degrading enzymes in the hepatocytes. This effect is largely due to the actions of catecholamines, but glucocorticoids also play a role. Corticosterone, dexamethasone, and cortisol increase the activity of glycogen phosphorylase, a glucose-liberating enzyme, in rat and chicken hepatocytes within 10 min of administration (see **Table 1**). Glucocorticoids act in this case via a Ca^{2+}-mediated signaling process, as the effect is diminished in Ca^{2+}-depleted medium. Other rapid effects of glucocorticoids in hepatocytes include increases in the phosphorylation of histone and nonhistone proteins and general activation of translational machinery, including increased synthesis of intracellular glucocorticoid receptors (see **Table 1**). These rapid effects may facilitate long-term, genomic responses to glucocorticoids.

Glucocorticoid Receptors in Lymphocytes

The immune system is another major target of glucocorticoid hormones. Membrane-mediated effects of glucocorticoids and membrane-associated forms of the intracellular glucocorticoid receptor have been demonstrated in various lymphocytes. In rat mast cells and basophils, cortisol inhibits the antigen-induced release of histamine and attenuates the antigen-induced release of Ca^{2+} from intracellular stores (see **Table 1**). This effect may be related to the potent antiallergic actions of glucocorticoids.

Studies with antibodies have demonstrated that a population of human lymphoma cells possesses a membrane-associated form of the intracellular glucocorticoid receptor (see **Table 2**). Cells that possess this form of the receptor are particularly sensitive to glucocorticoid-induced cytolysis.

Glucocorticoid Receptors in Adrenal Gland

Both the adrenal cortex and the adrenal medulla are targets of rapid glucocorticoid hormone action. Rapid effects in both areas appear to be related to the feedback regulation of adrenal hormone release. Corticosterone decreases the secretion of adrenal steroids from frog interrenal gland by 45–80%. This effect is not mimicked by dexamethasone and is not blocked by the specific glucocorticoid receptor antagonist RU43044 (see **Table 1**), indicating that this ultra-short feedback regulation of adrenal steroid secretion is mediated by another type of glucocorticoid receptor.

A membrane glucocorticoid-binding site in bovine adrenal cortex has high affinity ($K_D = 77$ nM) for corticosterone and very low affinity ($IC_{50} = 25\text{--}50$ μM) for dexamethasone, triamcinolone, and cortisol (see **Table 2**).

Chromaffin cells of the adrenal medulla secrete catecholamines in response to a variety of neurotransmitters, including acetylcholine. These cells are exposed to very high concentrations of glucocorticoids in venous blood from the adrenal cortex. At high concentrations (up to 10 μM), glucocorticoids modulate the responses of adrenal chromaffin cells to acetylcholine and to K^+-induced depolarization rapidly (see **Table 1**). Dexamethasone immediately diminishes the acetylcholine-induced current when applied extracellularly to dispersed guinea pig chromaffin cells, but has no effect when applied intracellularly. In PC12 cells from rat medullary tumors, corticosterone and corticosterone–BSA inhibit depolarization-induced intracellular Ca^{2+} release by a mechanism that involves G-protein-mediated calcium signaling.

Glucocorticoid Receptors in Pituitary

Several hypothalamic peptide hormones can cause cells of the anterior pituitary to release adrenocorticotropic hormone (ACTH), which in turn stimulates the release of glucocorticoid hormones from the adrenal cortex. Glucocorticoids regulate pituitary production/secretion of ACTH in a complex system of feedback inhibition. This inhibition occurs on rapid (seconds to minutes), delayed intermediate (10–15 min to hours), and delayed slow (hours to days) time courses. Rapid feedback inhibition of pituitary ACTH secretion by

Table 1 Selected membrane-mediated effects of glucocorticoids

Hormone	Effect	Tissue	Dose (EC_{50})[a]	Organism	Reference
Liver					
Corticosterone/ dexamethasone	↑ glycogen phosphorylase activity	Hepatocytes	1–10 μM B; 10–1000 nM Dex	Rat	Gomez-Munoz et al. (1989). *Biochem. J.* **262**, 417–423
Cortisol	↑ glycogen phosphorylase activity	Hepatocytes		Chicken	Sancho et al. (1986). *Biochim. Biophys. Acta* **88**, 249–255
Adrenal					
Corticosterone	↓ depolarization-induced calcium release	PC12 cells	100 nM–10 μM	Human	Lou and Chen (1998). *Biochem. Biophys. Res. Commun.* **244**, 403–407
Dexamethasone	↓ acetylcholine-induced current	Chromaffin cells	10 μM	Guinea pig	Inoue and Kuriyama (1989). *Am. J. Physiol.* **257**, C906–C912
Corticosterone	↓ steroid release	Interrenal tissue	10 μg/ml	Frog	Netchitailo et al. (1991). *J. Mol. Endocrinol.* **6**, 249–255
Intestine					
Cortisol	↑/↓ GABA-induced contractility	Ileum	1–10 pM (↑);10–1000 nM (↓)	Guinea pig	Ong et al. (1987). *Neurosci. Lett.* **82**, 101–106.
Endometrium					
Dexamethasone	↑ actin assembly	Endometrial cells	0.1 μM	Human	Koukouritaki et al. (1997). *J. Cell. Biochem.* **65**, 492–500
Immune system					
Cortisol	↓ histamine release	Mast cells	3 μM	Rat	Dukhanin et al. (1996). *Inflamm. Res.* **45**, S15–S16
Pituitary					
Corticosterone, cortisol, dexamethasone	↓ CRF-stimulated ACTH release	Pituitary	100 nM	Rat	Widmaier and Dallman (1984). *Endocrinology* **115**, 2368–2374
Dexamethasone	↓ AVP-stimulated ACTH release	Anterior pituitary	1 μM	Rat	Nicholson and Gillham (1989). *J. Endocrinol.* **122**, 545–551
Corticosterone	↓ CRF-stimulated ACTH release	Pituitary	45 μg/kg	Dog	Keller-Wood and Bell (1988). *Am. J. Physiol.* **255**, R344–R349
Cortisol/dexamethasone	↓ prolactin release	Rostral pars distalis	10 nM–1 μM	Tilapia	Borski et al. (1991). *Proc. Natl. Acad. Sci. USA* **88**, 2758–2762
Brain/neuronal tissue					
Corticosterone	↑ Ca^{2+} uptake	Synaptosomes	130 nM	Rat	Sze and Iqbal (1994). *Neuroendocrinology* **59**, 457–465
Cortisol/corticosterone	↑ tryptophan uptake ↓ calcium current	Hippocampal CA1 neurons	1 pM–100 nM (F) 10 pM–100 nM (B)	Guinea pig	Neckers and Sze (1975). *Brain Res.* **93**, 123–132 ffrench-Mullen (1995). *J. Neurosci.* **15**, 903–911
Corticosterone	↓ vasopressin release	Hypothalamic slices	100 nM–100 μM	Rat	Liu and Chen (1995). *Brain Res.* **704**, 19–22
Corticosterone	↑/↓ somatostatin release	Hypothalamic neurons	100 nM–1 μM	Rat	Estupina et al. (1997). *Exp. Brain Res.* **113**, 337–342

Compound	Effect	Tissue/cell	Dose/concentration	Species	Reference
Cortisol/corticosterone	↓ CRF release	Hypothalamic synaptosomes	750 nM (B) 6–60 nM (F)	Sheep	Edwardson and Bennett (1974). *Nature* **251**, 425–427
Cortisol	↑/↓ single-unit activity	Medial preoptic septal neurons	Iontophoresis	Rat	Kelly et al. (1977). *Exp. Brain Res.* **30**, 53–64
Corticosterone	↑/↓ firing rate	Pontine reticular neurons	2.5–3 mg/kg	Rat	Dubrovsky et al. (1985). *J. Neurosci. Res.* **14**, 117–128
Corticosterone	↑/↓ spontaneous and evoked activity	Hypothalamus, amygdala, midbrain	25–33 mg/kg	Rat	Feldman et al. (1983). *Exp. Neurol.* **80**, 427–438
Corticosterone	↓ population spike amplitude	Hippocampal pyramidal cells	100 nM–10 μM	Rat	Vidal et al. (1986). *Brain Res.* **383**, 54–59
Corticosterone	↓ population spike amplitude	Hippocampal pyramidal cells	0.05–5 nM	Rat	Talmi et al. (1992). *Neuroendocrinology* **55**, 257–263
Corticosterone	↑/↓ amplitude of sciatic-evoked responses	Pontine reticular neurons	2.5–3 mg/kg	Rat	Dubrovsky et al. (1985). *J. Neurosci. Res.* **14**, 117–128
Corticosterone/cortisol	↑/↓ activity	Hypothalamic neurons	Iontophoresis	Rat	Saphier and Feldman (1988). *Brain Res.* **453**, 183–190
Cortisol	↑/↓ sciatic-evoked responses	Hypothalamic neurons (MBH)	Iontophoresis	Rat	Mandelbrod et al. (1981). *Brain Res.* **218**, 115–130
Corticosterone/cortisol	↑/↓ TBPS binding	Synaptosomes	10–100 nM (↑); >100 nM (↓)	Rat	Majewska et al. (1985). *Brain Res.* **339**, 178–182; Majewska (1987). *Brain Res.* **418**, 377–382
Cortisol	↓ GABA-induced depolarization	Spinal ganglion neurons	5 μM–1 mM	Bullfrog	Ariyoshi and Akasu (1986). *Brain Res.* **367**, 332–336; Ariyoshi and Akasu (1987). *Brain Res.* **435**, 241–248
Corticosterone	↑/↓ activity	Medullary neurons	11–25 μg/animal	Newt	Rose et al. (1993). *Neuroendocrinology* **57**, 815–824; Rose et al. (1995). *Neuroendocrinology* **62**, 406–417
Behavioral effects					
Corticosterone	↓ courtship behavior		0.6 nM	Newt	Orchinik et al. (1991). *Science* **252**, 1848–1851; Moore and Miller (1984). *Horm. Behav.* **18**, 400–410
Corticosterone	↑ perch hopping		26 ng/ml	Sparrow	Breuner et al. (1998). *Gen. Comp. Endocrinol.* **111**, 386–394
Corticosterone	↑ locomotor response to novelty		2.5–5 mg/kg	Rat	Sandi et al. (1996). *Eur. J. Neurosci.* **8**, 794–800
Corticosterone	Stimulation of behavior during social challenge		2 mg/kg	Rat	Haller et al. (1997). *J. Neuroendocrinol.* **9**, 515–518
Corticosterone	↑ lordosis		200 μg/animal	Rat	Kubli-Garfias (1990). *Horm. Behav.* **24**, 443–449
Cortisol	↑/↓ aggression		1–10 μM	Hamster	Hayden-Hixson et al. (1991). *J. Neuroendocrinol.* **3**, 613–622

[a]B, corticosterone; F, cortisol; Dex, dexamethasone.

Table 2　Selected glucocorticoid-binding sites associated with plasma membranes

Hormone	K_D	Organism	Reference
Liver			
Cortisol	12 nM, 344 nM	Rat	Ibarrola et al. (1996). *Biochim. Biophys. Acta* **1284**, 41–46[a]
Dexamethasone	7 nM, 90 nM	Rat	Howell et al. (1989). *Biochem. J.* **260**, 435–441[a]
Cortisol	1.4 nM	Rat	Suyemitsu and Terayama (1975). *Endocrinology* **96**, 1499–1508
Corticosterone	None available	Rat	Spindler et al. (1991). *J. Steroid Biochem. Mol. Biol.* **39**, 315–322
Cortisol	4.5 nM	Chicken	Trueba et al. (1987). *Int. J. Biochem.* **19**, 957–962
Pituitary			
Corticosterone	3.2 nM	Rat	Koch et al. (1978). *J. Endocrinol.* **79**, 215–222
Corticosterone	None available	Mouse (AtT-20 cells)	Harrison et al. (1979). In: Leavitt and Clark (eds.) *Steroid hormone receptor systems*, pp. 423–443. New York: Plenum
Adrenal cortex			
Corticosterone	77 nM	Calf	Andres et al. (1997). *Cell. Mol. Life Sci.* **53**, 673–680
Brain			
Corticosterone	120 nM	Rat (synaptosomes)	Towle and Sze (1983). *J. Steroid Biochem.* **18**, 135–143
Corticosterone	6 nM (via CBG)	Vole (synaptosomes)	Orchinik et al. (1997). *J. Steroid Biochem. Mol. Biol.* **60**, 229–236
Corticosterone	0.5 nM	Newt (synaptosomes)	Orchinik et al. (1991). *Science* **252**, 1848–1851
Corticosterone	24.2 nM	Sparrow (synaptosomes)	Breuner et al. (1997). *Soc. Neurosci. Abst.* **23**, 1076
Lymphocytes			
Corticosterone	None available	Human (leukemic cells)	Gametchu et al. (1993). *FASEB J.* **7**, 1283–1292

[a]Indicates that the glucocorticoid-binding protein has been purified.

glucocorticoids is thought to be mediated by membrane receptors. The stimulation of ACTH release by CRF, oxytocin, vasopressin, and insulin is diminished rapidly by glucocorticoids, including corticosterone, cortisol, and dexamethasone (see **Table 1**). These effects are not completely understood, but appear to involve the attenuation of secretagogue-induced increases in second messenger accumulation. Some fast feedback effects, with latencies of 15–20 min, have been attributed to rapid protein synthesis.

Glucocorticoid-binding sites have been characterized in plasma membranes from rat and mouse pituitary cells (see **Table 2**). The rat membrane receptor has high affinity (K_D = 3.2 nM) for corticosterone and does not bind dexamethasone. Mouse pituitary tumor (AtT-20) cell membranes specifically bind corticosterone, but not dexamethasone or triamcinolone. This binding site appears to be a glycoprotein, as treatment of cells with proteases abolishes glucocorticoid binding and treatment with neuraminidase enhances binding.

The release of other pituitary hormones can also be modulated by glucocorticoids. In pituitaries of the teleost fish tilapia, cortisol inhibits the release of prolactin rapidly, apparently via the membrane-mediated modulation of Ca^{2+} and cAMP levels (see **Table 1**).

Glucocorticoid Receptors in Brain

Stress effects on neuronal activity and animal behavior are widely varied, stressor specific, and dependent on the endocrine/sensory history of the organism. Rapid glucocorticoid actions on neurophysiology and behavior show the same variability. In the brain, glucocorticoids can modulate both spontaneous and evoked neuronal activity rapidly. The direction of this modulation (increase or decrease) depends on the identity of the target neuron and is often context dependent. In the rat hypothalamus, for instance, corticosterone increases the activity of oxytocin-secreting neurons, but is mainly inhibitory to vasopressin neurons and neurons projecting to the median eminence (see **Table 1**). In the newt, corticosterone inhibits the responses of naive medullary reticular neurons to sensory stimuli, but it potentiates sensory responses of the same neurons when they have been previously exposed to vasotocin (see **Table 1**). Glucocorticoid-induced increases in sparrow perch-hopping behavior are dependent on photoperiod.

The best correlations between glucocorticoid-binding characteristics of membrane receptors and doses of glucocorticoids necessary for rapid physiological/behavioral effects have been demonstrated in the brains of rats and newts. In rat brain synaptosomes, corticosterone causes an increased uptake of Ca^{2+} and tryptophan (see **Table 1**). The EC_{50} for this effect (130 nM) is almost identical to the K_D (120 nM) determined for glucocorticoid binding to synaptic plasma membranes from the rat brain. In newts, corticosterone causes a rapid inhibition of male courtship behavior (see **Table 1**). This effect has an EC_{50} of 0.6 nM and is not mimicked by dexamethasone.

The K_D for corticosterone binding to newt synaptic plasma membranes is 0.5 nM, and dexamethasone does not compete with corticosterone for this binding site.

Other effects of glucocorticoids in the brain include rapid modulation of neuropeptide release by hypothalamic neurons, modulation of spontaneous neuronal activity in various brain regions, and modulation of neuronal responses to sensory stimuli (see **Table 1**). It is likely that these rapid neuronal responses to glucocorticoids mediate rapid changes in behavior during stress.

Glucocorticoid Transport Proteins

There is still debate over the mechanisms by which glucocorticoid hormones cross plasma membranes. Certain membrane glucocorticoid-binding proteins also transport the steroids across the plasma membrane. One major membrane steroid transporter, P-glycoprotein, binds corticosterone, cortisol, and dexamethasone and transports them out of cells. This protein is expressed at high levels in epithelia of adrenal cortex, kidney proximal tubule, biliary hepatocytes, brain capillaries, small intestine, and colon.

Rat liver plasma membranes possess a bidirectional glucocorticoid transporter that is specific for corticosterone and cortisol. Immunochemical methods demonstrate that this binding site is distinct from P-glycoprotein. Specific transmembrane transport of glucocorticoids has also been demonstrated in membrane vesicles from pituitary and placenta.

Corticosteroid-Binding Globulins

Of the pool of glucocorticoid hormones circulating in the blood, a substantial fraction occurs bound to plasma proteins. Adrenal steroids (cortisol, corticosterone, and deoxycorticosterone) bind specifically and with high affinity to corticosteroid-binding globulin (or transcortin). While its functions are still unclear, CBG does interact specifically with a plasma membrane receptor. Specific, high-affinity CBG receptors have been purified from plasma membranes of rat and human liver and human endometrium and trophoblast cells. The interaction of the CBG–cortisol complex with trophoblast cell membranes causes activation of adenylate cyclase and accumulation of cAMP.

High affinity ($K_D = 6$ nM) binding of corticosterone to vole synaptic plasma membranes appears to involve one form of CBG. Specific binding to vole membranes was abolished by the saline perfusion of brains before binding studies, and vole plasma displayed a corticosterone-binding profile similar to that of synaptic plasma membranes (see **Table 2**).

Signal Transduction by Membrane Glucocorticoid Receptors

Pharmacological manipulations of nongenomic glucocorticoid effects (see **Table 1**) have revealed some aspects of the signal transduction mechanisms by which the hormones modulate cell physiology rapidly. These signaling mechanisms are nearly as diverse as the hormone effects. Existing data indicate that glucocorticoids can initiate rapid responses via (1) modulation of intracellular Ca^{2+}, often via G-protein-mediated pathways, and (2) activation/ inhibition of other signal transduction systems.

Modulation of Calcium Signaling

A large body of evidence indicates that glucocorticoids initiate rapid responses in many target cells by the modulation of intracellular calcium signaling. Cortisol inhibits N- and L-type Ca^{2+} currents in hippocampal neurons via a pertussis toxin-sensitive G-protein and protein kinase C (see **Table 1**). In rat brain synaptosomes, corticosterone enhances depolarization-induced Ca^{2+} influx rapidly and potentiates calmodulin-induced activation of voltage-sensitive calcium channels (see **Table 1**). Fish pituitary cells, rat lymphocytes, and PC12 cells respond to glucocorticoid treatment with rapid decreases in intracellular Ca^{2+} accumulation. In PC12 cells, this effect is diminished by pertussis toxin and by inhibitors of protein kinase C.

Many rapid effects of glucocorticoids are modulated by changes in extracellular calcium concentration. For example, the corticosterone-induced inhibition of vasopressin release from hypothalamic slices is potentiated in Ca^{2+}-rich medium and decreased in Ca^{2+}-depleted medium (see **Table 1**). The same manipulation of extracellular Ca^{2+} concentration attenuates/ enhances the corticosterone-induced decrease in population spike amplitude in hippocampal neurons (see **Table 1**). The corticosterone-induced increase in hepatocyte glycogen phosphorylase activity is diminished in Ca^{2+}-depleted medium.

Other Signaling Pathways

A variety of other signal transduction pathways have been implicated in the mediation of rapid glucocorticoid actions. The diversity of these pathways reflects the diversity of rapid glucocorticoid actions. Roles have been proposed for rapid glucocorticoid signaling via the $GABA_A$ receptor system, the cytoskeleton, the cAMP and cGMP pathways, and the nitric oxide system. Certain rapid effects of glucocorticoids result from the interaction of the hormones with other membrane proteins. One such protein is the GABA$_A$ receptor, a membrane protein complex that forms an agonist-gated chloride channel. Most studies indicate that metabolites of adrenal steroids, rather than the hormones themselves, modulate GABA$_A$ receptor function. However, there are reports of interactions between glucocorticoids and GABA$_A$ receptors. Glucocorticoids alter physiological responses to GABA and modulate agonist binding to the GABA$_A$ receptor (see **Table 1**). Other intracellular signaling pathways have been implicated in mediating the rapid effects of glucocorticoids. In human endometrial cells, dexamethasone induces rapid actin polymerization without concomitant changes in actin synthesis, implicating the cytoskeleton as another rapid glucocorticoid effector system (see **Table 1**). Cortisol inhibits cAMP phosphodiesterase in bovine testis and cardiac muscle homogenates and enhances guanylate cyclase activity in various tissues, indicating other possible mechanisms of rapid glucocorticoid signaling. Inhibitors of nitric oxide synthase prevent corticosterone-induced increases in the locomotor activity of rats in a novel environment (see **Table 1**).

See Also the Following Articles

Corticosteroid-Binding Globulin (Transcortin); GABA (Gamma Aminobutyric Acid); Glucocorticoids, Overview.

Further Reading

Antoni, F. A., Hoyland, J., Woods, M. D. and Mason, W. T. (1992). Glucocorticoid inhibition of stimulus-evoked adrenocorticotropic release caused by suppression of intracellular calcium signals. *Journal of Endocrinology* **133**, R13–R16.

Fant, M. E., Harbison, R. D. and Harrison, R. W. (1979). Glucocorticoid uptake into human placental membrane vesicles. *Journal of Biological Chemistry* **254**, 6218–6221.

Gee, K. W., McCauley, L. D. and Lan, N. C. (1996). A putative receptor for neurosteroids on the GABA$_A$ receptor complex: the pharmacological properties and therapeutic potential of epalons. *Critical Review of Neurobiology* **9**, 207–227.

Grote, H., Ioannou, I., Voigt, J. and Sekeris, C. E. (1993). Localization of the glucocorticoid receptor in rat liver cells: evidence for plasma membrane bound receptor. *International Journal of Biochemistry* **25**, 1593–1599.

Harrison, R. W. and Yeakley, J. (1979). Evidence for glucocorticoid transport into AtT-20 cells. *Molecular and Cellular Endocrinology* **15**, 13–18.

Howie, J. G. R., Hopton, J. L., Heaney, D. J. and Porter, A. M. D. (1992). Attitudes to medical care. The organization of work and stress among general practitioners. *British Journal of General Practice* **42**, 181–185.

Lackner, C., Daufeldt, S., Wildt, L. and Allera, A. (1998). Glucocorticoid-recognizing and-effector sites in rat liver plasma membrane: kinetics of corticosterone uptake by isolated membrane vesicles. III. Specificity and stereospecificity. *Journal of Steroid Biochemistry and Molecular Biology* **64**, 69–82.

Majewska, M. D. (1987). Antagonist-type interaction of glucocorticoids with the GABA receptor-coupled chloride channel. *Brain Research* **418**, 377–382.

Mechanic, D. (1972). General medical practice: some comparisons between the work of primary care physicians in the United States and England and Wales. In: *Public expectations and health care.* New York: Wiley.

Orchinik, M., Moore, F. L. and Rose, J. D. (1994). Mechanistic and functional studies of rapid corticosteroid actions. *Annals of the New York Academy of Sciences* **746**, 101–114.

Richardsen, A. M. and Burke, R. J. (1991). Occupational stress and job satisfaction among physicians: sex differences. *Social Science and Medicine* **33**, 1179–1187.

Riska, E. and Wegar, K. (1993). Women physicians: a new force in medicine? In: Riska, E. & Wegar, K. (eds.) *Gender, work and medicine.* London: Sage.

Rose, J. D., Kinnaird, J. R. and Moore, F. L. (1995). Neurophysiological effects of vasotocin and corticosterone on medullary neurons: implications for hormonal control of amphibian courtship behavior. *Neuroendocrinology* **62**, 406–417.

Schmidtke, J., Wienker, T., Flugel, M. and Engel, W. (1976). *In vitro* inhibition of cyclic AMP phosphodiesterase by cortisol. *Nature* **262**, 593–594.

Strel'chyonok, O. A. and Avvakumov, G. V. (1991). Interaction of human CBG with cell membranes. *Journal of Steroid Biochemistry and Molecular Biology* **40**, 795–803.

Sutherland, V. J. and Cooper, C. L. (1993). Identifying distress among general practitioners: predictors of psychological ill-health and job dissatisfaction. *Social Science and Medicine* **37**, 575–581.

Swanson, V., Power, K. G. and Simpson, R. J. (1998). Occupational stress and family life: a comparison of male and female doctors. *Journal of Occupational and Organizational Psychology* **71**, 237–260.

Winefield, H. R. and Anstey, T. J. (1991). Job stress in general practice: practitioner age, sex and attitudes as predictors. *Family Practice* **8**, 140–144.

Memory and Stress

S J Lupien
McGill University and Geriatric Institute of Montreal,
Montreal, Canada
F S Maheu
National Institute of Mental Health, Bethesda, MD, USA

This article is a revision of the previous edition article
by S J Lupien and S Brière, volume 2, pp 721–727,
© 2000, Elsevier Inc.

Emotion, Stress, and Memory
Emotion and Stress: Two Different Entities?
Memory for Emotionally Arousing Events
Memory after Stress
Conclusion

Glossary

Acute stress	Mental or bodily tension resulting from internal or external factors that tend to alter the existing equilibrium.
Arousal	A condition that varies in a continuum from a low point in sleep to a high point represented by intense excitement.
Emotion	A state of excited feeling of any kind. Basic emotions presumably are universal, are biologically based, are present from infancy, and have associated facial expressions and primitive action scripts. Basic emotions include love, joy, anger, sadness, and fear.
Stress response	The total set of reactions to the stressor.
Stressor	Any physical or psychological agent that causes the disequilibrium. Physical stressors are situations that can operate in the absence of consciousness and include disturbances of the internal environment (anoxia, hypoglycemia, etc.), external extremes (heat and cold), and physical strain (exercise or injury). Psychological stressors are situations for which there is a consciously perceived potential for harm and include stimuli that affect emotion and result in fear, anxiety, or frustration.

Emotion, Stress, and Memory

Emotionally arousing and stressful experiences are often cited as the cause of many psychological and physical problems. Many of us have experienced emotionally arousing and stressful experiences at one point or another of our life and have noted that these experiences can have important effects on our memory. Declarative memory, which is the type of memory we refer to during the course of this article, is defined as the conscious or voluntary recollection of previously learned information. We can have forgotten an important meeting or anniversary due to work overload, or else we can have a vivid recollection of a car accident or any other emotionally arousing experience. Because of their impact on our lives, we have a tendency to pay more attention to the negative effects of stress on our memory and to forget that, under certain conditions, emotionally arousing and stressful experiences can also have a positive impact on memory function. The goal of this article is to describe the positive and negative effects of emotionally arousing and stressful experiences on memory function and to delineate the psychological and biological determinants of these effects.

Emotion and Stress: Two Different Entities?

Emotion and stress share many characteristics. A stressful experience will often cause a particular emotion (e.g., surprise, fear, or joy), and particular emotions can create stressful situations (e.g., blushing due to extreme timidity can cause a stressful situation). Moreover, an emotion possesses many of the properties of a stressor. First, it often has an identifiable source. Second, it is usually brief and leads to an intense and conscious experience of short duration. Finally, an emotion creates bodily reactions (e.g., increase in heart rate or perspiration) that are similar to those induced by a stressor, and both states act by increasing arousal. Because of these similarities between emotion and stress, most of the literature on emotion, stress, and memory intermixes the effects of emotion and those of stress on memory function. However, emotion and stress are two different entities. Although a stressful experience will almost always trigger a specific emotion, a particular emotion does not always elicit a stress reaction. As far as laboratory setting is concerned, emotion and stress differ in the way they are induced and, thus, in the way they influence memory in humans. Hence, emotions are usually induced by the presentation of emotional words, films, or pictures, whereas stress is usually induced by putting the individual in a social situation known to create a stress (e.g., public speaking). Because of this important difference between the experimental paradigms used to measure the effects of emotion and stress on memory, different questions have been asked. The induction of emotion has been used to measure memory for emotionally arousing events, whereas the induction of stress has been used to measure the specific effects of stress on subsequent memory function.

Memory for Emotionally Arousing Events

It is well known that what we encode and remember from an event depends primarily on the attention that we devoted to this event and its components. If we do not pay attention to what we are reading right now, there is less chance that we will remember it at a later time than if we gave all our attention to a lecture. This is because the more attention given to an event, the higher the probability that this event will be elaborated (relating the information from this event to other situations and related concepts in memory) at the time of encoding. Research on memory has shown that events that are poorly elaborated (shallow processing) at the time of encoding are remembered less well than events that are deeply elaborated (deep processing) at the time of encoding.

The level of attention devoted to an event at the time of encoding will greatly depend on the emotional salience of this event. Most of us remember what we were doing and with whom we were at the time we learned about the World Trade Center attacks, but the majority of us may have difficulty remembering what we were doing and with whom we were 13 days before or after the attacks. This flashbulb phenomenon may be explained by the fact that the emotion (e.g., surprise or anger) that was triggered by the announcement of the World Trade Center attacks directed the totality of our attention to the event, leading to a deeper elaboration and, thus, to an optimization of our memory for this event.

Memory for Central versus Peripheral Details

Studies of trauma victims have reported how vividly the traumatic event is recalled in the absence of any memory for information surrounding the traumatic event. A closely analogous situation appears in the field of law enforcement and describes the weapon focus phenomenon. Witnesses to violent crimes demonstrate a weapon focus effect in which the weapon captures most of the victim's attention, resulting in a reduced ability to recall other details of the scene and to recognize the assailant at a later time. This phenomenon has been explained by Easterbrook's cue utilization theory, which suggests that emotionally

arousing events narrow subjects' attention and lead them to attend only to the center of an event and to exclude more peripheral information. In general, laboratory experiments have confirmed this hypothesis. For example, as reported by Christianson, subjects viewed a series of slides in which the emotional valence of one critical slide in the series was varied. In the neutral version, the critical slide showed a woman riding a bicycle. In the emotional version, the same woman was seen lying injured on the street near the bicycle. In both versions, a peripheral car was seen in the distant background. The results showed that the central detail information (woman and bicycle) was retained better in the emotional condition but that the peripheral information (car in background) was retained better in the neutral event. In general, the pattern of results obtained from various studies shows that the central aspects of an emotional event (those events in the scope of attention) are well retained in memory, whereas memory for peripheral details (out of the scope of attention) are poorly remembered. Recently, Cahill and collaborators pushed this analysis further and reported gender-related influences in the recall of central versus peripheral information from an emotional story. Men and women with high male-related traits on the Bem Sex-Role Inventory show better memory for central aspects of an emotional story, as opposed to peripheral details. On the other hand, women and men with high female-related traits on the Bem Sex-Role Inventory have a better memory for peripheral details of an emotional story, as opposed to central information.

Immediate versus Delayed Memory for Emotional Events

Studies have examined the relation among emotion, retention interval, and memory. What these studies have shown so far is that emotionally arousing events delay forgetting. In a highly cited 1963 study, Kleinsmith and Kaplan presented subjects with pairs of words to learn. Some of the words were neutral, whereas others had a strong emotionally negative component (e.g., rape, mutilation). The memory of the word pairs was tested 2 min or 1 week after presentation. Memory performance tested shortly after learning (i.e., short-term declarative memory) generally refers to consolidation processes occurring within the first 3 h after learning (i.e., early phase), whereas memory performance tested after an extensive delay (i.e., long-term declarative memory) generally refers to the consolidation processes taking place 3 h post-learning (i.e., late phase) and that persist for at least a day and involve gene transcription and protein synthesis. Kleinsmith and Kaplan's study showed that at short intervals memory was poorer for emotional words, but at long intervals memory was better for emotional words. These results have been replicated many times, and the majority of studies have shown enhanced memory for emotionally arousing material, provided that memory is tested at longer retention intervals.

Possible Mechanisms Underlying the Increased Memory for Emotionally Arousing Events

Psychological as well as biological mechanisms have been suggested to explain how emotionally arousing events might enhance memory. At the psychological level, one of the most frequently cited references on the relation between emotionally arousing events and memory is the Yerkes–Dodson law. In a series of studies published in 1908, Yerkes and Dodson reported that arousal improved performance in a linear manner for easy tasks, whereas for difficult tasks they found that an inverted-U-shaped curve related better performance with medium arousal and worse performance with low or high arousal. However, many field and laboratory studies suggest that individuals retain information from high arousing events quite well, a finding that goes against the Yerkes–Dodson law predictions. Thus, Easterbrook nuanced Yerkes–Dodson arousal hypothesis, suggesting the cue utilization theory. According to this theory, increased arousal due to emotionally arousing events acts by narrowing attention to the central details of a scene, leading to better recall of central details compared to peripheral details. Based on this model, Cahill recently suggested that men's ability to better remember central emotional information was attributable to their higher use of the right amygdala when processing emotional material (the right brain hemisphere being biased for a global/holistic analysis of the information). On the other hand, women's remembering more precisely peripheral emotional information was attributable to their higher use of the left amygdala during the processing of emotional material (the left brain hemisphere being biased for local, finer analysis of the information).

Finally, Walker used the arousal hypothesis in conjunction with Hebb's concept of reverberating circuits in order to explain the retention interval effect of emotional memory. He suggested that emotional information, because it creates a high level of arousal at the time of learning, produces a more active consolidation process and leads to a stronger memory trace and better recall at longer intervals. In contrast, because it creates a high level of arousal, emotional information also acts by inhibiting recall at shorter interval due to the fact that the process of consolidation is active (and thus inaccessible) at this time.

Contrary to psychological explanations, biological explanations of memory for emotionally arousing events have presented extensive data indicating that emotionally arousing experiences produce a retrograde enhancement of memory for that experience via a variety of hormones released during these experiences. Hence, during emotionally arousing events, there is a secretion of the peripheral catecholamines epinephrine and norepinephrine by the adrenal medulla, a secretion of central norepinephrine by the locus ceruleus and a secretion of corticosteroids by the adrenal glands. The peripheral catecholamines enhance memory by reaching the vagus nerve, nucleus of the solitary tract, and locus ceruleus. Central norepinephrine is then secreted by the locus ceruleus, activating noradrenergic neurons throughout the brain. Significantly, central norepinephrine is also triggered as soon as an emotionally arousing event occurs, independently of peripheral catecholamines. Corticosteroids, being liposoluble, enhance memory by easily crossing the blood–brain barrier and reaching the brain. Adrenergic hormones and corticosteroids may facilitate memory consolidation for emotional information through their interactions with noradrenergic and corticosteroid receptors located in the amygdala, which, in turn, modulates hippocampal activity and enhances consolidation for emotionally arousing material.

Animal and human studies have confirmed the role of these hormones in the memory-modulating effects of emotionally arousing events. Thus, in rodents postlearning stimulation of the noradrenergic system enhances (but postlearning blockade inhibits) long-term declarative memory of an inhibitory avoidance task. Likewise, posttraining injections of moderate doses of synthetic corticosteroids enhance and pretraining corticosteroid synthesis inhibition impairs long-term expression of inhibitory avoidance in animals. In humans, prelearning blockade of central β-adrenergic receptors or prelearning corticosteroid synthesis inhibition impairs long-term declarative memory for emotionally arousing material, whereas prelearning or postlearning stimulation of the noradrenergic or corticosteroid systems enhances it. Although psychological and biological explanations of the arousal hypothesis were used to explain the positive effects of emotion on memory function, research performed to this day shows that arousal is significant as an intervening variable only when the source of the arousal (in this case, the emotionally arousing event) is directly related to the information to be remembered. As we will see next, when the source of emotion is not directly related to the information to be remembered, other psychological and biological mechanisms come into play and have a stronger impact on memory function than arousal itself.

Memory after Stress

Influences of Acute Stress on Subsequent Memory Function and Possible Psychological Effects Underlying These Influences

Remembering with great accuracy a particular emotionally arousing event is very different from performing various tasks involving memory in a day-to-day situation when we are faced with stress. We may remember with great accuracy the events in our lives surrounding the World Trade Center attacks, but we may also have forgotten the anniversary of a loved one due to work stress. Originally, the effects of a stressor on subsequent declarative memory for material unrelated to the source of stress were studied using noise as a stressor. Indeed, human beings possess a limited amount of attention that can be allocated to a particular task at any one time. Information overload is said to occur when this capacity is exceeded, that is, when there is too much information to process at the same time. When this happens, the individual may have difficulty discriminating between and attending to the relevant and irrelevant information to encode new events in memory. Studies measuring the effects of noise on memory reported that noise impairs the recall of the information encoded at the time of noise stress. This result has been interpreted as showing that noise acts by overloading the limited processing capacity of the individual, leading to impairments in processing task-relevant stimuli because of an increased distraction induced by task-irrelevant stimuli (in this case, noise). Because the individual is unable to discriminate between relevant and irrelevant information when under noise stress, memory impairment appears and is represented by a poorer recall of task-relevant stimuli.

Effects of Acute Stress on Subsequent Memory Function and Possible Physiological Mechanisms Underlying These Effects

In order to better understand the mechanisms by which stress might modulate subsequent memory processing of material unrelated to the source of the stressor, researchers aimed at defining and understanding, more specifically, memory processing, stress-related physiological activation, and the links between these two. Research over the past 40 years revealed that memory is not a unitary and passive process. In the field of cognitive psychology, the individual is viewed

as being active, constructive, and organized, not as being a passive recipient of environmental stimulation or overstimulation. Thus, the individual is seen as actively constructing a view of reality, as selectively choosing some aspects of experience for further attention, and as attempting to commit some of that information to memory. Hence, to better understand the influence of stress on subsequent memory processing of information unrelated to the stressor, it is thus necessary to determine the series of stages that make up the given act of memorization and to measure the exact effects of stress on specific components of this information processing system. Declarative memory is temporally defined in three phases; information must first be attended to (arousal and attentional processes) and encoded (short-term/working memory; phase 1) before it is consolidated (phase 2) into long-term memory and recalled (phase 3).

Physiological mechanisms have been suggested to explain the effects of stress on memory phases. The brain is the organ that gives an interpretation to a stressful experience, and it is also responsible for mounting the physiological response to the stressor. Important physiological components of the stress response include the hypothalamic-pituitary-adrenal (HPA) axis (with corticosteroids being the end product), the sympathoadrenal system, and the central noradrenergic system. The HPA axis, along with the sympathoadrenal system, governs metabolic responses to the slings and arrows of everyday life. Both these systems support a range of metabolic responses that serve to ensure the availability of sufficient energy substrates in circulation during periods when there is inevitably increased cellular activity in vital organs and an accompanying increase in the requirement for fuel. The corticosteroid system and the central noradrenergic system have been studied in relation with the memory-modulating effects of stress because these two systems, when activated, can modulate activity in noradrenergic and corticosteroid receptors in the frontal lobes, hippocampus, and amygdala, three brain structures involved in declarative memory processes.

Rodent studies have shown that when a laboratory stressor (e.g., tail shocks, water immersion, or restraint stress) is administered at various times before or after learning, as well as before recall, stress-induced elevations in corticosteroid levels modulate declarative memory according to an inverted-U-shaped function. Optimal declarative memory for material unrelated to the stressor (e.g., inhibitory avoidance protocols or spatial water-maze tasks) occur at moderate levels of stress and stress-induced increases in circulating corticosteroid levels, whereas lower (i.e., boredom or drowsiness) or higher stress levels and stress-induced increases in circulating corticosteroid levels are less effective or may even impair declarative memory performance on these tasks.

In humans, when a laboratory stressor (e.g., a public speaking task combined with a public arithmetic task) is administered before learning or retrieval, high corticosteroid levels following stress are associated with memory impairments for material unrelated to the stressor, such as neutral words lists. Recently, studies measuring the influence of stress on memory for emotional material unrelated to the stressor reported more heterogeneous findings. Thus, when a laboratory stressor was presented before learning or retrieval of emotional and neutral information unrelated to the stressor, high corticosteroid levels following stress were associated with memory impairments for emotional information (whether positive or negative), whereas they had no influence on memory for neutral material. However, two other studies showed that stress administered before or after learning enhanced memory for emotional material, whereas it had no impact or impaired subsequent memory for neutral information.

Altogether, these results show that stress-related elevations in corticosteroids can have different effects on subsequent memory for material unrelated to the stressor. The effects of emotionally arousing and/or stressful events on declarative memory vary according to the nature of the material to be remembered, with elevated levels of corticosteroids enhancing memory for the emotionally arousing event itself but leading, more often than not, to memory impairments for material unrelated to the source of the stressor.

The time of day (morning vs. afternoon) and levels of circulating corticosteroids at the time of testing could also be important factors influencing the effects of stress-related elevations in corticosteroids on subsequent memory for material unrelated to the stressor. Corticosteroid receptors differ in terms of their affinity for circulating levels of corticosteroids. Mineralocorticoid receptors (MRs) have a 6- to 10-time higher affinity for corticosteroids than glucocorticoid receptors (GRs). A wealth of evidence now demonstrates that the activation of MRs is mandatory for the successful acquisition of environmental cues necessary to encode information, whereas the activation of GRs is necessary for the long-term memory consolidation of this information.

Endogenous levels of corticosteroids and, thus, the activation of the MRs and GRs, significantly vary during the day, with higher endogenous levels of corticosteroids in the morning (AM) phase than in the evening (PM) phase. Consequently, the addition of a stressful and emotionally arousing event, which

by itself will trigger a significant increase in the endogenous levels of corticosteroids, should have a differential impact on the activation of MRs and GRs as a function of time of day. In the AM phase, most of the MRs and approximately half of the GRs are activated, whereas, in the PM phase, most of the MRs and about one-tenth of the GRs are activated. If we apply a stressor in the AM phase, the endogenous increase in corticosteroid levels will act by saturating GRs, but the same stressor applied in the PM phase will act by activating approximately half of the GRs. Because stress-induced elevations in corticosteroid levels have been shown to modulate declarative memory for material unrelated to the stressor according to an inverted-U-shaped function, the differential activation of MRs and GRs at different times of the day imply that a stressor applied in the morning should impair memory function (right-hand-side of the inverted U-shaped curve), whereas the same stressor applied in the PM phase should increase or have no impact on memory (left-hand-side or top of the inverted-U-shaped curve). Moreover, given that stress has differential effects as a function of the emotional valence of the material to be learned, it can be suggested that the application of a stressor in the AM versus PM phase should have a different effect on memory for emotionally arousing or neutral information unrelated to the source of the stressor.

Individual differences could also be an important factor explaining the discrepancy in the effects of stress-related elevations in corticosteroids on subsequent memory for material unrelated to the stressor. Indeed, high and low corticosteroid responders can show different memory performance following stress. Individual differences could be attributable to genetic factors, corticosteroid sensitivity differences and lifespan cortisol exposure differences, gender, or personality.

Finally, very few studies measured the influence of the central noradrenergic system, activated following stress, on subsequent memory for material unrelated to the stressor. Animal studies reported that stress-induced elevations in norepinephrine levels (following foot shocks) modulate declarative memory according to an inverted-U-shaped function, with optimal levels enhancing (and lower or higher levels of norepinephrine impairing) memory for information unrelated to the source of stress (e.g., passive aversive conditioning). In humans, one recent study showed that the blockade of peripheral and central noradrenergic β receptors before the administration of a stressor did not impair memory for material unrelated to the source of stress. These results suggest that the β-adrenergic system is not implicated in the effects of stress on subsequent declarative memory function, contrasting with the well-established role of this system during the memorization of events that are emotionally arousing in nature. Further studies in humans are needed to determine the exact role played by the central noradrenergic system in the effects of stress on subsequent memory for information unrelated to the stressor.

Conclusion

In sum, important differences in mnemonic performance exist between memory for emotionally arousing events and memory for material unrelated to a stressor that is processed after stress. Interestingly, whether the subject is memorizing the emotionally arousing event itself or material unrelated to the stressor, both the central noradrenergic system and the corticosteroid system are at play, although they seem to act differently in the recall of neutral and emotional information. Experimental factors (e.g., nature of material to remember and time of day) and individual differences (e.g., personality and genetics) are also important components to consider because they can all influence the direction of the effects of emotion and stress on memory. Future studies considering and controlling for these factors and measuring the interactive and/or differential effects of the noradrenergic and corticosteroid systems should prove highly valuable to our understanding of the effects of emotionally arousing and stressful experiences on human declarative memory processes.

See Also the Following Articles

Cognition and Stress; Corticosteroids and Stress; Learning and Memory, Effects of Stress on; Self-Esteem, Stress and Emotion; Glucocorticoid Effects on Memory: the Positive and Negative.

Further Reading

Abercrombie, H. C., Kalin, N. H., Thurow, M. E., et al. (2003). Cortisol variation in humans affects memory for emotionally-laden and neutral information. *Behavioral Neuroscience* 117, 505–516.

Arnsten, A. F. T. (2000). Through the looking glass: differential noradrenergic modulation of prefrontal cortical function. *Neural Plasticity* 7, 133–144.

Buchanan, T. W. and Lovallo, W. R. (2001). Enhanced memory for emotional material following stress-level cortisol treatment in humans. *Psychoneuroendocrinology* 26, 307–317.

Cahill, L. (2003). Sex-related influences on the neurobiology of emotionally influenced memory. *Annals of the New York Academy of Science* 985, 163–173.

Cahill, L. and Alkire, M. T. (2003). Epinephrine enhancement of human memory consolidation: interaction with arousal at encoding. *Neurobiology of Learning and Memory* 79, 194–198.

Cahill, L., Gorski, L. and Le, K. (2003). Enhanced human memory consolidation with post-learning stress: interaction with the degree of arousal at encoding. *Learning and Memory* 10, 270–274.

Cahill, L., Gorski, L., Belcher, A., et al. (2004). The influence of sex versus sex-related traits on long-term memory for gist and detail from an emotional story. *Consciousness and Cognition* 13, 391–400.

Christianson, S. A. (1992). Emotional stress and eyewitness memory: a critical review. *Psychological Bulletin* 112, 284–309.

Domes, G., Heinrichs, M., Reichwald, U., et al. (2002). Hypothalamic-pituitary-adrenal axis reactivity to psychological stress and memory in middle-aged women: high responders exhibit enhanced declarative memory performance. *Psychoneuroendo-crinology* 27, 843–853.

Domes, G., Heinrichs, M., Rimmele, U., et al. (2004). Acute stress impairs recognition for positive words – association with stress-induced cortisol secretion. *Stress* 7, 173–181.

Easterbrook, J. A. (1959). The effect of emotion on cue utilization and the organization of behavior. *Psychological Review* 66, 183–201.

Elzinga, B. M., Bakker, A. and Bremner, J. D. (2005). Stress-induced cortisol elevations are associated with impaired delayed, but not immediate recall. *Psychiatry Research* 134, 211–223.

Golberger, L. and Breznitz, S. (1993). Handbook of Stress: Theoretical and Clinical Aspects (2nd Edition). New York: Free Press.

Jelicic, M., Geraerts, E., Merckelbach, H., et al. (2004). Acute stress enhances memory for emotional words, but impairs memory for neutral words. *International Journal of Neuroscience* 114, 1343–1351.

Kandel, E. R. (2001). The molecular biology of memory storage: a dialogue between genes and synapses. *Science* 294, 1030–1038.

Kleinsmith, L. J. and Kaplan, S. (1963). Paired associate learning as a function of arousal and interpolated interval. *Journal of Experimental Psychology* 65, 190–193.

Kuhlmann, S., Piel, M. and Wolf, O. T. (2005). Impaired memory retrieval after psychological stress in healthy young men. *Journal of Neuroscience* 25, 2977–2982.

Lupien, S. J., Fiocco, A., Wan, N., et al. (2005). Stress hormones and human memory function across the lifespan. *Psychoneuroendocrinology* 30, 225–242.

Maheu, F. S., Joober, R., Beaulieu, S., et al. (2004). Differential effects of adrenergic and corticosteroid hormonal systems on human short- and long-term declarative memory for emotionally arousing material. *Behavioral Neuroscience* 118, 420–428.

Maheu, F. S., Joober, R. and Lupien, S. J. (2005). Declarative memory after stress in humans: differential involvement of the β-adrenergic and corticosteroid systems. *Journal of Clinical Endocrinology and Metabolism* 90, 1697–1704.

Maheu, F. S., Collicutt, P., Kornik, R., et al. (2005). The perfect time to be stressed: a differential modulation of human memory by stress applied in the morning or in the afternoon. *Progress Neuropsychopharmacology and Biological Psychiatry* **29**(8), 1281–1288.

McGaugh, J. L. (2000). Memory – a century of consolidation. *Science* **287**, 248–251.

Milner, B., Squire, L. R. and Kandel, E. R. (1998). Cognitive neuroscience and the study of memory. *Neuron* **20**, 445–468.

Reul, J. M. H. M. and de Kloet, E. R. (1985). Two receptor systems for corticosterone in rat brain: microdistribution and differential occupation. *Endocrinology* **117**, 2505–2512.

Roozendaal, B. (2002). Stress and memory: opposing effects of glucocorticoids on memory consolidation and memory retrieval. *Neurobiology of Learning and Memory* **78**, 578–595.

Sauro, M. D., Jorgensen, R. S. and Teal Pedlow, C. (2003). Stress, glucocorticoids, and memory: a meta-analytic review. *Stress* **6**, 235–245.

Takahashi, T., Ikeda, K., Ishikawa, M., et al. (2004). Social stress-induced cortisol elevation acutely impairs social memory in humans. *Neuroscience Letters* **363**, 125–130.

Walker, E. L. (1958). Action decrement and its relation to learning. *Psychological Review* **65**, 129–142.

Wolf, O. T., Schommer, N. C., Hellhammer, D. H., et al. (2002). Moderate psychosocial stress appears not to impair recall of words learned 4 weeks prior to stress exposure. *Stress* **5**, 59–64.

Wust, S., Van Rossum, E. F., Federenko, I. S., et al. (2004). Common polymorphisms in the glucocorticoid receptor gene are associated with adrenocortical responses to psychological stress. *Journal of Clinical Endocrinology and Metabolism* **89**, 565–573.

Yerkes, R. M. and Dodson, J. D. (1908). The relation of strength of stimulus to rapidity of habit-information. *Journal of Comparative Neurology and Psychology* **18**, 459–482.

Memory Impairment

A J Parkin[†]
University of Sussex, Sussex, UK

This article is reproduced from the previous edition, volume 2, pp 728–731, © 2000, Elsevier Inc.

Memory in Posttraumatic Stress Disorder

Other Stress-Related Memory Disorders

Neurophysiological and Neuroanatomical Aspects of the Effect of Stress on Memory

Summary

Glossary

Declarative memory	Any memory task that requires a subject to retrieve a specific past event; used interchangeably with explicit memory and episodic memory.
Episodic memory	Any memory task that requires a subject to retrieve a specific past event; used interchangeably with explicit memory and declarative memory.
Explicit memory	Any memory task that requires a person to retrieve a specific past event; used interchangeably with declarative memory and episodic memory.
Flashback	Sudden reemergence of a traumatic memory that has previously been inaccessible; characteristic of posttraumatic stress disorder (PTSD).
Fugue	Stress-induced loss of memory in which the person loses personal identity and may even assume a new one.
Hippocampal formation	Name given to the hippocampus proper plus associated structures, including the dentate gyrus and entorhinal cortex.
Hippocampus	Region of the medial temporal lobes involved critically in the formation of new memories. Particularly vulnerable to the effects of cortisol but also to other neuromodulators that increase with the onset of stress.
Hysterical amnesia	Loss of memory for a specific period associated with trauma. Difficult to distinguish from PTSD.
Implicit memory	Any memory task that tests a person's memory for an event without direct reference to that event; used interchangeably with nondeclarative memory and sometimes with procedural memory.
Multiple personality	Memory disorder associated with history of abuse. If genuine, it is thought to be linked to stress, but many believe it has a strong iatrogenic component.

[†]Deceased.

Nondeclarative memory	Any memory task that tests a person's memory for an event without direct reference to that event; used interchangeably with implicit memory and sometimes with procedural memory.
Priming	A widely used measure of nondeclarative memory in which prior exposure of a stimulus can facilitate subsequent processing of that stimulus without the subject's awareness.
Procedural memory	Strictly speaking, this defines any form of memory that is not subject to conscious access but is sometimes used interchangeably with implicit memory and nondeclarative memory.
Trier social stress test	A widely used experimental manipulation for increasing stress in which subjects undertake a public-speaking exercise.
Wechsler memory scale revised	The most widely used instrument for assessing deficits in declarative memory. It tests both verbal and nonverbal memory.

Memory in Posttraumatic Stress Disorder

Posttraumatic stress disorder (PTSD) is now a recognized condition that presents in an individual following a traumatic event. It is observed most commonly in combat veterans but can also be found in people who have been involved in accidents, been the victim or witness of a violent event, or been subjected to sexual abuse as a child. The effects of PTSD on memory are somewhat complex. Typically the sufferer is amnesic for the traumatic experiences, but, from time to time, flashbacks occur in which the traumatic experience is recreated vividly in the individual's mind. It is not clear what determines the occurrence of a flashback, but one determining factor appears to be mood. Memory is known to be sensitive to state dependency in that a memory is more likely to be retrieved if the individual's mood state matches that experienced at the time of the traumatic experience. There is also some suggestion that the recall of traumatic memories has a dissociative quality in that the person attributes the traumatic recall to an aspect of their self that is in some way detached from their normal ongoing self.

There is now abundant evidence that PTSD victims also have an impaired ability to remember new information. For example, Vietnam veterans with PTSD performed more poorly than controls on components of the Wechsler Memory Scale, and this type of effect has been shown on a variety of other tests of memory. Adolescent victims of violence in Beirut with PTSD

have been shown to achieve lower academic performance than their counterparts without PTSD. Victims of PTSD also exhibit memory gaps ranging from minutes to hours. Examples include one person who remembered nothing between walking down a street in Boston and waking up in Texas and another who disappeared from a psychiatric unit and then awoke to find himself in battle dress in the woods. Also, consistent with the state dependency view of PTSD, victims of PTSD show a greater recall of trauma-related words but a poorer recall of neutral and positive affect words.

Other Stress-Related Memory Disorders

While PTSD is the most prominent psychiatric disorder of memory linked to stress, there are other conditions that have rather different qualities. The first of these is what has been termed hysterical amnesia. There are great similarities here with PTSD in that the patient has a temporary loss of memories for a particular adverse event. The only difference is that the disorder appears associated with less overall psychiatric morbidity than PTSD.

Far less common, although a great favorite with fiction writers, is the fugue state. In this dissociative disorder the patient loses his or her identity and, in many cases, assumes a new one. There are very few detailed studies of fugue because the condition can ameliorate quite quickly and a number of cases turn out be malingering. However, in a well-documented case, a young man was deeply disturbed by the death of his grandfather and remained in a fugue state for some time, exhibiting only fragments of memory about his own past. However, while watching the funeral scene in the film *Shogun*, his memory of himself came back, again stressing the importance that state dependency may play in the mediation of stress-related memory dysfunction.

Stress can also be implicated in perhaps the strangest of memory disorders – multiple personality disorder (MPD). Here the person assumes a number of different personalities that have differing relationships with one another. Thus, personality A may know about personality B but not vice versa, and so on. There is massive controversy about MPD, and many clinicians believe that the condition is essentially iatrogenic – generated by clinicians in suggestible clients and also faked by knowledgeable individuals, a good example being the famous case of the hillside strangler. Taking a more moderate view, it is possible to argue that in genuine cases of MPD, various personalities absorb different aspects of a stressful past. In one case, for example, a young woman had a history of sexual abuse and drug taking. Discussion of these different aspects of her past was only possible via different personalities that she presented.

Neurophysiological and Neuroanatomical Aspects of the Effect of Stress on Memory

There is now a great deal of knowledge about why stress can cause a loss of memory function. Stress is known to increase the levels of glucocorticoids, which in turn has adverse effects on memory. There is a disorder known as the Morbus-Cushing syndrome that results in abnormally high levels of cortisol production; patients with this disorder exhibit memory dysfunction as one of their primary symptoms. Cortisol is widely held to exert its adverse effects on a brain region known as the hippocampus. This structure, located bilaterally in the medial temporal lobes, is critically involved in the initial consolidation of memory and is also thought to mediate the storage of memories for some time after their initial registration. Animal studies have shown that increased cortisol levels result in a loss of hippocampal neurons and in a decrease in dendritic branching. This loss is thought to be attributable to an increased vulnerability of the hippocampus to endogenously generated amino acids. Further evidence for the effects of cortisol on the hippocampus comes from studies showing that a major physiological index of hippocampal function, long-term potentiation, is affected by the administration of cortisol.

Further evidence for cortisol involvement in stress-related memory dysfunction comes from work involving the endogenous indole isatin, which exists in particularly high levels in the hippocampus and cerebellum. At relatively low levels it has an anxiogenic effect and results in an increase in circulating levels of cortisol. It also negates the anxiolytic effects of atrial natriuretic peptide and its associated memory enhancement effects.

Other research also points toward a critical relationship between stress and hippocampal function. Monkeys exposed to stress as a result of overcrowding were found to have hippocampal damage, and there is similar evidence in humans. One study used magnetic resonance imaging to compare hippocampal volume in Vietnam veterans with PTSD and healthy subjects. The PTSD veterans were found to have an 8% reduction in the volume of the right hippocampus, with no changes in adjacent brain structures. Similarly, with positron emission tomography, Vietnam veterans with PTSD were found to have a reduced blood flow in the hippocampus, again indicating a degree of malfunction. The same research group has found a selective 17% reduction in the left hippocampus of adult survivors of sexual abuse.

The just-mentioned studies point to permanent changes in brain structure caused by stress and are presumably mediated, at least in part, by prolonged exposure to elevated cortisol levels. However, there is also evidence that increased cortisol levels can also cause temporary memory impairment. In one study, human volunteers were administered the synthetic steroid dexamethasone. The volunteers were then given two types of memory test involving either declarative memory or nondeclarative memory. Declarative memory is what we typically think of as memory – the ability to remember lists of words, recognize faces, and so on. The effect of dexamethasone was to reduce the performance on this type of memory dramatically. Unlike declarative memory, where the individual has to reflect directly on a previous event, nondeclarative memory tests an individual's retention indirectly. A favorite method is known as priming. Here a subject is exposed to a list of words and is asked, for example, to rate each word for pleasantness. No mention is made of having to remember any of the words. Subsequently, the subject is given a test, such as "Tell me the first word that comes to mind beginning with the letters PL." If the word placid was in the previous word list, there is a strong probability that this word will be generated in preference to other possibilities. This indicates that the subject has retained information about the word list. Interestingly, these effects appear independent of subjects' declarative memory and are shown reliably by people who have a dense amnesia for declarative information. The administration of dexamethasone did not affect nondeclarative memory. This type of effect has been reported in other studies and indicates that the effects of glucocorticoids are limited to declarative memory and, by implication, that the hippocampus, with its vulnerability to enhanced cortisol levels, is not involved in nondeclarative memory performance.

Aging has been associated with an increased vulnerability to stress, which has led to the possibility that the effects of age on memory may, in part, be mediated by cortisol levels. One study employed the Trier social stress test. Essentially, this test involves subjects being asked to speak in public as a means of inducing variable amounts of stress depending on the individual. Fear of public speaking was found to enhance cortisol levels in varying degrees, which in turn predicted recall performance, with higher cortisol levels predicting poorer recall. A comparable nonstressful task had no effect on performance. Interestingly, the best predictor of the relation between cortisol levels and memory performance was a measure obtained 60 min before the stressful event, thus indicating that the anticipation of stress is a crucial factor in determining memory performance.

While this account has emphasized the role of stress on memory via changes in cortisol levels, a variety of other neurotransmitters and neuropeptides are released during stress. These include adrenocorticotropic hormone (ACTH), dopamine, acetylcholine, endogenous opiates, vasopressin, oxytocin, and γ-aminobutyric acid. Of these, vasopressin and oxytocin are of particular interest in relation to the occurrence of flashbacks in PTSD. One study used a structured imagery technique designed to solicit the retrieval of traumatic memories in Vietnam veterans. The administration of vasopressin enhanced the recall of trauma, whereas oxytocin inhibited trauma recall, relative to the placebo.

A final issue is whether the available research on stress and memory has any bearing on the false memory debate. This debate has caused enormous controversy – the central point being whether memories of abuse could remain buried for years and then suddenly reemerge. Available evidence certainly makes an *a priori* case that the stress caused by continual abuse would be expected, via the mediation of cortisol, to have a deleterious effect on an individual's recall for the period of abuse. What is less clear is whether the mechanism used to account for flashbacks in PTSD could be adapted to explain recovered memory. It is a very problematic issue, not in the least because there is abundant evidence that so much recovered memory is generated by inappropriate hypnosis-based memory work induced by very biased therapists.

Summary

Stress has a range of effects on memory, ranging from minor lapses of memory in normal individuals to the sometimes devastating effects of PTSD. The major change in brain anatomy associated with prolonged exposure to stress is shrinkage of the hippocampus.

This is widely attributed to increased cortisol levels experienced during stressful periods.

PTSD, the most notable stress-related memory disorder, is characterized by impaired declarative memory and normal nondeclarative memory. Other stress-related memory disorders are hysterical amnesia, fugue, and multiple personality disorder. Transient increases in cortisol levels induced either synthetically or via stress induction procedures result in impaired declarative memory but normal nondeclarative memory. The sudden and vivid availability of traumatic memories in PTSD may be due to the special influence of vasopressin, which is also released during periods of stress.

See Also the Following Articles

Amnesia; Cognition and Stress; Hippocampus, Overview; Multiple Personality Disorder; Posttraumatic Stress Disorder, Neurobiology of.

Further Reading

Bremner, J. D. and Narayan, M. (1998). The effects of stress on memory and the hippocampus throughout the life cycle: implications for childhood development and aging. *Developmental Psychopathology* **10**, 871–885.

Bremner, J. D., et al. (1995). Functional neuroanatomical correlates of the effects of stress on memory. *Journal of Traumatic Stress* **8**, 527–553.

Lupien, S. J., et al. (1997). Stress-induced declarative memory impairment in healthy elderly subjects: relationship to cortisol reactivity. *Journal of Clinical Neuroendocrinology and Metabolism* **82**, 2070–2075.

McGaugh, J. L. (1989). Involvement of hormonal and neuromodulatory systems in the regulation of memory storage. *Annual Review of Neuroscience* **12**, 255–287.

Parkin, A. J. (1997). *Memory and amnesia* (2nd edn.). Hove, UK: Psychology Press.

van der Kolk, B. A., et al. (eds.) (1996). *Traumatic stress: the effects of overwhelming experience on mind, body and society*. New York: Guildford Press.

Menopause and Stress

N E Avis
Wake Forest University School of Medicine,
Winston-Salem, NC, USA

This article is a revision of the previous edition article by
N E Avis, volume 2, pp 732–735, © 2000, Elsevier Inc.

Menopause as a Stressful Life Event
Impact of Stress on Menopause Symptomatology
Stress and Ovarian Function
Conclusions

Glossary

Menopause	The permanent cessation of menses. The standard epidemiological definition of natural menopause is 12 consecutive months of amenorrhea, in the absence of surgery or other pathological or physiological cause (e.g., pregnancy, lactation, excessive exercise).
Perimenopause	That period of time immediately prior to menopause when the endocrinological, biological, and clinical features of approaching menopause begin through the first year after the final menstrual period. It is characterized by increased variability in menstrual cycles, skipped menstrual cycles, and hormonal changes. Early perimenopause is defined as menses in the previous 3 months, but changes in regularity. Late perimenopause is defined as no menses in the previous 3 months, but menses in the preceding 11 months.
Premenstrual syndrome (PMS)	A disorder characterized by a set of hormonal changes that trigger disruptive physical and emotional symptoms in a significant number of women for up to 2 weeks prior to menstruation.
Surgical menopause	Menopause induced by a surgical procedure that stops menstruation. Women who have both ovaries or the uterus with or without removal of the ovaries are generally included in this category.

Menopause as a Stressful Life Event

Whether or not menopause is viewed as a stressful life event can be looked at in two ways: (1) women's attitudes toward menopause, and (2) women's affective responses to menopause.

Attitudes toward Menopause

Cross-cultural and anthropological studies provide evidence that the meaning of menopause varies greatly across cultures. How a society views menopause is influenced by how it views aging and women in general. Menopause is often viewed as a positive event in women's lives in non-Western cultures, where menopause removes constraints and prohibitions imposed upon menstruating women. In countries where women have low status or are not allowed to show sexuality (such as in India), menopause is seen positively, as it provides freedom to go out in public and do things usually forbidden to women. Among South Asian women, the end of childbearing and the menstrual cycle is welcomed. While social status is tied to motherhood, it is motherhood that is valued and not biological fertility itself.

Among both Mayan and Greek women, menopause is seen as a positive event, although for different reasons. Mayan women marry young, do not practice birth control, and spend most of their reproductive years either pregnant or lactating. Pregnancy is viewed as dangerous and stressful, and menopause frees women from restrictions and pregnancy. While Greek women attempt to curtail family size and often use abortion as a means of birth control, menopause also frees Greek women from taboos and restrictions. A postmenopausal Greek woman is allowed to participate fully in church activities, as she is no longer viewed as a sexual threat to the community. Both Mayan and Greek women report better sexual relationships with their husbands following menopause, as the fear of pregnancy is eliminated. In other cultures, women give menopause little thought. In Papago culture, menopause may be completely ignored, to the extent that the language contains no word for menopause. In Japan there is no word to describe hot flashes. As Lock points out, the lack of a Japanese word to describe hot flashes is remarkable in a language that is infinitely more sensitive than English in its ability to describe bodily states (e.g., there are more than 20 words to describe the state of the stomach).

In Western societies, women are valued for sexual attractiveness and do not face restrictions found in other cultures. Aging, especially among women, is not revered, but rather is viewed quite negatively. In these societies menopause takes on a very different meaning. Despite these negative societal views, women themselves do not hold such negative attitudes.

A review of research on women's attitudes toward menopause conducted across a wide range of populations and cultures shows that women consistently feel relief about the cessation of menses and do not agree that they become less sexually attractive following menopause. Women consistently report that they are glad to no longer deal with menstruation, accompanying PMS or menstrual cramps, fear of pregnancy, and purchase of feminine products. Thus, the end of menstruation, rather than bringing on a sense of psychological loss, is often met with relief. While women may feel a decrease in sexual desire or frequency, which they attribute to aging as much as to menopause, women overwhelmingly disagree with the statement that postmenopausal women are less feminine or attractive. Studies consistently show that postmenopausal women generally have a more positive view of menopause than premenopausal women. Thus, women's own attitudes toward menopause are not as negative as those of the medical profession or Western societies as a whole.

Women's Response to Menopause

Another way to examine whether menopause can be viewed as a stressful life event is to look at the impact of menopause on mental health. Earlier reports based on patient or clinic populations often perpetuated the perception that women become depressed and irritable and suffer a host of other symptoms during menopause. These studies, however, suffered from numerous methodological problems. First, such patient-based samples are highly biased. Fewer than half of menopausal women seek treatment, and those who do tend to report more stress in general and suffer more from clinical depression, anxiety, and psychological symptoms than nonpatient samples. Second, these studies often did not differentiate between women who experienced surgical and those who experienced natural menopause. Women who undergo surgical menopause have a very different experience of menopause, in that they experience more sudden hormonal changes, as well as a surgical procedure. A number of studies have found that women who have had a surgical menopause report more distress than women who experience a natural menopause. Finally, these studies often used menopausal checklists that asked women to check off symptoms that they experienced due to menopause. When asked in this way, women will check off any symptom they have that fits their beliefs about what women experience during menopause. This method thus perpetuates existing stereotypes of the menopause experience.

Cross-sectional epidemiological studies of community-based samples of women do not show consistent evidence of a relation between menopause and depression or other negative moods in the general population. More recently, several longitudinal studies have shown an increased risk of depressive symptoms during perimenopause. However, it is important to note that only a minority of women appear to experience an increase in negative mood or depression during perimenopause, and other factors, such as stress and socioeconomic factors, are more related to depressed mood than hormones or menopausal status. Longitudinal data suggest that prior depression is the primary factor related to depression during menopause. Studies have also found that women who report greater mood disturbances at menopause also report menstrual cycle or reproductive-related problems. These include previous or current premenstrual symptoms or complaints, dysmenorrhea, and postpartum depression. Researchers have also found that social circumstances and stress account for much of the mood effects during the menopause transition. Studies that have included measures of stress or life changes have typically found that social factors are highly related to mood, and often more so than menopause status.

Thus, for the majority of women, menopause does not appear to be a stressful life event. However, like other life events or changes, this does not mean that menopause is not stressful for some women. It has been hypothesized that women who find menopause stressful are those who see it as the end of reproduction or a sign of old age. Women with less education or knowledge about menopause generally have more negative attitudes, as do women who have more symptoms in general or worse mental health.

Impact of Stress on Menopause Symptomatology

Vasomotor symptoms (hot flashes/flushes and night sweats) are the primary symptoms associated with menopause. Estimates of the incidence of hot flashes from population studies in the United States and worldwide have ranged from 24 to 93%. Studies of menopause in different cultures reveal wide cultural variation in symptom reporting. For example, hot flashes are uncommon in Mayan women, and Japanese and Indonesian women report far fewer hot flashes than women in Western societies. Because women across cultures differ in terms of their diet, physical activity, number of pregnancies, use of contraception, as well as attitudes toward menopause, it has been difficult to assess the reason(s) for this variation. However, even within a culture, a high degree of variability of symptom reporting is found among women, suggesting considerable individual variation in symptom experience. What differentiates symptomatic from asymptomatic women is not well understood.

Women experiencing other sorts of stress are likely to notice or amplify menopausal symptoms, as they would any symptom. Epidemiological studies have shown greater vasomotor symptoms associated with less education, interpersonal stress, more general symptom reporting, and negative attitudes toward menopause. A relationship between stress and hot flashes has been shown in several correlational and treatment studies. One study has shown that laboratory-induced stressors correlate with women's objectively measured hot flashes. However, hot flashes did not concentrate around the actual stressor, suggesting that stress may potentiate (rather than cause) hot flashes by decreasing the threshold for the triggering of hot flashes at the hypothalamic level. Findings that women who report more symptoms premenopause also report more menopausal symptoms are consistent with the notion that some people have greater sensitivity to symptoms.

Thus, consistent with other research on stress and symptoms, there is some evidence that women experiencing stress for other reasons may have a tendency to notice or report greater menopausal symptoms. However, stress is only one of many factors that appear to impact menopausal symptoms.

Stress and Ovarian Function

Impact of Stress on Ovarian Function

Appropriate secretion of hypothalamic gonadotropin-releasing hormone (GnRH) is necessary for ovarian cyclicity. Decreased GnRH is a common cause of anovulation. Research in both humans and monkeys suggests that stress desynchronizes the GnRH neuronal network. High levels of stress have been shown to lead to altered menstrual function in premenopausal women. The impact of stress on perimenopausal women has not been well studied, but there is some evidence that marked increases in stress may alter menstrual cycles in the short term. It has also been hypothesized that high levels of stress may accelerate menopause. Recent research, however, has shown conflicting findings, with one study finding some evidence that stress accelerated menopausal age among women who were already experiencing irregular cycles or who were African-American, and another study finding that women who reported more psychological symptoms had a longer perimenopause.

Ovarian Function and Stress Responsivity

It has also been hypothesized that reproductive hormones influence the response to stress. Several researchers have examined the impact of ovarian function on reactivity to stress. These studies have largely examined cardiovascular reactivity in response to laboratory stresses among women in differing stages of ovarian functioning. While studies have shown greater responses among postmenopausal or surgically menopausal women as compared to premenopausal women, more recent research among women with experimentally suppressed ovarian function has not shown greater responses to stress. This remains an area of investigation.

Conclusions

Although menopause itself is a physiological event, a woman's response to menopause depends on cultural, behavioral, psychosocial, as well as physiological factors. How an individual woman responds to menopause is a complex interaction of physiology, her current life circumstances, attitudes/concerns about fertility, the culture in which she lives, and her history of responding to physiological changes/symptoms. On the whole, menopause is not a stressful event for most women. Concurrent stresses from other sources, however, may exacerbate a woman's response to menopausal symptoms.

See Also the Following Articles

Menstrual Cycles and Stress; Premenstrual Dysphoric Disorder; Stress Induced Anovulation.

Further Reading

Avis, N. E. (1996). Women's perceptions of the menopause. *European Menopause Journal* 3(2), 80–84.

Avis, N. E. (2000). Is menopause associated with mood disturbances? In: Lobo, R. A., Kelsey, J. & Marcus, R. (eds.) *Menopause: biology and pathobiology*, pp. 339–352. New York: Academic Press.

Avis, N. E., Crawford, S. L. and McKinlay, S. M. (1997). Psychosocial, behavioral, and health factors related to menopause symptomatology. *Women's Health: Research on Gender, Behavior, and Policy* 3(2), 103–120.

Barsom, S. H., Mansfield, P. K., Kock, P. B., Gierach, G. and West, S. G. (2004). Association between psychological stress and menstrual cycle characteristics in perimenopausal women. *Women's Health Issues* 14, 235–241.

Berga, S. L. (1996). Stress and ovarian function. *The American Journal of Sports Medicine* 24(6), S36–S37.

Berga, S. L. and Louks, T. L. (2005). The diagnosis and treatment of stress-induced anovulation. *Minerva Ginecologica* 57, 45–54.

Beyene, Y. (1986). Cultural significance and physiological manifestations of menopause, a biocultural analysis. *Culture, Medicine & Psychiatry* 10, 47–71.

Bromberger, J. T., Matthews, K. A., Kuller, L. H., et al. (1997). Prospective study of the determinants of age at menopause. *American Journal of Epidemiology* **145**, 124–133.

Freeman, E. W., Sammel, M. D., Liu, L., et al. (2004). Hormones and menopausal status as predictors of depression in women in transition to menopause. *Archives of General Psychiatry* **61**(1), 62–70.

Freeman, E. W., Sammel, M. D., Lin, H., et al. (2005). The role of anxiety and hormonal changes in menopausal hot flashes. *Menopause* **12**(3), 258–266.

Freeman, E. W., Sammel, M. D., Lin, H. and Nelson, D. B. (2006). Associations of hormones and menopausal status with depressed mood in women with no history of depression. *Archives of General Psychiatry* **63**(4), 375–382.

Gold, E. B., Colvin, A., Avis, N. E., et al. (2006). Longitudinal analysis of vasomotor symptoms and race/ethnicity across the menopausal transition: Study of Women's Health Across the Nation (SWAN). *American Journal of Public Health* **96**(7), 1226–1235.

Kronenberg, F. (1990). Hot flashes: epidemiology and physiology. *Annals of the New York Academy of Sciences* **592**, 52–86.

Lock, M. (1986). Ambiguities of aging: Japanese experience and perceptions of menopause. *Culture, Medicine & Psychiatry* **10**, 23–46.

Nicol-Smith, L. (1996). Causality, menopause, and depression: a critical review of the literature. *British Journal of Medicine* **313**, 1229–1232.

Pearlstein, M. D., Rosen, K. and Stone, A. B. (1997). Mood disorders and menopause. *Endocrinology and Metabolism Clinics of North America* **26**(2), 279–294.

Shively, C. A., Watson, S. L., Williams, J. K., et al. (1998). Stress-menstrual cycle and cardiovascular disease. In: Orth-Gomer, K., Chesney, M. A. & Wenger, N. K. (eds.) *Women, stress, and heart disease*. Mahwah, NJ: Lawrence Erlbaum Associates, Inc.

Sommer, B., Avis, N., Meyer, P., et al. (1999). Attitudes toward menopause and aging across ethnic/racial groups. *Psychosomatic Medicine* **61**, 868–875.

Swartzman, L. C., Edelberg, R. and Kemmann, E. (1990). The menopausal hot flush: symptom reports and concomitant physiological changes. *Journal of Behavioral Medicine* **13**(1), 15–31.

World Health Organization Scientific Group. (1996). Research on the menopause in the 1990's. *WHO Technical Services Report Series* 886.

Menstrual Cycles and Stress

R Suri
UCLA Neuropsychiatric Institute and Hospital, Los Angeles, CA, USA
L Altshuler
UCLA Neuropsychiatric Institute and Hospital and West LA Veterans Administration Medical Center, Los Angeles, CA, USA

This article is a revision of the previous edition article by R Suri and L Altshuler, volume 2, pp 736–741, © 2000, Elsevier Inc.

The Menstrual Cycle

Biological Effects of Stress on Menstruation

Anorexia Nervosa and Amenorrhea

Exercise, Stress, and the Menstrual Cycle

Effects of Menstrual Cycle on Stress, Mood, and Psychiatric Symptoms

Consequences of Amenorrhea

Treatment Issues

Glossary

Amenorrhea	The absence of menses for 3 months or longer.
Anorexia nervosa	An eating disorder characterized by the refusal to maintain a minimally normal body weight; symptoms also include the absence of at least three consecutive menstrual cycles.
Corticotropin releasing hormone (CRH)	A 41-amino-acid peptide secreted by the paraventricular nucleus of the hypothalamus, which stimulates pituitary secretion of adrenocorticotropic hormone and, consequently, cortisol secretion by the adrenal cortex.
Functional hypothalamic amenorrhea	Amenorrhea associated with factors such as psychogenic stressors, excessive exercise, or weight loss.
Gonadotropin-releasing hormone (GnRH)	A decapeptide hormone that plays a significant role in reproductive physiology through stimulation of follicular stimulating hormone and luteinizing hormone by the pituitary. GnRH is secreted by neurons of the preoptic and arcuate

Secondary amenorrhea

nuclei of the hypothalamus in a pulsatile manner, with the amplitude and frequency of its secretions under the regulation of estrogen, progesterone, catecholamines, and neuropeptides.

Amenorrhea that occurs when the patient has menstruated in the past but has stopped for at least 3–6 months. Causes can include pregnancy, lesions of the hypothalamus or pituitary (from surgery, infection, irradiation, chemotherapy, infarction, or tumor), emotional stress, endocrine disease (e.g., thyroid, adrenal, or diabetes), or medications.

Stress can be conceptualized as a state of disharmony or threatened homeostasis, with the patient's adaptive response being specific to the stressor or being more generalized. Although the demands and complexity of society continue to increase, the physiological mechanisms for coping with adversity have not changed appreciably over the past thousands of years, and the physiological responses to social pressures, rapid changes, and increased information are often similar to responses to physical danger and threats to survival. The effects of stress can be profound, resulting in the mobilization of adaptive behaviors and peripheral functions and the inhibition of biologically costly behaviors such as reproduction. For many animals, environmental stress, or conditions of high population density, are associated with chronic anovulation and infertility. During unfavorable circumstances, the lack of reproduction allows females to focus scarce resources on survival, improvement in overall condition, and investment in existing offspring. Although animal studies have provided information on the hormonal pathways through which stressors impact reproductive function, these mechanisms are poorly understood in humans. Nevertheless, for women, psychosocial stressors such as bereavement or separation from family, in the absence of a psychiatric diagnosis, have been linked to abnormalities of the menstrual cycle. Rates of menstrual irregularities increase in proportion to chronic stress, which, if severe enough, can completely inhibit the female reproductive system. Although the nature of the actual stressor can be significant, the response of the individual to the stressor, as well as certain cognitive, behavioral, or personality traits, may cause some women to be more vulnerable to the stress of daily living than other women and may play a more significant role in affecting menstruation than the actual stressor itself. The impact of stress can range from a lack of menstrual cycles to persisting cycles of marginal quality.

The Menstrual Cycle

The menstrual cycle is defined by the regular, repetitive monthly occurrence of ovulation throughout a woman's reproductive life. Menarche, defined as the onset of the first menses, occurs in the United States between the ages of 9 and 12, with a mean of 12.6 years. The mean duration of the cycle is 28 days, and the cycle is divided into two functional phases: the follicular (or proliferative) phase and the luteal (or secretory) phase. Polymenorrhea refers to menstrual cycles that occur at intervals of less than 21 days, whereas oligomenorrhea describes menstrual cycles occuring at intervals greater than 35 days. Menstrual cycles tend to be most irregular in the first 2 years after menarche and in the 3–5 years before menopause (perimenopause).

The follicular phase of the menstrual cycles starts at the first day of menses, continues until ovulation, and is characterized by a variable length, low basal body temperature, development of ovarian follicles, vascular growth of the endometrium, and the secretion of estrogen from the ovary. The luteal phase begins with ovulation, continues until the beginning of menses, and is characterized by a relatively constant duration of 12–16 days, an elevated basal body temperature, the formation of the corpus luteum in the ovary with the secretion of progesterone and estrogen, and preparation of the endometrium for implantation of an embryo.

Regular menstrual cycles occur as a result of complex, coordinated interactions among the central nervous system, the hypothalamus, the pituitary, and the ovary. Specifically, menstrual cyclicity occurs as a result of the pulsatile secretion of gonadotropin-releasing hormone (GnRH) by neurons in the preoptic and arcuate nuclei of the hypothalamus. GnRH then acts on the pituitary to stimulate release of the gonadotropins luteinizing hormone (LH) and follicular stimulating hormone (FSH), which influence the selection and maturation of the follicle for ovulation as well as secretion of ovarian steroid hormones that act on the genital tract. GnRH is secreted in a pulsatile manner at approximately 1 pulse per h in the follicular phase and 1 pulse per 2–3 h in the luteal phase, and the amplitude and frequency of secretions are influenced by feedback from estrogen and progesterone as well as catecholamines, dopamine, and norepinephrine within the brain. Estrogen levels rise in the follicular phase, reaching a peak approximately 24–36 h before ovulation. LH increases steadily until the midcycle when there is a surge, and ovulation occurs approximately 10–12 h after the LH peak. In the absence of pregnancy, decreasing steroid levels result in the constriction of the arteries supplying the upper two-thirds of the endometrium, with subsequent shedding of the degraded endometrial tissue.

Biological Effects of Stress on Menstruation

Amenorrhea is defined by the absence of menses for 3 or more months. The failure of menarche to occur is referred to as primary amenorrhea; secondary amenorrhea refers to the discontinuation of menses after the onset of menarche. Prevalence rates for secondary amenorrhea range from 8.5% among women ages 13–18 years, 7.6% among women ages 15–24 years, and 3% among women ages 25–34 years.

Identifiable or organic causes of secondary amenorrhea and anovulation include a pituitary adenoma or hypothalamic tumor; however, the most common cause of amenorrhea is not the result of an identifiable organic source but is, rather, associated with psychological and lifestyle variables, including excessive exercise, low weight, affective and eating disorders, substance use, and stress. This condition is known as functional hypothalamic amenorrhea (FHA). The function of the hypothalamus is to maintain homeostasis and promote adaptation by regulating the neuroendocrine axis. It receives afferent neural information from other brain areas, as well as signals from the periphery that cross the blood–brain barrier, and then releases hormones that influence the synthesis and release of specific pituitary hormones in an integrated fashion, coordinating endocrine responses with internal and external demands. Changes in activity at one hypothalamic area can result in profound changes in the function of other areas. Psychophysiological factors, for instance, affect central neuroregulatory networks that subsequently disrupt the GnRH pulse generator and impact reproductivity. Specifically, stress can result in a decrease in GnRH drive, with the frequency and amplitude of the pulsatile release of GnRH falling out of the normal range. In general, catecholamines, epinephrine, and norepinephrine increase GnRH release, whereas β-endorphins decrease GnRH release. Although plasma concentrations of GnRH are too low to measure, LH levels correlate well with those of GnRH, and its secretory patterns can be used for information on hypothalamic-pituitary-gonadal (HPG) activity. LH pulses normally have a constant amplitude with a frequency of 2–6 h in the follicular phase and a more variable amplitude with a frequency of 2–6 h in the luteal phase. Studies have shown that, in women with the presence of both a stressful life event and a psychiatric diagnosis, spontaneous LH pulse

frequency is inhibited. A study of 67 patients with hypothalamic secondary amenorrhea found that the onset of the menstrual disorder was correlated with a psychosocial stressor in close to half of the patients. When both a psychiatric diagnosis and a stressful life event are present, LH pulse frequency can be reduced by as much as 50% of that for normally menstruating women. Studies have also demonstrated that the presence of an anxiety or depressive disorder reduces pulse amplitude significantly. However, for women with amenorrhea without a psychiatric disorder or a stressful life event, the pulsatile release of LH is similar to that in normally menstruating women in the follicular phase. Thus psychogenic factors appear to influence LH release, reflecting effects on HPG activity and GnRH secretion. With significant declines in pulsatile GnRH secretion, the pituitary secretion of LH and FSH is reduced, compromising folliculogenesis and ovulation.

A possible mechanism that may link the GnRH pulse generator and stress involves the hypothalamic-pituitary-adrenal (HPA) axis, which is activated by stress. Women with secondary amenorrhea often display hypercortisolism, and in monkeys and rats, the administration of corticotropin releasing hormone (CRH) results in an acute decrease in pulsatile GnRH and gonadotropin release. CRH also inhibits LH by central effects, partially mediated by central endogenous opiates. Stress stimulates the expression of CRH and vasopressin. In monkeys, vasopressin has been shown to decrease LH secretion acutely when administered intracerebroventricularly.

Further evidence suggesting involvement of the HPA axis has been provided by Berga, who demonstrated that cortisol concentrations, which reflect HPA activity, are elevated in women with FHA. In women with other causes of anovulation, cortisol concentrations were found to be comparable to those observed in women who were eumenorrheic with biochemical evidence of ovulation. Women with FHA who resumed ovulation had cortisol concentrations similar to eumenorrheic women and lower than women with persistent FHA.

Anorexia Nervosa and Amenorrhea

Much of the literature on stress and menstruation focuses on women with anorexia nervosa. Anorexia nervosa is characterized by a refusal to maintain body weight at or above the minimally normal weight for age and height, an intense fear of gaining weight even though underweight, disturbance in the way in which one's body weight or shape is experienced, and the absence of at least three consecutive menstrual cycles.

The disorder has a prevalence rate of 0.5–1.0% among females of late adolescence and early adulthood, although individuals with eating disorders that do not meet the full criteria for anorexia are more common. Anorexia accounts for 15–34.5% of patients with amenorrhea.

Clinical traits of anorexia often include an obsessive preoccupation with dieting, a desire to regress to prepubertal body habits to disguise femininity, and intense, obsessive-compulsive personality traits that result in hyperachievement. Mean age of onset for the disorder is 17 years, with possible bimodal peaks at ages 14 and 18. The onset of illness is often associated with a stressful life event, such as leaving home for college or the breakup of a relationship. The onset of dieting may be related to the stressor or may begin more insidiously, and amenorrhea can precede or be associated with weight loss. Unless the psychological stress is also addressed, menstrual cycles can remain abnormal, despite adequate weight gain. Follow-up studies at 2 years have found that psychological impairment persists in one-third to one-half of patients, with one-third of patients experiencing recurrent affective disorders and one-fourth of patients not regaining menses or attaining 75% of ideal body weight.

Females with anorexia nervosa demonstrate a pattern of 24-h gonadotropin secretion that is similar to prepubertal girls, with reversion to adult patterns following adequate weight gain and a change in behavior. Compared with normally menstruating women, the LH response to GnRH is diminished in the follicular phase. For women with secondary amenorrhea or infertility and weight loss, but without anorexia, similar but less severe changes in LH are seen.

Exercise, Stress, and the Menstrual Cycle

Strenuous, regular physical activity has also been associated with menstrual irregularities, oligomenorrhea, amenorrhea, or delayed menarche. Up to 50% of competitive runners, 25% of recreational runners, and 12% of cyclists and swimmers demonstrate amenorrhea. Both weight loss and stress have been implicated in the cause of exercise-associated amenorrhea through the disruption of GnRH secretion. Stress can be metabolic, psychological, or a combination of both, and its effects may be partly mediated by the increased β-endorphin levels that impact the amplitude and frequency of LH pulses. In addition, the release of CRH in endurance exercise can inhibit gonadotropin secretion and activate the release of corticosteroids and androgenic steroids.

Although psychological stress may result in erratic menstrual cycles, its role in exercise-related amenorrhea appears to involve initiation more than continuation.

Effects of Menstrual Cycle on Stress, Mood, and Psychiatric Symptoms

In addition to the influence of stress on the menstrual cycle, monthly fluctuations of reproductive hormones can impact a woman's vulnerability to the experience of stress. Some studies, for example, reported a four-fold increase in the prevalence of suicide attempts and allergic bronchial asthma attacks in the late luteal phase of the menstrual cycle.

The levels of estrogen, progesterone, and their metabolites fall during the late luteal phase of the menstrual cycle and remain low during the early follicular phase. These gonadal steroids modulate the central neurotransmitter function of serotonin, dopamine, norepinephrine, and γ-aminobutyric acid and thus, as their levels vary across the menstrual cycle, may influence symptoms of irritability, anxiety, depression, and fatigue. For example, the progesterone metabolites allopregnanolone and pregnanolone may have anxiolytic properties through their barbiturate-like effect on γ-aminobutyric acid receptors, with decreased levels of these metabolites correlating with increased tension and anxiety.

Premenstrual asthma, or the worsening of asthma symptoms and pulmonary function in relation to menstruation, has been described in approximately one-third of women. A number of studies reported increases in asthma prior to menstruation and, to a lesser extent, during menstruation. Mirdal suggested a relationship among lowered resistance to stress, lowered resistance to infections, and increased bronchial hyperreactivity as background etiological factors for the occurrence of premenstrual asthma.

The premenstrual and menstrual phases of the menstrual cycle have been associated with an increased vulnerability to an exacerbation of psychiatric symptoms, as well as a peak in psychiatric admissions. Literature in this area is limited to case reports and small studies, which have found evidence of premenstrual exacerbation in schizophrenia, depression, bulimia nervosa, anxiety disorders, and substance abuse. For example, in a prospective study of 27 women with research diagnostic criteria for major, minor, or intermittent depression responding to treatment with imipramine or phenelzine, one-fourth of the women experienced premenstrual recurrence of symptoms of low mood, anhedonia, anxiety, increased appetite, and hypersomnia, which remitted following menses. For some women, an increased consumption of alcohol and marijuana occurs premenstrually. A study of 14 women with alcohol dependence found an association between alcohol intake and severity of premenstrual symptoms. Similar findings were reported in a prospective study of 21 women with a history of regular marijuana use. Smoking frequency has also been shown to vary across the menstrual cycle, with approximately 70% of women reporting an increase in the 7–10 days before their menstrual period. Researchers postulate that reproductive hormones may influence psychiatric symptoms by direct effects on central neurotransmitter function, as well as by causing the serum concentrations of medication to vary across the menstrual cycle.

Consequences of Amenorrhea

The hypoestrogenism associated with secondary amenorrhea can have long-term effects, the most significant of which is osteoporosis. Osteoporosis results from an imbalance between bone formation and bone resorption. Rapid increases in bone density are seen during puberty, with peak bone density of the spine and hip occurring by age 20. Females ages 14–18 with amenorrhea, especially if associated with weight changes, anorexia, or excessive exercise, risk decreased bone mineral density compared with normally menstruating young women. Amenorrheic athletes, for instance, have a significantly reduced spinal bone mineral content compared with controls with normal menstrual cycles. The peak bone density of premenopausal women influences the onset of osteoporosis later in life; thus, as life expectancy increases, the potential morbidity from osteoporosis also increases.

Treatment Issues

Stress can have a profound impact on menstruation and reproduction, ranging from cycles of marginal quality to chronic anovulation. Although mediated through biological actions on the hypothalamus, GnRH, and the HPA axis, these effects are potentially reversible. In managing women with functional hypothalamic amenorrhea, the psychological, behavioral, and psychiatric variables that influence hypothalamic function must be considered. Although pharmacological interventions can supply appropriate sex steroid exposure, restore hormonal balance, or induce ovulation, hormonal treatments can prevent the recognition of important emotional, behavioral, or psychiatric symptoms. Many women with FHA may have a potentially reversible condition that can be addressed with education, changes in lifestyle, psychotherapy, assistance in identifying and coping with stressors, or attention to a psychiatric condition. Cognitive-behavioral therapy, for instance, has been shown to result in the recovery of ovarian function for women with FHA who do not have a psychiatric disorder or engage in excessive exercise. Such interventions can help ameliorate the long-term consequences of stress and anovulation, as well as the health hazards associated with relative hypoestrogenism.

Finally, in evaluating a woman of reproductive age, the relationship between her symptoms and her menstrual cycle should be considered. Emotional symptoms can vary across the menstrual cycle because reproductive hormones can influence vulnerability to stress as well as mood changes and anxiety. With an awareness of these fluctuations, women may benefit from a greater sense of predictability and control over their symptoms. In addition, overmedication or undermedication with pharmacological agents can be avoided.

See Also the Following Articles

Amenorrhea; Eating Disorders and Stress; Estrogen; Menopause and Stress; Premenstrual Dysphoric Disorder.

Further Reading

Barnea, E. R. and Tal, J. (1991). Stress-related reproductive failure. *Journal of In Vitro Fertilization and Embryo Transfer* 8, 15–23.

Berga, S. L. (1996). Functional hypothalamic chronic ovulation. In: Adashi, E. Y., Rock, J. A. & Rosenwaks, Z. (eds.) *Reproductive endocrinology, surgery and technology* (vol. 1), pp. 1061–1075. Philadelphia: Lippincott-Raven.

Berga, S. L. (1996). Stress and ovarian function. *American Journal of Sports Medicine* 24, S36–S37.

Berga, S. L., Daniels, T. L. and Giles, D. E. (1997). Women with functional hypothalamic amenorrhea but not other forms of anovulation display amplified cortisol concentrations. *Fertilization and Sterilization* 67, 1024–1030.

Berga, S. L. and Girton, L. G. (1989). The psychoneuroendocrinology of functional hypothalamic amenorrhea. *Psychiatric Clinics of North America: Women's Disorders* 12, 105–116.

Berga, S. L., Marcus, M. D., Loucks, T. L., et al. (2003). Recovery of ovarian activity in women with functional hypothalamic amenorrhea who were treated with cognitive behavioral therapy. *Fertilization and Sterilization* 80, 976–981.

Buskirk, E. R., Mendez, J. and Durfee, S. (1985). Effects of exercise on the body composition of women. *Seminars in Reproductive Endocrinology* 3, 9–16.

Carpenter, S. E. (1994). Psychosocial menstrual disorders: stress, exercise and diet's effect on the menstrual cycle. *Current Opinion in Obstetrics and Gynecology* **6**, 536–539.

Christia, J. S., Loyd, J. A. and Davis, D. E. (1965). The role of endocrines in the self regulation of mammalian population. *Recent Progress in Hormone Research* **21**, 501–578.

Chrousos, G. P. and Gold, P. W. (1992). The concepts of stress and stress system disorders. *Journal of the American Medical Association* **267**, 1244–1252.

Collins, A., Eneroth, P. and Landgren, B. M. (1985). Psychoneuroendocrine stress responses and mood as related to the menstrual cycle. *Psychosomatic Medicine* **47**, 512–527.

Dalton, K. (1964). The influence of menstruation on health and disease. *Proceedings of the Royal Society of Medicine* **57**, 18–20.

Drinkwater, B. L. (1984). Bone mineral content of amenorrheic athletes. *New England Journal of Medicine* **311**, 277–281.

Facchinetti, F., Fava, M., Fioroni, L., et al. (1993). Stressful life events and affective disorders inhibit pulsatile LH secretion in hypothalamic amenorrhea. *Psychoneuroendocrinology* **18**, 397–404.

Feingold, K. R., Gavin, L. A., Schambelan, M., et al. (1990). Female endocrinology. In: Andreoli, T. E., Carpenter, C. C., Plum, F. & Smith, L. H. (eds.) *Cecil essentials of medicine* (2nd edn., pp. 478–486). Philadelphia: Saunders.

Freeman, E. W., Purdy, R. H., Coutifaris, C., et al. (1993). Anxiolytic metabolites of progesterone: correlation with mood and performance measures following oral progesterone administration to healthy female volunteers. *Neuroendocrinology* **58**, 478–484.

Fries, H., Nillius, S. and Pettersson, F. (1974). Epidemiology of secondary amenorrhea. II: A retrospective evaluation of etiology with special regard to psychogenic factors and weight loss. *American Journal of Obstetrics and Gynecology* **118**, 473–479.

Glick, R., Harrison, W., Endicott, J., et al. (1991). Treatment of premenstrual dysphoric symptoms in depressed women. *Journal of the American Medical Women's Association* **46**, 182–185.

Hendrick, V., Altshuler, L. L. and Burt, V. K. (1996). Course of psychiatric disorders across the menstrual cycle. *Harvard Review of Psychiatry* **4**, 200–207.

Herzog, D. B. and Copeland, P. M. (1985). Eating disorders. *New England Journal of Medicine* **313**, 295–303.

Marshall, J. (1989). Regulation of gonadotropin secretion. In: Degroot, L., Besser, G., Marshal, J., et al. (eds.) *Endocrinology*. Philadelphia: Saunders.

Melo, N. K., Mendelson, J. H. and Lex, B. W. (1990). Alcohol use and premenstrual symptoms in social drinkers. *Psychopharmacology* **101**, 448–455.

Melo, N. K., Mendelson, J. H. and Palmieri, S. L. (1987). Cigarette smoking by women: interactions with alcohol use. *Psychopharmacology* **93**, 8–15.

Mirdal, G. M., Petersson, B., Weeke, B., et al. (1998). Asthma and menstruation: the relationship between psychological and bronchial hyperreactivity. *British Journal of Medicine and Psychology* **71**, 47–55.

Nepomnaschy, P. A., Welch, K., McConnell, D., et al. (2004). Stress and female reproductive function: a study of daily variations in cortisol, gonadotropins, and gonadal steroids in a rural Mayan population. *American Journal of Human Biology* **16**, 523–532.

Podolsky, E. (1963). The woman alcoholic and premenstrual tension. *Journal of the American Medical Women's Association* **18**, 816–818.

Reame, N., Sauder, S., Kelch, R., et al. (1984). Pulsatile gonadotropin secretion during the human menstrual cycle: evidence for altered frequency of gonadotropin-releasing hormone secretion. *Journal of Clinical Endocrinology and Metabolism* **59**, 328–337.

Rivier, C. and Vale, W. (1984). Influence of corticotropin releasing factor on reproductive function in the rat. *Endocrinology* **114**, 914–921.

Sapolsky, R. M., Romero, L. M. and Munck, A. U. (2000). How do glucocorticoids influence stress responses?: integrating permissive, suppressive, stimulatory, and preparative actions. *Endocrine Reviews* **21**, 55–89.

Schachter, M. and Shoham, Z. (1994). Amenorrhea during the reproductive years: is it safe? *Fertilization and Sterilization* **62**, 1–16.

Shalts, E., Xia, L., Xiao, E., et al. (1994). Inhibitory effects of arginine-vasopressin on LH secretion in the ovariectomized rhesus monkey. *Neuroendocrinology* **59**, 336–342.

Shangold, M. M. (1985). Exercise and amenorrhea. *Seminars in Reproductive Endocrinology* **3**, 35–43.

Taylor, J. W. (1974). The timing of menstrual-related symptoms assessed by a daily symptom rating scale. *Acta Psychiatrica Scandinavica* **60**, 87–105.

Tilbrook, A. J., Turner, A. I. and Clarke, I. J. (2000). Effects of stress on reproduction in non-rodent mammals: the role of glucocorticoids and sex differences. *Reviews of Reproduction* **5**, 105–113.

Tilbrook, A. J., Turner, A. I. and Clarke, I. J. (2002). Stress and reproduction: central mechanisms and sex differences in non-rodent species. *Stress* **5**, 83–100.

Warren, M. P. (1996). Clinical review 77: evaluation of secondary emenorrhea. *Journal of Clinical Endocrinology and Metabolism* **81**, 437–442.

Xiao, E. and Ferin, M. (1997). Stress-related disturbances of the menstrual cycle. *Annals of Medicine* **29**, 215–219.

Mental Stress Testing

P G Saab
University of Miami, Coral Gables, FL, USA
K A Kline
Virginia Military Institute, Lexington, VA, USA
J R McCalla
University of Miami, Coral Gables, FL, USA

This article is a revision of the previous edition article by P G Saab and K A Kline, volume 2, pp 742–746, © 2000, Elsevier Inc.

Introduction
Conducting Mental Stress Testing
Task Differences in Responses to Mental Stressors
Individual Differences in Responses to Mental Stressors
Other Considerations
Conclusion

Glossary

α-Adrenergic activity	Reflecting activity of sympathetic nervous system receptors located in the vasculature; stimulation leads to constriction of the blood vessels.
β1-Adrenergic activity	Reflecting activity of sympathetic nervous system receptors located in the heart; stimulation leads to increases in heart rate and contraction of the heart muscle.
Cardiac output	Quantity of blood ejected from the heart in liters per minute.
Endothelin-1	Potent vasoconstrictor peptide released by vascular endothelial cells.
Hemodynamic	Pertaining to changes in blood flow reflecting changes in the underlying components of blood pressure, cardiac output, and total peripheral resistance.
Left ventricular mass	Size of the heart muscle of the left ventricle; enlargement of the left ventricle is a risk factor for cardiovascular morbidity and mortality.
Nitric oxide	Potent vasodilator substance released by vascular endothelial cells.
Psychophysiological	Pertaining to the study of physiological responses to psychological stimuli (e.g., stressors).
Serotonin transporter gene Promoter polymorphism (5HTTLPR)	A coding variant in the promoter of the human serotonin transporter gene which results in low transcriptional activity of this gene and is thought to be a genetic susceptibility factor for depression.
Total peripheral resistance	The resistance to blood flow in the systemic blood vessels.
Vagal tone	Index of parasympathetic nervous system influences on the cardiovascular system.

Introduction

Mental stress testing is typically used to examine the physiological effects of exposure to acute stressors, i.e., tasks, presented in the laboratory. Widely used as a research technique, mental stress testing is usually intended to distinguish groups with varying risk for cardiovascular diseases. To this end, mental stress testing functions as a provocative tool for unmasking information that is not available from assessments made under static conditions alone. As such, the psychophysiological adjustments that occur in the context of mental stress testing can enhance understanding of regulatory adjustments due to exposure to stress. Furthermore, these adjustments have implications for the reactivity hypothesis, which states that individuals who consistently display exaggerated cardiovascular responses (i.e., reactivity) to stressors may be at increased risk for the development of hypertension and/or coronary heart disease. The present discussion is limited to cardiovascular responses, although mental stressors also affect other systems such as those pertaining to neuroendocrine and immune function.

Conducting Mental Stress Testing

Baseline, Stress, and Recovery Periods

Mental stress testing requires assessment during resting baseline as well as during stress conditions. Regulatory mechanisms operative under resting conditions become modified as individuals are exposed to stressors. Examination under baseline conditions in the laboratory is requisite since it provides a comparison against which stressor-induced responses can be evaluated. Baseline measures may be affected by a variety of factors, including level of consciousness, habituation to the laboratory and procedures, time of day, posture, and prior substance ingestion (e.g., cardioactive agents such as caffeine, nicotine, and certain medications). As such, the baseline serves as a control level; a true basal level is not likely to be achieved under these circumstances. In relation to control levels, stressor-induced responses provide a sample of dynamic adjustments under varying conditions. In addition, recovery to baseline levels following the termination of the stressor is often examined, as it provides further information about homeostatic mechanisms. To minimize extraneous influences and to ensure precise stimulus control, procedures for acquiring the baseline, stressor, and recovery data must be highly standardized. Efforts to enhance standardization have included scripted and/or taped instructions and computer presentation of stressor stimuli.

Types of Laboratory Stressors

Laboratory studies have utilized a wide range of stressors that differ to the extent that they elicit psychological versus physical stress. Social stressors include speech stressors (preparing and presenting a speech), interviews designed to elicit general or specific emotional responses, and tasks intended to mimic real-world social interactions, such as discussions of current events and role-play involving interpersonal conflict. Nonsocial psychological stressors include, but are not limited to, mental arithmetic (e.g., serial subtractions), mirror tracing (tracing a star looking only at its reflection in a mirror), reaction time (e.g., rapidly pressing a button in response to specific stimuli), the Stroop color-word interference test, video games, puzzle-solving tasks, and films (often consisting of graphic footage). Another commonly used stressor, the cold pressor test, is a physical stressor with a measurable psychological component. This task typically involves immersing a limb in ice water or placing an ice pack on the forehead. Finally, tasks such as static (e.g., squeezing a handgrip device) or dynamic (e.g., walking on a treadmill, riding a stationary bicycle) exercise are generally regarded as pure physical stressors and, thus, are not the focus of this article.

Several methods of classifying tasks have been proposed. A classic categorization scheme is Lacey's notion of sensory intake versus sensory rejection. Sensory intake tasks (e.g., reaction time) refer to stressors that require attention to visual or auditory cues in the external environment, while sensory rejection tasks (e.g., mental arithmetic) require mental work facilitated by blocking out external distractions. The most widely used classification system was proffered by Obrist, who distinguished laboratory stressors on the basis of the behavioral dimensions required for task completion, i.e., active versus passive coping. Active coping tasks provide an opportunity to influence the outcome of the situation by performing a specific behavior, while passive coping tasks require passive endurance of the stressor. Tasks such as shock avoidance reaction time, mental arithmetic, speech, video games, and the Stroop color-word interference test are considered active coping stressors. Examples of passive coping tasks include the cold pressor test and film viewing.

Task Selection

Mental stress testing may involve presenting individuals with one or more laboratory stressors. It is recommended that task selection be guided by the specific questions that the research intends to address. For example, the research question would determine whether a stressor that elicits responses that are variable or uniform in magnitude is chosen. An explicit rationale for stressor choice also requires articulation. Selection decisions are often made on the basis of the behavioral demands associated with the stressors. To illustrate, an investigator may wish to compare responses to stressors involving active coping with those requiring passive coping. This would be particularly critical for studies comparing Black and White Americans. The literature indicates that Blacks, who as a group have a higher prevalence of hypertension than Whites, are more responsive to passive coping stressors, whereas Whites are more reactive to active coping stressors.

The relevance of stressors to the groups under study also requires consideration. Stressors, by virtue of the domains they tap, may hold differential relevance for one group relative to another. For example, a large body of research comparing males and females (children and adults) and employing cognitive and/or achievement-oriented stressors demonstrated that males show exaggerated physiological responses compared to females. Given the differential gender-related expectancies for performance that are likely in such situations, it is probable that those types of tasks may have been less relevant for the females. Therefore, it is essential to select stressors that are expected to be equally pertinent to participants.

When there is interest in the relationship between mental stress and a particular psychosocial variable, a fair test requires the inclusion of a task that is relevant to the specific construct. To illustrate, if one is interested in the relationship between trait anger and responses to mental stress, it is incumbent upon the investigator to include an anger-relevant task. This situation will provide an opportunity for individual differences to emerge.

Consideration also needs to be given to the response patterns evoked by the stressor when making stressor choices. Investigators often wish to compare stressors that elicit different hemodynamic responses. Such decisions are aided by the availability of noninvasive methods (e.g., impedance cardiography) to assess hemodynamic parameters such as cardiac output and total peripheral resistance during mental stress testing.

Task Differences in Responses to Mental Stressors

Research indicates that mental stressors evoke integrated response patterns across several parameters rather than an isolated response in a sole parameter. Consequently, a vast array of stressors elicits relatively few response patterns. Situational stereotypy, the propensity for a specific type of mental stressor to elicit a particular response pattern, is well known. Pattern 1 and Pattern 2 response patterns have been identified. Pattern 1 is characterized by skeletal muscle vasodilation, elevated heart rate, augmentation of blood pressure primarily as a function of increases in cardiac output, enhanced β1-adrenergic activity, and decreased vagal tone. This myocardial response pattern is thought to characterize mental stressors involving active coping, sensory rejection, or mental work. Pattern 2 is associated with skeletal muscle vasoconstriction, smaller changes in heart rate, increases in blood pressure largely due to augmented total peripheral resistance, heightened α-adrenergic activity, and increased vagal tone. Stressors thought to elicit this vascular response pattern include those that involve passive coping, passive avoidance, inhibition, sensory intake, and vigilance. The use of adrenergic pharmacologic blockade has been informative with respect to clarifying the degree to which mental stressor response patterns are mediated by β-adrenergic and α-adrenergic receptor activity.

While Pattern 1 and Pattern 2 responses are often associated with active and passive coping stressors, respectively, some active coping tasks such as certain versions of mental arithmetic and speech (i.e., presentation period, not preparation) stressors are often associated with more of a mixed response pattern, composed of myocardial and vascular responses. It is well known that several variables influence and alter hemodynamic response patterns. A Pattern 1 response can be modified by a variety of factors, including instructional sets, expectations, appraisals, controllability, incentives, effort, predictability, individual differences, and the like, resulting in mixed response patterns.

Individual Differences in Responses to Mental Stressors

Responder Types

In addition to situational stereotypy, response stereotypy, which reflects the propensity for an individual to display a consistent response pattern across stressors, is also operative. A promising approach to the investigation of individual differences in reactivity to stressors has been the identification of participants on the basis of their response patterns. The literature shows that some individuals respond in a consistent hemodynamic manner across active coping and passive coping mental stressors. In this regard, among men, Black Americans are more prevalent among vascular responders, whereas White Americans are more prevalent among myocardial responders across various stressors. Alternatively, evidence also supports the view that individuals may respond in a variable manner across myocardial and vascular dimensions to specific stressors. It should be noted, however, that for certain stressors, due to their stimulus characteristics, situational stereotypy might overwhelm the response stereotypy of the individual. For example, the cold pressor test typically elicits a Pattern 2 response pattern despite an individual's response stereotypy. Nonetheless, there is considerable individual variability with respect to how that stressor is tolerated and experienced.

Psychosocial Variables

The literature linking psychosocial variables to individual differences in cardiovascular reactivity assumes that when confronted with a stressor, individuals possessing certain psychosocial characteristics display exaggerated cardiovascular responses. The most commonly studied constructs include Type A behavior pattern and hostility/anger. A meta-analysis of the Type A reactivity literature concluded that Type A males, but not females, exhibit greater heart rate and systolic blood pressure reactivity to a variety of tasks than their Type B counterparts. These findings were dependent upon the type of task used, and the strength of findings varied with the method of Type A behavior pattern assessment (i.e., interview or questionnaire). Numerous studies have examined relationships among hostility and/or anger and cardiovascular reactivity. Qualitative and quantitative reviews of this literature conclude that hostility/anger is consistently related to reactivity to social/interpersonal stressors (e.g., involving provocation) but not to reactivity to standard nonsocial stressors.

Other Considerations

Prolonged Recovery

There is growing support for the notion that prolonged recovery has pathophysiological consequences. Evidence of delayed blood pressure recovery is available for hypertensives, as well as for groups at risk for future hypertension, such as borderline hypertensives, Blacks, and individuals with a family history of hypertension. Furthermore, prolonged recovery from mental stress in borderline hypertensives has been shown to predict future sustained hypertension. Several recent studies have provided evidence of concurrent and prospective associations between recovery and outcome measures in adults and adolescents. Overall, research indicates that blood pressure and/or heart rate recovery may contribute uniquely to the prediction of ambulatory or resting cardiovascular measures.

Given increased recognition of the importance of recovery, investigation of the psychosocial correlates of post stressor responses is of interest. While a number of psychosocial factors have been examined in this regard, a promising variable is post stressor rumination, particularly when it involves the experience of anger. Studies have demonstrated delayed recovery from tasks involving harassment relative to nonharassment conditions, as well as more rapid recovery when participants are distracted and, thus, prevented from ruminating following emotionally provocative tasks.

Individual–Task Interactions

Understanding the potency of the mental stressor requires considering the interaction of the individual with the mental stressor. Although it is assumed that the stressor is perceived as stressful by the participants, in practice, this may not be the case. Appraisal of the stressor may be influenced by several situational variables, including the social context of the experiment, task ease, controllability, and novelty. In addition, subject variables such as experience, ability, involvement, and fatigue are also likely to impact perceptions. The individual's preexisting attitudes toward, experience with, and ability to perform similar tasks in real-life situations may also influence perception of the stressor. Stressor appraisal consequently will affect the extent to which the individual is engaged by the stressor. Engagement and involvement with the stressor are key in determining its efficacy and may reciprocally influence the effort that the individual expends when confronted with the stressor.

Stability

The notion that cardiovascular responses to mental stressors are relatively stable across tasks and over time is a critical assumption of the reactivity hypothesis. To make the case that exaggerated stress-induced responses have a detrimental impact on the cardiovascular system, it is first necessary to demonstrate that reactivity is a reproducible phenomenon. With regard to the stability of reactivity, there is increasing evidence of adequate test-retest reliability for cardiovascular responses to laboratory stressors, particularly with task standardization, presentation of alternate forms of the stressor, aggregation of responses across tasks and testing sessions, and relatively short test-retest intervals. Furthermore, meta-analytic reviews report stability of responses over periods of years in adult and pediatric-aged samples.

The adequate evaluation of the health implications of recovery also requires reliable recovery measures. Research shows that the test-retest reliability of recovery using definitions, such as the time required to return to baseline levels following stressor termination, does not yield adequate test-retest reliabilities. Other findings suggest that the reliability of recovery scores might be improved by aggregating measures across tasks. Future research needs to be directed at identifying factors that affect long-term stability of both reactivity and recovery.

Laboratory-to-Field Generalization

A second implicit assumption of the reactivity hypothesis is that an individual's cardiovascular responses to laboratory stressors are representative of responses to stressors encountered in everyday life. Evidence for the laboratory-to-field generalizability of reactivity remains marginal. Critics maintain that generalizability is adversely affected by the failure to utilize ecologically valid tasks in mental stress testing protocols. Given the lack of accepted standards to demonstrate that a stressor is ecologically valid, the ecological validity of a stressor is typically based on face validity rather than on psychometric characteristics. For example, it has been suggested that the use of interpersonal or social stressors might improve generalization, as real-life stressors are likely to involve social factors; the data on this issue remain mixed. Future research needs to be directed at specifying the properties that determine a stressor's ecological validity. When making choices about whether a laboratory stressor should be used as a predictor, it is likely that the investigator would be best served by selecting a task that elicits stable cardiovascular responses over the long term. Given the chronicity of naturally occurring stressors, predictability might be enhanced when prolonged laboratory stressors, rather than the typically brief stressors, are employed.

Left Ventricular Mass

While definitive support for the reactivity hypothesis would require demonstrating an association for cardiovascular reactivity and the development of hypertension and/or coronary heart disease, establishing a relationship with proximal medical endpoints would support the validity of the reactivity construct. The use of proximal endpoints, however, would not obviate the need for definitive longitudinal studies, which are not without their own limitations. Nonetheless, increasing attention needs to be directed at examining the association of cardiovascular reactivity evoked by mental stressors and proximal endpoints, such as increased left ventricular mass, a potent predictor of coronary heart disease. To date, the literature suggests that the relationship is modest at best. Further research examining this association is warranted, particularly as it pertains to left ventricular modeling and the contributions of responder type, ethnicity, and gender.

Genetic Contributions

The potential contributions of heritable factors to individual differences in cardiovascular reactivity have long been recognized. It has recently been proposed that future studies should involve systematic consideration of genetic, as well as environmental, factors as moderators or mediators of the association between reactivity and health outcomes. Technological advances are enabling the exploration of the role of specific genes in the determination of individual differences in reactivity. Some of the more promising candidates include, but are not limited to, the adrenergic receptor genes (i.e., $\beta 1$, $\beta 2$, $\alpha 1$, and $\alpha 2$), the endothelin-1 and endothelin-1 receptor A genes, nitric oxide synthase genes, and the serotonin transporter polymorphism, i.e., 5HTTLPR. For instance, a few studies have demonstrated associations of polymorphisms of the $\beta 1$- and $\beta 2$-adrenergic receptor genes with blood pressure reactivity and/or resting or stress levels. Similarly, the 5HTTLPR polymorphism has been associated with greater heart rate and/or blood pressure responses. There is, however, conflicting evidence regarding whether greater reactivity is observed in individuals with one or two long 5HTTLPR alleles or in individuals with two short alleles, as well as whether such relationships are moderated by gender.

Conclusion

Mental stress testing typically involves the assessment of physiological responses in a laboratory setting during exposure to mental stressors and baseline and recovery conditions. Stressors range from psychological to physical and social to nonsocial. Stressors differ in the behavioral demands required of participants. Tasks also elicit certain well-defined physiological response patterns. Researchers should employ stressors that most effectively address their research questions, taking into consideration the appropriateness of behavioral task demands, the significance of tasks for the groups being studied, and the relevance of tasks to psychosocial variables or response patterns of interest.

With few exceptions, there may be considerable individual variability in responses to mental stressors. Sources of variability include individual differences in the propensity to exhibit a particular response pattern, psychosocial characteristics, and a variety of preexisting and situational factors influencing individual–task interactions. In conducting mental stress testing, a number of additional areas of inquiry are worthy of consideration. These include the reproducibility of responses across stressors and testing sessions, the generalizability of laboratory responses to field settings, the predictability of proximal medical endpoints, and genetic contributions.

See Also the Following Articles

Autonomic Nervous System; Blood Pressure; Cardiovascular System and Stress; Hypertension; Type A Personality, Type B Personality.

Further Reading

Blascovich, J. and Katkin, E. S. (eds.) (1993). *Cardiovascular reactivity to psychological stress and disease*. Washington, D.C: American Psychological Association.

Kamarck, T. and Lovallo, W. R. (2003). Cardiovascular reactivity to psychological challenge: Conceptual and measurement considerations. *Psychosomatic Medicine* 65, 9–21.

Krantz, D. S. and Manuck, S. B. (1984). Acute psychophysiological reactivity and risk of cardiovascular disease: A review and methodologic critique. *Psychological Bulletin* 96, 435–464.

Lacey, J. I., Kagan, J., Lacey, B. C., et al. (1963). The visceral level: Situational determinants and behavioral correlates of autonomic response patterns. In: Knapp, P. H. (ed.) *Expression of the emotions in man*, pp. 161–196. New York: International Universities Press.

Manuck, S. B. (1994). Cardiovascular reactivity in cardiovascular disease: "Once more unto the breach" *International Journal of Behavioral Medicine* 1, 4–31.

Obrist, P. A. (1981). *Cardiovascular psychophysiology: a perspective*. New York: Plenum Press.

Saab, P. G., Llabre, M. M., Hurwitz, B. E., et al. (1992). Myocardial and peripheral vascular responses to behavioral challenges and their stability in black and white Americans. *Psychophysiology* 29, 384–397.

Schneiderman, N., Weiss, S. M. and Kaufmann, P. G. (eds.) (1989). *Handbook of research methods in cardiovascular behavioral medicine*. New York: Plenum Press.

Schwartz, A. R., Gerin, W., Davidson, K. W., et al. (2003). Toward a causal model of cardiovascular responses to stress and the development of cardiovascular disease. *Psychosomatic Medicine* **65**, 22–35.

Snieder, H., Harshfield, G. A., Barbeau, P., et al. (2002). Dissecting the genetic architecture of the cardiovascular and renal stress response. *Biological Psychology* **61**, 73–95.

Treiber, F. A., Kamarck, T., Schneiderman, N., et al. (2003). Cardiovascular reactivity and development of preclinical and clinical disease states. *Psychosomatic Medicine* **65**, 46–62.

Turner, J. R., Sherwood, A. and Light, K. C. (eds.) (1992). *Individual differences: Cardiovascular response to stress.* New York: Plenum Press.

Metabolic Syndrome

L Keltikangas-Järvinen
University of Helsinki, Helsinki, Finland

What Is Metabolic Syndrome?
Origins of MetS
MetS and Environmental Stress
Development of MetS in Childhood
MetS and Inherited Temperament

Glossary

Innate temperament	A biologically rooted behavioral disposition that is stable across time and situations.
Metabolic syndrome (MetS)	A constellation of physiological and metabolic abnormalities.

What Is Metabolic Syndrome?

Metabolic syndrome (MetS), also called insulin resistance syndrome, is a cluster of various physiological and metabolic abnormalities including hyperinsulinemia, hyperglycemia, hypertension, a decreased plasma concentration of high-density lipoprotein (HDL) cholesterol, an increased plasma concentration of very low density lipoprotein (VLDL) triglyceride, glucose intolerance, and abdominal obesity. Insulin resistance is the primary metabolic defect of this syndrome, with compensatory hyperinsulinemia being the common denominator ultimately responsible for other changes of this constellation. In addition to insulin resistance, abdominal obesity is a key contributor to the development of MetS (see **Figure 1**).

MetS is a huge public health problem worldwide that is responsible for a growing number of premature deaths throughout the world. Its prevalence is approximately 16% among Caucasians. However, comparison across different countries is difficult as there are different age structures of the population, and even though a World Health Organization (WHO) expert committee published a definition of MetS, there are other, differing definitions available.

MetS is significant because it plays an important role in the etiology of coronary heart disease (CHD) and non-insulin-dependent diabetes mellitus (type II diabetes). Type II diabetes is one of the most prevalent and serious metabolic diseases in the world, and among middle-aged men, CHD is still the leading cause of mortality in Western countries.

Origins of MetS

The exact cause of MetS is not known. It is generally accepted that a genetic predisposition, possibly an interaction of several genes, is an essential factor in the genesis of this disorder. In addition to a genetic predisposition, lifestyle factors such as physical inactivity, habitual alcohol drinking, and smoking play a role in the development of MetS. There is also compelling evidence that stress of diverse origins has a significant role in the development of MetS. It is well established that the development of MetS is indisputably related to activity and/or dysregulation in the two major physiological and neuroendocrine stress systems, the sympathetic-adrenomedullary (SA) system and the hypothalamic-pituitary-adrenomedullary (HPA) system, a key component being the activation of the HPA axis.

The primary role of SA and HPA systems is increasing the energy available for action; activity of these systems is needed in everyday performance. The label of stress systems is based on the fact that they are very sensitive to physical and mental stress. Stress usually refers to overactivity or dysregulation of those systems, not to their ordinary functioning.

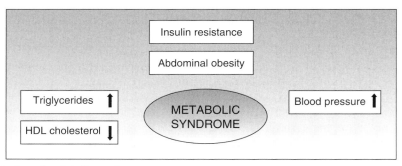

Figure 1   Contributing factors of metabolic syndrome.

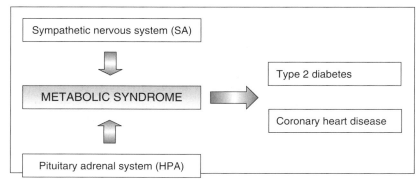

Figure 2   Stress contributes to the development of diabetes and coronary heart disease through metabolic syndrome.

SA and HPA systems are both known to exert marked insulin resistance. This is especially true with responses of serum cortisol, as it regulates glucose levels in the blood, with all of the accompanying consequences. To summarize, mental stress might contribute to the development of MetS and subsequently increase the risk of CHD and diabetes via the SA and HPA axes, with increased cortisol secretion being of basic importance (see **Figure 2**).

MetS and Environmental Stress

Evidence of the contribution of environmental stress to MetS via increased reactivity of the stress axis was first derived from animal experiments. It was shown that in standardized experimental stress situations, macaque monkeys reacted with helplessness and loss of control (i.e., with a behavioral stress reaction) and responded with an increased level of cortisol and detached MetS symptoms, especially body fat. Comparable findings have been reported with rats exposed to chronic, uncontrollable environmental stress.

In line with animal studies, it was shown in laboratory experiments with human beings that persons with a high level of MetS symptoms were likely to express elevated responses of serum cortisol during task-induced mental stress.

Research has predominantly emphasized the role of the HPA axis when searching for the mechanism mediating the relationship between stress and MetS. Enhanced sympathetic activity (SA activity) is, however, important as well because chronic sympathetic overactivity with hemodynamic consequences (increased heart rate and pulse pressure) may have pathogenic importance in the development of MetS.

It is also known that long-lasting stress predisposes a person to stronger acute stress reactions, both mental and physical; that is, chronically stressed individuals are likely to show greater reactivity to and prolonged recovery from short-term challenging tasks.

Evidence of the influence of stress on MetS has mostly been based on laboratory experiments, whereas real-life situations, that is, the influence of everyday mental stress, especially long-lasting stress, have not been well studied. The risk characteristic that has been systematically shown to be related to both reactivity of the HPA axis and MetS is vital exhaustion. Vital exhaustion is seen as an indicator of long-lasting mental stress and is characterized by feelings of excessive fatigue, loss of energy, increased irritability, and demoralization. It is also well established that vital exhaustion is a risk factor for CHD, especially for myocardial infarction. The highest risk here, however, is not related to a high level of cortisol but to hypocortisolemia, a state in which both mental and physiological reservoirs are unavailable. This questions the common argument that high risk would be related to high cortisol secretion.

We also know that several coronary-prone personality characteristics, such as type A behavior (i.e., a behavior pattern consisting of aggression, impatience, high striving for achievement, ambitiousness, competitiveness), hostility, and anger, are related to perceived stress and reactivity of SA and the HPA axis. They are also related to components of MetS, even though the empirical findings have not been consistent.

If environmental stress is likely to increase the level of MetS, there is also an inverse effect: environmental support is able to decrease the level of MetS. It is known that changes in perceived social support are associated inversely with changes in the MetS level; that is, increasing support decreases the level of MetS and vice versa. The effect of social support in stress and diseases is widely documented. It increases the overall positive effect, feelings of self-worth and acceptance. It may exert stress-buffering effects by affecting the appraisal of potential stressors or by bolstering coping efforts.

Development of MetS in Childhood

It is generally accepted that atherosclerosis, the underlying process of CHD, originates in childhood and adolescence and that CHD risk factors are already present then. In addition, fasting insulin levels in early adolescence have been shown to predict type II diabetes in young adulthood.

The MetS precursors also appear to be present as early as childhood. It has been shown that the essential parameters of MetS express strong clustering and high tracking, even in healthy children and adolescents. Consequently, the potential effect of stress on the parameters of MetS even in childhood and adolescence has evoked interest. Until recently, the studies were few in number. There are, however, findings that suggest that a stress-prone and inappropriate childhood environment predisposes a child to a high level and early tracking of the parameters of MetS. Sources of environmental childhood stress are, of course, likely to stem from the family environment, especially from parental child-rearing practices. It is well established that a mother's hostile child rearing, consisting of a strict disciplinary style, a tendency to emotionally reject the child, and a feeling that the child is a burden on her, preventing her self-fulfillment, indicates an environmental stress that, in some studies, has been shown to be correlated with an elevated level of a child's MetS parameters.

With regard to the child's own characteristics, some components of type A behavior in adolescence predict changes in the level of MetS, with aggressive competitiveness being especially associated with an increase of that syndrome. In addition, some findings suggest that childhood temperament, especially hyperactivity and negative emotionality, is associated with and predict a later elevated level of MetS (see Figure 3).

MetS and Inherited Temperament

The findings previously described are related to the question of whether inherited temperament could play a role as a stress buffer or make a person vulnerable to stress and consequently explain a variance of MetS. Temperament refers to biologically rooted individual differences in behavioral reactions and dispositions that are present early in life and are relatively stable across time and situations. Temperament

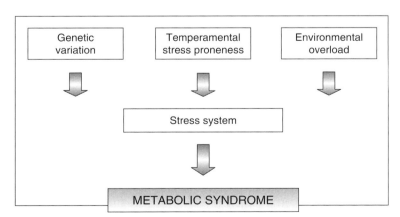

Figure 3   Origins of metabolic syndrome.

is an inherited core of personality; personality is developed by the interaction of inherited temperament and environment, mostly parental child-rearing practices.

Temperament has its origins in brain structures, and individual differences in temperament reflect innate differences in neuroendocrine and autonomic nervous system functions. Therefore, a biologically determined temperament has been viewed as one of the sources responsible for individual differences in stress proneness. It has been suggested to explain the variance in events that are experienced as stressful, and especially why daily troubles have greater health consequences for some individuals than others. There is, indeed, increasing evidence that differences in SA and HPA systems, i.e., differences in major stress systems, are attributable to different temperament profiles.

Findings suggest that childhood temperament plays a direct and indirect role in a development of MetS; that is, it interacts with the environment, meaning that some childhood temperamental factors (e.g., hyperactivity and negative emotionality) are related to an adulthood risk for MetS. In addition, childhood temperament also has an indirect effect. It has been suggested that the influence of hostile maternal child-rearing practices on the child's MetS level may be mediated by the child's temperament. Children with a difficult temperament, conceptualized in terms of negative emotionality (aggression and anger prone-ness), high activity, and low sociability, are especially vulnerable. Children with this type of temperament are especially prone to high levels of MetS when faced with hostile child rearing.

Interest in the role of adulthood temperament in individual stress reactions has been increasing of late. Findings have conflicted slightly with previous opinions on risk personality. A coronary-prone personality has traditionally been described in terms of hostility, depression, social aloneness, and type A behavior. In contrast, risk temperament is not primarily related to these kind of features; the most vulnerable individuals (i.e., persons who expressed systematically high levels of MetS) are those dealing with oversocialization and overresponsibility. These persons are highly sensitive to social cues of approval or the praise of others, have a strong tendency to conform to peer pressures, and are sensitive to the rejection of others, leading to excessive reward-seeking behaviors such as overworking in response to social rejection or frustration. As workers, they are persistent overachievers who frequently push themselves to exhaustion.

Issues concerning the role of temperament in physiological and neuroendocrine stress reactivity are still new and thus in process. The findings, however, have been promising for explaining the complicated relationship between mental stress and MetS. The findings also suggest that psychological and physiological stress symptoms might have the same source – it may be possible in the future to find a solid neurobiological basis for both psychological and physiological stress reactions.

See Also the Following Articles

Atherosclerosis; Heart Disease/Attack; Stress, Insulin Resistance and Type II Diabetes; Environmental Stress, Effects on Human Performance; Type A Personality, Type B Personality; Hypothalamic-Pituitary-Adrenal.

Further Reading

Björntorp, P. (1991). Metabolic implications of body fat distribution. *Diabetes Care* **14**, 1132.

Björntorp, P. (1992). Regional fat distribution: implications for type II diabetes. *International Journal of Obesity* **16** (supplement 4), S19–S27.

Björntorp, P. and Rosmond, R. (2000). The metabolic syndrome – a neuroendocrine disorder? *British Journal of Nutrition* **83**(supplement 1), S49–S57.

Black, P. H. (2003). The inflammatory response is an integral part of the stress response: implications for atherosclerosis, insulin resistance, type II diabetes and metabolic syndrome X. *Brain, Behavior, and Immunity* **17**, 350–364.

DeFronzo, R. A. and Ferrannini, E. (1991). Insulin resistance: a multifaceted syndrome responsible for NIDDM, obesity, hypertension, dyslipidemia, and atherosclerotic vascular disease. *Diabetes Care* **14**, 173–194.

Hansel, B., Giral, P., Nobecourt, E., et al. (2004). Metabolic syndrome is associated with elevated oxidative stress and dysfunctional dense high-density lipoprotein particles displaying impaired antioxidative activity. *The Journal of Clinical Endocrinology and Metabolism* **89**, 4963–4971.

Hjemdahl, P. (2002). Stress and the metabolic syndrome: an interesting but enigmatic association. *Circulation* **106**, 2634–2636.

Julius, S. and Gudbrandsson, T. (1992). Early association of sympathetic overactivity, hypertension, insulin re-sistance, and coronary risk. *Journal of Cardiovascular Pharmacology* **20**, S40–S48.

Keltikangas-Järvinen, L., Räikkonen, K., Hautanen, A., et al. (1996). Vital exhaustion, anger expression, and pituitary and adrenocortical hormones. *Arteriosclerosis, Thrombosis, and Vascular Biology* **16**, 275–280.

Lteif, A. and Mather, K. (2004). Insulin resistance, metabolic syndrome and vascular diseases: update on mechanistic linkages. *Canadian Journal of Cardiology* **20**(supplement B), 66B–76B.

Ravaja, N. and Keltikangas-Järvinen, L. (1995). Temperament and metabolic syndrome precursors in children: a three-year follow up. *Preventive Medicine* 24, 518–527.

Rosmond, R. (2005). Role of stress in the pathogenesis of the metabolic syndrome. *Psychoneuroendocrinology* 30, 1–10.

Räikkönen, K., Matthews, K. A. and Kuller, L. H. (2002). The relationship between psychological risk attributes and the metabolic syndrome in healthy women: antecedent or consequence? *Metabolism* 51, 1573–1577.

Seematter, G., Binnert, C., Martin, J. L., et al. (2004). Relationship between stress, inflammation and metabolism. *Current Opinion in Clinical Nutrition and Metabolic Care* 7, 169–173.

Metabolic Syndrome and Stress

R Rosmond
Björndammsterrassen 41, Partille, Sweden

This article is a revision of the previous edition article by P Björntorp and R Rosmond, volume 2, pp 747–749, © 2000, Elsevier Inc.

The Impact of Stress in Animal Studies
Effects of Stress in Humans
The Physiology of Stress
The Long-Term Effect of Stress on the Human Body
Concluding Remarks

Glossary

Metabolic syndrome	A well defined group of metabolic risk factors such as insulin resistance, atherogenic dyslipidemia, central (abdominal) obesity and hypertension.
Hypothalamic-pituitary-adrenal axis	The hormonostatic endocrine axis that regulates cortisol production and secretion.
Sympathetic nervous system	A division of the autonomic nervous system which mediates the response of the body to stress.

In recent years, scientists have recognized that some risk factors for cardiovascular disease and type 2 diabetes cluster together in certain people. The causal risk factors involved in the significant increase in cardiovascular disease and type 2 diabetes stem mostly from a now well-defined group of multiple metabolic risk factors called the metabolic syndrome (MetS). These risk factors include elevated insulin levels (insulin resistance), central (abdominal) obesity, atherogenic dyslipidemia, and hypertension. While these combined risk factors do not usually cause overt disease symptoms, it is obvious that persons with at least several of these correlated factors greatly increase the likelihood of atherosclerosis, heart disease, stroke, diabetes, kidney disease, and ultimately even premature death. Complicated genetic factors such as race, age, family weight, and diabetes history that interact equally with complicated cultural, dietary, psychosocial stress, exercise, and smoking factors, result in a heterogeneous at-risk patient group yet surprisingly consistent poor prognosis.

As MetS is gaining wider recognition in the clinic as a serious life-threatening condition, researchers and doctors are struggling to formalize the connections among all the diverse symptoms, risk factors, and correlated conditions. Of all the factors influencing MetS, chronic psychosocial stress is likely the most pervasive and controllable. Stress has long been recognized as a major contributor to hypertension, endocrine dysfunction, diabetes, and elevated cortisol-related conditions such as gluconeogenesis, increased serum glucose levels, decreased insulin production, perpetuation of catecholamine vasoconstriction, increased arterial blood pressure, fat and protein mobilization, and centralization of body fat. Considering the overlap in symptomatology between stress-correlated conditions and MetS, connecting the two, at least heuristically, is not a stretch. Indeed, solid evidence now exists that suggests the two conditions have reciprocal effects, with chronic stress including MetS and increased intra-abdominal fat and other hormonal dysfunction augmenting cortisol-induced stress and somatopsychic effects.

The Impact of Stress in Animal Studies

The activity of the hypothalamic-pituitary-adrenal (HPA) axis has been studied in several animal species in a variety of models of psychosocial stress. Not surprisingly, the majority of studies indicate that the HPA axis is activated in low-ranking animals in hierarchical social groups and in animals that have been defeated by a conspecific. However, activity and reactivity of the HPA axis has been shown to be modulated by a variety of different factors, including the species, gender, and behavioral style of the individuals.

Socially subordinated animals are generally more reactive to a novel stressor compared to their dominant counterparts, as shown in social groups of mice, rats, hamsters, guinea pigs, squirrel monkeys, and olive baboons. Taken together, these data indicate that social subordination and defeat appear to be stressful and lead to HPA axis activation. Chronic social stress can lead to long-term changes in HPA axis activity, including persistent elevations in basal glucocorticoids, abnormal responses to subsequent stressors, and impaired feedback regulation. For the most part, these effects are seen most clearly in subordinated animals housed in stable social groups; however, similar responses have been observed in dominant animals in such groups, and also in animals of all ranks in unstable social grouping.

Effects of Stress in Humans

Social stress is generally viewed as a major factor in the etiology of a variety of psychopathologies such as depression and anxiety, in addition to its effects on male and female reproduction, immune functioning, heart disease, etc. Social stress in people is often evaluated in terms of the number and magnitude of life events that an individual experience, and a general conclusion from this approach is that a plethora of moderately stressful events can have as great an impact as a few major events. Another important index that is strongly associated with the number of stressful events that are likely to be experience is social status. Low social status is regarded as having an impact on almost every area of the individual's life. Furthermore, the ranking difference itself, and the meaning assigned by the individual to his or her status with reference to others, may provide stress that is additional to (or interactive with) the material consequences of low status.

The Physiology of Stress

The stress response occurs through two major pathways in the human body: the central nervous system (CNS) and the endocrine system. The sympathetic nervous system (SNS) of the CNS that is involved when a stressor is encountered is the SNS stimulation of the adrenal glands, which, releases the catecholamines epinephrine (adrenaline) and norepinephrine (noradrenaline). The resulting fight-or-flight response via catecholamine release from end target neurons has an immediate effect by increasing heart rate, force of myocardial contraction and cardiac output, arterial blood pressure, blood coagulation, and serum glucose.

Simultaneously with nervous system stimulation, the hypothalamus and the pituitary glands secrete hormones into the general circulatory system. Once in the bloodstream, they arrive at the adrenal glands, which then secrete glucocorticoids, mainly cortisol, into the bloodstream to assist meeting the demands of the stressors. This endocrine pathway of hormones increases body metabolism, increases fatty acids in blood, increases blood pressure, and retains extra sodium, which results in increased water retention.

The Long-Term Effect of Stress on the Human Body

Since the early 1980s, a wealth of information has accumulated which illustrates that activation of the HPA axis leads to suppression of both the growth axis and the reproductive axis including activation of the sympathetic system. Chronic increase in cortisol, catecholamines, and chronic suppression of the growth and reproductive axes leads to a number of adverse health effects, and their sequelas result in increased morbidity and mortality.

Cortisol interferes at several levels of insulin action. In addition, cortisol inhibits insulin secretion from pancreatic β-cells. In primary cultured adipocytes, synthetic glucocorticoids (dexamethasone) induce progressive insulin resistance by sequentially regulating multiple aspects of the insulin-responsive glucose transport system. In the early stages, dexamethasone impairs the ability of insulin to translocate intracellular glucose transporters (GLUT 4) to the cell surface. Some, but not all, studies indicate that glucocorticoids may increase hepatic glucose metabolism. This diabetogenic effect of glucocorticoids is well characterized at least in animal models. In skeletal muscle, cortisol inhibits the glycogen synthase. Recent data indicate that subjects with insulin resistance do have an increased number of glucocorticoid receptors (GRs) in muscle.

In summary, initially hyperglycemia is accompanied by an increased insulin response to a glucose load, but eventually β-cell response becomes insufficient, and the unopposed actions of stress-related counterregulatory catabolic hormones (cortisol, catecholamines) serve to exacerbate the metabolic disturbances and contribute to the biochemical changes seen. This simplified account provides a framework within which the association between stress and insulin resistance can be understood.

Cortisol regulates adipose-tissue differentiation, function, and distribution, and in excess, causes visceral obesity. Glucocorticoids exert their cellular action by complexing with a specific cytoplasmic GR, which in turn translocates to the nucleus and binds to specific sites on chromatin. GRs belong to the superfamily of nuclear transcription factors. Cortisol exerts chronic effects on lipid metabolism. One of the most striking effects in humans is the centralization of body fat seen in Cushing syndrome, exhibited as severe truncal obesity. Excess cortisol promotes the activity of lipoprotein lipase (LPL), the primary enzyme responsible for conversion of lipoprotein triglyceride into free fatty acids and accumulation of triglycerides in adipocytes. The density of GRs, assessed by ligand-binding techniques and hybridization techniques with GR cRNA probes, is particularly high in intra-abdominal adipose tissue as compared to other regions. Furthermore, the antilipolytic action of insulin during the prevailing hyperinsulinemic state causes a blunted lipid mobilization, resulting in a condition with increased lipid accumulation. Moreover, in the presence of insulin, cortisol has a marked stimulatory effect on LPL activity in human adipose tissue *in vitro*. This effect involves both an increased level of LPL mRNA, leading to increased relative LPL synthesis, and additional posttranslational regulation.

The primary reason for considering stress as an etiologic factor relates to the influence of the SNS and neuroendocrine factors in hypertension, although high salt intake in some subjects may contribute through volume expansion. The principal hypothesis is that the stress-induced activation of hypothalamic, sympathohormonal regions occurs repeatedly over time, leading to cardiovascular adjustments that increase hypertension risk. Evidence relevant to this hypothesis derives from both animal and human experimental studies. Complications such as myocardial infarction and stroke are not directly due to elevated pressures, but to the resulting structural changes in the heart and blood vessels. One of the structural consequences of hypertension, hypertrophy of the left ventricle, is the strongest predictor, other than advancing age, of cardiovascular morbidity and mortality.

Concluding Remarks

The human body has many effector systems including the SNS and the HPA axis for maintaining homeostasis and connecting the brain with the periphery. Overall these systems interact both indirectly and directly. The HPA axis determines most of the acute and prolonged effects of stressors. The secretory end product of the HPA axis, cortisol, is kept within an optimal range through the feedback action of cortisol interacting with neural control mechanisms. Distressing events or situations evokes these two pathways of the stress response. However, each person's unique combination of heredity, life experience, personality, and ability to cope are all involved in the perception of an event and the meaning attached to it. Rather than confronting life-threatening stressors, life today centers around events that hold symbolic meaning; an upcoming test, a disagreement with a friend, or the boredom of a job.

Individuals with persistent psychosocial and socioeconomic handicaps such as anxiety and depression, poor economy, low education, and unemployment are more likely to suffer from frequent challenges of the SNS and the HPA axis. Thus, psychosocial stress preceded by genetic susceptibility that result in a disruption of central regulatory systems all adds up to less coping ability, followed by insulin resistance, atherogenic dyslipidemia, central (abdominal) obesity, and hypertension, that is, the metabolic syndrome.

Further Reading

Björntorp, P. and Rosmond, R. (2000). Obesity and cortisol. *Nutrition* 16, 924–936.

Björntorp, P., Holm, G., Rosmond, R., et al. (2000). Hypertension and the metabolic syndrome: closely related central origin? *Blood Pressure* 9, 71–82.

Charmandari, E., Tsigos, C. and Chrousos, G. (2005). Endocrinology of the stress response. *Annual Reviews in Physiology* 67, 259–284.

Dallman, M. F., Pecoraro, N. C. and la Fleur, S. E. (2005). Chronic stress and comfort foods: self-medication and abdominal obesity. *Brain Behavior and Immunity* 19, 275–280.

Henry, J. P. (1992). Biological basis of the stress response. *Integrative Physiological and Behavioral Science* 27, 66–83.

Hjemdahl, P. (2002). Stress and the metabolic syndrome: an interesting but enigmatic association. *Circulation* 106, 2634–2636.

Miller, D. B. and O'Callaghan, J. P. (2002). Neuroendocrine aspects of the response to stress. *Metabolism* 51, 5–10.

Rosmond, R., Dallman, M. F. and Björntorp, P. (1998). Stress-related cortisol secretion in men: relationships with abdominal obesity and endocrine, metabolic and hemodynamic abnormalities. *Journal of Clinical Endocrinology and Metabolism* 83, 1853–1859.

Metals, Oxidative Stress, and Brain Biology

D I Finkelstein, T Lynch, S Wilkins, R A Cherny and A I Bush
The Mental Health Research Institute of Victoria, Victoria, Australia

Introduction
Biometals in the Developing Organism
Biometals in the Adult
Parkinson's Disease
Alzheimer's Disease

Glossary

Alzheimer's disease (AD)	A progressive form of dementia with symptoms that include impaired memory, usually followed by impaired thought and speech. AD is histologically characterized by the deposition of extracellular amyloid plaques, the major constituent being the amyloid-β peptide (A-β).
Biometals	Metals found in living organisms that have defined physiological functions that serve to maintain normal cellular processes. These include copper (Cu), zinc (Zn), iron (Fe), and manganese (Mn).
Dopamine (DA)	A neurotransmitter that normally acts to reinforce behavior. Drugs of addiction act by causing dopamine release; a lack of dopamine results in the symptoms of Parkinson's disease. L-Dopa treatment provides the precursor for DA that partially compensates for the reduction of DA observed in Parkinson's disease.
Oxidative stress	The damage to cells caused by reactive oxygen species (ROS; e.g., hydrogen peroxide). Metals such as iron and copper are capable of redox chemistry in which a single electron may be accepted or donated by the metal, reacting with oxygen and thereby producing radicals and ROS. Oxidative stress is imposed on cells as a result of an increase in oxidant generation, a decrease in antioxidant protection, or a breakdown in oxidative damage-repair mechanisms.
Parkinson's disease (PD)	A debilitating disease occurring only in humans and resulting from a predominant loss of dopamine neurons. The symptoms include muscle rigidity, tremor, slow and shuffling gait, masklike facial expressions, and eventually cognitive decline and death. Some neurons
	contain Lewy bodies that consist of intracellular inclusions of α-synuclein.
Reactive oxygen species (ROS)	Natural by-products of the normal metabolism of oxygen that have important roles in cell signaling. During times of biological stress, ROS levels can increase, resulting in significant damage to, or death of neurons.
Substantia nigra (SN)	A specific part of the brain that is made up of neurons that contain the chemical neurotransmitter dopamine; loss of these cells occurs in Parkinson's disease.
Toxicological metals	Metals with no known normal biological function; these include lead and aluminum. These metals can interact with many proteins, resulting in the dysfunction of many biological processes.

Introduction

The brain is an exceptional tissue in that it concentrates biometals (copper, zinc, iron, and manganese) for its normal functional metabolism. Some of these processes include maintaining enzymatic and mitochondrial function, immunity, myelination, learning and memory, co-release with neurotransmitters, and binding with prion proteins. The importance of metals in antioxidant defense mechanisms should also be highlighted; for example, Cu/Zn superoxide dismutase protects against oxidative stress. The concentration of biometals in the brain, together with the brain's high levels of oxygen, appears to make the central nervous system vulnerable to a host of metal-centered pathologies.

Biometals in the Developing Organism

Deficiencies in biometals result in increased mortality, abnormal development, and poor growth. The accumulation of iron in the brain appears to be handled differently than the other biometals. Whereas copper, zinc, and manganese can be absorbed by the brain after the organ has developed, the neonatal period is critical for the establishment of normal iron content in the adult brain. Iron accumulates in the brain only while it is still growing; for rats and mice this occurs in the first few postnatal weeks, whereas in humans the period begins during the third trimester of pregnancy and is maintained throughout the first year of life. Iron, copper, zinc, and manganese are found in the milk of humans and other mammals. Mammalian milk meets the crucial supply requirements needed for the normal development of the neonate, with these biometals varying in concentration during the course of lactation. Interestingly, the iron content of milk is not reduced even when the iron status of the mother is poor, indicating tight regulation of the iron content of milk. Toxic milk syndromes have been observed in mice that have genetic defects in the copper or zinc pathways resulting in the abnormal delivery of these biometals, with significant biological consequences. Deliberately increasing the exposure of neonates to iron in this critical period has been shown to elevate iron levels in the adult brain.

Biometals in the Adult

Early studies used the term "trace element" to designate elements that are essential for normal function, including zinc, manganese, copper, iodine, iron, cobalt, molybdenum, tin, selenium, and chromium. The minimum nutritional requirements for individuals are hotly debated in the popular and scientific literature and are not discussed here. What is clear is that various genetic mutations can cause a disruption in the homeostasis of these elements, resulting in dramatic biological consequences (e.g., Segawa's syndrome and iron; Wilson's disease and copper). Biometals normally bind to a range of specific proteins (e.g., Cu/Zn and Mn bind to superoxide dismutase; Cu binds to the prion protein). Poisoning occurs when the levels of biometals exceed the body's capacity to bind them to specific metal-binding proteins. Two outcomes likely to result from this are that (1) the metal binds to an incorrect protein, causing dysfunction in a biological system or (2) the presence of such metals in an unbound form causes oxidative stress, which damages cells.

Parkinson's Disease

Parkinson's disease (PD) is characterized by the loss of dopaminergic neurons of the substantia nigra (SN) and the deposition of intracellular inclusion bodies. The principal component of these deposits is the α-synuclein protein that is expressed throughout the brain, and mutations in this protein (A30P and A53T) are responsible for familial forms of the disease. The association between iron and PD is multifaceted and complex; too little iron leads to neurological deficits, yet too much appears to result in neuronal loss. There is long-standing evidence of a selective increase in iron in the SN of patients with PD as well as an accumulation in animals following artificially induced lesions to the SN. Iron is required for the synthesis of dopamine (DA): tyrosine hydroxylase, a nonheme

iron-containing enzyme uses molecular oxygen to hydroxylate tyrosine, resulting in the formation of L-Dopa, the natural biochemical precursor of DA and the most common medication for the treatment of PD. Mutations in the iron-binding site of tyrosine hydroxylase have been identified in cases of L-dopa-responsive PD and Segawa's syndrome (a rare hereditary progressive dystonia with diurnal fluctuation). Other redox-active metals such as manganese have been associated with neurological disorders. Among the neurological effects of manganese poisoning (linked to occupational exposure) is an irreversible Parkinsonian-like syndrome. The specific mechanisms of the toxicity are not known.

Redox-active iron, α-synuclein, and DA are abundant in the SN. The three elements colocalized at one anatomical location can interact to generate toxic reactive oxygen species (ROS). It is apparent, however, that none of these elements alone is sufficient to perpetuate the neurodegeneration of PD: rather, the combination of iron, α-synuclein, and DA together generates toxic products. For instance, DA is a potent chelator of transition metals and can generate hydrogen peroxide in the presence of iron (or copper) and α-synuclein. Under these conditions, α-synuclein molecules link to form soluble aggregates known as oligomers. These oligomers are thought to be deposited as the microscopically visible intracellular inclusion bodies called Lewy bodies. This pathological mechanism has parallels with Alzheimer's disease, in which current theory suggests that soluble oligomeric intermediates, rather than the visible aggregates (plaques), are the cause of neurodegeneration.

Alzheimer's Disease

Alzheimer's disease (AD) is characterized by the deposition of extracellular amyloid plaques, the major constituent being the amyloid-β protein (A-β) that is cleaved from the membrane-bound amyloid precursor protein. There is considerable evidence for an imbalance in the homeostasis of biometals in AD, which is reflected by specific alterations in metal levels in the brain (in areas such as the hippocampus, amygdala, neocortex, and olfactory bulb). These observations take into account the varying background of biometals that exists throughout life. Not only do the levels of biometals change with age, but so do the concentrations of different metal transport and storage proteins. Whereas metal levels in the brains of laboratory mice rise dramatically with age, studies of brain-metal content in aging humans are less conclusive. Interestingly, of the major biometals only zinc appears to be elevated in tissue from the human AD brain. However, copper, zinc, and iron are present in very high concentrations, bound to the aggregated A-β that makes up the amyloid plaques. Although the normal function of A-β is unknown, it has been proposed that the biochemical environment of the aging brain provides conditions in which the A-β protein pathologically binds to copper and zinc, causing it to form oligomers that foster unregulated redox activity and toxic free-radical formation. A paradoxical consequence of the buildup of metals in the amyloid plaques is that the brain cells become deficient in these crucial biometal components, rendering them more susceptible to oxidative stress.

Further Reading

Barnham, K. J., Masters, C. L. and Bush, A. I. (2004). Neurodegenerative diseases and oxidative stress. *Nature Reviews Drug Discovery* 3(3), 205–214.

Berg, D., Gerlach, M. B., Youdim, K. L., et al. (2001). Brain iron pathways and their relevance to Parkinson's disease. *Journal of Neurochemistry* 79(2), 225–236.

Blennow, K., de Leon, M. J. and Zetterberg, H. (2006). Alzheimer's disease. *Lancet* 368(9533), 387–403.

Huang, X., Atwood, M., Hartshorn, G., et al. (1999). The A peptide of Alzheimer's disease directly produces hydrogen peroxide through metal ion reduction. *Biochemistry* 38(24), 7609–7616.

Lynch, T., Cherny, R. A. and Bush, A. I. (2000). Oxidative processes in Alzheimer's disease: the role of abeta-metal interactions. *Experimental Gerontology* 35(4), 445–451.

Lonnerdal, B., Keen, C. L. and Hurley, L. S. (1981). Iron, copper, zinc, and manganese in milk. *Annual Review of Nutrition* 1, 149–174.

Religa, D., Strozyk, R. A., Cherny, I., et al. (2006). Elevated cortical zinc in Alzheimer disease. *Neurology* 67(1), 69–75.

Metastasization

M K Demetrikopoulos
Institute for Biomedical Philosophy, Atlanta, GA, USA

This article is a revision of the previous edition article by M K Demetrikopoulos, volume 2, pp 750–751, © 2000, Elsevier Inc.

Glossary

Interferon	Glycoproteins produced by cells infected with a virus which inhibit viral growth and may be useful to treat tumors.
Metastasis	The spread of malignant tumor to a distant site.
Natural killer (NK) cell	A white blood cell that can kill certain types of cancer cells.
Prospective	An experimental design which is forward-looking.
Retrospective	A design which looks back and reviews aspects of a clinical situation.
Rotational stress	Physical stressor whereby subject's cage is gently, but continuously, moved in a circle on a horizontal plain.
Tumor progression	A measure of the cancer's metastasis, size, and/or weight.

While there is ample evidence which suggests that stress can have immunomodulatory effects, prediction of disease outcome based on generalizations from studies which examine *in vitro* immune function is difficult since the direction and degree of immunomodulation has been shown to be dependent on both the stimulus parameters employed and the immune variables under study. Therefore, research has been directed at examining disease-specific outcomes such as the effects of stress on cancer. This article will provide a brief overview of the effect of stress on cancer by examining how a variety of physical and psychological factors can effect tumor progression in both animal subjects and human patients. Additionally, the article will suggest possible mechanisms for this phenomena by presenting several known modifiers of tumor progression (i.e., hormones and neurochemicals) that are relevant in a discussion of the physiological consequences of stress. While it is well beyond the scope of this article to fully review this topic, several illustrative examples will be presented which were selected in order to demonstrate the complexity of this subject or because of their clinical relevance.

Physical Stress and Tumor Progression in Animals

Physical stressors are generally more easily defined than psychological stressors since they involve the imposition of a specific external condition or stimulus. It is important to be aware, however, that the imposition of these conditions will likely initiate a cascade of both physiological and psychological reactions to the stimulus.

There are a variety of physical stressors that have been shown to effect tumor growth in animal subjects including exposure to cold, changes in light/dark cycles, dietary restrictions, rotation, restraint, forced swim, and surgery. The complexity of the physiological and psychological cascade that follows the imposition of a rather simplistic physical stressor, such as rotation, is illustrated by a study by Zorzet et al. (2002: 368). Similar to their findings with restraint stress, they found a circannual rhythm in the expression of metastasis with rotational stress increasing metastasis volume in June and decreasing it in February compared to controls. The antitumor agent cyclophosphamide was able to block metastasis in the control mice but not in the mice in the rotational stress condition. Furthermore, the survival time of control mice in February was twice as long as in June. In all groups, survival time was inversely correlated with number of metastases, and number of CD3+ and CD4+ splenic T lymphocytes. The authors suggested that T-lymphocyte-mediated immune responses that vary seasonally were modulated by the rotational stress.

Psychological Stress and Tumor Progression in Animals

Psychological stress models provide a mechanism for studying the effects of psychological phenomena on tumor progression and serve as potential models for the effects of stress and psychiatric illness on cancer since the physical components of the stressors are either minimal or appropriately controlled for. A variety of psychological stressors have been shown to be important modifiers of tumor progression including handling, inescapable shock, housing, and social dominance. An important test of the psychological component of a physiological reaction is whether or not the response can be conditioned.

For example, Wu et al. (2001: 1) examined the effects of social isolation on liver metastasis in mice. Metastasis formation was quicker in the isolation stress condition such that isolated mice had five times the incidence of metastasis on day 7. The effect of isolation was evident across several measures such that metastasis was more likely in the isolated stress condition even with a smaller tumor challenge; survival time was shorter in the stress mice; and stressed mice did not respond as well to cisplatin chemotherapy. The fact that there was an effect on survival is particularly important since it would suggest that the effects are biologically meaningful to cancer development.

Psychological Stress and Tumor Progression in Humans

The relationship of psychological phenomena with cancer in human subjects has been reviewed in a series of papers presented in *Social Science Medicine* special issue *Cancer and the Mind*, 1985. Geyer (1993: 1545) found more severe life events and chronic difficulties in women with malignant breast cancer compared to women with benign lumps. Similarly, Hatch et al. (1990: 397) presented data which suggested that an increased rate of cancer living near the Three Mile Island nuclear accident was due to the stressfulness of the event and not due to the minimally increased radioactivity levels. While these studies suggest that a possible relation between psychological phenomena and tumor initiation may occur, the results are difficult to interpret given the fact that the data are mostly retrospective in nature. A prospective intervention by Spiegel et al. (1989: 888) examined the effect of a psychosocial intervention on survival time of women with metastatic breast cancer and found that survival time was essentially doubled in the intervention group compared to the control group. While this study did not address the effects of psychological phenomena on the early stages of cancer development, it demonstrated that psychosocial factors can modify the progression of cancer in patients and effect the survival time of patients with advanced disease. A more recent study by Butow et al. (2000: 469) demonstrated similar findings in that they showed that patients, who reported that they had minimized the impact of cancer in their lives, survived metastatic breast cancer longer.

Modifiers of Tumor Progression

A variety of factors are important in stress-induced tumor progression including hormonal modulation, neurochemical modulation, and the use of psychiatric pharmaceuticals. However, determining the influence of any particular variable is difficult due to the interrelationships of these systems. Additionally, many of these compounds are known to have diurnal, monthly, and yearly cycles which may interact in various ways with their stress-induced patterns of expression thus contributing to the difficulty of elucidating their individual contribution to mediating stress-induced changes in tumor progression.

In spite of the complexity just suggested, it has been demonstrated that a variety of hormonal factors contribute to stress-induced tumor progression including corticosterone, melatonin, estrogen, and prolactin among others. For example, the effects of estrogen have been suggested to be important for some forms of breast cancer. Experimental evidence by several investigators have begun to explore the underlying mechanism of this phenomenon including examination of the effects of tumor exposure during different phases of the menstrual cycle.

In addition to the contribution of hormonal factors on tumor progression, a variety of neurochemical factors act as modifiers of tumor progression including opiates and catecholamines. This line of research is especially clinically relevant since pain management is an important consideration in cancer patients. Gaining an understanding of the central nervous system pathways which can effect stress-induced changes in tumor progression will likely lead to improvements in pain management that do not contribute to tumor development. For example, a study by Gaspani et al. (2002: 18) demonstrated that the analgesic drug tramadol blocked the increased metastatic effect of surgery stress in rats. They suggested this was mediated by natural killer (NK) cells since tramadol increased NK cell activity in nonoperated subjects. This is in marked contrast to the typical suppression in NK activity that has been repeatedly demonstrated with morphine and other opiates used for patients undergoing surgery for cancer.

Furthermore, since the effects of stressors on tumor progression are likely due to the activation of psychological modifiers, it may be possible to intervene by the use of anxiolytic or antidepressant agents. In fact, stress models often demonstrate an amelioration of the detrimental effects of short-term stressors by anxiolytic agents and an amelioration of the effects of long-term or uncontrollable stressors by the use of antidepressant agents.

Hormonal and neurochemical agents may effect tumor progression directly by causing changes in tumor growth and also indirectly by modification of immune-related functioning. In fact, the majority of hormonal and neurochemical changes that occur following stress have known consequences on immune cells. For example, the effects of opiates on tumor progression have been shown to be related to changes in NK cell functioning. In addition to this, stress effects on tumor progression may be due to changes in NK number as well as due to changes in T and B cell number and/or functioning. Additionally, Wu et al. (2000: 1) have demonstrated that factors such as vascular endothelial growth factor, hepatocyte growth factor, and tumor necrosis factor α may be involved in metastasis by mediating the overexpression of normal endothelial cell functions such as migration, invasion, and tube formation.

Conclusion

The relation of stress to cancer has been suggested since at least the time of Galen and there have been many experimental studies which have attempted to elucidate this phenomenon since then. In testimony to the complexity of the subject, two earlier reviews came to vastly different conclusions as to the role of stress in cancer. In the first review, Sklar and Anisman (1981: 369) present a hypothesis that seems to be well supported by recent findings such that the chronicity of the stressor, the prior experience of the subject, controllability, and social context seem to be the major determining factors in predicting the direction of tumor progression. Additionally, the exact timing of an acute stressor in relation to the presentation of the tumor can dramatically effect the experimental outcome. They suggest that these factors may be producing enhanced tumor development by depleting brain catecholamines and increasing acetylcholine. In the second review, Justice (1985: 108) focused on the types of tumors studied and suggested that tumors be differentiated into viral and nonviral tumors; and the stress response could be thought of as having stages including a rebound or recovery stage following the presentation of an acute stressor. Justice hypothesized that viral tumors were enhanced during stress, were diminished during rebound or recovery to stress, and were the only type of tumors mediated through the immune system. Conversely, nonviral tumors were regulated outside of the immune system and were diminished during stress and enhanced during the rebound to stress. While there continues to be some studies which support this hypothesis, there are many studies that are contradictory. Yet, his review is an important reminder that it is necessary to understand the nature of the tumor understudy when designing and interpreting experimental studies. Another review by Demetrikopoulos et al. (1999: 417) presents a more thorough discussion of the relevance of these older reviews to the more recent findings and presents an overview of the current literature. A review by Ben-Eliyahu (2003: S27) examines a subset of this literature in detail and examines the effects of surgical stress on metastasis. This review explores the effects of cell-mediated immunity and explores possible therapeutic approaches that could be employed to reduce the effects of the surgical stress.

Overall, both physical and psychological stressors have been shown to effect tumor progression with most enhancing tumor growth and/or development. The mediators of this phenomenon are many and include a variety of both hormonal and neurochemical factors that are most likely utilizing central nervous system pathways that are important in anxiety and depression. Furthermore, the mechanisms underlying the effects of hormonal and neurochemical mediators on cancer include direct effects on tumors as well as modification of immunological functioning.

Further Reading

Ader, R., Felten, D. L. and Cohen, N. (eds.) (2001). *Psychoneuroimmunology* (3rd edn.). New York: Academic Press.

Ben-Eliyahu, S. (2003). The promotion of tumor metastasis by surgery and stress: immunological basis and implications for psychoneuroimmunology. *Brain Behavior and Immunity* 17, S27–S36.

Butow, P. N., Coates, A. S. and Dunn, S. M. (2000). Psychosocial predictors of survival: metastatic breast cancer. *Annals of Oncology* 11, 469–474.

Demetrikopoulos, M. K., Weiss, J. M. and Goldfarb, R. H. (1999). Environmental factors: stress and disease. In: McEwen, B. S. (ed.) *Handbook of Physiology: Coping with the Environment*, pp. 417–512. Oxford: Oxford University Press.

Gaspani, L., Bianchi, M., Limiroli, E., et al. (2002). The analgesic drug tramadol prevents the effect of surgery on natural killer cell activity and metastatic colonization in rats. *Journal of Neuroimmunology* 129, 18–24.

Geyer, S. (1993). Life events, chronic difficulties and vulnerability factors preceding breast cancer. *Social Science and Medicine* 37, 1545–1555.

Hatch, M. C., Beyea, J., Nieves, J. W., et al. (1990). Cancer near the Three Mile Island nuclear plant: radiation emissions. *American Journal of Epidemiology* 132, 397–412.

Justice, A. (1985). Review of the effects of stress on cancer in laboratory animals: importance of time of stress application and type of tumor. *Psychological Bulletin* 98, 108–138.

Sklar, L. S. and Anisman, H. (1981). Stress and cancer. *Psychological Bulletin* 89, 369–406.

Speigel, D., Bloom, J. R., Kraemer, H. C., et al. (1989). Effect of psychosocial treatment on survival of patients with metastatic breast cancer. *Lancet* 2, 888–891.

Vallejo, R., Hord, E. D., Barna, S. A., et al. (2003). Perioperative immunosuppression in cancer patients. *Journal of Environmental Pathology, Toxicology and Oncology* 22, 139–146.

Wu, W., Murata, J., Hayashi, K., et al. (2001). Social isolation stress impairs the resistance of mice to experimental liver metastasis of murine colon 26-L5 carcinoma cells. *Biological and Pharmaceutical Bulletin* 24, 772–776.

Wu, W., Murata, J., Murakami, K., et al. (2000). Social isolation stress augments angiogenesis induced by colon 26-L5 carcinoma cells in mice. *Clinical and Experimental Metastasis* 18, 1–10.

Zorzet, S., Perissin, L., Rapozzi, V., et al. (2002). Seasonal dependency of the effects of rotational stress and cyclophosphamide in mice bearing Lewis lung carcinoma. *Brain Behavior and Immunity* 16, 368–382.

Social Science and Medicine: Cancer and the Mind. (1985). 20. [A series of reviews].

Methylation of Genes/Imprinting, Stress Induced *See:* Early Environment and Adult Stress.

Metyrapone: Basic and Clinical Studies

E A Young
University of Michigan, Ann Arbor, MI, USA

This article is a revision of the previous edition article by E A Young, volume 2, pp 752–756, © 2000, Elsevier Inc.

Clinical Uses
Clinical Research Studies
Basic Science Studies

Glossary

11-Deoxycortisol	The immediate steroid precursor for cortisol.
11-β-Hydroxylase	The enzyme responsible for the conversion of 11-deoxycortisol to cortisol.
Cushing's disease/ syndrome	An endocrine disease due to excessive cortisol secretion. The syndrome may be due to a pituitary adenoma secreting intact adrenocorticotropic hormone as well as the larger precursor forms (Cushing's disease; pituitary-dependent Cushing's) or to an adrenal adenoma secreting cortisol (pituitary-independent Cushing's syndrome).
Depression	Major depression as defined by DSM-IV, consisting of a collection of symptoms of at least two weeks duration leading to impairment in day to day functioning.
Hypercortisolemia	Increased plasma cortisol, which occurs in Cushing's patients and in a subset of patients with depression.
Ovine corticotropin releasing hormone (oCRH)	The protein sequence of the hypothalamic CRH found in sheep, in which the hormone was initially isolated.
Panhypopituitarism	A disease characterized by the failure of multiple endocrine systems at the pituitary level, usually secondary to the injury of the pituitary.

Metyrapone is an 11-β-hydroxylase enzyme inhibitor that consequently blocks the last step in the synthesis of cortisol in the adrenal, which results in the secretion of 11-deoxycortisol, an inactive adrenal steroid (**Figure 1**). By blocking cortisol synthesis, metyrapone leads to the inhibition of glucocorticoid negative feedback, and this opens up the closed feedback loop of the hypothalamic-pituitary-adrenal (HPA) axis, leading to rebound adrenocorticotropic hormone (ACTH) secretion. The presence of an open feedback loop allows the researcher to investigate the hypothalamic and pituitary components of the axis under controlled conditions. Metyrapone is used primarily in human studies, whereas adrenalectomy is generally used in studies of experimental animals to accomplish the same goals. However, a few studies have investigated the effects of metyrapone in rodents.

Clinical Uses

In clinical endocrinology, metyrapone is used primarily in the diagnosis of Cushing's syndrome to distinguish excessive cortisol secretion secondary to excessive ACTH from an adrenal cause for cortisol hypersecretion in the absence of ACTH hypersecretion. In cases of a pituitary adenoma, the ACTH response is augmented tremendously with metyrapone blockade of cortisol synthesis, whereas hypercortisolemia from an adrenal adenoma is accompanied by a lesser ACTH response. With the advent of newer, more sensitive ACTH assays, as well as magnetic resonance imaging technology, this test may be less critical to the diagnosis of Cushing's syndrome than previously thought. In addition, metyrapone is used in the diagnosis of panhypopituitarism to determine if the patient is capable of responding to a stimulus to the HPA axis. In the past, metyrapone has been used as a treatment for hypercortisolemia in Cushing's disease, but the blockade of cortisol is too short term and the side effects limit its usefulness. In addition, one open-label study suggested that it was helpful in patients with depression. A recent placebo-controlled study suggested its potential usefulness in the treatment of refractory cases of major depression; these patients did not necessarily manifest baseline hypercortisolemia. Currently, ketoconazole is the preferred glucocorticoid synthesis inhibitor for the treatment of hypercortisolemia.

Clinical Research Studies

In addition to its standard clinical use, metyrapone is a useful research tool. In normal subjects given metyrapone between 8 a.m. and 2 p.m., brisk rebound ACTH secretion is observed 2 h following metyrapone administration, at which point cortisol levels have fallen to 3–4 $\mu g\ dl^{-1}$ (**Figure 2**). In normal subjects, the administration of metyrapone in the late afternoon and evening (between 4 and 10 p.m.) does not lead to rebound ACTH secretion. This is an indication that hypothalamic drive (endogenous

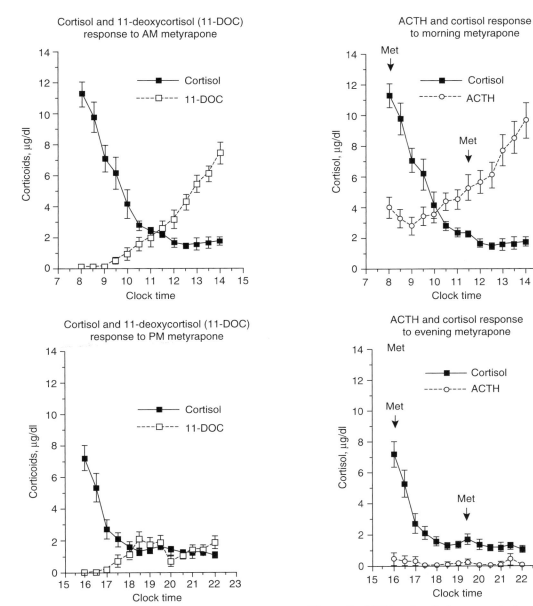

Figure 1 Administration of metyrapone leads to the blockade of cortisol production and secretion of 11-deoxycortisol, shown for both morning and evening administration in normal subjects.

Figure 2 ACTH and cortisol response to the administration of metyrapone in the morning and evening in normal subjects. Following the blockade of cortisol production, rebound ACTH secretion is observed in the morning but not in the evening.

corticotropin releasing hormone, CRH) is inactive during this time. Alternatively, it may be that the low levels of cortisol still present under metyrapone blockade (between 1 and 2 µg dl^{-1}) are able to exert the necessary inhibitory effect through high-affinity mineralocorticoid receptors. Using this same approach in depressed patients, we were able to demonstrate increased hypothalamic drive in the evening in depressed patients, whereas their ACTH response to metyrapone in the morning is relatively the same as controls. These studies suggest that depressed patients demonstrate increased brain CRH in the

evening. A recent report of ours also found a link between excessive response to metyrapone and failure to respond to a 6-week course of fluoxetine. In addition to studies of major depression, metyrapone has been used as a probe of HPA axis function in anxiety disorders, in which the data are mixed. One study of posttraumatic stress disorder showed increased ACTH secretion, but two other studies showed a normal ACTH response. One study of panic disorder also demonstrated a normal response.

Metyrapone has been used by a number of investigators to block glucocorticoid negative feedback in conjunction with CRH challenge studies. Metyrapone is particularly useful in reducing the effects of high baseline cortisol on the response to CRH and thus evaluating the true corticotroph response. The original studies by de Bold and colleagues demonstrated an increased ACTH response to oCRH in normal subjects given metyrapone compared to the same subjects given oCRH without metyrapone pretreatment. De Bold and colleagues were further able to characterize the effects of cortisol infusion following metyrapone plus oCRH challenge, thus demonstrating that the rise in cortisol induced by oCRH plays a significant role in terminating the ACTH response to oCRH. From these studies, it appears that both baseline cortisol and oCRH-induced increases in cortisol affect the ACTH response to oCRH.

Because patients with major depression demonstrate increased baseline cortisol, their ACTH response to oCRH is decreased. This has been observed in all studies. A number of investigators have examined the response to oCRH challenge under metyrapone in depressed patients. Studies by von Bardeleben and colleagues compared the response to oCRH under metyrapone in depressed patients to that of normal and depressed subjects given oCRH alone and concluded that elevated baseline cortisol was responsible for the diminished response to oCRH in depressed patients. However, these studies did not include normal subjects given oCRH plus metyrapone. Subsequent studies by Young and coworkers and Lisansky and coworkers using controls treated with metyrapone plus CRH confirmed a normal-to-augmented response to oCRH, thus arguing against CRH receptor downregulation in depression.

Metyrapone has also been used to evaluate the kinetics of ACTH inhibition by cortisol following cortisol infusion. Using metyrapone to augment the ACTH response, investigators have infused cortisol to study the fast feedback regulation of ACTH, although metyrapone pretreatment is not necessary to demonstrate fast feedback in humans.

Basic Science Studies

As stated previously, the majority of basic studies used adrenalectomy as a stimulus to ACTH secretion. However, in attempts to reduce the surgical stress involved in adrenalectomy, a few investigators have used metyrapone as a pharmacological adrenalectomy. These studies confirmed that metyrapone administration leads to an increase in both CRH and arginine vasopressin (AVP) in the hypophysial portal blood. Following treatment with metyrapone, a short-term rise was observed in plasma ACTH and β-endorphins

in rats, with a return to normal levels within 4 h. Plasma levels remained low at 24 h. However, by 72 h, ACTH secretion was again elevated. This same pattern was observed to be independent of whether metyrapone was administered during the peak of circadian activation (the evening) or the trough of activation (the morning). The measurement of pro-opiomelanocortin (the ACTH precursor) mRNA in the anterior pituitary and CRH mRNA in the paraventricular nucleus of the hypothalamus also demonstrated at least a 24-h lag time in the effects of metyrapone on steady-state mRNA levels. This lag in the plasma secretory response to the removal of negative feedback in rodents was also observed by Jacobson and colleagues using a different model. This finding contrasts to studies in humans (described earlier) in which rebound ACTH secretion was observed relatively promptly following the removal of glucocorticoid negative feedback during the peak of circadian activation.

See Also the Following Articles

Adrenocorticotropic Hormone (ACTH); Corticotropin Releasing Factor (CRF); Cushing's Syndrome, Medical Aspects; Cushing's Syndrome, Neuropsychiatric Aspects.

Further Reading

de Bold, C. R., Jackson, R. V., Kamilaris, T. C., et al. (1989). Effects of ovine corticotropin-releasing hormone on adrenocorticotropin secretion in the absence of glucocorticoid feedback inhibition in man. *Journal of Clinical Endocrinology and Metabolism* **68**, 431–437.

Jacobson, L., Akana, S. F., Cascio, C. S., et al. (1989). The adrenocortical system responds slowly to removal of corticosterone in the absence of concurrent stress. *Endocrinology* **124**, 2144–2152.

Jahn, H., Schick, M., Kiefer, F., et al. (2004). Metyrapone as additive treatment in major depression: a double-blind and placebo-controlled trial. *Archives of General Psychiatry* **61**, 1235–1244.

Kellner, M., Otte, C., Yassouridis, A., et al. (2004). Overnight metyrapone and combined dexamethasone/metyrapone tests in post-traumatic stress disorder: preliminary findings. *European Neuropsychopharmacology* **14**, 337–339.

Kellner, M., Schick, M., Yassouridis, A., et al. (2004). Metyrapone tests in patients with panic disorder. *Biological Psychiatry* **56**, 898–900.

Lisansky, J., Peake, G. T., Strassman, R. J., et al. (1989). Augmented pituitary corticotropin response to a threshold dose of human corticotropin releasing hormone in depressive pretreated with metyrapone. *Archives of General Psychiatry* **46**, 641–649.

Plotsky, P. L. M. and Sawchenko, P. E. (1987). Hypophysial-portal plasma levels, median eminence content, and immunohistochemical staining of corticotropin-releasing factor, arginine vasopressin, and oxytocin after pharmacological adrenalectomy. *Endocrinology* **120**, 1361–1369.

von Bardeleben, U., Stalla, G. L. K., Mueller, O. A., et al. (1988). Blunting of ACTH response to CRH in depressed patients is avoided by metyrapone pretreatment. *Biological Psychiatry* **24**, 782–786.

Young, E. A., Altemus, M., Lopez, J. F., et al. (2004). HPA axis activation in major depression and response to fluoxetine: a pilot study. *Psychoneuroendocrinology* **29**, 1198–1204.

Young, E. A., Haskett, R. F., Grunhaus, L., et al. (1994). Increased circadian activation of the hypothalamic pituitary adrenal axis in depressed patients in the evening. *Archives of General Psychiatry* **51**, 701–707.

Young, E. A., Lopez, J. F., Murphy-Weinberg, V., et al. (1997). Normal pituitary response to metyrapone in the morning in depressed patients: implications for circadian regulation of CRH secretion. *Biological Psychiatry* **41**, 1149–1155.

MHC (Major Histocompatibility Complex) *See:* Lymphocytes.

Migraine

N M Ramadan
Rosalind Franklin University of Medicine and Science, North Chicago, IL, USA

This article is a revision of the previous edition article by N M Ramadan, volume 2, pp 757–770, © 2000, Elsevier Inc.

Introduction
Epidemiology
Neural Basis of Head Pain
Genetics
Migraine Mechanisms
Classification of Headache Disorders
Clinical Presentations and Differential Diagnosis of Migraine
Management
Summary

Glossary

Cephalad	Toward the head.
Channelopathy	A condition resulting from many scenarios (membrane ion channels that open when they should not, channels that do not open very well or at all, channels that stay open too long, misplaced channels, and a lack of channels or too many channels) that potentially can be deleterious.
Comorbidity	The association between migraine and another condition that is unlikely to be random or causal.
Cortical spreading depression	A local neuronal phenomenon that is elicited by chemical, physical, or electrical stimuli; characterized by a short burst of neuronal electrical activity and followed by a short-lived (minutes) marching wave of slow neuronal suppression.
Incidence	The proportion of new cases of an illness in a defined population over a set time period.
Migraine	A primary headache disorder manifesting as episodic, usually unilateral severe head pain with nausea, vomiting, and light and noise sensitivity.
Neurogenic inflammation	A sterile inflammatory response that is caused by an injurious stimulus of peripheral neurons and that leads to the release of substances (e.g., neuropeptides) that alter vascular permeability.
Phonophobia	An unpleasant feeling when exposed to noise.
Photophobia	An unpleasant feeling when exposed to light.
Prevalence	The proportion of a given population with a disease over a defined period of time. Lifetime prevalence of migraine is the proportion of individuals in the general population who have ever had migraine during their life. Prevalence is the

Trepanation An old surgical procedure in which a hole is drilled or scraped into the skull, leaving the membrane around the brain intact.

average disease incidence multiplied by its duration.

Introduction

Migraine is a painful and disabling headache disorder that has plagued humanity for thousands of years. Julius Caesar, England's Queen Mary, Thomas Jefferson, Claude Monet, Vincent van Gogh, Georges Seurat (visual disturbances of migraine aura, the Seurat effect), Alexander Graham Bell, Friedrich Nietzsche, Peter Tchaikovsky, and Sigmund Freud all suffered from migraine. Over the centuries, migraine has been transformed from a disease that is caused by evil spirits to a vascular and then a neurovascular disorder with well-defined epidemiology, pathology, pathophysiology, pharmacology, therapeutics, and genetics. Several thousand years BC, trepanation was a common practice used to relieve migraine by releasing demons from the head. Egyptians bound a clay crocodile, holding grain in its mouth, to the head of headache patients, using a strip of linen that bore the Gods' names. Galen considered migraine a visceral pain disorder when he said, "How constantly do we see the head attacked with pain when yellow bile is contained in the stomach: as also the pain forthwith ceasing when the bile has been vomited." (Koehn, 1826) Tenth century Arabian physicians used garlic and hot iron on temple incisions (two-site venesection) to relieve head pain.

More recently, Sir Thomas Willis believed that migraine was caused by vasodilatation, arguing that headache symptoms were related to slowly ascending spasms beginning at the peripheral ends of the nerves. Similarly, Erasmus Darwin (Charles Darwin's grandfather) believed in vasodilation-induced migraine and proposed to treat it with centrifugation in order to force the blood from the head to the feet. Edward Liveing commented in "On Megrim, Sick-headache, and Some Allied Disorders" that the migraine, similar to epilepsy, is a malady of the nervous system caused by nerve-storm, which may be the first account of cortical spreading depression (CSD) as an initiator of migraine. Sir William Gowers proposed dividing the treatment of headache into prophylactic and episodic. He advocated continuous treatment with drugs to render attacks less frequent and treatment of the attacks themselves. In the late 1800s, the potent neurotoxin ergot, which comes from a fungus that grows on rye, was used to treat unilateral headache. Later in the early 1900s, the active chemical ergotamine was discovered and became the preferred treatment for migraine.

The modern understanding of migraine started with the work of Harold Wolff, a migraine sufferer himself, who performed elegant clinical experiments that supported the vascular theory of headache. Wolff and Ray published in 1940 a detailed map of pain-sensitive structures in the brain, which provided the basis for the link between arterial pathology and referred head pain. Contemporaneously, Leao discovered CSD in animals, which later was equated with human visual aura. Today, this phenomenon can be imaged and measured, and it is forming the backbone for the development of several classes of potential antimigraine drugs. To this end, it is important to mention seminal research from Boston (Cutrer and Sanchez del Rio), Detroit (Welch and Cao), Los Angeles (Woods), and elsewhere, which provided us with a window for analyzing and quantifying CSD in humans.

In the 1960s and beyond, Sicuteri, Lance, and Anthony stressed the role of serotonin in migraine. Their work was later amplified by Saxena, Humphrey, Martin, and others, who discovered the triptans. Also, the Copenhagen group led by Olesen drew attention to a mismatch between cerebral blood flow (CBF) changes and symptoms of migraine, which challenged the vasoconstriction–vasodilation theory. The same group evaluated the role of nitric oxide (NO) in inducing headache, and now NO synthase (NOS) inhibition is becoming a prime target in averting migraine.

The understanding of migraine mechanisms and therapeutics evolved over the last 2 decades with experiments that Moskowitz and fellow researchers conducted. The activation of the trigeminal system in animals was shown to induce plasma protein extravasation and neurogenic inflammation, and many antimigraine therapies blocked this response. Similarly, the initial work of Edvinsson and Goadsby was amplified in the last 10–15 years, culminating in advancing calcitonin gene-related peptide (CGRP) antagonists for migraine. Also, important work from Detroit, Michigan, and Bologna, Italy, supported the theory that the brain-energy metabolism in migraine sufferers is defective and that magnesium deficiency may contribute to the disease. These observations opened the field to testing magnesium, co-enzyme Q10 (CoQ10), and riboflavin (B2) for migraine prevention. Apropos, John Graham modernized the preventive treatment of migraine with the introduction of methysergide, Oscar Reinmuth's group drew attention to the role of propranolol in migraine, and recent studies from Welch and colleagues and Ferrari and coworkers suggested that migraine may be a progressive disorder that may warrant early and aggressive preventive therapy.

Finally, the potential role of peripheral and central sensitization in migraine, which Burstein and colleagues are unfolding, is opening new windows into migraine therapeutic strategies.

Migraine is not an orphan in the era of genomic discoveries. French and Dutch researchers led the effort demonstrating that some forms of migraine result from defective calcium trafficking across its channels and provided a new avenue for exploring migraine mechanisms and therapies. A knockin model of abnormal mutations now provides a model of familial hemiplegic migraine and susceptibility to CSD. Also, the discovery of mutations in the Na-K adenosine triphosphatase (ATPase) gene is steering us to new pathophysiological and pharmacological directions. Indeed, excessive synaptic glutamate (Glu) is a by-product of these mutations, which predisposes the migraine brain to hyperexcitability, sensitization, and/or neuronal cell death.

Epidemiology

Prevalence estimates of headaches vary significantly among studies. For example, the prevalence of headache disorders in Europe and the United States ranges from 13% (1-year prevalence in people with serious headaches) to 93% (lifetime prevalence in the United Kingdom, based on a telephone interview). Several factors contribute to the observed variability, including the time periods used for estimating prevalence (e.g., 1-year vs. lifetime), targeted age range and other sociodemographic factors, methods of ascertaining headache diagnoses, and cooccurrence of different headache types. Regardless of the study methods, the majority of population-based studies of headache disorders in adults indicate a female preponderance, which is not unexpected because most chronic pain disorders with a remitting and relapsing course (e.g., fibromyalgia and irritable bowel syndrome) are more prevalent in women.

Rasmussen et al. conducted a large 1991 epidemiological study (1000 people, 25–64 years old) on the prevalence of headache disorders in Copenhagen County, Denmark. Tension-type headache was the most common, followed by fasting headache, migraine, and headache attributed to nose or sinus disease (**Table 1**).

Epidemiology of Migraine

Few longitudinal studies have investigated the incidence of migraine. A 12-year follow-up of a Dutch general population sample ($n = 549$) determined that the incidence of migraine was 8.1 per 1000 person-years (male : female = 1 : 6). Data from a 2005 prevalence

Table 1 Lifetime prevalence of headache disorders in Denmark[a]

Type	Prevalence (%)
Primary headache disorders	
Tension-type headache	78.0
Migraine	16.0
Secondary headache disorders	
Fasting	19.0
Nose and sinus disease	15.0
Head trauma	4.0
Nonvascular intracranial disease (e.g., brain tumor)	0.5

[a]From Rasmussen, B. K., Jensen, R., Schroll, M., et al. (1991), Epidemiology of headache in a general population – a prevalence study, *Journal of Clinical Epidemiology* **44**, 1147–1157.

study in people 12–29 years old revealed slightly higher numbers – the incidence of migraine with aura was 14.1 per 1000 person-years and that of migraine without aura was 18.9 per 1000 person-years.

The incidence of migraine is two to three times higher in females than in males, and the peak age of onset is 5–9 years in males and 12–13 years in females for migraine with aura. For migraine without aura, the figures are 10–11 years for males and 14–17 years for females. The incidence of migraine may be increasing, particularly in women 10–49 years old.

In contrast to the paucity of studies of migraine incidence, several reports from various countries across the globe addressed migraine prevalence and established that it is a common disorder with particular predilection to Whites and women. Prior to 1988, population estimates of migraine prevalence varied from 3 to 35%. The application of the International Headache Society (IHS) 2004 diagnostic criteria led to more robust and consistent data on migraine epidemiology and allowed a better assessment of demographic influences such as race, socioeconomic status, gender, and geographical location. Indeed, several studies have now provided gender-dependent estimates of the 1-year prevalence of migraine: approximately 3–22% in women and 1–16% in men. The prevalence of migraine is highest in North America and lowest in Africa (**Figure 1**).

Population studies have confirmed that migraine is more prevalent in females than in males older than 12 years (female : male = 2–3 : 1), regardless of race or geographical location. Migraine in children is almost as prevalent in boys as it is in girls.

The prevalence of migraine follows an inverted-U curve with advancing age (**Figure 2**). This phenomenon is significantly more pronounced in females. The peak prevalence of migraine is in the fourth and fifth decades; it declines substantially thereafter.

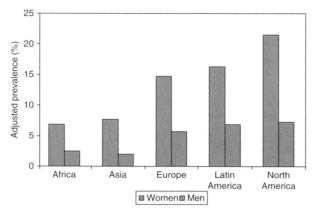

Figure 1 Prevalence of migraine across continents. From Lipton, R. B. and Bigal, M. E. (2005), Migraine: epidemiology, impact and risk factor for progression, *Headache* **45**(supplement 1), S3–S13.

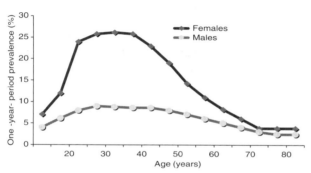

Figure 2 Prevalence of migraine by age. From Stewart, W. F., Lipton, R. B., Celentano, D. D., et al. (1992), Prevalence of migraine headache in the United States: relation to age, income, race, and other sociodemographic factors, *Journal of the American Medical Association* **267**, 64–69.

Migraine varies with race. Whites are more commonly affected (prevalence = 20.4% in women and 8.6% in males) than African Americans (16.2% in women and 7.2% in men) or Asian Americans (9.2% in women and 4.2% in men). Contrary to a widely held belief, migraine is more common in low-socioeconomic groups and in less-educated individuals. The use of care data indicate, however, that people in higher social strata and better-educated migraine sufferers are more likely to seek medical advice.

Neural Basis of Head Pain

Triggers of head pain in different headache disorders may vary, but the substrates for pain generation, stimulus conduction through the peripheral and central nociceptive pathways, recognition and perception of the experience, and memory and reaction to pain are largely similar whether the type of headache is primary (e.g., migraine) or secondary (e.g., trauma).

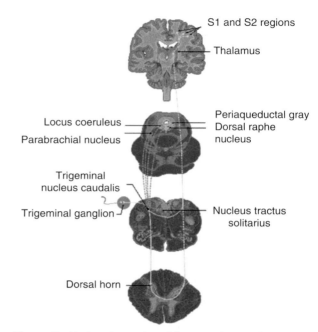

Figure 3 Nociceptive and modulatory pathways. Pathways in yellow represent afferent projections subserving pain; pathways in orange represent descending, mainly inhibitory projections.

A discussion of trigger mechanisms is beyond the scope of this article, but a brief overview of the final common pathways in pain are described next.

Neuroanatomy

The pathways of head pain can be anatomically dissected into four distinct locales (**Figure 3**):
1. Sensing organs such as the skin and blood vessels.
2. Sensory-discriminative regions, which include the trigeminal nucleus caudalis (TNC), thalamus, and the primary (S1) and secondary (S2) sensory cortices.
3. Emotion, memory, and behavioral response networks. These include the insula and hippocampus, which encode the memory and recognition of pain; cingulate, which modulates the affective and motivational aspects of pain; and precentral cortex, cerebellum, and cingulated, which are involved in the reaction to the painful experience.
4. Modulatory, predominantly inhibitory regions such as the hypothalamus, basal forebrain, and various brain-stem structures.

Head pain is generated when pain-sensitive intracranial structures are stimulated. These include vascular structures such as the circle of Willis and proximal middle cerebral arteries, neuronal structures including the trigeminal and glossopharyngeal nerves, and the cranial meninges, particularly the perivascular components of the dura. Pain signals are transmitted from these nociceptive structures cephalad, mostly via Aδ and C fibers that contain neurotransmitters such as Glu, CGRP, substance P (SP), and neurokinin A (NKA). Middle meningeal artery nociceptive fibers travel through the first division of the trigeminal nerve (V1) to the ipsilateral trigeminal ganglion (TG), whereas fibers from the middle cranial fossa dura run in V3 to the ipsilateral TG. First-order neuron fibers in TG then project centrally onto secondary sensory neurons in the TNC, which in turn send their projections to the contralateral nucleus ventralis posteromedialis (VPM) of the thalamus. Projections of the nociceptive pathway from the trigeminal brainstem nuclear complex include the trigeminal lemniscus, hypothalamic projections, pontine parabrachial nucleus (PBN), reticular formation, and the nucleus of the tractus solitarius (NTS). PBN feeds back into the trigeminal brain-stem nuclear complex and is involved in nociceptive control. Central processing of incoming pain signals beyond the thalamus include cortical areas such as the cingulate, insular, S1, and S2, as well as the cingulated gyrus and insula. Cortical neurons that are activated during head and peripheral pain include localizing and discriminating pain neuronal pools, which receive afferents from VPM, and those involved in the effective components of pain, which receive afferents from the medial thalamus.

Descending, predominantly inhibitory neuronal fibers project from the frontal lobe cortex to the hypothalamus and the periaqueductal gray (PAG) and from there descend to the rostral ventromedial medullary nuclear complex (RVM, the raphe magnus and adjacent reticular formation), which ultimately projects to the medullary and spinal dorsal horns.

Neurochemistry

The PAG–RVM system contains serotonin (5-HT) excitatory neurons that activate inhibitory interneurons of the substantia gelatinosa and lamina II of the spinal trigeminal nucleus. Electrical stimulation of either PAG or RVM or the exogenous injection of opioids, which activate the 5-HT system, results in inhibitory activity in the nociceptive neurons in the dorsal horn. Independently of PAG–RVM, a diffuse noxious inhibitory control (DNIC) system (not shown in **Figure 3**) directly reduces the firing of wide-dynamic range (WDR) neurons of the medullary dorsal horn cells following noxious stimulation from parts of the body that are remote from their receptor field.

The neurochemicals that are involved in pain derive from the vascular endothelium of nociceptive structures, which contains both vasoconstrictive (e.g., thromboxane, superoxide ions, and endothelin) and vasodilator substances (e.g., NO and prostacyclin), and from the adventitia–media junction of intracranial vessels, which are rich in neuropeptide-positive terminals (e.g., CGRP and SP).

Neurophysiology

Nociceptive activation induces peripheral sensitization, which is predominantly mediated by enhanced Na channels opening. This process perpetuates discharges along the nociceptive terminals and into TG with an ongoing cycle of enhanced Na-channel opening, excitatory neurotransmitter release, and further neuronal activation. With time, peripheral sensitization, perhaps through excessive N-methyl-D-aspartate (NMDA) Glu receptor activation, leads to a central sensitizing process initially at the TNC level and subsequently at the thalamic level and beyond. The phenomenon of central sensitization manifests physiologically as spontaneous activity in otherwise quiescent neurons, reduced threshold to activation, and expansion of the neuronal receptor field following distal stimulation.

Peripheral and central sensitization could continue unless various protective neuromodulatory mechanisms become operant. Modulation is mediated peripherally through the presynaptic inhibition of neurotransmitter release or centrally through several possible mechanisms, including the inhibition of afferent input. At the peripheral level, serotonergic presynaptic receptors of the 5-HT_{1D} and 5-HT_{1F} types and some metabotropic Glu receptors participate in suppressing neurotransmitter release. Centrally, TNC neurons are inhibited by local inhibitory interneurons (e.g., GABAergic), by activation of presynaptic inhibitory receptors (5-HT_{1D}, 5-HT_{1F}, 5-HT_{1B}, and metabotropic), or by descending inhibitory fibers (e.g., noradrenergic, adenosinergic, glutamatergic, serotonergic, and GABAergic). The descending modulatory system itself is under the control of various hypothalamic-pituitary outputs, such as estrogen levels, and melatonin cycles, which have direct relevance to the roles of sleep and menstrual cycles in migraine and other painful disorders.

Genetics

The genetics of most headache disorders remain elusive. On the other hand, some major advances in the genetics of migraine have been published in the last decade or so.

There is mounting evidence that a subform of migraine (familial hemiplegic migraine, FHM) is due to a membrane ion channelopathy or ionopathy (**Table 2**). A net gain of function of the calcium

Table 2 Some genetic defects in familial hemiplegic migraine that might predispose to hyperexcitable neurons[a]

Chromosome	Gene mutations locale	Potential biological or physiological consequence
19p13	CaCNA1A ($Ca_v2.1$)	↑ Ca^{2+} into presynaptic neuron, causing neurotransmitter release (e.g., glutamate)
1q23	$\tilde{\alpha}_2$ subunit of Na^+/K^+ ATPase	Defective clearing of glutamate from synaptic cleft
2q24	Neuronal Na channel	Enhanced EPSP
5p13	EAAT1 glutamate transporter	Defective clearing of glutamate from synaptic cleft

[a]CaCNA1A, α_1 subunit of calcium channel gene; ATPase, adenosine triphosphatase; Na, sodium; EPSP, excitatory postsynaptic synapse; EAAT1, excitatory amino acid transporter type 1.

channel leads to an excessive intracellular calcium influx into the presynaptic glutamatergic terminal, Glu release, and persistent postsynaptic activation that predisposes to cortical spreading depression (CSD). Indeed, a knockin mouse model of a CACNA1A mutation that predisposes animals to CSD and transient hemiplegia has been developed. Alternatively, a defective Na pump reduces the efficiency of Glu transporters in clearing Glu, resulting in excessive Glu at the synaptic cleft and subsequently in continued postsynaptic excitation. Interestingly, a heterozygous mutation on the gene encoding for the Glu transporter excitatory amino acid transporter type 1 (EAAT1) was discovered in 2004 in a patient with seizures, migraine, and alternating hemiplegia. Last, hyperexcitability can be caused by a neuronal Na-channel mutation, reported in 2005.

Genetic defects in FHM might not be extrapolated to the more common forms of migraine with and without aura, especially with the absence of consistent evidence of genetic mutations or functional polymorphism at the known FHM sites, but nearby loci are implicated. Furthermore, a 2005 genomewide scan of people with common forms of migraine confirmed genetic susceptibility at sites previously reported with FHM. In addition, new susceptibility loci were reported (3q and 18p11), which deserve further exploration.

Migraine Mechanisms

The mechanisms of migraine pain and its associated neurological, gastrointestinal, and autonomic manifestations are multiple and complex. Attacks could manifest as an isolated symptom (e.g., migraine aura without headache) or a sign and symptom complex (e.g., migraine with aura), which could take on a range of phenotypic expressions (e.g., emotional lability as part of a premonitory symptom complex followed by pain or a full-blown multiphasic attack manifesting as depressive symptoms, followed by a visual aura followed by pain with nausea and photophobia and phonophobia, and terminating with social-withdrawal feelings and tiredness). Therefore, deciphering migraine mechanisms requires a

comprehensive understanding of the isolated manifestations and explanations for the event sequences.

Migraine is a neurobiological disorder of altered neuronal excitability and defective adaptive mechanisms to stressors of the system. The susceptibility to migraine is an interplay between genetic factors and environmental elements (e.g., stress and weather change). The migraine cascade can be conceptualized as a sequence of events occurring in a series, starting with the activation of hypothalamic pathways that trigger the premonitory symptoms and followed by cortical neuronal activation and CSD. Neuronal activation releases various substances such as hydrogen ions and NO, which in turn activate nociceptive terminals that, on the one hand, cause the release of substances such as CGRP and, on the other hand, transmit neuronal impulses into the medulla to the thalamus and up to the cortex for perception and reaction to the headache. CGRP, SP, and NKA participate in neurogenic vasodilation and inflammation, leading to peripheral sensitization and an abnormal response to previously innocuous stimuli (e.g., blood-vessel pulsations becoming painful). Often, peripheral sensitization can culminate in central sensitization with the activation of ancillary trigeminal nociceptive (e.g., allodynia in the distribution of the first division of the trigeminal nerve) and paratrigeminal pathways (e.g., photophobia and phonophobia).

The female preponderance of migraine sufferers provides some insight into the mechanisms of headache and pain. A discussion of the role of sex hormones and migraine mechanisms is quite complex and beyond the scope of this article, but a few highlights are noteworthy. Women detect trigeminal pain at a lower threshold than men, and their tolerance for the painful stimulus may be lower. Some researchers observed that these gender differences may be related to higher sensory-receptor density on the peripheral nerve terminals in women. Furthermore, estrogen receptors (ERs) are distributed on various neuronal pools that participate in migraine pain trafficking (e.g., TNC, hypothalamus, amygdala, PBN, and PAG). Lastly, ERs modulate neuropeptides in the trigeminal system that are involved in migraine (e.g., CGRP, SP, and NKA).

Table 3 Comorbidity of migraine and systemic and psychiatric disorders

System	Condition
Gastrointestinal	Irritable bowel syndrome
Neurological	Epilepsy
	Multiple sclerosis
Psychiatric	Affective disorders
	Anxiety disorders
	Neuroticism
	Sleep disorders
	Substance abuse
	Suicide
Pulmonary	Asthma
Vascular and cardiovascular	Hypertension
	Hypotension
	Ischemic stroke
	Myocardial infarction
Others	Allergies
	Raynaud's phenomenon

Migraine is comorbid with psychiatric conditions such as generalized anxiety disorders and depression (Table 3), and migraine attacks often are triggered by stress and lack of sleep. It has been suggested that bidirectional signal transmission through the trigeminovascular system accounts for both the migraine symptoms and the induction of these symptoms by triggers such as stress. Also, migraine shares similar mechanisms with chronic pain when comorbid psychiatric conditions such as depression could result from functional alterations in the reward–aversion pathways.

Migraine patients have some personality traits such as neuroticism, which could lead to altered coping mechanisms. Indeed, one study suggested that a migraine sufferer's coping mechanisms include amplified physical symptoms, social litigation, and preoccupation with stress. Also, migraine patients are less calm, more irritable, do not relax as well as a nonmigraine healthy controls, and often respond to physical symptoms, including pain, with internal tension.

Classification of Headache Disorders

The development of a headache disorder classification that is intuitive, psychometrically robust, and easy-to-use enables a better understanding of conditions associated with headache, improves patients' management, and provides a standardized approach to headache research. Headache disorders can be classified broadly as primary (e.g., migraine), and secondary (e.g., posttraumatic). Indeed, the *International Classification for Headache Disorders* (2nd edn.;

ICHD-II) recognizes this dichotomy (Table 4). Primary headaches are classified largely on the basis of symptoms, whereas secondary headaches are grouped etiologically. Both acute and chronic forms of primary and secondary headache disorders are recognized (e.g., chronic migraine and chronic posttraumatic headache).

Clinical Presentations and Differential Diagnosis of Migraine

Migraine is characterized by episodes of head pain that is aggravated by movement, with associated nausea, photophobia, and phonophobia. Head pain in migraine is unilateral in approximately 60% of patients and throbbing in many but not all. Up to one-third of migraine patients experience transient neurological symptoms (i.e., aura) that herald or accompany the pain. Most migraine attacks last approximately 1 day (4–72 h in adults; they are of shorter duration in children), and their frequency is quite variable. The frequency of migraine is approximately once per month in population-based studies and three times per month in clinic-based cohorts. In the general population, 2–3% suffer chronic migraine, which is defined as attacks that recur more than 15 times per month. Last, the majority of migraine sufferers are disabled with their attacks.

A careful history and appropriate physical and neurological examination establish most causes of headache disorders. For example, the presence of associated symptoms (e.g., nausea and photophobia) helps to differentiate migraine from tension headache. Important elements of the history that help in establishing the diagnosis include (1) age of onset; (2) duration; (3) time to peak severity; (4) severity and headache-related disability; (5) frequency; (6) location; (7) preceding and accompanying symptoms, if any; (8) precipitating and aggravating factors; (9) circadian or diurnal patterns; and (10) relieving factors. It is also crucial to obtain a full headache medication history, including over-the-counter remedies.

The clinical presentations of migraine with and without aura are often characteristic (Table 5). On the other hand, the clinical presentations of secondary headache types mimicking migraine with aura are not unique (Table 6), with a few exceptions (e.g., benign or idiopathic intracranial hypotension). Also, the symptom complex of migraine and that of other primary headaches and secondary headaches overlap (Table 7). An algorithm that helps in the differentiation between primary and secondary headache disorders uses red flags (called SSNOOPs, an acronym based on the first letter of items in the

Table 4 Second International Classification for Headache Disorders (ICHD-II)[a]

Category	Type
Primary headache disorders (categories 1–4)	Migraine, tension-type headache, cluster headache and other trigeminal cephalgias, other primary headache (e.g., primary stabbing headache, primary cough headache)
Secondary headache disorders (categories 5–12)	Posttraumatic headache; headache attributed to cranial or cervical vascular disorders; headache attributed to nonvascular intracranial disorder; headache associated with substances or their withdrawal; headache attributed to infection; headache attributed to disorder of homeostasis; headache or facial pain associated with disorder of cranium, neck, eyes, ears, nose sinuses, teeth, mouth, or other facial or cranial structures; headache attributed to psychiatric disorder
Cranial neuralgias and central causes of facial pain (category 13)	Trigeminal neuralgia; glossopharyngeal neuralgia; nervus intermedius neuralgia; superior laryngeal neuralgia; nasociliary neuralgia; supraorbital neuralgia; occipital neuralgia; neck-tongue syndrome; external compression headache; cold stimulus headache; constant pain caused by compression, irritation or distortion of cranial nerves or upper cervical roots by structural lesions; optic neuritis; ocular diabetic neuropathy; head and facial pain attributed to herpes zoster; Tolosa-Hunt syndrome; ophthalmoplegic migraine; anesthesia dolorosa; central poststroke pain; facial pain attributed to multiple sclerosis; persistent idiopathic facial pain; burning mouth syndrome
Other headache, cranial neuralgia, central or primary facial pain	Headache unspecified

[a]From the Headache Classification Subcommittee, International Headache Society (2004), *Special issue on the international classification of headache disorders (2nd edn.), Cephalalgia* **24**(supplement 1).

Table 5 Diagnostic criteria for migraine[a]

Migraine without aura	A. At least five attacks fulfilling B–D B. Headache attacks lasting 4–72 h (untreated or unsuccessfully treated) C. Headache has at least two of the following characteristics: unilateral location, pulsating quality, moderate or severe pain intensity, aggravation by or causing avoidance of routine physical activity (e.g., walking or climbing stairs) D. During headache at least one of the following: nausea and/or vomiting, photophobia and phonophobia E. Not attributed to another disorder
Migraine with typical aura	A. At least two attacks fulfilling B–C B. Aura consisting of at least one of the following, but no motor weakness: fully reversible visual symptoms including positive features (e.g., flickering lights, spots, or lines) and/or negative features (i.e., loss if vision), fully reversible sensory symptoms including positive features (e.g., pins and needles) and/or negative features (i.e., numbness), fully reversible dysphasic speech disturbance C. At least two of the following: headache [1.21] fulfilling criteria B–D for migraine without aura; begins during the aura or follows aura within 60 min; headache [1.22] that does not fulfill criteria B–D for migraine without aura; begins during the aura or follows aura within 60 min; headache [1.23] does not occur during aura nor follows aura within 60 min D. Not attributed to another disorder

[a]From the Headache Classification Subcommittee, International Headache Society (2004), *Special issue on the international classification of headache disorders (2nd edn.), Cephalalgia* **24**(supplement 1).

following list) as the major branching point (**Figure 4**). SSNOOPs are:

- Systemic symptoms (fever or weight loss)
- Secondary risk factors: underlying disease (HIV or systemic cancer)
- Neurological symptoms or abnormal signs (confusion, impaired alertness or consciousness, neck stiffness, clumsiness, or weakness)
- Onset: sudden, abrupt, or split-second (first or worst)

- Older: new onset and progressive headache, especially in middle age (>50 years old)
- Previous headache history or headache progression: pattern change, first headache or different (change in attack frequency, severity, or new clinical features).

A variation of SSNOOP is SSNOOPP, which considers pain with local tenderness (e.g., jaw or temporal artery) as an additional red flag.

Table 6 Differential diagnosis of headache with transient neurological symptoms mimicking migraine with aura[a]

Cerebrovascular disease	Dissection, ischemic stroke and transient ischemic attacks, hemorrhagic stroke, AVM, primary CNS vasculitis, cerebrovenous sinus/dural thrombosis, postpartum angiopathy
Drug-induced	Nitric oxide-releasing compounds (e.g., nitroglycerin, sildenafil), illicit drugs
Endocrine/metabolic disorders	Hypoglycemia
Inherited/genetic disorders	CADASIL, MELAS, OTC deficiency
Nonvascular intracranial disorders	Focal encephalitis and aseptic meningitis, primary or metastatic brain tumors, idiopathic intracranial hypertension, HANDL (PLP), systemic vasculitis (e.g., SLE and aPL syndrome), HIV
Traumatic disease	Posttraumatic headache, postwhiplash injury
Others	Ictal headaches, whiplash injury, cervicogenic headache, chiari malformation type I, glaucoma

[a]aPL, antiphospholipid; AVM, arteriovenous malformation; CADASIL, cerebral autosomal dominant arteriopathy with subcortical infarcts and leukoencephalopathy; CNS, central nervous system; HANDL, headache, neurologic deficits, and cerebrospinal fluid lymphocytosis; HIV, human immunodeficiency virus; MELAS, mitochondrial encephalopathy with lactic acidosis and strokelike episodes; OTC, ornithine transcarbamylase; PLP, pseudomigraine with lymphocytic pleocytosis; SLE, systemic lupus erythematosus.

Table 7 Overlap in symptoms of migraine pain and secondary headaches

Symptom	Some examples of headache conditions
Unilateral headache	Trauma, cluster headache, trigeminal autonomic cephalgia, migraine, cerebrovascular disease, idiopathic jabbing headache, sinusitis, eye/jaw disease, cervical spine disease, giant cell arteritis
Throbbing pain	Migraine, cerebrovascular disease, hypertensive headaches
Exacerbation with movement	Migraine, headache attributed to conditions that increase intracranial pressure, posttraumatic headache, Chiari malformation type I, benign cough headaches
Photophobia	Migraine, cluster headache, meningitis, posttraumatic headache, subarachnoid hemorrhage
Nausea, vomiting	Headache attributed to conditions that increase intracranial pressure, meningitis, intracranial hemorrhage, trauma

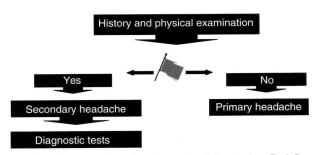

Figure 4 Approach to the diagnosis of headache. Red flag represents any of the SSNOOPs. Adapted from the Neurology Ambassador Program with permission.

General medical and surgical histories, social and family histories, medications intake, and review of systems may provide clues to the diagnosis. For example, transient visual obscuration and intracranial noises may point to idiopathic intracranial hypertension. An antecedent motor vehicle accident within 6–12 months of the headache onset may indicate posttraumatic headache or whiplash headache. General and neurological examinations are an integral component of the assessment of patients with headaches. Papilledema, carotid bruits, neck limitation of motion, second trigeminal nerve branch or occipital triggers, tender temporal artery, and focal

or lateralizing signs can all provide important clues to the diagnosis.

Once the characteristic symptoms of a migraine headache are identified and red flags are not elicited, imaging studies are likely to reveal a significant intracranial abnormality in only approximately 0.2% of patients. A magnetic resonance imaging (MRI) study is the preferred test when imaging is indicated.

Management

General Principles

General management strategies for migraine follow the TEEM© principles, which are:
- Trust and establish a strong rapport with the patient.
- Educate the patient about the disease/condition, treatment plan, and compliance. A major reason for failed therapy in headache disorders is noncompliance and/or unmatched or unrealistic expectations (e.g., expecting a cure for migraine).
- Empower the patient.
- Measure.

It is crucial to establish an accurate diagnosis based on a detailed history and physical examination and aided in special circumstances by neuroinvestigative techniques such as an MRI. It is also very important to systematically assess and follow up on the disease severity and disease-related disability by encouraging patients to maintain headache diaries in order to identify headache patterns, triggers, associated symptoms, response to intervention, and so on. The elicitation during the history of migraine comorbid conditions (**Table 3**) provides either opportunities to simplify treatment regimens (e.g., valproate for migraine and bipolar disease) or limitations on the use of certain medications (e.g., propranolol for migraine sufferers with asthma).

Pharmacotherapy of Migraine

Migraine pharmacotherapy can be divided into (1) the treatment of acute pain, (2) the treatment of associated symptoms, (3) traditional preventive agents, and (4) preemptive approaches when attacks have predictable triggers (e.g., menstruation). Preventive therapy for migraine is indicated for patients with (1) frequent or disabling attacks, (2) a prolonged aura, or (3) a poor response or intolerance to acute therapy.

Current acute therapy (**Table 8**) for migraine includes simple analgesics (e.g., acetaminophen) and compound analgesics (e.g., combined acetaminophen, aspirin, and caffeine; acetaminophen with codeine), nonsteroidal anti-inflammatory drugs (NSAIDs, e.g., ibuprofen), migraine-specific therapies such as ergots (ergotamine and dihydroergotamine, DHE) and triptans (serotonin type-1B and 1D, $5\text{-HT}_{1B/D}$, agonist), and adjuvant therapies such as metoclopramide for gastrointestinal disturbances. Over-the-counter nonspecific therapies are well suited for low-severity migraine, but patients with more disabling attacks are better served by using migraine-specific agents. When at-home therapy fails, parenterally administered drugs such as DHE, which is often combined with other drugs such as prochloperazine or metoclopramide, may be needed. The choice of acute or preventive therapy should be guided by evidence, when available.

Preventive therapy is ideally aimed at reducing attack frequency, severity, duration, and overall impact and at achieving synergy with abortive therapy to improve its effectiveness. Pharmacological prevention includes β-adrenergic blockers, anticonvulsant or antiepileptic drugs, antidepressants, calcium channel blockers, and NSAIDs. Evidence supports the use of group 1 drugs (**Table 9**) as the first-choice therapies in migraine prevention.

Nonpharmacological complementary and alternative (integrative) migraine therapy includes trigger-avoidance and physical and behavioral interventions.

Table 8 Acute migraine pharmacotherapy[a]

Drug class/mechanism	Drug/compound	Daily dose range (mg)
Analgesics, simple	Acetaminophen	1000
Analgesics, compound	Acetaminophen + ASA + caffeine	600 + 400 + 200
	Acetaminophen + codeine	(250–500) + 30
	Isometheptane + dichloralphenazone + acetaminophen	(65–130) + (100–200) + (325–650)
Ergots	Nasal dihydroergotamine	2–4
	Ergotamine	1–6
Nonsteroidal anti-inflammatory drugs	Aspirin (ASA)	650–1000
	Diclofenac	50–100
	Flurbiprofen	100
	Ibuprofen	400–1200
	Ketoprofen	75–150
	Mefenamic acid	500
	Naproxen	750–825
	Rofecoxib	25–50
	Tolfenamic acid[b]	200
Triptans	Almotriptan	6.25–12.5
	Eletriptan	40–80
	Frovatriptan	2.5–5.0
	Naratriptan	1.0–2.5
	Rizatriptan	5–10
	Sumatriptan	25–100
	Zolmitriptan	2.5–5.0

[a]Oral and nasal therapies with at least one randomized controlled trial demonstrating efficacy of the active compound versus either placebo or another comparator. Reprinted from Ramadan, N. M. and Buchanan, T. M. (2006), New and future migraine therapy, *Pharmacology & Therapeutics* **112**(1), 199–212, with permission from Elsevier.
[b]Not available in the United States.

Table 9 Migraine preventive therapy[a]

	Group				
	1	2	3	4	5
Efficacy	+++	+ to ++	+++	+++	−
Evidence	Good	Limited	Consensus	Good	Good
Adverse events	Mild to severe	Mild to moderate	Mild to concerning	Concerning	
Examples	Amitriptyline, valproate, propranolol, topiramate, timolol	Verapamil, vitamin B$_2$, candesartan	Nortriptyline, phenelzine	Methysergide	Nifedipine

[a]+ indicates efficacy established (+++ is highest); − indicates that there is no evidence for efficacy as migraine prophylaxis. Adapted from Buchanan, T. M. and Ramadan, N. M. (2006), Prophylactic pharmacotherapy for migraine headaches. *Seminars in Neurology* **26**(2), 188–198. Reprinted by permission.

A systematic review in 2000 led to the conclusion that relaxation training, biofeedback, and cognitive-behavioral therapy are proven treatments for migraine, but the evidence for physical treatments such as cervical manipulation and transcutaneous electrical nerve stimulation (TENS) is not as strong. Largely uncontrolled clinical trials support a role for acupuncture in migraine prevention, but two recent randomized trials failed to demonstrate that acupuncture is more effective than sham intervention.

Summary

Significant advances in the acute and prophylactic management of migraine headaches have emerged in recent years, providing relief for millions of migraine sufferers. Given that approximately 6% of men and 17% of women experience migraines, many untreated patients may benefit from proper diagnosis and treatment. Various treatment regimens for the prevention of migraines have proved effective, but long-term prognosis remains less well delineated.

Acknowledgment

The authors wish to thank Ms. Joyce Lenz for her editorial assistance in preparing this manuscript.

See Also the Following Article

Pain.

Further Reading

Aizenman, E. and Sanguinetti, M. C. (2002). Channels gone bad: reflections from a Tapas bar. *Neuron* **34**, 679–683.

Borsook, D., Becerra, L., Carlezon, W. A., Jr., et al. (2006). Reward-aversion circuitry in analgesia and pain: implications for psychiatric disorders. *European Journal of Pain* **11**, 7–20.

Buchanan, T. M. and Ramadan, N. M. (2006). Prophylactic pharmacotherapy for migraine headaches. *Seminars in Neurology* **26**(2), 188–198.

Burstein, R. (2001). Deconstructing migraine headache into peripheral and central sensitization. *Pain* **89**, 107–110.

Burstein, R. and Jakubowski, M. (2005). Unitary hypothesis for multiple triggers of the pain and strain of migraine. *Journal of Comparative Neurology* **493**, 9–14.

Buzzi, M. G. and Moskowitz, M. A. (2005). The pathophysiology of migraine: year 2005. *Journal of Headache Pain* **6**, 105–111.

Dichgans, M., Freilinger, T., Eckstein, G., et al. (2005). Mutation in the neuronal voltage-gated sodium channel SCN1A in familial hemiplegic migraine. *Lancet* **366**, 371–377.

Goadsby, P. (1997). Pathophysiology of migraine: a disease of the brain. In: Goadsby, P. J. & Silberstein, S. D. (eds.) *Headache*, pp. 5–24. Boston: Butterworth-Heinemann.

Headache Classification Subcommittee, International Headache Society (2004). *Special issue on the International Classification of Headache Disorders* (2nd edn.) *Cephalalgia* (supplement 1).

Hu, X. H., Markson, L. E., Lipton, R. B., et al. (1999). Burden of migraine in the United States: disability and economic costs. *Archives of Internal Medicine* **159**, 813–818.

Jen, J. C., Wan, J., Palos, T. P., et al. (2005). Mutation in the glutamate transporter EAAT1 causes episodic ataxia, hemiplegia, and seizures. *Neurology* **65**, 529–534.

Koehn, C. G. (ed.) (1826). *Claudii Galeni opera omnia. vol. xii. De loci affectis.* Leipzig: In officina Car. Cnoblochii.

Lea, R. A., Nyholt, D. R., Curtain, R. P., et al. (2005). A genome-wide scan provides evidence for loci influencing a severe heritable form of common migraine. *Neurogenetics* **6**, 67–72.

Lipton, R. B. and Bigal, M. E. (2005). Migraine: epidemiology, impact and risk factor for progression. *Headache* **45**(supplement 1), S3–S13.

Lyngberg, A. C., Rasmussen, B. K., Jorgensen, T., et al. (2005). Incidence of primary headache: a Danish epidemiologic follow-up study. *American Journal of Epidemiology* **161**, 1066–1073.

Martin, V. T. and Behbehani, M. M. (2001). Toward a rational understanding of migraine trigger factors. *Medical Clinics of North America* **85**, 911–941.

Quality Standards Subcommittee, American Academy of Neurology (1994). The utility of neuroimaging in the evaluation of headache patients with normal neurologic examinations. *Neurology* **44**, 1353–1354.

Ramadan, N. M. and Buchanan, T. M. (2006). New and future migraine therapy. *Pharmacology & Therapeutics* **112**(1), 199–212.

Rasmussen, B. K., Jensen, R., Schroll, M., et al. (1991). Epidemiology of headache in a general population – a prevalence study. *Journal of Clinical Epidemiology* **44**, 1147–1157.

Stewart, W. F., Lipton, R. B., Celentano, D. D., et al. (1992). Prevalence of migraine headache in the United States: relation to age, income, race, and other sociodemographic factors. *Journal of the American Medical Association* **267**, 64–69.

Stovner, L. J. and Scher, A. I. (2006). Epidemiology of headache. In: Olesen, J., Goadsby, P. J., Ramadan, N. M.,

Tfelt-Hansen, P. & Welch, K. M. A. (eds.) *The headaches* (3rd edn., pp. 17–25). Philadelphia: Lippincott Williams & Wilkins.

van den Maagdenberg, A. M., Pietrobon, D., Pizzorusso, T., et al. (2004). A Cacna1a knockin migraine mouse model with increased susceptibility to cortical spreading depression. *Neuron* **41**, 701–710.

Relevant Websites

Campbell, J. K., Penzien, D. B. and Wall, E. W. (2000). Evidence based guidelines for migraine headache: behavioral and physical treatments. http://www.aan.com.

Frishberg, B. M., Rosenberg, J. H., Matchar, D. B., et al. (2000). Evidence-based guidelines in the primary care setting: neuroimaging in patients with non-acute headache. http://www.aan.com.

Mineralocorticoid Receptor Polymorphisms

R H DeRijk and E R de Kloet
Leiden University Medical Center and Leiden University, Leiden, Netherlands

Mineralocorticoid Receptor Gene
Genetic Variants in the Mineralocorticoid Receptor

Glossary

Aldosterone	The classic salt-retaining steroid hormone secreted from the zona glomerulosa of the adrenal cortex; its release is stimulated by the renin–angiotensin system and rising plasma potassium concentrations.
Glucocorticoid hormones	Hormones synthesized and secreted from the zona fasciculata by the adrenal gland in response to stress and also during the diurnal rhythm. The main endogenous glucocorticoids are corticosterone in rodents and cortisol in humans.
Haplotypes	Combinations of several single-nucleotide polymorphism (SNP) alleles on the same chromosome. Here an allele is one variant of a sequence on the DNA, for example, a certain SNP. Often several haplotypes can be found in a gene due to unique combinations of SNPs.
Mineralocorticoid receptors (MRs)	Intracellular receptors by which aldosterone acts in epithelial cells to promote sodium transport while mediating the glucocorticoid-like effects in nonepithelial cells. In the brain, MRs bind the glucocorticoid hormones (corticosterone and cortisol) and mediate the effect of these steroids on appraisal processes and the onset of the stress response.
Single-nucleotide polymorphism (SNP)	A variation in DNA sequence that occurs with a frequency of at least 1%. SNPs can result in amino acid changes, if they are located in the coding region. If they are not in the coding region, they can influence gene regulation by effects on, for example, gene splicing or the promoter region or through the introduction of a stop codon.
Splice variant	mRNA splicing occurs following transcription leading to alternative different mature mRNA molecules, so-called splice variants. Splicing can be tissue specific and context dependent with effects on mRNA expression levels and potentially leading to alternative different proteins.

Transacti-vational properties
Zinc fingers

Effects different factors have on the control of gene expression.

A highly conserved protein domain consisting of about 30 amino acid residues enabling corticosteroid receptors to bind DNA. Steroid receptors have typically two of these domains, encoded by exon 3 and 4. Each domain contains four cysteine residues interacting with one zinc ion, which is crucial for the stability of this domain.

Mineralocorticoid receptors (MRs) have similar affinity for the naturally occurring glucocorticoids (corticosterone and cortisol) and the mineralocorticoid aldosterone. In the epithelia, such as in the kidney, colon, sweat glands and circumventricular organ of the brain, these MRs selectively bind aldosterone, in spite of the approximately 100- to 1000-fold higher concentrations of glucocorticoid hormone in humans. MR selectivity for aldosterone is maintained through the activity of 11β-hydroxysteroid dehydrogenase (11βHSD) type 2, which converts cortisol and corticosterone to inactive metabolites. Through this mechanism, aldosterone can regulate the electrolyte balance, blood volume, and blood pressure. In nonepithelial cells residing in the heart, blood vessels and brain, the MRs are nonselective due to virtual absence of 11βHSD type 2. Accordingly, MRs are exposed to both aldosterone and excess glucocorticoid hormone.

In addition to the regulation of the electrolyte balance, aldosterone and MRs have been implicated in vascular inflammation and damage and in fibrosis in the heart. These actions seem to be relatively independent from the regulation of blood pressure and electrolyte balance. In the brain, the activation of MRs can induce drinking behavior, salt craving, and other effects aimed at reestablishing the electrolyte balance. However, MRs also play a crucial role in the maintenance of cellular stability, regulation of the hypothalamic-pituitary-adrenal (HPA) axis, behavioral adaptation, and cell homeostasis. The MRs involved in the latter functions are predominantly located in the hippocampus, where the receptors are activated by cortisol or corticosterone, due to the relative absence of 11βHSD type 2. Finally, recent data indicate the expression of the MRs in adipose tissue, regulating adipocytes differentiation and thermogenesis.

On the binding of the ligand, aldosterone or cortisol/corticosterone, MRs translocate from the cytosol to the nucleus and bind as a homodimer to hormone responsive elements (HREs). Transcriptional activation occurs through direct interactions with transcription factors and recruitment of co-regulator proteins. This recruitment is governed in part by the ligand and by the HRE. Co-regulator complexes are involved in chromatin remodeling and the recruitment of numerous other factors that are part of the transcriptional machinery.

Genetic variants of the MR gene (i.e. splice variants, deletions, insertions, or SNPs) probably have effects on these functions. These effects include not only an action on the electrolyte balance and cardiovascular control but also on vascular inflammation, behavior, HPA axis control, and homeostatic control mechanisms.

Mineralocorticoid Receptor Gene

The MR (NR3C2) is a member of the nuclear receptor family and resembles the glucocorticoid receptor (GR; NR3C1). In the DNA-binding domain, amino acid identity between MR and GR is approximately 94%, in the C-terminus 57%, and in the N-terminus less then 15%. Transcriptional regulation is mediated by the N-terminal part (exon 2, region AF-1a and AF-1b), plus a small part of the ligand-binding domain (C-terminus, AF-2). DNA binding involves residues in exons 3 and 4. Furthermore, exons 5–9 are involved in ligand binding, dimerization (with exons 3–4), heat shock protein (Hsp)90 binding, nuclear localization, and transcriptional regulation.

The MR gene is located on chromosome 4 (4q31.1) and has a size of approximately 350 kbp (this can be viewed on the Ensembl website). On a regular basis, new SNPs are being identified. The full protein contains 984 amino acids and has a size of approximately 107 kDa. Two (possibly three) exon 1s exist, which can join exon 2 (see **Figure 1**).

Genetic Variants in the Mineralocorticoid Receptor

Genetic Variability

Genetic variants can result from mutations causing deletions, insertions, or just changes of the nucleotide at a given position. Depending on the position in the genome, different effects on the phenotype can be observed. Genetic variants can affect protein structure or regulation through different mechanisms. Even single base pair substitutions can cause dramatic changes to the phenotype; however, the vast majority of such changes which reach appreciable frequencies in the population (referred to as single nucleotide polymorphisms, SNPs) are benign.

The number of different SNPs in the human genome is probably in the range of 3–4 million out of

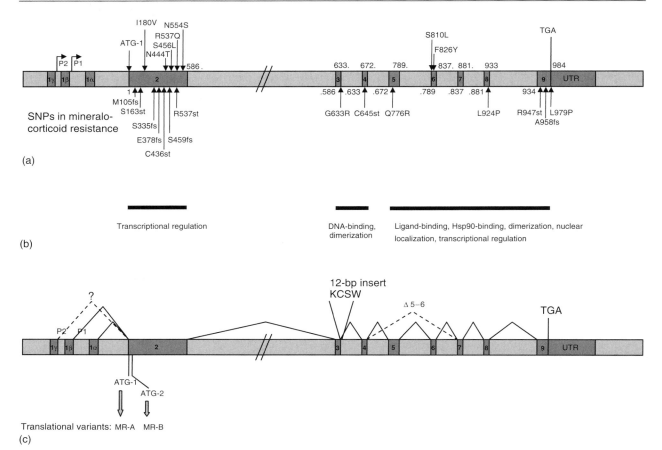

Figure 1 Human MR variants. a, Reported single-nucleotide polymorphisms (SNPs) leading to amino acid changes; b, the three functional domains; c, splice variants and translational variants. The number of the exon is in bold: **1α, 1β, 1γ, 2–9**. The exons are flanked by upper and lower numbers, which indicate the codon (or amino acid), ending with 984 in exon 9. If the number is followed by a dot, the codon spans both exons. Translation starts in the beginning of exon 2 and ends in exon 9 (TGA), followed by an untranslated region (UTR). In a (upper part), the indicated SNPs leading to amino acid changes are shown (from the Ensembl website), with the addition of S810L (associated with hypertension in pregnancy). In a (lower part), specific SNPs are shown that are found to be associated with mineralocorticoid resistance. These have a very low frequency and are only found in specific kindreds. The effects of these SNPs can involve a frameshift (fs) or the introduction of a premature stop codon (st). In b, the three functional domains are shown: the transcriptional active domain, the DNA-binding domain, and the ligand-binding domain (which has several other functions). In c, although both exon 1α and 1β can join exon 2, this is not clear for exon 1γ. In addition to most common annealing pattern (exons 2–9), exon skipping of exons 5 and 6 occurs, resulting in a frameshift with a new termination codon ending in exon 7 (position 2836). At the end of exon 3, 12 extra base pairs can be inserted due to alternative splicing (coding for Lys-Cys-Ser-Tyr), and joined with exon 4; this form is designated MR4+. KCSW, lysine-cysteine-serine-tryptophan.

a total of approximately 3 billion base pairs, counting only SNPs with a minor allele frequency of more then 1%. SNPs make up 90% of all human genetic variations, and two of every three SNPs substitute cytosine (C) with thymine (T), due to a high level of deamination of cytosine. These changes in nucleotide sequence give rise to alternative forms of a gene, named alleles. Combinations of several alleles on the same chromosomes are called haplotypes. However, not all possible combinations of the variants in a stretch of DNA are observed because of specific allele association or so-called linkage disequilibrium (LD). Often blocks of several SNPs are found, giving rise to several haplotypes in a gene.

SNPs are increasingly used to study the involvement of a certain gene and its protein product, in a complex phenotype, as is presented in psychiatric diseases. The association of an SNP in a given gene with a certain phenotype indicates the involvement of the gene. Alternatively, the carriers of a certain SNP/haplotype could represent a vulnerable (or protected) phenotype. Moreover, the determination of genetic variants could be used for more individual treatment of patients based on their specific needs, with respect to treatment efficacy and side effects.

However, several pitfalls are encountered when using variants in genetic research. Phenotyping is crucial because the effect of genetic variants are often moderate, which also calls for the use of large numbers of subjects in association studies. The elucidation of the molecular mechanism of a functional variant will strengthen the *a priori* hypothesis and will also help identify which genetic variant in a given haplotype causes the observed phenotype. Finally, the replication of an association in an independent cohort of subjects will overcome the often observed false-positive associations.

Variants of the Human Mineralocorticoid Receptor Gene

Splicing variants Several alternative splicing variants exist at the 5' end of the gene: exon 1α, exon 1β, or exon1γ can join exon 2 (**Figure 1c**). The existence of exon 1γ is still not completely clear. Upstream of exon 1α and 1β, many regulatory sites have been identified, and this region (P2 and P1) is considered the proximal promotor. The effect of the alternative use of exon 1s is still unresolved. However, during development a differential regulation and response to adrenalectomy of 1α, 1β, or 1γ is observed in the rat hippocampal CA1, CA2, and CA3 pyramidal cell fields and the dentate gyrus (DG) neurons.

In the human MR, a 12-bp insert directly adjacent to the 3' end of exon 3, as a result of alternative splicing, has been found. The result is four extra amino acids (lysine-cysteine-serine-tryptophan; KCSW) in between the two zinc (Zn)-fingers involved in DNA binding. No clear effect of this splice variant, especially on DNA binding, was found. It is, however, expressed in most human tissues, with relative levels varying from 5 to 50%, compared to the most common MR.

Another human MR isoform is derived from skipping exons 5 and 6 with a resultant premature stop, giving rise to a protein of 75 kDa, retaining DNA-binding capacity and ligand-independent transcriptional activity. The high level of expression of this splice variant makes it a potential important modulator of MR effects.

Translational variants also exist as a result of the alternative use of different translational start sites. Two different forms of the MR, designated MR-A and MR-B have recently been described, with different transcriptional activities.

Cardiovascular control Research into the molecular mechanism of mineralocorticoid resistance or pseudohypoaldosteronism (PHA1), characterized by urinary salt wasting and hypotension, has revealed several inactivating mutations in the MR gene. Two forms of PHA1 exist: an autosomal dominant form

that is mild and a recessive form that is more severe due to defects in the epithelial sodium channel. In the autosomal dominant form, the target organ defect is confined to the kidney and clinical expression varies from asymptomatic to moderate. It may be severe at birth, with a failure to thrive, but symptoms often remit with age. The frequency of these mutations, including frameshifts, splice-site mutations, and premature stop codons, is quite low, which accords with the fact that PHA1 is a relatively rare disease. The usefulness of these mutations lies primarily in the understanding of MR protein activity with respect to DNA binding, translocation, and transactivational properties.

An activating mutation in the MR has been detected in patients with severe hypertension, which is exacerbated in pregnancy. The mutation, serine to leucine (S810L; **Figure 1a**), was found to alter the MR ligand specificity; progesterone and other steroids lacking the C-21-OH group became agonists.

Stress responsiveness Mutations of the MR may compromise the role of this receptor in the control of neuronal stability and stress responsiveness. Indeed Brown Norway (BN) rats are, compared to Fisher rats, insensitive to adrenalectomy because there is no weight loss and resistance to saline intake. In the BN-rat MR gene, a tyrosine to cysteine (Y73C) substitution was detected. This mutation revealed a greater transactivational activity of aldosterone and, interestingly, also of progesterone, suggesting that the MR is constitutively more active in the BN rat. It is of interest to note that BN rats have a long life span and seem to have a relatively stable HPA axis, compared to other rat strains.

In humans, some SNPs have a high enough frequency to be potentially important for stress-related disorders, such as anxiety and depression. We found the MR 180V (MRI180V, isoleucine to valine; allele frequency 11%) to be associated with measures of depression in an elderly cohort. In human 180V carriers (i.e., the heterozygote I180V and the homozygote V180V genotypes), cortisol levels and heart rate were enhanced in response to psychological challenge evoked in the Trier Social Stress Test (**Trier Social Stress Test**), whereas the SNP was not associated with changes in blood pressure in response to salt loading as part of the Weinberger's test. Moreover, *in vitro* the response of the MR 180V allele to cortisol was attenuated, which was not observed with aldosterone. The finding suggests that such a subtle SNP can have profound effects on stress responsiveness with potentially important consequences for stress-related pathology.

See Also the Following Articles

Aldosterone and Mineralocorticoid Receptors; Corticosteroid Receptors; Steroid Hormone Receptors; Genetic Polymorphisms in Stress Response; Trier Social Stress Test.

Further Reading

Arriza, J., Weinberger, C., Cerelli, G., et al. (1987). Cloning of human mineralocorticoid receptor complementary DNA: structural and functional kinship with the glucocorticoid receptor. *Science* **237**, 268–275.

de Kloet, E. R., Joëls, M. and Holsboer, F. (2005). Stress and the brain: from adaptation to disease. *Nature Reviews Neuroscience* **6**(6), 463–475.

DeRijk, R. H., Wust, S., Meijer, O. C., et al. (2006). A common polymorphism in the mineralocorticoid receptor modulates stress responsiveness. *Journal of Clinical Endocrinology and Metabolism* Oct. 3 [Epub ahead of print].

Geller, D. S. (2005). Mineralocorticoid resistance. *Clinical Endocrinology* **62**, 513–520.

Vazquez, D. M., Lopez, J. F., Morano, M. I., et al. (1998). Alpha, beta, and gamma mineralocorticoid receptor messenger ribonucleic acid splice variants: differential expression and rapid regulation in the developing hippocampus. *Endocrinology* **139**, 3165–3175.

Zennaro, M.-C. and Lombes, M. (2004). Mineralocorticoid resistance. *Trends in Endocrinology and Metabolism* **15**(6), 264–270.

Relevant Website

Ensembl website.http://www.ensembl.org.

Mineralocorticoids, Overview *See:* Adrenal Cortex; Aldosterone and Mineralocorticoid Receptors.

Minorities and Stress

I Mino
Harvard University, Cambridge, MA, USA
W E Profit
Los Angeles, CA, USA
C M Pierce
Harvard University, Cambridge, MA, USA

This article is a revision of the previous edition article by I Mino, W E Profit, and C M Pierce, volume 2, pp 771–776, © 2000, Elsevier Inc.

Basic Issues
Disadvantaged Minorities
Treatment Considerations

Glossary

Culture	Refers to the dominant set of symbolic codes (linguistic, moral, aesthetic) and material practices (dietary, behavioral) that characterize a group. Culture may refer to an entire society's codes and practices, as when reference is made to the American or Japanese culture.
Deculturated	When people lose their culture or cannot use it because of changed circumstances.
Discrimination	A negating selection and differential comparison not based on merit.
Ethnicity	Refers to the particular reference group for individuals with a shared heritage, e.g., Puerto Rican, American Jewish. Some reference groups may be voluntary, such as those based on religion. Others may be involuntarily ascribed to the persons, such as those based on race.
Minority	A part of a population, numerically less than 50%, differing from others in some characteristics and often subjected to different treatment.
Prejudice	An injurious and intolerant preconceived judgment.
Racism	Intentional or unintentional bias directed at individuals or groups based upon notions of the superiority or inferiority of skin color.

Stress   In minority communities, stress occurs when an individual or group's resources are overextended, even to the point of causing paralysis, apprehension, disintegration, and ineffectiveness from perceived and/or actual duress and assaults from the majority community.

Basic Issues

The basic issues in discussing minorities and stress include defining minority, differentiating the individual's stress from the stress of his or her minority group, and deciding which minority variables are best studied.

Who Is a Minority?

Everyone can claim multiple minority memberships. In fact, an individual may only or best be described in terms of such memberships. For instance, there are over 6000 languages in the world. Everyone's native language is a minority language. No one can claim majority status in terms of nationality, age, occupation, religion, avocation, or talent. Some minority memberships bring honor, others dishonor. Minority memberships may be forced or sought. They can be voluntary or involuntary. Many memberships are visible, often relating to appearance, including bodily features, uniforms, and insignia. Language usage can suggest a minority status. However, many minority memberships are invisible and can even be kept secret, such as migrant status, transnational allegiance, racial identity, and political and social affiliations.

Cultural and social forces determine the saliency of minority memberships. Humans create hierarchies, which in turn breed class distinctions, whereby minorities are made through a process of exclusion or inclusion. Rules of membership can be flexible or rigid, fluid or static. In a given community one might be in the most favored economic group but the least favored social group. Many minority memberships find favor or disfavor from legal regulations.

No matter which minority memberships one has, there are two conditions that must be negotiated for each minority membership. On the one hand, an accommodation for being acculturated and/or deculturated is made. On the other hand, some people or agency has to accept you as a member of the group. Such certification, written or unwritten, can be meticulous or arbitrary. The evaluation may not be accurate, complete, or satisfying to either the assessor or the assessed. Furthermore, certification of legitimacy may vary from the vantage point of various individuals, groups, and organizations.

Most individuals probably give little thought to most of their minority memberships. Therefore, they have not rank-ordered them. Yet, they are aware that the saliency and importance in their lives for any such membership is in a constant state of flux. The importance of a minority membership depends on the combination of specific, general, immediate, and far-flung circumstances at any moment and place.

These ever-shifting interpersonal interactions and intrapersonal considerations mean that in some sense an individual's minority status is situational. Furthermore, the situation depends both on what the individual perceives and on what other persons and groups perceive, even when there is agreement about exactly what minority membership is being scrutinized. Misperceptions between parties can range from being innocuous to being life-threatening. A common cause for misperceptions comes from different opinions about the speed, type, and quantity of acculturation. Also, views may differ significantly about how much a person or group is acculturated, should be acculturated, or can be acculturated.

Seldom is it possible to address these misperceptions among parties without the withering burden of stereotypical thinking by all participants. Thus, an obstacle in contemplating or negotiating a minority or majority issue is that all parties have confusion about what is unique to the individual versus what is a stereotype about a collective group.

The importance of and investment in any minority membership varies from person to person and even from time to time, whether or not one is a member of the in-group. Therefore, even with unequivocal certainty that one is a minority or one is dealing with a minority, the same stressors do not exert uniform force among the actors. Everyone attaches different valences to any minority status, even those that occupy his or her most intense concern. Furthermore, it is usually not possible to ascertain how much any participant identifies with, accepts, or knows about any minority membership that is under discussion.

Is Stress the Same for the Individual and the Group?

Stress results when resources are overextended and overwhelmed. There is the threat of dissolution with accompanying fears of abandonment and inability to escape. Stress is the reciprocal of support. Theoretically, perfect biological, sociological, and psychological support would equal no stress. Stress may be acute, chronic, or intermittent, with dimensions of intensity and duration.

Individuals in a group under stress will have varying perceptions and adjustments. These differences are mediated by both existing background factors and factors peculiar to the stress. For instance, age, state of health, prior relevant experience, and faith are examples of attributes that help govern response to stress.

The number and general condition of a group under stress, as well as the quality of its leadership and its ability to be cohesive and cooperative, are important determinants of the group's outcome. Resourcefulness and a fierce will to survive increase the odds for a favorable outcome. The ability to take decisive, independent action is important.

In groups under stress, behavior of individuals speaks to the important aspect of group morale. Among such behaviors are the willingness to share, carefulness never to endanger the group, and the ability to perform multiple tasks.

Some individuals in any group thrive better than others. This seems true even when all the participants have similar backgrounds and quality of health. These individuals, for whatever reasons, may have more tolerance for uncertainty and ambiguity. Likewise, they may be more able to consider the consequences of the uncontrollable, the unpredictable, and the unexpected, with a more sanguine philosophy. In a mundane extreme environment such as a racial group living under oppression, such individuals may be more accepting of high risk and low reward, as the price for their own and their group's survival. Such persons are the group's everyday heroes, who demonstrate the greatest hope in the group that relief and amelioration are in the future.

Stressful events, due to their limited duration and more discrete circumstances, may be easier to study than stressful backgrounds. Groups and individuals in a railroad crash may be more easily understood and supported than individuals undergoing daily stress. In stressful events the individuals are more conscious of and willing to work for the common survival of the group. This shared specific stressful event will become another minority membership for each participant.

However, individual minority background experiences are filled with so much randomness, variability, and strategy that they are not easily delineated for study. There is a wide range of responses by individual members exposed to the same general trauma. Proximate factors such as personal loss and pain, differences in exactly what was witnessed, and the quantity of available and accessible resources required are never identical. This alone determines a plethora of heterogeneous responses by minority individuals under stress.

Which Minority Variables Are Best Studied?

The great bulk of minority studies are performed on populations considered disadvantaged. They verify in detail that, in general, life is more terrible for these subjects. The data are abundant in this verification, whether addressing health disparities, inequalities in the law, unfair housing and employment, discrepancies in educational opportunity and achievement, harshness in the criminal justice system, insensitivity to the needs of children, etc. The studies focus on vulnerable populations and indicate negative patterns of service, response, and rates of problems. They document that under all manner of geographic, demographic, and political climates these minorities fare poorly.

There is an awareness of, but underpublished interest in, the strengths of individuals in these groups. The strengths the groups had to have in order to survive are less emphasized. Probably methodologies have not evolved that can capture the extensiveness of life events that permit and sustain the host of strengths that differentiate disadvantaged minority people.

A related issue is the huge thrust on aspects of resiliency in these populations, without much consideration of resistance. Studies of resilience imply posttraumatic phenomena. Resistance inquiries seek to understand the defenses against the offenses delivered to the disadvantaged populations, in which trauma continues to accumulate but is deflected, minimized, or diluted.

Disadvantaged Minorities

Social, cultural, economic, and political pressures determine what minority memberships are designated as disadvantaged. They may share features as the result of such designation, but each majority community would elect, in its own manner, which groups are targeted and what form of disenfranchisement and handicap is appropriate.

General Characteristics

A society may have written and unwritten rules that designate a group as disadvantaged. Such groups are disenfranchised in numerous ways. It is permitted and expected that the group will be abused and exploited. They occupy the margins of the society, often fractionated and segregated. The groups are likely to be the source of both amusement and wrath for the general population. While given substantially less in the community, it is demanded that they do more for less reward.

Petitions for succor by the disadvantaged prompt exasperation, perplexity, and astonishment. Social machinery is elaborated and sustained that is designed to control, dominate, and disrespect the unworthies. As such, the designated disenfranchised group struggles for its security, safety, and livelihood.

The disadvantaged are tyrannized and easily disregarded, discounted, and trivialized. Even so, they are feared as social or economic competitors. Regardless of their powerlessness, they are dismissed as unproductive noncontributors. They may be resented on grounds of their standards and values. They are given blame but little sympathy for an improper identity. Often they are accused of inviting their own catastrophe. In many cases, such as being female or having colored skin, there is no way the person can banish that identifier.

An individual member of a disadvantaged minority may live a lifetime with little or no direct, overt discrimination. Of course, many are victims of hatred, including physical assault, destruction of possessions, deliberate neglect, and even death.

More common are everyday minor, but cumulative, aggressions and insults. For instance, a White couple approaches a well-dressed Black male in a luxury hotel lobby and requests a taxi. They assume, incorrectly, that the man is an employee. The lifelong toll from these microaggressions, both physiologically and psychologically, remains unstudied.

An abundance of comparative data demonstrates the hardship and adversity suffered by disadvantaged minorities. For instance, between 1996 and 2002, the gap between American White and Black wealth grew from 10:1 to 14:1. In the United States, White family wealth now is 14 times the median net worth of Black families. Blacks make twice as many emergency room and outpatient visits as Whites. They make a third fewer visits to a doctor's office, however. In 2003, the percentage of Whites with advanced degrees was twice that of Blacks with advanced degrees. The same numbers hold in the comparison of White and Black college graduates.

There are clear burdens and risks imposed on groups designated as disadvantaged. In general, they are treated unfairly, and their efforts to improve their conditions generate a significant portion of the world's stress and violence.

The historical circumstances of each country determine which groups are disadvantaged and what efforts are made to promote intergroup peace and prosperity. In the United States, as elsewhere, there are numerous disadvantaged minorities. Due to demographic considerations, the most important issue for the United States in the twenty-first century may relate to disadvantaged minorities. It is expected that during this century Whites will become the minority population. The reduced proportion of Whites probably will be accompanied by significant alterations in the influence and hegemony of Whites. How Whites, especially White males, respond to this shift, may be the defining activity of the United States in this century.

Typological Classification

Any classification scheme is both arbitrary and limited. It follows that there can be no complete agreement, since every citizen can use his or her own system. Overall, in the United States, those generally considered by the general public to be disadvantaged minority groups meet a few broad criteria. First, there is evidence, usually with academic credibility, that the designated status does bring uncommon burdens to both the designated member and the general society. Second, the designated minority usually has a long and continuous history regarding getting legal relief from specified ills. Third, in the view of the public, sometimes including members of the minority itself, the designated group inspires fear, requires restraint, and often is deserving of mild to severe punitive actions.

There are those who are constitutionally handicapped. People are born into this category. These include women as well as selected racial/ethnic groups. The groups selected by the United States government include Blacks, Hispanics, Asians, and Native Americans.

The other large category, which most of the public considers disadvantaged, makes up a disparate miscellany. In this general group are migrants, the disabled, criminals, religious and cult community groups, especially those distant from core Christian organizations, and people with a variety of conditions in which there is some disagreement as to how much genetics is at fault. These conditions include obesity, homosexuality, alcohol and drug addiction, and sexual deviations.

All the groups in this classification scheme have been persecuted. For instance, Blacks were enslaved, Native Americans were objects for official genocide, and Hispanics lost large tracts of land to the United States. In general, in the United States, cross-racial interactions, particularly between White and colored races, has brought conflict and stress.

Special Obstacles

Designated minorities meet ongoing stress in an attempt to overcome obstacles in pursuing an occupation, finding adequate housing, and attracting political benefits. Always they remain sensitive as to whether they are welcome or merely tolerated. There is the ceaseless focus on how much, how fast, and in which ways the person and the group accommodate to or resist oppression.

All the separate disadvantaged minorities in the categorization have their own issues. For instance, in the racial/ethnic group there is enormous ambivalence about the cost of integration in such terms as increased intermarriage and loss of unity and leadership as segregated housing diminishes.

As another example, many migrants remain closely tied to their country of origin. The economy of entire countries would be seriously impaired without the input of dollars remitted by migrant workers in the United States. Some migrants in the United States exercise voting rights in other countries. Strong transnational loyalty has to be balanced against charges of diluted loyalty from host nationals.

In this age of wide and rapid communication, designated disenfranchised groups know, as studies show, that bad behavior by one of them has a disproportionate and negative impact on the memory and attitude of majority citizens. The problem of having little control over portrayal by the media becomes a vexing issue of some magnitude.

All the disadvantaged groups protest that the rules are constantly and covertly altered. The fundamental belief is that their space, time, energy, and mobility should be limited and serve majority purposes. This makes the quest for equality all the more elusive, since rules once learned and a system once understood become mystifying and obfuscating.

An advantaged population tends not to see any special, unmerited, or unjustified privilege in what it does. Similarly, it may not calculate any disadvantage from having privilege. Not counting the cost to themselves of disenfranchising whole groups brings serious consequences to the majority. However, if the police have permission to exercise tactics in the disadvantaged community that would not be allowed in the advantaged community, it means that the entire community has elements of a police state. Well over 25% of Americans are in a disadvantaged group. The United States operates under the stress of a huge disadvantage. Any body politic that functions at less than 100% potential is handicapped. The oppressing portion of a society has an obstacle to its own achievement when it does not count the cost of oppressive behavior in everything from total gross national product to intellectual, cultural, and technical achievement, as well as personal freedom.

Treatment Considerations

History teaches that minority groups do best when they themselves are unrelenting in seeking redress from wrongs inflicted upon them. The broad societal pressures are exerted on and felt by all members of a disadvantaged minority. Yet it is hard to imagine how any one-on-one process, even if achieved, could eliminate a minority group's stress. Accordingly, treatment possibilities must be conceived on a grand scale. Only a broad approach can be sketched.

In the foreseeable future, direct medical interventions seem less promising than possible sociological and psychological approaches. The aim in these approaches is to provide increased hope and increased esteem to both the whole disadvantaged group and its individual members. In order to accomplish this objective, the groups themselves must somehow articulate and agree upon who is in their group and what the group cherishes. It must decide what to preserve and what to relinquish in accomplishing intergroup amity. The tactics required to reach these goals involve decreasing stress and increasing adaptation. Political and social action is obligatory.

Decreasing Stress

The disadvantaged minorities and their allies will need to continue and enlarge concerted, dedicated, social, and political actions to decrease stress. Diverse, multiple means must be instituted to teach the group, especially its youngsters, to anticipate the future. To do this, the group will have to mobilize structures at home, in community organizations, at schools, and at churches. All media channels, especially the Internet, TV, and radio, must be enlisted to help. The substantive debate about the details of the subject matter needs participation by persons who will inform themselves, seek input from the community, and be mindful of the history of the group.

Stress research would predict that supplying ways to help oneself and securing more support would be curative. Among topics, for instance, for colored groups would be propaganda analysis to learn to modulate messages that promote defeatism, futility, and loss of self-respect; lifestyle education to indicate the available steps that need to be and can be taken to increase the quality and quantity of life; and cross-racial interactions to emphasize aspects of group dynamics that aid or hinder interpersonal relations.

Perhaps special focus for many groups needs to be on networking and applying demographic remedies. For instance, in the United States, the racially/ethnically disadvantaged compared to the general population tend to be younger, more segregated, and more urban. A firm command of information of this sort will allow framing the future in terms of possible strengths and weaknesses.

Increasing Adaptation

Hopelessness and helplessness are the chief enemies to those under stress. The overall need is to supply support. Corollary to this need is to maximize adaptation. That is, one must cope.

For members of disadvantaged groups and the group as a whole, adaptation, historically, has required education as the critical step toward opportunity.

Acquisition of exploitable skills and unquestioned competency in these skills are more difficult to obtain by disadvantaged minorities. Therefore, much of their social action and networking has to be aimed at securing education.

Community members can facilitate adaptation for each other by countermeasures against noxious environmental stimuli: simple acts of encouragement, providing positive feedback, and giving credit for coping. Similarly, coping is facilitated by encouraging the members under stress, particularly youngsters, to explore options and to be cautious about foreclosing on any opportunity. Community members in a cohesive, cooperative community can augment coping by helping their community provide proper sites and environment for relaxation, another requirement for those in need of surcease. A community may underestimate its ability to contribute to coping. Yet by finding ways to make the community as stable as possible and by trying to reduce feelings of isolation the coping process is facilitated.

People cope better when they do not romanticize the past; when they have a present, clear, and certain mission; and when they appreciate the importance and urgency of that mission. Community members, by their positive attitudes and expectations, can contribute to the individual's enthusiasm for the direction of his or her future.

In coping, helplessness and hopelessness are to be avoided. Their presence may be manifested clinically, particularly by depression and anxiety. Furthermore, depression and anxiety may be comorbid with addiction, violence, obesity, diabetes, and cardiovascular disease. Medical surveillance to prevent illness and medical intervention to treat illness are important considerations in helping disadvantaged minorities to cope.

It is here that ongoing research holds promise to help disadvantaged populations. Advances in molecular biochemistry, endocrinology, genetics, and neurobiology can bring great relief to individuals and families of disadvantaged minorities. Being sure that medical care is accessible will depend somewhat on the political and social activities of the group itself.

See Also the Following Articles

Cultural Factors in Stress; Cultural Transition; Ethnicity, Mental Health; Racial Harassment/Discrimination.

Further Reading

Bell, C. C. (2004). *The sanity of survival: reflections on community mental health and wellness.* Chicago, IL: Third World Press.

Cohen, S., Kessler, R. C. and Gordon, L. U. (eds.) (1995). *Measuring stress: a guide for health and social scientists.* New York: Oxford University Press.

Cornish, E. (2004). *Futuring: the exploration of the future.* Bethesda, MD: World Future Society.

Green, B. L., Lewis, R. K. and Bediako, S. M. (2005). Reducing and eliminating health disparities: a targeted approach. *Journal of the National Medical Association* 97, 25–30.

Gruenewald, T. L., Kemney, M. E., Aziz, H., et al. (2004). Acute threat to the social self: shame, social self-esteem and cortisol activity. *Psychosomatic Medicine* 66, 915–924.

Hobfoll, S. E. (1998). *Stress, culture, and community: the psychology and philosophy of Stress.* New York: Plenum Press.

Jackson, J. S. and Volckens, J. (1998). Community stressors and racism: structural and individual perspectives on racial bias. In: Arriaga, X. B. & Oskamp, S. (eds.) *Addressing community problems: psychological research and interventions*, pp. 19–51. Thousand Oaks, CA: Sage Publications.

National Geographic Society. (2004). *Atlas of the world* (8th edn.). Washington, D.C: National Geographic Society Press.

Smedley, B. D., Stith, A. Y. and Nelson, A. R. (2003). *Unequal treatment: confronting racial and ethnic disparities in healthcare.* Washington, D.C.: National Academy Press.

Special Report. (2004). The state of African American health. *The Crisis* 111, 17–35.

U.S. Census, Bureau. (2004). *Statistical abstract of the United States: 2004–2005* (124th edn.). Washington, D.C.: U.S. Government Printing Office.

Mitochondria

I Manoli
National Institutes of Health, Bethesda, MD, USA, and University of Athens, Athens, Greece
S Alesci
National Institutes of Health, Bethesda, MD, USA
G P Chrousos
University of Athens, Athens, Greece

Background on Mitochondria

Mitochondria as Targets for Stress Hormones and Mediators

Mitochondrial Adaptation and Dysfunction during Acute and Chronic Stress

Seeking Mitochondrial Anti-stress Treatments

Glossary

Apoptosis	The active process of controlled cellular self-destruction, which is intrinsically programmed. It plays an important role in the development of multicellular organisms and in the regulation and maintenance of cell populations in tissues depending on physiological and pathological conditions. It can be initiated by the mitochondrion in response to energy deficiency, oxidative stress, and increased Ca^{2+}, among other stimuli.
Mitochondria	Intracellular organelles containing their own genetic material and the enzymatic machinery for major metabolic pathways, including the citric acid cycle, fatty acid oxidation, and oxidative phosphorylation, and for apoptosis.
Oxidative phosphorylation	The coupling of electron transport in the respiratory chain to ATP synthesis via the proton gradient and ATP synthase in the presence of oxygen, which occurs at the inner mitochondrial membrane.
Oxidative stress	The imbalance between reactive oxygen species production and antioxidant defenses, resulting in cellular damage.
Reactive oxygen species (ROS)	Oxygen-containing chemical species with unpaired electrons that are highly reactive and function in cell-signaling processes but also, at higher level, can damage cellular macromolecules and participate in apoptosis.

Background on Mitochondria

Mitochondria play a pivotal role in cell homeostasis, housing multiple metabolic pathways (including the tricarboxylic acid-, β-oxidation- and urea cycle) and the oxidative phosphorylation machinery that generates energy in the form of ATP. Research during the last decade has extended the prevailing view of mitochondrial function well beyond their critical role in supplying energy. Mitochondria synthesize heme and steroid hormones; are important for intracellular Ca^{2+} metabolism and signaling; generate the majority of cellular reactive oxygen species (ROS); and serve as the cell's gatekeeper for apoptosis. They contain multiple copies of circular mitochondrial DNA (mtDNA) and function under dual genetic control. Both nuclear and mtDNA encode genes that modulate mitochondrial protein synthesis and import, enzymatic activities, biogenesis, and apoptosis.

Most of the ATP necessary to supply energy to tissues and organs is generated by the mitochondrial oxidative phosphorylation system (OXPHOS). Under aerobic conditions, electrons derived from the oxidation of glucose or fatty acids are transferred through the respiratory chain complexes I–IV. At each of the enzymatic complexes I, III, and IV, protons are pumped out of the mitochondrial matrix into the intermembrane space, generating an electrochemical gradient used by the fifth enzymatic complex (ATP synthase) to drive ATP synthesis.

Mitochondria consume more than 90% of the cell's oxygen and are therefore the main site of ROS production. ROS, including superoxide, hydrogen peroxide, and hydroxyl radicals, are generated as a by-product of mitochondrial activity, primarily at complexes I, II, and III of the respiratory chain. Normally, 2–5% of O_2 used in the mitochondria is metabolized into superoxide. The superoxide radicals are converted to hydrogen peroxide by superoxide dismutase (SOD), which can further form the highly reactive hydroxyl radical. Mitochondrial (Mn-SOD and glutathione peroxidase) and cytosolic (Cu-SOD and catalase) antioxidant enzymes help to scavenge the ROS and limit their toxicity.

ROS play a significant role in the regulation of cell-signaling processes and in cytoprotection; thus their controlled generation is necessary for cell survival. On the other hand, when produced in excess of cellular antioxidant reserves, lipid peroxidation, mtDNA damage, OXPHOS dysfunction, and damage to Fe–S-containing enzymes ensue. Oxidative stress to nuclear or mtDNA results in strand breaks and base modifications, followed by cellular dysfunction, mutagenesis, and carcinogenesis.

Mitochondria are involved in cell death by at least three general mechanisms: the release of proteins that trigger the activation of the caspase family of proteases, the disruption of oxidative phosphorylation and ATP production, and the modification of the cellular reduction–oxidation (redox) potential. Each of those mechanisms can result in programmed cell death (apoptosis) or cell necrosis. The initiation of apoptosis occurs via the opening of the permeability transition pore (mtPTP) located in the inner mitochondrial membrane. The mtPTP is composed of the adenine nucleotide translocator (ANT), voltage-dependent anion channel (VDAC), Bax, Bcl2, cyclophilin D, and benzodiazepine receptor. The opening of the mtPTP leads to swelling of the mitochondrial inner membrane and the rupture of the outer membrane, followed by the release of cytochrome c, procaspases 2,3,4, and caspase-activated deoxyribonuclease (CAD) into the cytoplasm. Cytochrome c activates apoptotic protease activating factor (Apaf-)1, which first activates procaspase 2 and 9, and subsequently caspases 3, 6, and 7, inducing apoptosis. Another caspase-activating protein released by mitochondria is the apoptosis-inducing factor (AIF). AIF and endonuclease G are transported to the nucleus and initiate chromatin condensation and degradation. Depending on the amount of cytochrome c and caspase inhibitors available, the cell undergoes either necrosis or apoptosis. The Bcl-2 family proteins exhibit pro- and/or anti-apoptotic properties (**Figure 1**).

Given their critical role in cell physiology, it is obvious that mitochondria are among the first responders to various stressful stimuli challenging cell homeostasis. They are responsible for meeting the enormous energy demands of the fight-or-flight response in vital tissues. Among other equally important effects, they control the fever response by the modulation of thermogenesis, balance the host immune

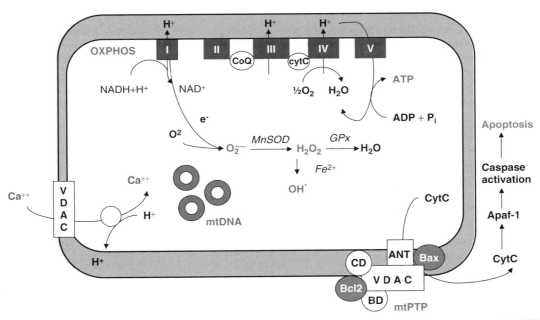

Figure 1 Mitochondrial functions. The figure illustrates (1) energy (ATP) production at the oxidative phosphorylation chain (OXPHOS) in the inner mitochondrial membrane, (2) reactive oxygen species (ROS) generation in the mitochondrial matrix and the enzymes Mn superoxide dismutase (MnSOD) and glutathione peroxidase (GPx), and (3) induction of apoptosis through the opening of the mitochondrial permeability transition pore (mtPTP). The OXPHOS complexes are complex I (NADH–ubiquinone oxidoreductase), complex II (succinate–ubiquinone oxidoreductase), complex III (ubiquinol–cytochrome c oxidoreductase), complex IV (cytochrome c oxidase), and complex V (ATP synthase). Ca^{2+} defuses through the outer membrane via the voltage-dependent anion channel (VDAC). The VDAC together with adenine nucleotide translocator (ANT), Bax, and cyclophilin D (CD) are components of the mtPTP. The release of cytochrome c (CytC) in the cytoplasm activates apoptotic protease activating factor (Apaf-)1 and subsequently caspases that eventually lead to proteolysis and apoptosis.

response during infection by deciding on the fate of the affected cells, and adjust the oxidative stress response for cytoprotective and signaling purposes.

Mitochondria as Targets for Stress Hormones and Mediators

Several important mediators of the stress response, namely hormones (glucocorticoids, GCs, and catecholamines), immune mediators (cytokines), and heat shock proteins (Hsps), among other factors, exert multiple effects on mitochondrial biogenesis, metabolism, ROS generation, and apoptosis.

Glucocorticoids

GCs play a major role in survival during stress. Increased cortisol levels raise the resting energy expenditure and metabolic rate by as much as 200% during acute stress. Despite the significant hyperglycemia, the observed decrease in the respiratory quotient (the ratio of the carbon dioxide produced to oxygen consumed) suggests that a significant portion of that energy comes from the oxidation of lipids. GCs also stimulate protein degradation in muscle and lymphoid tissue to provide amino acids for gluconeogenesis in the liver.

In addition to the well-described molecular mechanism of GC action, via binding to glucocorticoid receptors (GRs) in the cytoplasm, and subsequent translocation of the GC–GR complexes to the nucleus for the trans-activation or -repression of nuclear gene targets, nongenomic mechanisms, such as the activation of phosphatidylinositol 3 (PI3) kinase and other cytosolic signaling pathways are increasingly recognized. Mitochondrial function can be affected directly or indirectly through both these mechanisms. Furthermore, GRs were recently described inside the mitochondria of several cell types, and mtDNA contains nucleotide sequences that are highly similar to the nuclear DNA GR binding consensus sequences. Thus, it is possible that GCs stimulate mtDNA transcription by direct interaction via the mitochondrial GR.

Indeed dexamethasone, a synthetic GC, stimulates the transcription of mtDNA-encoded genes (COX II and cyt-b) in hepatoma cell lines; a rise of mitochondrial transcripts (COX I, II, and III) was also found in colon epithelium of rats after dexamethasone injection. A recent study of rat skeletal muscle suggests an increase in mitochondrial biogenesis, mtDNA transcription (COX II and III), and cytochrome c activity after treatment with dexamethasone for 3 days. The mechanism underlying the observed transcriptional induction remains unclear because no increases in mitochondrial transcription factor A (Tfam) or nuclear respiratory factor (NRF-)1 and 2 have been observed in these studies.

Several studies suggest the modulation of mitochondrial metabolic activities by GCs in a biphasic mode. Low doses of or early exposure to GCs induce mitochondrial biogenesis and the enzymatic activity of selected subunits of the respiratory chain complexes, whereas higher doses or prolonged exposure cause increased ROS generation and respiratory chain dysfunction. Those effects depend on the target organ and developmental stage of the organism. Our recent transcriptional screening for mitochondrial targets of GC action in the human skeletal muscle revealed the induction of mitochondrial translation and energy metabolism-related genes after a shorter exposure to dexamethasone and the down-regulation of genes involved in lipid metabolism, induction of ROS, and apoptosis after prolonged exposure.

Clinical studies of the effects of chronic exposure to GCs have shown increased lactate production following aerobic exercise (suggesting anaerobic glycolysis due to mitochondrial dysfunction), decreased complex-I activity and oxidative damage-induced alterations in skeletal muscle mtDNA and nuclear DNA after long-term GC treatment. Moreover clinical symptoms resembling mitochondrial disorders, such as external ophthalmoplegia, have also been described under such conditions.

ROS generation follows exposure to GCs in different tissues. Hydrogen peroxide is described as a potent mediator of glucocorticoid effects in skeletal muscle cells, stimulating myogenesis and myotube formation at low doses while inducing apoptosis and cell death at higher concentrations or after prolonged treatment. GCs increase oxidative stress damage to neurons, in part by increasing glutamate and calcium and in part by decreasing antioxidant enzymes, specifically in the hippocampal neurons. Hydrogen peroxide is also synthesized in large amounts by neutrophils and macrophages during the oxidative burst, when it aids in destroying engulfed microorganisms. Moreover, various apoptotic stimuli, such as tumor necrosis factor (TNF-)α, have been shown to increase the levels of mitochondria-derived hydrogen peroxide. The increased production of hydrogen peroxide or superoxide after prolonged exposure to GCs in various tissues leads to mtDNA oxidative damage and apoptosis.

Interestingly, antioxidant compounds (i.e., N-acetyl-cysteine, vitamin C, and vitamin E) and enzymes (i.e., SOD and catalase) can prevent those adverse effects in skeletal muscle and vascular endothelium, both *in vitro* and *in vivo*. Those findings suggest a primary pathogenetic role of ROS in GC-induced tissue damage.

GCs are important regulators of T-cell growth, differentiation, and apoptosis. Their profound anti-inflammatory and immunosuppressive activities place synthetic GCs among the most commonly prescribed drugs worldwide, especially for the treatment of hematological malignancies, such as leukemia and lymphoma.

The current evidence suggests that GC-induced cell death is linked to the *de novo* synthesis of one or several gene products. Genes described as being up- or downregulated during GC-induced apoptosis include c-myc139 and T-cell-death-associated gene (TDAG)8, Bcl-x_L, IkB, GILZ, and GITR. Interaction with other transcription factors, such as nuclear factor (NF-)κB, activator protein (AP-)1, nuclear factor of activated T cells (NF-AT), cAMP response element binding protein (CREB), and signal transducer and activator of transcription (STAT)5 is also critical. On the other hand, GC binding to its receptor rapidly induces ceramide generation via the activation of the phosphatidyl-inositol-specific phospholipase C (PIPLC) and acidic sphingomyelinase (aSMase) enzymes, which is necessary for caspase 9 activation.

A vast amount of data indicates that the disruption of mitochondrial integrity is a prerequisite for GC-induced apoptosis. This is tightly regulated by the balance between pro-(the BH-3 only: Bim, Bid, and Bad) and anti-apoptotic (Bcl-2 and Bcl-x_L) Bcl-2 family members, resulting in the activation of Bax and Bak, the opening of the mtPTP in the outer mitochondrial membrane, and the release of cytochrome c. The multimeric complex containing cytochrome c, caspase 9, and Apaf-1 (called the apoptosome) activates caspase 3, which finally leads to apoptosis.

Catecholamines

Catecholamines are the primary mediators of the fight-or-flight response. Norepinephrine is the major neurotransmitter in the peripheral sympathetic nervous system, whereas epinephrine is the primary hormone secreted by the adrenal medulla. The release of both is increased during stress. Their effect on target tissues is mediated by 6α- and 3β-adrenoceptor subtypes.

Epinephrine affects mitochondrial metabolism mainly by mobilizing body energy stores to augment the availability of substrates for oxidation. Epinephrine stimulates both lipolysis and glycogenolysis (most notably in the skeletal muscle) by interacting with the β_1- and β_2-adrenoceptors. It also acts through the G_s-protein-coupled β_2-adrenergic receptor to stimulate adenyl cyclase activity and cAMP production, leading to the activation of the protein kinase A (PKA). This signaling pathway is responsible for the modulation of numerous processes and notably gene transcription through the phosphorylation of CREB.

Another major mitochondria-targeted effect of catecholamines is the enhancement of thermogenesis, which occurs primarily in the brown adipose tissue, which is highly innervated by sympathetic nerve terminals. During this process, energy derived from the oxidation of fuel substrates is dissipated as heat rather than being stored as ATP (uncoupling). Uncoupling occurs via β_3-adrenergic stimulation and the downstream regulation of specific uncoupling proteins (UCPs). The inner mitochondrial membrane in brown adipose tissue contains UCP-1. Other known UCPs include UCP-2, which is widely expressed, and UCP-3, which seems to be expressed primarily in the skeletal muscles, heart, and brown adipose tissue, which are controlled by thyroid hormone and leptin. Several pharmaceutical companies have worked on the development of β_3-adrenoceptor agonists to stimulate UCP-1 in brown adipocytes and increase energy expenditure in obese patients. Unfortunately, these drugs often have adverse side effects on the cardiovascular system and poor bioavailability.

The peroxisome proliferator-activated receptor γ co-activator (PGC-)1α controls adaptive thermogenesis in adipose tissue and skeletal muscle by stimulating mitochondrial biogenesis and oxidative phosphorylation. Stress, fasting, and exercise activate the PGC-1α through different signaling pathways, including β-adrenergic (β_3/cAMP), Ca^{2+}-dependent, NO and mitogen-activated protein kinase (MAPK) pathways. PGC-1α, in turn, activates the expression of nuclear respiratory factor (NRF)-1 and-2, estrogen-related receptor (ERR-)α, and PPAR-α, which regulate the mitochondrial biogenesis and fatty acid oxidation pathways. NRF-1 and NRF-2 regulate the expression of Tfam, a nuclear-encoded transcription factor that binds regulatory sites on mtDNA and is essential for the replication and transcription of the mitochondrial genome. Furthermore, NRF-1 and NRF-2 regulate the expression of nuclear genes encoding respiratory chain subunits and other proteins required for mitochondrial function.

Cytokines

The overproduction of inflammatory cytokines, with the subsequent induction of NO, platelet activating factor, and prostaglandins have been implicated in the changes leading to the multiorgan failure associated with, for example, sepsis. This pro-inflammatory state is described as the systemic inflammatory response syndrome (SIRS).

Cytokines like TNF-α can induce apoptosis in several cell populations, whereas other cytokines such as interleukin (IL)-1 and IL-6 often inhibit apoptosis. The release of these pro-inflammatory cytokines is a major component of the stress response to infection, ischemia/reperfusion injury, and trauma. The intracellular signaling pathways involved in TNF-α- or Fas ligand (FasL)-induced apoptosis appear to be caspase 3-dependent.

Exciting new findings describing mitochondria localization of functional proteins required for the activation of interferon 1 expression in response to viral infections highlight the central role played by mitochondria in balancing the host immune response to viral infection and possibly to other pathogens.

Heat Shock Proteins

Hsps constitute a highly conserved and functionally interactive network of chaperones, some of which are constitutively expressed and others that are induced by various environmental, physical, and chemical stressors that challenge the intracellular milieu and cause damage to DNA and proteins. Chaperones are proteins that disaggregate, refold, and renature misfolded proteins, thus protecting the cell from the damage imposed by stressful stimuli. If the stressor is heat shock, the induced chaperones are called heat shock proteins.

The induction of Hsps following cellular damage can prevent apoptosis. Hsp27, 70, and 90 have been implicated in protection against apoptosis induced by multiple signals, such as heat shock, nutrient withdrawal, ROS, endoplasmic reticulum stress, proteasome inhibition, UV radiation, and chemotherapy-induced DNA damage. Hsps promote cell survival by preventing mitochondrial outer-membrane permeabilization and subsequent cytochrome c release, caspase activation, and apoptosome assembly. In addition, Hsp60 and Hsp70 interact with the outer mitochondrial membrane-specific translocase (TOM), contributing to the importing of nuclear-encoded proteins into the mitochondrial matrix. It may well be that the beneficial effects of fever initially described by Hippocrates actually relate to increased Hsp expression and their protective effects.

Mitochondrial Adaptation and Dysfunction during Acute and Chronic Stress

The acute response to stressful stimuli is characterized by the massive release of stress mediators. Their coordinated interaction aims at (1) maintaining the effective circulation (and hence oxygenation) of the brain, cardiac muscle, and skeletal muscle; (2) increasing energy generation by the release of substrates (i.e., glucose, fatty acids, and amino acids) from body fuel storages (i.e., the liver, adipose tissue, and skeletal muscle); and (3) optimizing ATP availability to vital tissues at the expense of others (i.e., the gonads and gastrointestinal tract).

Tissue oxygen consumption and total energy expenditure are profoundly increased during the initial phase of the acute stress response. Rapid elevations in GC and catecholamine levels stimulate mitochondrial oxygen consumption and ATP formation to sustain the substantial hypermetabolic state. Mitochondria respond by modulating the expression and activity of certain OXPHOS subunits, or by increasing significantly their size and numbers (mitogenesis). Yet the exact mechanisms by which mitochondria fulfill this increased energy demand remain poorly understood.

Although the initial burst in mitochondrial function is necessary for survival, excessive mitochondrial activation during critical illness, such as trauma, surgery, or sepsis, can be detrimental to the cell (**Figure 2**). Stress-induced hyperglycemia, resulting from increased glucose mobilization and insulin resistance, is a common finding in these conditions, and its severity correlates strongly with increased mortality risk. Several lines of evidence support the concept that mitochondrial impairment, caused by glucose toxicity, is the underlying mechanism for the disturbance in oxygen use, called cytopathic hypoxia. Cellular glucose overload can exceed the capacity of the respiratory chain leading to (1) increased ROS generation and oxidative damage to the mitochondrial complexes I and IV, and the antioxidant enzyme MnSOD; (2) the impaired detoxification of superoxide and other free radicals; (3) the shunting of glucose into toxic pathways (i.e., polyol and hexosamine); and (4) increased apoptosis. Recent studies show that strict glycemic control with insulin therapy can prevent and correct mitochondrial ultrastructural and functional abnormalities in surgical intensive-care patients.

Prolonged physical and, interestingly, psychological stress can induce oxidative damage. In a recent study, psychological stress, both perceived stress and chronicity of stress, in mothers of children suffering from chronic illness was shown to be associated with increased markers of oxidative stress in their circulation (F_2-isoprostanes levels and isoprostanes/vitamin E ratio), in addition to telomere shortening. Telomeres are DNA sequences necessary for DNA replication, which shorten at cell division at a rate related to the levels of oxidative stress. Once telomeres are

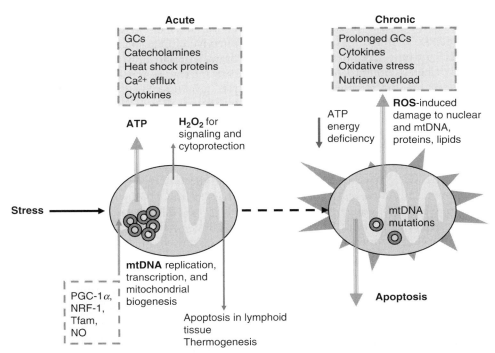

Figure 2 Mitochondrial stress response under acute and chronic stress. Early exposure to glucocorticoids (GCs) or other stressful stimuli and their respective mediators induce mitochondrial biogenesis and the enzymatic activity of selected subunits of the respiratory chain complexes to meet the increased energy demands of the cell. Controlled production of reactive oxygen species (ROS), apoptosis, and thermogenesis serve as protective mechanisms against infection or other cell damage. Prolonged stress can exceed mitochondrial reserves, leading to respiratory chain dysfunction and decreased ATP production, increased ROS generation, and significant apoptosis and/or necrosis. mtDNA, mitochondrial DNA; NRF, nuclear respiratory factor; PGC, peroxisome proliferator-activated receptor γ coactivator; Tfam, mitochondrial transcription factor A.

shortened to a critical length, cells enter a stage of replicative senescence; hence, telomere length is a determinant of cell senescence and longevity. Although not examined in the study, it is expected that changes in the mtDNA, which is far more prone to oxidative damage, could also arise under those conditions. These findings have implications for the molecular mechanisms at the cellular level by which stress may promote the earlier onset of age-related diseases.

Psychological stress can lead to oxidative stress, but the opposite seems to hold true also. An intriguing recent study in an animal model showed a strong positive correlation between the expression levels of two antioxidant enzymes, glyoxalase and glutathione reductase 1, and anxiety levels. To determine whether those genes have a causal role in the genesis of anxiety, genetic manipulation was performed to induce or inhibit their activity. The local overexpression of these genes in the mouse brain resulted in increased anxiety-like behavior that was decreased with their inhibition. The authors propose oxidative stress as a new and unsuspected player in the complex control of anxious behavior, which, if exaggerated, in humans can be expressed as panic disorder, obsessive-compulsive disorder, posttraumatic stress disorder,

social and other specific phobias, and generalized anxiety disorder.

The metabolic syndrome (central/visceral obesity, insulin resistance, dyslipidemia, hypertension, pro-inflammatory, and prothrombotic syndrome) has been associated with hyperactivity of the hypothalamus-pituitary-adrenal axis. The pathogenesis remains unknown, but both genetic and environmental factors have an important share. It is proposed that underlying genetic polymorphisms or alterations in nuclear and, potentially more important, in mitochondrial DNA, in combination with exposure to environmental stresses such as excessive caloric intake, exhaust mitochondrial reserves and lead to the imbalance and failure of energy metabolism.

Support for this theory comes from numerous animal studies, across several species, which demonstrate the strong beneficial effects of calorie restriction on life expectancy. Reduced workload on the respiratory chain leads to improved energy output and decreased oxidative stress and subsequent damage. In this regard, a study that selected rats for their low versus high intrinsic capacity to run on a treadmill over 11 generations – hence, rats with low-versus high-power mitochondria – demonstrated that cardiovascular risk factors, such as obesity, hyperglycemia, hyperlipidemia, hypertension, and insulin resistance, segregate with low aerobic capacity and reduced expression of genes required for mitochondrial biogenesis and oxidative phosphorylation.

Defects in mitochondrial fatty acid oxidation can lead to the intracellular accumulation of fatty acid metabolites that disrupt insulin signaling and possibly also secretion from the pancreatic β-cells, leading to insulin resistance and ultimately failure. Defects of mitochondrial oxidative phosphorylation and mitochondrial copy number are indeed observed in the skeletal muscle of elderly subjects and of healthy relatives of individuals with type 2 diabetes. Moreover, alterations in mtDNA, specific mutations in mitochondrial tRNA, or decreased expression of genes regulating mitochondrial function, such as PGC-1α, are all associated with type 2 diabetes.

Transgenic animal models, in which antioxidant enzymes are overexpressed, such as manganese superoxide dismutase (MnSOD) or Cu,ZnSOD in *Drosophila*, exhibit a significantly extended life span. To the contrary, in knockouts for MnSOD, a 100% increased incidence of cancer was observed, whereas knockouts for mtDNA polymerase γ (POLG), the enzyme responsible for mtDNA proofreading, experience a significant acceleration in their aging process, with cardiomegaly, lipoatrophy, osteoporosis, anemia, and alopecia – but, interestingly, an absence of oxidative stress. The later study and others challenge the free-radical theory of aging and pose further questions in the fascinating field of mitochondrial pathology.

Seeking Mitochondrial Anti-stress Treatments

Therapeutic options for mitochondrial dysfunction are currently very limited. Strategies are being developed for mitochondria-targeted therapeutics, using their distinct biophysical and biochemical properties. The high negative potential of the mitochondrial matrix allows for selective targeting of positively charged compounds. Furthermore, the presence of specific transporter-dependent delivery for pro-drugs that can be subsequently activated by mitochondrial enzymes enable the design of highly specific agents.

The most effective of such attempts to date has been the development of mitochondria-targeted antioxidants. Mito-vitamin E and mito-coenzyme Q are coupled to a triphenylphosphonium cation, which accumulates several hundredfold in the mitochondrial matrix due to the large membrane potential, which is negative inside. First-line evidence from *in vitro* applications and initial animal studies on cardiac

ischemia-reperfusion injury have been very promising. Further support for mitochondria-targeted antioxidants comes from a transgenic mouse model, in which the overexpression of the antioxidant enzyme catalase targeted specifically to mitochondria (vs. to peroxisomes or the nucleus) significantly reduced oxidative damage in both nuclear and mitochondrial DNA, resulting in increased murine life span and delayed cardiac pathology and cataract development.

We can envision a rapid increase in the efforts to exploit the unique properties of mitochondria for the development of selective therapeutic agents aimed at increasing mitochondrial biogenesis and energy output while concomitantly minimizing mitochondrial Ca^{2+} overload, ROS production, and oxidative stress.

Acknowledgments

This work was supported by the Intramural Research Programs of the National Human Genome Research Institute and by the National Institute of Mental Health. The authors have no conflicts of interest related to this work.

Further Reading

Balaban, R. S., Nemoto, S. and Finkel, T. (2005). Mitochondria, oxidants, and aging. *Cell* **120**(4), 483–495.

Chinopoulos, C. and Adam-Vizi, V. (2006). Calcium, mitochondria and oxidative stress in neuronal pathology: novel aspects of an enduring theme. *FEBS Journal* **273**(3), 433–450.

Chrousos, G. P. (1998). Stressors, stress, and neuroendocrine integration of the adaptive response: the 1997 Hans Selye memorial lecture. *Annals of the New York Academy of Sciences* **851**, 311–335.

Chrousos, G. P. (2004). The HPA axis and the stress response. *Endocrine Research* **26**(4), 513–514.

Epel, E. S., Blackburn, E. H., Lin, J., et al. (2004). Accelerated telomere shortening in response to life stress. *Proceedings of the National Academy of Sciences USA* **101** (49), 17312–17315.

Goldenthal, M. J. and Marin-Garcia, J. (2004). Mitochondrial signaling pathways: a receiver/integrator organelle. *Molecular and Cellular Biochemistry* **262** (1–2), 1–16.

Jezek, P. and Hlavata, L. (2005). Mitochondria in homeostasis of reactive oxygen species in cell, tissues, and organism. *International Journal of Biochemistry and Cell Biology* **37**(12), 2478–2503.

Kino, T., Charmandari, E. and Chrousos, G. P. (eds.) (2004). *Special issue on glucocorticoid action: basic and clinical implications*. Annals of the New York Academy of Sciences. 1024.

Lee, S. H. K. D., Tanaka, M. and Wei, Y. (eds.) (2004). *Special issue on mitochondrial pathogenesis: from genes* and apoptosis to aging and disease. *Annals of the New York Academy of Sciences.* 1011.

Lemasters, J. J. and Nieminem, A. L. (2001). *Mitochondria in pathogenesis.* New York: Kluwer Academic/Plenum.

Lowell, B. B. and Shulman, G. I. (2005). Mitochondrial dysfunction and type 2 diabetes. *Science* 307(5708), 384–387.

Manoli, I., Le, H., Alesci, S., et al. (2005). Monoamine oxidase-A is a major target gene for glucocorticoids in human skeletal muscle cells. *FASEB Journal* 19(10), 1359–1361.

Oberholzer, C., Oberholzer, A., Clare-Salzler, M., et al. (2001). Apoptosis in sepsis: a new target for therapeutic exploration. *FASEB Journal* 15(6), 879–892.

Pacak, K., Aguilera, G., Sabban, E., et al. (eds.) (2004). *Special issue on stress: current neuroendocrine and genetic approaches. Annals of the New York Academy of Sciences.* 1018.

Psarra, A. M., Solakidi, S. and Sekeris, C. E. (2006). The mitochondrion as a primary site of action of steroid and thyroid hormones: presence and action of steroid and thyroid hormone receptors in mitochondria of animal cells. *Molecular and Cellular Endocrinology* 246(1–2), 21–33.

Scheffler, I. E. (1999). *Mitochondria.* New York: Wiley-Liss.

Sheu, S. S., Nauduri, D. and Anders, M. W. (2006). Targeting antioxidants to mitochondria: a new therapeutic direction. *Biochimica et Biophysica Acta* 1762(2), 256–265.

Wallace, D. C. (2005). A mitochondrial paradigm of metabolic and degenerative diseases, aging, and cancer: a dawn for evolutionary medicine. *Annual Review of Genetics* 39, 359–407.

Monoamine Oxidase

P Huezo-Diaz and I W Craig
King's College London, London, UK

Stress and the Cycle of Violence
Genetic Factors in Aggression and Violence
MAOA as a Candidate Gene
The Role of Stress and Abusive Upbringing in Aggression and Violence
Conclusion

Glossary

Allele	One of two or more possible forms of a gene. An individual may possess two identical, or two different, alleles, except for those of the genes on the X chromosome in males because they possess only a single copy of this chromosome.
Antisocial behavior (ASB)	A pervasive pattern of disregard for and violation of the rights of others occurring since age 15 years old.
Cycle of violence	The observed relationship between violent parenting and violence in the parents' offspring.
Major effect gene	A gene whose influence can be detected without the need to control for environmental factors.
Null mutation	A mutation that completely eliminates the function of the gene.
Promoter	The section of DNA that precedes a gene and controls its activity.

Stress and the Cycle of Violence

A common observation in studies of ASB and aggression in humans is the cycle of violence, in which there is a tendency for individuals who were exposed to abusive parents and/or difficult childhoods to manifest antisocial personalities in adulthood. Not all individuals exposed to abusive childhoods, however, develop antisocial and violent tendencies. The challenge is, therefore, to establish the extent to which genetic predispositions and the extent to which stressful environments are responsible for eliciting the violent behavior. Recent research suggests that there is an interaction between the two that may underpin this repeating pattern.

Genetic Factors in Aggression and Violence

Results from more than 50 behavioral genetic studies indicate that, on average, approximately 41% of the variance of ASB is due to genetic factors, approximately 16% is due to shared environmental factors and approximately 43% is due to nonshared environmental factors. The same overall pattern appears to hold for violence. Epidemiological studies have also consistently shown that the risk of aggression is greater in males than in females, and this raises the possibility that genetic and environmental influences contribute differentially to the risk of aggressive behavior depending on gender. Twin studies indicate that common environmental factors, sex-specific genes, and the interaction between the two play an important role in increasing liability toward aggressive behavior in males, even though females have a higher heritability and males a higher common environmental liability.

Evidence for a direct role of testosterone levels, which could be genetically determined, in promoting aggression in humans is not clear-cut. This leaves open the possible influence of other specific genetic factors that may contribute to increased aggression in males; recent interest has focused on the monoamine oxidase A gene, *MAOA*, in this regard.

MAOA as a Candidate Gene

The main role for the monoamine oxidase (MAOA) enzyme is thought to be in degrading serotonin following its reuptake from the synaptic cleft, although it is also capable of degrading both norepinephrine and dopamine. It therefore plays a key role in the regulation of nerve transmission, and alterations in its activity produced by pharmacological intervention or through genetic variants are likely to have profound effects on behavior. Indeed, drugs inhibiting its activity have long been employed in the treatment of behavioral disorders, particularly depression.

A wide range of genetic variants of the *MAOA* gene exists in the general population. One of the most significant is a DNA motif localized in the promoter 1.2 kb upstream from the *MAOA* coding region, comprising a 30-bp repeat existing in 3, 3.5, 4, or 5 copies (**Figure 1**). It has been shown that the copy number has a significant effect on the level of the gene's expression. The two predominant forms observed in the population are those with three or four repeats of the motif, with the three-copy version having reduced transcriptional activity compared to the four-copy allele. The gene is located on the X chromosome, which means that females have two copies but males have only one. Any defect in the gene in males

is therefore exposed because they are unaffected by the status of a second copy.

A possible direct role for *MAOA* in predisposing violence, ASB, and conduct disorders was suggested by studies of males from a Dutch pedigree who exhibited a complex behavioral syndrome (including impulsive aggression). All affected individuals suffered from a mutation in the *MAOA* gene that resulted in zero activity of the enzyme. A role for *MAOA* deficiency in promoting aggression is further supported by studies on mutant mice that had deletions of portions of their monoamine oxidase gene, resulting in the lack of enzyme activity in the brain and liver. Behavioral studies on the adult male mice indicated heightened aggression in response to intruders and also increased inappropriate courtship behaviors. These have been the only reports to date of the phenotypic consequences of null mutations. The existence of high- and low-activity *MAOA* alleles in the human population, however, raises the intriguing possibility that lower levels of the enzyme may predispose male individuals to ASB and/or violent behavior.

There have been a variety of reports suggesting a role for variants at the *MAOA* locus in the context of violence and/or ASB, particularly in relation to subgroups of males with alcoholism and attention deficit and hyperactivity disorders. Generally, it appears that individuals with the low-activity allele are at risk, but there is no overall consensus concerning its possible status as a major effect gene. Nevertheless, a significant and intriguing interaction between stressful environments and low-activity variants of *MAOA* in promoting violence and ASB has recently emerged.

The Role of Stress and Abusive Upbringing in Aggression and Violence

Given the observed relationship between abusive environments and antisocial outcomes, the *MAOA*

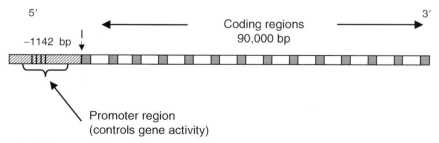

Figure 1 Representation of the monoamine oxidase gene (*MAOA*). The promoter region (in diagonal lines) controls the levels of gene activity and contains a 30-bp repeat (often referred to as a variable-number tandem repeat, VNTR). Different copy numbers of the basic motif have different effects on transcription. Three- and four-copy motifs are the most common in the population, with the former conferring lower activity than the latter. Rare alleles with 2-, 3.5-, and 5-copy motifs are also observed. I indicates position of transcription initiation (RNA synthesis). Exons (coding regions) are in gray (not to scale).

gene became a candidate for a genetic predisposing factor that may interact with stress induced by adverse early rearing experiences to promote ASB. Caspi and associates, in 2002, were the first to study the interactions between environment and *MAOA* activity variants in the etiology of ASB in males by investigating the patterns of antisocial outcomes in a range of male children who had been maltreated. A broad range of measures for ASB was followed in the males from a longitudinal cohort of approximately 800 individuals who were age 26 at the time of data collection. The information available relevant to ASB included the commission of violent crimes, a personal disposition toward violence, and adolescent conduct disorder (assessed according to *Diagnostic and Statistical Manual*, 4th edn., criteria). Whichever measure of antisocial outcomes was examined, a significant association between maltreatment and ASB conditional on the individual's *MAOA* genotype was observed. Whereas maltreated males with low-activity alleles were significantly at risk of conviction for violent crime or of exhibiting other ASB, those with high-activity alleles were not. An increasing tendency to antisocial acts by those with more extreme childhood maltreatment was observed for males with the low-activity allele, but not for those protected by a high-activity allele.

Similar observations have since been reported in studies employing data from white male twins from the community-based longitudinal Virginia Twin Study for Adolescent Behavioural Development. Several other studies have been completed, and an analysis of all the information currently available is broadly supportive of an interaction between variants of this gene and stressful environments in predisposing ASB.

It is of interest that an analogous promoter variant system of this X chromosome gene has been discovered in rhesus macaque monkeys. A variable-repeat motif of 18 bp has been identified and shown to regulate the expression of *MAOA*. Of particular relevance to the putative role of functional *MAOA* variants in humans is that male macaques with the low-activity form were found to be more aggressive in competing for food.

The physiological relationship between the stress caused by abusive upbringing and the apparent protection provided by the high-activity allele for *MAOA* is not yet clear. Stress is known to elicit an increase in levels of transcription factors, such as c-Fos. These factors, in turn, may upregulate genes encoding components of neurotransmitter pathways, and it is possible that the apparent risk conferred by the low-activity allele of *MAOA* reflects a relative inability to respond to the effects of stress arising from maltreatment.

Conclusion

The lack of a functional copy of the *MAOA* gene in humans and mice results in ASB and aggression, and the less-functional fundamental variation of the gene appears to have related behavioral consequences. In particular, there is a complex interaction between the response to chronic stress and functional variants of the gene and the likelihood of individuals developing ASB or violent behavior. Longitudinal studies of the effects of childhood maltreatment and its interaction in males with high- or low-activity genetic variants of the *MAOA* gene suggest that the high-activity allele may confer protection in males because carriers are much less likely to develop ASB and aggressive behavior than are those with low-activity alleles.

See Also the Following Articles

Aggression; Domestic Violence; Gene Environment Interactions in Early Development.

Further Reading

Brunner, H. G., Nelen, M., Breakefield, X. O., et al. (1993). Abnormal behavior associated with a point mutation in the structural gene for monoamine oxidase A. *Science* **262**, 578–580.

Cases, O., Seif, I., Grimsby, J., et al. (1995). Aggressive behaviour and altered amounts of brain serotonin and norepinephrine in mice lacking MAOA. *Science* **268**, 1763–1766.

Caspi, A., McClay, J., Moffitt, T. E., et al. (2002). Role of genotype in the cycle of violence in maltreated children. *Science* **297**, 851–854.

Craig, I. W. (2005). The role of monoamine oxidase A, MAOA, in the aetiology of antisocial behaviour: the importance of gene environment interactions. In: Bock, G. & Goode, J. (Eds.) *Molecular mechanisms influencing aggressive behaviours* (Novartis Foundation Symposium 268), pp. 227–237. New York: John Wiley & Sons.

Deckert, J., Catalano, M., Syagailo, Y. V., et al. (1999). Excess of high activity monoamine oxidase A gene promoter alleles in female patients with panic disorder. *Human Molecular Genetics* **8**, 621–624.

Denney, R. M., Koch, H. and Craig, I. W. (1999). Association between monoamine oxidase A activity in human male skin fibroblasts and the genotype of the MAO promoter-associated variable number tandem repeat. *Human Genetics* **105**, 541–551.

Foley, D. L., Eaves, L. J., Wormley, B., et al. (2004). Childhood adversity, monoamine oxidase A genotype, and risk for conduct disorder. *Archives of General Psychiatry* **61**, 738–744.

Kim-Cohen, J., Caspi, A., Taylor, A., et al. (in press). MAOA, early adversity, and gene-environment interaction predicting children's mental health: new evidence and a meta-analysis. *Molecular Psychiatry*.

Moffitt, T. E., Caspi, A., Rutter, M. and Silva, P. A. (2001). *Sex differences in antisocial behaviour: conduct disorder, delinquency and violence in the Dunedin Longitudinal Study*. Cambridge, UK: Cambridge University Press.

Newman, T. K., Syagailo, Y. V., Barr, C. S., et al. (2005). Monoamine oxidase A gene promoter variation and rearing experiences influences aggressive behaviour in rhesus monkeys. *Biological Psychiatry* 57, 167–172.

Sabol, S. Z., Hu, S. and Hamer, D. (1998). A functional polymorphism in the monoamine oxidase A gene promoter. *Human Genetics* 103, 273–279.

Vierikko, E., Pulkkinen, L., Kaprio, J., et al. (2003). Sex differences in genetic and environmental effects on aggression. *Aggressive Behaviour* 29, 55–68.

Relevant Website

http://www.ojp.usdoj.gov/bis.

Motor Vehicle Accidents, Stress Effects of

T C Buckley
Boston VA Medical Center and Boston University School of Medicine, Boston, MA, USA
E B Blanchard
University at Albany–State University of New York, Albany, NY, USA

This article is reproduced from the previous edition, volume 2, pp 777–780, © 2000, Elsevier Inc.

Introduction
Psychological Disorder Following MVAs
What Predicts Psychopathology Following MVAs?
What Predicts Remission of Psychological Disorder?
Conclusion

Glossary

Comorbidity	The simultaneous presence of two disorders in the same individual.
Longitudinal studies	Studies that assess individuals at multiple points in time in a prospective manner.
Prevalence	Total number of cases of a particular disorder over a given period of time.
Psychopathology	Difficulty with psychological functioning (e.g., depression, anxiety, alcohol abuse).
Spontaneous remission	The alleviation of signs and symptoms of a particular disorder in the absence of formal treatment.

Introduction

The negative impact that motor vehicle accidents (MVAs) have on society is staggering. Total property damage, health-care expenditure, and hours lost from employment have a cost to the U.S. economy of over 150 billion dollars each year. Moreover, the individual psychosocial consequences of MVAs can be very debilitating. Motor vehicle accident survivors often deal with complicated issues for the rest of their lifetime subsequent to an accident that may have lasted a total of 3 s. It is not uncommon for MVA survivors to face such complicated issues as bereavement, chronic pain, permanent disability, financial problems, loss of employment, depression, a variety of anxiety problems, and legal difficulties. Space limitations prevent us from covering all of these topics in detail. This article does not cover such interesting topics as the role that litigation plays in posttrauma recovery, the experimental investigation of posttrauma psychiatric symptoms, and the role of psychosocial treatments for MVA survivors. This article summarizes the literature on the chief behavioral problems that follow MVAs: specific phobia, posttraumatic stress disorder (PTSD), and major depression.

Psychological Disorder Following MVAs

Specific Phobia

A specific phobia is a behavioral disorder in which individuals manifest an excessive and unrealistic fear of a situation or object. Exposure to the feared situation will invariably provoke an anxiety response (e.g., situationally bound panic attack) from the phobic individual. Phobic individuals will deliberately avoid their feared situation or else endure the situation with great distress. Phobic fears can be seen in individuals with seemingly no traumatic history with the feared object or situation. Phobic fears can also develop via classical conditioning when aversive conditions are paired with the phobic object (which would not have been the target of phobic behavior at the time of conditioning). MVAs can serve as a strong, single-trial conditioning event that leads to a phobic fear of driving-related situations in some individuals.

The experience of a MVA can be very frightening. Quite often, individuals will report that they experienced an extreme sense of life threat during the course of their accident. Thus, MVAs can serve as a single-trial conditioning event that will come to elicit anxiety responses (e.g., panic attacks) in future driving-related situations. For some individuals, the conditioned response is so severe that driving becomes exceedingly difficult. A small set of MVA survivors will discontinue driving following their MVAs, whereas others restrict their driving behavior relative to pre-MVA driving behavior.

The prevalence of a specific phobia of driving-related situations following MVAs is difficult to estimate. Some investigators have adopted a strict definition of driving phobia, wherein a complete elimination of driving or severe restriction of driving (i.e., only drives to work) defines phobic driving behavior. Others have adopted less restrictive criteria, defining driving phobias (sometimes termed driving reluctance) as a change in postaccident driving behavior characterized by increased anxiety related to some or all aspects of travel and a reduction in total number of miles traveled. Estimates of severe driving phobia (i.e., elimination or near-elimination of driving) are about 10–15% of MVA survivors. Estimates of less severe driving phobia or driving reluctance are between 38 and 77%.

Despite the general lack of diagnostic and prevalence data, one thing is clear: MVAs change the driving behavior of MVA survivors greatly. In countries where dependence on a private automobile is great, this can be a costly issue. Fortunately, exposure-based behavioral treatments can be very efficacious ways to treat driving phobia and reluctance to drive.

Posttraumatic Stress Disorder

PTSD is currently classified as an anxiety disorder by the American Psychiatric Association. It is a condition that follows exposure to an event that involves severe threat to one's life or physical integrity (e.g., wartime trauma, rape, MVAs). Following such life-threatening events, some individuals meeting the diagnostic criteria for PTSD will continue to reexperience their traumatic event in one of the following ways: psychological distress upon exposure to trauma-reminiscent cues, physiological arousal upon exposure to trauma-reminiscent cues, intrusive recollections of the trauma, trauma-related dreams that disrupt sleep, and flashbacks of the event. They also will evidence behavioral avoidance of trauma-related stimuli in much the same way that phobic individuals

will, as well as cognitive avoidance (trying not to think about the MVA). Depressive-type symptoms such as a restricted range of emotional experience and a loss of interest in pleasurable activities are also part of the symptomatic criteria. Finally, individuals meeting the diagnostic criteria for PTSD may have chronic hyperarousal, evincing such symptoms as sleep disturbance, exaggerated startle response, and difficulty concentrating.

Given the fear, sense of life threat, and extent of physical injury associated with severe MVAs, it is not surprising that a certain number of MVA survivors will develop PTSD. Prevalence estimates of PTSD among MVA survivors range from 1 to 46%. These discrepancies are due in large part to sample recruiting methods and diagnostic procedures. Self-referred clinical populations yield prevalence estimates of 40% or higher. However, more representative samples of consecutive accident admissions in hospital settings (i.e., emergency rooms) consistently yield prevalence rates near 20%. After reviewing the literature during the course of our work with MVA survivors, it is our impression that the most accurate prevalence estimate of PTSD following accidents is about 20%.

Studies that have examined this prevalence issue have varied in terms of time post-MVA that the patients were assessed. It is clear from longitudinal research that prevalence rates can vary greatly as a function of time postaccident. While many individuals will meet the criteria for PTSD in the first 1–4 months post-MVA, approximately 50% of those cases will spontaneously remit without formal intervention over the course of 6–12 months posttrauma. Thus, for MVA survivors who meet symptomatic criteria for PTSD shortly following trauma, many will experience a remission of symptoms without formal intervention. This spontaneous remission phenomenon is similar to that seen in PTSD populations subsequent to other traumas such as rape and wartime atrocity. What distinguishes those who remit vs. those who do not is covered in a later section of this article.

Major Depressive Disorder

Unipolar major depression is the most common mood disorder. Major depressive episodes are discrete periods of time (usually months to years) when individuals experience a variety of cognitive, affective, and physiological symptoms such as depressed mood, anhedonia, difficulty with concentration, feelings of worthlessness, sleep disturbance, appetite disturbance, psychomotor agitation/retardation, fatigue, and suicidal ideation or attempts.

Individuals often experience major depressive episodes in the months following their MVA. One empirical question is whether the depression is a consequence of the MVA or whether the presenting individuals had problems with major depression prior to their MVA. Longitudinal studies suggest that a large number of individuals who experience major depressive episodes following MVAs are experiencing depression for the first time in their life. The incidence of depression during the time periods of these studies is greater than one would expect in non-MVA representative population samples during the same period of time. In addition, the onset of episodes is quite often close in time to the occurrence of the MVA. Considering these two findings, it is tempting to attribute causal status to MVAs for inducing major depressive episodes in some individuals. In addition, individuals who have had difficulties with major depression prior to their accident quite often experience another episode of depression following their MVA.

Thus, a large portion of the cases of major depression noted are a direct consequence of the MVA itself. Not surprisingly, major depression is a common comorbid condition with PTSD. The limited amount of research on the impact of comorbid depression with PTSD indicates poorer outcomes in major role functioning in individuals with comorbidity relative to individuals with one condition or the other.

What Predicts Psychopathology Following MVAs?

Phobic avoidance, PTSD, and major depression are more likely to occur post-MVA in individuals who are in more severe accidents. The severity of MVAs has generally been judged in two ways. First, subjective ratings of perceived life threat have been used as an index of severity of accident. Individuals who report a greater fear of death at the time of the MVA generally have more post-MVA psychopathology than those with a lower sense of life threat.

Second, the severity of MVAs has been assessed via more objective methods by quantifying the extent of physical injury incurred during the accident. Some studies have found this variable to have predictive power, in that the more severe the physical injuries, the more likely the individuals were to have behavioral problems. Other studies have failed to find such a relationship. Measurement differences may account for a large part of this variation. Some studies simply dichotomize the presence or absence of injury to predict psychological outcome in their data analyses, whereas other studies have quantified physical injury in a dimensional manner, assessing the range and severity of injuries through the use of instruments with good psychometric properties. Studies that use

these more reliable and valid physical assessment instruments are those that demonstrate the predictive utility of assessing physical injury. It is our impression that the degree of physical injury is a valid predictor of post-MVA psychopathology.

Consistent with research in other areas of trauma (i.e., rape trauma, wartime trauma), a history of previous trauma seems to be predictive of who will develop post-MVA psychopathology and who will not. Those with histories of previous trauma are more likely to have post-MVA psychopathology than those without previous trauma histories. The mechanisms that drive this cumulative trauma phenomenon are not known. Suffice it to say that previous trauma indicates a poor prognosis for survivors of serious MVAs.

Also consistent with the non-MVA trauma literature is the fact that previous psychopathology (preexisting depression, obsessive-compulsive disorder, etc.) indicates a poor prognosis for survivors of MVAs. Preexisting axis I disorders increase the likelihood of trauma-related diagnoses such as PTSD, specific phobia with traumatic onset, and major depression. This could be due to similar predispositions such as biological vulnerability, poor coping skills, and/or a lack of social support systems. It does appear that high levels of perceived social support are protective against the development of post-MVA psychopathology. These findings are entirely consistent with the literature that has assessed the relationship between social support and a variety of stress-related difficulties ranging from behavioral problems to immune functioning.

Gender has consistently been found to be predictive of psychopathology following MVAs. Women develop PTSD, major depression, and specific phobia at greater rates than men following MVAs. It may be that men are likely to cope with their problems by self-medicating with alcohol or drugs and thus present with different psychiatric diagnoses. The epidemiological literature as a whole would suggest that men are more likely to use alcohol and drugs as coping mechanisms.

What Predicts Remission of Psychological Disorder?

At a time when health-care resources are at a premium, a question of great interest to clinical researchers is, among MVA survivors with psychopathology shortly following an MVA, what variables will identify those individuals whose psychiatric symptoms will remit without intervention? Because treatment resources may not be available to all MVA victims (especially with accidents involving large numbers of individuals, i.e., bus accidents), the identification of predictors of recovery is a very important applied question.

Not surprisingly, the degree of psychiatric symptomology present shortly after the occurrence of MVA is predictive of remission of symptoms. Individuals with greater numbers of symptoms and more severe symptoms are less likely to show remission of diagnostic status than those who meet diagnostic criteria for disorder in the months post-MVA but have lower levels of symptomatology. The level of initial physical injury is also predictive of the remission of psychiatric symptoms. Those who are injured more severely at the time of MVA are less likely to show remission of psychiatric symptoms over time.

The rate of physical recovery, as assessed by self-report measures, is also predictive of psychiatric symptom remission. Those whose physical injuries recover at a slower rate also show a slower remission of psychiatric symptoms. The causal relationship between these variables is unknown. Some investigators have speculated that physical injury status, especially pain, exacerbates and maintains psychiatric symptoms, whereas others have argued that the presence of psychiatric symptoms makes people more sensitive to pain and thus more likely to inflate self-report scores of pain. This is a particularly vexing dilemma when trying to assess the rate of physical and emotional recovery in MVA survivors because many of their injuries are soft tissue injuries (e.g., cervical and lumbar spine strains), which do not lend themselves to quantifiable measurement other than by self-report methods.

Finally, the presence of behavioral avoidance shortly after trauma signifies a poor prognosis. Individuals who show a high degree of driving reluctance or avoidance shortly after their MVA are less likely to show a remission of psychiatric problems such as PTSD than those who force themselves to drive. It may be the case that self-administered exposure helps break the cycle of anxious responding in the presence of trauma-reminiscent cues that characterize PTSD.

Conclusion

Empirical investigation of the psychosocial consequences of MVAs is a growing field of research. Unfortunately, MVAs are a ubiquitous phenomenon in industrialized countries. The psychosocial consequences of MVAs are severe and many. Blanchard and Hickling is a valuable reference for clinicians who seek information about the psychosocial treatment of MVA survivors.

See Also the Following Articles

Acute Stress Disorder and Posttraumatic Stress Disorder; Acute Trauma Response; Avoidance; Major Depressive Disorder; Posttraumatic Stress Disorder, Delayed.

Further Reading

Blanchard, E. B. and Hickling, E. J. (1997). *After the crash: assessment and treatment of motor vehicle accident survivors*. Washington, D.C.: American Psychological Association.

Buckley, T. C., Blanchard, E. B. and Hickling, E. J. (1996). A prospective examination of delayed onset PTSD secondary to motor vehicle accidents. *Journal of Abnormal Psychology* 105, 617–625.

Ehlers, A., Mayou, R. A. and Bryant, B. (1998). Psychological predictors of chronic posttraumatic stress disorder after motor vehicle accidents. *Journal of Abnormal Psychology* 107, 508–519.

Kessler, R. C., Sonnega, A., Bromet, E., Hughes, M. and Nelson, C. B. (1995). Posttraumatic stress disorder in the National Comorbidity Survey. *Archives of General Psychiatry* 151, 888–894.

Kuch, K., Cox, B. J. and Evans, R. J. (1996). Posttraumatic stress disorder and motor vehicle accidents: a multidisciplinary overview. *Canadian Journal of Psychiatry* 41, 429–434.

Taylor, S. and Koch, W. J. (1995). Anxiety disorders due to motor vehicle accidents: Nature and treatment. *Clinical Psychology Review* 15, 721–738.

Mourning *See:* Bereavement.

Mucosal Secretory Immunity, Stress and

J A Bosch
University of Birmingham, Birmingham, UK and
University of Illinois at Chicago, Chicago, IL, USA
D Carroll
University of Birmingham, Birmingham, UK

This article is a revision of the previous edition article by
D Carroll, C Ring, and A Winzer, volume 2, pp 781–785,
© 2000, Elsevier Inc.

Introduction

An Outline of Mucosal Secretory Immunity

Neuroendocrine Regulation of Salivary S-IgA Secretion

Stress and S-IgA

Stress and Innate Secretory Immunity

Stress and Microbial Colonization

Conclusion and Future Perspectives

Glossary

Antigen	Molecule that initiates a response of the immune system; abbreviation of antibody generator.
Immunoglobulin or antibody	Protein that is produced by a specialized set of white blood cells (B lymphocytes) that has the capacity to specifically bind to antigens. This binding labels antigens for destruction by molecules and cells of the immune system.
Infection	Invasion and multiplication of microorganisms, which may lead to tissue damage and disease.
Mucosa	The mucus-coated lining of all body cavities and passages that form the interface with the outside world.
Secretory immunity	Protection against infection and noxious substances that is provided by the proteins present in the mucous secretions that coat the mucosa.

Introduction

Both human and animal studies have provided convincing evidence that psychosocial stress is associated with increased susceptibility to infectious disease. It has been estimated that 90 to 95% of all infections initiate at the mucosa; the mucus-secreting lining of all body cavities and passages that form the interface with the outside world. Examples are the soft oral tissues, the respiratory, gastrointestinal, and genitourinary tracts, and the eyes. Hence, investigating the effects of stress on the immunological protection of the mucosa is an obvious starting point for research attempting to explain the link between stress and susceptibility to infectious diseases.

The mucosal surfaces are protected by the secretory immune system, which entails the secretions of a large number of local glands, including the salivary glands, the lacrimal glands, and the glands of the respiratory and gastrointestinal tracts. These glands secrete a wide variety of protective proteins (e.g., immunoglobulins, mucins, cystatins, lysozyme, lactoferrin) that constitute a first line of defense that prevents infection and disease by interfering with the entry and multiplication of microorganisms and noxious substances. This mucosal secretory immune system is under autonomic nervous system control, and it is well established that both acute and protracted psychological stress perturb autonomic nervous system activity. Thus, autonomic nervous system regulation of mucosal secretory immunity affords a plausible pathway by which psychological stress may increase disease susceptibility.

This article provides an overview of the research on stress and mucosal secretory immunity. Most research in this area has used saliva as a model system for studying mucosal secretory immunity. Moreover, of the many protective proteins that constitute secretory immunity, one protein, secretory immunoglobulin A (S-IgA), has attracted particular attention.

An Outline of Mucosal Secretory Immunity

The Secretory Immunoglobulins

Immunoglobulins (also called antibodies) are proteins that are secreted by specialized cells of the immune system, the B lymphocytes. Antibody production by the B lymphocytes is induced by foreign elements (called antigens), such as toxins, allergens, bacteria, and viruses. Upon interaction with an antigen, B lymphocytes rapidly divide and transform into immunoglobulin-producing plasma cells. A unique feature of immunoglobulins is that they have the capacity to bind (i.e., recognize) specific antigens, which helps with neutralizing or destroying this antigen. The most abundant immunoglobulin found in mucosal secretions is secretory immunoglobulin A (S-IgA).

S-IgA is produced locally by plasma cells that have migrated into the glandular tissues. Plasma cells in the salivary glands produce a polymeric form of IgA (as opposed to IgA found in plasma, which is monomeric). This polymeric IgA (pIgA) is transported and secreted into saliva as S-IgA. The formation and secretion of S-IgA is a two-step process. First, the pIgA locks on to a receptor molecule, referred to as the polymeric-immunoglobulin receptor (pIgR), present on the basolateral surface of a glandular cell. The pIgR is translocated from the basolateral to the apical surface of the glandular cell, where it is cleaved off and secreted into saliva as S-IgA. Accordingly, both IgA secretion by the plasma cells and the availability of pIgR for translocation by the glandular cells are rate-determining steps in the secretion of S-IgA. The pIgA receptor itself can also be translocated and is subsequently secreted as secretory component (SC).

Human IgA occurs in two isotypic forms, IgA1 and IgA2. The most notable difference between the two is that IgA1 is more vulnerable to degradation by bacteria, which makes this IgA isotype less effective. This may explain why the less vulnerable IgA2 subclass is more abundant in mucosal secretions; whereas the IgA1 subclass makes up some 90% of the total IgA in serum, it comprises 60% of S-IgA in saliva and only 35% of S-IgA in the lower gastrointestinal tract.

Innate Secretory Immunity

S-IgA is only one of many protective proteins secreted in the fluids covering the mucosa. The secretion of these other, innate immune factors (e.g., mucins, cystatins, lysozyme, lactoferrin) is also under strong neurohormonal control. Accordingly, these antimicrobial secretory proteins are also good candidates for psychoneuroimmunological investigation, although they currently received insufficient attention. **Table 1** lists several innate secretory factors that have been studied in this arena.

Neuroendocrine Regulation of Salivary S-IgA Secretion

As indicated, the synthesis and release of the secretory proteins by salivary glands and other mucosal secretory exocrine glands is under autonomic nervous system control, providing a sound neurobiological basis for anticipating an effect of stress on salivary secretory immunity. The preganglionic autonomic centers in the brain stem that regulate salivary gland activity receive direct inhibitory and excitatory inputs from brain areas that are part of recognized stress circuits and centers for homeostatic regulation. Studies with rats have shown that stimulation of both the sympathetic and parasympathetic autonomic nerves that innervate the salivary glands gives a rapid increase of S-IgA secretion into saliva, although the effect of sympathetic stimulation appears more robust than that of parasympathetic stimulation. Similar rapid

Table 1 Measures of innate secretory immunity that have been used in stress studies

Secretory protein	Where found	Functions
MUC5B (also denoted as MG1)	Saliva, nasal fluid, bronchial mucus, middle ear secretions, gall bladder epithelia	A mucin, i.e., a high-molecular-weight glycoprotein that consists largely (>75%) of carbohydrate. MUC5B is a major constituent of mucous gels covering the mucosa, where it protects against noxious substances and desiccation. Binds to a limited number of microorganisms. Host defense functions of MUC5B are enhanced by the formation of complexes with other secretory proteins.
MUC7 (also denoted as MG2)	Saliva, bronchial mucus	A mucin; binds and aggregates a large number of bacteria and fungi. Possibly also inactivate viruses.
Lactoferrin	Breast milk, nasal fluid, bronchial mucus, saliva, ocular fluid, and gastrointestinal secretions; also secreted by neutrophils	Inhibits microbial growth by binding iron, thereby depleting microorganisms from this essential substrate. Has anti-inflammatory effects and kills bacteria and fungi.
Lysozyme	Present in nearly all mucosal secretions including nasal fluid, bronchial mucus, saliva, ocular fluid, and gastrointestinal secretions; also secreted by neutrophils	Bacteriocidal by breaking down a cell wall component of gram-positive bacteria. Has also antimicrobial functions (growth-inhibiting, antiviral) through other mechanisms.
Cystatin S	Saliva, bronchial mucus	Cystatin S is a cystatin, i.e., protein that inhibits the activity of cysteine proteinases, thereby inhibiting enzymes that, among other things, are involved in virus replication and tissue invasion by bacteria.
α-Amylase	Saliva and pancreatic secretion. Low concentrations have also been demonstrated in other bodily fluids, including blood plasma, bronchial secretions, and tears	Starch-degrading enzyme. Influences the growth and tissue adhesion of streptococcal bacteria. Salivary α-amylase has been proposed as a measure of adrenergic activity, although this claim is still controversial.

increases in S-IgA secretion are observed in the gastrointestinal tract after stimulation of the local autonomic nerves. Autonomic stimulation of the salivary glands primarily affects the IgA translocation process and has little, if any, effect on IgA release by B lymphocytes.

It is still unclear whether the classic sympathetic transmitter norepinephrine is a major factor in the sympathetic stimulation on salivary S-IgA secretion. For example, the enhanced S-IgA output during moderate physical exercise, a strong sympathetic stimulus, is not attenuated by either alpha- or beta-adrenergic blockade in humans. An effect of sympathetic neuropeptides, which are coreleased with norepinephrine, has been demonstrated in animals. Other pharmacological studies in animals suggest that parasympathetic stimulation of S-IgA secretion may involve the classic parasympathetic transmitter acetylcholine and various neuropeptides.

Whereas autonomic stimulation may rapidly affect S-IgA levels, slower effects ($>$24 h) have been reported for glucocorticoids. The release of glucocorticoid hormones is considered central to the stress response. In rats, the synthetic glucocorticoid dexamethasone reduces both total salivary S-IgA and antigen-specific S-IgA levels. In contrast to salivary S-IgA levels, serum IgA levels are increased. Moreover, the expression of SC, the molecule that transports S-IgA into the secretions, is also increased. The effects of glucocorticoids on S-IgA secretion in humans remain to be studied, and since human and rodent S-IgA systems differ in several ways, findings for rodents should be generalized with caution.

In addition to direct stimulation of glandular S-IgA secretion, autonomic transmitters and glucocorticoids may indirectly affect the secretion of S-IgA by affecting immunological processes in the lymphoid tissues. Lymphoid organs are innervated by the autonomic nerves, and the residing immune cells carry functional receptors for the various autonomic transmitter substances. Indeed, autonomic nervous system activation has been shown to influence various aspects of local immune processing, including antigen presentation, antibody production, and cell migration. Thus, autonomic transmitters may also affect the S-IgA response by influencing the immunological priming of B lymphocytes in the lymphoid organs.

Stress and S-IgA

The Critical Distinction between Acute and Protracted Stress

The results of research on stress and S-IgA appear inconsistent at first glance. For example, some studies

Table 2 Results of academic examination studies that measured S-IgA[a]

	S-IgA concentration (μg/ml)	S-IgA secretion (μg/min)
Samples taken during or close to a single exam (i.e., acute stress)		
McClelland et al., 1985	↑	
Evans et al., 1994		↑
Bosch et al., 1996, 1998	↑	↑
Bristow et al., 1997	↑	↑
Spangler et al., 1997	↑	
Huwe et al., 1998	↑	↑
Samples taken during the extended exam period (i.e., protracted stress)		
Jemmott et al., 1983	↓	↓
Kiecolt-Glaser et al., 1984	↔	
Jemmot et al., 1988	↓	↓
Mouton et al., 1989	↓	↓
Li et al., 1997	↓	
Deinzer et al., 1998	↓	↓
Deinzer et al., 2000	↔[b]	↔

↑, increase; ↓, decrease; ↔, no change; empty cells indicate not determined.
[a]Studies are separated on the basis of whether samples were taken close to (i.e., during, or minutes before or after) a single exam or sometime during the extended exam period. For complete references, see Bosch et al., 2004.
[b]In this study a decrease was observed 1 and 2 weeks after the exam period.

report that S-IgA decreases during academic examination stress, whereas other studies report an increase. Research within psychoneuroimmunology has repeatedly demonstrated that acute and protracted stressors can generate opposing results on the same immunological parameters, and this also seems to apply to S-IgA. To illustrate this, **Table 2** categorizes academic examination studies on the basis of whether saliva samples were collected close to (i.e., during, or minutes before or after) a single examination or sometime during the extended examination period. Sorting studies according to this single criterion reveals a remarkably consistent picture: all studies in which the samples were collected close to an actual examination were associated with increases in S-IgA, whereas nearly all of the remaining studies found decreases. Clearly, the acute stress of an imminent exam increases salivary S-IgA levels, whereas protracted academic stress is associated with a decrease. Note that these distinct S-IgA responses are independent of when the nonstress reference, or baseline, measurement is taken.

S-IgA and Chronic Stressors

There is a robust association between protracted (i.e., weeks to years) forms of stress, impaired immune function, and health. Typical examples of such stressors are marital disruption, bereavement, caregiving for a severely ill spouse, and unemployment. Given the association between these types of stressors, immunity, and health, it is surprising that very few studies have examined S-IgA in this context. Nonetheless, a fairly consistent picture emerges from those that have. For example, lower salivary S-IgA levels have been observed in individuals distressed by living in parts of the United States stricken by environmental disasters (e.g., the Three Mile Island nuclear power plant, toxic waste sites in Delaware) than in individuals living in safer environments. Likewise, the academic stress studies cited previously (see **Table 2**) indicate that protracted academic pressures can lower salivary S-IgA levels.

A number of S-IgA studies have investigated chronic stress exposure by using self-report inventories. Such questionnaires typically request subjects to check a list of recent major life events (e.g., death of a spouse, divorce, loss of job) or minor daily hassles (e.g., minor conflicts and annoyances at home or work), or require subjects to give a general assessment of the stressfulness of their lives. The validity of this approach is established by prior research demonstrating that individuals scoring highly on such questionnaires exhibit increased susceptibility to a variety of infectious and inflammatory conditions, including respiratory infections and oral infectious diseases. The evidence provided by these questionnaire-based S-IgA studies also tends to support the hypothesis that higher levels of stress exposure and perceived stress are associated with lower levels of salivary S-IgA.

Despite consistent indications that chronic stressors lower S-IgA levels, methodological considerations temper a firm conclusion at this stage. For example, none of the studies controlled for potential sources of confounding, such as health behaviors (e.g., smoking, alcohol consumption), oral health, or medication usage. Further, many of the studies, including those with null results, tested small samples and/or used questionnaires with inferior psychometric properties. Thus, although largely supportive of the hypothesis that chronic stress lowers salivary S-IgA, there is a pressing need for a large-scale, well-controlled study to accurately assess the impact of perceived chronic stress on salivary S-IgA.

S-IgA and Acute Stress

Examination stress and other naturalistic stressors
The results of the academic examination studies summarized in **Table 2** indicate that the acute stress (of an imminent or ongoing examination) is associated with increased S-IgA levels. The fact that acute forms of

stress increase S-IgA levels is also confirmed by research using other stress paradigms. For example, S-IgA secretion is elevated in air traffic controllers following a stressful work shift. Also, S-IgA secretion is elevated in soccer coaches watching their team play. It should be noted that that such acute increases are transient; S-IgA returns to baseline values typically within 1 h after acute stress exposure.

Laboratory stressors Further support for the hypothesis that acute stress increases salivary S-IgA is provided by studies that used conventional laboratory stressors such as computer games, mental arithmetic, and time-paced memory tests. These experiments, which are performed under highly controlled conditions, use stressors of short duration (5–30 min) that typically require mental effort and elicit robust sympathetic nervous system activation. The results consistently show increases in S-IgA concentrations (µg/ml) but tend to be somewhat less consistent regarding increases in S-IgA secretion rate (µg/min). This indicates that concomitant reductions in saliva flow rate contribute to the concentration increases during acute stress.

More recent studies have demonstrated that under some conditions, which include specific emotional states (e.g., disgust) and stimuli (e.g., pain, cold), S-IgA levels may transiently decrease. The mechanisms causing these rapid decreases have yet to be elucidated. Hedonic tone per se does not seem to determine the direction of the acute changes in S-IgA; both positive and negative emotional states (induced by imagery, listening to music tapes, or watching humorous sketches) have been associated with increases in S-IgA. Thus, apart from a few studies using painful stimuli or stimuli that induce disgust, virtually all types of acute states and virtually all experimental manipulations elicit an acute and transient rise in salivary S-IgA.

Stress and Oral Immunization

The research described thus far has concerned the effects of stress on total S-IgA levels. A few studies also investigated the effects of psychosocial stress on the daily variation in specific S-IgA, i.e., S-IgA that binds to a specific antigen. In these studies, participants were required to swallow a capsule containing rabbit albumin each morning for 8–12 weeks, and the daily variations in specific S-IgA (i.e., S-IgA directed against the rabbit protein) in saliva were measured in association with variations in daily mood and events. Antigen-specific S-IgA levels were lower on days with higher levels of negative mood and undesirable events and were elevated on days with more positive moods and desirable events. Considering the pivotal role of the secretory immune defenses in protecting against infection, oral immunization provides an important and underutilized model for studying the effects of psychosocial factors on immune function.

The validity of the conventional method of measuring total S-IgA levels (as opposed to antigen-specific S-IgA levels described previously) has been a topic of heated debate. This debate, however, rests on the assumptions that S-IgA is a readout parameter for specific immune responses directed toward a particular antigen. If this were the case, only the levels of S-IgA molecules that are specifically directed against particular antigens would matter for host protection, rendering the measurement of total S-IgA levels less meaningful. However, total S-IgA for a large part consists of polyreactive antibodies (i.e., recognizing many different antigens). This broad specificity of S-IgA antibodies implies that total immunoglobulin levels, and not just antigen-specific levels, are important to mucosal protection. This idea is consistent with the evidence showing that total S-IgA levels predict the risk for respiratory and oral infections. Thus, the measurements of total and antigen-specific S-IgA levels seem to be immunologically meaningful ways of determining mucosal protection.

Effects on Secretory Component and S-IgA Subclasses

During acute stress in humans, the secretion of S-IgA appears to be regulated independently from the secretion of its transporter molecule, SC. For example, the passive stress induced by viewing a surgical video produced a rapid decrease in S-IgA secretion but an increase in the secretion of SC. During conventional active stress, a time-paced memory task, both S-IgA and SC secretion increased. It is as yet unclear whether these acute increases are due to increased endothelial transport or to a combination of increased IgA availability and transport into saliva. Both stress and physical exercise studies show that the rapid increases in S-IgA mainly reflect increases in the IgA1 subclass. The mechanism responsible for this subclass-specific effect is unknown.

Stress and Innate Secretory Immunity

Stress and Mucins

Two human studies have shown that acute stress enhances the secretion in saliva of the mucins MUC5B and MUC7. These findings are in line with the results of animal studies showing that increased gastrointestinal and respiratory mucin secretion

occurs in response to water immersion and restraint stress. These animal experiments also found effects on related biological processes, such as mucin synthesis and posttranslational processing (e.g., sulfatation, glycosylation). Pharmacological studies show that synthesis, posttranslational modification, and secretion of salivary mucins results, at least in part, from beta-adrenergic stimulation.

Stress-induced increases in salivary mucin may have consequences that benefit the host by enhancing mucosal barrier function, but also some that benefit microorganisms. For instance, the acute stress-induced increase in salivary MUC5B secretion enhances the adherence (*in vitro*) of *Helicobacter pylori,* a causative agent of duodenal ulcers and stomach cancer. Again, the effects of acute and protracted stressors may be quite different. For example, protracted stress decreases colonic mucin secretion in rats. This decrease in mucin secretion enhances mucosal permeability, thereby potentiating reactivation of experimental colitis induced by a chemical irritant.

Stress and α-Amylase

Studies in the early 1980s reported that salivary α-amylase concentration increases during relaxation and decreases with acute stress. However, later studies were unable to replicate these findings and instead found that acute stress increases salivary α-amylase concentration and secretion rate. These effects are again thought to result from stress-induced sympathetic activation, which would be consistent with the findings of studies showing that α-amylase secretion is increased by administration of adrenergic agonists, electrical stimulation of the local sympathetic nerves, and physical exercise. Moreover, increases in salivary α-amylase correlate with serum norepinephrine and cardiac left ventricular ejection time, a measure of cardiac sympathetic drive. Nonetheless, recent claims that salivary α-amylase is a valid noninvasive measure of adrenergic activity should be regarded with caution. First, α-amylase is also secreted in response to nonadrenergic sympathetic transmitters, i.e., various neuropeptides. Second, α-amylase secretion is also stimulated by parasympathetic stimulation, and parasympathetic stimulation augments the effects of sympathetic stimulation.

Stress and Other Mucosal Secretory Proteins

In humans, acute stressors that elicit sympathetic-parasympathetic coactivation increase the secretion of salivary cystatin S and lactoferrin, but no or only minimal effects are seen in response to a stress exposure that evokes sympathetic activation in conjunction with a vagal withdrawal (a time-paced memory test). This finding is consistent with the notion that the two branches of the autonomic nervous system have a synergistic effect on secretory gland activity; that is, although sympathetic activation is the main stimulus for glandular protein secretion, the effects are strongly augmented by concurrent parasympathetic activity. As for more protracted stress, a decrease in salivary lysozyme secretion is observed during an examination period. The association between self-reported stress and salivary lysozyme levels appears inconsistent: one study found a negative correlation, whereas another did not find any association.

Stress and Microbial Colonization

A remaining, and critical, issue is whether the effects of stress on secretory immunity translate into functional changes, such as affecting processes that are involved in microbial colonization. Such functional effects might explain the alterations in mucosal microflora, seen in both humans and animals, under various forms of psychological strain, such as depression, space flight simulations, maternal separation, familial strains, animal fighting and relocation, and life events. Such effects may also explain the close association between stress and oral diseases with a bacterial etiology, such as periodontal disease and dental caries.

Aggregation is a process by which bacteria are clumped together through interactions with the host's secretory proteins so that these microorganisms cannot effectively adhere to the mucosal surfaces. Hence, a decreased bacterial aggregation indicates a decreased capacity for mucosal microbial clearance. Examination stress reduces the aggregation by saliva of the oral bacterium *Streptococcus gordonii*. A reduced streptococcal aggregation is also observed in rats administered physiological doses of the beta-adrenergic agonist isoproterolol for 1 week. This indicates that both brief and prolonged sympathetic activation can negatively affect the capacity of saliva to aggregate oral bacteria.

Microbial adhesion is a process by which microbes gain a stable foothold in the host; it constitutes a first and essential step in infection. Acute laboratory stress in humans enhances saliva-mediated adhesion of oral bacteria (viridans streptococci) and non-oral bacteria (*Helicobacter pylori*). Laboratory stress also affects the saliva-mediated adhesion of microorganisms to each other. Animal studies demonstrate that glucocorticoid administration is associated with an increased bacterial adherence to the intestinal mucosa and a

reduced luminal S-IgA. Similarly, in rats, 1 week of physiological doses of the beta-agonist isoprotenol increased the salivary adherence of *Streptococcus mutans*. Thus, stress, sympathetic activation, and elevated glucocorticoid levels promote the adhesion of microorganisms to mucosal surfaces.

Conclusion and Future Perspectives

Psychological stress has a variety of effects on mucosal salivary secretory immunity in humans, including altered secretion of adaptive and innate immune factors, reduced bacterial aggregation, increased bacterial adherence, and altered microbial coadherence. There is still little known about the effects of stress on secretory immunity in secretions other than saliva. The scant research in this area, mostly in rodents, confirms and extends the salivary findings in humans; there are effects on protein secretion, synthesis, and posttranslational modification, as well as on functional changes such as enhanced bacterial adherence and increased intestinal permeability.

In addition to an emphasis on salivary immunity, there has been a disproportional focus on S-IgA. The fact that individuals deficient in S-IgA, the most common form of immunodeficiency, are, for the most part, in good health suggests that other secretory factors may be important.

More attention also needs to be paid also to the effects of protracted stress exposure on secretory immunity. Knowledge about the effects of chronic stress on innate secretory immunity is practically absent, and the studies on chronic stress and S-IgA, although painting a fairly consistent picture, suffer from several methodological shortcomings. Further, the underlying mechanisms have yet to be fully elucidated. A promising model for studying the effects of chronic stress on adaptive secretory immunity is mucosal immunization.

Finally, researchers should extend their horizons to include the study of the functional implications of stress-induced changes in mucosal protein secretion. A number of microbiological methods are available to investigate the effects of immunosecretory changes on microbial colonization processes, which include viral invasion, bacterial adherence, bacterial growth, and bacterial aggregation. This approach, rarely considered in the realm of psychoneuroimmunology, may reveal the mechanisms by which immunosecretory changes affect the mucosal microflora and susceptibility to infection. Moreover, this methodology will help to strengthen the proposition that stress, via its effects on secretory immunity, has important health consequences.

Acknowledgment

Support for this work was provided by grant 1-RO3-DE-16726-01 from the National Institute of Dental and Craniofacial Research to J. A. B.

See Also the Following Articles

Acute Stress Response: Experimental; Autonomic Nervous System; Immune Function, Stress-Induced Enhancement; Immune Response; Immune System, Aging; Lymphocytes; Sympathetic Nervous System.

Further Reading

Bosch, J. A., Ring, C., de Geus, E. J. C., Veerman, E. C. I. and Amerongen, A. V. (2002). Stress and secretory immunity. *International Review of Neurobiology* 52, 213–253.

Bosch, J. A., Turkenburg, M., Nazmi, K., et al. (2003). Stress as a determinant of saliva-mediated adherence and coadherence of oral and non-oral microorganisms. *Psychosomatic Medicine* 65(4), 604–612.

Bosch, J. A., de Geus, E. J. C., Veerman, E. C. I., Hoogstraten, J. and NieuwAmerongen, A. V. (2003). Innate secretory immunity in response to laboratory stressors that evoke distinct patterns of cardiac autonomic activity. *Psychosomatic Medicine* 65(2), 245–258.

Bosch, J. A., de Geus, E. J. C., Ring, C., NieuwAmerongen, A. V. and Stowell, J. R. (2004). Academic examinations and immunity: academic stress or examination stress? *Psychosomatic Medicine* 66(4), 625–626.

Brandtzaeg, P. and Johansen, F. E. (2005). Mucosal B cells: phenotypic characteristics, transcriptional regulation, and homing properties. *Immunological Reviews* 206, 32–63.

Norderhaug, I. N., Johansen, F. E., Schjerven, H. and Brandtzaeg, P. (1999). Regulation of the formation and external transport of secretory immunoglobulins. *Critical Reviews in Immunology* 19(5–6), 481–508.

Proctor, G. B. and Carpenter, G. H. (2002). Neural control of salivary S-IgA secretion. *International Review of Neurobiology* 52, 187–212.

Schenkels, L. C. P. M., Veerman, E. C. I. and Nieuw Amerongen, A. V. (1995). Biochemical composition of human saliva in relation to other mucosal fluids. *Critical Review in Oral Biology and Medicine* 6(2), 161–175.

Soderholm, J. D. and Perdue, M. H. (2001). II. Stress and intestinal barrier function. *American Journal of Physiology Gastrointestinal and Liver Physiology* 280(1), G7–G13.

Teeuw, W., Bosch, J. A., Veerman, E. C. and Amerongen, A. V. (2004). Neuroendocrine regulation of salivary IgA synthesis and secretion: implications for oral health. *Biological Chemistry* 385(12), 1137–1146.

Multi Drug Resistance P Glycoprotein and other Transporters

E C M de Lange
Leiden University, Leiden, Netherlands

ATP-Binding Cassette Transporter Superfamily

Multidrug Resistance Transporter Proteins

Multidrug Resistance Transporter Proteins and Pharmacokinetics

Other Physiological Functions of Multidrug Resistance and Other ATP-Binding Cassette Transporters

Multidrug Resistance: ATP-Binding Cassette Transporter Modulation and Regulation of Expression

Glossary

ATP-binding cassette (ABC) transporters	A large and multifunctional family of structurally related membrane proteins. ABC transporters use the energy of ATP hydrolysis to pump substrates across cell membranes and are involved in the transmembrane transport of various substances.
Multidrug resistance (MDR)	The ability of cells to develop resistance to a broad range of structurally and functionally unrelated drugs after being exposed to (one of) these drugs. The mechanism is that the efflux transport by these proteins leads to lower intracellular concentrations, thereby protecting the cells and tissues from potential toxic compounds from the external milieu.
Multidrug resistance-related proteins (MRPs)	A group of MDR ABC transporters that are structurally related to but distinct from P-glycoproteins; mainly transports anionic derivatives of drugs when conjugated to glutathione/glucuronide. This family of MRP proteins comprises nine members in humans, designated MRP1–MRP6.

P glycoprotein (Pgp)	The first discovered MDR transporter and most well-known ABC transporter; has been shown to transport a variety of structurally unrelated compounds across cellular membranes.

ATP-Binding Cassette Transporter Superfamily

The ABC transporters comprise a large and multifunctional family of structurally related membrane proteins that are located in the plasma membrane of the cells or in the membrane of various cellular organelles. ABC transporter proteins use the energy of ATP hydrolysis to translocate various molecules across these barriers, and some other ABC transporters use ATP to form specific membrane channels. The ABC transporters serve a variety of physiological roles, and also some inherited diseases appear to be linked to mutations in the genes encoding for the ABC transporters.

At present, approximately 50 ABC transporters are known. Many synonyms exist for these transporters due to their history of discovery. Recently, a consistent nomenclature has been introduced on the basis of the organization of domains and amino acid homology of these ABC transporters. In the new nomenclature, the ABC transporters are divided into seven distinct subfamilies: ABCA, ABCB, ABCC, ABCD, ABCE, ABCF, and ABCG. **Table 1** presents the classification of these families and their members (including the synonyms), together with their expression, endogenous and exogenous substrates, functions, and relation to human disorders. It is clear that the ABC transporters govern the kinetics of chemical communication in the body, which makes the knowledge of their specific actions in homeostatic and feedback mechanisms extremely important for further insight into the body's functioning at the molecular level under normal and challenged (stress) conditions.

Multidrug Resistance Transporter Proteins

ABC transporters have been the subject of intense scrutiny as potential mediators of clinical drug resistance. The identification of the MDR1-encoded P-glycoprotein (Pgp) approximately 20 years ago, allowed us to recognize that reduced intracellular accumulation of anticancer agents can result in significant degrees of drug resistance. Over the years, Pgp has become the prototype of the MDR transporters. Among the ABC transporters, two other major groups can be identified as being involved in intrinsic and/or acquired MDR of cells: the multidrug resistance-related protein (MRP) family and the breast cancer resistance protein (BCRP). Many drugs that have been developed for the treatment of human diseases are substrates for these multidrug transporters. Because of that, the degree of expression and the functionality of these transporters can directly affect the therapeutic effectiveness of such agents. Treatment failure due to MDR was first found in connection with cancer, but later in time it was also found in connection with other conditions such as some autoimmune disorders and infectious diseases (**Table 1**).

P-Glycoprotein

Pgp is the most well-known of the ABC transporters and was the first to be identified in humans, in which it plays a critical role in drug resistance in the treatment of cancers. Numerous investigations with many drugs have demonstrated that Pgp has an important role in determining the concentration–time profiles of Pgp substrates in the different parts of the body. In general, Pgp preferentially extrudes large hydrophobic, positively charged molecules. This transporter also is involved in the transport of certain cytokines. Pgp may even play a role in allograft rejection and in the inhibition of apoptosis. Another possible role of Pgp lies in the pathogenesis of Alzheimer's disease by the direct interaction of Pgp on amyloid-β40 and amyloid-β42 or by Pgp's influencing the accumulation of these proteins. Also, an interesting role for Pgp is indicated in the neuroendocrine functioning and regulation of the hypothalamic-pituitary-adrenocortical (HPA) axis because Pgp is involved in the efflux of certain natural and synthetic glucocorticoids from the brain.

Multidrug Resistance-Related Protein Family

The MRPs (or the ABCCs) have a broad tissue distribution and are able to extrude negatively charged anionic drugs and neutral drugs conjugated to glutathione, glucuronate, or sulfate. Some MRPs are able to transport neutral drugs if co-transported with glutathione. The total MRP family now includes MRP1–MRP9 (and ABCC7 and ABCC8). MRP1 was the first to be discovered and is actually a prototype glutathion conjugate pump that transports a variety of drugs conjugated to glutathione, sulfate, or glucuronate; anionic drugs and dyes; neutral-basic amphiphatic drugs; and even oxyanions. The most important substrate of MRP1 is the endogenous leukotriene LTC4. MRP1 also contributes to the blood–cerebrospinal fluid (CSF) barrier at the level of the choroid epithelial cells. MRP2 and MRP3 have overlapping substrate specificities with MRP1 but different tissue distributions, and they appear also to exhibit drug resistance.

Table 1 ATP binding cassette transporter families and members[a]

Family	Member (synonyms); most common name	Tissue expression	Physiological substrates; other substrates;[b] inhibitors/modulators	Function	Genetic mutations related to human disease
ABCA	ABCA1 (ABC1, TGD, HDLDT1, CERP)	Ubiquitous (plasma membrane)	Phospholipids, cholesterol	Removal of phospholipids and cholesterol on to high-density lipoprotein particles	Tangier disease, artherosclerosis
	ABCA2 (ABC2)	Brain, kidney, lung, heart, lysosomal membrane	*Estramustine?*	Steroid transport?	
	ABCA3 (ABC3, ABCC)	Lung			
	ABCA4 (ABCR, ABC10, STGD)	Retina (rod photoreceptors)	*N-retinylidene-phosphatidyl-ethanolamine, retinaldehyde*		Stargardt disease, retinitis pigmentosa, macular dystrophy, cone–rod dystrophy
	ABCA5	Muscle, heart, testes			
	ABCA6	Liver			
	ABCA7	Spleen, thymus			
	ABCA8 (ABCR)	Ovary			
	ABCA9	Heart			
	ABCA10	Muscle, heart			
	ABCA11	Stomach			
	ABCA12	Low in all tissues			
ABCB	ABCB1 (MDR1, PGP, PGY1, GP170) P-Glycoprotein	Epithelial cells of kidney, liver, choroid plexus, intestine; endothelial cells of brain capillaries	IL-2, IL-4, IFN-γ, amyloid β-40, amyloid β-42, glucosylceramide, platelet-activating factor *Actinomycine D, aldosteron, amprenavir, bisantrene, calcein-M, citalopram, colchicine, corticosterone, cortisol, cyclosporin A, dexamethasone, digoxin, domperidone, doxorubicin, daunorubicin, enaminonen, erythromycine, etoposide, FK506, indinavir, loperamide, lovastatin, morphine, nelfinavir, ondansetron, paclitaxel (taxol), phenytoin, prednisolone, quinidine, rifampin, ritonavir, sanquinavir, sparfloxacin, teniposide, terfenadine, (99m)-Tc-tetrofosfine, valspodar (PSC833), verapamil, vinblastine, vincristine Inhibitors: Agosterol A, amiodarone, amitryptilin, amprenavir, biricodar (VX-710), chlorpromazin, cyclosporin A, diltiazem, dipyridamol, fluphenazin, GF120918, gramicidine D, LY335979, mefipriston, midazolam, nelfinavir, pimozin, pluronic L61, progesterone, promethazin, propafenone, propanolol, quinidine, reserpine, ritonavir, saquinavir, spironolactone, staurosporin, tamoxifen, trifluoperazin, triflupromazin, V-104, valinomycine, valspodar (PSC 833), verapamil*	Multidrug resistance	

Family	Gene	Localization	Substrates	Function	Phenotype/Disease
	ABCB2 (TAP1, PSF1, RING4, ABC17)	Ubiquitous (ER)	Peptides	Peptide transport (into the ER)	Juvenile-onset psoriasis; immune deficiency
	ABCB3 (TAP2, PSF2, RING11, ABC18)	Ubiquitous (ER)	Peptides	Peptide transport (into the ER)	Immune deficiency
	ABCB4 (PGP3, MDR3(2), PFIC-3)	Liver (hepatocytes)	Long-chain phosphatidyl-choline	Phosphatidylcholine transport	Progressive familial intrahepatic cholestasis-3, intrahepatic cholestasis of pregnancy
	ABCB5 (MTABC3)	Ubiquitous			
	ABCB6 (ABC14, UMAT, MTCA3)	Ubiquitous in mitochondria	Iron?	Iron transport	
	ABCB7 (ABC7, ATMIP, ASAT)	Ubiquitous in mitochondria	Iron?	Fe/S cluster transport	Sideroblastic anemia with ataxia
	ABCB8 (MABC1)	Mitochondria			
	ABCB9	Lysosomes			
	ABCB10 (MTABC2)	Mitochondria	Intermediates in heme/biosynthesis?		
	ABCB11 (sPGP, BSEP, PGY4)	Liver (hepatocytes)	Bile salts (e.g., taurocholate) *Paclitaxel (taxol)*	Bile salt transport	Progressive familial intrahepatic cholestasis-2
ABCC	ABCC1 (MRP1, MRP) Multidrug resistance related protein	Ubiquitous in normal tissues (mainly lung and choroid plexus epithelial cells) and brain capillary endothelial cells	17-β-glucuronyl estradiol, S-glutathionyl prostaglandin A2, glutathione disulfide, 4-hydroxynonenol-GS, leukotriene C4 (LTC4)-GS, leukotriene D4 (LTD4)-GS, leukotriene E4 (LTE4)-GS, NNAL-O-glucuronide lipid peroxidation products, nitroquinoline 1-oxide-GS *Aflatoxin B1-epoxide-GS, arsenite, arsenate (sodium), BCECF, calcein, chlorambucil-GS, colchicine, CPT-14, daunorubicin, DHEAS, 2,4-dinitrophenyl-GS doxorubicin, epirubicin, ethacrunic acid-GS, etoposide, fluorescein, flutamide, hydroxyflutamide, glucuronosyl etoposide, herbicides, heavy metals, indomethacin (-GS), melphalan-GS, methotrexate, rhodamine, ritonavir, sequinavir, 99Tc-Sestambi, SN-38, SN-38-GS, SNARF, tobacco nitrosamines, 99Tc-tetrofosmin, vinblastine, vincristine* Inhibitors: Agosterol A, benzbromarone, budesonide, biricodar (VX-710), cyclosporin A, indomethacin, probenecid, genistein, quercetin, sulfinylpyrazone, verapamil	Drug resistance, ubiquitous GS-X pump, immune response involving cysteinyl leukotrienes	
	ABCC2 (MRP2, cMOAT)	Liver, intestine, kidney, brain endothelial cells (plasma membrane)	Bilirubin-glucuronides, GSSH, GSH, including cotransport, estradiol-17-β-D-glucuronide, acidic bile salts *Anionic drug conjugates, cisplatin, doxorubicin, epirubicin, etoposide, indinavir, phenytoin, ritonavir, saquinavir, sulfinpyrazone, vinblastine* Inhibitors/modulators: Leukotriene C4, probenecid	Organic anion efflux, hepatobiliary extrusion of amphiphatic ions	Dubin–Johnson syndrome

Continued

Table 1 Continued

Family	Member (synonyms); most common name	Tissue expression	Physiological substrates; other substrates;[b] inhibitors/modulators	Function	Genetic mutations related to human disease
	ABCC3 (MRP3, cMOAT-2)	Liver, bile ducts, gut, adrenal cortex of kidney, intestine, placenta	Bile salts, leukotriene C4 Anionic drug conjugates, acetaminophen glucuronide methotrexate, etoposide, teniposide Inhibitors/modulators: Probenecid	Drug resistance	
	ABCC4 (MRP4, MOAT-B)	Many tissues (plasma membrane)	Cyclic nucleotides, conjugated steroids and bile acids, DHEAS nucleotide analogs, 9-(2-phosphophenyl methoxylethyl)-adenine, prostaglandins, taurolithocholate 3-sulfate, thiopurine monophosphates Nucleotide analogs, organic anions, nucleosides, monophosphates, zidovudin, other antiretroviral agents Inhibitors/modulators Probenecid	Nucleoside transport	
	ABCC5 (MRP5, MOAT-C)	Ubiquitous	Cyclic nucleotides, nucleotide analogs, 9-(2-phosphono-methoxyethyl) adenine, thiopurine monophosphates Nucleotide analogs, organic anions nucleoside monophosphates, mitoxantrone, topotecan, doxorubici Inhibitors/modulators: Probenecid fumitremorgin C, GF120918	Nucleoside transport	
	ABCC6 (MRP6)	Kidney, liver (plasma membrane)	BQ-123? (acidic peptide)	Elastic tissue homeostasis	Pseudo-xanthoma elasticum
	ABCC7 (CFTR)	Exocrine tissues		Cystic fibrosis transmembrane conductance regulator (cAMP-dependent chloride channel)	Cystic fibrosis, CBAVD, pancreatitis, bronchiectasis
	ABCC8 (SUR1)	Pancreas		K(ATP) channel regulation	Familial persistent hyperinsulinemia hypoglycemia of infancy
	ABCC9 (SUR2)	Heart, muscle		Sulfonurea receptor	Dilated cardiomyopathy
	ABCC10 (MRP7)	Ubiquitous (low)			
	ABCC11 (MRP8)	Testis and breast, lower in all other tissues			
	ABCC12 (MRP9)	Brain and testis, lower in all other tissues			

		Tissue	Substrates[b]	Function	Disease
ABCD	ABCD1 (ALD, ALDP)	Many tissues (peroxisomes)	VLCFA	VLCFA transport regulation	Adrenoleukodystrophy
	ABCD2 (ALD1, ALDR)	Many tissues (peroxisomes)	VLCFA		
	ABCD3 (PMP70, PXMP1)	Many tissues (peroxisomes)	VLCFA		
	ABCD4 (PMP69, P70R)	Many tissues (peroxisomes)	VLCFA		
ABCE	ABCE1 (OABP)	Ovary, testes, spleen		Oligoadenylate-binding protein	
ABCF	ABCF1	Ubiquitous			
	ABCF2 (ABC50)	Ubiquitous			
	ABCF3	Ubiquitous			
ABCG	ABCG1 (ABC8, human white)	Ubiquitous		Cholesterol transport	
	ABCG2 (ABCP, MXR, BCRP) Breast cancer resistance protein	Mainly in liver, placenta, small intestine; also in heart, lung, skeletal muscle, kidney, spleen, thymus, brain capillaries	Heme, porphyrins, flavanoids, pheophorbide, sulfated estrogens *Anthracyclines, bisantrene, diflomotecan, etoposide, flavopiridol, imatinib mesylate (STI-571, Gleevec), imatrib, irinotecan, SN-38, methotrexate, mitoxantrone, lamivudine, rhodamine 123, teniposide, topotecan, zidovudine, Inhibitors/modulators CI1033, futremorgirin C, GF120918, hammerhead ribozyme, HIV protease inhibitors, imatinib (STI-571, Gleevec) pantoprazole, prazosin, reserpine, ZD1839 (Iressa)*	Drug resistance, stem-cell differentiation, survival of stem cells (under hypoxic conditions).	HIV treatment?
	ABCG4 (white2)	Liver			
	ABCG5 (steroline 1)	Liver, intestine		Sterol transport, biliary cholesterol secretion/absorption	Sitosterolemia, sterol accumulation, artherosclerosis
	ABCG8 (steroline 2)	Liver, intestine		Sterol transport, biliary cholesterol secretion/absorption	Sitosterolemia, sterol accumulation, artherosclerosis

[a]BCECF, 2',7'-bis(carboxyethyl)-5(6)-carboxyfluorescein; CBAVD, congenital bilateral absence of the vas deferens; CFTR, cystic fibrosis transmembrane conductance regulator; DHEAS, dehydroepiandrosterone; ER, endoplasmic reticulum; GSH, glutathione; GSSH, glutathione persulfide; GS-X, GSH conjugate; HIV, human immunodeficiency virus; IFN, interferon; IL, interleukin; PMEA, 9-(2-phosphophenyl methoxylethyl)-adenine; VLCFA, very long-chain saturated fatty-acyl-CoA.
[b]Other substrates appear in italics.

MRP4 and MRP5 broaden the spectrum of drug resistance to nucleotide analog drugs; MRP6 plays a role in elastic tissue homeostasis. The functions of MRP7–MRP9 are largely unknown.

Breast Cancer Resistance Protein

BCRP (or ABCG2) is an ABC half transporter that displays drug resistance. In general, the BCRP transporter preferentially extrudes large hydrophobic, positively charged molecules. BCRP is involved in MDR in cancer, especially with regard to acute myeloid leukemia. Also, it plays a role in the survival of stem cells under hypoxic conditions and might play a role in regulating stem-cell differentiation.

Multidrug Resistance Transporter Proteins and Pharmacokinetics

Both the absorption and body distribution of drugs depend on their passage through diverse barriers. A number of MDR transporters limit the absorption of drugs via the gastrointestinal tract and the distribution of drugs into the brain via the blood–brain barrier; excretion is also governed by these transporters.

Oral Absorption

Efflux transporters such as Pgp and the MRPs in the intestinal may form the rate-limiting barrier to oral drug absorption. The poor bioavailability characteristics of many chemotherapeutic agents for cancer and human immunodeficiency virus (HIV) protease inhibitors may be explained by the fact that those drugs are among the best substrates for these transporters. The co-administration of the relevant substrates with the inhibitors/modulators of these transporters is a possible route to enhancing bioavailability. Of interest is the systematic site-specific expression of Pgp and MRPs along the various parts of the gastrointestinal tract.

Brain Distribution

The brain is the tissue most frequently targeted by drugs. To be effective, drugs must be transported to the site of action. The interface between the blood and brain is composed of the blood–brain barrier (brain capillary endothelial cells) and the blood–CSF barrier (choroid plexus epithelial cells).

The presence of these efflux transporters at the blood–brain/CSF barriers explains the fact that many drugs exhibit poor brain distribution despite their favorable lipophilic character; the barriers are substrates for the efflux transporters. Thus, in many studies Pgp, especially (expressed at the luminal face of the brain capillary endothelial cells), has been shown to be responsible for lowering the brain distribution of many drugs. MRP1 is more specifically localized in the basolateral membrane of the choroid epithelial cells, preventing CSF penetration of its substrates. Pgp is also expressed at the choroid epithelial cells, but in a manner that governs influx transport. Other ABC transporters, such as MRP2 and BCRP, have also been implicated in protecting the brain tissue against exogenous compounds.

Drug Excretion

The liver and kidneys play an important role in the excretion of drugs, the main routes being through the biliary tract and renal proximal tubule, respectively. In both the liver and kidneys, Pgp and other multidrug transporter proteins are variably expressed in the different suborgan structures and cell linings.

Functional Genetic Polymorphism

In addition, functional genetic polymorphisms, as have been identified for the Pgp gene, may influence the absorption, distribution, and excretion of the transporters substrates.

Other Physiological Functions of Multidrug Resistance and Other ATP-Binding Cassette Transporters

The ABC transporters govern a broad spectrum of physiological functions because they are involved in the transmembrane transport of various substances that exhibit a wide variety of chemical structures; examples are endogenous compounds such as ions, amino acids, peptides, sugars, vitamins, steroid hormones, bile acids, and phospholipids and also many exogenous compounds. Next we briefly describe a number of these physiological roles.

Defense against Oxidative Stress, Cancer, and Inflammation

Adequate glutathione (GSH) levels are essential to life and needed to fight infections and cancer cells. The MRPs that have been functionally characterized so far act as ATP-dependent export pumps for conjugates with glutathione, glucuronate, or sulfate. The most important substrate of MRP1 is the endogenous glucuronide conjugate leukotriene C4 (LTC4), a *de novo* synthesized mediator of inflammation. MRP1 and MRP2 also mediate the co-transport of unconjugated amphiphilic compounds, together with free glutathione. MRP3 preferentially transports glucuronides but not glutathione S-conjugates or free GSH. In addition, MRP1 and MRP2 contribute to the control of the intracellular glutathione disulfide levels and may thereby play an essential role in the response to oxidative stress when the activity of glutathione disulfide reductase becomes rate limiting. Thus, the members of the MRP family serve as export pumps that prevent the accumulation of anionic conjugates and glutathione disulfide in the cytoplasm, and they therefore play an essential role in detoxification and defense against oxidative stress.

Lipid Metabolism

The transport of specific molecules across lipid membranes is also an essential factor in the physiology of all living organisms, and a large number of specific transporters have evolved to carry out this function. Many ABC genes play a role in the maintenance of the lipid bilayer and in the transport of fatty acids and sterols within the body. Actually, the ABCA1 transporter is responsible for delivering cholesterol to nascent high-density lipoprotein (HDL) particles, a process known as reverse cholesterol transport. Enhancing ABCA1 activity, either through changes in gene expression or activity, is a plausible therapeutic strategy for increasing HDL levels. Dietary cholesterol is the primary contributor to the risk of developing cardiovascular disease for a subset of patients. The half-transporters ABCG5 and ABCG8 form a heterodimer responsible for regulating intestinal cholesterol absorption and the excretion of cholesterol in the liver. Increasing ABCG5/G8 expression or activity is a viable strategy for reducing dietary cholesterol. The expression of a large number of ABC transporters in monocytes/macrophages and their regulation by cholesterol flux indicate that these transporter molecules are potentially critical players in chronic inflammatory diseases such as atherosclerosis.

Antigen Presentation

The transporter associated with antigen processing 1 (TAP1; ABCB2) and TAP2 (ABCB3) are half-transporters that serve to transport peptides into the endoplasmatic reticulum. At that site, they can be complexed with class I human leukocyte antigen (HLA) molecules for presentation on the cell surface. TAP expression is required for the stable expression of the HLA class I proteins. The TAP complex transports amino acid peptides with a preference for Phe, Leu, Arg, and Tyr at the C-terminus, similar to the specificity of the HLA class I proteins. Several DNA viruses such as herpes simplex virus express molecules that interfere with antigen expression by disrupting the function of the TAP complex. TAP2 (ABCB3) functions as a heterodimer with TAP1.

Regulation of Insulin Secretion

Mutations in ABCC8 may result in familial persistent hyperinsulinemic hypoglycemia of infancy, demonstrating its role in the regulation of insulin secretion. Actually ABCC8 forms ATP-sensitive potassium channel together with an inwardly rectifying potassium channel. The closure of ATP-sensitive potassium channels in pancreatic islet β-cells initiates a cascade of events that leads to insulin secretion. ABCC8 therefore seems to be responsible for regulating glucose metabolism by insulin secretion.

Chloride Secretion

Chloride is the most abundant anion and the predominant permeating species. The chloride channels are crucial for transepithelial transport and the control of water flow, and they often provide unexpected permeation pathways for a large variety of anions. ABCC7 (CFTR, cystic fibrosis transmembrane) is a cAMP-dependent chloride channel and is responsible for chloride secretion in the gastrointestinal mucosa. The major toxins that cause secretory diarrheas act by increasing the levels of cAMP or cGMP. This results in a secondary increase in active chloride secretion through ABCC7, whereas sodium and water follow passively. Compounds that inhibit ABCC7 appear to be well suited as treatments for both secretory diarrhea and cholera.

Potassium Channel Regulation

ATP-sensitive potassium (KATP) channels, as inhibited by intracellular ATP, play key physiological roles in many tissues. KATP channels set membrane excitability in response to stress challenge and preserve cellular energy-dependent functions. ABCC9, together with an inwardly rectifying potassium channel, forms a KATP channel. This complex may have a vital role in securing cellular homeostasis under stress. Mutations in ABCC9 may lead to KATP channel dysfunctions and have been related to susceptibility to dilated cardiomyopathy.

Bile Salt Transport

Canalicular bile secretion is the rate-limiting step in bile formation. The canalicular membrane contains ABC proteins that transport biliary compounds against steep concentration gradients across the canicular membrane. Pgp excretes hydrophobic cationic compounds, whereas ABCB4 (Pgp3 or MDR3) acts as a phospholipid flippase for phosphatidyl choline. In addition to biliary excretion of phospholipids, bile is also the major pathway for the elimination of cholesterol, mostly derived from HDLs in plasma.

ABCC2 (MRP2) is an important (bilirubin) conjugate export pump. A major liver bile-salt transporter in the liver is ABCB11 (BSEP, bile salt export pump). The production of bile is also critically dependent on the coordinated regulation and function of this BSEP. The endothelin antagonist bosentan inhibits BSEP and leads to the intracellular accumulation of cytotoxic bile salts, and bile-salt-induced liver damage. Similarly, troglitazone, an insulin sensitizer, induces cholestasis and hepatotoxicity via competitive inhibition of the BSEP-mediated bile salt transport.

Multidrug Resistance: ATP-Binding Cassette Transporter Modulation and Regulation of Expression

Modulation

MDR modifying agents, which inhibit the function of the MDR transporters by either competitive or noncompetitive mechanisms, are good candidates for the pharmacological modulation of transporter functionality, currently still mostly focused on cancer treatment. The modulators are intended to increase the cytotoxic action of MDR-related drugs by preventing the extrusion of anticancer drugs from the target cells to significantly improve the treatment effectiveness.

To date, three generations of modulators/inhibitors exist, mostly acting on Pgp. The first generation comprises calcium channel blockers (verapamil, diltiazem, and azidopine), quinine derivatives, calmodulin inhibitors (trifluoroperazine and chlorpromazine), and the immunosuppressive agent cyclosporin A. The modulators of the second generation consists of derivatives of the first-generation compounds, for example R-verapamil and PSC-833 (from cyclosporin). Because of differences in the substrate-specificities and inhibitor-sensitivities of the different MDR proteins expressed in different tumor cells, proper therapeutic intervention requires an advanced diagnosis and targeted modulator agents. The third generation of MDR modifiers was devised to specifically interact with a particular MDR transporter. One example is the reversins, which are small hydrophobic peptide derivatives that are supposed to interact with Pgp with high affinity and selectivity; their clinical efficiency has yet to be proven.

Regulation of Expression

A number of environmental stimuli are known to affect the expression of the Pgp (*mdr1*) genes. In humans, it has been suggested that *mdr1* may function as a heat shock gene and its expression may be modulated by the numerous agents that trigger these signaling pathways. It seems likely that cellular stress and Pgp expression are closely linked because this transporter plays a crucial role in the protection of cells from toxic products released during environmental stress. More specifically, it has been found that certain steroid hormones enhance Pgp expression. Enhanced expression does not necessarily lead to enhanced efflux functionality because examples also exist of enhanced expression but decreased functionality.

See Also the Following Articles

Aging and Stress, Biology of; Cancer Treatment; Cholesterol and Lipoproteins; Corticosteroids and Stress; Cytokines, Stress, and Depression; Dexamethasone Suppression Test (DST); Environmental Factors; Genetic Factors and Stress; Hippocampus, Corticosteroid Effects on; Immune Response; Metabolic Syndrome; Oxidative Stress; Stress, Definitions and Concepts of; Synthetic Glucocorticoids; Perinatal Dexamethasone.

Further Reading

Borst, P. and Oude Elferink, R. (2002). Mammalian ABC transporters in health and disease. *Annual Review of Biochemistry* 71, 537–592.

Dean, M., Rzhetsky, A. and Allikmets, R. (2001). The human ATP-binding cassette (ABC) transporter superfamily. *Genome Research* 11(7), 1156–1166.

Glavinas, H., Krajcsi, P., Cserepes, J., et al. (2004). The role of ABC transporters in drug resistance, metabolism, and toxicity. *Current Drug Delivery* 1, 27–42.

Haimeur, A., Conseil, G., Deeley, R. G., et al. (2004). The MRP-related and BCRP/ABCG2 multidrug resistance proteins: biology, substrate specificity and regulation. *Current Drug Metabolism* 5(1), 21–53.

Kerb, R., Hoffmeyer, S. and Brinkmann, U. (2001). ABC drug transporters: hereditary polymorphisms and pharmacological impact in MDR1, MRP1 and MRP2. *Pharmacogenomics* 2(1), 51–64.

Liscovitch, M. and Lavie, Y. (2002). Cancer multidrug resistance: a review of recent drug discovery research. *IDrugs* 5, 349–355.

Meijer, O. C., Karssen, A. M. and de Kloet, E. R. (2003). Cell- and tIssue-specific effects of corticosteroids in relation to glucocorticoid resistance: examples from the brain. *Journal of Endocrinology* 178(1), 13–18.

Müller, M. B., Keck, M. E., Binder, E. B., et al. (2003). ABCB1 (MDR1)-type P-glycoproteins at the blood-brain barrier modulate the activity of the hypothalamic-pituitary-adrenocortical system: implications for affective disorder. *Neuropsychopharmacology* 28, 1991–1999.

Renes, J., de Vries, E. G., Jansen, P. L., et al. (2000). The (patho)physiological functions of the MRP family. *Drug Resistance Update* 5, 289–302.

Schmitz, G. and Kaminski, W. E. (2001). ABC transporters and cholesterol metabolism. *Frontiers in Bioscience* **6**, D505–D514.

Štefkova, J., Poledne, R. and Hubacek, J. A. (2004). ATP-binding cassette (ABC) transporters in human metabolism and diseases. *Physiology Research* **53**, 235–243.

Stein, W. D. (2002). Reversers of the multidrug resistance transporter P-glycoprotein. *Current Opinion in Investigative Drugs* **3**(5), 812–817.

Sukhai, M. and Piquette-Miller, M. (2000). Regulation of the multidrug resistance genes by stress signals. *Journal of Pharmacy and Pharmaceutical Sciences* 268–280.

Tan, B., Piwnica-Worms, D. and Ratner, L. (2000). Multidrug resistance transporters and modulation. *Current Opinion in Oncology* **12**(5), 450–458.

Wijnholds, J., Evers, R., van Leusden, M. R., et al. (1997). Increased sensitivity to anticancer drugs and decreased inflammatory response in mice lacking the multidrug resistance-associated protein. *Nature Medicine* 1275–1279.

Multiple Personality Disorder

R P Kluft
Temple University, Philadelphia, PA, USA

This article is a revision of the previous edition article by R P Kluft, volume 2, pp 786–790, © 2000, Elsevier Inc.

Introduction
History
Definition and Characteristic Findings
Etiology
Diagnosis
Treatment
Miscellaneous Concerns
Concluding Remarks

Glossary

Alter	A distinct identity or personality state with its own characteristic and relatively enduring pattern of perceiving, relating to, and thinking about the environment and self. An alter has its own identity, self-representation, autobiographic memory, and sense of ownership of its own thoughts, feelings, and actions. Some synonyms are personality, personality state, subpersonality, alter personality, and disaggregate self-state.
Dissociation	"Disruption in the usually integrated functions of consciousness, memory, identity, or perception" (American Psychiatric Association, 2000: 519); the segregation of some subsets of information from other subsets of information in a relatively rule-bound manner (Spiegel, 1986: 123).
Ego state	"An organized system of behavior and experience whose elements are bound together by some common principle but that is separated from other such states by boundaries that are more or less permeable" (Watkins and Watkins, 1993: 278).
Iatrogenesis	The creation (or worsening) of a problematic condition as a result of the interventions of a helping professional.
Integration	The unification of all personalities into a single coherent identity; the cessation of separateness of a particular personality or group of personalities; the interventions made by a therapist to bring together two or more personalities at a particular point in time.
Personality	An enduring pattern of behavior, adaptation, and inner experience that is pervasive over time and across situations (in general psychology); synonym for alter (in dissociative disorders).
Resolution	An outcome in which a multiple personality patient has achieved smooth function, continuity of contemporary memory, and the relief of distressing symptoms due to the more facile cooperation and collaboration of the remaining personalities. Some personalities may have integrated.
Shift	A change in the personality system such that while the personality or alter in apparent executive control has not changed or been replaced, it is being influenced by different alters behind the scenes than it had been, leading to minor changes in the appearance, actions, and speech of the alter in apparent executive control.
Switch	A transition from one personality being in apparent executive control to another personality being in apparent executive control.

Introduction

Multiple personality (dissociative identity disorder in the United States) has been described as difficult to understand, difficult to diagnose, difficult to treat, and difficult to discuss objectively not only because of its complexity, but also because of the controversies that often surround it. Its study draws upon the literatures of dissociation, hypnosis, memory, cognitive psychology, social psychology, development, trauma, attachment and psychoanalysis, among others, requiring researchers and clinicians to grapple with concerns and issues that often appear remote and obscure.

History

Conditions in which an individual's customary personality or way of being is replaced by an alternative (and often very different) personality or way of being, whose activities are unknown to the customary personality, were virtually worldwide and commonplace prior to the modern scientific era. Possession states were attributed to the intrusion of various forces, spirits, angels, demons, gods, or ancestors. Judeo-Christian possession states included forms in which the intruding entity took over completely, leaving the possessed person without memory for the intruding entity's actions, and forms in which both customary personality and intruding entity were aware of one another and contended for control (somnambulistic and lucid possession, respectively).

As possession was discredited (circa 1775–1800), cases with these phenomena were reported and described in secular terms (e.g., exchanged identity, doubling of the personality). By the 1830s, French physician Antoine Despine and his physician son and nephew had observed and treated series of such patients. Utilizing contemporary methods and magnetism, a precursor of hypnosis, successful treatments and integrations were achieved. Throughout the nineteenth century there was considerable interest in multiple personality.

However, rising forces in psychiatry and psychology eclipsed its study. Bleuler subsumed multiple personality under schizophrenia. Freud abandoned dissociation for repression. Janet was marginalized by psychoanalysis and the discrediting of his mentor, Charcot. Behaviorism disregarded multiple personality. Within a generation, multiple personality was largely forgotten except as a historical curiosity.

Two books, *The Three Faces of Eve* and *Sybil*, brought multiple personality to the attention of North American readers. A small but increasing number of North American clinicians began to report numbers of such patients (1970s–80s). Sensitized by feminism and the plight of Viet Nam veterans to the sequelae of abuse for women, children and combat veterans, they understood multiple personality as a chronic posttraumatic dissociative condition. Cases were recognized with increasing frequency. This experience was duplicated in The Netherlands and elsewhere.

In the 1990s there were highly polarized debates about whether multiple personality was iatrogenic, instigated and sustained by clinicians' interest in motivating patients to demonstrate the condition's phenomena, and whether the abuses alleged by patients, often recalled after years of apparent amnesia, were false, suggested by leading questions or subtle expressions of interest.

It remains unclear whether multiple personality can be created by iatrogenic factors alone. Some reports indicate that efforts to create conditions similar to multiple personality have been undertaken by various intelligence agencies. Some social psychology manipulations can cause subjects to demonstrate some characteristics of multiple personality under experimental conditions. However, no evidence demonstrates that clinicians exert influences similar to the interventions of either covert agencies or laboratory experiments. While some individuals are subject to develop false memories, many memories that became available after long absence from awareness have proven accurate.

Definition and Characteristic Findings

Criteria

The American Psychiatric Association's *Diagnostic and Statistical Manual of Mental Disorders,* 4th edition, text revision (DSM-IV-TR) offers four diagnostic criteria for dissociative identity disorder (multiple personality) (**Table 1**).

Phenomena

Multiple personality involves problems with identity, memory, thinking, containment, cohesive conation, and the switch process. Problems of identity may include the presence of other identities (alters), depersonalization, an absence of or confusion about identity, alters' impingements on one another, and the combined presence of two or more alters. Problems of memory may include amnesia for past events, losing blocks of contemporary time, uncertainty about whether events did or did not occur, fragmentary recall, and experiencing events as dream-like, unreal, or of uncertain reality. There are often amnesia barriers across the alters, which may be aware or

Table 1 DSM-IV diagnostic criteria for dissociative identity disorder[a]

A. The presence of one or more distinct identities or personality states (each with its own relatively enduring pattern of perceiving, relating to, and thinking about the environment and self).
B. At least two of these identities or personality states recurrently take control of the person's behavior.
C. Inability to recall important personal information that is too extensive to be explained by ordinary forgetfulness.
D. The disturbance is not due to the direct physiological effects of a substance (e.g., blackouts or chaotic behavior during alcohol intoxication) or a general medical condition (e.g., complex partial seizures). Note: in children, the symptoms are not attributable to imaginary playmates or other fantasy play.

[a]From the American Psychiatric Association (2000), p. 529. Reprinted with permission from the Diagnostic and Statistical Manual of Mental Disorders, Copyright 2000. American Psychiatric Association.

unaware of one another or display directional amnesia. In directional amnesia, alter A may know about alter B and be aware of B's thoughts and activities, while B knows little or nothing about A, is unaware of A's thoughts, and has no recall of what happens when A is in control.

Problems of thinking include cognitive errors, magical thinking, and the toleration of mutually incompatible ideas and perceptions without appreciating the impossibility of their coexisting (trance logic). They stem from distortions of reality made to accommodate to intolerable childhood circumstances.

Problems of containment include the intrusions of alters into one another and leakage of the memories, feelings, and sensations of one alter into the awareness and experience of another.

Problems of cohesive conation (will and intentionality) refer to difficulties in the distribution of executive control across the alters. Patients' sense of control of themselves and their actions may be compromised, along with their sense of ownership, responsibility, and voluntary control of themselves and their actions.

Problems of the switch process refer to changes of executive control that are jarring, incomplete, or so frequent that the person cannot concentrate or pay attention consistently enough to accomplish necessary functions and tasks.

Personalities

Personalities, personality states, subpersonalities, personifications, self-states, and alters are synonyms. They are relatively stable and enduring entities with fairly consistent ways of perceiving, relating to, and thinking about the environment and self. They are experienced as having their own identities, self-images, personal histories, and senses of ownership of their own activities and mental contents. Personalities usually but not inevitably have names. Some names may refer to attributes or emotions or humiliating insults. Usually a rather passive, guilt-ridden, dependent, masochistic, and depressed personality in apparent control most of the time bears the legal name. Alternate personalities may differ in name, age, race, gender, sexual orientation, areas of knowledge, predominant affect, vocabulary, and apparent intelligence. Alters may or may not be aware of one another. Alters may relate to one another in a potentially complex inner world. They constitute ongoing sets of parallel processes; that is, as one alter is dealing with the outside world, another may be making comments on or to the first, while others are interacting with one another, oblivious to external events. Neuropsychophysiological studies often demonstrate significant differences in different types of personality.

Personalities arise as desperate coping strategies, initially serving adaptive and defensive purposes. Achieving a degree of autonomy and persisting beyond the situations to which they were responses, they may become increasingly problematic and disruptive. Alters are formed by repudiating a sense of self and a representation of self in interactions with others that have become intolerable, severing empathic connection and erecting boundaries between the self that has become intolerable and a more adaptive identity created to manage the adaptation believed to be required. This new alter, envisioned and experienced as real, is accepted and interpreted as real. Its alternate autobiographic memories are endorsed as real.

For example: Lois, a 5-year-old girl, is molested by her previously warm and loving Uncle Ben. She is deeply attached to her uncle and does not want to lose him, afraid of the consequences of telling her parents, confused about the feelings and sensations arising in her, wishing this molestation had never occurred, and wanting someone to rescue her. **Table 2** illustrates numerous coping strategies and alters that might be created to embody them. Strategies strongly influence the transformations of identity and autobiographic memory that alters will embody. For example, Bad Lois must repudiate knowledge that would demonstrate that Lois is an innocent victim. Louis not only must disregard attributes and experiences that would compel him to acknowledge he is a little girl, but also may need to hallucinate having a male body with appropriate musculature, facial hair, and genitalia.

Alters often experience themselves as having relationships with one another in an inner world that

Table 2 Coping strategies and alter formation of 'Lois'[a]

Cognitive coping strategy	Alter created
This did not happen	A Lois who knows, and a Lois who does not
I must have deserved it	Bad Lois, whose behavior would explain trauma as punishment
I must have wanted it	A sexual alter, Sherrie
I can control it better if I take charge	An aggressively sexual alter, Vickie
I would be safe if I were a boy	Louis, Lois' male twin
I wish I were a big man	Big Jack, based on some person of power who could prevent this
I wish I were the one who could hurt someone and not be hurt	Uncle Ben, or a more disguised identification with the aggressor
I wish I could feel nothing	Jessie, who endures all yet feels nothing
I wish someone could replace me	The Girls, who encapsulate specific experiences of trauma unknown to Lois
I wish someone would comfort me	Angel, with whom Lois imagines herself to be while the body is being exploited and the Girls are experiencing the trauma

[a]From Kluft (1999), p. 5.

may be experienced as possessing reality and importance that is equally or more compelling than the external world. Inner world events may be reported as if they had occurred in external reality, and vice versa.

Comorbidity

Multiple personalities commonly suffer additional mental disorders. It may be difficult to be sure whether the diagnostic criteria for some of these other disorders are satisfied by symptoms emerging from multiple personality or whether they indicate co-occurring diagnoses that require treatments of their own. Posttraumatic stress disorder, major depression, various substance abuses, borderline personality disorder, other anxiety and affective disorders, somatoform disorders, sexual dysfunctions, eating disorders, and other personality disorders commonly co-occur. Symptoms of another disorder may be found in all or most of the personalities, but sometimes only in particular personalities. Distinguishing between comorbidities and look-alike epiphenomena can prove challenging.

Prognosis may be determined more by the treatability of comorbid conditions than by the multiple personality. For example, a multiple personality with posttraumatic stress disorder and a depression that responds well to medication has a much better prognosis than one with posttraumatic stress disorder, anorexia nervosa, rapid-cycling bipolar disorder, and borderline personality disorder.

Etiology

The predominant theory of the etiology of multiple personality holds that this condition comes into being when a child with high hypnotic potential and problematic support from caretakers and/or attachment issues experiences overwhelming traumatic stress, usually on a repeated basis, and is not protected,

comforted, and supported in a way that alleviates the child's distress. The iatrogenesis hypothesis was noted previously. Many scholars consider both alternatives plausible and do not assume that either precludes the possibility of the other.

Data consistent with the predominant theory include the high hypnotizability of this patient group, documentation of abuse in 95% of two cohorts of young dissociative patients, and epidemiological studies in many nations using reliable and valid screening and diagnostic instruments finding a similar incidence of multiple personality (4–6% of psychiatric inpatients) in many nations with very different degrees of awareness of and sympathy toward the diagnosis of multiple personality. If clinicians with special interest in multiple personality act in such a way as to create it, an assumption of the iatrogenesis hypothesis, significantly higher percentages should be encountered in countries in which clinicians are accused of applying such pressures.

Observations consistent with the iatrogenesis hypothesis are the development of transient multiple personality-like phenomena in laboratory settings, reports of the creation of artificial multiple personality by intelligence agencies, and the fact that multiple personality patients have been known to create additional personalities in response to therapists' suggestions. Those most experienced with multiple personality hold that multiple personality cannot be created by therapists under normal clinical circumstances, but that additional personalities can be created in response to perceived pressures from a therapist.

Diagnosis

It was long thought that multiple personality was rare and sufficiently flamboyant to make its presence self-evident. Multiple personality has proven to be far from rare, usually covert, and commonly misdiagnosed for an average of 6.8 years. With the demonstration of widespread false negative diagnoses, diagnostic efforts were accorded greater importance.

The Natural History of Multiple Personality

While a small percentage (6%) of adult multiple personalities are florid and overt most of the time, the vast majority either take pains to avoid drawing attention to their situations and/or have only windows of overtness, usually in the context of psychosocial stress or encountering situations that in some way are analogous to overwhelming childhood events or that force them to contend with an abusive figure from their childhood (or someone who is perceived as similar to such a figure). Usually personalities either are relatively quiescent or exert their influence from behind the scenes by shifting or intruding into or otherwise influencing (by persuasion or threat) the personality in apparent executive control. They may contrive to pass as the usually apparent personality.

Multiple personality usually is clandestine in children and difficult to distinguish from various turmoils and early manifestations of psychotic disorders in adolescents. Young adults often work to avoid detection and deny manifestations of the condition. As individuals mature, they usually enter a complex matrix of work, family, and relationships and are less closely connected with important figures of their childhood. Less immediately pressured to keep childhood issues out of awareness and increasingly experiencing situations that are related to or analogous to childhood experiences (including intercurrent adult trauma), they often become symptomatic and seek treatment for what appears to be anxiety or depression. Treating clinicians may recognize or suspect dissociative phenomena.

Diagnostic Approaches

Considering the usually covert nature of multiple personality, it cannot be assumed that it will declare itself in typical clinical interviews or mental status examinations, or even in therapy sessions. Clinicians have derived lists of suggestive signs of multiple personality. Experience-derived suggestive signs include common findings in multiple personalities' histories and indications of dissociated behavior (i.e., having been given many different diagnoses, being told by others of disremembered out-of-character behavior, finding objects, productions, or writing in one's possession that one cannot recall acquiring or creating). Loewenstein developed a mental status that studies six relevant symptom clusters: (1) indications of

multiple personality processes at work (e.g., differences in behavior, linguistic indications, switching/shifting); (2) signs of the patient's high hypnotic potential (e.g., enthrallment, trance logic, out-of-body experiences); (3) amnesia; (4) somatoform symptoms; (5) posttraumatic stress disorder symptoms; and (6) affective symptoms.

Instruments have been developed to screen patients for dissociative phenomena; high scores or particular patterns of response suggest that further evaluation is needed. Structured diagnostic interviews have enabled actual diagnostic assessment. The most well-known of these are the Dissociative Experiences Scale (Bernstein and Putnam) for screening and the Structured Clinical Interview for the Diagnosis of DSM-IV Dissociative Disorders – Revised (Steinberg) for diagnostic purposes.

Differential Diagnosis

The differential diagnosis includes other dissociative disorders, psychotic disorders, affective disorders, borderline personality disorder, partial complex seizures, factitious disorders, and malingering. Evaluators knowledgeable about all of these disorders usually find differential diagnosis to be straightforward. Evaluators unfamiliar with dissociative disorders commonly encounter difficulties because phenomena of many of these conditions overlap.

Treatment

Approaches and Modalities

Treatment resembles a stage-oriented trauma therapy, modified to include work with alters. However, work with some alters and issues may be quite advanced and work with others may be just beginning while still others have not yet been discovered. The treatment may be understood as a series of short-term therapies imbricated within the process of a long-term psychotherapy. Virtually every therapeutic model and modality has been applied to multiple personality. In practice, advocates of different theoretical models and treatment approaches find themselves making many similar interventions. In successful treatments, the pragmatic realities of dealing with multiple personality tend to determine what is done.

Treatment Stages

In the three-stage model of modern trauma therapy outlined by Herman, a phase of safety, in which the patient receives sanctuary and support and is strengthened, is followed by a phase of remembrance and mourning, in which the mind's representation of its traumatic experiences is explored, processed, and mastered and in which the losses and consequences associated with traumatization are grieved. The mind is reintegrated, and roles and functions are resumed in a phase of reconnection.

In the nine-stage treatment of multiple personality (Kluft, 1999a,b) with multiple personality (1) the psychotherapy is established and (2) preliminary interventions are made to establish safety, develop a therapeutic alliance that includes the alters, and enhance the patient's coping capacities. Then follows (3) history gathering and mapping to learn more about the alters, their concerns, and how the system of alters functions. Then is it possible to begin (4) the metabolism of trauma within and across the alters. As the alters share more, work through more, communicate more effectively with one another, and achieve more mutual awareness, identification, and empathy, their conflicts are reduced, as is contemporary amnesia. They increasingly cooperate and experience some reduction of their differences and senses of separateness. This is called (5) moving toward integration/ resolution. More solidified stances toward one's self and the world are reached in (6) integration/resolution. Smooth and functional collaboration among the alters, usually including the blending of several personalities, is called a resolution. Blending all alters into a subjective sense of smooth unity is an integration. Then the patient focuses on (7) learning new coping skills, working out alternatives to dissociative functioning, and resolving other previously unaddressed concerns. Issues continue to be processed, and mastery without resort to dysfunctional dissociation is pursued in (8) solidification of gains and working through. Finally, treatment tapers, and the patient is seen at increasingly infrequent intervals in a stage of (9) follow-up.

Typical Issues

Treatment may prove arduous and challenging to patient and therapist alike. Work with traumatic material can be upsetting and destabilizing. Worse than the material itself is the pain of integrating what patients learn into their perceptions of their relationships with significant others who may appear to have been perpetrators of previously unremembered mistreatment. This is complicated by the fact that it is usually not possible to either validate or invalidate most of the traumatic memories that emerge. Patients should be informed about the possibility that material that emerges and may be useful for treatment may not prove to be accurate.

Processing traumatic memories has been controversial because the accuracy of initially unavailable memories has been challenged and the affects experienced in association with this processing may cause upset and trigger self-destructive impulses. Occasionally decompensation occurs. Some multiple personalities cannot tolerate such work. However, thus far, reported successful recoveries to the point of integration have involved processing traumatic memories. Studies have demonstrated that many recovered memories of multiple personality patients have been confirmed, and some have been proven inaccurate. Current opinion suggests that deliberate processing of traumatic memories should not proceed unless patients have demonstrated adequate strength and stability for such work. All others should be treated supportively, addressing traumatic memories only when they are intrusive, are disruptive, and cannot be put aside.

Patients typically have periods of wanting to disavow everything said in therapy, trying to banish painful memories of trauma, betrayal, and loss associated with important people in their lives in order to retain relationships and a sense of safety within those valued relationships. Tact, containment, and circumspection are required from therapist and patient alike. The patient should be protected from becoming overwhelmed by and lost in the traumatic material, and treatment should be paced to safeguard the patient's safety and stability. All pressures to get everything out and over with must be resisted.

The alter system is designed to facilitate escape from pain and difficulty or, failing that, to reframe or disguise it. Alters often reenact scenarios that (in their perceptions) are tried and true methods of keeping pain at bay, even if they disrupt the patient's treatment, life, and relationships. Containing and/or minimizing such events is an ongoing challenge to the treatment, rarely completely successful until therapy is well advanced.

Some have advised against working with alters lest separateness be reified and reinforced by their being addressed directly and individually, and recommend speaking in ways that always convey that the patient is a single person. In practice, working directly with alters often may make them more prominent transiently, but as they are worked with, empathized with, and helped to communicate with other alters, their separateness is eroded. All published series of successful integrations have been contributed by authors who work directly with alters.

The therapist should treat all of the personalities with respect, simultaneously appreciating the immediacy, forcefulness, and defensive aspects of their entrenched and subjectively compelling senses of separateness, and that all express aspects of a single individual, whose personality structure is to have multiple personalities. Interventions to contain alters' dysfunctional behaviors, aggressiveness toward other personalities, self-destructiveness, and irresponsible autonomy (e.g., failing to care for children, who may be seen as belonging to another personality) may prove necessary. The therapist may call upon personalities to work on their particular issues in the treatment and to facilitate their cooperation with the treatment and one another.

Treatment must respect the entirety of the patient's concerns. Specific multiple personality treatment may be deferred repeatedly to address pressing concerns and other mental health issues. For example, a woman with multiple personality whose child develops cancer is not in a position to pursue trauma work.

Patient Subgroups

Some multiple personality patients cannot achieve the goals of the early stages of treatment and move on to process traumatic events and bring personalities together. Those with severe comorbidity and maladaptive character issues may never achieve enough stability to follow that path. Their treatment will involve ongoing efforts to enhance safety and strength and will defer trauma work unless material is intrusive and unavoidable. Therapy prioritizes better coping strategies and enhanced cooperation among alters. An intermediate group will go through phases in which trauma work can be done and phases in which it cannot be tolerated. Therapists should be flexible and err on the side of caution whenever uncertain about the safety of trauma work.

Hypnosis

Multiple personality is associated with high hypnotizability, a stable trait. Hypnosis may occur because a clinician performs an induction procedure, because an individual induces self-hypnosis, or because spontaneous trance is triggered by some stimulus or activity, such as strong emotion or meditation. Therefore, therapists cannot control whether hypnosis occurs in the course of a therapy. Bearing this in mind, therapists should avoid making remarks that might suggest that particular events have taken place or that particular persons were involved in doing harmful things, because they may be heard as powerful hypnotic suggestions.

Notwithstanding such concerns, hypnotic interventions can play a major role in stabilizing multiple personality patients, managing abreactions, containing powerful emotions, accessing alters for therapeutic work, and promoting integration.

Miscellaneous Concerns

Forensic Aspects of Multiple Personality

The relevance of multiple personality as a defense varies tremendously depending upon (1) diverse requirements for the insanity defense in different jurisdictions and (2) the phenomenology in particular multiple personalities. Criminal acts may have taken place because of the impact of multiple personality upon a person's capacity to know his or her own mind and control its various aspects, without thereby satisfying legal definitions of insanity.

The assessment of defendants claiming to have or thought to have multiple personality should proceed with a keen eye toward discerning both factitious and malingered presentations, informed by a state-of-the-art knowledge of multiple personality drawn from the modern clinical literature.

The Impact of Controversy

Controversy magnifies the burden of having, treating, or researching multiple personality. Multiple personality patients must contend with the impact of efforts to deny the reality of their condition and the credibility of what they believe to be their autobiographic memories, attacks on the competence and credibility of those who treat them, and criticism and rejection from those who believe, either accurately or inaccurately, that the multiple personality patient is revealing their secrets or making scandalous accusations against them or those they love in treatment. Therapists treating such patients must contend with ongoing questioning of their efforts, methods, and intentions and accusations that they are encouraging iatrogenesis and confabulated false memories. Researchers have difficulty obtaining funds to expand our knowledge of this condition and may be endangering the trajectory of their careers by working in this area.

Concluding Remarks

Notwithstanding the complexity and difficulty associated with multiple personality, this disorder often proves treatable to a satisfactory outcome and offers unique insights into the impact of overwhelming stressors upon human memory and identity and into the neuropsychophysiology of mental structures and functions. It is moving into the mainstream of the mental health professions and should be of concern to all mental health professionals.

See Also the Following Articles

Coping Skills; Dissociation; Hypnosis.

Further Reading

Bernstein, E. and Putnam, F. W. (1986). Development, reliability, and validity of a dissociation scale. *Journal of Nervous and Mental Disease* **174**, 727–734.

Boon, S. and Draijer, N. (1993). *Multiple personality in the Netherlands: a study on reliability and validity of the diagnosis.* Amsterdam: Swets & Zeitlinger.

Coons, P. M. (1980). Multiple personality: diagnostic considerations. *Journal of Clinical Psychiatry* **141**, 330–336.

Kluft, R. P. (1999a). Current issues in dissociative identity disorder. *Journal of Practical Psychiatry and Behavioral Health* **5**, 3–19.

Kluft, R. P. (1999b). An overview of the psychotherapy of dissociative identity disorder. *American Journal of Psychotherapy* **55**, 289–319.

Kluft, R. P. (2005). Diagnosing dissociative identity disorder. *Psychiatric Annals* **35**, 633–643.

Kluft, R. P. and Fine, C. G. (eds.) (1993). *Clinical perspectives on multiple personality disorder.* Washington, D.C.: American Psychiatric Press.

Loewenstein, R. J. (1991). An office mental status examination for complex chronic dissociative symptoms and multiple personality disorder. *Psychiatric Clinics of North America* **14**, 567–604.

Putnam, F. W. (1989). *Diagnosis and treatment of multiple personality disorder.* New York: Guilford.

Putnam, F. W. (1997). *Dissociation in children and adolescents: a developmental perspective.* New York: Guilford.

Ross, C. A. (1997). *Dissociative identity disorder: diagnosis, clinical features, and treatment of multiple personality.* New York: Wiley.

Spiegel, D. (1986). Dissociating damage. *American Journal of Clinical Hypnosis* **29**, 123–131.

Steinberg, M. (1994). *Structured clinical interview for DSM-IV dissociative disorders, revised.* Washington, D.C.: American Psychiatric Press.

Tutkun, H., Sar, V., Yargiuc, I., Ozpulat, T., Yanik, M. and Kiziltan, E. (1998). Frequency of dissociative disorders among psychiatric inpatients in a Turkish university clinic. *American Journal of Psychiatry* **155**, 800–805.

Watkins, H. and Watkins, J. (1993). Ego-state therapy in the treatment of dissociative disorders. In: Kluft, R. P. & Fine, C. G. (eds.) *Clinical perspectives on multiple personality disorder*, pp. 277–299. Washington, D.C.: American Psychiatric Press.

Multiple Sclerosis

A T Reder
University of Chicago, Chicago, IL, USA

This article is a revision of the previous edition article by A T Reder, volume 2, pp 791–795, © 2000, Elsevier Inc.

Multiple Sclerosis – Overview

Immune Abnormalities in Multiple Sclerosis

Neuroendocrine and Sympathetic Nervous Systems in Multiple Sclerosis

Stress Inhibits Experimental Allergic Encephalomyelitis

Could Stress Affect Immune Function?

Do Neurosurgical Lesions or Physical Trauma Incite Multiple Sclerosis Plaques?

Does Stress Cause Multiple Sclerosis? Actual Data from Multiple Sclerosis Patients

Medical-Legal Implications

Glossary

Cytokine	A protein secreted by the immune cells that affects immune responses.
Experimental allergic encephalomyelitis (EAE)	An autoimmune disease caused by the injection of brain proteins (myelin oligodendrocyte protein, MOG; proteolipid protein, PLP; myelin basic protein, MBP); in some ways, a model of multiple sclerosis.
Human leukocyte antigen (HLA)	A protein on the membrane of most cells that is recognized by immune cells.
Interferon (IFN)-γ	A cytokine secreted by lymphocytes that is involved in Th1 immune responses. Treatment with this IFN causes exacerbations of multiple sclerosis.
Oligoclonal bands	Immunglobin G of restricted heterogeneity, which forms several discrete bands on electrophoresis of cerebrospinal fluid.
Oligodendroglia	Myelin-forming cells of the central nervous system.
Plaque	Inflammatory and scarred (gliosis) central nervous system lesions in multiple sclerosis.
T helper 1 (Th1) cells	T helper lymphocytes that secrete IL-2 and IFN-γ and mediate delayed-type hypersensitivity immunity.
T helper 2 (Th2) cells	T helper lymphocytes that secrete IL-4 and IL-10 and amplify humoral immunity.

Ask a roomful of multiple sclerosis (MS) patients whether MS attacks are caused by stress, and 9 out of 10 will say "of course." However, objective and quantitative measurement is difficult for both MS exacerbations and stress. Could stress affect immunity and could immune changes in turn affect MS? More important, does stress directly affect MS?

Multiple Sclerosis – Overview

Multiple sclerosis is a disease caused by intermittent perivenular inflammation of areas of the central nervous system (CNS). These plaques affect every function controlled by the brain and spinal cord.

MS usually appears between the age of 20 and 50, in women twice as often as men, and is most common in people of northern European ancestry. A complex interaction of multiple genes and the environment may lead to MS. HLA-DR2 predisposes to MS in northern Europeans, but other HLA types are linked to MS in Sardinia, Turkey, and the Middle East. MS is more common in areas far from the equator. Migration studies suggest that an environmental influence before puberty also affects the development of MS. Viruses are the main environmental culprits, but no single virus has been convincingly linked to MS.

Three factors consistently increase MS exacerbations: (1) virus infections (there may also be some effect of prostate, bladder, and sinus infections, which provoke MS symptoms and possibly cause exacerbations), (2) delivery of a baby (there are more exacerbations during the several months postpartum than during pregnancy), and (3) IFN-γ (injections of IFN-γ causes a fourfold increase in MS flares).

Immune Abnormalities in Multiple Sclerosis

The immune system is abnormal in MS. Inflammatory cells destroy oligodendroglia and some neurons in MS plaques. Macrophages far outnumber lymphocytes in these lesions. The inflammation in brain tissue is reflected by small numbers of activated immune cells in the cerebrospinal fluid (CSF; T cells outnumber B cells and macrophages in CSF) and excessive levels of immunoglobulins (IgG; seen in oligoclonal bands). Some T cells and some antibodies recognize virus or brain antigens (myelin oligodendrocyte protein, MOG; proteolipid protein, PLP; myelin basic protein, MBP; heat shock proteins; S-100 protein; and αB-crystallin), but most recognize other targets (e.g., nonsense antibodies). Cytokines in the CSF such as tumor necrosis factor (TNF)-α and interleukin (IL)-6 correlate with disease activity and blood–brain barrier (BBB) damage. In culture, very high doses of IFN-γ and

TNF-α kill oligodendroglia; at lower doses, TNF-α still interferes with oligodendroglial function.

The peripheral blood is also abnormal in MS. Changes in the blood sometimes precede clinical attacks. Several weeks before exacerbations, mitogen-activated white blood cells secrete excessive amounts of IFN-γ and TNF-α, and lymphocytes show more IFN-γ-induced $[Ca^{2+}]_i$ influx. All of these peripheral immune changes could amplify the antibrain immune response.

During attacks, suppressor cell function drops, IL-12 increases and is likely to induce IFN-γ, and expression of the costimulatory CD80 (B7.1) protein increases on lymphocytes. These changes may lead to antibrain immune reactions. Treatments for MS partially reverse immune abnormalities, and reduce exacerbations by 33%. Interferon-beta reduces inflammatory cytokines, increases suppressor cell function, and prevents immune cells from entering the brain. Glatiramer acetate shifts cells from pro-inflammatory (Th1) to anti-inflammatory (Th2) immunity. Both agents may also induce neurotrophic factors in lymphocytes.

Neuroendocrine and Sympathetic Nervous Systems in Multiple Sclerosis

There are other abnormalities in MS possibly linked to stress responses. MS and Crohn's disease occur together more often than expected. Both are relapsing/remitting diseases with possible viral/bacterial triggers, show similar immune abnormalities, and have anecdotal links to stress. However, typical autoimmune diseases such as systemic lupus erythematosus are not linked to MS.

There is an increased incidence of depression in MS patients and possibly in their families. The diagnostic laboratory test for depression – the dexamethasone suppression test – is abnormal in active MS, at least as often as in depression.

Some patients have elevated cortisol and enlarged adrenal glands. Steroids do not inhibit proliferation and do not induce glucocorticoid receptor translocation in MS lymphocytes compared to normal lymphocytes. Responses to corticotropin releasing hormone (CRH) are normal, but arginine vasopressin (AVP) stimulation of the pituitary is subnormal. These abnormalities may all be a consequence of chronic high cortisol levels caused by stress or inflammation, which could change the set point for steroid responses. (Rats susceptible to EAE have similar neuroendocrine abnormalities; EAE-sensitive strains are less responsive to steroids.)

Glucocorticoid therapy curtails acute inflammation in MS plaques. Steroid therapy may correct the abnormal endogenous glucocorticoid feedback that otherwise allows unchecked immune responses. As a corollary, some MS patients may need higher levels of steroid therapy than normal subjects to inhibit immune functions. Note that a sudden drop in steroid levels may enhance immunity.

The sympathetic nervous system (SNS) is abnormal in MS, especially in patients with progressive disease. MS patients with progressive disease often have cold purple legs, reflecting decreased control of blood vessel tone. These patients have diminished R-R wave variation on an electrocardiograph (EKG) during inspiration and reduced sympathetic skin responses. This response is a sympathetic discharge after a peripheral stimulus. All these abnormalities are likely to be from a loss of sympathetic control caused by MS plaques in the spinal cord.

The SNS innervates immune organs. The loss of sympathetic tone may have consequences for the immune system in MS. When nerves are cut, the target tissue develops denervation supersensitivity to the relevant neurotransmitter. In MS, β-adrenergic receptors (β-AR) and responses to adrenergic agonists (which induce cAMP) are increased in CD8$^+$, CD28$^+$ T lymphocytes (suppressor T cells). These cells are responsible for the reduced concanavalin A-induced suppressor function seen during the exacerbations and progression of MS. Stress elevates catecholamines and could theoretically destabilize immune regulation if MS lymphocytes were overly sensitive to adrenalin.

Muscarinic receptors are increased on CD4$^+$ lymphocytes (T helper cells). Vagal output could potentially affect the development of thymic tolerance or activate T helper cells. Stress effects on the parasympathetic nervous system are not well studied.

Stress Inhibits Experimental Allergic Encephalomyelitis

Immunization with brain proteins (MBP, PLP, and MOG) causes autoimmune EAE in one animal model of MS. Some stress effects on EAE could therefore be instructive. However, the murine immune system has significant differences from the human immune system, the initial antigenic trigger in MS is unknown, and some drugs have completely opposite effects in EAE and MS. For these reasons, the effects of stress in EAE may not always correspond to the effects in MS.

Glucocorticoids suppress EAE. Merely picking up a rat ameliorates EAE. Handling stress triggers a surge of corticosterone, the rat homolog of human cortisol. Restraint stress also suppresses acute EAE, but it does not affect established EAE. In parallel with these

endogenous steroid effects, treatment with dexamethasone markedly inhibits all stages of EAE. Extending these data to humans suggests that stress should inhibit MS. Anecdotal reports that MS improves after skydiving fit into this line of thought, but remain anecdotes.

When stress is stopped, there is a rebound of severe inflammation in EAE. Similarly, if the dexamethasone used to suppress EAE is suddenly withdrawn, rats develop very severe disease within 5 days. This rebound worsening is seen following a 3-day pulse of dexamethasone even in rats that have recovered from EAE. A pulse of high-dose steroids is a standard treatment for MS exacerbation, yet clinical rebound is seldom seen in MS. Again, EAE differs from MS.

Catecholamines also inhibit EAE through β$_2$-adrenergic receptors on lymphocytes. Terbutaline, a β$_2$-adrenergic agonist; misoprostal, a prostaglandin E analog; and pentoxifylline, a phosphodiesterase III inhibitor, all elevate cAMP. These agents increase levels of cAMP in lymphocytes, inhibit Thl responses, and reduce EAE severity.

Could Stress Affect Immune Function?

Stress appears to inhibit the immune system. After intense studying for final exams, medical students are more likely to develop upper respiratory tract infections. Similarly, bereavement (loss of a loved one), divorce, caring for a spouse with Alzheimer's disease, and surgery for breast cancer are associated with excess infections and decreased *in vitro* immune function.

Acute stress and chronic stress both affect immunity. Acute stress causes a rise in serum catecholamines and cortisol; these suppress immune function and also affect immune cell distribution and trafficking. Chronic stress enforces the hypothalamic AVP response to stress, but reduces steroid responses, and so may increase cellular immunity. Products of this stress response affect immunity. Agents that elevate cAMP in lymphocytes inhibit EAE. When used to treat MS exacerbations, glucocorticoids speed up recovery from exacerbations but have no long-term benefit. Steroids cause apoptosis of T cells that are in contact with astrocytes in inflammatory sites. This argues that stress should prevent MS exacerbations. However, although terbutaline does decrease fatigue, treatment of MS patients with cAMP elevators has no significant effect on disease activity.

Two factors could boost immune function after stress. A rebound in immune function is possible after stress is withdrawn. Second, virus infections appear to trigger MS exacerbations. One of three upper respiratory tract infections is followed by an

MS flare, possibly because viruses induce IFN-γ and other inflammatory cytokines. It therefore seems logical to invoke a chain of events that ultimately cause attacks of MS – stress, immunosuppression, virus infection, and then an exacerbation of MS.

Do Neurosurgical Lesions or Physical Trauma Incite Multiple Sclerosis Plaques?

Theoretically, direct trauma to brain tissue damages the BBB and could be a nidus for an MS plaque. Stress, frequently associated with surgery or injury could also potentially affect inflammation at the site of trauma. What is the evidence?

One to 2 days after direct trauma to a rat brain or spinal cord, mononuclear cells invade the damaged area. Seven days after injury, lymphocytes isolated from lymph nodes induce adoptive-transfer EAE. At later times, lymph node cells are not encephalitogenic, indicating that endogenous suppressor mechanisms prevent further immune reactivity to the brain. Thus, there is a critical period following trauma when immune cells are predisposed to attack the brain. A critical period is more difficult to define in MS, but some studies have looked at exacerbations during the period following trauma.

EAE is prone to develop at an electrolytic lesion – damage to the BBB, heat (releasing heat shock proteins), hemorrhage (including white blood cells), and inflammation are potential mechanisms. Moreover, trauma can induce diffuse changes in the brain. At 4–7 days after trauma, the BBB becomes leaky in the gray matter contralateral to the insult.

Early reports suggested that trauma caused the onset of MS. Contrary to a few case reports, anesthesia or spinal taps do not trigger attacks of MS. Most experts now believe that there is no convincing connection between trauma and exacerbations of MS. There remains some debate, although it mainly takes place in courtrooms.

MS plaques are twice as frequent in the cervical spinal cord as other cord sites. It has been argued that flexion and extension of the neck stretch the cord and predispose to MS lesions. Some also suggest that the effect would be more pronounced at the level of a herniated disk. All of these arguments are irrelevant in the thoracic area, which is only slightly mobile compared to the cervical cord and is infrequently the site of herniated disks. The thoracic cord is a relatively frequent site of MS lesions, but is thinner than the cervical cord so the number of plaques per gram of tissue is not so different. A related condition, transverse myelitis, is actually more common in the thoracic area. Because two diseases can have additive effects, the removal of a symptomatic disk in an MS patient can decrease some neurological symptoms.

Direct trauma to the CNS under controlled conditions was studied in MS patients with severe tremors. In the 1970s, several patients treated with thalamic ablation developed MS plaques along the needle track. Other patients, however, had similar surgery but had no lesions along the track. More recent treatment of tremor with thalamic lesions or stimulation has not been reported to cause MS plaques. The discrepancy between old and new studies may lie in the neurosurgical technique. Hot electrodes could generate heat shock proteins (B. G. W. Amason, personal communication), which cross-react with MBP. However, the older studies were anecdotal and at the time imaging was nonexistent; plaques may have been present before the needle was inserted.

The biopsy of a large, active MS plaque should be a provocateur of nearby inflammation. As with other recent neurosurgical procedures in MS patients, there are no reports of biopsies being followed by exacerbations.

Does Stress Cause Multiple Sclerosis? Actual Data from Multiple Sclerosis Patients

All the arguments described so far suggesting that stress and immunity cause MS exacerbations, are theoretical. The only way to resolve these speculations is through controlled studies of the effect of stress on the course of MS.

There is a large literature on the effect of physical and psychological stress on MS. In one of the first recorded cases of MS, Augustus d'Este wrote in 1822 (Murray 2005) that decreased vision followed the funeral of "a relative for whom I had the affection of a son." Much of the early literature is anecdotal or is based on retrospective, uncontrolled studies.

MS symptoms are intermittent, have highly variable severity, and involve disparate areas of the nervous system. Moreover, even without new active inflammation, MS symptoms can be mimicked if old subclinical lesions are compromised. Elevation of body temperature, external heat or humidity, and infections (e.g., upper respiratory, urinary tract, lung, prostate) lower the safety factor for electrical impulses along a nerve and amplify the prior loss of function in plaques. There are also many patient reports of acute worsening with menses, anxiety, stress, fatigue, malaise, and depression. Thus, various forms of stress could make MS symptoms worse without changing immunity or immune function.

These pseudoexacerbations are likely to confound the clinical exam and history of true MS exacerbations. MS symptoms are also quite subject to selective memory in the patient's search for the cause of the exacerbation. The best way to examine any connection between stress and MS is with controlled prospective studies by investigators with extensive MS experience. Only a few have been performed.

For example, in controlled prospective studies Sibley and Siva showed that emotional stress is not linked to MS exacerbations. They also found no convincing link between physical trauma and MS exacerbations. Buljevac and Ackerman reported a link, but recall bias may have contributed to this result. Severe stress, such as gunshot wounds and SCUD missile attacks, actually seemed to reduce exacerbations.

Medical-Legal Implications

Stress or trauma often coincides with MS exacerbations. Trauma to the brain can cause CNS dysfunction, and it is often difficult to sort out whether trauma or MS is responsible for a given symptom. Moreover, stress or trauma could amplify the effects of prior MS lesions. Confounding factors such as elevated temperature, infections, and fatigue could also intensify MS symptoms.

Some argue that in some patients, at some times, stress could modify immunity and possibly trigger attacks of MS. However. this position is highly speculative and probably wrong in a disease with very complex clinical symptoms. There is no clear evidence that stress or trauma causes the onset of MS or that stress or trauma triggers attacks of MS.

See Also the Following Articles

Brain Trauma; Central Stress Neurocircuits; Immune Suppression.

Further Reading

Ackerman, K. D., Heyman, R., Rabin, B. S., et al. (2002). Stressful life events precede exacerbations of multiple sclerosis. *Psychosomatic Medicine* **64**, 916–920.

Andersen, B. L., Farrar, W. B. and Golden-Kreutz, D. (1998). Stress and immune responses after surgical treatment for regional breast cancer. *Journal of the National Cancer Institute* **90**, 30–36.

Anlar, B., Karaszewski, J. W., Reder, A. T., et al. (1992). Increased muscarinic cholinergic receptor density on CD4$^+$ lymphocytes in progressive multiple sclerosis. *Journal of Neuroimmunology* **36**, 171–177.

Arnason, B. G. W. and Reder, A. T. (1994). Interferons and multiple sclerosis. *Neuropharmacology* **17**, 495–547.

Buljevac, D., Hop, W. C. J., Reedeker, W., et al. (2003). Self reported stressful life events and exacerbations in multiple sclerosis: prospective study. *British Medical Journal* **327**, 646–651.

Burgerman, R., Rigamonti, D., Ranelle, J. M., et al. (1992). The association of cervical spondylosis and multiple sclerosis. *Surgical Neurology* **38**, 265–270.

Karaszewski, J. W., Reder, A. T., Anlar, B., et al. (1993). Increased high affinity beta-adrenergic receptor densities and cyclic AMP responses of CD8 cells in multiple sclerosis. *Journal of Neuroimmunology* **43**, 1–7.

Levine, S., Strebel, R., Wenk, E. J., et al. (1962). Suppression of experimental allergic encephalomyelitis by stress. *Proceedings of the Society for Experimental Biology and Medicine* **109**, 294–298.

Michelson, D. and Gold, P. W. (1998). Pathophysiologic and somatic investigations of hypothalamic-pituitary-adrenal axis activation in patients with depression. *Annals of the New York Academy of Sciences* **840**, 717–722.

Murray, T. J. (2005). *Multiple sclerosis: The history of a disease*. New York: Demo.

Popovich, P. G., Stokes, B. T. and Whitacre, C. C. (1996). Concept of autoimmunity following spinal card injury: possible roles for T lymphocytes in the traumatized central nervous system. *Journal of Neuroscience Research* **45**, 349–363.

Poser, C. M. (1994). The role of trauma in the pathogenesis of multiple sclerosis: a review. *Clinical Neurology and Neurosurgery* **96**, 103–110.

Reder, A. T. and Arnason, B. G. W. (1985). Immunology of multiple sclerosis. In: Vinken, P. J., Bruyn, G. W., Kiawans, H. L. & Koetsler, J. C. (eds.) *Handbook of clinical neurology: demyelinating diseases*, pp. 337–395. Amsterdam: Elsevier Science Publishers.

Reder, A. T., Thapar, M. and Jensen, M. (1994). A fall in serum glucocorticoids provokes experimental allergic encephalomyelitis: implications for treatment of inflammatory brain disease. *Neurology* **44**, 2289–2294.

Sibley, W. A., Bramford, C. R., Clark, K., et al. (1991). A prospective study of physical trauma and multiple sclerosis. *Journal of Neurology, Neurosurgery & Psychiatry* **54**, 584–589.

Siva, A., Radhakrishnan, K., Kurland, L. T., et al. (1993). Trauma and multiple sclerosis: a population-based cohort study from Olmsted County, Minnesota. *Neurology* **43**, 1878–1882.

Multiple Trauma

P N Soucacos
University of Athens School of Medicine, Athens, Greece
E O Johnson
University of Ioannina School of Medicine, Ioannina, Greece

Multiple Trauma: Background
Physiological Responses to Trauma
The Neuroendocrine Stress Response to Trauma
Time-Dependent Changes in the Stress Response
Immune System Response to Trauma
Posttraumatic Psychological Complications

Glossary

Hemorrhagic shock	Significant acute blood loss leading to hypovolemia and hypotension.
Open fracture	A compound fracture with an open wound down to the bone; usually associated with severe vascular impairment.
Posttraumatic stress disorder (PTSD)	The development of characteristic symptoms after a traumatic event, including numbed responsiveness to stimuli, autonomic and cognitive dysfunction, and dysphoria.

Multiple Trauma: Background

In most Western societies, traumatic injuries represent the third leading cause of death after cardiovascular diseases and tumors. Of the accidents that occur, approximately 60% take place at home or during sport activities, 27% take place at work, 9% are related to traffic accidents, and approximately 4% are the result of violent actions. However, of the polytraumatic injuries, over 70% are attributed to traffic accidents, followed by accidents at home (20%) and work (10%). More than one-half of the patients with multiple trauma have fractures, dislocations, or both.

In the polytrauma patient, the management of orthopedic injuries can have profound effect on the patient's ultimate functional recovery and may be life- or limb-saving. Life- and limb-threatening musculoskeletal problems include hemorrhage from wounds and fractures, infections from open fractures, limb loss from vascular damage and compartment syndrome, and loss of function from spinal or peripheral neurological injuries. The frequency of pulmonary complications, adult respiratory distress syndrome (ARDS), fat emboli, and pneumonia has been correlated to the timing and type of treatment of long bone fractures, with a statistically significant increase in morbidity, pulmonary complications, and length of hospitalization when stabilization of a major fracture was delayed. Consequently, since the early 1990s, emphasis has been on early total care of multiply injured patients, including fracture stabilization.

Multiple trauma injuries are frequently complicated with open fractures. Open fractures types IIIB and IIIC are extremely severe injuries that often may lead to limb amputation. These fractures are usually caused by a high-energy impact that results in extensive bony comminution or segmental bone loss, pronounced soft tissue injury including extensive skin loss, tendon and nerve damage, muscular and periosteal stripping from the bone (type IIIB), and severe circulatory compromise of the extremity related to the complete ischemia produced secondary to trauma of the major vessels (type IIIC).

The incidence of amputation rate of type IIIC fractures ranges from 60 to 100%. The aim today is not just to salvage the limb that has sustained this compound injury but to produce a functional painless extremity with at least protective sensation. Several variables play a decisive role in determining the outcome and success of preserving a limb. These include the extent and severity of vascular injury, the bone and soft tissue damage, the type and duration of limb ischemia, the patient's age, the time elapsed from the initial injury to surgery, and concomitant organ injuries. To determine which limbs can be salvaged and which should be amputated primarily, numerous scales using a variety of criteria have been proposed assessing the severity of injury. They include the mangled extremity syndrome, the mangled extremity severity score, and NISSSA (N = nerve, I = ischemia, S = soft tissue injury, S = skeletal injury, S = shock, and A = age of patient).

Patients with multiple injuries pose a significant challenge. Optimal management is essential early on after trauma to avoid long-term complications, sepsis, organ failure, and subsequent increased late mortality. The principles of management now include simultaneous assessment and resuscitation, with complete physical examination and diagnostic studies as appropriate to establish priorities for life-saving surgery. Trauma management can be divided into four periods (**Table 1**). The primary goal during the acute

Table 1 Periods of trauma management

	Time after trauma
Acute or resuscitation period	1–3 h
Primary or stabilization period	1–72 h
Secondary or regeneration period	3–8 days
Tertiary or rehabilitation period	after 8 days

Table 2 Primary and secondary physiological insults

Primary insults	Secondary insults
Hypoxia	Ischemia
Hypotension	Reperfusion injury
Organ and soft tissue injury	Compartment syndrome
Fractures	Operative interventions infections

Table 3 Acute and prolonged responses to traumatic stress

Acute responses	Prolonged responses
Activation of blood-clotting mechanisms	Immunological alterations: mobilization of leukocytes, increased T cells and macrophages, increased acute-phase plasma proteins
Shift of body fluids from extravascular compartment to restore blood volume	
Blood flow redistributed to ensure perfusion of vital organs	Inflammatory cells invade injured area
Respiratory and renal functions compensate acid–base balance	Increased fibroblasts for collagen scaffolds for wound repair

or resuscitation period is to establish adequate ventilation, maintain circulation (intravascular volume and cardiac function), and assess neurological state. The primary or stabilization period of treatment starts when all vital functions have been stabilized by achieving adequate ventilation, hemodynamic stability, and control of intracranial or internal hemorrhage. During this stage, priorities for surgical treatment after resuscitation are given to brain injuries, eye and facial injuries, progressive compression of the spinal cord, visceral injuries, open fractures, fractures with concomitant injuries to major vessels, pelvic ring fractures, and unstable spine fractures. The secondary period is a phase of regeneration. Reconstructive treatments during this phase include secondary wound closure and soft-tissue reconstruction, osteosynthesis of upper extremity fractures, and complex joint reconstruction. After eight days, in the tertiary period, the prognosis of the polytrauma patient is usually apparent. If recovery continues, final reconstructive operations can be performed, including bone grafting at sites of massive bony defects, special soft-tissue reconstructions, definitive closure of amputation sites, and any remaining procedures that were postponed. In cases with organ dysfunction or respiratory distress (e.g., ARDS), further surgical procedures cannot be considered.

Physiological Responses to Trauma

Early death following multiple traumatic injuries is usually attributed to primary brain injury or significant blood loss (hemorrhagic shock), whereas late traumatic death is usually the result of secondary brain injury and host defense failure. The host defense response system is triggered by a series of insults that occur primarily or secondarily (**Table 2**). The host defense response is characterized by the local and systemic release of various factors (hormonal mediators, pro-inflammatory cytokines, acute phase proteins, etc.) that make up the systemic inflammatory response.

Adjustments in homeostatic mechanisms occur following trauma in an effort to maintain homeostasis and ensure wound healing. Multiple factors, including diminished blood volume, tissue underperfusion, extensive tissue damage, and invasive infections initiate the stress-response cascade via the neuroendocrine system. As a result of these initial physiological adjustments, tissue perfusion is maintained, and vital organ function and wound repair are supported.

Major traumatic injury is associated with rapid blood loss, tissue underperfusion, massive cellular damage, and disturbances to vital organ function. Response to the traumatic stress include local changes at the injury site and system changes that occur either acutely or gradually with have a prolonged responses (**Table 3**).

The events that take place following trauma are generally graded – the more severe the injury, the greater the response. In addition, the responses to trauma change over time and can be divided into acute-phase and chronic-phase changes. The acute-phase changes occur immediately after injury and are characterized by a fall in metabolic functions and a decrease in core temperature and by increased levels of stress response hormones. Many of the changes observed acutely are related to hypovolemia. With the restoration of blood flow and with time, the patient's responses change. In the chronic phase, the metabolic rate rises, body temperature increases, and blood insulin levels reach normal or can be increased (**Table 4**). The chronic phase following injury is characterized by a hypermetabolic state. The degree of hypermetabolism (increased oxygen production) is generally related to the severity of the injury. Patients

Table 4 Time course in responses to multiple trauma

	Acute phase	Chronic phase
Blood glucose	Elevated	Normal or slightly elevated
Glucose production	Normal	Increased
Free fatty acids	Elevated	Normal
Insulin levels	Low	Normal or elevated
Catecholamines	Elevated	High to normal
Blood lactate	Elevated	Normal
Oxygen consumption	Low	Elevated
Cardiac output	Low	Increased
Core temperature	Low	Elevated

with long-bone fractures exhibit a 15–25% increase in metabolic rate, whereas those with multiple injuries increase metabolic needs by 50%. Patients with severe burn injures covering over 50% of their body may demonstrate a resting metabolic rate that is twice basal levels.

Multiple trauma injury is a clinical condition that results in a marked activation of neuroendocrine stress response aimed at restoring hemodynamic and metabolic hemeostasis. The stress response is activated by diverse physical conditions (e.g., ischemia and glucopenia) and is primarily mediated by the hypothalamic-pituitary-adrenal (HPA) axis and sympathetic systems. The activation of the stress response system appears to be critical for survival from injury.

The Neuroendocrine Stress Response to Trauma

Traumatic injury poses a significant psychological and physiological threat, and it provokes an immediate neuroendocrine response. Neural input from the cerebral cortex, injured tissues, and receptors detecting fluid loss results in increased adrenocorticoptropic hormone (ACTH), growth hormone (GH), prolactin, and arginine vasopressin (AVP) release from the pituitary and in a general activation of the sympathetic nervous system with increases in epinephrine and norepinephrine concentrations. Secondary changes include the stimulation of cortisol and aldosterone. The duration of these responses generally depend on the severity of the injury and varies among hormones. The autonomic nervous system provides a rapidly responding mechanism to control a wide range of functions, including cardiovascular, respiratory, gastrointestinal, renal, endocrine, and other systems.

The stress system consists of three central and two peripheral components. The central components of the stress system comprise the locus ceruleus in the

reticular formation, which regulates arousal; the brain-stem centers of the autonomic system, which regulates sympathetic/adrenomedullary function; and the hypothalamic paraventricular nucleus (PVN), which regulates adrenocortical function. The peripheral components consist of the sympathetic/adrenomedullary system and the pituitary-adrenal axis. The interactions among the various components of the stress system are numerous and complex. Corticotropin releasing hormone (CRH)-secreting neurons of the lateral paraventricular nucleus project toward the arousal and sympathetic system in the hindbrain, and conversely, catecholaminergic fibers from the locus ceruleus and central sympathetic system project via the ascending noradrenergic bundle to the PVN in the hypothalamus. The activation of the CRH neurons in the PVN results in the release of CRH into the hypophysial portal system and the stimulation of the arousal and sympathetic centers in the brain stem in a positive reverberating feedback loop.

Both endorphins and ACTH secreted by the proopiomelanocortin (POMC) neurons of the arcuate nucleus exert inhibitory effects on CRH secretion. As POMC neurons are stimulated by CRH, they provide another negative feedback control loop on the HPA axis. ACTH stimulates the release of cortisol from the adrenal cortex, the later which feeds back in a negative fashion, both at the level of the pituitary and of the hypothalamus, forming the long feedback loops. The activation of the stress system has direct consequences on the function of other major systems, particularly those responsible for reproduction, growth, and immunity.

Today, the role of AVP in the control of ACTH secretion and its involvement in various stress response paradigms is generally accepted. AVP is released from two sites in the hypothalamus; the parvicellular division of the PVN, where CRH is also formed, and from the magnocellular neurons of the supraoptic nucleus (SON) and the PVN. Recent evidence supports an intricate interaction of AVP with CRH and with glucocorticoids, the inhibitory feedback component of the HPA axis.

It is clear that AVP plays an important role in the stress response. Chronic stress paradigms have shown with relative consistency a shift in the CRH: AVP ratio that may relate to a differing feedback sensitivity of AVP to glucocorticoid feedback restraint or a greater responsivity of AVP, over CRH, to chronic stimulatory stress input. AVP serum concentrations significantly increase in the critically ill patient population. However, the lack of a correlation between AVP concentrations and hemodynamic parameters suggests a complex dysfunction of the vasopressinergic system in critical illness.

Extremely low corticosteroid-binding globulin (CBG) levels in early-stage multitrauma is reflected in a concomitant higher free cortisol index, indicative of higher free cortisol levels. This suggests that CBG plays an active role in the glucocorticoid response to severe stress and the regulation of cortisol availability to target tissues.

Time-Dependent Changes in the Stress Response

It appears that the hypothalamus and anterior pituitary function may be altered differently in the first few hours or days (acute phase) compared to 7–10 days (chronic phase) after disabling multiple traumatic injuries. During the first few hours or days after multiple traumatic insult, circulating GH levels become elevated and the normal GH profile is altered (peak GH levels and interpulse concentrations are high, and the GH pulse frequency is elevated). After a prolonged period, the changes observed with the somatropic axis change; GH secretion pattern becomes random or chaotic, with a considerable reduction in pulses.

Within a couple of hours after trauma, serum $3,5,3'$ triiodothyronine (T_3) levels decrease, whereas thyroxine (T_4) and thyroid-stimulating hormone (TSH) levels rise briefly. Later, in the chronic phase, TSH levels are low to normal, and T_3 and T_4 concentrations are low. Prolactin levels show a pronounced increased following trauma. In the chronic phase, on the other hand, prolactin secretion is blunted. It has been suggested that this may play a role in the anergic immune dysfunction and in the increased susceptibility to infection observed at this time.

The stress-induced hypercortisolism triggered by trauma is associated with elevated ACTH release, which, in turn, is augmented by CRH, cytokines, and the noradrenergic system. Circulating aldosterone also rises markedly, and this may be attributed, at least in part, to the activated renin–angiotensin system. Hypercortisolism acutely shifts carbohydrate, fat, and protein metabolism, so that energy becomes available to the vital organs, such as the brain, and so that anabolism can be delayed. Intravascular fluid retention and enhanced AVP response provide hemodynamic advantages for the fight-or-flight stress response. Finally, the hypercorisolism induced by acute trauma may reflect an attempt by the organism to dampen its own inflammatory response. There is some evidence of a biphasic time course with the eventual dissociation of ACTH and cortisol concentrations following major trauma or surgery. Although there is some evidence of a possible role of endothelin

and/or atrial natriuretic peptide (ANP) in this dissociation of concentrations of cortisol and ACTH, the mechanism or significance of this in the regulation of HPA axis function in the critically ill or stressed is not clear.

In the chronic phase, serum ACTH levels drop and are low, whereas cortisol levels remain high. This suggests that cortisol release in this later stage may be driven by a different pathway. On the other hand, circulating levels of adrenal androgens (dehydroepiandrosterone sulfate, DHEAS), which has an immunostimulatory effect on T helper (Th-)1 cells are low during the chronic state. Some suggest that sustained hypercortisolism in the presence of low levels of DHEAS and prolactin in the chronic phase could provoke an imbalance between immunosuppressive and immunostimulatory pathways, which could increase susceptibility to infections.

Taken together, the neuroendocrine stress response differs in the acute and chronic phases following traumatic injury. Initially following trauma, the anterior pituitary actively releases hormones into the circulation, whereas anabolic target organ hormones are inactivated in the periphery. In the chronic state, the pulsatile release of anterior pituitary hormones becomes reduced, presumably because of reduced hypothalamic stimulation. The end result is diminished activity of target tissues and impaired anabolism.

Immune System Response to Trauma

The increased stress response after traumatic injury is associated with altered immune function and decreased immunity. The immune function of most patients is suppressed as a result of their traumatic injuries. Immunological changes after multiple trauma correlate with the degree of tissue damage, as well as with severity of hemorrhage and ischemia. Trauma has been found to significantly depress polymorphonuclear and monocyte functions, with both the phagocytic and bactericidal functions of these cell types being depressed. For the most part, immune changes are attributed to excessive cortisol levels.

Corticosteroids represent one of the most potent endogenous anti-inflammatory agents known. They have the capacity to inhibit and suppress virtually all critical inflammatory and immune cell functions, even at physiological concentrations and particularly during the early development of the immune/inflammatory response. At the molecular level, they inhibit the production of most inflammatory mediators, including interleukin (IL-)1, tumor necrosis factor (TNF), phospholipase A2, and prostaglandins. Hence, the stress-induced enhanced production and secretion of glucocorticoids appears to counterregulate and suppress excessive immune/inflammatory cell activation and mediator production that could otherwise result in self-induced tissue injury. This suggests a critical role for the corticosteroids in maintaining physiological homeostasis during the adaptive response to noxious stressors.

Several neurohormonal systems and immunological factors appear to play a fundamental role in these communicatory links, which enable the peripheral immunological apparatus to signal and interact with the brain and participate in maintaining immunological homeostasis. This is facilitated by an extensive coexpression of receptors and overlap of the synthesis of a multitude of hormonelike molecules that regulate cell function. In this regard, IL-1, a major product of activated macrophages, has been extensively studied. IL-1 receptors are expressed not only on peripheral T lymphocytes but also in the brain, where, in addition, it is synthesized. In addition to regulating a wide range of neural functions, including arousal, body temperature, sleep, food intake, reproductive behavior, and mood, that appear to be under direct central nervous system (CNS) control, some of the actions of IL-1 on peripheral immune function also appear to mediated by IL-1 in the CNS. However, the relation of CNS IL-1 to peripheral immune system-derived IL-1 remains to be elucidated. IL-1 is also a potent stimulator of the HPA axis, resulting in the release of corticosteroids. Corticosteroids, in turn, feed back to inhibit macrophage release of IL-1. Other examples of this intricate communication between the immune and nervous system are rapidly being characterized.

Recent evidence suggests that there are two major pathways by which the CNS can regulate the immune system. The first pathway is through neurohormonal systems, particularly the HPA, or stress, axis. Other neurohormonal systems that appear to also play important roles include the hypothalamic-pituitary-gonadal (HPG) axis, the hypothalamic-pituitary-thyroid (HPT) axis, and the hypothalamic-growth hormone axis. The second major pathway is the autonomic nervous system and the release of norepinephrine and acetylcholine. Glucocorticoids inhibit the functions of virtually all inflammatory cells via the alteration of transcription of cytokine genes (TNF, IL-1, and IL-6) and inhibition of the production of arachidonic acid-derived pro-inflammatory substances, such as leukotrienes and prostaglandins.

Conversely, the immune system modulates CNS function through various factors, particularly cytokines, which can act independently or synergistically. The CNS contains IL-1 receptors in areas that control the acute-phase response. In addition, IL-1 stimulates the production of endothelia cell prostaglandins, which in turn, induce CRH release from the median eminence. In contrast, IL-6 acts as a potent stimulator of ACTH and cortisol release. In healthy individuals, this bidirectional regulatory system forms a negative feedback loop, which keeps the CNS and immune system in balance.

The efferent sympathetic/adrenomedullary system apparently participates in an important way in the interactions of the adrenal axis and the immune/inflammatory reaction by being reciprocally connected with the CRH system, by receiving and transmitting humoral and nervous immune signals from the periphery, by innervating lymphoid organs, and by reaching all sites of inflammation via the postganglionic sympathetic nerve fibers.

Posttraumatic Psychological Complications

Multiple trauma injury poses a significant challenge to patients' perception of control over their environment. The various and multiple stressors presented not only by the traumatic episode itself but from the sequelae of events following the accident (multiple surgeries, diagnostic tests, etc.) diminish patients' perception of control, resulting in additional, although subjective, activation of the stress response.

Psychological complications are an important and persistent factor after injury and are associated with adverse effects on the daily activities of the patient. Multiple-trauma patients have been reported to suffer from loss of initiative, irritability, mood swings, feelings of guilt, among others, assessed using the State/Trait Anxiety Scale. The prevalence of posttraumatic stress disorder (PTSD) and symptoms of depression and anxiety in severely injured polytrauma patients is not clear. It appears, however, that the incidence of PTSD is low following multiple traumatic injuries in victims who were healthy before experiencing the trauma. Nonetheless, a substantial proportion of severely injured accident victims develop some form of psychiatric morbidity.

During the first few hours and days following a serious multitraumatic injury, most patients have at least short periods of anxiety with dissociative symptoms, such as derealization, occurring for a short duration in approximately 15% of the patients. Over the following weeks and months, the rates of PTSD reported range from 8 to 39%. A few long-term follow-up studies (28 months) report psychiatric morbidity, mostly depressive disorders, in approximately 22% of trauma victims and PTSD in 8% after 5 years.

Further Reading

Barton, R. N. (1987). The neuroendocrinology of physical injury. *Baillières Clinical Endocrinology and Metabolism* 1(2), 355–374.

Johnson, E. O., Kamilaris, T. C., Chrousos, G. P., et al. (1992). Mechanisms of stress: a dynamic overview of hormonal and behavioral homeostasis. *Neuroscience and Biobehavioral Reviews* 16, 115–130.

Keel, M. and Trentz, O. (2005). Pathophysiology of polytrauma. *Injury* 236(6), 691–705.

Smith, E. M. and Blalock, J. E. (1989). A molecular basis for interaction between the immune and neuroendocrine systems. *International Journal of Neuroscience* 38, 455–465.

Soucacos, P. N., Beris, A. E., Xenakis, T. A., et al. (1995). Open type IIIB and IIIC fractures treated by an orthopaedic microsurgical team. *Clinical Orthopaedics* 314, 59–66.

Van den Berghe, G. (2000). Novel insights into the neuroendocrinology of critical illness. *European Journal of Endocrinology* 143, 1–13.

Willmore, D. W. (1991). Homeostasis: bodily changes in trauma and surgery. In: Sabiston, D. C. (ed.) *Textbook of surgery.* Philadelphia: W. B. Saunders.

Muscular Dystrophy   *See:* Myopathy.

Musculoskeletal Problems and Stress

S Svebak
Norwegian University of Science and Technology, Trondheim, Norway

This article is a revision of the previous edition article by S Svebak, volume 2, pp 796–802, © 2000, Elsevier Inc.

Epidemiology of Musculoskeletal Pain

Muscle Fiber Contraction, Hardness, and Pain

Sperry's Principle: Brain Control of Muscle Tension

Motivation, Emotion, Muscle Tension, and Performance

Personality and Sensitivity to Emotional versus Ergonomic Loads

Central Nervous System Mechanisms of Pain Sensitivity

Coping with Musculoskeletal Problems: Prevention and Rehabilitation

Glossary

Brain neuro- transmitters	Biochemical substances that modulate the efficacy of nerve-impulse transmission in the brain.
Emotional load	The psychosocial causes of unpleasant and enduring emotions induced by the perceived or extrinsic nature of workload, inducing psychobiological changes that can cause bodily complaints and illness.
Ergonomic load	The physical causes of biomechanical strain induced by frequent or enduring postural work demands.
Fear avoidance	Passivity due to fear of the pain expected from movements.
Myalgia	Pain from the skeletal muscles.
Myofascial pain	Pain from the fasciae that cover the skeletal muscles.
Striate muscles	Skeletal muscles named after their microscopically observable striated pattern of muscle fiber arrangements. These fibers are of two major kinds: one is designed for aerobic metabolism and the other for anaerobic metabolism (in which oxygen is not involved). Individuals differ in their proportion of fiber types, mainly due to genetic disposition.
Tendonitis	Pain from the tendons of the skeletal muscles.

Skeletal muscles represent the only case in which the brain can exert some degree of volitional control over the activity level of an organ. Despite this fact, much pain, stiffness, and discomfort are presented to the health-care system as originating in the skeletal muscles. It is perceived by the patient as beyond control.

Epidemiology of Musculoskeletal Pain

Most musculoskeletal problems present as nonspecific pain, that is, pain that has no obvious and verifiable cause. Often it is due to a complex constellation of ergonomic, physiological, motivational, and emotional load factors that act on biological mechanisms involved in pain perception. Not all pain is attributable to a particular body area. A major diagnostic criterion in fibromyalgia is the presence of widespread pain. However, the most prevalent types of muscle pain involve the neck, shoulders, and lower back; the extremities may also be involved (mostly the gastrocnemius muscle of the legs and the flexor muscles of the forearms).

A major proportion of muscle pain is due to myalgia, myofascial pain, and pain from the tendons of muscles, referred to as tendonitis. In the lower back, the muscles involved are the musculus (m.) erector spinae, m. iliocostalis lumborum, and m. glutaeus medius. In the neck and shoulders, the m. trapezius, m. deltoideus, and muscles covered by these superficial muscles are also prevalent sources of pain.

Muscle pain is not always taken to the health-care system. In most cases, the pain and related discomfort is mild and involves transient disability or the pain is treated by the consumption of over-the-counter analgesics. It has been estimated that, on average, 30–40% of musculoskeletal pain relates to work and that severe episodes of low back pain may occur in less than 5% of the population. However, the 1-year prevalence of musculoskeletal pain may be as high as 50% among adults in Western societies. In a recent study involving 70% of a county population ages 20 and above ($N = 64,690$), the 1-year prevalence, including less severe episodes of muscle pain, was as high as 50.1% in females and 42.6% in males. Continuous pain and discomfort for at least 3 months were most prevalent in the neck, shoulders, and lower back (females: neck = 19.4%, shoulders = 21.1%, lower back = 17.4%; males: neck = 14.5%, shoulders = 16.8%, lower back = 14.2%). In preadolescents, persistent pain may be as prevalent as 15%, with pain in the neck and lower extremities accounting for a major proportion of this pain, particularly among the girls.

There was a shift toward multidisciplinary paradigms in musculoskeletal pain research after 1985 with the increasing acknowledgment of psychological and psychosocial factors. On the behavioral side, more children and adults are physically inactive in everyday life than ever before, although mental activity may be high in front of a visual display unit or television screen. On the other end of this skewed distribution of physical activity level is a small percentage of the adolescent and young adult population that is extremely active in competitive sports. Both lifestyles increase the risk of musculoskeletal pain but for different reasons. Inactivity causes the atrophy of skeletal muscle and poor circulation, resulting in poor workload tolerance; sport injuries cause pain due to physical overload, mishaps, and accidents.

Muscle Fiber Contraction, Hardness, and Pain

Human muscles are of three kinds. They are distinguished mainly by the anatomical microstructure that can be microscopically observed by histological inspection. (1) Striate (skeletal) muscles have a striated pattern, reflecting the special arrangement of muscle fibers side by side; they contract on stimulation by nerves in the pyramidal and extra-pyramidal systems. (2) Smooth muscles induce movements in internal organs, including the digestive tract and blood vessels; they lack a striated pattern and contract on stimulation by the autonomic nervous system. (3) The heart muscle has a semi-structured arrangement of fibers and is stimulated by nerves in a special section of the autonomic nervous system. A number of other factors modulate the neural stimulation of muscles, including neurotransmitters, hormones, and the acid–base balance of the body.

Muscles can also be classified according to the dimensionality of their movements. Skeletal muscles induce one-dimensional movements due to the attachment of their tendons to the skeleton across joints. In contrast, smooth muscles induce two-dimensional movements by the compression of the diameter of a tube (e.g., blood vessel); the heart muscle fiber contractions induce three-dimensional movements to reduce the globular volume and act as a pump.

Skeletal muscles harden with contraction. Activation from complete relaxation to maximum voluntary contraction (MVC) presents a substantial change in muscle hardness that is easily palpable, whereas a shift from relaxation to 5% of MVC can be accurately assessed only by the use of modern pressure technology and electromyography (EMG). In EMG, surface and implanted electrodes pick up neuroelectrical impulses generated by motor nerve activation. Research has supported a relationship between hardness and tenderness in the trapezius muscle of patients with chronic tension-type headache. This relationship is present also on days without pain and, therefore, indicates a permanent alteration of muscle hardness and tenderness that is different from that of healthy controls. Also, the mechanism is more enduring and extensive than those responsible for the perception of pain from these muscles.

Skeletal muscles are composed of a mixture of aerobic and anaerobic fibers (see **Figure 1**). There are remarkable individual differences in the ratio of aerobic (type 1) to anaerobic (type 2) fibers among individuals. These differences are genetically given. A subset of the type 2 fibers, the type 2A fibers, can perform aerobic metabolism when forced to do so, whereas the type 2 B fibers are nearly always anaerobic. Oxygen is needed in aerobic metabolism, and carbon dioxide is a waste product. Oxygen is not involved in anaerobic metabolism, and lactic acid is a waste product that can be used by type 1 fibers for aerobic metabolism. This is to say that the blood circulation brings oxygen to the aerobic fibers and washes out harmful carbon dioxide from the local tissue, whereas the waste product from type 2 fibers, lactic acid, can be exploited by neighboring aerobic fibers and, therefore, puts less demand on the systemic circulation. Aerobic fitness training makes aerobic fibers more efficient at aerobic metabolism, but it does not increase the number of genetically given aerobic fibers. Elite marathon runners may have 80% of aerobic fibers in their leg muscles, whereas elite sprint runners have around 80% of anaerobic fibers in their leg muscles.

The genetic differences are often forgotten when people explain why they intuitively feel they are not made for aerobic activities such as long-distance running, cross-country skiing, and other endurance activities at a moderate intensity. Conversely, they also shed light on why others display an intuitive distaste for anaerobic activities such as sprinting and downhill skiing. Most individuals have a good balance between type 1 and 2 muscle fibers and, therefore, are capable of performing aerobic as well as anaerobic work to a reasonable degree. Some individuals are strongly genetically biased toward a high tolerance for anaerobic work only, whereas others have a remarkable tolerance for aerobic work production without experiencing muscle pain.

Sperry's Principle: Brain Control of Muscle Tension

The sole product of brain function, including our thinking mechanism and the related mental functions of motivation, emotion, attention, and memory, is muscular coordination. Skeletal muscles make up most of the body mass in humans. Consequently, perceptual-motor control of the skeletal muscles presents the most extensive challenge to the brain's capacity for information processing. The perceptual component in motor control is a less extensive challenge than is the challenge of motor coordination. This perspective on the brain's control of body functions is named Sperry's principle.

The musculoskeletal system is the biological substrate for volitional behavior in the common sense. The dynamics of motor activity is also the basis for displays of expressive behavior, despite the often unintended nature of such displays, and other elements of body language including body posture. The way we sit on a chair and stand by the desk involves a much more automatic coordination of complex muscle tension patterns than is involved in the volitional movement of a finger to release a button. Walking toward a good friend involves the activation of a whole range of muscle coordination, including automated control of walking, the expression of a friendly display as well as raising a hand to say hello. The ballistic smoothness of such movements in space is taken care of by integrated input from the cerebellum.

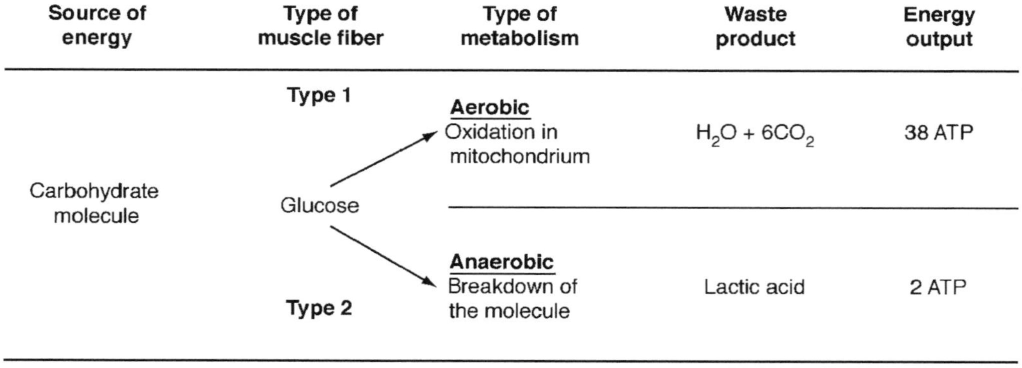

Source of energy	Type of muscle fiber	Type of metabolism	Waste product	Energy output
Carbohydrate molecule	Type 1	**Aerobic** Oxidation in mitochondrium	$H_2O + 6CO_2$	38 ATP
	Glucose			
	Type 2	**Anaerobic** Breakdown of the molecule	Lactic acid	2 ATP

Figure 1 Major differences in metabolic energy production between aerobic (type 1) and anaerobic (type 2) muscle fibers. Note that lactic acid is a waste product from type 2 fibers and can be available for subsequent aerobic metabolism in type 1 fibers. ATP, adenosine triphosphate (the work horse in muscle contractions).

The Pyramidal Pathway of Muscle Control

The most remarkable connection between the cortex of the brain and the skeletal muscles is called the pyramidal tract. Nerve fibers in this tract originate in the motor cortex and synapse with a second nerve fiber in the spinal tract to make the nerve impulse from the cortex initiate contraction in a group of skeletal muscle fibers. There is no other example of a monosynaptic connection from the cortex of the brain to a target organ in the body. This arrangement is responsible for the precise control of intended movements with minimal interference from other parts of the brain. The brilliance of this volitional control can become remarkable with practice, as professional musicians, and in elite athletes.

A motor nerve fiber from the brain to the muscle terminates by splitting up into several endings to stimulate simultaneously a group of muscle fibers in a single motor unit (SMU). All fibers in one SMU are of the same kind (type 1 or 2). The number of fibers may vary between approximately 10 and 200, with small SMUs in muscles involved in precise motor control, such as in the muscles of the fingers, and with large SMUs involved in the postural muscles of the trunk.

The Extra-Pyramidal Pathways to the Skeletal Muscles

Body posture is regulated via the extra-pyramidal pathways from the brain to the skeletal muscles. These influences originate subcortically and, therefore, are subject to automated induction of tension patterns. Several such pathways are integrated as parts of the basal ganglia between the thalamus and the cortex. One extra-pyramidal pathway originates in the reticular formation of the medulla oblongata and is a powerful modulator of skeletal muscle tension levels throughout the body. This pathway provokes muscle tension with increasing anxiety, alertness, and levels of effort to assure a stabilizing platform for intended actions as part of the attentional demands and flight-or-fight adaptive mechanisms of the hypothalamus and limbic system.

All extra-pyramidal pathways to the skeletal muscles are multisynaptic and can receive input from several other subcortical connections. This fact explains the chronic nature of many tension-related muscle problems and why they are influenced by a number of psychological processes that are beyond volitional control. It also explains the frequent need for an adjustment of lifestyle, including physical exercise habits and interpersonal competence, in the rehabilitation of musculoskeletal-pain patients, as well as why it is a time-consuming challenge to recover from musculoskeletal-pain problems.

Motivation, Emotion, Muscle Tension, and Performance

Brain activation of muscle tension is often due to task involvement, which is influenced strongly by motivational processes. Long ago, Malmo demonstrated that the intensity of motivational involvement in perceptual-motor tasks provokes increasingly higher tension levels in muscles that are not strictly involved in the demands that are extrinsically given by the nature of the task. One example is the operation of a joystick by the dominant forearm; muscle tension gradients build up in the nondominant forearm, which is never called on by the extrinsic nature of that task. He demonstrated that such generalized gradients of muscle tension tend to become more marked with increasing interest, anxiety, and effort. The quality of the performance may also improve with the increasing gradients of tension.

Quality versus Intensity of Motivational States

Apter and Svebak reviewed a series of EMG experiments on muscle tension patterns provoked by the performance of a perceptual-motor task in a playful versus serious-minded motivational state. They concluded from these experiments that playful task involvement with high effort provokes a pattern biased toward high pyramidal activation of muscles called on by the extrinsic nature of the task and low extra-pyramidal tension gradients in background muscles. Serious-minded task involvement consistently provoked gradients of high tension buildup in the seemingly passive muscles of the nondominant forearm, the legs, and the neck when the dominant forearm was actively performing a perceptual-motor task. These states of motivational involvement can be manipulated with some success by the use of extrinsic incentives such as the promise of a monetary bonus for a good performance or the threat of aversive electric shock for a poor performance. Incentives improve performance, whereas the qualitative distinction between serious-mindedness and playfulness has been reflected less clearly in the quality of perceptual-motor performance.

Playfulness and serious-mindedness are facets of personality. Some individuals are dominated more of the time by one of these motivational states, whereas others reside in the opposite state. When extrinsic incentives are not manipulated, motivational dominance explains why some people present with enduring and seemingly unprovoked muscle tension patterns that are not present in others performing the same type of perceptual-motor task. When extrinsic incentives are manipulated, they may interact with aspects of personality, which explains some of the, often paradoxical, differences of workload tolerance across individuals. The incentive that is perceived as a threat by one person may be welcomed as an exciting challenge by another.

Personality and Sensitivity to Emotional versus Ergonomic Loads

Patients with chronic low back pain (i.e., daily pain for more than 3 months) have elevated scores on somatization disorder without meeting the *Diagnostic and Statistical Manual of Mental Disorders*, 4th edition (DSM-IV) criteria for this diagnosis. Some of these pain patients also tend to report the incidence of lifetime major depression as well as alcohol dependence. Other personality factors can increase the risk of back pain when challenged by the nature of the workload. One example is a high emotional load. Hospital staff members in some wards are exposed to high emotional loads when working with chronically ill children and their parents or when employed as a midwife, situations in which a life-threatening crisis can present without much warning. Employees who score high on neuroticism, with a tendency to overrespond with anxiety, worry, and other dysphoric moods when faced with emotional stressors, are at increased risk of suffering from pain in the neck and shoulders. In contrast, staff members in wards with a predominantly high ergonomic load are at increased risk of low back pain. This risk is mediated, provided they score high on personality traits reflected in habitual impatience and the willingness to respond on impulse with a high motor effort when coping with such a load.

Personality can increase the risk of musculoskeletal pain in ways that distinguish ergonomic from emotional load factors. They can also add to local tissue damage and cause muscle pain as a result of nested vicious circles of algogenic processes (see **Figure 2**). With ergonomic load, the brain activates muscles predominantly via the pyramidal pathways to induce intentional movements. The speed and force components can induce muscle and tendon ruptures as well as pain from a high spinal load on disks, which respond with hernias that may irritate local nerves and give rise to irradiating pain. An increased risk of such ruptures occurs when high force is provoked by an impulsive brain discharge into the striate muscles with a composition of fibers designed for low enduring loads (type 1 fibers). Ruptures of tendons can be provoked, and pain from inflammatory processes may be provoked as secondary consequences of these ruptures also involving the fasciae of muscles.

With emotional load, the extra-pyramidal pathways from the brain to the muscles become more

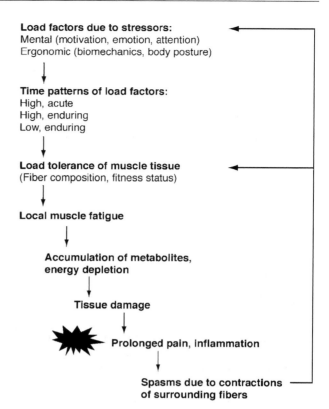

Figure 2 Relationship among factors in musculoskeletal load, their time and intensity parameters and their tissue tolerance. Arrows indicate hypothesized patterns of nested vicious circles in musculoskeletal pain.

activated and induce enduring tension in muscles not strictly called on by the extrinsic nature of motor tasks. These activation patterns are likely to have side-effects on blood circulation through the muscles, resulting in local ischemia. The brain activation pattern may also be in conflict with the local tolerance for enduring a low workload due to a bias toward anaerobic type 2 muscle fibers, which are quickly exhausted. The resulting tissue damage provokes inflammation that gives rise to pain.

Central Nervous System Mechanisms of Pain Sensitivity

Several brain processes can significantly influence pain sensitivity. The perception of pain is always subjective. Pain can be perceived with no biologically definable cause. In contrast, large tissue damage may not always give rise to the perception of severe pain. Also, pain thresholds tend to fluctuate throughout the day and over weeks. One reason for these poor relationships between the degree of tissue damage and pain perception is purely due to a shift in the focus of attention. Pain is mediated in unemployment where body awareness can be facilitated in the lack of extrinsic attentional demands. Hypnotic and meditative techniques guide a shift in the focus of attention away from pain and may also induce relaxation.

Brain Neurotransmitters

Several neural pathways and chemical neurotransmitters of the brain modulate sensitivity to pain. Until recently, most brain research on pain sensitivity concentrated on the thalamus; now it has become evident that many areas of the brain modulate pain perception. The spinothalamic tract is the most predominant nociceptive pathway for this cortical input, but the spinoreticular pathway is also acknowledged to be important, and they both terminate in the somatosensory cortex where there are small receptive areas that explain the perception of pain in discrete areas of the body but not the diffuse nature of most clinical pain. A third pathway is the spinomesencephalic pathway that terminates in the periaqueductal gray matter of the midbrain, an area rich in opioid receptors. All these pathways modulate pain perception.

The main neurotransmitters in the cortex are glutamate (pyramidal cells that are excitatory) and γ-aminobutyric acid (GABA; nonpyramidal cells that are inhibitory). Anxiolytic medication acts on GABA to facilitate neuroelectric inhibition. The cortical degeneration of glutamate receptors is a monotonous process from birth to the onset of puberty. Early onset means there will be a higher density of glutamate receptors than late onset. Subcortical serotonergic neurons inhibit pain perception. Serotonergic hyposecretion tends to provoke dysphoric moods such as irritability and depression. Endorphins act like morphine and moderate pain sensitivity (via the opioid receptors). Their secretion is believed to increase with good moods and to decrease with bad moods. However, personality factors may play a more important role than moods in the psychological regulation of the endorphins, and personality as well as mood states may influence other pain-modulating transmitters more than they influence endorphin secretion. Enkephalins are also endogenous opioids and decrease pain sensitivity.

In 1992, the endogenous cannabinoid (cannabis-like molecules) brain system was discovered and, since then, has attracted much research due to its ubiquitous receptor in the brain. These molecules bind to the CB_1 receptor that is densely distributed in areas related to motor control, emotional control, cognition and motivated behavior. These new insights may provide cannabinoid receptor antagonists and improve clinical approaches to a diversity of problems including pain, obesity, anxiety and drug addiction.

Spinal and Peripheral Mechanisms

The gate control theory of pain sensitivity was proposed by Melzack and Wall in 1965 to include free nerve endings in the deeper layers of the skin. These nerve endings respond to touch by inhibiting the spinal transmission of pain signals from the body to the brain. The pleasant component of being touched can also induce a shift in mental state that, subsequently, induces increased pain thresholds via changes in pain neurotransmitters of the brain. A therapeutic circle of events is indicated by the fact that the spinal pain-transmission peptide, substance P, is regulated via the secretion of serotonin in the brain. All mental influences that raise the secretion of brain serotonin also increase the concentration of substance P in the brain, which, again, increases spinal serotonin, which, in turn, reduces spinal substance P and therefore reduces pain sensitivity.

Coping with Musculoskeletal Problems: Prevention and Rehabilitation

There is probably no better way to prevent nonmalignant musculoskeletal pain and discomfort than to develop sensory-motor competence from early childhood and to maintain this competence throughout life. And yet there is no guarantee. A healthy ego development is based on the acquisition of sensory-motor skills. Through play, work, and sports, experience gradually builds to provide a solid basis for the individual to define those motor activities that are intrinsically felt to be right. There is no better way to find out what one's own skeletal muscles are good at and where their tolerance limits are. It is more important to health for an individual to maintain a level of physical fitness that is felt to be intrinsically rewarding than to meet some socially mandated standard prescription such as jogging three times a week for at least 20 min. Not all individuals are genetically equipped with skeletal muscles made for aerobic exercise, but all are made to be active.

Work-related musculoskeletal pain and discomfort often reflect a mixture of biomechanical (postural), physical (climatic factors and lightening noise), and psychosocial (mental demands and psychosocial relationships) exposures. An extensive review of ergonomic intervention studies by Westgaard and Winkel concluded that successful outcomes are due to (1) organizational culture interventions with high commitment of the stakeholders, (2) the use of multiple interventions to reduce identified risk factors, and (3) the modification of risk factors for the individual workers at risk, using measures that ensure the active involvement and support of the worker.

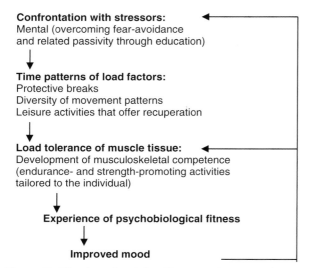

Confrontation with stressors:
Mental (overcoming fear-avoidance
and related passivity through education)

Time patterns of load factors:
Protective breaks
Diversity of movement patterns
Leisure activities that offer recuperation

Load tolerance of muscle tissue:
Development of musculoskeletal competence
(endurance- and strength-promoting activities
tailored to the individual)

Experience of psychobiological fitness

Improved mood

Figure 3 The dynamic relationship among important elements in rehabilitation of musculoskeletal pain. Arrows indicate hypothesized patterns of nested self-rewarding benign circles in the psychobiological development of musculoskeletal competence.

Multidisciplinary intervention programs have been recommended for nonmalignant musculoskeletal pain since the 1970s. A review of 65 treatment outcome studies for back pain was published in 1992. These studies included a diversity of treatments across the psychological, medical, physical, and occupational fields. They lasted, on average, 7 weeks with a range of from 1 to 31 weeks. Hours spent in treatment ranged from 4 to 264, with an average of 96 h. The site of pain in most studies was reported to be the back or in heterogeneous locations. The results from a meta-analysis clearly support the conclusion that multidisciplinary treatments for nonmalignant chronic musculoskeletal pain are superior to single-discipline treatment, waiting list, and no treatment. And the effects have proven to be stable over time. Interestingly, the effects also extend beyond the reduction of pain. Patients report improved mood, a high frequency of return to work, and a reduced need for support from the health-care system after multidisciplinary treatments (**Figure 3**). These early findings are strongly supported in recent research.

Patients must be encouraged to be physically active; the recommendation of a passive lifestyle is not a professional treatment. In this encouragement, fear avoidance may be the major obstacle. This concept was introduced in 1983 by Lethem et al. to account for a passive lifestyle in patients with chronic musculoskeletal pain, in which the avoidance of movements that are expected to give rise to pain leads to the maintenance or exacerbation of fear. The effectiveness of rehabilitation is improved when the patient learns to orient him- or herself away from patterns of passive avoidance and toward active confrontation with pain and the related fear. Multidisciplinary

treatments of groups of outpatients with various diagnoses, of various ages, and of both genders are best at overcoming pain-related fear. And professionals, beyond being academically skilled, also should be socially competent to provide emotional security as well as facilitate motivation and fun.

Further Reading

Apter, M. J. and Svebak, S. (1992). Reversal theory as a biological approach to individual differences. In: Gale, A. & Eysenck, M. W. (eds.) *Handbook of individual differences: biological perspectives*, pp. 323–353. Chichester: John Wiley.

Ashima, M., Bendtsen, L., Jensen, R., et al. (1999). Muscle hardness in patients with chronic tension-type headache: Relation to actual headache state. *Pain* 79, 201–205.

Bru, E., Mykletun, R. and Svebak, S. (1993). Neuroticism, extraversion, anxiety and Type A behaviour as mediators of neck, shoulder and lower back pain in female hospital staff. *Personality and Individual Differences* 15, 485–492.

Bruehl, S., Carlson, C. R., Wilson, J. F., et al. (1996). Psychological coping with acute pain: an examination of the role of endogenous opioid mechanisms. *Journal of Behavioral Medicine* 19, 129–142.

Flor, H., Fydrich, T. and Turk, D. C. (1992). Efficacy of multidisciplinary pain treatment centers: a meta-analytic review. *Pain* 49, 221–230.

Lethem, J., Slade, P. D., Troup, J. D. G., et al. (1983). Outline of fear avoidance model of exaggerated pain perceptions. *Behavior Research and Therapy* 21, 401–408.

Malmo, R. B. (1975). *On emotions, needs, and our archaic brain*. New York: Holt, Rinehart and Winston.

Mikkelsson, M., Salaminen, J. J. and Kantiainen, H. (1999). Non-specific musculoskeletal pain in preadolescents: prevalence and 1-year persistence. *Pain* 73, 29–35.

Norton, P. J., Asmundson, G. J. G., Norton, G. R., et al. (1999). Growing pain: 10-year research trends in the study of chronic pain and headache. *Pain* 79, 59–65.

Sperry, R. W. (1952). Neurology and the mind-brain problem. *American Scientist* 40, 291–312.

Svebak, S., Hagen, K. and Zwart, J.-A. (in press). One-year prevalence of chronic musculoskeletal pain in an adult Norwegian county population: relations with age and gender. The Nord-Trøndelag Health Study. *Journal of Musculoskeletal Pain* 14 (in press).

Storrø, S., Moen, J. and Svebak, S. (2004). Effects on sick-leave of a multidisciplinary rehabilitation programme for chronic low back, neck, or shoulder pain: comparison with usual treatment. *Journal of Rehabilitation Medicine* 36, 12–16.

Vlaeyen, J. W. and Linton, S. J. (2000). Fear-avoidance and its consequences in chronic musculoskeletal pain: a state of the art. *Pain* 85, 317–332.

Westgaard, R. H. and Winckel, J. (1997). Ergonomic intervention research for improved musculoskeletal health: a critical review. *International Journal of Industrial Ergonomics* 20, 463–500.

Music Therapy *See:* Integrative Medicine (Complementary and Alternative Medicine).

Myopathy

G A Small
Drexel University of Medicine, Philadelphia, PA, USA

This article is a revision of the previous edition article by G A Small, volume 2, pp 803–809, © 2000, Elsevier Inc.

Glossary

Electro-diagnosis	A method of evoking electrical responses or recording spontaneous electric responses from nerves and muscles, as well as from the neuromuscular junction, in order to localize pathology to one or more of these specific regions.
Fatigue	A diminishing in muscle strength that is measurable but often without clear anatomic or organic explanation.
Muscular dystrophy	A progressive, untreatable muscle disease defined by scarring and inflammation on histology. The condition is generally recognized as inherited.
Myalgia	Pain attributed to a muscular origin.
Myositis	The inflammation of muscle creating pain, fatigue, and weakness. It is generally proximally predominant.

Myopathy defines a category of neurological diseases affecting muscle proteins and muscle cell substructure, muscle membrane, and other subcellular chemical constituents involved in the transduction of carbon-bond energy into muscle contraction.

Muscle Structure

Skeletal muscle contracts voluntarily, requiring the transduction of a nerve action potential to a chemical message at the neuromuscular junction. This elicits an end-plate potential in the muscle membrane, bringing the membrane to its electrical threshold, which results in calcium release throughout the muscle cell, initiating conformational changes in subcellular proteins (actin, myosin, and troponin) and shortening of the muscle cell, generating force.

Muscle tissue histochemically is a mosaic of muscle proteins surrounded by a muscle membrane, called endomysium, and grouped into fascicles by perimysial connective tissue. The entire muscle is enclosed by a connective tissue cocoon continuous with the perimysium, known as the epimysium, which in turn is continuous with tendon tissue. This bonding of the entire muscle substructure across joints directs the vector of contractile force of each muscle cell in a similar direction, resulting in a coordinated contraction of muscle and flexion or extension of a limb.

Muscle histologically appears as a mosaic due to the dark or light staining characteristics of subcellular proteins involved in fast or slow muscle contraction. Whereas some muscles are dominated by one type and twitch quickly, others are dominated by slower contracting cells, conserving energy. The adaptive advantage of fast- or slow-twitch muscle fibers has a teleological explanation in the response of the organism to threats in the environment. Muscles that have a predominance of fast-twitch fibers are the limb and eye muscles, allowing the organism to respond quickly either toward prey or away from predators, determining whether the organism survives by getting nourishment or avoiding danger. These muscle cells twitch with a great force, but they cannot sustain that force for long. Slow-twitch fibers can contract with reasonable force indefinitely, as long as the pathways for the energy breakdown of fatty acids exist. Such muscles are involved in sustained activity and not necessarily in fight, fright, or flight activity.

Electrical impulses generate neurotransmitter release into the neuromuscular junction, resulting in electrical responses at the muscle membrane, which are carried to all parts of the muscle cell through a complicated system of invaginations of the muscle membrane known as the T tubule system and sarcoplasmic reticulum. These electrical responses are then transduced into the release of calcium from the sarcoplasmic reticulum into the cytoplasm of the muscle cell, known as the sarcoplasm. The interaction of calcium ions with filaments of the muscle proteins actin and myosin allow these strands, lying parallel, to be drawn against one another longitudinally along the muscle cell axis to shorten it. This is an ATP-dependent process. Damage to signal transduction along this pathway results in weakness that may be abrupt and permanent, fluctuating, or relentlessly progressive, depending on the pathophysiology and location of the damage.

Fatigue can result from the functional breakdown at any one of these levels, even at the mental or central nervous system level. Fatigue implies that normal forces are being initially generated and cannot be maintained. It can be measured more easily than its cause can be specifically elicited. Stress to any part of the nerve, neuromuscular junction, and muscle, as well as muscle subcellular structure, can exceed the capacity of the system elements to work synergistically, resulting in diminished muscle strength, which is perceived as fatigue by the individual.

Diseases of Muscle

The variety of muscle diseases reflects the specific localization of pathology in the muscle substructure. Scores of separate muscular dystrophies, inflammatory, and metabolic conditions have been described.

Muscular Dystrophies

Dystrophinopathies   Dystrophinopathies are defined by abnormalities of the large structural protein dystrophin, which was first described in the late 1980s, revolutionizing the study of Duchenne muscular dystrophy. Abnormalities of the structural protein depend on genetic problems in the gene for dystrophin at Xp21. Duchenne and Becker muscular dystrophies fall into this category.

Duchenne muscular dystrophy, the most common muscular dystrophy in children, is inherited in an X-linked recessive manner. Females carry the gene, and their male offspring have a 50% chance of manifesting the disease, depending on whether they inherit the abnormal X chromosome. Although the symptoms generally do not appear until early childhood, serum muscle enzymes are frequently elevated

in infancy. The upper extremities are usually affected later than the lower ones in a proximal to distal fashion. Walking is generally not possible by puberty. During late adolescence, the respiratory muscles are significantly compromised and the cardiac muscle is affected. These two manifestations, as well as the general danger of immobility, resulting in deep vein thrombosis, pneumonia, and skin breakdown, are the general causes of mortality. Dystrophin is absent from muscle tissue.

Becker muscular dystrophy differs from Duchenne muscular dystrophy in that the age of onset is later, the rate of progression slower, and the disease is not terminal. Abnormal dystrophin occurs in muscle. Becker muscular dystrophy refers to numerous abnormal dystrophy subtypes. The lethal disturbance in the dystrophin gene, resulting in the low or abnormal translation of effective dystrophin, is unique for each subtype. The muscle substructure is then prone to inflammation, scarring, and the general pathological characteristics necessary for histological diagnosis.

Myotonic muscular dystrophy   This is the most common muscular dystrophy in adults. The pathophysiology is unclear; however, the genetics of this very commonly underdiagnosed condition is different from the dystrophinopathies. Myotonic dystrophy is inherited in an autosomal dominant pattern. It is a multisystem disease that includes cardiomyopathy, cataracts, endocrine problems, and central neurogenic hypoventilation. The prevalence is 1 in 20,000. Variations in the phenotype of the disease occur despite the classical description of individuals with this syndrome as having neck flexor atrophy along with ptosis; some patients have a normal physiognomy. Some patients endure muscle cramps, whereas others have a disease incompatible with a normal life span due to cardiopulmonary problems. All suffer cataracts by age 40. It is very slowly progressive in most patients.

By definition, myotonia is a problem of impaired muscle relaxation secondary to the depolarization of the muscle membrane and impaired repolarization. Characteristic electrodiagnostic findings are waxing and waning repetitive motor-unit action potentials with the characteristic audible sound of a dive bomber. This electrodiagnostic finding is not specific for myotonic muscular dystrophy but is present in all the myotonic diseases, suggesting that the disease itself is a muscle membrane disorder. In the early 1990s, the gene for myotonic dystrophy was mapped to chromosome 19, but the gene product has not been identified clearly. The likely candidate is a protein kinase involved in the function of numerous tissues within the body, thus explaining the pleiotropism of the disorder. Myotonic muscular dystrophy is one of the trinucleotide repeat sequence diseases. The repetitive appearance of three nucleotides in sequence may occur up to thousands of times within the gene, resulting in genomic instability.

Congenital forms This designation includes obscure, slightly progressive, or nonprogressive diseases clearly present at birth. Patients may manifest mental retardation, seizures, and anatomical brain abnormalities. Muscle pathology is variable, including rodlike structures and central cores. Heritability is varied.

Inflammatory Myopathies

Polymyositis Polymyositis is an inflammatory T-cell-mediated dysfunction of muscle cells, with high serum creatine phosphokinase (CPK), white cell invasion of muscle cells, and progressive proximal weakness. It responds well to steroids.

Dermatomyositis Dermatomyositis is a B-cell-mediated disease of muscle and muscle vasculature, also affecting the skin. It is associated controversially with underlying malignancy.

Inclusion body myositis Patients with clinical manifestations of polymyositis who do not respond to prednisone probably have inclusion body myositis (IBM). With more advanced pathological examinations, many victims of steroid unresponsive polymyositis have been found to have vacuolated muscle fibers, mononuclear cell invasion, and amyloid deposits and tubular filaments by electron microscopy. The discovery of amyloid in muscle fibers, along with inflammation, prompted a trial of immunosuppression to determine whether the suppression of the inflammatory response would result in improved strength; this did not occur. The amyloid degeneration in victims of this disease may be similar to the amyloid degeneration seen in the brains of patients with Alzheimer-type dementia. Therefore, IBM may indeed be a primary degenerative disease, such as amyotrophic lateral sclerosis or Alzheimer-type senile dementia. If the theory is correct, this does not bode well for immunomodulating therapeutic trials.

Metabolic Myopathies

Metabolic myopathies are separated predominantly into glycogen-storage diseases and mitochondrial disorders; these genetically determined abnormalities of glucose and fatty acid metabolism result in myoglobinuria, severe muscle weakness, and disordered acid–base homeostasis. They are a cause of occult fatigue in numerous patients and can be difficult to diagnose. The fact that the mitochondrion possesses its own genome complicates heritability further and underscores the relationship between cytoplasmic inheritance and nuclear inheritance in many of these disease states.

Glycolytic pathway pathology Abnormal metabolism of the stored form of glucose (glycogen) is determined by numerous heritable defects in glycolytic and glycogenolytic enzyme pathways. The lack of phosphofructokinase, phosphoglycerate kinase, lactate dehydrogenase, and phosphoglycerate mutase results in myoglobinuria with exercise. In these conditions, glucose cannot be used efficiently as fuel for muscular contraction, and cramps and myalgia occur with exertion. When the exertion is significant, muscle breakdown occurs and serious systemic consequences can result, such as acidosis and renal failure. An outmoded method of diagnosing glycogen-storage diseases involved exercising a muscle under ischemic conditions and failing to record an appropriate rise in venous lactate; the sophisticated enzymatic analysis of muscle biopsy specimens has supplanted this test. Exercise intolerance is generally the rule in these disorders, and hypoglycemia can occur as well. Therapy is largely related to altering the patient's level of activity and ratio of protein to complex carbohydrate intake.

Mitochondrial myopathies Mastery of the evolving field of mitochondrial myopathies is complicated by almost monthly discoveries and supplantation of previous ones. Abnormalities in mitochondrial function result in disordered fatty acid metabolism. Patients with fatigue and exercise intolerance have abnormal aggregations of mitochondria in their muscle tissue. Patients with weakness, mild or severe, are found to have elevated of lactic acid levels in the serum and cerebrospinal fluid (CSF) due to the reliance of the body on glycolytic function for the production of ATP rather than on the breakdown of the fatty acids. There is no effective treatment for any of the mitochondrial disorders. Attempts to supplement the diet with a variety of respiratory chain constituents, such as coenzyme Q, have met with only anecdotal success. The predominant importance of defining a syndrome of muscle weakness, exercise intolerance, and fatigue is to differentiate an organic from a psychiatric cause of impaired function in patients. Fatigue and myalgia are the predominant complaint of patients who present to the neurologist or their general physician with these diseases. It is likely that the vast majority of patients with these symptoms are initially diagnosed to have stress-related psychiatric conditions – a disservice foisted on a small subgroup who may suffer from mitochondrial pathology.

Toxic Myopathy

Numerous toxins affect the muscle protein matrix. The most common exogenous muscle toxins are ethanol, hydroxymethylglutaryl coenzyme A (HMG-CoA) reductase inhibitors, and steroids.

Ethanol   Ethanol causes a direct toxic effect, raising serum CPK and causing electromyographic changes of myopathy and proximal as well as distal muscle weakness. In severe cases, myoglobinuria occurs; cardiotoxicity is common. Alcohol itself may not be the lone offender; other electrolyte disturbances and vitamin deficiencies are contributory. Abstinence from ethanol is mandatory.

HMG-CoA reductase inhibitors   HMG-CoA reductase inhibitors are used commonly for lipid- and cholesterol-lowering effects, having proved to decrease the incidence of fatal myocardial infarction in patients with elevated cholesterol. Unfortunately, these drugs may also interfere with fatty acid metabolism, and muscle damage occasionally occurs with severe elevations in serum CPK, renal failure, and muscle weakness. A specific pathology has not been clearly delineated; however, abnormal energy metabolism within muscles is blamed for muscle breakdown in susceptible patients.

Steroids   A number of endocrinological conditions such as thyrotoxicosis and Cushing's syndrome, as well as hypoparathyroidism and vitamin D deficiency, cause myopathy. The most common endocrinologically induced myopathy represents the toxicity of large doses of endogenous glucocorticoids to the muscle milieu.

Acute steroid myopathy   Acute steroid myopathy has only recently been distinguished from chronic steroid myopathy. Groups of asthmatic patients given high doses of steroids with or without the concomitant use of nondepolarizing muscle relaxants in intensive care units were found to develop static weakness and myosin-deficiency myopathy by muscle biopsy. Weakness occurring in these conditions is independent of prolonged neuromuscular blockade. It improves. At the present time, there is only supposition as to why the combined use of high doses of steroids and the critical illness state or neuromuscular blockade prompts myosin loss. The trophic influence of the electrochemical message sent through the neuromuscular junction to muscle combined with the catabolic effects of glucocorticoids probably combine to create this pathology.

Chronic steroid myopathy   Unlike acute steroid myopathy, patients on low to medium doses of steroids for any of a number of medical conditions can become progressively weak over weeks to months. The problem tends to be proximally predominant, and the pathology of the condition involves type II muscle fiber atrophy, a similar pathology seen in patients who are chronically bedridden and not exposed to steroids.

Differential Diagnosis of Myopathy

Central Nervous System Disease

It is distinctly uncommon for diseases of the brain, brain stem, or spinal cord to cause weakness bilaterally without other accompanying symptoms, whereas muscle weakness can occur in isolation without myalgia, sensory loss, or clear serum elevations of CPK. Bilateral brain disease resulting in bilateral limb weakness or bilateral cranial nerve abnormalities generally impairs the mental status. It is this preservation of mental status in patients with myopathy that makes distinguishing myopathy from brain or brain-stem diseases simple. It is only slightly more problematic to distinguish spinal cord causes of weakness from myopathy. Mental status is preserved in spinal cord disease unless respiratory muscle function is compromised severely and hypoxemia causes delirium. Sensory loss is the rule in myelopathic disease, as well as severe bowel and bladder dysfunction. The bowel and bladder dysfunction occurring in myopathy is due more to immobilization and the inability of the patient to physically get to a bathroom than it is to any primary pathology of the detrusor or anal sphincter muscles.

Neuropathy

Neuropathy can cause unilateral or bilateral muscle weakness generally with a distal predominance; however, sensory loss occurs in most neuropathies. Very rare neuropathies, such as multifocal motor conduction block neuropathy or primary motor neuropathy from motor neuron disease or lead intoxication, can mimic myopathy, but reflexes are absent or depressed. Patients with severe myopathy may have decreased or even absent reflexes, but this is extremely rare. In difficult cases, distinguishing neuropathic from myopathic weakness depends on electrodiagnosis and muscle biopsy. It is not unusual for an individual undergoing a workup for amyotrophic lateral sclerosis, which affects the lower motor neuron, to undergo a muscle or nerve biopsy to help distinguish benign myopathic disease from the devastating diagnosis of anterior horn cell disease. However, the majority of neuropathies cause greater distal than proximal weakness, with profound sensory loss early in the course of the syndrome, thus allowing the clinician to distinguish neuropathy from myopathy in most cases.

Neuromuscular Junction Diseases

Patients with neuromuscular junction disease may have a predominant disease of the cranial innervated musculature and present with double vision, lid drooping, dysphagia or dysarthria, or problems with neck extension. Isolated respiratory muscle weakness has also been reported, but not commonly. Extracellular calcium, responding to the action potential reaching the end of the motor nerve, enters the presynaptic nerve through voltage-sensitive channels, causing the vesicles of acetylcholine to couple with the nerve membrane, releasing acetylcholine as the chemical message; this results in muscle contraction in the postjunctional area. Botulinum toxin envenomation creates a condition in which toxin enters the prejunctional membrane, preventing acetylcholine vesicles from coupling with the prejunctional nerve membrane, aborting the message for the muscle to contract. This condition results in the degeneration of this part of the nerve; in a sense, botulinum toxin envenomation not only causes a neuromuscular junction short circuit, but actually causes a distal motor neuropathy. Patients generally need months to regrow this part of the nerve.

Lambert–Eaton syndrome is the prototypic autoimmune disease in which antibodies are raised to voltage-gated calcium channels. Molecular mimicry among moieties on small-cell carcinomas and the prejunctional neuromuscular junction membrane creates a situation whereby the host raises antibodies both to small-cell cancer and the prejunctional membrane, resulting in an attack on the cancer and the fluctuating weakness seen as calcium inefficiently enters the prejunctional neuromuscular junction membrane due to competitive inhibition by these antibodies.

Most postjunctional neuromuscular diseases are the result of abnormalities induced in the coupling of acetylcholine to its receptor in the postjunctional membrane or in abnormalities of the acetylcholine receptor itself. Iatrogenic neuromuscular junction blockade occurs with the use of depolarizing or nondepolarizing muscle relaxants. The autoimmune disease myasthenia gravis results in inefficient neuromuscular transmission and weakness due to abnormalities in the acetylcholine receptor through competitive inhibition by autoantibodies. Similar to the Lambert–Eaton syndrome, myasthenia gravis can be treated with a number of immunomodulating agents such as steroids or with the removal of exogenous antibody through plasma exchange or through other forms of nonspecific immunosuppression. Many patients have been thought to have conversion reaction because weakness can be subtle. Exogenous stressors such as the flu can stress the neuromuscular junction and cause even more inefficient neuromuscular communication, resulting in fluctuating weakness. Some victims are treated for psychiatric disease, delaying proper treatment.

Myopathy

Myopathy is generally characterized by mild to moderate elevations of the CPK level, greater proximal than distal muscle weakness, with the preservation of deep tendon reflexes and no sensory loss. The varieties of myopathy have already been discussed.

Electrodiagnosis

The proper designation of weakness as originating in the muscle can be made noninvasively through clinical examination and then confirmed through the electrodiagnostic capabilities of electromyography and nerve conduction studies. Using our knowledge of the anatomy of the muscle and recruitment of muscle fibers in the development of muscle contractions, we can evoke patterns of responses from muscles with a needle electrode for quick and efficient disease localization.

Using the principle of differential amplification, a needle electrode with two active recording surfaces separated by an insulator is introduced superficially into muscle. Recording the difference in voltage between the two active surfaces, a simple wave form is generated during contraction. The muscle cell group that contracts, innervated by one particular motor neuron, is termed the motor unit. As the muscle contraction is maintained voluntarily by the patient, a repeating waveform appears on the oscilloscope. Minimal contraction is necessary for this waveform to appear repetitively, up to 5–15 times s^{-1}. As the individual increases the force of the contraction, another motor unit is recruited to increase muscle tension, and another waveform appears on the screen, twitching between 5 and 15 Hz. Because there are hundreds of motor units in a typical muscle, hundreds of motor units appear and create a pattern of discharge on the oscilloscope. In patients with nerve disease, the number of motor neurons is decreased. Therefore, the number of motor units recorded on the screen is decreased. If the nerve disease has been occurring

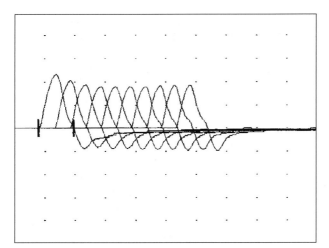

Figure 1 Successive decreases in waveform amplitude during repetitive stimulation testing in a patient with myasthenia gravis.

long enough, the muscle cells that were served by the damaged nerve in question will have been reinnervated by the remaining normal nerves; then each of the waveforms seen will be larger than generally expected. In addition, the rate at which each motor unit contracts is much faster than the normal 5–15 Hz. Neuropathy is then the likely diagnosis.

In contrast, in myopathy the number of motor units remains the same, but the number of muscle cells contracting effectively decreases. Assuming that a random distribution of muscle cells either have died or are damaged significantly, then each resulting motor unit creates a smaller waveform on the electromyographer's oscilloscope. In addition, because a contraction of the weak muscle, even to a moderate extent, necessitates the recruitment of motor units to maintain the same force as in a normal muscle, the contraction pattern appearing on the oscilloscope appears to be that of a maximum voluntary contraction, even though full voluntary contraction has not yet been achieved. Myopathy is then the likely diagnosis.

The repetitive stimulation method may distinguish myopathy from disorders of the neuromuscular junction. Repetitive nerve stimulation results in numerous recorded compound motor action potentials (**Figure 1**). In the case of neuromuscular junction disease, however, either too little or varying amounts of acetylcholine are released at the neuromuscular junction and fewer muscle cells contract. Less force is generated in the muscle, which expresses itself as weakness clinically and as a decrease in waveform amplitude, as shown in **Figure 1**.

Muscle Biopsy

It is through sophisticated staining methods of muscle tissue that our understanding of the myopathic

conditions has shifted since the mid-1980s. This has resulted in more accurate diagnoses and in the discovery of new forms of myopathy. Undoubtedly, additional forms of myopathy and a further subspecification of disorders now lumped together under one designation will be discovered in the near future. One example of this is IBM, which was previously thought to be a steroid-unresponsive form of polymyositis and now enjoys its own designation as a separate disease entity, largely due to sophisticated histopathological techniques.

Therapy

Muscular dystrophies by definition are designated untreatable. Gene therapy trials will probably remove this untreatable designation. At the present time, physical rehabilitation is really our only means of keeping patients with muscular dystrophy as strong as possible. In the case of myotonic muscular dystropy, in which weakness is generally not the worst problem, the avoidance of late-stage complications such as heart block and respiratory compromise from central neurogenic hypoventilation is the rule. In the case of glycogen-storage diseases, in which the avoidance of sudden exertion and dehydration helps best, genetic counseling is our only other means of prevention. The therapeutic armamentarium in myopathy, however, is greatly widened when we address inflammatory myopathy.

Corticosteroids

Corticosteroids prevent the mobilization of plasma cells and communication among a variety of white blood cells by decreasing interleukin production, minimizing inflammatory reactions and subsequent muscle destruction. This form of immunosuppression is still considered nonspecific in that no one particular process of the immune response is knowingly targeted. Prednisone is the mainstay of treatment for dermatomyositis, polymyositis, and the immune-mediated myopathies accompanying collagen vascular diseases such as systemic lupus erythematosus and rheumatoid arthritis.

However, the previous discussion of steroid-induced myopathy, whether acute or chronic, should not be taken lightly. The very treatment for these myopathies may precipitate a chronic form of weakness and, therefore, the steroid dosage necessary to prevent weakness should be titrated downward to the lowest effective dose. Alternate day therapy may slightly decrease the incidence of steroid myopathy and other abnormal side effects such as ulcer disease, cataract formation, glaucoma, hypertension, diabetes, and aseptic necrosis of the hip, as well as severe weight gain from lipogenesis. Many inflammatory myopathies burn out and do not need to be treated for more than 2–3 years. Even this length of time may create enough of an opportunity for untoward side effects to occur.

Intravenous Immunoglobulin

Intravenous immunoglobulin (IgG) has failed to show significant results in polymyositis; however, some cases of dermatomyositis stabilize or improve with the use of pooled IgG. Perhaps it is because dermatomyositis is a B-cell-, plasma-cell-, and antibody-mediated disease that the application of large quantities of anti-idiotypic and nonspecific antibodies act as competitive and noncompetitive inhibitors, blocking pathogenic host antibodies from destroying muscles. IgG is used more for other causes of weakness at other locations in the neuraxis, such as the neuromuscular junction in the case of myasthenia gravis, and for Guillain–Barré syndrome, an inflammatory proximal neuropathy.

Plasmapheresis

The removal of plasma proteins, cytokines, and immunoglobulins and their replacement either with another individual's plasma or with an albumin and saline solution has been used in other immune-mediated conditions, both neurological and non-neurological. A controlled trial of plasma exchange in patients with polymyositis and dermatomyositis failed to show any benefit, however.

Conclusion

Current medications are helpful but are also toxic when used chronically, so although medical science can provide benefits for some clearly defined myopathic syndromes, we can expect more clinical trials of other pharmaceuticals. The variety of myopathies mirrors the variety of diseases in other parts of the neuroaxis. Genetic influences, environmental influences, immunological influences, and toxic causes of weakness clearly illustrate the vulnerability of muscle tissue to a variety of stressors. However, psychic stress does not cause weakness. It can create fatigue, but clearly it does not create a consistently measurable abnormality of force generation due to muscle damage or neuromuscular junction disease. Therefore, weak patients need to be worked up for organic diseases. The complicated structure of nerve, neuromuscular junction, and muscle allows for breakdowns at any point along the way, and many diseases result, some of which have been clearly defined; all of which are measurable as weakness at the bedside, in the electrophysiology laboratory, and pathologically.

The physiological muscle response to numerous exogenous and endogenous stimuli may be normal contraction, paralysis, or anatomic disruption. The most explicit exposition of stress affecting muscle occurs in acute steroid myopathy, in which normal contraction may be affected to the point of paralysis without anatomic disruption of the muscle membrane and intracellular contents. In addition, acute steroid myopathy may also express its severity in myosin dissolution and the eventual anatomic disruption of the muscle membrane. This form of toxic myopathy best illustrates the effects of stress on muscle.

Further Reading

Engel, A. and Franzini-Armstrong, C. (1994). *Myology* (2nd edn.). New York: McGraw-Hill.

Griffin, J., Low, P. and Poduslo, J. (1993). *Peripheral neuropathy* (3rd edn.). Philadelphia: Saunders.

Kimura, J. (1981). *Electrodiagnosis in diseases of nerve and muscle: principles and practice* (2nd edn.). Philadelphia: Davis.

Rowland, L. (1995). *Merritt's textbook of neurology* (9th edn.). Baltimore, MD: Williams & Wilkins.

Sethi, R. and Thompson, L. (1989). *The electromyographer's handbook* (2nd edn.). Boston: Little, Brown and Company.

N

Natural Disasters *See:* Community Studies; Disasters and Mass Violence, Public, Effects of.

Natural Killer (NK) Cells

T L Whiteside, M Boyiadzis and R B Herberman
University of Pittsburgh Cancer Institute and
University of Pittsburgh School of Medicine,
Pittsburgh, PA, USA

This article is a revision of the previous edition article by
T L Whiteside, A Baum, and R B Herberman, volume 3, pp 1–7,
© 2000, Elsevier Inc.

Characteristics of Natural Killer Cells
Biological Importance of NK Cells
Measurement of NK Cells
NK Cells in Human Disease
NK Cells and Aging
Stress and NK Cells

Glossary

Activated NK cells	A subset of NK cells responding to stimulatory signals that have upregulated expression of receptors for interleukin-2 as well as other surface molecules and have acquired new functional attributes that facilitate cellular interactions.
Antibody-dependent cellular cytotoxicity	A form of cell death mediated by NK cells in the presence of an antibody that is specific for an antigen expressed on the surface of target cells and decorates the NK cell through binding to a receptor for immunoglobulins. This antibody forms a bridge between effector and target cells.
Cytotoxicity	One of the functions of NK cells commonly used for assessing the level of NK activity in the peripheral blood, other body fluids, or mononuclear cells isolated from tissues.
Effector cells	NK cells that induce lysis of target cells.
NK cells	A subpopulation of lymphocytes characterized by the expression of surface markers that are distinct from those present on T or B lymphocytes. NK cells have a unique capability to recognize and eliminate a broad range of abnormal cell targets without prior sensitization. They are components of innate immunity responsible for immune surveillance against infectious agents and transformed cells.
NK-cell assay	An assay used to measure NK activity by coincubation of effector (E) with radioactively labeled target (T) cells at several different E : T ratios. The assay estimates the percentage of specific lysis attributable to NK cells based on levels of radioactivity released from a defined number of target cells.

Characteristics of Natural Killer Cells

NK cells are effectors of the innate immune system that play an important role in host response against viruses and tumor cells through the production of cytokines and direct cytolytic activity. Unlike other effector cells, NK cells are able to kill these targets spontaneously, without having had prior encounters with them. NK cells also appear to be highly sensitive to stress, exhibiting dramatic changes in function in response to acute or chronic stress. Because they appear to be involved in important immunological defense against infectious agents and against cancer, and because they are affected so readily by stress or emotional state, NK cells have been a well-studied variable in the stress–illness relationship.

Natural killer cells were first described in the early 1970s based on their functional capability to lyse tumor cells in the absence of prior stimulation. This characteristic of NK cells was considered to fit their role as mediators of immune surveillance. Since then, NK cells have been shown to mediate other biologically important functions. NK cells are now known to produce cytokines that regulate the development of acquired specific immunity, play a role in the rejection of bone-marrow grafts, be responsible for the selective elimination of abnormal cells, and be implicated in the development of autoimmune diseases and the graft versus host disease (GVHD).

NK cells make up from 10 to 15% of human peripheral blood lymphocytes, as determined by phenotyping using labeled monoclonal antibodies (MAbs). NK cells can home to secondary lymphoid organs. It is estimated that approximately 5% of mononuclear cells in uninflamed lymph nodes are NK cells, and they constitute 0.4–1% of the lymphoid cells found in inflamed tonsils and lymph nodes. Thus, the extravascular lymphoid tissues represent a large pool of innate effector cells because, in aggregate, lymph nodes harbor 40% of all lymphocytes, whereas peripheral blood contains only 2%.

NK Cell Development and Subsets

NK cells originate in the bone marrow from CD34+ hematopoietic progenitor stem cells and require the bone marrow microenvironment for complete maturation. In the presence of stromal cell-derived growth factors, c-kit ligand and flt-3 ligand, the CD34+ stem cells acquire the surface receptor for the cytokines interleukin (IL)-15/IL-2. The acquisition of the IL-15/IL-2 receptor renders the NK progenitors (NKP) responsive to IL-15, a critical cytokine for NK cell development. The next steps of development involve the acquisition of the unique NK cell receptor repertoire and proliferation into phenotypically and functionally mature NK cells.

Two subsets of NK cells are present in the peripheral blood of healthy adults. The majority of NK cells express low levels of CD56 (CD56^{dim}) and high levels of Fcγ receptor III (FcγRIII, CD16^{high}), whereas 10% of NK cells are CD56^{bright} CD16$^{dim/-}$. In the lymph nodes, the majority of NK cells belong to the NK-cell bright subset. These two NK subsets differ in receptor expression, trafficking, cytokine production, and the ability to mediate cytotoxicity. CD56^{dim} NK cells are more cytotoxic and mediate higher antibody-dependent target cell lysis but produce low levels of cytokines (**Table 1**). In contrast, CD56^{bright} NK cells can produce abundant cytokines, but exert low natural cytotoxicity and antibody-dependent cellular cytotoxicity (ADCC).

Table 1 Subsets of natural killer cells in humans[a]

	CD56^{bright}	CD56^{dim}
CD56	++	+
CD16	-/+	++
NK receptors		
KIR	-/+	++
CD94	++	-/+
NKG2A	+	-/+
Cytokine and chemokine receptors		
IL-2 R$\alpha\beta\gamma$	+	-
IL-2 R $\beta\gamma$	+	+
c-Kit	+	-
CCR7	++	-
CXCR1	-	++
CX$_3$CR1	-	++
Adhesion molecules		
CD2	++	+
CD44	++	+
CD62L	++	-/+

[a]++ denotes high-density expression; + denotes low-density expression; -/+ denotes variable expression; - denotes no expression. CCR7, chemokine receptor C7; CX, chemokine receptor; IL, interleukin; KIR, killer immunoglobulin-like receptor.

Receptors

The triggering of NK cell cytotoxicity is determined by the balance of activating and inhibitory signals received via the broad repertoire of receptors found on individual NK cells. These receptors monitor the interactions of NK cells with other effector cells of the immune system and with cellular targets (**Figure 1**). In humans, there are three main classes of receptors: natural cytotoxicity receptors (NCRs), killer immunoglobulin-like receptors (KIRs), and killer C-type lectin receptors.

The NCRs, which bind to as yet unidentified tumor antigens, are all activating receptors and have been demonstrated to be involved in the NK-cell-mediated killing of various cancer cell lines. Three NCRs (NKp46, NKp44, and NKp30) have been identified. NKp46 and NKp30 are constitutively expressed by all peripheral blood NK cells and are not found on other immune cells. NKp44 is not expressed by resting NK cells, but is upregulated by IL-2 stimulation.

The KIRs belong to the immunoglobulin superfamily. There are two functionally distinct sets of KIRs: inhibitory and activating. KIRs specifically recognize major histocompatibility complex (MHC) class I alleles, including groups of HLA-A, -B, and -C molecules. Each specific set of inhibitory and activating KIRs has an identical extracellular domain and, consequently, each set binds to identical ligands. However, because of differences in their cytoplasmic domains, one set of KIRs signals an inhibitory response and the other set signals an activating response following their

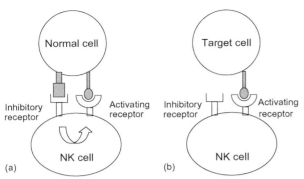

Figure 1 Natural killer cell cytotoxicity. a, No lysis; b, lysis. NK cell cytotoxicity depends on a delicate balance between activating and inhibitory receptors. The presence of activating receptors and inhibitory receptors on the surface of NK cells is necessary to protect normal cells from lysis. Inhibitory signals normally predominate over activating receptors, and a cell able to induce such signals (e.g., through expression of abundant MHC molecules) avoids lysis. This process occurs constantly as NK cells survey normal host tissues. However, when activating receptors engage their ligands on target cells in the absence of inhibitory receptor–ligand interactions, a net activating signal is generated, resulting in lysis of the target. Virally infected or tumor cells downregulate ligands that are recognized by the NK-cell inhibitory receptors (i.e., MHC molecules) and, thus, NK cells are able to recognize these targets as nonself and to kill them.

binding to identical MHC class I alleles. Inhibitory KIRs usually have a higher affinity for MHC-class ligands and, therefore, coligation of both activating and inhibitory receptors results in a net negative signal. Presumably, this double set of receptors with opposing signaling properties exists to regulate NK activity and to protect normal cells from being eliminated.

The killer C-type lectin receptors include inhibitory heterodimers of CD94 complexed with NKG2A or NKG2B and activating heterodimers complexed with NKG2C or NKG2E. These receptors all recognize the overall expression of MHC class I, in that they bind to HLA-E, which is expressed only in association with MHC leader peptides. Another activating C-type lectin receptor, NKG2D, is expressed as a homodimer that binds to peptides associating with the stress-inducible molecules MIC-A, MIC-B, or ULBPs.

In addition to the various activating and inhibitory receptors, NK cells express several receptors that play an important role in enhancing their interaction with target cells and enhancing the NK-cell-mediated cytotoxicity (**Table 2**).

Mechanisms of Cytotoxicity

NK cells possess a unique capacity for recognizing and killing a broad range of abnormal targets such as virally infected or transformed cells and certain allogeneic targets. Although the molecular events involved in the process of target recognition and

Table 2 NK-cell receptors and ligand specificity[a]

	Activating	Inhibitory	Ligand specificity
KIRs	+	+	MHC class I alleles including groups of HLA-A, -B, -C
NCRs	+		Unknown
C-type lectin receptors			
CD94/ NKG2A/B		+	HLA-E
CD94/NKD2C	+		HLA-E
NKG2D	+		MICA, MICB, ULBP-1, -2, -3
Coreceptors			
CD16 (FcγRIII)			Fc of IgG
CD2			CD58
2B4			CD48
CD 40 ligand			CD40

[a]KIRs, killer immunoglobulin-like receptors; MHC, major histocompatibility complex; NCRs, natural cytotoxicity receptors.

signaling are not fully known, the cellular alterations that result from effector (E) cell–target (T) cell interactions have been identified. NK cells can use two different mechanisms for killing, and several distinct sequential steps are involved in the process of target cell lysis.

• *Perforin-mediated cytotoxicity.* NK cells can lyse target cells through a calcium-dependent release of intracytoplasmic granules containing perforin or granzymes A and B. This secretory activity mediated by perforin/granzyme release results in necrosis and is directed primarily at NK-sensitive targets, such as K562 tumor cells. Perforin forms pores in target cells, whereas the granzyme release is necessary for target cell killing.

• *Induction of apoptosis through death receptors.* Activated NK cells express the Fas ligand (FasL) and can kill Fas+ (CD95+) targets through the activation of enzymes that fragment DNA. In addition, NK cells express tumor necrosis factor (TNF)-related apoptosis-induced ligand (TRAIL) and can thereby activate apoptosis in cells that express TRAIL receptors, including death receptor 4 and death receptor 5. Nonsecretory NK activity (surface receptor-mediated apoptosis) is preferred for NK-resistant targets such as fresh tumor or solid tissue cells.

Activated NK cells can rapidly kill a number of targets by combining these two mechanisms. NK cells that survive a lytic event are able to recirculate and can bind to another susceptible target and kill it. The efficiency of NK cell-mediated lysis (killing) is dependent on the ratio of NK cells to abnormal cells and on the level of NK-cell activation.

Biological Importance of NK Cells

NK cells participate either directly or indirectly in a variety of essential biological processes, ranging from reproduction to immunoregulation (**Table 3**).

Defense against Infections

The major function of NK cells appears to be defense against infection. They have been shown to mediate antiviral, antifungal, and antibacterial activities *in vitro*. NK cell importance in the control of infections *in vivo* is supported by studies of experimental viral infections in mice and by reports correlating low NK activity with increased sensitivity to frequent and severe viral infections in humans, including herpes simplex virus (HSV), Epstein–Barr virus (EBV), and cytomegalovirus (CMV) infections. *In vivo* responses of NK cells to a viral challenge involve increases in cytotoxicity, proliferation, migration of NK cells to infected tissues, and production of interferon (IFN)-γ by NK cells. Virus-induced interferons increase NK cell functions and also modulate IL-12 expression, contributing to the development of an antiviral milieu early on during infection and prior to the appearance of virus-specific T cells. Activated NK cells may reduce viral replication by killing infected host cells, and they are able to produce a variety of cytokines that can inhibit viral replication as well as facilitate antigen processing or antigen presentation by increasing the expression of MHC molecules.

Antitumor Effects

NK cells were first discovered because of their ability to kill *in vitro* certain tumor cell lines. Subsequently, NK cell antitumor activity has been convincingly demonstrated in several animal models of cancer and metastasis. These experimental studies suggest that activated NK cells play an important role in limiting both local tumor growth and dissemination of metastases. In particular, activated NK cells are thought to be responsible and ideally suited for antitumor surveillance because they appear to be able to enter solid tissues, migrate to sites of metastasis, and eliminate malignant targets while sparing normal tissue cells. The depletion of NK cells from animals enhances the *in vivo* growth of implanted tumor cells, whereas the administration of NK cells to animals with metastatic cancer eliminates the tumor and prolongs survival. In a prospective study following 3500 Japanese over 11 years, the incidence of cancer was significantly increased in those with lower initial NK cytotoxic activity. In gastric and colon cancer patients, lower NK cytolytic activity at diagnosis correlated with higher tumor volume, metastases, and a worse prognosis. These data suggest that an adequate NK cell number and levels of NK activity are needed to mediate immune surveillance against malignancy.

Regulation of Immunity

NK cells can exert immunoregulatory activity through their interactions with other immune effector cells and by producing several cytokines, bridging innate immunity with adoptive immunity. Recently, dendritic cells (DC) have been implicated in the activation of NK cells. The activation of NK cells by DCs may play a role in shaping the emerging adaptive responses.

NK cells are constantly primed for activation by normal host cells, but their activation is negatively balanced by the inhibitory receptors that recognize self MHC class I antigens. A loss of this self-inhibitory mechanism could lead to both cytotoxicity and cytokine release by NK cells and may play a role in autoimmunity. Alterations in NK cell functions have been described in patients with autoimmune diseases. Such patients may have low levels of natural killing due to both reduced levels of circulating NK cells and defects in lytic activity.

Measurement of NK Cells

The measurement of NK cells in body fluids or cell suspensions consists of determinations of the NK cell number and NK activity. Both are necessary for an adequate evaluation of natural immunity or for following its changes during disease or in response to stress. In most instances, the level of NK activity per cell is the best estimate of the functional potential of NK cells.

NK cell numbers are generally measured using monoclonal antibodies specific for NK cell-associated markers (e.g., CD56 and CD16 in humans, NKR-P1 in rats, and NK1.1 in mice), which are labeled with a fluorescent dye. Following staining, the percentage of positive cells in a population is determined by flow cytometry; this percentage value is then converted into the absolute number of NK cells based on the simultaneously obtained differential lymphocyte count. Or, in a single-platform flow cytometry method, fluorosphere beads are used to allow for the direct calculation of the stained NK cells in a tube.

Natural killer activity has been traditionally measured in short-term (4-h) ^{51}Cr release assays, in

Table 3 Biological significance of NK cells

Elimination of intracellular pathogens: viruses, fungi, and bacteria
Surveillance against cancer and elimination of metastases
Regulation of immunity
Involvement in pregnancy and fertility
Regulation of liver growth and regeneration
Regulation of hematopoiesis
Interactions with the neuroendocrine system

which a standard number (5×10^3) of cultured K562 cells is used as radiolabeled targets (T) and peripheral blood mononuclear cells as effectors (E). The latter are adjusted in number to give at least four different E : T ratios in the assay. This allows for the generation of a lytic curve by plotting the percentage of specific lysis against the E : T ratio. More recently, flow cytometry methods have been introduced that simultaneously measure NK-cell cytotoxicity and NK-cell phenotype. These methods are gaining acceptance because they dispense with radioactivity, are cost effective, and offer an opportunity to evaluate several distinct characteristics of effector cells. However, these methods have not yet been validated against the Cr-release assay, which remains the gold standard for measuring NK activity. The results of NK-cell assays are usually expressed as lytic units (LU) calculated from the lytic curve and defined as the number of E required to kill 5×10^3 targets in a batch of tested cells. Computer programs are available to facilitate the transformation of these data.

NK Cells in Human Disease

NK cell abnormalities either in NK-cell number or activity have been described in human diseases. In either case, only chronic abnormality in NK cell activity or number is considered to be pathological because transient changes accompany a variety of physiologically normal events (e.g., circadian variations, daily stress, exercise, or a common cold). Although the absolute number of NK cells in the peripheral circulation may be significantly below or above a normal range, this does not mean that NK activity is also abnormal. Often, individuals with a low number of NK cells have normal NK activity because their NK cells are activated. Conversely, some individuals with a high NK cell number may have little NK activity due to a lack of or low function of these cells. Therefore, to evaluate the functional potential of NK cells appropriately, it is necessary to measure both NK-cell number and NK activity and to express NK-cell functions on a per cell basis.

Chronically low levels of NK cell activity are seen in cancer, acquired or congenital immunodeficiency diseases (e.g., AIDS), severe life-threatening viral infections (HSV, EBV, and CMV), a subset of patients with chronic fatigue syndrome (CFS), certain autoimmune diseases (e.g., connective tissue diseases), and behavioral disorders (e.g., depression). Persistently elevated NK cell activity is relatively rare, being reported in autoimmune liver disease (including viral hepatitis) and in NK-cell lymphoproliferations. The latter present as elevations in the number or activity of NK cells or both and are characterized by a benign course,

lymphocytosis of large granular lymphocytes (LGL), cytopenias, and splenomegaly. Rare acute proliferations of LGL have been reported and are consistent with aggressive leukemia/lymphoma.

Persistently low levels of the NK-cell number or activity in patients with advanced metastatic or other diseases may be associated with more severe symptoms or an increased risk of disease progression. Therefore, it may be advantageous for patients with chronically low NK cell activity to receive therapy designed to augment NK cell functions. Such therapies are available and consist of the administration of agents known to upregulate endogenous NK activity (e.g., interferons, IFNs; IL-2) or an adoptive transfer of autologous A-NK cells, either systemically or regionally. These therapeutic strategies have not been extensively evaluated, however. More recently, adoptive transfers of NK-92, an NK-cell line established from a patient with non-Hodgkin's lymphoma, have been used in the therapy of hematological malignancies and solid tumors with acceptable toxicity and the goal of providing the host with an excess of antitumor effector cells able to eliminate tumor cells.

NK Cells and Aging

The cells of the immune system are constantly renewed from hematopoietic stem cells. With age, a reduction in the overall capacity for the renewal of these stem cells as a whole has been observed. Unlike T and B cells, the absolute number of NK cells is increased in older individuals compared to young or middle-aged groups, and IFN-γ production and phagocytosis are also increased. Total NK-cell cytotoxicity is stable, however, so the NK-cell cytotoxicity on a per cell basis is impaired in older individuals, as is the response of NK cells to IL-2. The age-associated increases in the number of NK cells and in T cells expressing NK receptors might reflect an alteration in regulatory mechanisms that favors NK-cell functions associated with the regulation of immune responses at the expense of antitumor functions, for example.

Stress and NK Cells

Interactions between NK cells and neuroendocrine systems have received increasing attention. NK cells express receptors for neuropeptides, opioids, prolactin, and other neurohormones, which regulate interactions between the brain and the immune system. Therefore, NK cells are highly responsive to changes in the serum levels of these hormones. Stress often involves all these hormones, and the effects of stress on the immune response can be monitored by serially following changes in NK cell activity.

For example, major stressful life events in otherwise healthy individuals are generally associated with low NK cell activity. However, this effect of stress on NK cells is dependent on several other variables, including the duration of a stressful event, how long afterward responses are measured, and variables that affect the intensity of stress experienced.

Several studies have addressed effects of stress on NK cells and have begun to identify mechanisms underlying these effects. These studies have examined stress effects on overall NK activity, on the number of NK cells in circulation, and on the level of activity per NK cell. NK cell numbers tend to change as NK cells leave the bloodstream and migrate into tissue or lymph nodes. Stress-related changes in cell numbers and activity reflect this process, and thus NK activity per cell is the most reliable way of measuring the effects of stress on these cells.

Two primary systems are involved in the regulation of stress: the sympathetic nervous system (SNS) and the hypothalamic-pituitary-adrenocortical (HPA) axis. SNS activation is initially achieved through neural stimulation and is more or less immediate. Measurable increases in organ or system function tied directly to SNS activation (e.g., heart rate) can be detected within 1 min after the onset of a stressor. Endocrine activity, principally catecholaminergic, intensifies and extends the duration of neural stimulation, and the release of epinephrine and norepinephrine from the adrenal medullae and sympathetic neurons is reliably associated with stress.

The effects mediated by the HPA axis, which culminate in the increased release of glucocorticoids (i.e., cortisol) from the adrenal cortexes, are slower to act or to recover. Ordinarily, changes in HPA activity are not detectable for several minutes, but once initiated, they may persist for hours. This suggests that initial or acute stress responses are governed principally by the SNS, which may have a stimulatory effect on NK activity or may affect cell migration (more NK cells released into circulation). In general, acute stress lasting as little as a few minutes is associated with large, rapid increases in NK-cell number in peripheral blood circulation and a corresponding increase in overall cytotoxicity. Chronic stress lasting days, weeks, or months appears to be associated with the suppression of NK-cell number and cytotoxicity (**Table 4**). Differences in how acute and chronic stress affect NK cells provide some insight into the mechanisms, functions, and consequences of stress modulation of NK activity, as outlined briefly in the following section.

NK Cells and Acute Stress

Acute stress is almost always associated with a rapid release of catecholamines, leading to an immediate increase in NK-cell number in the peripheral

Table 4 Summary of the effects of acute and chronic stress in human NK cells[a]

	Acute stress	Chronic stress
Cell number	+ +	− −
Cell cytotoxicity	+	−
Overall cytotoxicity	+ +	−
Cytokine production	+	+ + (pro-inflammatory)
Possible mechanisms	SNS, HPA axis	SNS, EOPs, HPA axis

[a]+ and + +, highest/increased effects; − and − −, lowest/decreased effects; EOPs, endogenous opioid peptides; HPA, hypothalamic-pituitary-adrenal; SNS, sympathetic nervous system.

circulation, probably due to changes in NK-cell trafficking (i.e., increased movement from lymphoid or nonlymphoid tissue into the peripheral circulation as a result of a reduction in NK cell adherence to endothelial cells combined with an increase in blood flow). This increase in the number of NK cells is accompanied by increases in individual cell function, as observed in some studies but not in others. However, an acute elevation of glucocorticoids within 10–20 min after stress causes immune cells to marginate and subsequently to enter target tissues, probably as a result of the local release of cytokines, which act as chemoattractants. Hence, the enhancing effect of acute stress on immune cells is short-lived and is followed by a suppression of NK cell activity that may be unrelated to changes in NK-cell number. These effects have been observed in naturalistic studies of tandem parachute jumpers and in laboratory studies using far less severe stressors. In numerous studies, the time course of acute stress on NK-cell number appears to be biphasic, increasing on the initial encounter with stress and decreasing rapidly to the baseline resting level or below as soon as the stressor is terminated. Thus, NK-cell-enhancing effects of acute stress are reversible. Age, social support, time of day, and other variables appear to modulate the influence of acute stress on NK cells. The acute reactivity of NK cells during or shortly after an acute stressor may be correlated with levels of SNS activation (e.g., epinephrine and norepinephrine levels) and varies across the time of day. It has been observed that the most labile responses in NK cell activity occur late in the afternoon. A variety of measures thought to completely or partly reflect sympathetic arousal, including blood pressure and stress hormone levels, have been correlated with changes in NK-cell number and function.

The available studies underscore the complexity of acute stress responses and factors determining NK activity. They also suggest that the regulation of immune responses to acute stress depends on both catecholamine and cortisol phases of the response.

Furthermore, there may be several other pathways (e.g., those involving modulation by endogenous opioids) by which acute stress might affect the activity of NK cell.

NK Cells and Chronic Stress

Chronic stress, involving the repeated or sustained elevation of stress hormones, appears to suppress NK cell activity as well as the number of cells in circulation. For example, studies of medical students at the time of low and higher stress periods confirmed that NK cells were suppressed during prolonged stress. Similarly, studies of caregivers for Alzheimer's disease patients and of bereaved populations also provide evidence of chronic suppression of NK cell activity. In one study, bereaved women exhibited lower NK cell activity than nonbereaved participants, and in another study, caregivers were observed to have lower NK cell activity and increased plasma cortisol concentrations than controls. Studies of disasters, such as earthquakes or nuclear accidents, have also provided evidence of a lower number of NK cells in stressed groups, particularly if participants reported greater worry, intrusive thoughts about the disaster, or general persistent distress. Depression in young adults is associated with depressed NK activity. The effects of chronic stress on NK cells are clearly different from those of more short-lived acute stress, and it is possible that the suppression of cytotoxicity, cytokine release, and/or the NK-cell number observed in chronic stress is due to more slowly acting hormonal systems. It appears that long-term (i.e., chronic) responses to stress are also likely to be characterized by SNS and HPA activity, but the latter is thought to exert predominantly suppressive, nonreversible influences on the immune system. Lasting stress also appears to deplete the number of NK cells in blood, although it is not clear where these cells go when they have left the bloodstream or how these changes differ from the reversible effects of acute stress. The potential mechanisms responsible for these long-term effects are presently unknown. Nevertheless, the potential consequences of having persistently low NK cell activity related to chronic stress may represent a health hazard, although no direct relationship has been established so far between disease development and chronically low NK activity.

NK Cells and Cancer

Based on NK cell responsiveness to stress, many studies have used NK activity as a biomarker of stress, attempting to correlate it with health, disease, and the ability to cope with life. This is particularly evident in studies linking stress and depression with development of cancer. By and large, these studies were performed with small cohorts of patients and yielded conflicting results. Although the literature dealing with the involvement of stress in cancer development, cancer progression, or response of cancer to treatment is extensive, few large-cohort investigations of immune surveillance and stress are available. In one such study of 6284 Jewish Israelis who had lost an adult son, there was an increased incidence of melanoma in the parents of accident victims and war casualties relative to nonbereaved members of the population. Unfortunately, no NK-cell numbers or activity was measured in this study. Because stress and depression have been linked with the altered cytokine profile (e.g., increased pro-inflammatory cytokine production), downregulation of MNC class I and class II molecules, and reduced NK activity in numerous studies and because the same biological effects accompany cancer progression, the tendency has been to seek correlations among stress, NK activity, and cancer and to speculate that NK activity may be a surrogate marker linking stress to cancer. However, inconsistent preliminary data and a lack of prospective long-term studies in large cohorts of humans do not at this time permit the conclusion that NK activity can be considered a biomarker of stress or a biomarker of cancer development progression.

See Also the Following Articles

Depression Models; Industrialized Societies; Lymph Nodes; Immune Surveillance – Cancer, Effects of Stress on; Immunity; Immune Response; Immune Cell Distribution, Effects of Stress on; Immune Function, Stress-Induced Enhancement.

Further Reading

Bryceson, Y. T., March, M. E., Barber, D. F., et al. (2005). Cytolytic granule polarization and degranulation controlled by different receptors in resting NK cells. *Journal of Experimental Medicine* 202, 1001–1012.

Hamerman, J. A., Ogasawara, K. and Lanier, L. L. (2005). NK cells in innate immunity. *Current Opinion in Immunology* 17, 29–35.

Lanier, L. L. (2003). Natural killer cell receptor signaling. *Current Opinion in Immunology* 15, 308–314.

Rajagopalan, S. and Long, E. O. (2005). Understanding how combinations of HLA and KIR genes influence disease. *Journal of Experimental Medicine* 201, 1025–1029.

Reiche, E. M. V., Nunes, S. O. V. and Morimoto, H. K. (2004). Stress, depression, the immune system, and cancer. *Oncology* 5, 617–625.

Whiteside, T. L. and Herberman, R. B. (1995). The role of natural killer cells in immune surveillance of cancer. *Current Opinion in Immunology* 7, 704–710.

> **Necrotic Neural Injury** *See:* Brain Trauma; Glucocorticoids – Adverse Effects on the Nervous System.

Negative Affect

A A Stone and A A Gorin
State University of New York, Stony Brook, NY, USA

This article is reproduced from the previous edition, volume 3, pp 8–11, © 2000, Elsevier Inc.

Definition of Negative Affect
Role of Negative Affect in Stress Research
Conceptual Issues
Measurement

Glossary

Arousal	A state of activation, surprise, and intensity.
Circumplex model	A dimensional approach to mood wherein two independent dimensions are crossed to form a two-dimensional space encompassing all mood states.
Negative affectivity	A stable personality characteristic associated with high levels of negative mood; sometimes referred to as trait negative affect or neuroticism.
Positive affect	Experiences high in the qualities of joyfulness, happiness, pleasantness, and cheerfulness.
Specific affect model	Position that there is a limited set of distinctive moods that do not fall along one or two dimensions.

Definition of Negative Affect

Negative affect refers to a set of states that fall into the broad class of phenomena known as mood, emotion, and affect. Emotions and affects sometimes refer to shorter fluctuations than mood (minutes versus hours), although these terms are often used interchangeably. These terms all refer to constructs that include subjective feelings, behavioral changes, and physiological states, and the majority of research on negative affect has focused on subjective states. Surprisingly, there are only weak to moderate associations among subjective, behavioral, and physiological indicators of mood. Research in the field of psychophysiology, for instance, has found that facial expressions associated with an affective state (say anxiety) are only moderately correlated with the subjective experience of either anxiety or physiological activation. This suggests that the three domains of mood may be measuring somewhat different aspects of the construct.

The functions of moods and emotions have been debated since Darwin, but most theorists agree that emotions have a strong biological basis, assisting in the preparation, shifting, and maintenance of action. In everyday life, individuals often assign emotions a primary role when describing the causes of their behavior. In addition to action, emotions and mood can also influence attention and memory. Emotional arousal, for example, may narrow attentional focus, and the recall of certain memories may be mood-dependent. While there is considerable debate about the function and definition of mood, for this article, we will largely focus on the subjective component of negative affect because this is the most common and useful definition available. Also, using a multidimensional definition of mood results in a tremendous overlap with other components of the stress model (namely, the environmental and physiological aspects of stress).

Role of Negative Affect in Stress Research

In order to understand the importance of negative affect in stress research, we first place it in the context of a general model of stress. As earlier articles of this work have shown, there are different conceptual models for thinking about stress. One model states that environmental changes interact with individuals' predisposing psychological states to produce a subjective experience and a concurrent set of physiological changes. Some stress theorists focus entirely on alterations in the environment to define stress, for example, using life events to define stress. Other theorists focus on the resulting physiological states; a good example of this is the seminal work of Hans Selye. Still other theorists base their definition of stress on the subjective perception of stress, which is the underlying conceptualization used in the Perceived Stress Scale.

Clearly, the latter definition of stress is closely linked to the construct of negative affect. It is difficult to imagine an individual reporting that they are feeling stressed, out of control, and unable to cope, yet not feeling high levels of negative affect at the same time. In a similar vein, it is difficult to imagine how the undesirable events that environmentalists use to define stress would not invoke negative affect. Death of a loved one is a major life event that has been used to define stress, and certainly negative affect is associated with mourning the death of a loved one. However, theorists who define stress as any alterations in one's environment (even positive ones) would not necessarily require associated alterations in negative moods.

Conceptual Issues

Behavioral scientists have devised several ways of measuring negative affect and the more general concept of mood. These range from single-item measures that are anchored with positive and negative descriptors at opposite ends of the scale to much more complicated, multidimensional adjective checklists. Several conceptual issues need to be discussed to place assessment methods in an appropriate context.

Structure of Negative Affect

The first issue pertains to the structure of mood. Two opposing views have emerged about how to best represent structure, namely, the specific affect approach and the dimensional approach. The specific affect approach views mood as being made up of a number of distinct states that, though related to one another, have distinguishing characteristics. According to this approach, different negative affects are associated with unique patterns of physiological activation, for example, the type of arousal associated with fear differs from that associated with anger. Both of these states are considered negative affect, yet each is associated with a distinctive pattern of subjective, physiological, and facial characteristics. In contrast, the dimensional approach rejects the idea of specific affects in favor of a limited number of core affective dimensions. One of the dimensions often discussed concerns the degree of negativity. The most developed dimensional model is based on two affective dimensions that are crossed to yield a two-dimensional space. Like primary colors mixed together in order to create a vast array of hues, the moods in this two-dimensional space are each composed of a mixture of positive and negative affect. Within the dimensional

approach to mood, there are differing viewpoints concerning how to label the dimensions and create the two-dimensional space. Watson and Tellegen advance the position that positive affect and negative affect are the two core dimensions, whereas Russell advances the position that a single bipolar dimension of positive/negative is crossed with a unipolar activation dimension. Both viewpoints have support in the literature and scales based on each approach are currently in use.

Regardless of the specific dimensional labels used, poles of the dimensions are typically anchored with representative adjectives. The pleasant pole is generally indicated with adjectives such as happy, delighted, glad, cheerful, warm-hearted, and pleased, whereas the unpleasant pole is often marked with adjectives such as unhappy, miserable, sad, gloomy, and blue. Proponents of the activation dimensional construct label the high activation end with words such as aroused, astonished, stimulated, surprised, active, and intense, whereas the low activation end is marked with words such as quiet, tranquil, still, inactive, idle, and passive.

Content of Negative Affect

The second conceptual issue concerns the way people experience and recall their moods. When asked to report about their moods over a distinct period of time, for example, the last day or week, do people report about the frequency of their moods or do they report about the intensity of their moods? This question was addressed in a study by Diener and colleagues. By varying instructions on a mood checklist, they found that reports of mood intensity were not related to reports of mood frequency, indicating that frequency and intensity are two different ways of conceptualizing mood. From an applied perspective, when people are asked in a more general way how their mood was over the last day or over the last week, it is not clear whether they are reporting about the frequency or intensity. This ambiguity requires future research in order to facilitate interpretation of mood assessments.

Recall of Negative Affect

A third conceptual issue concerns individuals' abilities to recall mood states and whether reports of mood over long periods of time are accurate. Research on autobiographical memory has shown that there are a number of biases that occur in retrospective recall. For example, comparisons of momentary (immediate) and retrospectively recalled moods suggest that rather than providing an accurate summary of moods, retrospective reports are heavily based on more recent experiences. Several other biases in the recall of mood have been identified, leading some experts to advocate that a summary of momentary moods may be most appropriate for characterizing mood over longer periods of time.

Stability of Negative Affect

A fourth issue concerns the stability of negative affect over time, an issue related to the prior two points. A distinction has been drawn in the literature between state negative affect, which refers to transient fluctuations in negative emotions, and trait negative affect, which refers to enduring and stable levels of negative affect over extended periods time. Trait negative affect, also known as negative affectivity and neuroticism, is associated with trait anxiety, poor self-esteem, introspective and ruminative behaviors, and negative views of the world and others. Important to the conceptualization of negative affect, recent studies have revealed that state negative affect and negative affectivity have differential influences on health. A study by Cohen and colleagues, for example, measured the impact of negative affect on symptoms of respiratory viral infection. Levels of state and trait negative affect were both associated with amount of subjective health complaints; however, only state negative affect was predictive of objective measures of illness (i.e., mucus weight). This study highlights the need to consider the stability of negative affect in conceptualizations of mood. As discussed below, decisions made about the stability of negative affect influence its measurement.

Measurement

There are numerous methods for measuring negative affect and mood. Among the single-item self-report measures of negative affect available, the use of a simple 0 to 7 point scale has often been used. The ends of such scales are often marked with not at all and extremely, and people simply rate where their current mood (state) and/or their general mood (trait) falls along the continuum. This measurement strategy has been used by proponents of both the specific affect and dimensional approach. Other single-item scales include bipolar scales marked with adjectives such as happy at one end of the scale and sad at the other end, and graphical approaches that use adjective labeled grids and circles based on a circumplex model of emotion. While single-item measures are available, by far the most commonly used approach to the self-report measurement of mood is the multi-item adjective checklist. This type of scale presents a participant with a number of adjectives

that are selected to represent either the specific or dimensional approach to mood. Each adjective is rated by the participants as to how well it represents either their current mood (state) or typical mood (trait). Linear combinations of adjectives are created (usually a simple summation of responses to selected groups of adjectives representing scales or dimensions) that index the level of mood. The psychometric properties (reliability, validity) of these questionnaires are excellent, and participants and patients have little difficulty completing them.

Examples of well-established mood-adjective checklists include the Nowlis Mood Adjective Checklist, which has a brief, 36-adjective version; the Profile of Mood States, which is composed of 65 adjectives and is rated for how the subjects felt over the past week; the Multiple Affect Adjective Checklist, which uses 132 adjectives to measure depression, anxiety, and hostility; and the Positive and Negative Affect Schedule, which taps the positive and negative dimensions of mood with 10 adjectives for each scale.

Observational methods for the measurement of mood are also available, although they are usually much more cumbersome and difficult to employ. Observational coding of facial expressions is a highly complex, labor-intensive, yet reliable method for measuring negative emotion. Theories of emotion involving facial feedback have been proposed, with some evidence supporting the utility of the observational measurement. While not often used in the stress literature, facial expression measurement of affect might be profitably employed in laboratory-based experiments.

In terms of negative affectivity, perhaps the most widely employed measure is the Neuroticism, Extraversion, and Openness to Experience Personality Inventory (NEO-PI). The NEO-PI is a self-report personality inventory that assesses negative affectivity and other dimensions of personality. In addition to the NEO-PI, several other measures are available that can be used to assess either state or trait negative affect, depending on the instructions given regarding the time frame of focus.

There is, then, an impressive assortment of measures for the investigator interested in measuring negative affect. Choice of an instrument for a given study will depend upon the nature of the task and the researcher's decision about the model of affect that best suits their needs.

See Also the Following Articles

Affective Disorders; Anger; Anxiety; Depression Models; Hostility; Stress Generation.

Further Reading

Cohen, S., Doyle, W. J., Skoner, D. P., Fireman, P., Gwaltney, J. M. and Newsom, J. T. (1995). State and trait negative affect as predictors of objective and subjective symptoms of respiratory viral infections. *Journal of Personality and Social Psychology* **68**, 159–169.

Diener, E., Larsen, R. J., Levine, S. and Emmons, R. A. (1985). Intensity and frequency: dimensions underlying positive and negative affect. *Journal of Personality and Social Psychology* **48**, 1253–1265.

Leventhal, H. and Tomarken, A. J. (1986). Emotion: today's problems. *Annual Review of Psychology* **37**, 565–610.

Oatley, K. and Jenkins, J. M. (1992). Human emotions: function and dysfunction. *Annual Review of Psychology* **43**, 55–85.

Stone, A. A. (1995). Measurement of affective response. In: Cohen, S., Kessler, R. C. & Underwood, L. U. (eds.) *Measuring stress: a guide for health and social scientists*, pp. 148–171. New York: Oxford University Press.

Watson, D. and Clark, L. A. (1984). Negative affectivity: The disposition to experience aversive emotional states. *Psychological Bulletin* **96**, 465–490.

Watson, D. and Tellegen, A. (1985). Toward a consensual structure of mood. *Psychological Bulletin* **98**, 219–235.

Negative Life Events *See:* Community Studies; Life Events Scale; Life Events and Health.

Neighborhood Stress and Health

A V Diez Roux
University of Michigan, Ann Arbor, MI, USA

Neighborhoods and Health
Neighborhood Stressors and Their Measurement
Evidence Linking Neighborhood Stressors and Health

Neighborhoods and Health

Neighborhoods have recently received increasing attention as relevant to health. A large body of work has documented associations of neighborhood socioeconomic characteristics (or measures of neighborhood deprivation) with a variety of health-related outcomes, including health behaviors as well as physical and mental health outcomes. For example, neighborhood disadvantage has been associated with higher prevalence of smoking, unhealthy diets, and greater incidence and prevalence of cardiovascular disease. Although the strength of the associations is often small compared to those observed for individual-level socioeconomic characteristics, they are consistent across studies and tend to persist after statistical controls for person-level measures of social position, suggesting an independent effect of neighborhood context on health.

The extent to which associations between neighborhood socioeconomic characteristics and health reported in observational studies reflect causal mechanisms remains a subject of research and debate. An important limitation of existing work pertains to the use of neighborhood deprivation or neighborhood disadvantage as a proxy for the specific neighborhood characteristics that may be relevant to the health outcome being studied. The use of aggregate measures of neighborhood disadvantage also raises questions regarding whether residual confounding by person-level socioeconomic position could explain some of the associations observed. An important consideration in interpreting results to date is that neighborhood constructs are grossly misspecified in existing research because of its reliance on very crude proxies for neighborhoods (usually administrative areas such as wards in the UK or census tracts in the United States) and limitations in the neighborhood-level measures used. Hence, neighborhood effects are likely to be underestimated compared to the effects of individual-level variables, for which measurement strategies are much better developed.

Several specific mechanisms through which neighborhood contexts may affect health have been proposed. Some of these mechanisms involve features of the physical environment of neighborhoods and others involve features of the social environment.

The physical environment includes not only traditional physical exposures such as environmental toxins and noise, but also features of the man-made environment such as street layout, transportation availability, land use, presence and design of public spaces, and other aspects of urban design. These man-made physical features of neighborhoods have recently been referred to as the built environment. The social environment includes social norms, social cohesion, and social capital and features such as violence or social disorder. The proximate individual-level pathways through which neighborhood physical and social environments may affect individual health include health behaviors and exposures to acute and chronic stressors. For example, it has been hypothesized that street connectivity and land use mix may promote walking in daily life and physically active lifestyles. It has also been proposed that certain features of neighborhoods may serve as chronic or acute stressors with consequent physiological responses that may impair health. An important focus of current research on neighborhoods and health is to empirically examine the presence and relative importance of these different pathways and the specific neighborhood characteristics linked to them.

Neighborhood Stressors and Their Measurement

Although exposure to neighborhood sources of acute and chronic stress is often hypothesized to play a role in the relationship between neighborhood context and health, empirical documentation of the health effects of neighborhood stressors remains limited. There is still scant information of what the most relevant stress-generating features of neighborhoods might be, or on the way in which these features should be measured in empirical investigations. The most common domains investigated as potential neighborhood stressors include neighborhood problems, neighborhood disorder, violence and safety, and physical ambient characteristics.

Neighborhood problems are generally assessed by asking residents to report on the extent to which they perceive that different issues are a problem in their neighborhood. Examples of the neighborhood domains assessed include violence, noise, traffic, litter, air quality, vandalism, drug use, and presence and quality of resources and services. Responses are typically added to construct an index of neighborhood problems. Cumulative exposure to neighborhood problems is hypothesized to be a source of chronic stress.

Neighborhood disorder refers to conditions and activities in the neighborhood that indicate a breakdown of social order. Scales to measure neighborhood disorder typically assess neighborhood markers of social incivility, disruption, and physical decay. Some researchers distinguish physical and social disorder. Signs of physical disorder include the presence of abandoned buildings, noise, graffiti, vandalism, and disrepair. Signs of social disorder include the presence of crime, loitering, public drinking or drug use, conflicts, and indifference. It is hypothesized that these signs of disorder signify a breakdown of social control and result in the experience of a threatening environment for all residents, regardless of whether they themselves have been victimized. Long-term exposure to neighborhoods with high levels of social and physical disorder is hypothesized to result in chronic stress.

Violence and perceived safety are among the most common neighborhood sources of stress investigated in empirical studies. Measures of neighborhood violence are constructed using survey responses to neighborhood violence scales or using crime statistics obtained from governmental agencies. Perceived safety is also assessed through surveys of residents. It is hypothesized that exposure to violence or to an unsafe residential environment is a source of chronic stress.

Physical ambient characteristics such as noise, crowding, housing characteristics, and proximity to environmental toxins have also been hypothesized to be sources of stress that vary across neighborhoods. These ambient characteristics are usually measured using census data or by linking residence data to other data sources, such as noise measurements or proximity to airports or environmental toxins. In contrast to neighborhood problems, neighborhood disorder, and violence/safety, which are hypothesized to affect health through psychosocial mechanisms, the factors investigated under the general rubric of physical ambient characteristics may affect health through pathophysiological mechanisms that do not involve psychological stress. For example, crowding may affect the probability of contracting infectious diseases through increased disease transmission, and environmental toxins may have direct carcinogenic or cardiovascular effects. However, it has also been argued that the perception of the presence of these physical environmental characteristics may have psychosocial consequences analogous to those observed for other stressors.

Evidence Linking Neighborhood Stressors and Health

The evidence linking neighborhood stressors to health remains limited. Most research has focused on self-reported health outcomes and health behaviors. For example, perceived neighborhood disorder has been found to be associated with poor self-reported health, poor physical functioning, adverse mental health outcomes, the presence of chronic health conditions, and heavy drinking. Although it has long been hypothesized that neighborhood sources of stress may contribute to physical health outcomes such as blood pressure, very few studies have linked neighborhood stressors to objectively measured physical health outcomes. Two physical health outcomes examined in relation to potential neighborhood stressors are blood pressure (or blood pressure reactivity) and low birth weight.

Causal inference from existing studies of neighborhood stressors and health is rendered complex by their observational design and the possibility of confounding by individual-level factors associated with place of residence. Most observational studies have only limited ability to control for these individual-level factors. Another important set of confounders includes other neighborhood attributes such as features of the built environment, which often covary with the measures of neighborhood stressors used. Measures of the physical and built environment of neighborhoods are often part of the neighborhood stressors scales used, making it difficult to determine whether it is the physical feature itself through its effects on health behaviors or the psychosocial consequence of the factor that results in the health effects. There is also little consensus on the conceptualization or the measurement of the features of neighborhoods that may be sources of stress. Thus, the extent to which neighborhood contexts affect health through the stress pathway and the relative importance of this pathway compared to pathways involving environmental influences on health behaviors or direct effects of environmental exposures (such as toxins or allergens) remain largely undetermined.

See Also the Following Articles

Community Studies; Crowding Stress; Cushing's Syndrome, Neuropsychiatric Aspects; Environmental Factors; Health and Socioeconomic Status.

Further Reading

Aneshensel, C. and Sucoff, C. (1996). The neighborhood context of adolescent mental health. *Journal of Health and Social Behavior* 37(4), 293–310.

Diez Roux, A. V. (2001). Investigating area and neighborhood effects on health. *American Journal of Public Health* 91(11), 1783–1789.

Diez Roux, A. V., SteinMerkin, S., Arnett, D., et al. (2001). Neighborhood of residence and incidence of coronary heart disease. *New England Journal of Medicine* 345, 99–106.

Evans, G. W. (2001). Environmental stress and health. In: Baum, A., Revenson, T. A. & Singer, J. E. (eds.) *Handbook of health psychology*, pp. 365–385. Mahwah, NJ: Lawrence Erlbaum Associates Inc.

Ewart, C. and Suchday, S. (2002). Discovering how urban poverty and violence affect health: development and validation of a neighborhood stress index. *Health Psychology* 21, 254–262.

Gee, G. and Payne-Sturges, D. C. (2004). Environmental health disparities: a framework integrating psychosocial and environmental concepts. *Environmental Health Perspectives* 112, 1645–1653.

Harburg, E., Erfurt, J. C., Chape, C., et al. (1973). Socioecological stressor areas and black white blood pressure: Detroit. *Journal of Chronic Diseases* 26, 595–611.

Hill, T. and Angel, R. (2005). Neighborhood disorder, psychological distress, and heavy drinking. *Social Science and Medicine* 61, 965–975.

Latkin, C. A. and Curry, A. D. (2003). Stressful neighborhoods and depression: a prospective study of the impact of neighborhood disorder. *Journal of Health and Social Behavior* 44, 34–44.

Morenoff, F. (2003). Neighborhood mechanisms and the spatial dynamics of low birth weight. *American Journal of Sociology* 108, 976–1017.

Perkins, D. D. and Taylor, R. B. (1996). Ecological assessments of community disorder: their relationship to fear of crime and theoretical implications. *American Journal of Community Psychology* 24(1), 63–107.

Ross, C. E. and Mirowsky, J. (2001). Neighborhood disadvantage, disorder, and health. *Journal of Health and Social Behavior* 42(3), 258–276.

Steptoe, A. and Feldman, P. M. (2001). Neighborhood problems as sources of chronic stress: development of a measure of neighborhood problems and associations with socioeconomic status and health. *Annals of Behavioral Medicine* 23, 177–185.

Wilson, K., Elliott, S., Law, M., et al. (2004). Linking perceptions of neighbourhood to health in Hamilton, Canada. *Journal of Epidemiology and Community Health* 58, 192–198.

Nelson's Syndrome

A Stathopoulou and K Dimitriou
General Hospital of Athens, Athens, Greece
G Kaltsas
University of Athens, Athens, Greece

This article is a revision of the previous edition article by G Kaltsas and A Grossman, volume 3, pp 12–13, © 2000, Elsevier Inc.

Pathogenesis
Incidence
Pathophysiology – Molecular Pathology
Predictive Factors
Clinical Features
Diagnosis and Treatment

Glossary

Adrenocorticotropin (ACTH)	A 39-amino-acid peptide hormone produced from the pituitary, from a larger precursor molecule (pro-opiomelanocortin) that stimulates the secretion of glucocorticoids, mineralocorticoids, and androgenic steroids from the adrenal cortex.
Cushing's disease	The most common cause of Cushing's syndrome as a result of ACTH hypersecretion from a pituitary tumor (usually a microadenoma 3–10 mm in diameter).
Cushing's syndrome	Chronic glucocorticoid excess that leads to skin, muscle, bone, neuropsychiatric, gonadal and metabolic abnormalities (glucose intolerance and hyperlipidemia), obesity, and hypertension.
Gamma knife	A stereotactic radiosurgery device that allows well-defined, deep-seated brain tumors (<3 cm in diameter) to be treated in a single session under local anesthesia, using the overlapping of narrow collimated beams from 201 cobalt-60 sources.
Transsphenoidal surgery	Treatment of choice for pituitary tumors; the pituitary is approached from the nasal cavity though the sphenoid sinus, the anterior–inferior sella is removed, and the dura layer is incised. The adenoma is removed selectively while normal pituitary tissue is identified and preserved.

Nelson's syndrome defines patients with pituitary-dependent Cushing's syndrome (CS), i.e., Cushing's disease (CD), who have undergone bilateral adrenalectomy and have developed pituitary expansion with increased plasma adrenocorticotropin (ACTH) levels and progressive pigmentation of the skin. Total adrenalectomy still offers the only definitive curative procedure to lower cortisol levels adequately in patients with persistent ACTH-dependent CS, in whom radiotherapy with or without medical adrenocortical enzyme-blocking therapy has been insufficient.

Pathogenesis

Plasma ACTH levels are either within the normal range or elevated modestly in patients with CD. After bilateral adrenalectomy, even during cortisol replacement therapy, plasma ACTH levels may rise as much as 20-fold, and this may be associated with tumor growth. Nelson's syndrome represents the clinical progression of a pre-existing ACTH-secreting adenoma following bilateral adrenalectomy and normalization of the hypercortisolism; the suppressive effect of excessive levels of cortisol is no longer present, ACTH secretion markedly increases, and the pituitary adenoma may thus progress. However, the exact underlying mechanism(s) leading to tumor development and excessive ACTH secretion is not well defined. Following corticotropin-releasing hormone (CRH) infusion, ACTH secretion is stimulated greater and for a longer period of time in patients with Nelson's syndrome than in those with CD. An increase in basal ACTH production and pulsatile secretion with significantly greater quantitative regularity of serial ACTH release patterns in Nelson's syndrome compared to untreated CD has been demonstrated.

Extremely high plasma ACTH levels and aggressive neoplastic growth might be explained by the lack of appropriate glucocorticoid negative feedback due to defective glucocorticoid signal transduction. At the transcriptional level, expression of pro-opiomelanocortin (POMC), the precursor molecule of ACTH, is under negative feedback control by glucocorticoids. Although mutations of the POMC promoter region that could lead to relative resistance to glucocorticoids have generally been excluded in patients with Nelson's syndrome, in one of four such tumors a mutation was found at the level of the glucocorticoid receptor, explaining the glucocorticoid resistance and probably contributing to the tumoral progression.

Incidence

Currently, bilateral adrenalectomy is rarely used to treat CD as primary surgery, with an initial cure rate of approximately 50% and an improvement rate of around 80%. Although longer follow up after primary surgery presents an increase in recurrences, there still remain some patients with CD who will benefit from bilateral adrenalectomy. Furthermore, bilateral adrenalectomy is still used after the failure of repeated transsphenoidal surgery or pituitary radiotherapy to cure CD, in patients in whom the source of ACTH cannot be determined easily, and when the medical control of hypercortisolemia cannot be achieved adequately. Such patients are at risk of developing Nelson's syndrome, which ranges from 8% to 38% in adults, mainly in patients treated at an early age. Approximately 30% of patients develop classical Nelson's syndrome following bilateral adrenalectomy with progressive hyperpigmentation and an obvious ACTH-secreting tumor with a time interval between adrenalectomy and the diagnosis of Nelson's syndrome ranging from 0.5 to 24 years. Another 50% develop evidence of a microadenoma without marked progression, while around 20% never develop a progressive tumor. The reason for these differences in clinical behavior is not well defined and difficult to be predicted currently prior to adrenal surgery.

Pathophysiology – Molecular Pathology

Although several candidate genes that control the cell cycle, apoptosis, angiogenic, and growth factors as well as other signaling pathways have been studied, no clear information unraveling the pathophysiology of corticotroph adenomas and/or Nelson's tumors has been established. It is not yet clear whether corticotroph adenoma formation is the result of a unique molecular mechanism or a constellation of many different possibilities. However, glucocorticoids, and therefore their deprivation also, might exert variable effects on tumor growth.

Predictive Factors

Neither the duration of disease before adrenalectomy, the preadrenalectomy cortisol levels, and the suppressibility to dexamethasone administration nor the duration of postadrenalectomy follow up has been found to be an important predictor. High basal ACTH levels after adrenalectomy in excess of 600 ng l^{-1}, particularly if found less than 1 year postoperatively, were predictive of subsequent Nelson's syndrome in some, but not all, studies suggesting that no unique threshold value can be established. Although several studies have suggested that the preadrenalectomy age was the most important predictive factor for developing Nelson's syndrome, as the great majority of patients who developed Nelson's syndrome underwent an adrenalectomy before the age of 35 years,

this was not confirmed from subsequent studies. Pregnant women and children also seem to be at higher risk for the disease. Subnormal dose or noncontinuous glucocorticoid replacement therapy has also been thought to be associated with increased risk of development of the syndrome. Although a clustering of clinical, biochemical, and radiological factors can be used to try to predict the development of Nelson's syndrome there is currently no unique factor with a strong predictive value. It is hoped that a detailed molecular analysis between the slowly and rapidly growing corticotroph adenomas following adrenalectomy might provide some answers and can be used as a predictive marker.

Clinical Features

Pituitary tumors in patients with classic Nelson's syndrome are among the most aggressive and rapidly progressive tumors. All patients with Nelson's syndrome present with hyperpigmentation similar to that in Addison's disease and often an expanding intra- and/or extrasellar mass lesion. Symptoms are a consequence of extension of the tumor and compression of surrounding structures; headaches, visual field defects, and extraocular nerve palsies are among the most common clinical signs. Cases of diabetes insipidus and hypopituitarism are exceptional. Malignant transformations with central nervous system and distant metastases, as well as behavioral changes, have been described; interestingly, a number of ACTH-secreting pituitary carcinomas have developed in the context of Nelson's syndrome. Pituitary apoplexy and hydrocephalus may also complicate the course of these tumors. In addition, complications related to increased ACTH levels have been reported. Paratesticular and paraovarian tumors producing cortisol or androgens in an ACTH-dependent manner as well as testicular adrenal rests with hyperplasia have been described.

Diagnosis and Treatment

The diagnosis is suspected clinically when hyperpigmentation and signs of other mass effects on adjacent tissues develop in a patient with previous bilateral adrenalectomy and is confirmed by measuring plasma ACTH levels, which are extremely high, often ranging from 220 pmol l^{-1} (1000 ng l^{-1}) to 2200 pmol l^{-1} (10 000 ng l^{-1}). However, ACTH levels do not reflect accurately the size or aggressiveness of the tumor.

It is important to note the prevailing cortisol level when measuring ACTH, as patients with CD postadrenalectomy often have considerably elevated ACTH levels before their morning hydrocortisone dose, whereas 1–2 h later the level may show a highly significant fall.

Thus, the diagnosis of Nelson's syndrome requires the presence of rising levels of ACTH in association with evidence of tumor growth and the presence of optimal hydrocortisone replacement therapy; pigmentation and high levels alone may simply indicate inadequate replacement therapy. The presence of tumor is confirmed by computered tomography (CT) and magnetic resonance imaging (MRI) scans; in contrast to CD, these tumors are usually macroadenomas.

Nelson's tumors are recognized for their large size and aggressive and invasive growth. Once the diagnosis of Nelson's syndrome is made, pituitary surgery is the initial mode of treatment. Most neurosurgeons approach the tumor by the transsphenoidal route and resect as much as possible. Pituitary surgery of Nelson's macroadenomas should be performed before extrasellar expansion of the tumor occurs, as it is probably more successful when Nelson's adenomas are relatively small. Parasellar expansion, especially cavernous sinus invasion, by the pituitary tumor has been related to low surgical cure rate. Moreover, in large Nelson's tumors, spontaneous hemorrhage in the tumor can occur, which can lead to severe neurological complications. However, complete excision is not always possible and adjuvant treatment is usually required, especially if the tumor has not been irradiated previously.

The role of external beam radiation either before or postoperatively in preventing Nelson's syndrome in CD treated with bilateral adrenalectomy has not been defined clearly; adequate doses of pituitary radiotherapy, particularly immediately postoperatively, appear to decrease such an occurrence. Following the application of conventional radiotherapy, 50% of patients with Nelson's syndrome obtained normalization of plasma ACTH levels at a median of 9.5 years. However, no prospective studies comparing the incidence of Nelson's syndrome between patients who had been irradiated with either conventional or focal radiotherapy with patients who have not received such treatment are currently available.

The role of adjuvant focal beam radiotherapy in cases of patients who had previously received conventional pituitary radiotherapy, either with stereotactic multiarc treatment (SMART) from a linear accelerator or the so-called gamma knife, is currently being investigated. A recent study failed to demonstrate any substantial response in tumor size in patients with Nelson's syndrome who received SMART.

The majority of these highly aggressive and infiltrating pituitary tumors in patients with Nelson's syndrome frequently respond poorly to (repeated) surgical and radiotherapeutic procedures with progressive tumor growth and rising ACTH levels. An alternative approach for such patients is medical treatment to suppress ACTH hypersecretion; bromocriptine, cyproheptidine, and sodium valpronate have all been used to transiently control ACTH secretion, but with minimal effect on pituitary tumor growth. Somatostatin analogs have also been used, obtaining some control of ACTH levels but not tumor size. The use of cytotoxic chemotherapy for highly aggressive tumors has also been advocated although this treatment modality is applied when no other therapeutic options are available. Recently it has been demonstrated that corticotroph adenomas express in higher density somatostatin receptor subtype 5 rather than subtype 2, which is the main target of currently available somatostatin analogs. It is believed that the newly developed somatostain analogs that selectively bind to somatostatin receptor 5 will be more efficacious. Following recent *in vitro* data demonstrating that rosiglitazone (a peroxisomal proliferator-activated receptor (PPAR)-γ agonist) may lead to enhanced apoptosis and decreased cell division, PPAR-γ agonists show new potential for the prevention and treatment of Nelson's syndrome. Retinoids are also under investigation as it seems that they directly suppress ACTH secretion by glucocorticoid tumors.

Further Reading

Andreassen, M. and Kristensen, L. O. (2005). Rosiglitazone for prevention or adjuvant treatment of Nelson's syndrome after bilateral adrenalectomy. *European Journal of Endocrinology* **153**, 503–505.

Assie, G., Bahurel, H., Bertherat, J., et al. (2004). The Nelson's syndrome . . . revisited. *Pituitary* **7**, 209–215.

Gaffey, T. A., Scheithauer, B. W., Lloyd, R. V., et al. (2002). Corticotroph carcinoma of the pituitary: a clinicopathological study. Report of four cases. *Journal of Neurosurgery* **96**, 352–360.

Herman-Bonert, V. and Fagin, J. A. (1995). Molecular pathogenesis of pituitary tumors. *Baillières Clinical Endocrinology and Metabolism* **9**, 203–223.

Jenkins, P. J., Trainer, P. J., Plowman, P. N., et al. (1994). The long-term outcome after adrenalectomy and prophylactic pituitary radiotherapy in adrenocorticotropin-dependent Cushing's syndrome. *Journal of Clinical Endocrinology and Metabolism* **79**, 165–171.

Karl, M., Von Wichert, G., Kempter, E., et al. (1996). Nelson's syndrome associated with somatic frame shift mutation in the glucocorticoid receptor gene. *Journal of Clinical Endocrinology and Metabolism* **81**, 124–129.

Kasperlink-Zaluska, A. A. and Jeske, W. (2005). Letters to the editors. *Clinical Endocrinology* **63**, 232–237.

Kasperlik-Zaluska, A. A., Nielubxicz, J., Wislawski, J., et al. (1983). Nelson's syndrome: incidence and prognosis. *Clinical Endocrinology* 19, 693–698.

Kemink, L., Pieters, G., Hermus, A., et al. (1994). Patient's age is asimple predictive for the development of Nelson's syndrome after total adrenalectomy for Cushing's disease. *Journal of Clinical Endocrinology and Metabolism* 79, 887–889.

Kemink, S. A., Grotenhuis, J. A., De Vries, J., et al. (2001). Management of Nelson's syndrome: Observations in fifteen patients. *Clinical Endocrinology* 54, 45–52.

Kelly, P. A., Samandouras, G., Grossman, A. B., et al. (2002). Neurosurgical treatment of Nelson's syndrome. *Journal of Clinical Endocrinology and Metabolism* 87, 5465–5469.

Nagesser, S. K., van Seters, A. P., Kievit, J., et al. (2000). Long-term results of total adrenalectomy for Cushing's disease. *World Journal of Surgery* 24, 108–113.

Oldfield, E. H., Schulte, H. M., Chrousos, G. P., et al. (1986). Corticotropin-releasing hormone (CRH) stimulation in Nelson's syndrome: response of adrenocorticotropin secretion to pulse injection and continuous infusion of CRH. *Journal of Clinical Endocrinology and Metabolism* 62, 1020–1026.

Pernicone, P. J., Scheithauer, B. W., Sebo, T. J., et al. (1997). Pituitary carcinoma: a clinicopathologic study of 15 cases. *Cancer* 79, 804–812.

Van Aken, M. O., Pereira, A. M., van den Berg, G., et al. (2004). Profound amplification of secretory-burst mass and anomalous regularity of ACTH secretory process in patients with Nelson's syndrome compared with Cushing's disease. *Clinical Endocrinology* 60, 765–772.

Van der Hoek, J., Lamberts, S. W. and Hofland, L. J. (2004). The role of somatostatin analogs in Cushing's disease. *Pituitary* 7, 257–264.

Neonatal Handling and Stress *See:* Stress Hyporesponsive Period; Eclampsia and preeclampsia; Fetal Stress; Pregnancy, Maternal and Perinatal Stress, Effects of; 11β-Hydroxysteroid Dehydrogenases.

Neonatal Maternal Deprivation *See:* Stress Hyporesponsive Period; Eclampsia and preeclampsia; Fetal Stress; Pregnancy, Maternal and Perinatal Stress, Effects of; 11β-Hydroxysteroid Dehydrogenases.

Nerve Growth Factors *See:* Neuroinflammation.

Nervous System *See:* Brain and Brain Regions; Hippocampal Neurons; Hippocampus, Overview; Neuroendocrine Systems.

Neural Stem Cells

U S Sohur, J G Emsley, B D Mitchell and J D Macklis
Massachusetts General Hospital, Harvard Medical School, and Harvard University, Boston, MA, USA

Introduction

Definitions: Neural Stem Cells, Progenitors, and Precursors

Functional Adult Neurogenesis Occurs in Nonmammalian Vertebrates

The Discovery of Constitutive Adult Mammalian Neurogenesis

The Location of Neural Precursor Cells and Their Isolation *in Vitro*

Neurogenic versus Nonneurogenic Regions in the Adult Brain

Factors That Stimulate Neurogenesis

Induction of Neurogenesis in Nonneurogenic Regions of the Adult Brain

Function of Adult Neurogenesis and Neural Precursor Cells in the Adult Brain

Consequences of Disturbed Adult Neurogenesis and the Reaction of Neurogenic Regions to Disease

Conclusions and Future Prospects

Glossary

Gliogenesis	The generation of neuroglia; glia were recognized about 150 years ago as connective elements in the nervous system. There are three main types of glial cells in the CNS: astrocytes, oligodendrocytes, and microglia. Astrocytes and oligodendrocytes both develop from neuroepithelial cells, while microglia develop from mesodermal hemapoietic precursors. Glial cells are estimated to occupy about half the brain and outnumber neurons by about 10 to 1. Glia are involved in most aspects of neural function. Thus, during development, radial glia guide neuronal migration. Microglia are immune cells and are involved in neuroinflammation. Oligodendrocytes myelinate axons. Astrocytes play a pivotal role in the blood–brain barrier.
Lineage-specific precursors or progenitors	Cells with restriction to one distinct lineage (e.g., neuronal, astroglial, glial, oligodendroglial).
Multipotent progenitors	Proliferative cells of the adult brain with only limited self-renewal that can differentiate into at least two different cell lineages.
Neurogenesis	The birth of new neurons.
precursor cell	A generic term encompassing both stem and progenitor cells.
Stem cells	Stem cells of the mammalian CNS are (1) self-renewing, with the theoretically unlimited ability to produce progeny indistinguishable from themselves, (2) proliferative, continuing to undergo mitosis (though perhaps with quite long cell cycles), and (3) multipotent for the different neuroectodermal lineages of the CNS, including the multitude of different neuronal and glial subtypes.
Subgranular zone (SGZ)	Zone of the dentate gyrus that is the origin of stem cells in the hippocampus.
Subventricular zone (SVZ)	Sometimes also called the subependymal zone, this zone lies immediately adjacent to the cells (ependymal) that line the walls of the lateral cerebral ventricles. In the adult, this zone gives rise to neural precursors/stem cells, the progeny of which are immature neurons that normally migrate to the olfactory bulb

Introduction

Over most of the past century of modern neuroscience, it was thought that the adult mammalian brain was incapable of generating new neurons or having neurons added to its complex circuitry. However, recent findings show that neurogenesis, the birth of new neurons, constitutively occurs in two specific regions of the adult mammalian brain (olfactory bulb and hippocampal dentate gyrus) and that there are significant numbers of multipotent neural precursors, or stem cells, in many parts of the adult mammalian brain.

The rise of precursor cell biology has brought new life to neural transplantation and the consideration of cellular replacement strategies to treat diseases of the brain. The idea of making new neurons is appealing for neurodegenerative diseases or selective neuronal loss associated with chronic neurological or psychiatric disorders. One goal of neural precursor biology is to learn from this regionally limited, constitutive neurogenesis how to manipulate neural precursors toward therapeutic neuronal or glial repopulation. Elucidation of the relevant molecular controls might allow both control over transplanted precursor cells and the development of neuronal replacement therapies based on the recruitment of endogenous cells.

This article deals with adult neurogenesis, cellular repair of the adult mammalian central nervous system (CNS), and what is known about the location, behavior, and function of precursor cells in the adult brain. In the context of CNS regeneration, this information lies at the core of all attempts to guide neuronal or glial development from neural precursors in the adult CNS for therapeutic purposes. These topics are also important for at least two other reasons. First, adult neurogenesis and precursor cell function might play an important role in the function of the healthy and diseased brain; specifically, they may underlie particular aspects of neuronal plasticity in response to functional demands. Second, neurogenesis and precursor cell biology in the adult CNS also appear to recapitulate some of the molecular, cellular, and other requirements for neuronal development in the developing brain. Neural repair is of potential importance for neurodegenerative disorders such as amyotrophic lateral sclerosis (ALS), Parkinson's disease, and Huntington's disease, as well as acquired damage such as with spinal cord injury and stress-induced neurodegeneration.

Definitions: Neural Stem Cells, Progenitors, and Precursors

Rigorously defined, adult CNS stem cells exhibit three cardinal features: (1) they are self-renewing, with the theoretically unlimited ability to produce progeny indistinguishable from themselves; (2) they are proliferative, continuing to undergo mitosis (though perhaps with quite long cell cycles); and (3) they are multipotent for the different neuroectodermal lineages of the CNS, including the multitude of different neuronal and glial subtypes. Multipotent progenitors of the adult brain are proliferative cells with only limited self-renewal that can differentiate into at least two different cell lineages (multipotency). Lineage-specific precursors or progenitors are cells with restriction to one distinct lineage (e.g., neuronal, astroglial, glial, oligodendroglial). Together, CNS stem cells and all precursor/progenitor types are, broadly defined, precursors. It is preferred to use the term stem cell as rigorously defined previously, and to use precursor or progenitor for most forms of multipotent or lineage-restricted mitotic cells. This article uses precursor cell as a generic term encompassing both stem and progenitor cells.

Adult neurogenesis comprises the entire set of events of neuronal development, beginning with the division of a precursor cell and ending with the presence and survival of a mature, integrated, functioning new neuron. Neurogenesis is sometimes incorrectly used only in the sense of precursor cell proliferation, but this definition clearly falls short. Precursor cell proliferation is not predictive of net neurogenesis. True neuronal integration depends on many complex variables and progressive events.

Even in the absence of a fully detailed molecular characterization, neural precursor cells of the adult brain clearly possess features that justify a view of these cells as extremely promising for the goals of CNS cellular repair. They are undifferentiated, often highly mobile cells, relatively resistant to hypoxia and other injury, proliferatively active, and able to produce mature neurons and glia. The most critical caveat, however, is that precursor cells in the adult mammalian brain are heterogeneous, and, while all of these criteria might apply in many cases, it is not clear how many of the sometimes site-specific and condition-specific observations in neural precursor biology can be broadly generalized, and how many reflect particulars of a certain brain region or a certain condition.

While the identity of true CNS stem cells is as yet unknown, the heterogeneity of neural precursor cells is also an important aspect of the promise of such cells. Their variable specialization and differentiation competence provides great promise for application in medicine. The idea that one cell fits all might turn out to be as unrealistic as it is unnecessary. Adult neural precursors with partial fate restriction may, in some cases, allow for more efficient production of desired cell types. The brain itself may provide the environmental determinants for the different forms and sequelae of adult neurogenesis and gliogenesis and may powerfully enable and direct specific lineage development.

Functional Adult Neurogenesis Occurs in Nonmammalian Vertebrates

Adult neurogenesis occurs in many nonmammalian vertebrates. The medial cerebral cortex of lizards, which resembles the mammalian dentate gyrus, undergoes postnatal neurogenesis and can regenerate in response to injury. Newts can regenerate their tails, limbs, jaws, and ocular tissues and the neurons that occupy these regions. Goldfish undergo retinal neurogenesis throughout life and, impressively, can regenerate surgically excised portions of their retina in adulthood. Although some nonmammalian animals can undergo quite dramatic regeneration of neural tissue, it is unclear how relevant this phenomenon is to mammals. Indeed, it has been proposed that selective evolutionary pressures have led mammals to lose such abilities.

Birds, whose brains are much closer to mammals in complexity, also undergo postnatal neurogenesis.

Lesioned postnatal avian retina undergoes some neurogenesis, with the new neurons most likely arising from Müller glia. In songbirds, new neurons are constantly added to the high vocal center, a portion of the brain necessary for the production of learned song, as well as to specific regions elsewhere in the brain (but not all neuronal populations). It is possible to manipulate experimentally the extent to which new neurons are produced in at least one songbird, the zebra finch, which does not normally seasonally replace high vocal center (HVC-RA) projection neurons in the song production network. Inducing cell death of HVC-RA neurons in zebra finches leads to deterioration in song. Neurogenesis increases following induced cell death, and birds variably recover their ability to produce song coincident with the formation of new projections from area HVC to area RA, suggesting that induced neuronal replacement can restore a learned behavior.

The Discovery of Constitutive Adult Mammalian Neurogenesis

Ramon y Cajal (1928, p. 750) has been widely quoted as writing that "in the adult centers the nerve paths are something fixed, ended and immutable. Everything may die, nothing may be regenerated." The relative lack of recovery from CNS injury and neurodegenerative disease and the relatively subtle and extremely limited distribution of neurogenesis in the adult mammalian brain resulted in the entire field reaching the conclusion that neurogenesis does not occur in the adult mammalian brain. Joseph Altman was the first to use techniques sensitive enough to detect the ongoing cell division that occurs in adult brain. Using tritiated thymidine as a mitotic label, he published evidence that neurogenesis constitutively occurs in the hippocampus and olfactory bulb of the adult mammalian brain. These results were later replicated using tritiated thymidine labeling followed by electron microscopy. However, the absence of neuron-specific immunocytochemical markers at the time resulted in identification of putatively newborn neurons being made based on purely morphological criteria. These limitations led to a widespread lack of acceptance of these results and made research in the field difficult.

The field of adult neurogenesis was rekindled in 1992, when it was shown that precursor cells isolated from the forebrain can differentiate into neurons *in vitro*. These results, and technical advances such as the development of immunocytochemical reagents that could more easily and accurately identify the phenotype of various neural cells, led to an explosion of research in the field. Normally occurring neurogenesis

in the subventricular zone (SVZ)/olfactory bulb and the dentate gyrus subregion of the hippocampus have now been well characterized in the adult mammalian brain.

The Location of Neural Precursor Cells and Their Isolation *in Vitro*

If adult multipotent precursors were limited to the two neurogenic regions of the brain, the SVZ and dentate gyrus, it would severely limit the potential for neuronal replacement therapies based on *in situ* manipulation of endogenous precursors (**Figure 1**). However, *ex vivo* studies, in which precursors were isolated from the adult brain, provide evidence for cells with precursor cell properties in the adult brain. Such cells were first found embryonically, then in the adult hippocampus and the SVZ. Following these first reports, cells with similar properties have been isolated from many other adult mammalian brain regions as well. Neural precursor cells can be propagated in two main forms: in adherent cultures and under floating conditions, in which they aggregate to form heterogeneous ball-like structures, termed neurospheres. While it has become standard for some groups to use this so-called neurosphere-forming assay as a key criterion for neural stem cells, the ability to form a neurosphere, alone, is not a sufficiently reliable hallmark of stem cells and does not fully differentiate between various mitotic and precursor cell populations. Clonal analysis provides important additional information. By subcloning individual cells, one can test whether an individual cell from these spheres can again give rise to secondary spheres, which upon transfer into differentiation conditions can produce all neural lineages (see **Figure 1**).

In vitro, many such factors are likely to be present in the complex media used to culture neural precursors. Epidermal growth factor (EGF) and fibroblast growth factor 2 (FGF-2) are two key growth factors used in neural precursor cultures to maintain cells in their mitotic and undifferentiated state. The general effectiveness of both factors as mitogens for precursors has also been demonstrated *in vivo*, and they have been used more recently to enhance induced neurogenesis in the normally nonneurogenic CA1 region of the hippocampus after focal ischemia. However, their effects *in vivo* are not identical to those *in vitro*, and, consequently, their physiological relevance for normal neural precursor cell function of the adult brain is not known.

The efficacy of an individual growth factor *in vitro* does not prove that it plays a role in neurogenic permissiveness *in vivo*. Cell culture systems are highly artificial in many respects. *In vivo*, precursor cells

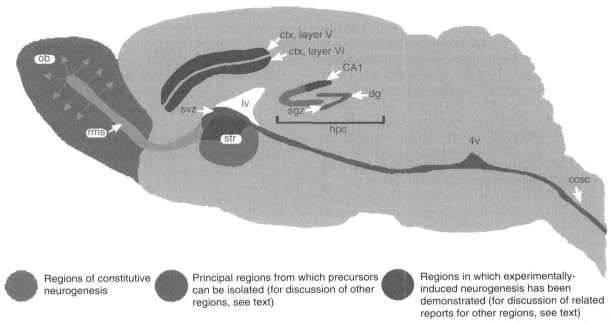

Regions of constitutive neurogenesis

Principal regions from which precursors can be isolated (for discussion of other regions, see text)

Regions in which experimentally-induced neurogenesis has been demonstrated (for discussion of related reports for other regions, see text)

Figure 1 From Emsley, J. G., et al. (2005). *Progress in Neurobiology* **75**, 321–341.

are never alone. Their relationship to a neurogenic microenvironment might be inseparable from their inherent properties. Regional differences *in vivo* reinforce the importance of the microenvironment for normal precursor cell function and neurogenesis. Nevertheless, *in vitro* studies are indispensable for many questions in neural precursor biology, including investigation of the transcriptional control of adult neurogenesis and neural differentiation.

Neurogenic versus Nonneurogenic Regions in the Adult Brain

In the adult mammalian brain, constitutive neurogenesis occurs only in the olfactory bulb and the dentate gyrus of the hippocampus. In the olfactory system, precursor cells reside in the anterior aspect of the SVZ in the walls of the lateral ventricles, migrate into the olfactory bulb, and differentiate into granule or periglomerular interneurons. In the dentate gyrus of the hippocampus, the precursor cell population is found in the subgranular zone (SGZ) of the dentate gyrus. Here, new hippocampal granule cell neurons are produced. These two brain regions are thus referred to as neurogenic regions of the brain. As is discussed in more detail later, reports of low-level and transient constitutive neurogenesis in the normal neocortex have been disputed, primarily for methodological reasons. Single reports have also appeared on constitutive adult neurogenesis in the amygdala, area CA1 of the hippocampus, the dorsal vagal complex of the adult brain stem, the spinal cord, and the substantia

nigra, although some of these results have been disputed and require further investigation.

Transplantation studies support the principle of defining neurogenic and nonneurogenic regions and provide evidence about the role of the microenvironment in influencing the potential of neural precursors. If precursor cells are transplanted into neurogenic regions, they can differentiate into neurons in a region-specific way. SVZ precursor cells generate hippocampal neurons when transplanted into the hippocampus, and SGZ precursor cells generate olfactory interneurons after transplantation into the rostral migratory stream of the olfactory ventricle (anterior extension of the lateral ventricle). When implanted outside the neurogenic regions, both types of precursor cells generate only glia. These data further support the interpretation that neurogenesis is dependent upon a permissive microenvironment, rather than on the regionally different properties of precursor cells. Local microenvironmental influences on the behavior of precursors and their ability to differentiate into neurons support the argument that it will be critical for the goal of neuronal repopulation to understand the cellular and molecular controls over cell type-specific precursor cell differentiation in the adult CNS.

It came as a surprise to many in the field that neurogenic regions are defined by the neurogenic permissiveness of the local microenvironment, rather than by the presence of neural precursor cells. Neural precursor cells have been found in a large number of brain regions, including white matter tracts. It is possible that the entire brain contains neural precursor cells (albeit at very low density), just as it contains partially restricted glial precursors that act as progenitor cells. These widely distributed neural precursor cells do not seem to differ fundamentally from one another, although they are far from homogenous, with notably different growth kinetics and differentiation potential. Their function outside the classical neurogenic regions is not known, nor is their relation to the precursor cells of the neurogenic regions. For example, neural precursor cells from the spinal cord behave *in vitro* much like their counterparts from the SGZ and SVZ. That is, they are multipotent after implantation into the hippocampus, producing granule cell neurons, but generate only glial cells and no neurons *in situ* or when transplanted back to their original site in the spinal cord. *In vivo*, no adult neurogenesis can be found in the rodent spinal cord. In sum, the extent of neurogenesis in a region is a function of the local microenvironment on precursor cells with (varying) neurogenic potential.

There is, therefore, an important conceptual distinction between neurogenic and nonneurogenic regions, which might reflect complex molecular and functional states rather than a fixed cellular environment. Can nonneurogenic regions be molecularly modified to promote neurogenesis? Could this change in neurogenic permissiveness be induced under certain pathological conditions? There are strong natural precedents in other vertebrate systems, such as the avian telencephalon and the olfactory epithelium, for the concept that selective neuronal death can alter the differentiation of precursors, thereby inducing or increasing neurogenesis. While not yet proven, it is hypothesized that this change in neurogenesis occurs via alterations in the local molecular microenvironment that resemble conditions seen during nervous system development and in adult neurogenic regions.

Factors That Stimulate Neurogenesis

Seizure Activity

Seizure activity can increase hippocampal neurogenesis. However, it appears that seizure-induced neurogenesis may contribute to inappropriate plasticity, highlighting the fact that newly introduced neurons need to be appropriately integrated into the brain in order to have beneficial effects. Chemically or electrically induced seizures induce the proliferation of SGZ precursors, the majority of which differentiate into neurons in the granule cell layer. However, some newborn cells differentiate into granule cell neurons in ectopic locations in the hilus or molecular layers of the hippocampus and form aberrant connections to

the inner molecular layer of the dentate gyrus, in addition to the CA3 pyramidal cell region. It is hypothesized that these ectopic cells, with their aberrant connections, might contribute to the phenomenon of hippocampal kindling.

Behavioral Environment

Events occurring in the hippocampus dramatically demonstrate that behavior and environment can have a direct influence on the brain's microcircuitry. Animals living in an enriched environment containing toys and social stimulation have more newborn cells in their hippocampus than control mice living in standard cages. Experiments to further assess which aspects of the enriched environment contribute to increased neurogenesis revealed that part of the increase can be attributed simply to exercise via running. Associative learning tasks that involve the hippocampus also appear to increase neurogenesis. While this is still quite speculative, it is possible that the processes mediating these effects on neurogenesis may underlie some of the benefits that physical and social therapies provide for patients with stroke and brain injury. IGF-I appears to be one of the factors that might mediate behavioral influences on hippocampal neurogenesis.

Stress and Neurotransmitter Effects

Stress increases systemic adrenal corticosteroid levels and reduces hippocampal neurogenesis. Conversely, adrenalectomy, which virtually abolishes adrenal corticosteroids, increases hippocampal neurogenesis, suggesting that adrenal hormones at least partially mediate the effects of stress on hippocampal neurogenesis. Serotonin is a strong positive regulator of adult hippocampal neurogenesis. Drugs that increase serotonin action, such as antidepressants, increase neurogenesis. Together, these results demonstrate that adult neurogenesis can be modified by systemic signals, suggesting that modifying such systemic signals in addition to local signals may be useful in developing potential future neuronal replacement therapies involving manipulation of endogenous precursors.

Transcription Factors and Signaling Pathway Effects

Transcription factors and chromatin proteins, such as the methyl-CpG binding protein and HMGB1 chromatin protein, may regulate adult hippocampal neurogenesis, and Wnt signaling might also play a critical role in controlling the fate of hippocampal neural stem cells. The developmentally critical basic helix-loop-helix (bHLH) transcription factor *NeuroD* has also been shown to be involved in adult hippocampal neurogenesis.

Depression and Neurogenesis

An interesting, but quite speculative and controversial, hypothesis concerning the role of hippocampal neurogenesis in human depression has been proposed and is outlined later in the article.

Induction of Neurogenesis in Nonneurogenic Regions of the Adult Brain

Induced neurogenesis in nonneurogenic regions can be envisioned in two basic forms: (1) local parenchymal precursor cells might be activated to generate new neurons upon a stimulus associated with a pathological event or with a set of directed molecular and/or genetic signals, or (2) precursor cells from normally neurogenic regions (e.g., the SVZ) might respond to either type of stimulus and migrate into the parenchyma. There are examples for both possibilities.

Several groups have recently demonstrated the induction of modest levels of neurogenesis in normally nonneurogenic regions in response to selective neuronal death or degeneration. As described later, Magavi et al. found that endogenous multipotent precursors normally located in the adult brain can be induced to differentiate into neurons in the normally nonneurogenic adult mammalian neocortex, a result recently extended to corticospinal motor neurons. More recently, other groups have reported similar and complementary results in a normally nonneurogenic region of the hippocampus and in the striatum, confirming and further supporting this direction of research. These reports of seemingly regenerative neurogenesis in the vicinity of targeted cortical neuron degeneration and cerebral ischemia suggest that the lack of normal neurogenic permissiveness in these regions is not unalterable. The controversial examples of reportedly extremely low-level constitutive neurogenesis outside the classical neurogenic regions might also support this possibility, potentially as leakage from normally tightly inhibited systems. Are precursor cells resident in nonneurogenic regions waiting for either instructive neurogenic signals or release from inhibition to awaken them to develop into new, function-restoring neurons?

Magavi et al in 2000 were the first to show that regenerative neurogenesis is possible in the neocortex. Induced synchronous apoptotic degeneration of corticothalamic neurons of layer VI of anterior cortex in adult mice led to the generation of new nerve cells in this region that projected to the thalamus. This work served as a proof of concept for the induction of adult mammalian neurogenesis in cortex that has been extended to the striatum, hippocampus, and corticospinal system (see below). Thus, although the density of multipotent precursors in adult brain outside the anterior SVZ and the dentate gyrus is exceedingly low, these precursors under an appropriate *in vivo* environment (such as that generated by apoptotic neurons) can differentiate into astroglia, oligodendroglia, and neurons: the latter can receive afferents and extend axons to their appropriate targets. That is, cerebral cortex undergoing targeted apoptotic degeneration can direct multipotent precursors to integrate into adult cortical microcircuitry. The population specificity of neuronal death was found to be essential, allowing for maintenance of local circuitry and survival of surrounding cells that alter gene expression to direct precursors. Other groups have reported similar and complementary results in hippocampus and striatum, confirming and further supporting this direction of research. Nakatomi and colleagues, using an *in vivo* ischemia model, found that repopulation of neurons in the CA1 region of the hippocampus is possible following the elimination of CA1 neurons. Recently, Chen et al. demonstrated induction of low-level neurogenesis of corticospinal motor neurons, with progressive extension of axons into the cervical spinal cord over 3 to 4 months. The critical challenge will be to assess true functional integration of recruited adult-born neurons.

Taken together, these results demonstrate that endogenous neural precursors can be induced to differentiate into CNS neurons in a region-specific manner and at least partially replace neuronal populations that do not normally undergo neurogenesis. It appears that these results may be generalized to at least several classes of projection neurons, including the clinically relevant striatal medium spiny neurons and corticospinal motor neurons. Microenvironmental factors appear capable of supporting and instructing the neuronal differentiation and axon extension of adult-born neurons derived from endogenous precursors.

Function of Adult Neurogenesis and Neural Precursor Cells in the Adult Brain

Given the restricted regional occurrence of constitutive neurogenesis in the adult mammalian brain, it is reasonable to hypothesize that there are specific contributions of adult neurogenesis to the functions of the hippocampus and the olfactory system. Possibly, these functions differ fundamentally from functions found elsewhere in the brain.

For the most part, the adult brain seems to do just fine without the ability to generate or regenerate neurons. Obviously, this characteristic of the mammalian CNS presents as a disadvantage in cases of neuronal loss, which cannot be replaced, but one theory is that this is the price paid during evolution for increasingly powerful and complex computing power. This reasoning posits that the cardinal requirement for stability in the system precludes the capability for neuronal replacement. Despite its appeal and clarity, this theory has for years been at odds with the fact that, even without considering actual cellular replacement or addition via neurogenesis, there is amazing structural and synaptic plasticity in the brain. Nonetheless, the fact remains that there is normally no (or extremely little) neurogenesis outside the two specific neurogenic regions of the adult brain. This striking restriction of neurogenesis to these two regions suggests that the question should be asked differently: What are the special functions of the dentate gyrus and olfactory bulb that require maintenance adult neurogenesis?

In simple terms, the hippocampus and olfactory system would appear to have little in common functionally. Whereas the hippocampus is one of the best-studied areas of the brain and has been named the gateway to memory because of its important and indispensable role in learning and memory, much less is known about the olfactory system. However, considering the evolutionary importance of olfactory perceptual learning, and the similar output modulatory roles of dentate gyrus granule neurons and olfactory bulb granule neurons that have been postulated, the functions of neurogenesis in each system might indeed be more closely related.

A gatekeeper theory has been proposed to help explain the potential function of adult-born dentate gyrus granule neurons. This theory hypothesizes that new granule cells allow for optimization of the mossy fiber connections between the dentate gyrus and CA3 in accordance with the level of complexity and novelty frequently encountered by an individual. Because adult neurogenesis occurs at a bottleneck connection, even a few new neurons could have a large impact. Selectively eliminating the adult-born neurons would be the method of choice to test this idea. However, both irradiation and treatments with cytostatic drugs as a means of killing dividing precursor cells are less selective than would be desired, with many structural and potentially functional side effects. Therefore, despite being highly intriguing, results of such studies have remained ambiguous and difficult to interpret.

Similarly, while the precise function of new neurons in the olfactory bulb is not yet known, recent evidence from Magavi, Macklis, and colleagues has identified an entirely novel function of adult-born olfactory bulb granule neurons – they are especially responsive to novel odorants and undergo experience-dependent modification in response to familiarization with novel odorants presented as the neurons are integrating into functional circuitry. Selective circuit integration of activated neurons might underlie at least some of this change in population response. These results indicate that adult-born granule neurons provide a novel form of synaptic plasticity via insertion of entirely new cellular units into existing functional circuitry.

Consequences of Disturbed Adult Neurogenesis and the Reaction of Neurogenic Regions to Disease

Because so little is known about the physiological function of adult neurogenesis, it has been difficult to evaluate the possible consequences of disturbed neurogenesis. Nevertheless, altered adult hippocampal neurogenesis has been proposed to play a role in a number of disorders. The most robust data that support this role come from studies of temporal lobe epilepsy.

Experimental seizures are a robust inducer of cell proliferation and net neurogenesis. Because of this, dysregulated adult neurogenesis might provide an explanation for the development of the granule cell dispersion found in many cases of temporal lobe epilepsy. There is some evidence that ectopic neurons can form in seizure-induced neurogenesis and that they might contribute to seizure activity. In addition, there have been recent reports of increased neurogenesis in Alzheimer's disease, as well as in Huntington's disease. Further, experimental depletion of dopamine in a rodent model of Parkinson's disease has been reported to decrease precursor cell proliferation in both the SVZ and dentate gyrus. The reproducibility and functional significance of these phenomena in neurological disorders have yet to be evaluated.

Several experimental data suggest another quite speculative hypothesis, that a failure of adult hippocampal neurogenesis might underlie major depression. Patients with long-lasting depression have global hippocampal atrophy. Consistent with this hypothesis, stress-related glucocorticoids are associated with a decrease in neurogenesis, and increased serotonin levels are associated with an increase in neurogenesis. If adult neurogenesis is blocked by irradiation, the behavioral effects of fluoxetine treatment (a serotonin reuptake inhibitor) have been found to be abolished. However, the hippocampus is generally thought to be involved in memory consolidation and less involved in the generation of mood, suggesting that altered hippocampal neurogenesis may be secondary to, rather than causative of, depression. Further, depression is not thought to be primarily a hippocampal disorder, and the presumed link to adult neurogenesis would need to depend strongly on the functional contribution of new dentate gyrus neurons to hippocampal function. The fact that neurogenesis occurs only in the dentate gyrus, while hippocampal atrophy in depression and positive effects of therapies are widespread throughout the hippocampus, argues that these phenomena are not directly linked. Thus a possible link between depression and neurogenesis remains speculative and in need of further rigorous analysis.

Conclusions and Future Prospects

Neurogenesis and neural precursor/stem cell biology suggest that the generation, insertion, and functional integration of new neurons is possible in the adult mammalian brain. From the point of view of fundamental neuroscience, it is important to learn about the normal role of precursor cells and the normal function of neurogenesis in the neurogenic regions of the adult CNS. This information might have immense implications for our understanding of brain function in development, normal adulthood, and disease states. Circuit plasticity at the level of individual cells, neuronal or glial, adds a new layer of complexity to our understanding of how brain structure and function interact. Better understanding of these issues may enable the prevention of disease and dysfunction, beyond the established goals of trying to repair neurons lost as a consequence of neurodegeneration and CNS damage. A better understanding of the cellular and molecular controls over differentiation of neural precursor cells along specific cellular lineages during development and in the adult CNS will be critical for the development of cellular therapeutic approaches for repopulating damaged or diseased areas of the nervous system. The future prospect of directing the development and integration of precursors in the adult mammalian brain toward the replacement of lost neurons or glia is exciting, and several recent lines of work provide remarkable progress toward this aim.

Acknowledgments

This article was updated and modified from a review article for a different readership (Sohur, U. S., Emsley, J. G., et al. (2006) Adult neurogenesis and cellular brain repair with neural progenitors, precursors, and stem cells. *Philosophical Transactions of the Royal Society of London. Series B, Biological Sciences* 361(1473), 1477–1497).

See Also the Following Articles

Neurogenesis; Hippocampal Neurons; Hippocampus, Overview.

Further Reading

Altman, J. (1969). Autoradiographic and histological studies of postnatal neurogenesis. IV. Cell proliferation and migration in the anterior forebrain, with special reference to persisting neurogenesis in the olfactory bulb. *Journal of Comparative Neurology* 137, 433–457.

Altman, J. and Das, G. D. (1965). Autoradiographic and histological evidence of postnatal hippocampal neurogenesis in rats. *Journal of Comparative Neurology* 124, 319–335.

Arlotta, P., Molyneaux, B. J., Chen, J., Inoue, J., Kominami, R. and Macklis, J. D. (2005). Neuronal subtype-specific genes that control corticospinal motor neuron development in vivo. *Neuron* 20, 183–185.

Chen, J., Magavi, S. S. and Macklis, J. D. (2004). Neurogenesis of corticospinal motor neurons extending spinal projections in adult mice. *Proceedings of the National Academy of Sciences USA* 101, 16357–16362.

Gage, F. H. (2000). Mammalian neural stem cells. *Science* 287, 1433–1438.

Jacobs, B. L., Praag, H. and Gage, F. H. (2000). Adult brain neurogenesis and psychiatry: a novel theory of depression. *Molecular Psychiatry* 5, 262–269.

Kempermann, G., Wiskott, L. and Gage, F. H. (2004). Functional significance of adult neurogenesis. *Current Opinions in Neurobiology* 14, 186–191.

Koketsu, D., Mikami, A., Miyamoto, Y. and Hisatsune, T. (2003). Nonrenewal of neurons in the cerebral neocortex of adult macaque monkeys. *Journal of Neuroscience* 23, 937–942.

Magavi, S. S., Leavitt, B. R. and Macklis, J. D. (2000). Induction of neurogenesis in the neocortex of adult mice. *Nature* 405, 951–955.

Magavi, S. S. P., Mitchell, B. D., Szentirmai, O., Carter, B. S. and Macklis, J. D. (2005). Adult-born and pre-existing olfactory granule neurons undergo distinct experience-dependent modifications of their olfactory responses in vivo. *Journal of Neuroscience* 25, 10729–10739.

Molyneaux, B. J., Arlotta, P., Hirata, T., Hibi, M. and Macklis, J. D. (2005). Fezl is required for the birth and specification of corticospinal motor neurons. *Neuron* 47, 817–831.

Nakatomi, H., Kuriu, T. and Okabe, S. (2002). Regeneration of hippocampal pyramidal neurons after ischemic brain injury by recruitment of endogenous neural progenitors. *Cell* 110, 429–441.

Parent, J. M., Vexler, Z. S., Gong, C., Derugin, N. and Ferriero, D. M. (2002). Rat forebrain neurogenesis and striatal neuron replacement after focal stroke. *Annals of Neurology* 52, 802–813.

Rakic, P. (2002). Neurogenesis in adult primate neocortex: an evaluation of the evidence. *Nature Reviews Neuroscience* 3, 65–71.

Ramon y Cajal, S. (1928). *Degeneration and regeneration of the nervous system.* Volume 2. Haffner Publishing Co., New York. p. 750.

Reynolds, B. A. and Weiss, S. (1992). Generation of neurons and astrocytes from isolated cells of the adult mammalian central nervous system. *Science* **255**, 1707–1710.

Richards, L. J., Kilpatrick, T. J. and Bartlett, P. F. (1992). De novo generation of neuronal cells from the adult mouse brain. *Proceedings of the National Academy of Sciences USA* **89**, 8591–8595.

Scharff, C., Kirn, J. R., Grossman, M., Macklis, J. D. and Nottebohm, F. (2000). Targeted neuronal death affects neuronal replacement and vocal behavior in adult songbirds. *Neuron* **25**, 481–492.

Seaberg, R. M. and van der Kooy, D. (2003). Stem and progenitor cells: the premature desertion of rigorous definitions. *Trends in Neuroscience* **26**, 125–131.

Neurodegenerative Disorders

M F Mendez and A M McMurtray
West Los Angeles Veteran's Affairs Medical Center and University of California, Los Angeles, CA, USA

Overview of Neurodegenerative Disorders

Neurodegenerative Dementias: Alzheimer's Disease

Neurodegenerative Movement Disorders: Parkinson's Disease

Conclusions

Glossary

Alzheimer's disease	A progressive neurodegenerative dementia affecting memory and other cognitive functions.
Hippocampus	Area of the brain concerned with encoding and storage of new declarative memory.
Neuron	Single cell functional unit of the nervous system.
Parkinson's disease	Progressive neurodegenerative disorder affecting movement, balance, and postural stability.
Substantia nigra	Area of the brain principally affected in Parkinson's disease containing a high concentration of dopaminergic neurons.

Overview of Neurodegenerative Disorders

Neurodegenerative disorders are characterized by a gradual loss of neurons, often leading to death. The term encompasses a broad range of clinical diseases, including progressive dementing conditions, of which the most common are Alzheimer's disease (AD), movement disorders, exemplified by Parkinson's disease (PD), and a range of other neurological disorders. Neurodegenerative disorders have in common a gradual loss of neurons and synaptic connections, usually occurring in later life. Specific diseases are distinguished by the presence of characteristic symptoms that depend on the location at which neuronal loss is occurring in the brain. Typically, the degree of neuronal loss correlates directly with the appearance and progression of the clinical symptoms. In AD, neuronal loss occurs early in the hippocampus, a brain region concerned with declarative episodic memory. In PD, the characteristic clinical triad of tremor, bradykinesia, and postural instability only become evident after 70–80% of dopaminergic neurons in the substantia nigra are lost.

The gradually progressive nature of these disorders, often combined with a long preclinical course before the development of symptoms, allows ample time and opportunity for environmental factors such as stress to contribute to disease development and progression. These features, however, make detection of environmental factors with disease-modifying effects by traditional epidemiological methods difficult. Prospective studies attempting to identify associations between stress beginning early in life and a clinical syndrome many years later in middle or even late life are hindered by the long length of time between exposure and disease onset, while retrospective studies are hampered by trying to quantitate environmental stress and account for the large fluctuations that occur over the course of a lifetime. Additionally, definitive diagnosis of most neurodegenerative disorders requires inspection of brain pathology after death, further complicating study of patients during life. Consequently, most knowledge concerning the relationship of stress to neurodegenerative disorders originates either from studies of animal models or from changes in stress-related hormones in those with neurodegenerative disorders compared to those without.

Despite the limitations, the scientific literature substantially supports an association of psychological and physiological stress with the risk of neurodegenerative disease. This article describes the clinical and neuropathological findings of AD and PD, as illustrative of the most common neurodegenerative disorders. It describes the effects of stress on animal models of neurodegenerative disorders and evidence for alterations in stress hormones in the setting of neurodegenerative disease.

Neurodegenerative Dementias: Alzheimer's Disease

AD is the most common neurodegenerative disorder and a major health-care problem that will continue to increase in importance as the U.S. population ages. Currently, more than 4 million Americans have a diagnosis of AD, resulting in enormous economic and social costs for their care, with a total in the United States alone approaching $100 billion per year.

AD occurs primarily but not exclusively in the elderly, with onset in most patients occurring after age 65. More rarely, onset may occur as early as the fourth decade of life, particularly in those with a familial form of the disease. Overall, prevalence for AD among the elderly (age 65 or greater) is about 6%, doubling approximately every 5 years after age 60, affecting between 26 and 45% of those age 85 or older. The annual incidence of new cases of AD per 100 000 people in the United States also rises with advancing age, one reason why investigators predict that AD will affect an increasingly large number of persons in the coming years, as the average age of the U.S. population increases. Some have predicted that in the United States the number of people with this disease may reach 14 million by the year 2050.

In the absence of a definitive clinical test or biomarker, the clinical diagnosis of AD depends on clinical criteria. The diagnosis of clinically probable AD by National Institute of Neurologic and Communicative Disorders and Stroke and the AD and Related Disorders Association Work Group (NINCDS-ADRDA) criteria requires impairment in at least two cognitive domains, progressive deterioration, absence of delirium, onset between 40 and 90 years of age, and lack of evidence for other dementing diseases after a standard work-up. Besides memory, other cognitive domains that may be affected include language, visuospatial perception or constructions, calculations, praxis, and executive functions. Patients meeting these criteria typically display progressive impairment in activities of daily living such as driving, buying groceries, preparing meals, doing laundry, and basic functions such as walking safely and maintaining personal hygiene. The diagnosis of clinically probable AD using NINCDS-ADRDA

criteria reportedly results in correct identification at autopsy in 85 in 95% of cases. Like other neurodegenerative disorders, gradual deterioration until death is typical, with a mean survival after symptom onset of 10.3 years.

The definitive diagnosis of AD requires clinicopathological correlation. One hallmark of the disorder is the presence of intracellular neurofibrillary tangles (NFTs) containing the microtubule associated tau protein in an abnormal phosphorylated state. Another hallmark of AD is the presence of extracellular senile or neuritic plaques greater than expected for the patient's age. The central core of these plaques is composed of β-amyloid peptides such as Aβ42. Around this amyloid core are degenerating dendrites and axons, some of which contain paired helical filaments like those found in NFTs. In addition to NFTs and neuritic plaques, the neuropathology of AD, like all neurodegenerative disorders, includes a progressive loss of neurons and their synaptic connections.

Both familial and environmental risk factors exist for development of AD. First, the development of AD at an early age (younger than age 65) often occurs as a result of autosomally dominantly inherited mutations in genes such as presenilin 1 and 2 and the amyloid precursor protein. Second, presence of an apolipoprotein E genotype with at least one ϵ4 allele results in an earlier age of onset of the disorder. Apolipoproteins are cholesterol-bearing proteins that mediate neuronal protection and repair and may participate in Aβ42 deposition. Third, women appear to be at slightly greater risk for AD, even when accounting for their greater longevity over men. Fourth, in addition to age, risk for AD increases with traumatic head injury, small head size, and low education, presumably on the basis of decreased neuronal reserve. Finally, later age of symptom onset, prominent psychiatric symptoms, and comorbidity such as cerebrovascular disease, heart failure, a history of heavy alcohol use, excessive weight loss, and institutionalization all may have a negative impact on clinical progression and eventually survival. In contrast, environmental and familial risk factors such as ethnic background and marital status are not proven to affect survival or rate of disease progression.

More recent evidence implicates psychological stress as an additional risk factor for the development of AD. Several studies show that patients with a high susceptibility to distress are more prone to AD in later life. When patients are followed to autopsy, those with a high susceptibility to distress as indicated by the personality trait of neuroticism are twice as likely as those without this susceptibility to have the NFTs and neuritic plaques of AD. Those with high distress proneness have a greater than 10-fold increase in episodic memory decline compared to those with low distress proneness. Other studies indicate that everyday hassles and challenging life events may exacerbate age-related declines on episodic memory tests. These findings implicate accelerated damage to the hippocampi as the mediator of the effects of stress on memory.

Much data indicate that the hippocampal region is involved in the response to stress. Animal and human studies indicate memory deficits associated with hippocampal damage after chronic stressful experiences. Corticosteroid receptors are abundant in the hippocampus, and high, stress-induced concentrations of glucocorticoids become toxic to the hippocampal neurons. Studies have reported high concentrations of cortisol in association with hippocampal atrophy in patients with dementia, as well as in posttraumatic stress disorder and major depression.

Many studies suggest abnormal function of the hypothalamic-pituitary-adrenal (HPA) axis in patients with AD. There are reports of increased serum cortisol levels and reduced feedback inhibition of cortisol secretion in patients with AD. Corticosteroid hypersecretion may downregulate the hippocampal corticosteroid receptors, which in turn dampens the feedback inhibition of the HPA, leading to further hypersecretion and eventual hippocampal neuronal loss. Other studies have focused on abnormal neuroendocrine responses to challenge with a chemical agent. Several studies report that AD patients demonstrate elevated cortisol levels relative to nondemented controls after challenge by a dexamethasone suppression test. In these studies, cortisol levels after administration of dexamethasone correlated directly with dementia severity. Another study compared cortisol and prolactin responses to administration of naltrexone, an opiate antagonist, in AD patients and normal elderly controls. In this study, normal control patients demonstrated a significantly greater increase in cortisol levels after a single dose of naltrexone compared to the AD patients, with no difference in prolactin response between the groups. Finally, cortisol levels have been shown to directly correlate with severity of cognitive decline and degree of hippocampal atrophy in AD patients.

One further mechanism for stress-induced injury in AD is vascular. The neuropathology of AD and the cerebrovascular changes may be synergistic. Higher stress-induced systolic and diastolic blood pressure (BP) reactivity, including variability in BP on 24-h ambulatory monitoring, has been associated with decreased performance in verbal memory and executive tests. The relation of BP reactivity to decreased cognitive function may be mediated by silent cerebrovascular changes from cerebral hypoperfusion. Repeated episodes of stress-induced BP reactivity can result in white matter changes or other silent cerebrovascular lesions on neuroimaging. Finally, life may also produce a hypercoagulable state that could contribute to cerebrovascular disease.

Neurodegenerative Movement Disorders: Parkinson's Disease

PD is an extrapyramidal movement disorder of unknown etiology, with onset between the ages of 50 and 65 years, and is more common in males than females with a ratio of 3:2. PD is fairly common, with a prevalence of approximately 100 to 180 per 100 000 population. Disease course is shorter on average than AD, with an 8-year mean duration of illness. Patients with PD have a two- to fivefold increased mortality compared to nondemented people in the same community. Risk of mortality directly relates to symptom severity, with death typically occurring due to aspiration pneumonia, urinary tract infection, or unrelated conditions of the elderly.

Clinically, PD has five primary characteristics: resting tremors, rigidity, bradykinesia, postural instability, and responsiveness to treatment with dopaminergic agents. In any particular patient some components may be evident and others not, and components are commonly asymmetric at onset. Of the primary clinical characteristics, presence of tremor is most suggestive of PD as opposed to other parkinsonian disorders. The tremor is classically present at rest, occurring at approximately four to eight cycles per second, and may develop in one upper extremity before spreading to involve all four limbs, face, and tongue. Bradykinesia contributes to the expressionless or masked face, sialorrhea, and micrographia. The gait is festinating, with abnormal righting reflexes and a slightly flexed posture. Eye movements may have subtle abnormalities in voluntary gaze, pursuit, and convergence. Many patients develop autonomic symptoms including postural hypotension, impotence, atony of the large bowel with constipation, and esophageal spasm.

Characteristic pathological changes of idiopathic PD typically occur in the pars compacta of the substantia nigra. Classically, there is marked depigmentation and neuronal loss, with presence of Lewy bodies in this region. As a consequence of these changes, dopaminergic neurons in the substantia nigra pars compacta are lost, affecting projections to the corpus striatum. Less pronounced changes are evident in a variety of other brain stem and diencephalic nuclei, including the locus ceruleus, dorsal vagal nucleus, and sympathetic ganglia. Although depletion of dopamine is the classic neurotransmitter deficit in PD, levels of norepinephrine, glutamate decarboxylase, GABA, methionine-enkephalin cholestokinin, and serotonin are also decreased in the substantia nigra of PD patients. No evidence supporting or suggesting a link between stress and neurotransmitter levels has been reported in PD.

Lewy bodies are characteristic of PD. Certain sites show a predilection for development of Lewy bodies, including the entorhinal region, the CA2 sector of the hippocampal formation, limbic nuclei of the thalamus, anterior cingulate, agranular insular cortex, amygdale, ventromedial divisions both of the basal and accessory basal nuclei, and central nucleus. Lewy bodies are composed of aggregates of α-synuclein, suggesting a possible central role for this protein in the pathogenesis of PD. Further evidence in the form of dopaminergic loss and inclusion body formation in α-synuclein mice reinforces a causal role for α-synuclein in this disorder. The proposed pathological mechanism starts with a reduction in the solubility of α-synuclein, resulting in the formation of filaments, which then aggregate into the cytoplasmic inclusions called Lewy bodies that contribute to the dysfunction or death of the glial cells and neurons in which they form in PD patients. However, no evidence for a relationship between degree of pathological changes or presence of Lewy bodies and stress has been reported in PD.

Environmental risk factors for PD include age, family history, and rural living possibly related to pesticide exposure. A genetic component to risk for development of PD is suggested by some studies reporting an increased prevalence rate of PD in relatives of PD patients compared to the general population. This has not been confirmed in twin studies, which failed to demonstrate increased concordance among identical twin pairs. Exposure to environmental toxins may be a rare cause of PD, such as from exposures to pesticides or herbicides and well water consumption. In contrast to AD, most studies do not find that APOE e4 is a risk factor for PD or PD dementia; however, PD patients show a trend toward slightly higher APOE e4 allele frequencies (12.5 to 17%) compared to normals (10 to 12.5%). One study showed that the APOE e4 allele frequency was significantly higher for PD dementia compared to PD and may affect an earlier age of onset for PD. Additionally, while female gender is associated with an increase risk of developing AD, male gender is associated with increased risk of PD.

Stress is probably an additional risk factor for PD. When compared to levels in unaffected spouses and siblings, cortisol levels in untreated patients with idiopathic PD are elevated. Other neuroendocrine abnormalities such as elevated levels of prolactin and decreased levels of growth hormone and adrenocorticotropic hormone have been demonstrated in patients with PD compared to normal controls. The clinical understanding of HPA axis dysfunction in PD, however, is often complicated by medical treatment, since selegiline, a medication used in treating patients with PD, may lower cortisol levels. Investigators have studied neuroendocrine abnormalities in a dog model of PD, using 1-methyl-4-phenyl-1,2,3,6-tetrahydropyridine (MPTP)-treated animals. After MPTP treatment, which damages neurons in the substantia nigra, plasma ACTH and cortisol are elevated in the treated dogs compared to untreated controls. In these animals, elevated cortisol levels result in excessive stimulation of neuronal glucocorticoid receptors, contributing to excitotoxic cell death. Excitatory stimulation of postsynaptic glutamate (NMDA) receptors in nigrostriatal neurons increases intracellular concentrations of calcium, possibly leading to disruption of the cell cytoskeleton or activation of caspase pathways leading to programmed cell death. Increased oxidative stress at the cellular level is also important in the pathogenesis of PD. Oxidative stress, through the depletion of glutathione and other free radical detoxificant enzymes, impaired mitochondrial complex I activity, or enhanced iron-mediated free radical production may contribute directly to neuronal loss in PD.

Conclusions

In summary, stress and its physiological effects may play a role in the progressive loss of neurons that occurs in neurodegenerative disorders. Increased cortisol levels due to both acute and chronic stress have demonstrated associations with hippocampal degeneration and memory impairment. This may be particularly relevant in the study of neuronal loss in AD, a disorder in which hippocampal degeneration occurs early in the disease course. Stress-induced alterations in BP and consequent vascular injury may further predispose to AD. In PD, elevated cortisol levels result from abnormalities of the function of the HPA axis, possibly contributing to loss of dopaminergic neurons in the substantia nigra by a variety of mechanisms, including excitotoxic cell death, increased intracellular calcium levels, and increased oxidative stress. Much more research is vitally needed in order to more clearly characterize and understand the contributions of stress to AD, PD, and the many other neurodegenerative disorders.

See Also the Following Articles

Aging and Stress, Biology of; Alzheimer's Disease; Behavior, Overview; Brain and Brain Regions; Glucocorticoids – Adverse Effects on the Nervous System; Parkinson's Disease.

Further Reading

Belanoff, J. K., Gross, K., Yager, A., et al. (2001). Corticosteroids and cognition. *Journal of Psychiatric Research* 35, 127–145.

Bremner, J. D. (1999). Does stress damage the brain? *Biological Psychiatry* 45, 797–805.

Deshmukh, V. D. and Deshmukh, S. V. (1990). Stress-adaptation failure hypothesis of Alzheimer's disease. *Medical Hypotheses* 32, 293–295.

Fratiglioni, L., Paillard-Borg, S. and Winblad, B. (2004). An active and socially integrated lifestyle ion late life might protect against dementia. *Lancet Neurology* 3, 343–353.

Kirschbaum, C., Wolf, O. T., May, M., et al. (1996). Stress- and treatment-induced elevations of cortisol levels associated with impaired declarative memory in healthy adults. *Life Science* 58, 1475–1483.

McEwen, B. S. (2002). Sex, stress and the hippocampus: allostasis, allostatic load and the aging process. *Neurobiology of Aging* 23, 921–939.

Meyer, J. S., Rauch, G., Rauch, R. A., et al. (2000). Risk factors for cerebral hypoperfusion, mild cognitive impairment, and dementia. *Neurobiology of Aging* 21, 161–169.

Nasman, B., Olsson, T., Viitanen, M., et al. (1995). A subtle disturbance in the feedback regulation of the hypothalamic-pituitary-adrenal axis in the early phase of Alzheimer's disease. *Psychoneuroendocrinology* 20, 211–220.

Sapolsky, R. M. (1999). Glucocorticoids, stress, and their adverse neurological effects: relevance to aging. *Experimental Gerontology* 34, 721–732.

Sapolsky, R. M., Romero, L. M. and Munck, A. U. (2000). How do glucocorticoids influence stress responses? Integrating permissive, suppressive, stimulatory, and preparative actions. *Endocrinology Review* 21, 55–89.

VonDras, D. D., Powless, M. R., Olson, A. D., et al. (2005). Differential effects of everyday stress on the episodic memory test performances of young, mid-life, and older adults. *Aging and Mental Health* 9, 60–70.

Waldstein, S. R. and Katzel, L. I. (2005). Stress-induced blood pressure reactivity and cognitive function. *Neurology* 64, 1746–1749.

Waldstein, S. R., Siegel, E. L., Lefkowitz, D., et al. (2004). Stress-induced blood pressure reactivity and silent cerebrovascular disease. *Stroke* 35, 1294–1298.

Wilson, R. S., Evans, D. A., Bienias, J. L., et al. (2003). Proneness to psychological distress is associated with risk of Alzheimer's disease. *Neurology* 61, 1479–1485.

Wilson, R. S., Barnes, L. L., Bennett, D. A., et al. (2005). Proneness to psychological distress and risk of Alzheimer disease in a biracial community. *Neurology* 64, 380–382.

Neurodevelopmental Disorders in Children

N J Rinehart and B J Tonge
Monash University, Clayton, Victoria, Australia

Autism and Asperger's Disorder
Attention-Deficit/Hyperactivity Disorder (ADHD)
Stress Associated with Autism and ADHD
Conclusion

Glossary

Pervasive developmental disorders (PDD)	A group of serious neuro-developmental disorders affecting communication and social skills and behaviour.
Autism (autistic disorder)	A PDD that involves delayed and deviant language development, impaired social skills and ritualistic and repetitive patterns of behaviour, usually associated with intellectual disability but a minority have normal IQ (high functioning).
Asperger's disorder	A PDD characterised by normal intellectual ability and language development but the presence of impaired social skills and ritualistic and repetitive patterns of behaviour.
Autism spectrum disorder	A term usually applied to represent autistic disorder, Asperger's disorder and atypical autism or PDD not otherwise specified (PDD-NOS) which share some common features of problems with communication and social skills and behaviour.
Attention-deficit/hyperactivity disorder (ADHD)	A neuro-developmental disorder presenting with inattention, impulsiveness and motor hyperactivity excessive for the developmental age and usually associated with learning problems.

Autism and Asperger's Disorder

Autistic disorder (referred to as autism here) and Asperger's disorder are classified under the umbrella term pervasive developmental disorders (PDDs). PDD applies to children who share the core features of severe and pervasive impairment in social and communication skills, together with the presence of restricted and repetitive patterns of behavior and interest. Other disorders that are categorized as PDDs include Rett's disorder, childhood disintegrative disorder, and pervasive developmental disorder, not otherwise specified (PDD-NOS). These disorders have their onset within the first 3 years of life. This section focuses on the two main PDDs, autism and Asperger's disorder. The term autistic spectrum disorders (ASDs) is frequently used to a describe a group of individuals with either autism or Asperger's disorder and is used accordingly in this article.

Epidemiology

The prevalence of autism is around 10–12 per 10 000. There is no evidence that prevalence varies between countries or racial groups, and social class and level of parental education are not associated with autism. Autism is more common in boys than girls (4:1), and this gender distribution is even more marked in Asperger's disorder (10–13:1).

Clinical Features of Autism

Autism presents with delays and abnormalities in the development of language and social skills and the presence of rigid, repetitive, stereotyped play and behavior, often in association with intellectual disability (i.e., an IQ below 70) and a variety of neurological conditions such as epilepsy. A reliable diagnosis can be made from the age of 2 years. Parents usually first seek help because their child has language delay and a lack of nonverbal communication. About 50% of children with autism fail to develop functional speech and only slowly learn to compensate with gesture. Language development is often abnormal in the remainder, with echolalia, self-directed jargon, and the repetition of irrelevant phrases, for example, from a television show. The correct use of pronouns and the related development of a sense of self and others are delayed. Poor comprehension, problems expressing needs by words and gesture, and difficulty in social understanding are frequently the causes of stress, frustration, and disturbed behavior. Children who do develop functional language usually have difficulty in using language socially and in initiating or sustaining reciprocal conversations. In contrast to children with autism, young people with Asperger's disorder have no delay in the development of normal expressive and receptive language, including the use of communicative phrases by the age of 3. However, children with Asperger's disorder have problems in their social use of language, for example, being verbose and preoccupied with a favorite topic. Their speech may appear odd due to the use of an unusual accent or the presence of abnormalities in pitch and volume, leading, for example, to a flat and monotonous delivery.

The play, behavior, and daily life of children with autism is usually rigid and repetitive. Their ritualistic play lacks imagination and social imitation. The older children may develop preoccupations with themes such as train timetables or dinosaurs, and this will be the focus of their play, drawing, and conversation. Change or unexpected events can be a significant source of stress: for example, the change of a school timetable.

Approximately 80% of children with autism also have intellectual disability, and a range of other emotional and behavioral disturbances is common. Children with autism who have intellectual (thinking) abilities within the normal range are referred to as high functioning. In contrast, all children with Asperger's disorder have normal intellectual abilities.

High levels of inattentiveness and behavioral hyperactivity are common problems in children with autism and Asperger's disorder; for example, at least 13% of children with autism also meet criteria for ADHD (although a diagnosis of ADHD cannot be made concurrently with a diagnosis of ASD). The overlap of these disorders suggests that ASDs and ADHD share areas of brain dysfunction.

The Neuropsychology of ASDs

There are three main brain theories of autism: theory of mind, the executive dysfunction theory, and the theory of weak central coherence. A poor theory of mind refers to problems with understanding that other people have their own perspectives and thoughts; it is believed to be a reason why people with ASDs have difficulties understanding and relating to other people. The executive dysfunction theory accounts for the problems that people with ASDs experience with timing and planning and producing appropriate and relevant behavior (e.g., coping with changes in the school timetable, planning homework). This breakdown in the ability to effectively direct one's behavior is also thought to be related to the repetitive, stereotyped, and restricted behavioral patterns of ASDs. Weak central coherence refers to a problem with being unable to see the forest for the trees and is thought to be responsible for why people with ASDs tend to be obsessed with details and often miss the bigger picture.

Standardized tests have demonstrated that the neuropsychological profile of autism is characterized primarily by deficient cognitive flexibility and planning, but without problems in the ability to sustain and direct attention (problems attributed to the prefrontal regions of the brain). Research suggests that the kinds of problems that individuals with Asperger's disorder have in directing their behavior may be different from those observed in autism, for example, their problem may be more one of initiating behavior than moving effectively from one behavior to another, perhaps suggesting that different parts of the prefrontal brain are involved in each disorder. Neuromotor testing has found that the walking and upper body postural alignment of people with ASDs is similar to that observed in patients who have Parkinson's disease and patients with cerebellar ataxia, indicating the role of the basal ganglia and cerebellum in these disorders. Again, autism and Asperger's disorder may be associated with different kinds of motor problems, which would suggest the differential involvement of these brain regions.

Neuroimaging Studies in ASDs

Neuroimaging techniques that enable us to look at the structure and function of the brain (e.g., computed tomography [CT], magnetic resonance imaging [MRI], and functional magnetic resonance imaging [fMRI]) have been unsuccessful in revealing a part or function of the brain that is consistently abnormal in all children diagnosed with ASDs. Structural changes in the brains of individuals with autism include a slightly increased average brain volume, a reduction in neuronal integrity in prefrontal areas (an area important for executive functioning – see preceding), decreased gray matter volume in the limbic system (an area important for social understanding), reduced neuron numbers in the vermis of the cerebellum, and gross structural changes in the cerebellum (an area important for motor and cognitive functioning) and the parietal lobes (an area important for efficient attention). fMRI studies have shown decreased activation in the highly interconnected cortical and subcortical frontal structures, suggesting a disconnection between thinking and motor processors in the brain. In summary, the brain imaging research data showing multiple brain region involvement and inconsistencies between people with ASDs fits with the clinical definitions of these disorders as being psychiatrically and neurologically complex and heterogeneous.

Genetics

The cause of the majority of cases of ASD remains unknown, but they are almost certain to have a multifactorial and complex genetic basis. Autism is associated with defined environmental causes, such as rubella and cytomegalovirus, fetal infections, perinatal brain injury, toxins, and specific genetic abnormalities such as tuberous sclerosis and fragile X syndrome in less than 10% of cases. A higher incidence of prenatal stressors occurring between 21 and 32 weeks of gestation has been associated with the later development of autism. A suggested link between measles, mumps, and rubella vaccination and the use of thiomerosol in vaccines as a cause of the increased prevalence of autism has been discounted by several comprehensive studies.

Attention-Deficit/Hyperactivity Disorder (ADHD)

The symptoms of ADHD may vary in different settings, and diagnosis is often subdivided into the number of symptoms in each of the dimensions of inattention or hyperactivity/impulsiveness. Thus, a child may be diagnosed as ADHD predominately hyperactive type or predominantly inattentive type. Estimates of the prevalence of ADHD vary widely, ranging from 20 to 1–2% depending on the application of diagnostic criteria. The combined inattentive-hyperactive subtype is the most common presentation.

Epidemiology

The childhood prevalence of ADHD is approximately three times higher in males than in females. Symptoms usually reduce with maturation, but at least 30% of children with ADHD will continue to suffer from the disorder in adulthood.

Clinical Features of ADHD

The diagnosis of ADHD is based on a clinical judgment that there are sufficient symptoms of inattention and hyperactivity/impulsiveness, together with the decision that these symptoms cause significant impairment in daily functioning in at least two settings and are not consistent with the developmental level of the child. Therefore, diagnosis requires a careful and comprehensive history of the child's development and behavior from the parents and other informants such as the teacher, together with observation of the child's behavior.

Apart from showing high levels of distractibility and inattention, children with ADHD are disorganized and are usually unable to follow routine or complete tasks. They have difficulty monitoring their behavior and therefore often interrupt others, have difficulty following rules, and display inappropriate and impulsive behavior. Those who also suffer from hyperactivity are constantly restless and fidgety, have difficulty remaining seated, and behave as if they are driven by a motor. These behaviors are influenced by aspects of the environment, such as the degree of external stimulation and sensory complexity. Therefore, observers may report differences in behavior depending upon the context. For example, a teacher in a busy, noisy classroom setting is more likely to observe inattention than a teacher's aide who meets with the child for individual teaching in a quiet library environment. However, the symptoms and impairments are usually observed, at least to some extent, in all aspects of the child's daily life.

The Neuropsychology of ADHD

In common with ASDs, neurocognitive testing has revealed that ADHD involves deficiencies within the prefrontal regions of the brain described under the umbrella term of executive dysfunction. However, the type of prefrontal executive dysfunction differs between ASDs and ADHD. The classic ADHD profile is characterized by inhibitory deficits and problems with sustained attention, compared to planning and cognitive flexibility deficits in the cognitive profile of children with autism.

Neuroimaging Studies of ADHD

As is the case with ASDs, no consistent structural abnormalities have been recorded for individuals affected by ADHD. ADHD has been associated in some but not all studies with smaller whole brain volumes, right prefrontal anomalies, and structural anomalies in the basal ganglia, cerebellum, and corpus callosum. As is the case with ASDs, fMRI studies have shown decreased activation in the highly interconnected cortical and subcortical frontal structures, particularly in neural regions that subserve key attentional and inhibitory functions.

Genetics and Stressors

The inherited basis for ADHD has been estimated in around 80% of cases, with perinatal brain injury (e.g., caused by stress, alcohol, tobacco, and other substance abuse during pregnancy) responsible for the remainder. The cause in the inherited cases is likely to be a complex interaction of multiple genes, while in some individuals there will also be an interaction with perinatal brain injury or other environmental stressors such as fetal alcohol exposure or postnatal malnutrition. As is the case with ASDs, there has been a large number of candidate gene and linkage studies of ADHD. Genetic screening for ASDs and ADHD is not yet possible.

Stress Associated with Autism and ADHD

Neurodevelopmental disorders present a considerable stress and burden for the affected individual, parents, siblings, and caregivers in the community. The particular stressors change over time and therefore need to be considered in the context of a human life span approach.

Stress Issues from Birth to Preschool

The trajectory of the stress and devastation that accompany a diagnosis of a neurodevelopmental disorder begins for the parents when their child is between 1 and 3 years of age, when parents realize, either through their own observations or through those of others (e.g., extended family, maternal health nurse, general practitioner), that something is not quite right with their child's developmental progress, for example, behavioral deficits in the form of language or social delays, inattentiveness, or behavioral excesses in the form of increased motor activity and hypervigilance. This realization usually triggers a string of subsequent referrals for pediatric, audiological, psychological, and speech and language assessment. Incumbent in each of these referrals is set of neurobiological and developmental test protocols to rule out various diagnoses. For example, a pediatrician may request a series of metabolic (e.g., phenylketonuria) and genetic tests (e.g., fragile X). The psychologist may undertake behavioral and cognitive standardized assessments, while the speech pathologist may request standardized assessments of receptive (i.e., understanding) and expressive (communicative) language. Investigation and testing may occur over a period of 3–12 months, at which time the family will be referred to a specialist (e.g., child psychiatrist, clinical psychologist) or specialist clinic for final diagnostic confirmation. The time length and uncertainty about their child's diagnostic status that parents experience during the assessment process is often stressful.

The formal diagnosis of a neurodevelopmental condition will often trigger a significant grief reaction in parents, who may mourn the loss of their perfect child and be required to reconsider future plans they may have had for their child, e.g., attending particular schools. In the case of ASDs, or when the child has additional severe intellectual disability, there may be a sense of loss about not having grandchildren, as many people affected by these disorders do not go on to partner and have their own children. Furthermore, research has shown that mothers of children with autism are more likely to suffer from depression than mothers of children with other physical conditions (e.g., cystic fibrosis) and mental disabilities.

Parents are typically provided with information about the genetic component of neurodevelopmental disorders at the time of diagnosis. For example, in the case of ASDs, if an older sibling has autism, the risk that a subsequent sibling will have autism is 2–8%. This information is stressful for parents because it has implications for younger siblings and for future family planning.

After a formal assessment has taken place, parents will play an important advocacy role throughout the child's life, a role that requires a significant emotional and financial commitment to ensure that a high quality of life is maintained for their child at each developmental stage. During the preschool years, parental advocacy typically involves organizing appropriate early interventions (e.g., speech and language, occupational therapy, behavioral management). The process of dealing with often lengthy waiting lists to access public services, or self-funding private interventions places a considerable emotional and financial burden on families and may place stress on the larger family unit by increasing work hours for caregivers and reducing time and resources for other family members, in particular, unaffected siblings. Surveys of maternal stress levels have estimated that approximately two-thirds of mothers of children with ASDs experience clinically significant levels of stress when their child is between 2 and 7 years of age. Stress levels are particularly high when a child with ASD has high levels of maladaptive and disruptive behaviors.

Children with ADHD often have hostile interactions with other children (e.g., hitting and biting) during the preschool years. This places a considerable stress not only on parents, but also on the broader preschool community (e.g., parents of other children and teachers). Compared to fathers, mothers have reported that they find these behaviors to be significantly more stressful.

Receiving education about the disorder and skills training in managing problem behaviors, learning relaxation and stress management techniques, and increased social support (e.g., respite care and community support groups) have been found to be useful for improving parental mental health and reducing parental stress associated with having a child with a neurodevelopmental condition.

Stress Associated with the Primary School Years

Interventions put in place during preschool years will typically continue into the primary school years depending on the availability of community and privately funded resources. During the school years, parents often become concerned about their child's education and adverse school experiences such as being teased. They focus on advocating for appropriate educational modifications and placements to promote their child's ability to reach individual academic potential and to experience a safe and supportive school environment. This usually involves families again seeking out the services of psychologists and speech pathologists so that their child can have updated assessments of language and cognitive ability. This process is a burden for children and parents because it is time consuming and costly. In some cases, at the end of such assessment processes, children are deemed ineligible for education aide support or special consideration because of bureaucratic and funding reasons (e.g., the child's IQ is 72 points rather than 70 points). This issue sometimes requires higher levels of advocacy from involved health professionals to assist parents with appeal processes.

For children with autism who have good early intervention, focused on the parent (e.g., behavior management training, psychoeducation) as well as the child, disruptive behaviors are manageable, and the quality of life for the child and family is generally improved. For children who do not receive good early interventions, or when standard interventions are inadequate, perhaps due to additional neurobiological comorbidity and ongoing disruptive behaviors (e.g., stubbornness, self-injury, and aggression), there is an increased risk of failure in school and community activities, in some cases leading to more restrictive care. When psychological and behavioral interventions have not been successful in the management of disturbed emotions and behaviors, which may be underpinned by high levels of anxiety, treatment with neuroleptic medication (e.g., haloperidol, risperidone, imipramine, clomipramine, fluoxetine) that targets specific symptoms might prove helpful.

While the antisocial behavioral tendencies (e.g., biting and hitting) of children with ADHD may subside with good management during the preschool years, for older children poor management and associated comorbidity (e.g., conduct disorder and oppositional defiant disorder, learning disorders) increase the chances of school failure and peer rejection. Comorbidity with oppositional defiant disorder (e.g., clashing verbally with authorities) has been suggested at between 32 and 60%, while comorbidity with conduct disorder (e.g., engaging in theft) has been estimated at anywhere between 12 and 25%. Stimulant medications (e.g., methylphenidate and dexamphetamine) are effective treatments for the symptoms of ADHD. Side effects, which may include decreased appetite, insomnia, fatigue, irritability, and increase in pulse rate and blood pressure, may be a source of stress for the individual and for parents. Tricyclic antidepressants (imipramine) clonidine, or atomoxetine (an inhibitor of the presynaptic norepinephrine transporter) are alternative treatments for children who have intolerable side effects or are unresponsive to stimulant medication. Parents may be stressed by the uncertainty of potential long-term effects of placing their child on medication. Currently there is a lack of good long-term evidence for the effectiveness of stimulant medication on learning, but they may decrease the risk of later substance abuse.

Stress Associated with the Secondary School Years

In the normal scheme of development, the transition from a relatively protected and highly structured primary school setting to secondary school is often a time of stress for children and families; these concerns and issues are magnified when a child has a neurodevelopmental disorder. In contrast to primary school, secondary school is often larger and requires the young person to be independent, navigate the school timetable, and engage in homework. All of these activities require good executive functions, e.g., planning, preparation, and anticipation, skills classically affected by neurodevelopmental disorders.

Adolescence is a developmentally complex time defined by social and sexual development and identity formation. Because social understanding and adaptability are innately reduced in ASDs it is an especially complex time for these young people. The affected young person may be more stressed than their nonaffected peers as they go through puberty and deal with changes in physical body shape, development in their thinking and insight, and emerging sexuality. Stress is also elevated for those individuals who develop comorbid psychiatric conditions, particularly depression, during this time. Depression may manifest as mood disturbance and irritability, sleep and appetite disturbance, and thoughts of suicide that may be enacted. The increased vulnerability to depression during adolescence may be associated with self-awareness of the disability, pubertal brain development, and a family history of depression. Stress and anxiety have been associated with the onset of tic disorder, or Tourette syndrome, in young people with ASDs. There is also an increased risk of developing psychosis during adolescence or early adult life, particularly for young people with Asperger's disorder. Individuals with associated intellectual disability are at greater risk for developing epilepsy during the adolescent and early adult years.

In addition to ongoing issues that first emerge in the primary school years (e.g., associated learning difficulties estimated in up to 50% of children with

ADHD) for young people affected by ADHD and their families, new hazards during secondary schooling revolve around ongoing and escalating child–parent conflicts, delinquent behavior, substance abuse (e.g., nicotine, alcohol, and illicit drug use), and an increased risk of being involved in car accidents, all of which may lead to school suspensions, community marginalization, and an increased risk of a breakdown of family relationships. It has been noted that increased marital discord when a child in the family has been diagnosed with ADHD may be influenced by the parents themselves having ADHD, given the associated genetic vulnerability. Young people who are treated with stimulant mediation for ADHD are less likely to use substances compared with adolescents with ADHD who are not receiving treatment.

In contrast to individuals with ADHD, individuals with ASDs often go to lengths not to use drugs and alcohol, an issue that may paradoxically cause stress and social conflict because the individual with ASD may feel driven to impose their rigid views about abstinence onto unsuspecting others, for example, taking a cigarette or alcoholic beverage out of the hand of a friend or restaurant patron.

Stresses during Adulthood

For people affected by ASDs, the adulthood stressors vary widely according the individual's intellectual ability, capacity for independent living, and provision of social, emotional, financial, and occupational support. It has been suggested that individuals with associated intellectual disability and epilepsy are at greater risk for deterioration during early adulthood, while there may be some improvement in functioning in normally intelligent young adults with ASDs. People with moderate to profound intellectual ability may be placed in special housing accommodation or residential care, depending on the family's emotional and financial ability to retain care within the family unit. This time of transition may be particularly stressful for the individual because it involves adaptation to a new environment and many changes in daily routine. Transition is stressful for family members involved in the decision-making process because they often feel a great sense of guilt and loss. Thus, the grieving process over the loss of the young person's potential, which begins for parents when they first come to terms with the diagnosis, is often revisited at this developmental point. Alternatively, the prospect of providing continuing care, without the hope of relief, is a source of anxiety for aging parents.

Even when young people with ASDs have relatively intact intellectual ability (e.g., ranging from mildly impaired to normally intelligent), they remain greatly impaired in their ability to process social information. Like the transition from primary school to secondary school, the transition to adulthood involves another leap of independence, involving a greater need for executive abilities (e.g., budgeting money, planning meals) and social adjustment. Indeed, the social rules may become even more perplexing for an adult with ASDs, as the immediate supports and supervision from parents, teachers, and school aides reduce or disappear as the young person is expected to live independently in the community. The transition to adulthood is perhaps more complex for individuals who have poorer adaptive and life skills, with a lack of early intervention and skills training and poor management of associated comorbid psychiatric conditions such as anxiety during the formative years.

Reduced social ability and obsessional characteristics associated with ASDs may put an individual at greater risk for being unwittingly involved in inappropriate or illegal behavior, for example, sexual offending or stalking, which may occur in the context of naive and inept attempts to make social contact. Similarly, there have been reports in the Australian and European media about individuals with ASDs stealing trams or trains to pursue an obsessional interest in the rail system. Interventions to manage these types of forensic issues may be punitive and inappropriate, particularly when the individual's diagnosis may not be known, leading to additional feelings of being rejected and further emotional and behavioral problems.

Adults with ADHD are usually less disruptive and hyperactive than children with ADHD, but usually remain somewhat impulsive, disorganized, inattentive, and restless or lack motivation. Young adults with comorbid conduct disorder and an inability to control their behavior are at increased risk for being in trouble with the law, ranging from accumulating multiple speeding fines to committing more significant crimes, such as robbery. The disinhibited, poorly focused, and overactive symptoms of those with ADHD may make it difficult to maintain employment and social and stable intimate relationships.

Conclusion

ASDs and ADHD are lifelong neurodevelopmental conditions, possibly involving overlapping brain regions, that are associated with numerous and accumulating individual stressors across the life span. Despite the many differences between ASDs and ADHD, there are many commonalities in the factors that may protect against or lessen the impact of these stressors. At the forefront of these is the availability of early interventions, parent support and guidance, and ongoing management at key developmental stages from health, education, and welfare services (e.g., general practitioners, psychologists, psychiatrists). These may prevent the accumulation of stressful events and related complications that significantly reduce the quality of life of the affected individual and family and are costly to society with an increased prospect of unemployment, family and relationship breakdown, legal issues, and psychiatric care.

See Also the Following Articles

Attention-Deficit/Hyperactivity Disorder, Stress and; Parenting, Stress of.

Further Reading

Barkley, R. A. (1998). *Attention deficit hyperactivity disorder: a handbook for diagnosis and treatment* (2nd edn.). New York: Guilford Press.

Bradshaw, J. L. (2001). *Developmental disorders of the frontostriatal system: neuropsychological, neuropsychiatric and evolutionary perspectives.* Hove, East Sussex, UK: Psychology Press Ltd.

Brereton, A. V. and Tonge, B. J. (2005). *Preschoolers with autism: an education and skills training program for parents.* London: Jessica Kingsley.

Cohen, D. J. and Volkmar, F. R. (eds.) (1997). *Handbook of autism and pervasive developmental disorders,* (2nd edn.). New York: Wiley & Sons.

Howlin, P. (2000). Outcome in adult life for more able individuals with autism or Asperger syndrome. *Autism* 4(1), 63–83.

Neuroendocrine Systems

G Fink
Mental Health Research Institute, Melbourne, Australia

This article is a revision of the previous edition article by G Fink, volume 3, pp 14–30, © 2000, Elsevier Inc.

Introduction

Hypothalamic-Pituitary Axis

Neurohemal Junctions and Circumventricular Organs

The Hypothalamo-Adenohypophysial System

The Hypothalamo-Neurohypophysial System

The Intermediate Lobe of the Pituitary Gland

Pineal Gland: Melatonin and Photoperiodic Control of Circadian Rhythms

Hormonal Effects on the Nervous System

Psychoneuroendocrinology

Glossary

Action potentials	Electrical impulses that propagate signals along nerve fibers. The potentials are produced by the flux of ions, in particular sodium and potassium ions, through ion channels along the nerve cell membrane.
Exocytosis	The release of a secretory product, including neurotransmitters, in packets or quanta. The secretory products are packaged by the Golgi apparatus of the cell in membrane-bound vesicles. Exocytosis involves fusion of the vesicular membrane with the cell membrane, resulting in the release of the quantum of product inside the vesicle. This is thought to be the major mechanism of secretion in most secretory cells, including neurons.
Limbic system	The system comprising a number of structures, all interconnected, to form a circuit that is concerned primarily with emotions, memory, olfaction, and neuroendocrine control; gets its name from the fact that it forms a border between the new and old (in evolutionary terms) brains.
Neurohemal junction	A specialized junction between nerve terminals and a plexus of capillaries that facilitates the transport of neurohormones from the nervous system into the bloodstream or *vice versa*.
Neurohormone	A chemical substance released from nerve terminals and transported to its target cells by the bloodstream. Neurohormones are often the same chemical substances as neurotransmitters.
Neurosecretion	The secretion of hormones by nerve cells.
Neurotransmitter	A chemical compound released by nerve cells (at nerve synapses or neuromuscular junctions) that either excites or inhibits a target cell. The target cell may be another nerve cell, glandular cell, or muscle fiber. Chemical neurotransmission is widely used in the nervous system and, because it is capable of analog functions, has a considerable advantage over electrotonic transmission, which is necessarily digital.
Portal vessels	The vessels that transport blood and solutes from one capillary bed to a second capillary bed before joining the systemic circulation. The hypophysial portal vessel system transports neurohormones released from hypothalamic nerve terminals into a primary capillary plexus in the median eminence to a secondary capillary–sinusoidal plexus in the pituitary gland.
Steroid hormones	Molecules composed of a basic fused unit of three 6-membered (cyclohexane) and one 5-membered (cyclopentane) carbon rings with a variety of functional groups attached. The large number of carbon–hydrogen bonds makes steroids nonpolar.
Stimulus secretion coupling	The link between a stimulus, usually membrane depolarization (axon potentials in the case of nerve cells), and the release of a neurotransmitter or neurohormone.
Synapse	A specialized junction between two nerve cells where signaling most commonly occurs by way of the release of neurotransmitters.

Introduction

The human pituitary gland weighs no more than one gram, but it nonetheless controls all the major endocrine systems and is indispensable for life. Located at the base of the brain and closely surrounded by protective dense bone and fibrous membranes, the gland is composed of the neurohypophysis or neural lobe and the adenohypophysis. Derived embryologically from a neural downgrowth, the neural lobe is composed of axons that project from nerve cells in the hypothalamus and terminate on capillaries of the inferior hypophysial artery. This is the site at which arginine vasopressin (AVP) (lysine vasopressin in pigs) and oxytocin are released into the systemic circulation. Synthesized in the supraoptic nucleus (SON) and paraventricular nucleus (PVN), AVP, also called the antidiuretic hormone, controls the volume of body water, whereas oxytocin is concerned mainly with stimulating milk ejection during lactation and contraction of the uterus (womb) during parturition.

The adenohypophysis is derived from an outgrowth of the roof of the mouth and, in subhuman species, is divided into the pars distalis and the pars intermedia. The pars distalis is more commonly called the anterior lobe, whereas the pars intermedia together with the neural lobe or pars nervosa forms the posterior lobe. There is no distinct pars intermedia in the human. The anterior pituitary gland secretes hormones that control the adrenal and thyroid glands, the gonads, body growth, and development of the breast and lactation. The hormones involved in this pituitary control are, respectively, adrenocorticotropic hormone (ACTH), thyrotropin (TSH, thyroid stimulating hormone), the gonadotropins, growth hormone (GH), and prolactin. In addition to being growth promoting (trophic) and stimulating immediate hormonal or cellular events (tropic), these hormones all affect metabolism. The loss of ACTH with the consequent loss of adrenocortical hormone secretion, and perhaps to a lesser degree GH and TSH, makes removal of the gland (hypophysectomy) lethal.

Although ACTH is considered to be the main anterior pituitary stress hormone, GH and prolactin are also released in response to stress and so receive special attention in this article. Thus, for example, insulin-induced hypoglycemia is a potent metabolic stress that, in humans, results in a massive and rapid release of GH. Stress-induced prolactin release may, under certain circumstances, be causally related to infertility.

Anterior pituitary hormone secretion is under central nervous system (CNS) control and is modulated by the feedback of hormones secreted by the pituitary target organs: the adrenal and thyroid glands, the gonads, and, as shown recently, fat tissue by way ofadipokines such as leptin and adiponectin. Neural control of the anterior pituitary hormones is mediated by the hypothalamic-pituitary regulatory neurohormones (formerly termed factors), which are released from the hypothalamus into the hypophysial portal vessels and transported by them to the anterior lobe, where they either stimulate or inhibit the release of the anterior pituitary hormones. The hypothalamic-pituitary regulatory factors are now termed neurohormones because, instead of being released at

synapses, they are released and transported to their target cells in the bloodstream.

The hypothalamic-pituitary system is the interface between the CNS and the endocrine system by which external factors, such as stress and day length, and internal factors, such as emotion, trigger endocrine responses. It was therefore termed the neuroendocrine system, and the pituitary gland is said to be under neuroendocrine control. In addition to the hypothalamic-pituitary system, the circumventricular organs also satisfy the criteria of neuroendocrine systems. The term neuroendocrine is also applied to interactions between nerve and endocrine cells in the periphery and especially the viscera, of which the gastrointestinal system and its appendages (especially the pancreas) are the most prominent. Of special relevance to stress is the sympathetic component of the autonomic nervous system and the adrenal medulla. Derived from the embryonic neural crest, the cells of the adrenal medulla are modified postganglionic neurons that secrete their neurotransmitters, mainly adrenaline (epinephrine) and opioids, directly into the bloodstream.

The present article focuses on the principles of neuroendocrine control of the pituitary gland and illustrates how the hypothalamic-pituitary system (1) was used to demonstrate that certain peptides satisfy the criteria of neurotransmitters or neurohormones; (2) played a significant role in our understanding of gene transcription, translation, and posttranslational processing; and (3) could be used as a window to study brain function in the conscious human (neuroendocrine window of the brain). Although only mentioned briefly in this article, neuroendocrinology is also concerned with the effects of pituitary target hormones on the brain-pituitary system, that is, on the way that hormones secreted by the anterior pituitary target glands play an important role in brain differentiation and plasticity; affect central neurotransmission and thereby mood, mental state, and memory; and exert feedback effects on the brain-pituitary system. These hormonal feedback systems constitute the afferent limb of homeostatic regulatory systems, which ensure that the output of pituitary hormones is maintained at a preset and functionally optimal level.

Hypothalamic-Pituitary Axis

Brief History

The central importance of the anterior pituitary gland as conductor of the endocrine orchestra was not understood until the early 1930s when P. E. Smith published his parapharyngeal method for removing the gland (hypophysectomy). The effects of hypophysectomy proved to be so dramatic that for a short period most scientists in the field, including the distinguished neurosurgeon, Harvey Cushing, thought that the pituitary gland was autonomous. However, around the same time, William Rowan, working in Alberta on the annual migration of birds, showed that day length had a potent effect on the growth of the gonads. Rowan's experiments, together with those on seasonal breeding in animals, the effects of stressful stimuli on endocrine organs, and the effects of brain lesions on pituitary hormone secretion led to the concept that the anterior pituitary gland must be under CNS control, a view that Cushing soon adopted. The observational and experimental evidence that supported this concept was summarized by F. H. A. Marshall in his 1936 Croonian lecture.

It had long been known that the pituitary gland and brain were connected by the pituitary stalk, but several lines of evidence suggested that neural control of the anterior pituitary gland was mediated not by nerve fibers in the pituitary stalk but by chemical substances released into the hypophysial portal vessels. These vessels, first described by G. T. Popa and U. Fielding in 1930, surround the pituitary stalk, linking a primary plexus of capillaries at the base of the hypothalamus with a second capillary plexus in the anterior pituitary gland. Throughout the 1930s and 1940s, a debate raged about the direction of blood flow in the hypophysial portal vessels. Based on histological evidence, this debate could have been avoided had someone read the 1935 report by Bernado Houssay and associates that in the living toad blood flowed from the hypothalamus down to the pituitary gland. But Houssay's paper was published in French.

The neurohumoral hypothesis of the control of the anterior pituitary gland was first formally advanced by H. B. Friedgood in 1936 and J. C. Hinsey in 1937. However, it was the elegant pituitary graft experiments of G. W. Harris and Dora Jacobsohn that showed beyond doubt that the anterior pituitary gland was controlled by substances released at nerve terminals in the median eminence at the base of the hypothalamus and transported to the pituitary gland by the hypophysial portal vessels. The characterization of the first three of these substances, thyrotropin-releasing factor (later thyrotropin-releasing hormone, TRH), luteinizing hormone-releasing factor (LRF; later, luteinizing hormone-releasing hormone, LHRH; or gonadotropin-releasing hormone, GnRH), and somatostatin, was to take a further 18–21 years of hard work in the laboratories of Roger Guillemin and Andrew Schally, for which they were awarded the 1977 Nobel Prize for Physiology and Medicine.

The sequence of corticotropin releasing factor-41 (CRF-41; later, corticotropin releasing hormone, CRH-41) was determined by Wylie Vale and associates in 1981, a breakthrough that had eluded many workers for more than 25 years.

Soon after its characterization as a decapeptide in 1971, G. Fink and M. Jamieson measured LHRH by radioimmunoassay in hypophysial portal blood of the anesthetized rat and showed that its release could be increased fivefold by a small electrical stimulus applied to the medial preoptic area of the hypothalamus. The neurohumoral hypothesis of neural control of the anterior pituitary control had been proved.

General Anatomy and Development

The pituitary gland is anatomically linked to the hypothalamus at the base of the brain by way of the pituitary stalk (**Figure 1**). The hypothalamus comprises a medial part adjacent to the third cerebral ventricle, in which are located the major hypothalamic nuclei, and a lateral part made up mainly of a large cable of nerve fibers that carries reciprocal fiber tracts between midbrain and forebrain, the medial forebrain bundle (**Figure 2**), in which are embedded aggregations of nerve cell bodies. Axons from nerve cell bodies located in the hypothalamic nuclei project to the median eminence, where they either terminate on the loops of primary capillaries of the hypophysial portal vessels in the external layer of the median eminence or form a cable that passes through the internal layer of the median eminence to form the bulk of the pituitary stalk and then the neural lobe (**Figure 3**). The median eminence, so called because it protrudes as a small dome in the midline from the base of the hypothalamus, forms the floor of the third ventricle and is delineated by the optic chiasm in front, the mamillary bodies behind, and a depression (hypothalamic sulcus) on either side. Arising from the median eminence is the neural stalk, which links the pituitary gland to the brain.

The pituitary gland is located in a fossa in the basisphenoid bone at the base of the skull, the sella turcica (so called because its shape resembles a Turkish saddle). The close proximity of the hypothalamus and pituitary gland to the optic chiasm means that tumors in either the hypothalamus or the pituitary gland may press on, or more rarely invade, the optic chiasm or tracts, thereby leading to visual defects.

The hypothalamic-pituitary axis is divided functionally into two systems (**Figure 4**): the hypothalamo-adenohypophysial axis (the hypothalamus, hypophysial portal vessels, and adenohypophysis) and the hypothalamo-neurohypophysial axis (the hypothalamus, neural stalk, and neural lobe). The neural stalk is made up of numerous nerve fibers that project

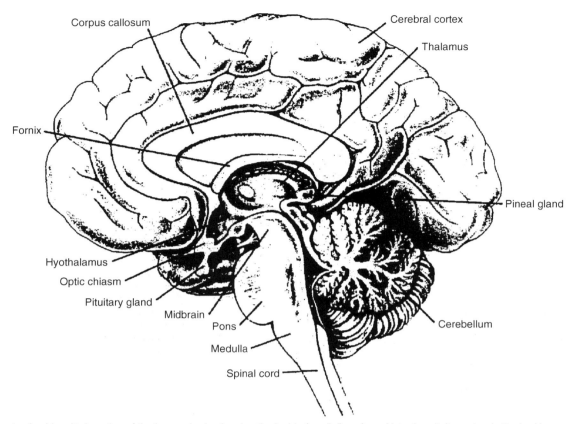

Figure 1 A midsagittal section of the human brain showing the inside (medial) surface. Note the pituitary gland attached by way of the pituitary stalk to the floor of the hypothalamus. The hypothalamus and the thalamus, which lies above it, form the wall of the third cerebral ventricle, at the posterior end of which is the pineal gland.

mainly from the PVN and SON of the hypothalamus to terminate on a capillary bed derived from the inferior hypophysial artery and located in the neural lobe of the pituitary gland. Nerve fibers in the neural lobe (or pars nervosa) are surrounded by pituicytes, the equivalent of glial cells. Also present in the neural stalk are nerve fibers of other types of chemical neurotransmitter (in addition to AVP and oxytocin), such as the endogenous opioids and dopamine, which are present in nerve fibers that project from the arcuate nucleus and innervate the pars intermedia. Because the stalk and median eminence are continuous, these dopaminergic neurons are a continuation of a dense palisade of dopaminergic fibers that also terminate on the primary plexus of the hypophysial portal vessels enmeshed with nerve fibers that contain other neurohormones. The pituitary stalk and median eminence are covered by a single layer of cells termed the pars tuberalis, which is continuous with the pars distalis.

The adenohypophysis develops from an outgrowth of the ectodermal placode, which forms the roof of the embryonic mouth (or stomadeum). This ectodermal outgrowth forms Rathke's pouch and meets the neurohypophysis, which grows down from the floor of the embryonic third ventricle. Rathke's pouch closes and separates from the roof of the mouth. The caudal (rear) part of the pouch remains thin to form the pars intermedia, which becomes tightly juxtaposed to the rostral surface of the neurohypophysis (**Figure 5**). The rostral part of the pouch develops into the pars distalis (**Figure 5**). Vascularization of the median eminence and the pituitary gland begins on approximately day 15 of embryonic life (E15) in the rat, and the hypophysial portal vessels become defined by E18. Nerve terminals in the median eminence with granular vesicles (presumably neurohormones) are first evident on E16 and the first secretory granules appear in pars distalis cells on E17. This sequence of embryonic development suggests that the development of secretory cells in the pars distalis may depend in part on the development of nerve terminals in the median eminence and the anlage of the hypophysial portal vessels.

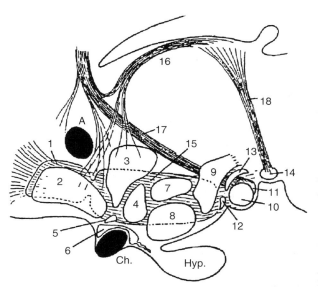

Figure 2 Diagram showing the relative positions in a sagittal plane of hypothalamic nuclei in a typical mammalian brain and their relation to the fornix, stria habenularis, and fasciculus retroflexus. (1) Lateral preoptic nucleus (permeated by the medial forebrain bundle). (2) Medial preoptic nucleus. (3) Paraventricular nucleus. (4) Anterior hypothalamic area. (5) Suprachiasmatic nucleus. (6) Supraoptic nucleus. (7) Dorsomedial hypothalamic nucleus. (8) Ventromedial hypothalamic nucleus. (9) Posterior hypothalamic nucleus. (10) Medial mamillary nucleus. (11) Lateral mamillary nucleus. (12) Premamillary nucleus. (13) Supramamillary nucleus. (14) Interpeduncular nucleus (a mesencephalic element in which the fasciculus retroflexus terminates). (15) Lateral hypothalamic nucleus (permeated by the medial forebrain bundle). (16) Stria habenularis. (17) Fornix. (18) Fasciculus retroflexus of Meynert (habenulopeduncular tract). A, anterior commissure; Ch., optic chiasma; Hyp., hypophysis (pituitary gland).

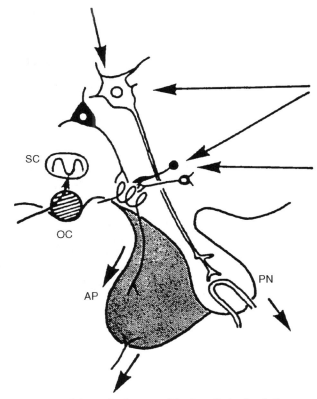

Figure 4 Schematic diagram of the hypothalamic-pituitary system showing the magnocellular (white) projections directly to the systemic capillaries of the pars nervosa (PN) and the parvicellular (black) projections to the primary plexus of the hypophysial portal vessels, which convey neurohormones to the pars distalis of the anterior pituitary gland (AP). Dorsal to the optic chiasm (OC) are suprachiasmatic nuclei (SC), which receive direct projections from the retina and play a key role in the control of circadian rhythms (indicated by the sinusoidal curve). Activity of the intrinsic neurons of the hypothalamus is influenced greatly by projections (arrows) from numerous areas of the forebrain, midbrain, and hindbrain, particularly the limbic system, as well as by hormones, mainly estrogen and progesterone in the case of the hypothalamic-pituitary-gonadal system.

Neurohemal Junctions and Circumventricular Organs

Neurohemal junctions are the fundamental functional modules of the major central neuroendocrine system, the median eminence. They are composed of nerve terminals and capillaries that are closely juxtaposed and thereby facilitate the transport of chemical messengers from nerve terminals into the bloodstream and *vice versa* (**Figure 6**). Neurohemal junctions are also the fundamental units of the neurohypophysis and of the circumventricular organs, such as the organum vasculosum of the lamina terminalis, the subfornical organ, and the pineal gland, which are located at various sites around the third

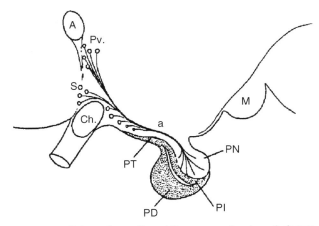

Figure 3 Schematic section of the mammalian hypothalamus and pituitary gland showing the neurohypophysial tract (labeled a) comprised mainly of fibers derived from the paraventricular (Pv.) and supraoptic (So) nuclei. A, anterior commissure; Ch., optic chiasma; M, mamillary bodies; PD, pars distalis; PI, pars intermedia; PN, pars nervosa; PT, pars tuberalis.

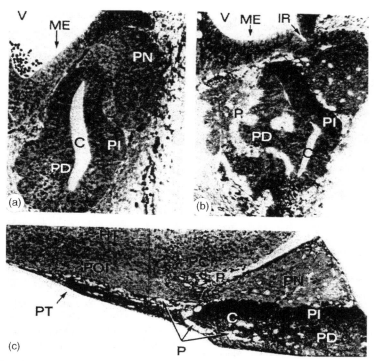

Figure 5 Photomicrographs of midline sagittal sections through the hypothalamic-pituitary complex showing the development of the pituitary gland in the rat. a, On embryonic day 15 (E15; × 120); b, on E17 (× 120); c, on E20 (× 80). In a, the pituitary anlage shortly after closure of Rathke's pouch, which migrates dorsally to meet neurohypophysial downgrowth from the floor of the hypothalamus. Rotation of the pituitary gland caudally through 135° with respect to the base of the diencephalon (hypothalamus) is seen, as is the invasion of the pars distalis (PD) by the leash of portal vessels (P) on E17. AS, anatomical stem; C, hypophysial cleft; HT, hypothalamus; IR, infundibular recess; ME, median eminence; PCI, pars caudalis infundibuli; PI, pars intermedia; PN, pars nervosa; POI, pars oralis infundibuli; PT, pars tuberalis; V, third ventricle. (1-μm Araldite sections, toluidine blue stain.) Reproduced with permission from Fink, G. and Smith, G. C. (1971), Ultrastructural features of the developing hypothalamo-hypophysial axis in the rat, *Zeitschrift für Zellforschung und mikroskopische Anatomie* **119**, 208–226.

cerebral ventricle, and the area postrema, located in the floor of the fourth cerebral ventricle. All the circumventricular organs are characterized by the fact that their vessels are fenestrated (**Figure 6**) and that the blood–brain barrier is inoperative at these sites. The neurohemal junctions in the median eminence, neurohypophysis, and pineal gland facilitate the transport of neurohormones from the nerve terminals or nerve cell derivatives (pineal) into the bloodstream, whereas at the other circumventricular organs, neurohemal junctions facilitate the transport of neurohormones from the blood to nerve cells. The latter mechanism has been implicated in the cross-talk between peripheral organs and the brain so that, for example, the hypertensive effect of the peptide, angiotensin, is due in part to its activation of neurons of the subfornical organ, which have a high density of angiotensin receptors. In addition to their importance as sites for the transfer of chemical messengers from nerve terminals into blood vessels, and *vice versa*, the neurohemal junctions of circumventricular organs are also sites at which drugs or toxins, which are

normally excluded by the blood–brain barrier, can penetrate the brain and affect brain function.

The Hypothalamo-Adenohypophysial System

Neurohormonal Control of Anterior Pituitary Hormone Secretion

The transmission of signals between the brain and the anterior pituitary gland is mediated by chemical messengers called neurohormones, which are transported by the hypophysial portal vessels from the hypothalamus to the anterior pituitary gland (**Figures 3–5**) where they either stimulate or inhibit the release of anterior pituitary hormones. Synthesized in nerve cells of the hypothalamic nuclei, the neurohormones are released from nerve terminals into the plexus of primary capillaries of the hypophysial portal vessel system. These capillaries are derived from the superior hypophysial arteries and coalesce to form the hypophysial portal veins, which run on the

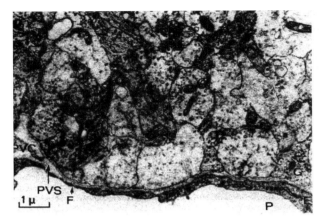

Figure 6 Electromicrograph of the external layer of the median eminence of a rat on the first postnatal day (× 13,200). Note the high density of nerve terminals around part of a primary portal capillary vessel (P), which is fenestrated (F). Note also the large number of agranular and granular vesicles in the nerve terminals. These vesicles contain the packets (quanta) of neurohormone or neurotransmitter that are released on nerve depolarization as a consequence of nerve action potentials. The neurohormones are released into the perivascular space and from there move rapidly into portal vessel blood for transport to the pituitary gland. This arrangement is typical of neurohemal junctions found in the several circumventricular organs of the brain. E, endothelial cell; G, glial process; PVC, perivascular cell; PVS, perivascular space. Reproduced with permission from Fink, G. and Smith, G. C. (1971), Ultrastructural features of the developing hypothalamo-hypophysial axis in the rat, *Zeitschrift für Zellforschung und Mikroskopische Anatomie* **119**, 208–226.

surface or through the pituitary stalk to the anterior pituitary gland, where they form a secondary plexus of vessels called the pituitary sinusoids. Vessels on the surface of the stalk are the long portal vessels, whereas those within the substance of the stalk are the short portal vessels.

Hypophysial Portal Vessels

The portal vessels are so called because they transport chemical messengers from one capillary bed (primary capillaries) to a second capillary bed before entering the general circulation. In principle, this is identical to the hepatic portal system, which transports substances from the primary bed of capillaries in the intestine and its appendages (e.g., the pancreas) to a second bed of capillaries or sinusoids in the liver. Fenestration of the primary and the secondary (sinusoids) plexus of capillaries (**Figure 6**) facilitates the transport of substances across the capillary wall. Hormones released from anterior pituitary cells are transported by pituitary veins into the systemic circulation by which they are transported to their major target organs, the gonads and the adrenal and thyroid glands.

Hypothalamic Neurohormones

Outline Most of the neurohormones that mediate the neural control of anterior pituitary hormone secretion are peptides that are synthesized in discrete hypothalamic nuclei. Neurohormone-secreting neurons are the final common pathway neurons for neural control of the anterior pituitary gland, a term borrowed by G. W. Harris from Sherrington's description of the alpha-motor neurons of the spinal cord that innervate and control the contraction of skeletal muscles. Like the alpha-motor neurons, hypothalamic neurons are controlled by inputs to the hypothalamus from the brain stem, midbrain, and higher brain centers. The hypothalamic neuroendocrine neurons are thus connected with many other regions of the nervous system and, in particular, the components of the limbic system, which is involved in higher brain functions, including emotion, olfaction, and memory.

The neural control of all established anterior pituitary hormones is mediated by at least one or more neurohormones. In some cases, two neurohormones may act synergistically, as is the case of ACTH, the release of which is stimulated by both the 41-amino-acid-residue peptide CRH-41 and the nonapeptide AVP. The control of ACTH secretion is further complicated by the fact that urocortins, relatively new members of the CRH-41 family of peptides, act mainly by way of CRH type 2 receptors in the PVN to modulate AVP and CRH-41 synthesis. Hypophysial portal blood and immunoneutralization studies suggest that ACTH secretion may be inhibited by atrial natriuretic peptide (ANP).

In other cases two neurohormones may act antagonistically, as is the case for GH, whose release is stimulated by the 44-amino-acid-residue peptide GH-releasing hormone (GHRH-44) and inhibited by the 14- or 28-residue peptide somatostatin-14 or -28. The neural regulation of pituitary GH secretion is even more complex than originally thought; Bowers and associates discovered in 1981 that a hexapeptide, referred to as GH-releasing peptide-6 (GHRP-6), is a potent GH secretagogue. Subsequent studies showed that GHRP-6 binds to a receptor, GH secretagogue receptor (GHS-R), that is distinct from the GHRH-44 receptor. The endogenous ligand for the GHS-R is ghrelin, a 28-amino-acid-residue peptide secreted mainly by neuroendocrine cells of the gastric mucosa, which also stimulates GH release.

Prolactin seems to be the only anterior pituitary hormone that is predominantly under the inhibitory control of the brain. Evidence for this came first from the studies of Everett and Nikitowitch-Winer, who showed that prolactotrophs were the only cell type that did not undergo atrophy in pituitary grafts underthe kidney capsule, where they are far removed from central neural control. This histological observation was confirmed by the finding that prolactin concentrations in plasma are increased in animals bearing pituitary grafts under the kidney capsule. There is substantial evidence that dopamine, released into hypophysial portal blood from tuberoinfundibular dopaminergic neurons, inhibits prolactin release. Indeed, dopamine agonists such as bromocriptine, cabergoline, and quinagolide are highly effective in treating hyperprolactinemia, a relatively common cause of infertility in women. Dopamine is now regarded as the prolactin inhibitory factor (PIF). Hyperprolactinemia is frequently due to benig tumors (adenomas) of the anterior pituitary gland, and these too can often be controlled by treatment with dopamine agonists. Stress is another common cause of hyperprolactinemia. Indeed, the prolactin response to stress in the human is as sensitive as that of ACTH and adrenal glucocorticoid response to stress.

The search for a prolactin-releasing factor (PRF) has continued for many years. Potential candidates have included TRH, vasoactive intestinal peptide, GnRH-associated peptide (GAP), and two novel, closely related hypothalamic peptides (termed PrRP31 and PrRP20) discovered in 1998 by Hinuma and associates when searching for a ligand for an orphan receptor (hGR3). Recent evidence suggests that the peptides intermedin and adrenomedullin may also release prolactin. However, although all these compounds are capable of stimulating prolactin release from pituitary cells *in vitro*, and in some cases under pharmacological conditions *in vivo*, robust proof that any of these compounds are the physiological PRF remains to be established.

The neural control of the gonadotropins, luteinizing hormone (LH) and follicle-stimulating hormone (FSH), is mediated by one and the same decapeptide, GnRH.

Criteria for neurohormones and neurotransmitters Werman, in 1972, summarized the criteria for classifying a candidate compound as a neurotransmitter or neurohormone thus: "If it can be shown that a substance is released into the extracellular space from presynaptic nerves in quantities consistent with the amount and rate of stimulation and the physiology of transmitter release at that junction, and if it can be shown that the material released acts on postsynaptic membranes by using molecular mechanisms identical with those used by the physiologically evoked transmitter, then that substance is a transmitter." Werman's two principal criteria – endogenous release (collectibility) and exogenous

mimicry (identity of action) – should be supplemented by a third criterion invoking the topochemistry of the mechanisms for the synthesis and inactivation of the transmitter.

The technique of collecting hypophysial portal blood in the anesthetized rat (developed by Fink and Worthington in 1966) has made it possible to satisfy these criteria for all the hypothalamic-pituitary neurohormones outlined here, as well to clarify the mechanism and physiological significance of post-translational processing. The measurement of neurohormone release into the hypophysial portal blood has also made it possible to ascertain whether newly discovered hypothalamic compounds could serve as hypothalamic-pituitary regulatory factors. This is exemplified by work in our laboratory, which showed that the concentrations of the cardiac peptide ANP were about four times greater in portal than in systemic blood, a finding that led to immunoneutralization studies that suggest that ANP is an ACTH-inhibiting factor. Studies of hypophysial portal blood can also exclude the neurohormonal role of a candidate neurotransmitter. Thus, for example, although immunohistochemistry suggests that angiotensin and cholecystokinin are both present in the median eminence, their concentrations in portal blood are not greater than in peripheral blood, which makes it unlikely that either plays a role as a neurohormone.

All the hypothalamic-pituitary regulatory neurohormones are present in regions of the nervous system outside the hypothalamus, where Werman's criteria for a neurotransmitter need to be proved by determining whether the neurohormones are released (by push–pull cannulae or dialysis), activate cells (e.g., electophysiologically), and are responsible for a behavioral effect. The functional significance of neurohormone action in areas of the CNS outside the hypothalamus is illustrated poignantly by CRH-41, which is believed to synchronize the endocrine, autonomic, immunological, and behavioral responses to stress.

Neurohormone receptors The hypothalamic neurohormones and their receptors, all members of the G-protein-coupled, seven transmembrane superfamily, underscore the adage that the evolution of hormones is less dependent on structural changes in the hormones than on the uses to which they are put. The latter depends entirely on the receptors and the signal transduction systems that mediate receptor activation, a point illustrated by the receptors that mediate the neurohormone control of ACTH and GH secretion.

The actions of CRH-41 in brain and periphery are mediated by two main receptor subtypes, CRH1 and

CRH2, with splice variants CRH2α and CRH2β. A third CRH receptor has recently been discovered in catfish pituitary. cAMP-linked CRH receptors also mediate the action of the urocortins, the mammalian homologs of urotensin in fish, and of sauvagine, a homolog of CRH-41 derived from the South American tree frog. In addition to mediating the neural control of ACTH release, CRH-41 and the urocortins exert actions on the brain and the cardiovascular system. CRH1 receptors (1) are localized predominantly in brain and pituitary, (2) have a high affinity for CRH-41, (3) are expressed by pituitary corticotrophs, and (4) are responsible for mediating the stress-induced CRH-41 stimulation of ACTH release. CRH2 receptors have a greater affinity for the urocortins than for CRH-41 and are present mainly in heart and skeletal muscle. However, the CRH2α splice variant is also present in brain and pituitary gland, where it is expressed by pituitary gonadotrophs, but not corticotrophs, leading to the suggestion that CRH2α may mediate stress effects on gonadotropin secretion. The ACTH-releasing action of CRH-41 is potentiated by AVP, which binds to the $V_{1\beta}$ receptor. The $V_{1\beta}$ receptor activates the inositol phospholipid cycle. Synergism between CRH-41 and AVP involves calcium-activated cAMP production. ACTH secretion is inhibited by ANP, an action mediated by two guanylyl cyclase-coupled receptor subtypes: A and B.

Human GHRH receptor cDNA was first cloned and sequenced in Mike Thorner's laboratory in 1993 and was found to be a member of a family of receptors that includes secretin, calcitonin, vasoactive intestinal peptide, and parathyroid hormone. The activity of the GHRH receptor (GHRH-R) promoter is enhanced by the pituitary-specific transcription factor POU1FI (formerly Pit-l). The importance of POU1FI, the prototypic POU-homeodomain transcription factor, for the development and activity of the GHRH-R is demonstrated by the fact that the GHRH-R is not present in the pituitary gland of dwarf mice (dw/dw) that lack POU1FI. Glucocorticoids stimulate, whereas estrogen inhibits, GHRH-R gene expression, actions that are likely to be mediated by the glucocorticoid and estrogen response elements present in the promoter and that explain in part the physiological effects of glucocorticoids and estrogen on GH secretion. The pituitary expression of GHRH-R mRNA in the rat increases with embryonic development to reach a peak at E19.5 (2 days before parturition), followed by a decline through to postnatal day 12 and then an increase to day 30, followed by a decline with age. If a similar pattern occurs at the corresponding times in humans, then that could be a major factor in the decline in plasma GH concentrations with age in the elderly. The GHRH-R is distinct from the GHS-R whose ligand is the 28-amino-acid-residue gastric peptide ghrelin. Both types of receptor are members of the seven-transmembrane helix, G-protein-coupled receptor family.

There are six receptors for somatostatin (SSTR), encoded by five distinct genes. All six receptors are present in the anterior pituitary gland; SSTR-5 is the most prominent on the somatotrophs, followed by SSTR-2 (which has splice variants A and B). Hypothalamic arcuate neurons that secrete GHRH express SSTR-2 and SSTR-1, supporting the proposition that the action of somatostatin may involve an effect on the release of GHRH. Relatively large amounts of somatostatin are also present in the cerebral cortex and hippocampus, regions that express the SSTR-2A. In the periphery, somatostatin secreted by pancreatic islet cells inhibits the secretion of insulin, glucagon, and a range of gut peptides.

The complexity of the receptors involved in the control of ACTH and GH secretion contrasts with the apparent simplicity of the gonadotropin control system, in which GnRH mediates the neural control of both LH and FSH, and the apparent simplicity of the thyrotropin and prolactin control systems, in which there is evidence, so far, for only one neurohormone each, TRH and the PIF dopamine, respectively. Dopamine inhibition of prolactin release is mediated by the dopamine 2 (D2) receptor. Alternative splicing results in a long and short form of the D2 receptor, and this allows coupling to different types of G-protein. When activated, the D2 receptor inhibits adenylyl cyclase.

Whether the complexity of the neurohormones and receptors involved in the neural control of GH and ACTH release is a consequence of evolutionary convergence of different regulatory systems that are not deleterious and are therefore retained or whether complexity has developed as a consequence of selective pressure to provide flexibility or increase the number of variables that can influence the two systems remains to be determined.

Clinical relevance All the hypothalamic neurohormones have been used extensively as tests of anterior pituitary function, or pituitary responsiveness. In addition, neurohormone agonists and antagonists have been deployed for a variety of diagnostic tests and therapeutic regimes. Thus, analogs of CRH-41 and urocortin have been developed with a view to their possible use in the treatment of depression, anxiety, anorexia nervosa, and stroke. The use of dopamine agonists, such as bromocriptine, cabergoline, and quinagolide, for the treatment of hyperprolactinemia and prolactin-secreting pituitary adenomata has been mentioned previously. GnRH superactive agonists and antagonists are used for chemical castration, as an adjunct treatment of cancer of the breast and prostate gland, for fertility control, and for the treatment of infertility and precocious puberty. Somatostatin, or its potent synthetic analogs such as Octreotride, has been used in the treatment of GH-secreting pituitary adenomas that lead to acromegaly and also ectopic GH-secreting tumors, most commonly small-cell carcinomas of the lung or tumors of the gastrointestinal system. The action of Octreotide in treating GH-secreting tumors can be potentiated by dopamine agonists such as bromocriptine and cabergoline.

Somatostatin and its agonists are also effective in the treatment of pancreatitis. Orally active, nonpeptide mimetics of GHRP-6, such as MK-677, have been developed and these may have therapeutic value in the treatment of children of short stature and adult GH deficiency. GHRH, GHRP-6, and its mimetics are also being explored as useful agents for the treatment of metabolic deficiencies that occur in aging.

Teleology of Neurohormonal Control

The hypothalamic-pituitary axis illustrates the remarkable economy of physiological systems. First, and perhaps most impressive, are the hypophysial portal vessels, which, by transporting the neurohormones from the hypothalamus to the pituitary gland, undiluted by mixture in the systemic circulation, ensure that hypothalamic neurohormones released in very small amounts from the hypothalamus reach the pituitary gland at concentrations several orders of magnitude greater than in the systemic circulation and therefore sufficient to exert their effects. The corollary of this is that relatively little neurohormone needs to be released to exert its effect and that therefore only a small amount of new neurohormone needs to be synthesized. The metabolic economy of the hypophysial portal system is brought into sharp relief by the fact that the hypothalamic concentration and total content of the hypothalamic-anterior pituitary regulatory neurohormones are three or more orders of magnitude lower than those of the neurohypophysial nonapeptides AVP and oxytocin, which reach their peripheral targets by the systemic circulation.

Second, the transport of neurohormones at effective concentrations by the hypophysial portal vessels also protects the body from the potential adverse effects of the high concentrations of neurohormones necessary to stimulate or inhibit pituitary hormone secretion. Thus, for example, the high portal blood concentrations of somatostatin may, in the systemic circulation, have adverse effects on the gut and on insulin secretion by the pancreatic islets. Similarly, as shown by Fink and associates, the portal plasma concentrations of ANP that inhibit ACTH secretion would, in the systemic circulation, cause a lethal drop in blood pressure.

Third, neurohormones in the hypothalamo-adeno-hypophysial system, by also serving as chemical messengers in several related systems or mechanisms, may serve to orchestrate appropriate physiological responses. Thus, for example, somatostatin, in addition to inhibiting GH secretion is also secreted by pancreatic islets and inhibits the secretion of insulin, glucagon, and a range of gut peptides. As mentioned earlier, CRH-41 is present in higher brain centers and in the periphery, and it has been implicated in stress-related behaviors, cardiovascular control, and the synchronization of the endocrine, autonomic, and immunological components of the stress response.

The Hypothalamo-Neurohypophysial System

Principles and Overview

The neural lobe is the site of release of the nonapeptides oxytocin and AVP into the systemic circulation. Presumably because a considerable distance removes the target cells of these peptides from their site of release in the neural lobe and because there is massive dilution in the systemic circulation, the rate and the amount of synthesis of oxytocin and AVP and their content in the hypothalamus are about three orders of magnitude greater than that of neurohormones concerned in anterior pituitary control. This fact, together with their synthesis in discrete hypothalamic nuclei, their ease of assay, and that both nonapeptides contain disulfide bridges that allow the incorporation of the radioactive tracer $[^{35}S]$-cysteine, contributed to four important landmarks in neuroendocrinology. First, oxytocin and AVP were the first of the hypothalamic neurohormones to be sequenced (by Du Vigneaud and colleagues). Second, the glycoprotein components of their precursor proteins led to their conspicuous histochemical staining and thereby to the concept of neurosecretion (the Scharrers), a term applied to neurons whose main purpose seemed to be to secrete neurohormones rather than transmit signals by propagated action potentials. Third, the fact that both peptides have disulfide bridges and that synthesis involves the incorporation of cysteine, which can be labeled with the relatively high-energy radionuclide ^{35}S, made them excellent models for the first studies of neuropeptide synthesis and transport (first shown by Sachs and associates). Fourth, oxytocin- and AVP-containing neurons were the first neuroendocrine neurons from which electrophysiological recordings were made (by J. Green and B. Cross in 1959).

The concept of neurosecretion was soon discarded because it was shown that the magnocellular neurons are no different from others – they propagate action potentials and release neurohormones or neurotransmitters. In fact, oxytocin- and AVP-containing neurons facilitate electrophysiological recording because they are large and because their axons terminate in the surgically accessible neural lobe. This makes it relatively easy to locate and verify by antidromic stimulation the identity of the neurons and record from them. Furthermore, the electrophysiological activity of the hypothalamic magnocellular neurons can be correlated with the secretion of AVP and oxytocin.

Finally, because the neural lobe is largely made up of nerve terminals, it proved to be a useful model for the study of exocytosis and stimulus-secretion coupling, the coupling between the cascade of ion fluxes through membrane channels (membrane depolarization) triggered by action potentials and the calcium-dependent release of neurohormones or neurotransmitters. Neurohormones, like all other known neurotransmitters and peptide and protein hormones, are packaged in secretory vesicles (**Figure 6**), which are released in packets or quanta.

Function

AVP (or the antidiuretic hormone) is concerned mainly with the control of body water. As its name implies, AVP also induces vasoconstriction and thereby can increase blood pressure, although this mechanism usually becomes operational only after a substantial loss of blood volume. AVP cells of the SON and PVN respond to osmotic stimuli. An increase in plasma osmolality triggers the release of AVP, which increases water reuptake in the nephron, which as a consequence causes an overall increase in body water with a fall in plasma osmolality. This is a perfect example of a homeostatic regulatory mechanism. In addition to its role in osmoregulation, AVP synthesized in the smaller (parvicellular) neurons of the PVN acts synergistically with CRH-41 to release ACTH.

Oxytocin, concerned mainly with milk ejection during lactation and parturition (the birth process), provides the perfect example of the role of neurohormones in neuroendocrine reflexes. Thus, oxytocin is the neurohormonal component of the milk-ejection reflex whereby suckling at the nipple of lactating mothers triggers volleys of impulses that travel through the mammary nerves to the spinal cord and, by way of a multisynaptic pathway, reach the hypothalamus where they trigger the release of oxytocin. Oxytocin transported by the systemic circulation stimulates the contraction of the myoepithelial cells of the breast, resulting in milk ejection. During parturition, oxytocin coordinates and reinforces uterine contractions. That is, as uterine contractions force the head of the fetus against the cervix, volleys of impulses are triggered that ascend through multisynaptic pathways involving the pelvic nerves and the spinal cord to the hypothalamus to trigger the release of oxytocin, which acts on the smooth muscle cells of the uterus. This is a classical positive feedback system, which is terminated by expulsion of the fetus and placenta.

The Intermediate Lobe of the Pituitary Gland

Model for Posttranslational Processing

The major secretion of the intermediate lobe of the pituitary gland is α-melanocyte-stimulating hormone (α-MSH), a 13-amino-acid-residue peptide that, together with ACTH and β-endorphin, is derived from the precursor proopiomelanocortin (POMC). In addition to α-MSH, the pars intermedia also contains other derivatives of POMC – β-MSH, γ-MSH, corticotropin-like intermediate lobe peptide (CLIP), and β-endorphin – which together with the ACTH make up the melanocortins. The fact that in the pars distalis ACTH is the major hormone derived from posttranslational processing of POMC, whereas in the pars intermedia α-MSH is the major active hormonal product of POMC processing, reflects the presence of different enzymatic processing pathways in the two parts of the gland. The release of α-MSH is inhibited by dopaminergic neurons that originate in the arcuate nucleus and reach the intermediate lobe by way of the neural stalk. Humans are conspicuous among mammals in that the pars intermedia is not defined as a separate lobe of the human pituitary gland.

Melanocortins

Although they are all derived from POMC, melanocortins have diverse physiological functions. α-MSH, first thought to stimulate the growth of melanocytes and pigment formation (melanogenesis), is also involved in fever, inflammation, and the immune response. Indeed, several of the melanocortins, including ACTH, affect cytokine-induced effects on thymocytes, T and B lymphocytes, and neutrophils. The actions of the melanocortins are mediated by five melanocortin receptor subtypes (MC1–5). Although all the melanocortin receptors are seven-transmembrane G-protein-coupled, the tissue distribution of the five receptors is quite distinct. Thus, the MC1 is located on melanocytes and mediates MSH-stimulated melanocyte proliferation and melanogenesis, while the MC2 receptor is located in the adrenal cortex, where it mediates the ACTH-induced secretion of glucocorticoids and mineralocorticoids. The MC3 and MC4 receptors are both located in the brain; the function of MC3 is unknown, but MC4 is involved, together with leptin (a protein produced by adipocytes) and neuropeptide Y, in the regulation of body weight. Studies on mutant *ob/ob* mice show that the action of leptin in regulating body weight is mediated, at least in part, by hypothalamic melanocortin activation, which results in decreased food intake. The importance of hypothalamic melanocortin activity for moderating food intake is illustrated by the agouti peptide, which is a high-affinity antagonist for the MC1 receptor and induces obesity in the mouse. The MC4 receptor is also involved in grooming behavior. The MC5 receptor, whose function remains unknown, is widely distributed in body organs, including the spleen, thymus, skin, and bone marrow. Cutaneous pigmentation is a function of the MC1 receptor, and MC1 gene variants may predispose to red hair and light skin color, which may make the individual susceptible to melanoma.

Pineal Gland: Melatonin and Photoperiodic Control of Circadian Rhythms

The pineal gland is a circumventricular organ (**Figure 1**) that secretes melatonin into the circulation and plays an important role in the photoperiodic control of reproduction in seasonal breeding animals. The gland deserves special mention here because it reinforces the principles of neuroendocrine control. Philosophers (e.g., Descartes, who called this the seat of the soul) and scientists have long been intrigued by the pineal. The secretion of melatonin is exquisitely sensitive to light. Pinealocytes in submammalian species are photoreceptors, and the gland offers an excellent experimental model for studies of the transduction of light into nerve impulses and neurohormone secretion.

The outer segment (sensory pole) of the pinealocyte in fish, amphibia, and reptiles has all the ultrastructural characteristics of a true photoreceptor, but these features are only vestigial in mammals and intermediate forms exist in birds. In fish, amphibia, and reptiles, the effector pole of the pinealocyte synapses with secondary pineal neurons that give rise to the pineal tract, which transmits signals to the CNS.

In birds and mammals, however, pinealocytes secrete melatonin directly into the circulation (or cerebrospinal fluid) in a neuroendocrine manner.

Melatonin, a derivative of serotonin, is synthesized within pinealocytes in two steps. First, serotonin is converted by N-acetyl-transferase (NAT) to N-acetyl serotonin, which is then converted to melatonin by hydroxyindole-O-methyltransferase. Because little if any melatonin is stored, the rate of melatonin secretion is tightly linked to its synthesis, which depends on NAT action, which in turn depends on norepinephrine release from the dense sympathetic innervation of the gland. In mammals, the control of melatonin secretion by light is mediated by a multisynaptic pathway that starts in the retina of the eye and successively involves synapses in the suprachiasmatic nuclei, the PVN, the intermediolateral column of the spinal cord, and the neurons of the superior cervical ganglion of the sympathetic nervous system. Sympathetic terminals in the pineal gland release norepinephrine, which stimulates melatonin secretion by an action on adrenoreceptors on pinealocytes. cAMP seems to be the main intracellular second messenger that mediates the action of norepinephrine in this system. The main point of regulation seems to be NAT, which, depending on the species, can be affected at the level of NAT gene expression as well by posttranslational modifications that alter the activity of the enzyme.

The secretion of melatonin starts with the onset of the dark period (night) and stops with the onset of the light period (day). The secretion of melatonin during the dark period is stopped abruptly by exposure to light. In blind people, the secretion of melatonin takes on the typical 25-h free-running period. Taken together, these and other data suggest that the secretion of melatonin is predominantly controlled by light exposure superimposed on the intrinsic rhythm of the major neural clock, the suprachiasmatic nuclei.

An interaction between melatonin and the hypothalamic-pituitary-adrenal stress response system has been suggested; indeed, melatonin has been implicated in glucocorticoid receptor-induced gene expression. However, the precise role of melatonin in the circadian rhythm of ACTH and adrenal corticosteroids, and in the stress response, has yet to be established. This applies equally to the long-researched but unanswered questions as to whether melatonin is a hypnotic or sedative and whether it can resynchronize circadian rhythms that have been disrupted by rapidly crossing time zones (jet lag). Melatonin is a powerful antioxidant, which may explain some of its alleged beneficial effects with respect to aging. So far, the most robust evidence regarding the function of melatonin in mammals relates to its inhibitory actions with respect to reproduction, especially in seasonal breeding animals such as the wallaby, hamster, vole, and sheep.

What is well established is that the suprachiasmatic nuclei constitute the central generator of circadian rhythms of the body, with one notable exception – the daily anticipation of a meal. That is, rats in which the suprachiasmatic nuclei have been lesioned are still able to anticipate one meal per day. This anticipation is associated with an increase in activity, core body temperature, and plasma corticosterone concentrations that occur 2–4 h before access to the meal. The precise nature and location of the feeding-entrained oscillator that presumably determines the daily rhythm of feeding anticipation have yet to be established. However, studies with c-Fos (early immediate gene) activation have implicated the nucleus accumbens and the limbic system. The relative importance of the pineal gland and its precise role in the photoperiodic control of circadian rhythms also wait to be determined. With the discovery of genes that regulate circadian rhythms and melatonin synthesis, the prospects of defining what is likely to be a remarkably elegant and robust molecular control system seem excellent.

Hormonal Effects on the Nervous System

The steroid and thyroid hormones, the secretions of the three major pituitary target organs, exert powerful effects on the brain. These effects may be classified in terms of (1) feedback actions, (2) brain differentiation and neural plasticity, (3) neurotransmission, and (4) membranes and ion channels. Feedback actions of the corticosteroids on the brain and pituitary gland are discussed in detail elsewhere. Many entries also deal with the specific effects of corticosteroids on brain that are mediated by corticosteroid receptors, but that are not necessarily related to the feedback control of ACTH release. For information on the actions of steroids on brain differentiation, neurotransmission, cell membranes, and ion channels, the reader is referred to the Bibilography.

Psychoneuroendocrinology

The recognition that the secretion of pituitary hormones reflects the activity of hypothalamic neurons, which in turn reflects neurotransmitter activity in the brain, provides the basis for the use of pituitary hormone secretion as a marker of disordered central neurotransmission that may underlie or be associated with mental disorders. The development of this discipline, psychoneuroendocrinology, has been impeded by our lack of fundamental knowledge about the precise neurotransmitter regulation of hypothalamic

neurons that regulate the anterior pituitary gland. Nonetheless, several robust findings have been made and these provide important clues for further research that might optimally be carried out in conjunction with human genetics and sophisticated brain imaging.

For example, it has long been known that plasma cortisol concentrations are abnormally high in patients with psychosis, especially severe depression. Furthermore, as shown by the groundbreaking work of Carroll and Rubin and their associates, in many psychotic patients it is not possible to suppress these high cortisol concentrations by injecting a glucocorticoid agonist such as dexamethasone (the dexamethasone suppression test). Although it cannot accurately discriminate among the different types of psychoses, the failure of dexamethasone to suppress cortisol levels provides robust biological evidence that a patient is suffering from a severe psychosis. The inability of dexamethasone to suppress cortisol levels in many patients with depressive psychosis points to a significant abnormality in the regulatory mechanism for ACTH release. The elucidation of the precise nature of this abnormality may help explain the central neurotransmitter dysfunction that leads to severe depression or other psychosis.

The growth hormone and prolactin responses to pharmacological challenge are also abnormal in certain psychotic states. In anorexia nervosa, for example, a life-threatening condition that occurs predominantly in young women, the normal GH surge that can be induced by the infusion of L-tryptophan, the precursor for serotonin synthesis, is completely absent. This cannot simply be attributed to a lack of food intake because the GH response to L-tryptophan infusion is enhanced, rather than suppressed, in women of a similar age who have been placed on a low-calorie diet. Again the precise explanation for this phenomenon, first shown by Guy Goodwin and associates, is not established, but points to an abnormality in central serotonin function that may underlie or be associated with anorexia nervosa.

The advantages of the psychoneuroendocrine investigation of mental disorders are that it is relatively inexpensive, only mildly invasive, and can be carried out in severely ill patients. Its power will depend on further fundamental research that may enable us to interpret accurately the neuroendocrine responses to pharmacological challenge.

See Also the Following Articles

Adrenal Medulla; Circadian Rhythms, Genetics of; Feedback Systems; Food Shift Effect; Primate Hierarchies and Personality; Reproductive Dysfunction in Primates, Behaviorally Induced; Secretagogue; Urocortins; Corticotropin

Releasing Factor (CRF); Corticotropin Releasing Factor-Binding Protein; Corticotropin-Releasing Factor Receptors; Anti-CRF; CRH Anxiety Circuitary in Brain; Dex-CRH Test; Corticotropin Releasing Factor Receptor Deficiency in Mice; Corticotropin-releasing factor (CRF) Family of Neuropeptides – Role in Inflammation.

Further Reading

Bale, T. L. and Vale, W. W. (2004). CRF and CRF receptors: role in stress responsivity and other behaviors. *Annual Reviews of Pharmacology and Toxicology* **44**, 525–557.

Balthasar, N., Dalgaard, L. T., Lee, C. E., et al. (2005). Divergence of melanocortin pathways in the control of food intake and energy expenditure. *Cell* **123**(3), 493–505.

Boorse, G. C. and Denver, R. J. (2006). Widespread tissue distribution and diverse functions of corticotropin-releasing factor and related peptides. *General Comparative Endocrinology* **146**(1), 9–18.

Cone, R. D. (2005). Anatomy and regulation of the central melanocortin system. *Nature Neuroscience* **8**(5), 571–578.

Ellacott, K. L., Halatchev, I. G. and Cone, R. D. (2006). Characterization of leptin responsive neurons in the caudal brainstem. *Endocrinology* **147**(7), 3190–3196.

Fink, G. (1988). The G. W. Harris Lecture: Steroid control of brain and pituitary function. *Quarterly Journal of Experimental Physiology* **73**, 257–293.

Fink, G. (1997). Mechanisms of negative and positive feedback of steroids in the hypothalamic-pituitary system. In: Bittar, E. & Bittar, N. (eds.) *Principles of medical biology*, pp. 29–100. Greenwich, CT: JAI.

Fink, G., Dow, R. C., Casley, D., et al. (1992). Atrial natriuretic peptide is involved in the ACTH response to stress and glucocorticoid negative feedback in the rat. *Journal of Endocrinology* **135**, 37–43.

Fink, G. and Smith, G. C. (1971). Ultrastructural features of the developing hypothalamo-hypophysial axis in the rat. *Zeitschrift für Zellforschung und Mikroskopische Anatomie* **119**, 208–226.

Fink, G., Sumner, B., Rosie, R., et al. (1999). Androgen actions on central serotonin neurotransmission: relevance for mood, mental state and memory. *Behavioral Brain Research* **105**, 53–68.

Ganguly, S., Weller, J. L., Ho, A., et al. (2005). Melatonin synthesis: 14-3-3-dependent activation and inhibition of arylalkylamine N-acetyltransferase mediated by phosphoserine-205. *Proceedings of the National Academy of Science USA* **102**(4), 1222–1227.

Getting, S. J. (2006). Targeting melanocortin receptors as potential novel therapeutics. *Pharmacology and Therapeutics* **111**(1), 1–15.

Goodwin, G. M., Shapiro, C. M., Bennie, J., et al. (1989). The neuroendocrine responses and psychological effects of infusion of L-tryptophan in anorexia nervosa. *Psychological Medicine* **19**, 857–864.

Guillermet-Guibert, J., Lahlou, H., Cordelier, P., et al. (2005). Physiology of somatostatin receptors. *Journal of Endocrinological Investigation* **28**(11 supplement), 5–9.

Hauger, R. L., Grigoriadis, D. E., Dallman, M. F., et al. (2003). International Union of Pharmacology. 36: Current status of the nomenclature for receptors for corticotropin-releasing factor and their ligands. *Pharmacological Reviews* **55**(1), 21–26.

Larsen, P. R., Kronenberg, H. M., Melmed, S. and Polonsky, K. S. (eds.) (2003). *Williams textbook of endocrinology* (10th edn.) Philadelphia: Saunders.

Luque, R. M., Kineman, R. D., Park, S., et al. (2004). Homologous and heterologous regulation of pituitary receptors for ghrelin and growth hormone-releasing hormone. *Endocrinology* **145**(7), 3182–3189.

Mayo, K. E., Miller, L. J., Bataille, D., et al. (2003). International Union of Pharmacology. 35: The glucagon receptor family. *Pharmacological Reviews* **55**(1), 167–194.

Mendoza, J., Angeles-Castellanos, M. and Escobar, C. (2005). Entrainment by a palatable meal induces food-anticipatory activity and c-Fos expression in reward-related areas of the brain. *Neuroscience* **133**(1), 293–303.

Schumacher, M., Weill-Engerer, S., Liere, P., et al. (2003). Steroid hormones and neurosteroids in normal and pathological aging of the nervous system. *Progress in Neurobiology* **71**(1), 3–29.

Turek, F. W., Joshu, C., Kohsaka, A., et al. (2005). Obesity and metabolic syndrome in circadian clock mutant mice. *Science* **308**(5724), 1043–1045.

Werman, R. (1972) CNS cellular level: membranes. *Annual Review of Physiology* **34**, 337–374.

Yoo, S. H., Ko, C. H., Lowrey, P. L., et al. (2005). A noncanonical E-box enhancer drives mouse Period2 circadian oscillations in vivo. *Proceedings of the National Academy of Science USA* **102**(7), 2608–2613.

Neurogenesis

P Tanapat and E Gould
Princeton University, Princeton, NJ, USA

This article is reproduced from the previous edition, volume 3, pp 31–36, © 2000, Elsevier Inc.

Development of the Dentate Gyrus
Stress Effects on Neurogenesis
Adrenal Steroids Affect Neurogenesis through NMDA
  Receptors
Functional Implications of Stress Effects on Neurogenesis

Glossary

Bromodeoxyuridine (BrdU) labeling	A nonradioactive method for labeling proliferating cells and their progeny. BrdU is a thymidine analog that is incorporated into cells that are in the DNA synthetic phase of the cell cycle. BrdU incorporation can be visualized using immunocytochemical methods and can be combined with stereological analyses to estimate the total numbers of new cells generated at a given time. Short survival times (e.g., 2 h) can be used to label proliferating cells. When combined with the use of immunohistological markers, longer survival times (e.g., several weeks) can be used to determine the cellular phenotype of the newly generated cells.
Dentate gyrus	A brain region that is part of the hippocampal formation. It consists of the following three major components: (1) the granule cell layer, densely packed with granule cell bodies; (2) the hilus, a region that contains the granule cell axons (mossy fibers), interneurons, and progenitor cells; and (3) the molecular layer, a region that contains the granule cell dendritic trees and interneurons.
Neurogenesis	The process of forming a new neuron. Neurogenesis involves the proliferation of neuronal progenitors and the subsequent differentiation of these cells into neurons.
[³H]Thymidine autoradiography	A method that labels proliferating cells and their progeny with radio-labeled thymidine, a molecule that is incorporated into cells that are in S phase. Cells that have incorporated [³H]thymidine can be visualized with autoradiography. However, because [³H]

thymidine autoradiography allows the detection only of labeled cells in the top 3 µm of a section, this technique cannot be used for stereological analyses.

Most neurons in the mammalian brain are produced during the embryonic period. In contrast, the granule cell population of the dentate gyrus of the hippocampal formation is produced during an extended period that begins during gestation and continues well into adulthood. Previously, it was shown that the production of new granule neurons is suppressed by stress. Taken together, these observations suggest that stressful experiences during postnatal development and adulthood have the potential to significantly alter both the structure and function of the hippocampal formation.

Development of the Dentate Gyrus

In most regions of the mammalian brain, the majority of neurons are produced during a discrete part of the embryonic period. In contrast, granule neurons in the dentate gyrus of the hippocampal formation are produced primarily during the postnatal period and throughout adulthood in mammalian species ranging from rodents to primates, including humans. During the embryonic period, the first granule neurons arise from progenitor cells located in the wall of the lateral ventricle that migrate across the hippocampal rudiment to reside in the developing granule cell layer (**Figure 1a**). A subpopulation of these progenitor cells does not undergo final division, is maintained in the hilus and subgranular zone of the dentate gyrus, and continues to give rise to new granule neurons. In the rodent, the majority of neurons in the dentate gyrus are produced during the first 2 postnatal weeks from this secondary proliferative zone; cells in the hilus and subgranular zone divide, migrate along radial glial fibers, and ultimately reside in the granule cell layer (**Figure 1b**). In addition, some granule neurons are also produced from cells within the granule cell layer during this period. Following the second postnatal week, cell proliferation and migration decrease and the granule cell layer is formed. In the primate, the formation of the granule cell layer occurs during the prenatal period, but the production of new granule neurons continues postnatally as well.

In both rodents and primates, new neurons are produced throughout adulthood from progenitor cells

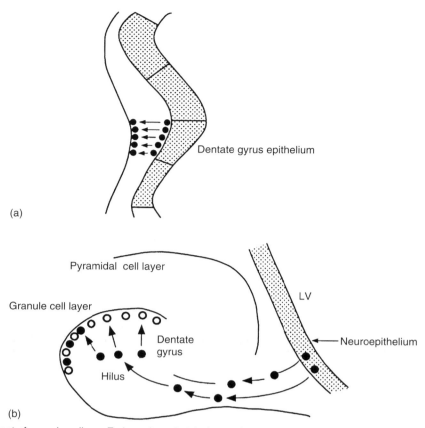

Figure 1 Development of granule cells. a, Embryonic period; b, late embryonic period. During the embryonic period, the first granule neurons arise from progenitor cells located in the wall of the lateral ventricle that migrate across the hippocampal rudiment to reside in the developing granule cell layer. During the late embryonic period and early postnatal development, granule cell precursors in the hilus divide and migrate to the granule cell layer. At the same time, precursor cells in the lateral ventricle continue to migrate into the dentate gyrus. The stippled area represents dentate gyrus neuroepithelium of the lateral ventricle (LV); solid circles represent migrating granule neuron precursors; open circles represent postmitotic immature granule neurons.

located in the hilus and subgranular zone (**Figure 2**). Studies using [³H]thymidine or bromodeoxyuridine (BrdU) molecules, which are incorporated by cells during S phase, and various histological markers of cell phenotype have revealed that cells divide, migrate, extend axons, become incorporated into the granule cell layer, and ultimately express the morphological and biochemical characteristics of mature granule neurons. Although the numbers of new cells produced are much fewer than those observed during development, stereological studies have demonstrated that several thousand new cells are produced each day in the adult rodent brain. Because the majority of neurons in the dentate gyrus are produced postnatally, this brain region is particularly sensitive to changes in the environment during both postnatal development and adulthood compared to other brain regions. Thus, factors that regulate the production of granule neurons are capable of exerting significant effects on both the structure and the function of the hippocampal

formation, which may extend throughout the life of the organism. The remaining part of this article focuses on the regulation of granule neuron production by stress, the factors likely to mediate this regulation, and the possible functional implications of stress-induced changes in postnatal neuron production.

Stress Effects on Neurogenesis

During the first 2 postnatal weeks, termed the stress hyporesponsive period, rat pups exhibit a diminished response to most stressors that are known to increase circulating levels of adrenal steroids in adulthood. However, male rat pups do exhibit an increase in circulating corticosterone levels following acute exposure to the odor of an unfamiliar adult male (adult males are a natural predator of rat pups). Using this paradigm, it has been shown that a single exposure to the odors of an unfamiliar adult male during the stress hyporesponsive period results in a significant

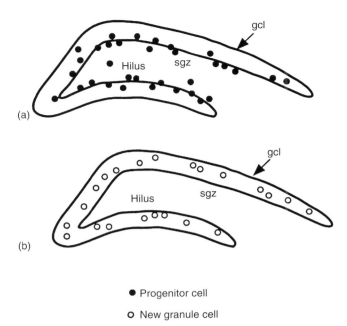

● Progenitor cell

○ New granule cell

Figure 2 Production of new neurons. a, Progenitor cells; b, incorporation into granule cells. In both rodents and primates, new neurons are produced throughout adulthood from progenitor cells located in the hilus and subgranular zone (sgz). Studies using [^{3}H]thymidine or bromodeoxyuridine, both of which are incorporated by cells during S phase, and various histological markers of cell phenotype have revealed that these cells become incorporated into the granule cell layer (gcl) and ultimately express the morphological and biochemical characteristics of mature granule neurons.

decrease in the proliferation of granule cell precursors in the developing dentate gyrus 24 h following exposure.

Acute stressful experiences also decrease the number of new granule neurons produced during adulthood in a number of different species, including rats, tree shrews (animals considered to be phylogenetically between insectivores and primates), and marmosets. In adult rats, exposure to the odors of natural predators, such as foxes or weasels, elicits a stress response characterized by increased serum corticosterone levels and a characteristic electrophysiological response in the dentate gyrus. A single brief exposure to trimethyl thiazoline, a component of fox feces, rapidly suppresses the proliferation of cells in the dentate gyrus.

Similar observations have been made in studies that have examined the effect of social stress in nonrodent species. In tree shrews, the introduction of two adult same-sex conspecifics immediately results in the establishment of an enduring dominant–subordinate relationship. During this time, the subordinate exhibits a robust stress response characterized by elevated cortisol levels, increased heart rate, hypoactivity, and vigilance. Although able to recover physically on removal from the presence of the dominant, the subordinate exhibits an immediate stress response during subsequent encounters with the dominant. A single

brief exposure to a dominant animal, without physical contact, results in a rapid decrease in the number of new cells produced in the dentate gyrus of subordinate tree shrews compared to control animals. Likewise, studies of marmosets using a resident intruder paradigm, a model of psychosocial stress similar to the dominant–subordinate paradigm used with tree shrews, have yielded similar results. In this paradigm, a male marmoset is introduced into the cage of another male. Immediately after being placed in the cage, the intruder exhibits a stress response characterized by elevated mean arterial blood pressure and a dramatically increased heart rate. A single brief exposure to a psychosocial stress in the resident–intruder paradigm results in a rapid decrease in the number of new granule neurons produced in the dentate gyrus compared to naïve control animals.

In addition to exerting an acute impact on granule cell production, stress has also been shown to produce prolonged suppression of this process with repeated exposure. It has been demonstrated that 28 days of exposure to a dominant animal for 1 h each day results in a chronic increase in cortisol levels in adult tree shrews. Furthermore, exposure to chronic stress using this paradigm also results in a decrease in new cell production in the dentate gyrus, which is associated with a decrease in the total volume of the granule cell layer.

Adrenal Steroids Affect Neurogenesis through NMDA Receptors

Although the factors that mediate the stress-induced suppression of granule cell production remain unknown, adrenal steroids are likely to play a significant role in this effect. Several lines of evidence have indicated that adrenal steroids naturally regulate the production of hippocampal granule neurons. First, throughout life, a negative correlation between circulating adrenal steroid levels and the rate of granule neuron production exists. During the late embryonic period, adrenal steroid levels are high and few granule cells are produced. Following parturition, basal levels of glucocorticoids are low during the stress hyporesponsive period. This 2-week period is characterized by a diminished response to stress and maximal rates of neurogenesis. By the third postnatal week and into adulthood, circulating adrenal steroid levels are relatively high and granule production is diminished compared to the levels observed during development. With aging, the levels of glucocorticoids are elevated further and the rate of granule cell production becomes minimal.

Consistent with these natural observations, several studies have demonstrated that the production of neurons can be altered by the experimental manipulation of circulating adrenal steroid levels both during development and adulthood. During the stress hyporesponsive period, the administration of corticosterone results in a significant decrease in the number of granule neurons produced. Similar suppressive effects of adrenal steroids on the proliferation of granule cell precursors have been observed in adulthood as well. The treatment of adult rats with corticosterone results in a decrease in the production of new cells, whereas the removal of adrenal steroids by adrenalectomy results in a rapid increase in the number of new cells produced and, ultimately, in the number of new granule neurons. Despite the dramatic effects of hormone manipulations on cell proliferation in the dentate gyrus, very few granule cell precursors express adrenal steroid receptors, suggesting that adrenal steroids influence neurogenesis indirectly.

In addition to increasing circulating adrenal steroid levels, stressful experiences stimulate hippocampal glutamate release and alter the expression of the NMDA subtype of glutamate receptor in the hippocampal formation. Several lines of evidence suggest that adrenal steroids affect cell proliferation in the dentate gyrus via excitatory input. First, the timing of perforant path development and increased expression of NMDA receptors in the developing dentate gyrus coincides with an observed decrease in granule neuron production. Second, experimental manipulation

of NMDA receptor activation during development or adulthood results in rapid changes in the numbers of new granule neurons. The administration of NMDA receptor antagonists increases the proliferation of granule cell precursors and the production of new granule cells during the early postnatal period and in adulthood in rats and tree shrews. It is likely that these effects are mediated by the perforant pathway, inputs that can involve NMDA receptor activation, because lesion of the entorhinal cortex enhances cell proliferation in the dentate gyrus in adulthood.

The regulation of granule cell production by adrenal steroids and NMDA receptor activation occur via a common pathway. Treatment with corticosterone and MK801 during adulthood results in an increase in cell proliferation that is similar to that observed with MK801 treatment alone. Conversely, adrenalectomized rats that are treated with NMDA demonstrate numbers of proliferating cells that are similar to animals treated with NMDA alone; both groups demonstrate a significant decrease in the numbers of proliferating cells compared to control animals. Collectively, these results indicate that adrenal steroids and NMDA receptor activation decrease cell proliferation via a common pathway. In addition, these results indicate that NMDA receptor activation exerts a more proximal effect on cell proliferation, as evidenced by the fact that the experimental manipulation of NMDA receptor activation can block the effects of corticosterone.

Although the mechanism by which adrenal steroids and NMDA receptor activation suppress cell proliferation is not known, it is possible that these factors initiate a cascade of events that result in a lengthening of the cell cycle. *In vitro* studies in nonneuronal systems have shown that glucocorticoids are capable of lengthening the G1 phase or G2/M phases of the cell cycle. Alternatively, these factors may induce changes that prevent precursor cells from progressing through the cell cycle. *In vitro* studies have also demonstrated that glucocorticoids can reversibly halt the progression of the cell cycle in nonneuronal systems. If adrenal steroids do in fact inhibit progenitor cells from dividing, the removal of adrenal steroids may result in the disinhibition of cells that are normally prevented from progressing through the cell cycle. Such an effect could account for the speed and magnitude of the increases in the number of cells in S phase following the removal of adrenal steroids.

Functional Implications of Stress Effects on Neurogenesis

The functional implications of the stress-induced suppression of neurogenesis are not known. However, the suppression of granule cell production during a time when the majority of granule neurons are produced is likely to have a significant effect on the structure of the adult hippocampal formation. The hippocampal formation has been implicated in learning and memory, raising the possibility that decreases in the production of granule neurons during development may have a negative impact on learning and memory in adulthood. Although there is some evidence to support the idea that stressful experience during development is correlated with impaired cognitive function, an involvement of stress-induced changes in granule neuron production has not yet been investigated.

Although the exact functional significance of adult-generated neurons is not known, evidence suggests a relationship between these new cells and hippocampal-dependent learning. Specifically, the survival of adult-generated cells appears to depend on learning hippocampal-dependent tasks at a critical time after their production. Taken together with the observation that stress suppresses the production of granule neurons, the finding that learning enhances the number of granule neurons suggests that stress-induced changes in neurogenesis may have a significant impact on learning. It is important to note that functional changes are not likely to be immediately evident. New cells require time to differentiate and become incorporated into functional circuitry. Thus, the period following stress-induced changes in cell proliferation is most likely to be functionally relevant. In addition, it is important to note that the functional changes attributable to acute changes in cell production are not likely to be of an observable magnitude. For this reason, the impact of stress-induced changes in neuron production is most likely to be of interest when considering conditions of chronic stress. Thus, although previous studies have demonstrated enhancements in learning as a result of conditions of acute stress, the mechanisms that underlie these effects are likely to involve processes other than changes in neuron production, such as changes in synaptic efficacy.

Several studies have demonstrated that chronic stress or corticosterone treatment exerts a significant impact on hippocampal-dependent learning. In addition, later studies have demonstrated that a stress-induced impairment of spatial learning on different tasks can be observed with both a shorter and a longer duration of stress; 8 days of psychosocial stress result in impaired performance on the hole board spatial discrimination task, and exposure to 6 months of psychosocial stress results in impaired performance on the Morris water maze spatial learning task. The stress-induced impairment observed is not permanent; rats that were tested on the radial arm maze 18 days following the termination of stress performed comparably to control rats. This observation is consistent with a possible involvement of adult-generated cells. If adult-generated cells are indeed necessary for normal performance on this task, an impairment may only persist as long as the production of these cells is altered. Once the stress-induced decrease is no longer present, we expect to observe normal levels of performance. However, stress-induced impairments during the early postnatal period, when the granule cell layer is forming, may have lasting effects.

In general, the degree to which the structure of the adult brain can be altered by experience is limited by the fact that neurons in most brain regions are produced during a discrete period of early embryonic development. Thus, the postnatal production of neurons in the dentate gyrus presents an unusual situation in which the experience of an organism may exert dramatic and potentially long-lasting effects on the structure and function of this brain region.

See Also the Following Articles

Glucocorticoids – Adverse Effects on the Nervous System; Glucocorticoid Effects on Memory: the Positive and Negative; Hippocampal Neurons; Hippocampus, Corticosteroid Effects on.

Further Reading

Altman, J. and Bayer, S. A. (1990). Migration and distribution of two populations of hippocampal granule cell precursors during the perinatal and postnatal periods. *Journal of Comparative Neurology* **301**, 365–381.

Gould, E. and Cameron, H. A. (1996). Regulation of neuronal birth, migration and death in the rat dentate gyrus. *Developmental Neuroscience* **18**, 22–35.

Gould, E., McEwen, B. S., Tanapat, P., et al. (1997). Neurogenesis in the dentate gyrus of the adult tree shrew is regulated by psychosocial stress and NMDA receptor activation. *Journal of Neuroscience* **17**, 2492–2498.

Gould, E., Tanapat, P., Hastings, N. and Shors, T. J. (1999). Neurogenesis in adulthood: a possible role in learning. *Trends in Cognitive Sciences* **3**, 186–191.

Gould, E., Tanapat, P., McEwen, B. S., et al. (1999). Proliferation of granule cell precursors in the dentate gyrus of adult monkeys is diminished by stress. *Proceedings of the National Academy of Sciences USA* **95**, 3168–3171.

Sapolsky, R. M. and Meaney, M. J. (1986). Maturation of the adrenocortical stress response: neuroendocrine control mechanisms and the stress hyporesponsive period. *Brain Research* **396**, 64–76.

Tanapat, P., Galea, L. A. and Gould, E. (1998). Stress inhibits the proliferation of granule cell precursors in the developing dentate gyrus. *International Journal of Developmental Neuroscience* **16**, 235–239.

Neuroimaging and Emotion

N A Harrison and H D Critchley
University College London, London, UK

Emotion
Definition of Emotion
Emotion Perception and Attention
Memory and Learning
Interoception and Subjective Feeling States
Social Interaction
Emotion Regulation
Emotion Dysregulation

Glossary

Amygdala	An almond-shaped cluster of inter-related nuclei and associated cortex in the anterior medial temporal lobe.
Arousal	A dimension of emotion that varies from calm to excitement and predicts behavioral activity level.
Blood–oxygen level-dependent (BOLD) signal	$T2^*$-weighted signal in functional magnetic resonance imaging (fMRI) that reflects hemodynamic changes in regional perfusion evoked by neural activity.
Functional magnetic resonance imaging (fMRI)	A non-invasive technique with good spatial resolution that detects changes in regional blood flow associated with neural activity.
Interoception	A representation of visceral activity; the afferent limb of homoeostatic neural control of bodily organs.
Magnetoence-phalography (MEG)	A non-invasive technique with high temporal resolution that detects the changing magnetic fields associated with neural activity.
Valence	A dimension of emotion that varies from unpleasant (negative) to pleasant (positive) to reflect motivational value.

Emotion

Emotion is central to our everyday human experience. Emotional events or objects within our environment are assigned value, bias our attention, and enhance our subsequent memory. Neuroimaging techniques, perhaps more than other approaches, have led to a growing awareness that emotion, unlike many other psychological functions, is relatively unencapsulated and interacts with and influences multiple other areas of functioning. In addition to effects on attention, perception, memory, and learning, emotion also forms the backbone of our social relationships and is an important component of empathetic understanding of others. Emotional cues also act as powerful reinforcers, have a marked influence on our thoughts and reasoning, and serve to bias our ongoing behavior. Although emotions come in many flavors that may equally serve to bias multiple psychological functions, much of the contemporary research on emotional neuroscience has focused on the processing of fear. For the purposes of this article, we follow this focus, which also accords with an emphasis on stress responses.

Consistent with a broad role in human functioning are the wide-ranging manifestations associated with disorders of emotion regulation. Emotion disequilibrium underlies not just anxiety and stress-related illness but the entire range of mental disorders and acts as the common denominator in much of human unhappiness. This article reviews the contributions of neuroimaging studies to our developing understanding of the neurobiology of human emotion. One particular aim is to highlight how emotion interacts with and influences other areas of cognition and to illustrate how an understanding of the mechanisms underlying these interactions can enable a greater understanding of stress-related disorders.

Definition of Emotion

Differences in definition can lead to markedly different conceptualizations of emotion and underlie seemingly contradictory theories of emotion in the literature. A prevalent view conceptualizes emotion as a transient perturbation in an organism's functioning evoked by a triggering (i.e., emotive) stimulus (either external or internal). Most accounts of emotion also subscribe to a multicomponent description with physiological arousal, motor expression, and subjective feelings forming the reaction triad of emotion. However, the extent to which changes in these various components are necessary and sufficient to define an episode as emotional is more controversial. For the purposes of this article, we use the following definition: emotions are transient events, produced in response to external or internal events of significance to the individual; they are typically characterized by attention to the evoking stimulus and changes in neurophysiological arousal, motor behavior, and subjective feeling state that engender a subsequent biasing of behavior.

Emotion Perception and Attention

Implicit within this definition is that events of significance to the individual (emotive stimuli) are susceptible to preferential perceptual processing. One mechanism through which this is achieved is through the emotional biasing of attentional processes. This is illustrated in behavioral studies using visual search paradigms, in which target items are discriminated from an array containing a variable number of distracter items. Emotionally valenced items or objects are indeed identified more rapidly than nonemotional items. Furthermore, in spatial tasks, the presentation of an emotional cue on one side of the visual space increases the speed of identification of nonemotional stimuli subsequently presented on the same side (i.e., attention is drawn to the location of the preceding emotive stimulus). Neuroimaging studies investigating the neural basis of this emotional capture of attention in spatial orientation tasks show that it is correlated with activity in regions of the frontal and parietal cortices as well as the lateral orbitofrontal cortex.

Evidence from patient studies, neuroimaging, and electroencephalography suggests that even unattended emotional stimuli are more likely to enter awareness, suggesting further mechanisms through which emotional stimuli influence perception. Neuroimaging studies continue to delineate the brain mechanisms through which unattended emotional stimuli gain enhanced access to awareness. One influential hypothesis suggests that the emotional salience of a stimulus is rapidly detected by the amygdala after cursory representational processing. The amygdala subsequently facilitates attention and perception via projections to the sensory cortices to enable more detailed sensory processing. Convergent anatomical studies suggest that this is mediated by both direct and indirect amygdala influences on sensory cortices; reciprocal direct connections exist between the amygdala and sensory cortices, and a projection from the central nucleus of the amygdala to the cholinergic nucleus basalis of Maynert enables indirect ascending cholinergic neuromodulatory influences to be exerted on the same cortical regions.

Functional neuroimaging studies have tested this hypothesis using visual backward-masking paradigms in which briefly presented visual targets are rendered invisible by subsequently presented stimuli. Unseen emotional stimuli, presented in this subliminal manner, can nevertheless still evoke neural responses in the amygdala, compared to nonemotional (neutral) stimuli. Moreover, masked presentations of face stimuli portraying fearful (vs. neutral) facial expressions enhances activation within the fusiform cortex (an extra-striate visual area containing a region implicated as being specialized for processing faces). This activation of the fusiform face area (FFA) is predicted by the magnitude of amygdala activation. Further evidence that emotional processing in the amygdala may enhance activity within sensory cortex comes from the observation that patients with amygdala damage fail to show this enhancement of activity within the face-processing visual cortex when tested on the same paradigm. The presentation of fearful face cues has also been shown to enhance even early perceptual functions such as contrast sensitivity, which is consistent with the suggestion that the amygdala may modulate even activity within the primary visual cortex.

Preattentive processing of emotional stimuli indicates early representational discrimination between emotional and nonemotional events. Studies in humans using magnetoencephalography (MEG), a neuroimaging technique with high temporal resolution, showed discriminatory responses to emotional faces as early as 100–120 ms. This compares to characteristic face-related responses that occurs much later, at 170 ms. Electrophysiological studies in humans using intracranial electrodes also showed an early, 120- to 160-ms response to aversive stimuli. The early recognition of emotionally valenced stimuli accords with animal data suggesting that the amygdala may be activated by a rapid subcortical pathway. Neuroimaging studies in both normal and brain injury subjects highlight subcortical amygdala activation in humans. One study exploited two separate findings: (1) that low- and high-spatial frequency information is processed by separate visual neural pathways and (2) that coarse emotional cues are carried in low-frequency components. When subjects were presented low-frequency (blurred) face stimuli fearful (vs. neutral face stimuli), enhanced activity was seen in the amygdala, pulvinar nucleus of the thalamus, and superior colliculus, components of a proposed subcortical circuit (**Figure 1**). In contrast, the presentation of the same faces at high spatial frequency activated the cortical regions, including the fusiform (face-identity-specific) cortex. Implicit processing of emotional valence can be demonstrated in patients with damage to the primary visual cortex, who are not consciously aware of stimuli presented in their blind hemifield (i.e., blindsight). These patients show amygdala activation to fearful faces presented in their blind hemifield, illustrating the presence of the subcortical visual processing of emotion to the level of the amygdala.

Together these lesion and functional imaging studies provide mechanistic insight into the role of amygdala, through interactions with the sensory cortices, in facilitating enhanced attention and perception of

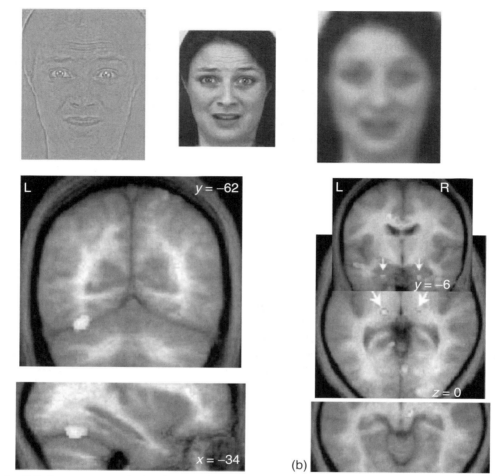

Figure 1 Neural activity in response to viewing facial expressions. a, High-spatial frequency information; b, low-spatial frequency information. High-spatial frequency images activated the fusiform cortex, specialized for the processing of facial identity. Fearful (vs. neutral) facial expressions activated the amygdala bilaterally (vertical arrows) with greater response to low-spatial frequency images. Low-spatial frequency fearful images also activated the posterior inferior thalamus bilaterally (diagonal arrows) and the superior colliculus on the right suggesting that low-spatial frequency images containing emotion information activate a subcortical pathway to the amygdala. Reprinted by permission from Macmillan Publishers Ltd: *Nature Neuroscience;* Vuilleumier, P., Armony, J. L., Driver, J., et al., Distinct spatial frequency sensitivities for processing faces and emotional expressions, **6**, 624–631, copyright (2003).

visually presented emotional stimuli. The preferential early processing of emotionally valenced material, illustrated most powerfully with fearful stimuli, sets up a primary bias in subsequent information processing that underpins the regulation of ongoing and prospective behavior.

Neuroscientific studies of human emotion have tended to focus on the visual processing of emotional facial expressions. Nevertheless, this visual communication of emotional state through changes in the facial musculature is only one part of a richer multimodal vocabulary of affect. Information signaling emotional state is also conveyed by autonomic changes in the skin (leading to color change and sweating) and pupils, by posture and bodily movements, and by content and prosody of speech. Low-level auditory

processing of emotional signals are the primary source of emotional information in speech. The prioritized processing of emotional sounds, particularly non-speech intonations of emotional state (gasps, screams, etc.), is illustrated within the primary and accessory auditory cortices. As with the visual system, amygdalo-cortical interactions are implicated in enhanced auditory attention to emotive sounds. Moreover, specificity in emotional processing may cross sensory modalities, such that ventral insular regions implicated in disgust-processing may be activated by auditory and visual expressions of disgust as well as by disgusting stimuli.

A degree of regional specialization in human emotional processing is suggested from the convergence of lesion and neuroimaging studies. Acquired damage to the amygdala impairs the recognition and behavioral experience of fear. Similarly, the neuroimaging literature emphasizes a predominant sensitivity of amygdala responses to threat and fear signals. As previously indicated, other studies implicate regions of insula and striatum in the selective processing of disgust. The impaired recognition of facial expressions of disgust was reported in a patient with damage to these regions, whereas the stimulation of the insula may evoke feelings of nausea or a perception of unpleasant tastes. These lines of evidence for specialized emotion-specific processing within different brain regions are generally circumscribed to fear/threat (amygdala), disgust (insula and striatum), and, to a lesser extent, sadness (subgenual cingulate activity). Many neuroimaging studies highlight a general sensitivity of amygdala responses to the emotional intensity of external emotional stimuli, for which threat is perhaps most arousing.

The insula cortex also appears to play a more complex role in emotion perception, apparently through relating perceptual information with interoceptive representations of bodily states. Thus, insula activity is engaged during the recognition and experience of disgust, sadness, happiness, and fear; during the learning and expression of threat; during the perception of noxious stimuli; and during the experience of phobic symptoms, hunger, and satiety; and even during explicit facial emotion categorization.

Memory and Learning

Emotion has a striking and well described impact on memory processes. Animal studies, particularly the work of LeDoux, highlight the central role of the amygdala in fear conditioning, a form of implicit memory. The same is true in humans, illustrated in many neuroimaging and lesion studies. Fear conditioning is a rapid form of learning that a stimulus is potentially harmful. If an adverse event (unconditioned stimulus, US; e.g., a painful shock) occurs after a relatively innocuous stimulus, the latter (the conditioned stimulus, CS) comes to predict the adverse event and will engender arousal responses associated with the presence of threat. Patients with bilateral amygdala damage do not acquire conditioned fear responses (autonomic or motor), despite having an intact explicit knowledge of the association between the CS and US. Functional neuroimaging studies also confirm the importance of the amygdala in fear conditioning (i.e., the learning of CS–US associations). However the role of the amygdala in the expression of threat responses is more time-limited and shows habituation. Consistent with animal data, neuroimaging studies also describe amygdala engagement in more general associative reinforcement learning,

including operant stimulus–reward learning and appetitive behavior.

In addition to simple associative responses, human memory is characterized by declarative richness in episodic and semantic memory. These domains of memory, typically supported both at encoding and recollection by activity within the hippocampus, are strongly modulated by emotional experience. Typically, emotional events and stimuli are remembered better than nonemotional occurrences. Animal studies highlight noradrenergic mechanisms enhancing amygdalo-hippocampal connectivity in preferential encoding of emotional objects. Brain-imaging studies in humans have gone much further, highlighting amygdala activation during encoding actually predicts the accuracy of subsequent declarative memory of positively or negatively valenced stimuli (**Figure 2**) and in delineating the functional architecture for mood-congruency effects (in which negative information is encoded and recalled to a greater extent when the subject is in a negative mood and, likewise, positive material is encoded and recalled to a greater extent in positive mood states). However, the role of the amygdala extends beyond encoding processes; it is also engaged during the retrieval of emotional items and contexts.

Interoception and Subjective Feeling States

Changes in bodily state, reflected in both physiological arousal and motor behavior, are obligatory defining characteristics of emotion. James and Lange, and more recently Damasio, argued that emotional feeling states must have their origin in the brain's representation of the bodily (arousal) state. Without changes in bodily arousal, there is no emotion. This peripheral account of emotion predicts that afferent feedback signals from muscles and viscera associated with physiological arousal are integral to emotional experience. These mechanisms have been illuminated in a number of neuroimaging experiments examining central representation and rerepresentation of autonomic arousal states and homoeostatic sensations, such as temperature.

The role of the insula cortex in this context is particularly interesting. In a positron emission tomography (PET) study, activation within the viscerosensory mid-insula cortex correlated closely with the actual stimulus temperature, yet the subjective ratings of the perceived intensity or pleasantness of hot and cold stimuli correlated with activity in the right anterior insula and orbitofrontal cortex. This finding suggests a dissociation between a primary central representation of viscerosensory information, within

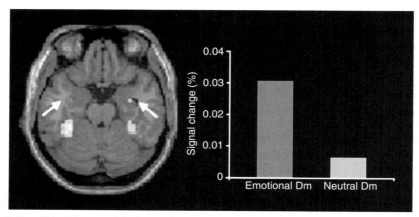

Figure 2 Level of activity within the amygdala (arrows) during the encoding of emotional images predicts whether a subject is subsequently able to recall emotional pictures (emotional Dm) but not neutral pictures (neutral Dm). Reprinted from *Neuron* **48**, E. A. Phelps & J. E. LeDoux, Contributions of the amygdala to emotion processing: from animal models to human behavior, pp. 175–187, Copyright 2005, and adapted from *Neuron*, **42**, F. Dolcos, K. S. LaBar & R. Cabeza, Interaction between the amygdala and the medial temporal lobe memory system predicts better memory for emotional events, pp. 855–863, Copyright (2004), with permission from Elsevier.

mid-insula, and subjective feelings of warmth or cold, represented in the right anterior insula and orbitofrontal cortex. A general role for these regions in the representation of emotional feelings is also supported by their activation observed during generated states of sadness and anger, anticipatory anxiety and pain, panic, disgust, sexual arousal, trustworthiness, and even subjective responses to music.

Behavioral and neuroimaging studies in patients with selective peripheral autonomic denervation (pure autonomic failure, PAF) lend further support to the importance of viscerosensory feedback to emotional feelings. These patients, who do not have autonomic (e.g., heart-rate or skin-conductance) changes in response to emotional stimuli or physiological stressors, show a subtle blunting of subjective emotional experience. In a fear conditioning study of PAF subjects and controls, both groups showed amygdala activity during the learning of threat (face stimuli, CS, were paired with an aversive blast of white noise, US). However, compared to controls, the right insula cortex showed attenuated responses to threat stimuli in the PAF patients, suggesting this region is sensitive to the presence and absence of autonomic responses generated during emotional processing. Moreover, when the threat stimuli were presented unconsciously (using backward masking), the same insula regions (including the right anterior insula) were sensitive to both the conscious awareness of emotion events and induced bodily arousal reactions. This study, particularly, suggests that the right insula is a neural substrate for the contextual integration of external emotional events with feeling states arising from bodily reactions.

The notion that subjective emotional feelings arise from central representations of bodily arousal states predicts that people who are more aware of their bodily responses may experience more intense emotions and feelings. Investigations examining individual differences in interoceptive awareness suggest that patients with anxiety disorders are more attuned to bodily reactions such as their own heartbeat or stomach motility. One such interoceptive task was translated into a neuroimaging study. Subjects were played a series of notes, presented in groups of 10, either synchronously or out of phase with their own heartbeats (see **Figure 3a**). In half the trials, subjects had to judge the timing of their heartbeat in relation to the notes (the control condition was a detection of a rogue note in the sequence). When subjects focused interoceptively to the timing of their own heartbeat, there was enhanced activity in the somatomotor, insula, and cingulate cortices. However, only one region, the right anterior insula cortex, reflected a conscious awareness of internal bodily responses (i.e., how accurately subjects performed the interoceptive task). Significantly, activity in this region, and even the relative amount of right anterior gray matter here (**Figure 3b**), predicted day-to-day awareness of bodily reaction and the subjective experience of negative emotions, particularly anxiety symptoms across individuals. Together these studies suggest that the right anterior insula is a principal neural substrate supporting conscious emotional feelings arising from interoceptive information concerning bodily arousal state (**Figure 4**).

Social Interaction

A characteristic of our social interactions is an intuitive ability to understand other people's mental and

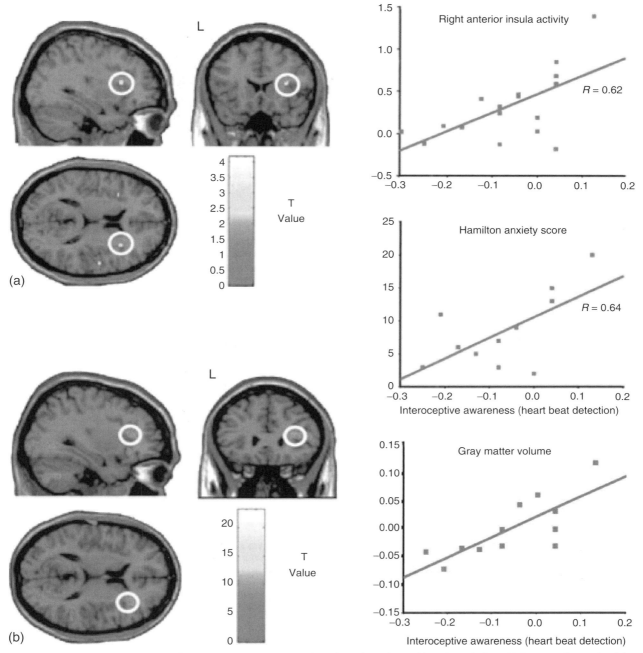

Figure 3 Interoceptive awareness (measured as accuracy on a heartbeat detection task). a, Association with increased neural activity in the right anterior insula/operculum; b, correlation with the gray matter volume of the right anterior insula region. Further subjects with greater interoceptive awareness also showed greater neural activity in this region during interoceptive trials. Activity in this region also correlated with anxiety scores, suggesting that emotional feeling states are supported by explicit interoceptive representations within right insula cortex. Reprinted by permission from Macmillan Publishers Ltd: *Nature Neuroscience*; Critchley, H. D., Wiens, S., Rotshtein, P., et al., Neural systems supporting interoceptive awareness, **7**(2), 189–195, copyright (2004).

emotional states. Humans show a marked tendency to mimic one another's gesticulations, emotional facial expressions, and body postures, suggesting that this mirroring of activity mediates and facilitates emotional understanding among individuals. At a neural level, cells in monkey premotor cortex have been described that respond to observing or performing the same motor actions. Corresponding human imaging studies of action observation also illustrate premotor cortical activity when observing the actions of others, and magnetoencephalography (MEG) studies report resynchronization in the primary motor cortex. Significantly,

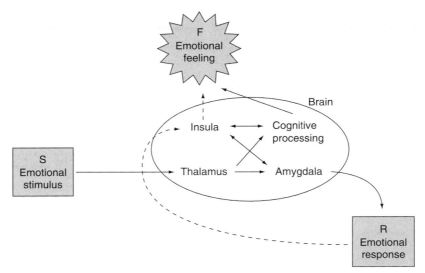

Figure 4 A functional neuroanatomical modification of William James's (1884) model of emotional responses. Emotional stimuli (S) elicit automatic emotional responses (R) via thalamus–amygdala pathways (solid line arrows). This low-level processing occurs independently of conscious cognitive processing. Peripheral autonomic responses are fed back to the mid-insula and then are remapped to the right anterior insula where they interact with higher-level cognitive processing. Emotional feeling states therefore result from peripheral-central interaction in the right anterior insula. Reprinted from *Trends in Cognitive Sciences*, **6**(8), J. S. Morris, How do you feel?, pp. 317–319, Copyright (2002), with permission from Elsevier.

these mirror activations are somatotopic with respect to the body part performing the action.

Accumulating evidence supports the extension of these action-perception mechanisms to emotions and feeling states. A common neural representation is proposed for the perception of actions and feelings in others and their experience in self. Thus, viewing emotional facial expressions in others activates automatically mirrored expressions on one's own face (surprisingly, even when the observed facial expressions are masked, hence unavailable to conscious awareness). Significantly, this automatic mimicking of emotional expressions also extends to autonomic expressions of emotional states such as pupil size in expressions of sadness. Neuroimaging studies show shared neural activation in the somatosensory cortex when a subject experienced or observed another being touched, right insula activity when a subject experienced disgusting odors or observed expressions of disgust, and the activation of a common matrix of regions when a subject experienced or observed pain. The imitation or observation of emotional facial expressions also activates a largely similar network of brain regions including the premotor areas that are critical for action representation. There is also selectivity; compared to nonemotional facial movements, emotional expressions activate the right frontal operculum and anterior insula, and regions such as the amygdala, striatum, and subgenual cingulate are differentially responsive when imitating happy or sad emotions.

Emotion Regulation

Understanding the adaptive mechanisms through which we can control the expression of our emotions is clinically and socially important. Unlearning established emotional reactions is difficult. Many studies have examined the modulation of previously learned emotional responses with experimental extinction; the repeated presentation of a previously CS without its associated US rapidly leads to a diminished emotional response. Nevertheless, the relationship between the two stimuli is not forgotten but inhibited and can be rapidly reinstated. Neuroimaging of extinction learning (or the inhibition of emotional responses) shows increased amygdala activity in early extinction; however, retention after a day was associated with activity in the subgenual anterior cingulate and ventromedial prefrontal cortices, which suggests a role for this region in the longer-term recall of extinction learning (**Figure 5**).

Emotional responses may also be regulated volitionally, using cognitive control or reappraisal. For example, an image of a woman crying may be interpreted as one of sadness, but, if the subject is then told that the picture was taken after her daughter's wedding, it may be reappraised as one of great joy. Neuroimaging studies of emotional reappraisal demonstrate an attenuation of activity in the amygdala associated with enhanced activity in the left middle frontal gyrus, suggesting that activity within the lateral

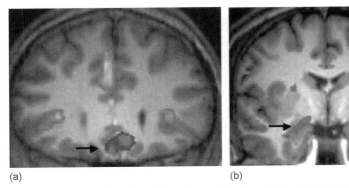

(a)   (b)

Figure 5 Regions activated in the extinction of conditioned fear. a, Ventromedial prefrontal cortex (arrow) showing less response to the conditioned stimulus (CS+) during acquisition; b, amygdala activation (arrow) in response to the CS+ during acquisition versus early extinction. During extinction training, ventromedial prefrontal cortex activity gradually increased, and the magnitude of this increase predicted the retention of extinction learning. Extinction training resulted in a reduction of amygdala activity in response to the CS+ and predicted the success of early extinction. Reprinted from *Neuron*, **48**, E A. Phelps & J. E. LeDoux, Contributions of the amygdala to emotion processing: from animal models to human behavior, pp. 175–187, Copyright (2005), and adapted from *Neuron*, **43**, E. A. Phelps et al., Extinction learning in humans: role of the amygdala and vmPFC, pp. 897–905, Copyright (2004), with permission from Elsevier.

prefrontal cortex modulates emotional reactivity of the amygdala, possibly via connections to medial prefrontal cortex. Similar cognitive emotion-regulation techniques can powerfully diminish responses acquired through fear conditioning, and neuroimaging studies using this paradigm again show increased activity in the left middle frontal gyrus with cognitive control. Taken together, these studies suggest that cognitive emotion regulation and lower-level extinction learning recruit similar overlapping neural mechanisms for the regulation of the amygdala to control primary emotional responses.

Emotion Dysregulation

The wide-ranging influences of emotion on other psychological functions may also be seen in the variety of symptoms and presentations associated with emotional disorders. Posttraumatic stress disorder (PTSD), resulting from exposure to a highly traumatic emotional event and usually associated with injury or risk of injury to self or others, is frequently associated with symptoms in multiple psychological domains. Enhanced arousal and startle responses to previously innocuous stimuli are common, as are intrusive traumatic memories (flashbacks) of the triggering event, the numbing of emotional feelings, and impairments to social relationships. The identification of brain regions that show increased activation associated with the enhanced perception and memory for emotional events and associated feeling states enables the linkage of psychological mechanisms in conditions such as PTSD and phobias with their underlying neural substrates.

Abnormal cortisol regulation and adrenergic stress responses are also seen in PTSD, as is a reduction in hippocampal volume. Imaging studies showing a similar reduction in hippocampal volume in endocrine disorders associated with chronically elevated cortisol levels, such as Cushing's disease, suggest an etiological role for stress hormones such as cortisol in this reduction in hippocampal volume. These conclusions are further supported by a recent study of healthy postmenopausal women, which showed a strong correlation between hippocampal volume and lifetime levels of perceived stress, suggesting an influence of stress on regional brain volumes even in the normal population.

Maladaptive cognitive interpretations of situations or events are central components of many emotional disorders such as depression and the anxiety disorders and are a feature focused on by many of the psychological therapies used in their treatment. Understanding the neural mechanisms mediating the modulation of emotional responses will be essential to developing a comprehensive neurobiological understanding of these disorders. Furthermore, a better understanding of these mechanisms offers the opportunity to develop more targeted approaches specifically focused on changing these maladaptive emotional reactions.

See Also the Following Articles

Amygdala; Brain and Brain Regions; Emotions: Structure and Adaptive Functions; Hippocampus, Overview.

Further Reading

Calder, A. J., Keane, J., Manes, F., et al. (2001). Impaired recognition and experience of disgust following brain injury. *Nature Neuroscience* 3(11), 1077–1078.

Craig, A. D. (2002). How do you feel? interoception: the sense of the physiological condition of the body. *Nature Reviews Neuroscience* 3, 655–667.

Critchley, H. D., Mathias, C. J. and Dolan, R. J. (2001). Neuroanatomical basis for first and second order representations of bodily states. *Nature Neuroscience* **4**(2), 207–212.

Critchley, H. D., Mathias, C. J. and Dolan, R. J. (2002). Fear conditioning in humans: the influence of awareness and autonomic arousal on functional neuroanatomy. *Neuron* **33**(4), 653–663.

Critchley, H. D., Wiens, S., Rotshtein, P., et al. (2004). Neural systems supporting interoceptive awareness. *Nature Neuroscience* **7**(2), 189–195.

Damasio, A. R. (1994). *Descartes error: emotion, reason and the human brain.* New York: Grosset/Putnam.

Damasio, A. R. (1999). *The feeling of what happens: body and emotion in the making of consciousness.* New York: Harcourt Brace.

Darwin, C. (1872). *The expressions of emotion in man and animals.* London: John Murray. (Reprinted 1998 (3rd edn.), Ekman, P. (ed.). London: Harper Collins.)

Dimberg, U., Thunberg, D. and Elmehed, K. (2000). Unconscious facial reactions to emotional facial expressions. *Psychological Science* **11**(1), 86–89.

Dolan, R. J. (2002). Emotion, cognition, and behavior. *Science* **298**, 1191–1194.

Dolcos, F., LaBar, K. S. and Cabeza, R. (2004). Interaction between the amygdala and the medial temporal lobe memory system predicts better memory for emotional events. *Neuron* **42**, 855–863.

Gallese, V. (2003). The manifold nature of interpersonal relations: the quest for a common mechanism. *Philosophical Transactions of Royal Society London B* **358**(1431), 517–528.

Gianaros, P. J., Jennings, J. R., Sheu, L. K., et al. (2007). Prospective reports of chronic life stress predict decreased grey matter volume in the hippocampus. *NeuroImage* **35**(1), 220–232.

Harrison, N. A., Singer, T., Rotshtein, P., et al. (2006). Pupillary contagion: central mechanisms engaged in sadness processing. *Social and Affective Neuroscience* **1**, 5–17.

James, W. (1884). Physical basis of emotion. *Psychological Review* **1**, 516–529.

LaBar, K. S. and Cabeza, R. (2006). Cognitive neuroscience of emotional memory. *Nature Reviews Neuroscience* **7**, 54–64.

Lange, C. (1885/1922). *The emotions.* Haupt, I. A. (trans.). Baltimore, MD: Williams & Wilkins.

LeDoux, J. E. (1996). *The emotional brain: the mysterious underpinnings of emotional life.* New York: Simon & Schuster.

Morris, J. S. (2002). How do you feel? *Trends in Cognitive Sciences* **6**(8), 317–319.

Morris, J. S., DeGelder, B., Weiskrantz, L., et al. (2001). Differential extrageniculostriate and amygdala responses to presentation of emotional faces in a cortically blind field. *Brain* **124**, 1241–1252.

Morris, J. S., Friston, K. J., Buchel, C., et al. (1998). A neuromodulatory role for the human amygdala in processing emotional facial expressions. *Brain* **121**, 47–57.

Morris, J. S., Ohman, A. and Dolan, R. J. (1998). Conscious and unconscious emotional learning in the human amygdala. *Nature* **393**, 467–470.

Ochsner, K. N. and Gross, J. J. (2005). The cognitive control of emotion. *Trends in Cognitive Sciences* **9**(5), 242–249.

Penfield, W. and Faulk, M. E. (1955). The insula: further observations on its function. *Brain* **78**(4), 445–470.

Phelps, E. A. and LeDoux, J. E. (2005). Contributions of the amygdala to emotion processing: from animal models to human behavior. *Neuron* **48**, 175–187.

Phillips, M. L., Young, A. W., Senior, C., et al. (1997). A specific neural substrate for perception of facial expressions of disgust. *Nature* **389**, 495–498.

Scherer, K. R. (2000). Psychological models of emotion. In: Borod, J. C. (ed.) *The neuropsychology of emotion*, pp. 137–162. New York: Oxford University Press.

Singer, T., Seymour, B., O'Doherty, J., et al. (2004). Empathy for pain involves the affective but not sensory components of pain. *Science* **303**(5661), 1157–1162.

Vuilleumier, P., Armony, J. L., Driver, J., et al. (2003). Distinct spatial frequency sensitivities for processing faces and emotional expressions. *Nature Neuroscience* **6**, 624–631.

Vuilleumier, P., Richardson, M. P., Armony, J. L., et al. (2004). Distant influences of amygdala lesions on visual cortical activation during emotional face processing. *Nature Neuroscience* **7**, 1271–1278.

Wicker, B., Keysers, C., Plailly, J., et al. (2003). Both of us disgusted in my insula: the common neural basis of seeing and feeling disgust. *Neuron* **40**, 655–664.

Neuroimmunomodulation

N R Rose
Johns Hopkins University, Baltimore, MD, USA

This article is reproduced from the previous edition, volume 3, pp 37–48, © 2000, Elsevier Inc., with revisions made by the Editor.

Communication between the Nervous System and the Immune System

Communication Channels between the Nervous System and the Immune System

Cytokine Interactions with the Nervous System

Clinical Implications of Neural-Immune Signaling

Glossary

Cytokines	Signal molecules released from immunocytes, supporting cells, or other cell types (endothelial cells) that can interact with other cells of the immune system and alter their intracellular capabilities.
Immunocytes	Cells of the immune system.
Innervation	The distribution of nerve fibers that end in association with a particular structure, region, or organ.
Neurohormone	A blood-borne signal of endocrine nature that is either derived from the brain directly or released from the pituitary gland due to neurally derived factors.
Neuro-modulation	The interaction of a neurally derived signal with a target cell that alters the intracellular capabilities of that cell through either genomic or nongenomic mechanisms.
Neuropeptides	Neural signal molecules derived from larger prohormones that consist of 3–100 or more amino acids; released from nerve endings, cells of neural origin, or cells of immune or endocrine origin.
Neuro-transmitter	A signal molecule released from nerve endings that can interact with specific receptors on target cells and alter either ion channels or second messengers following transduction.

Neuroimmunomodulation is the bidirectional signaling between the central nervous system (CNS) (the brain and spinal cord) and the cells and organs of the immune system. The CNS can send neuroendocrine signals that act on specific subsets of cells of the immune system and can also send direct neural connections into lymphoid organs, where released neurotransmitters act on specific cell subsets of the immune system. These subsets of immunological cells possess a variety of receptors for neurohormones and neurotransmitters that permit signal transduction, influencing the activities and synthetic capacities of those cells. This direct neural-immune signaling modulates individual cellular functions as well as collective immune responses. Thus, the CNS can modulate immune responses, including innate immunity, cell-mediated immunity, autoimmunity, and complex collective immune reactivity to infections, cancer, and other challenges. This neural-immune circuitry permits behavioral influences, including those resulting from physical and psychological stressors, to modulate the activities of the immune system. The immune system, in turn, through the release of cytokines from specific subsets of cells, can signal neurons in the CNS and peripheral nervous system (PNS) directly and indirectly. This signaling influences the visceral and neuroendocrine functions of the hypothalamus, as well as the cognitive and affective functions of the forebrain. Some of the inflammatory cytokines, acting through the hypothalamus, can influence the activation of two highly significant components of the stress axes profoundly, the hypothalamic-pituitary-adrenal (HPA) axis and the sympathetic component of the autonomic nervous system (ANS). Therefore, the two great memory systems and communication systems of the body, the CNS and the immune system, are in constant communication with one another through biological signaling using endocrine hormones, neurotransmitters, and cytokines.

Communication between the Nervous System and the Immune System

Since the time of Galen, an association has been suspected between the mind or emotions and the clinical course or outcome of disease, as in Galen's description of melancholia and breast cancer. Early studies in humans pointed toward an association between psychosocial factors, particularly psychological stressors and the response of humans to various diseases thought to involve the immune system, such as bacterial and viral infections, allergic disorders, autoimmune diseases, and cancer. However, early correlational studies were unable to identify the communication channels through which such interactions between the nervous system and immune system could take place. Early studies in rodents also demonstrated a link between psychological stressors and antibody responses, graft-versus-host responses, susceptibility to viral infections, and other reactions of the immune system, but, again, the neural communication channels were not elucidated in these early studies of the 1950s and 1960s.

Evidence for Neural-Immune Communication in Humans

Numerous studies of depressed individuals have reported diminished lymphocyte responses to proliferative stimuli (mitogens) or the diminution of other immune parameters such as natural killer (NK) cell activity or ratios of lymphocyte subsets. However, not all studies found such changes. Many variables influence the extent or presence of alterations in immunological parameters, including the type and severity of depression, time and treatment factors, and the age and gender of the patients. The most enduring findings reported that these diminished measures of immune response correlate best with the severity of depression and older age, particularly in men. The extent to which these diminished measures of immunological reactivity contribute to increased morbidity and mortality remains elusive.

Bereavement studies from the loss of a spouse also demonstrate diminished lymphocyte responses to mitogens and diminished NK cell activity, particularly in men. As in studies of other stressors in humans, the quality and extent of social support and the individuals' perception of control over their circumstances can act as buffers to ameliorate the stress-induced decline in measures of immunological reactivity.

The most extensive literature on neural-immune communications in humans is derived from studies of life stressors and psychosocial factors in selected groups of patients, particularly the studies of Janice Kiecolt-Glaser and Ronald Glaser. These investigators demonstrated diminished lymphocyte responses to mitogens, altered lymphocyte subsets, diminished NK cell activity, and increased antibody responses to viral epitopes on previously latent viruses in medical students during examination stress. Subsequent reports also demonstrated a diminished production of Th1 (cell-mediated) cytokines in medical students faced with examinations. Loneliness or lack of social support contributed to the presence and persistence of these alterations. Similar alterations in immune responsiveness (diminished mitogen responses and NK cell activity, and altered antibody or cytokine responses) have also been reported in a variety of other stressors, including marital separation and divorce, hostile behavior toward spouses in both recent and long-standing marriages, caregiving to a loved one with dementia (e.g., Alzheimer's disease),

and adaptation to a nursing home. In some of the marital studies, a significant impact of hostile behavior was noted on stress mediators, with the elevation of epinephrine and norepinephrine (NE), adrenocorticotropic hormone (ACTH), growth hormone (GH), and prolactin. These important studies indicate direct links between behaviors or psychosocial factors, neuroendocrine and neurotransmitter mediators, and altered immune responses. It now appears that these links have direct implications for health through the modulation of wound repair, inflammation, NK cell response and tumor metastases, lymphocyte functions, and collective cell-mediated (vs. humoral) immune responses to infectious challenges by viruses and bacteria.

Positive emotions and positive factors also can modulate immune reactivity, often in a direction opposite to that of stressors. Social support interventions in nursing home subjects demonstrated an enhancement of some of the immunological parameters that were diminished previously. Lee Berk and colleagues have shown that mirthful laughter is accompanied by a diminution of stress mediators such as NE and cortisol and by enhanced NK cell activity and other immunological measures. Exercise that does not exceed 70–80% of capacity results in enhanced NK cell activity, enhanced lymphocyte mitogen responses, and enhanced measures of cell-mediated activity; exercise that exceeds these limits depresses many of these same parameters substantially. Due to the nature of the measurements of immune responsiveness in humans, limited mainly to blood samples, the extent to which these changes reflect the direct effect of mediators on individual cell functions, or the indirect effects of such parameters as altered cell trafficking, is not known. Some studies of various relaxation responses report the enhancement of some measures of immune response as well.

Studies in women with breast cancer by David Spiegel and colleagues and in patients with malignant melanoma by Fawzy Fawzy and colleagues have reported that structured psychological interventions involving counseling and peer support can extend longevity and enhance the quality of life. These provocative studies have evoked great interest in both scientific and lay communities and await further confirmation in multicenter trials and in studies in which neural-immune mediators and immunological measures are carried out in the same patients.

Caution is needed in studies of immune responses that accompany various stressors, positive behavioral and emotional factors, or structured interventions. Specific measures of immunological reactivity imply specific health consequences. For example, enhanced NK cell activity appears to aid in the innate response to viral killing and in the killing of metastatic cancer cells, particularly when blood-borne. Enhanced cell-mediated immunity, production of Th1 cytokines such as interleukin (IL-2) and interferon (IFN-γ), boosts host responses to viral infections and appears to be protective in elderly individuals; human immunodeficiency virus (HIV)-positive individuals; and patients with a variety of cancers, including relatively nonimmunogenical cancers. However, enhanced cell-mediated T lymphocyte responses may be highly detrimental to an individual with an autoimmune disease such as multiple sclerosis; clinical trials with INF-γ showed an increased frequency of demyelinating attacks on the CNS. Thus, enhancing the immune system is a meaningless phrase unless we define (1) which parameters of immunological reactivity are enhanced, (2) which specific group of individuals is being studied, and (3) what specific immunological challenges the individuals are facing. The popular literature and lay understandings of this concept are virtually absent and need to be addressed.

Evidence for Neural-Immune Communication in Experimental Animals

A striking body of evidence for neural-immune communication in experimental animals comes from the conditioning studies of Robert Ader and Nicholas Cohen. Using a taste aversion model, they demonstrated that immune suppression from the administration of cyclophosphamide could be conditioned by a novel taste stimulus. This conditioned immune suppression was of sufficient functional magnitude that the conditioned rodents who were given the novel taste stimulus at a later time in their drinking water died of pneumonia; this agent had no effect in unconditioned animals. These investigators later studied conditioned immunosuppression in genetically autoimmune animals with a lupuslike syndrome that kills them early in life. These conditioned animals showed remarkably extended longevity without evidence of the lupus-related lymphadenopathy. As a further demonstration (one more pleasing to immunologists), Ader and Cohen demonstrated that an antigen itself (rather than a drug) could be paired with a novel taste stimulus to produce a conditioned enhancement of the magnitude of secondary antibody responses. Although the implications for application to humans facing difficult drug therapy with immune-reactive agents are highly promising, those studies are only now being pursued.

Studies in animals have investigated the immunological consequences of a wide range of physical and psychological stressors. In some circumstances, stressors such as extensive restraint result in suppressed NK cell activity, diminished lymphocyte proliferative responses to mitogens, and even diminished cell-mediated and humoral immune responses. However, many complications arise in these stress and immunity studies. Sometimes, a stressor elicits enhanced immune responses rather than suppressed immune responses. Subtle differences in shock paradigms, related to frequency, intensity, and repetitions of the shocks, can produce the opposite effects, or no change at all, in immunological measurements. Even more perplexing is the finding that some stressors elicit the enhancement of one form of cell-mediated immune response and the suppression of a closely related but different cell-mediated immune response.

Thus, the impression expressed frequently in the lay literature that all stressors are bad for the immune system is simply incorrect. Some intriguing findings related to the exposure of rodents to stressors such as mild foot shocks involve the controllability of the stressors. Rodents who could not control the termination of the shocks showed a greater extent of immunological impairment than their counterparts who were able to control the termination of the shock and had less ability to respond to challenges from viruses, bacteria, or tumors. In general, acute laboratory stressors result in a wider and more complicated array of changes in immunological reactivity than chronic stressors. It is the chronic stressors that appear to be most likely to result in suppressed immune reactivity across a wide range of responses. Perhaps one of the most intriguing findings related to stressors and immune responses is their consequence for the progression of autoimmune diseases in experimental animals. Physical and psychological stressors, in general, protect against the progression of autoimmune symptoms and consequences; however, in the poststress interval, that benefit is lost or reversed, sometimes worsening the disease progression. A recent fascinating finding is the ability of IL-1β to stimulate the corticotropin releasing hormone (CRH) system in the hypothalamus, thereby activating both the HPA axis (cortisol secretion) and the sympathetic nervous system (SNS; norepinephric, NE, neurotransmission). It appears that IL-1β is one of the most potent activators of both of these stress axes compared with other physical and psychological stressors. Perhaps the immunological reactivity that results in the production of systemic inflammatory mediators should be considered at the top of the list of potent stressors in both experimental animals and humans.

One additional area of investigation that demonstrates a link between the nervous system and the immune system is the immunological consequences of direct lesions placed in the CNS. In general, lesion sites that result in altered immune responses are found in the hypothalamus, the limbic forebrain (septum, hippocampal formation, amygdala, and some cortical regions), and brain-stem areas related to the regulation of autonomic outflow and processing or the reticular formation. These lesion studies suggest a complex array of circuitry that involves both excitatory and inhibitory neural connections that ultimately are able to alter the reactivity of specific portions of the immune system via neuroendocrine or autonomic outflow.

Communication Channels between the Nervous System and the Immune System

The CNS has two major routes of communication by which it can signal cells and tissues of the immune system. The first is the neuroendocrine channels that generally emanate from the hypothalamus and regulate the outflow of anterior and posterior pituitary hormones. Some of these hormones exert direct influences on immunocytes (cells of the immune system), whereas other anterior pituitary hormones act by stimulating additional hormones from target organs in the periphery. The second is the direct neural channels that provide anatomical nerve fiber connections between the CNS and lymphoid organs and tissues. These neural channels are either part of the ANS (and connect via a two classical two-neuron chain to the target structure) or part of the one-neuron sensory (afferent) connections from the periphery into the CNS. Some primary afferents are capable of releasing neurotransmitters both proximally, into the CNS, and distally, into the site of distribution of the sensory receptive elements. The autonomic nerve distribution to lymphoid organs and tissues derives principally from the sympathetic division of the ANS.

The immune system can signal neurons or supporting cells of the CNS and PNS principally via the release of cytokines. The cytokines can act on peripheral neuronal elements in the local paracrine environment and can act on CNS cells either through the actions of circulating cytokines or through the activation of primary afferents that activate central afferent autonomic circuitry.

Immunocytes Possess Receptors for Hormones and Neurotransmitters

Immunocytes, including lymphocytes (both B and T cells), macrophages/monocytes, granulocytes, thymocytes, stem cells, and other associated cell types, possess receptors for hormones and neurotransmitters. Some hormone receptors are present on the plasma membrane of immunocytes; their stimulation results in the altered activation of ion channels or the altered production of second messengers. Other

hormone receptors are found intracellularly and, when combined with a properly configured hormone (ligand), can exert genomic influences by acting as transcription factors or in combination with other transcription factors. The hormone–receptor complex can also alter intracellular transduction pathways. In addition, immunocytes possess neurotransmitter receptors on the plasma membrane. When activated by the appropriate ligand, these receptors on immunocytes can influence intracellular events through one or more second-messenger pathways. Some receptors for neurotransmitters (e.g., the β adrenoceptor) appear to be identical to their counterparts on neurons and peripheral target organs of the SNS, whereas other receptors (e.g., the substance P, SP, receptor) appear to be configured slightly differently from their neuronal counterparts. Immunocytes possessing this SP receptor respond more broadly to SP and substance K elements of the tachykinin family than does a neuron with its more narrowly responsive SP receptor.

Neurotransmitter and hormone receptors are not expressed by all immunocytes and, when expressed, are not distributed uniformly across all subsets or during all states of activation. For example, Virginia Sanders and others have demonstrated that β adrenoceptors, responsive to catecholamines such as NE and epinephrine, are expressed more abundantly on B lymphocytes than on T lymphocytes and more abundantly on T suppressor/cytotoxic (CD8) cells than on T helper/inducer (CD4) cells. Although β adrenoceptors are present on immature thymocytes, they increase in density during maturation. Activated T cells possess higher numbers of β adrenoceptors than resting T cells. Lymphocytes from aged animals possess higher numbers of β adrenoceptors than their younger counterparts. At first glance, this suggests an increasing sensitivity of these cells to catecholamines with age; however, these receptors on aged lymphocytes are poorly coupled with their G-protein and show a diminished transduction of cAMP via adenylate cyclase. Thus, many variables may influence the ability of neurotransmitters to influence immunocytes.

Immunocyte subsets possess receptors for a variety of neurotransmitters, including both α and β adrenoceptors, dopamine receptors, muscarinic cholinergic receptors, excitatory amino acid receptors, and peptidergic receptors (SP; calcitonin gene-related peptide, CGRP; somatostatin; vasoactive intestinal peptide, VIP; and opioid peptides, to name a few).

The signaling of immunocytes through neurotransmitter–receptor interactions may initiate direct intracellular changes that can be detected readily, or they may exert indirect effects that become apparent mainly during signaling from a second ligand. For example, activation of the T-cell receptor with anti-CD3 antibody will result in the more robust production of the second messenger cAMP when β adrenoceptor activation is present than when it is absent. It is likely that neurotransmitters often act in synergistic (or countersynergistic) fashion with other neurotransmitters, hormones, cytokines, growth factors, and other signals; in this way, they resemble the dual-signaling and modulatory capacities of cytokines.

Neurohormonal Signaling of Immunocytes

A wide range of hormones, including those of the anterior pituitary, the posterior pituitary, and peripheral glands, can signal cells of the immune system and exert profound effects on the ability of the immune system to mount an appropriate defense response. The best-known hormonal system with regard to immune function, the HPA system (acting via CRH, ACTH, and cortisol), plays such an important and integral role in basic immunophysiology that Hugo Besedovsky proposed that the HPA axis is an integral component of the immune system itself. Although even a basic review of the hormonal effects on immune reactivity is far beyond the scope of this article, a few highlights are mentioned in selected areas.

The hypothalamic-pituitary-adrenal axis CRH, produced mainly in the paraventricular nucleus (PVN) of the hypothalamus, is released from axons into the private vascular channel of the hypophysial-portal system. The resultant high concentration of CRH stimulates the release of ACTH from corticotrophs in the anterior pituitary. ACTH is released into the general circulation and activates cells in the adrenal cortex to release cortisol into the general circulation in humans (corticosterone in rodents). Both ACTH and cortisol exert effects on a variety of immunocytes. Interestingly, CRH is found in sites in addition to the PVN, such as macrophages, in a variety of peripheral organs. Thus, even CRH may exert hormonal influences on immunocytes directly, in addition to its contribution in activating ACTH and cortisol production.

CRH-producing neurons in the PVN are a major target of action for circulating inflammatory cytokines, especially IL-1β, acting either directly or indirectly to enhance the activity of the CRH neurons. CRH neuronal activation resulting from either peripheral or central IL-1β stimulation enhances the production of ACTH and cortisol via the HPA axis and, in addition, activates the hypothalamic-sympathetic axis, thus enhancing both of the major classical stress axes physiologically. Esther Sternberg

and colleagues showed that CRH hypothalamic neurons are important regulatory cells in autoimmune diseases. She studied genetically autoimmune-prone animals, such as the Lewis/N rat, to identify potential defects contributing to the susceptibility of these rats to autoimmune diseases. She found a lack of responsiveness of the hypothalamic CRH neurons following attempts to activate them by psychological stressors, neurotransmitter signaling, and the administration of cytokines. Sternberg concluded that the diminished apacity of these rats to activate the HPA axis following appropriate stimuli contributed to their inability to generate a cortisol-evoked suppression of unwanted cell proliferation during immune challenge, particularly by self-reactive clones of cells. When the hypothalamic CRH neurons in closely related autoimmune-resistant rat, the Fischer 344, were lesioned or blocked, these rats became as susceptible to autoimmune-provoking stimuli as Lewis/N rats. These important findings suggest that Besedovsky was correct in considering the HPA axis to be a vital physiological component of the immune system.

For many years, cortisol and other glucocorticoids were thought to be major immunosuppressive hormones. Dexamethasone and other such steroids were often given to patients for their anti-inflammatory or immune suppressing effects, including the treatment of autoimmune diseases. Studies of glucocorticoid effects on immunocytes have reported lymphocyte and thymocyte apoptosis; inhibition of T-cell proliferation; inhibition of cytokine production, such as IL-1 and IL-2; and suppression of a host of innate and acquired immune responses. Interestingly, work by Daynes and Araneo noted that physiological concentrations of glucocortocoids, in contrast to the massively suppressive effects of pharmacological doses of these agents, shifted the balance of cytokine production in T-helper lymphocytes from Th1 (diminished IL-2 and IFN-γ) to Th2 (enhanced IL-4 and IL-10), thus altering acquired immune responses away from cell-mediated immunity (Th1) and toward humoral immunity (Th2). Many researchers and clinicians have proposed that the maintenance of robust cell-mediated immunity is critical for protection against viral infections and some tumors and is necessary for maintaining a relative state of health in patients with HIV infection, some cancers (including some that are relatively nonimmunogenic), and immunosenescence in the elderly. ACTH has also been noted to exert a wide range of immune effects, including reduced IFN-γ production, increased NK cell activity, and complex effects on antibody production.

Dehydroepiandrosterone (DHEA) is an adrenal hormone that some investigators have reported as countering the effects of cortisol. DHEA can enhance some cell-mediated immune responses, restore some immune responses in aged animals, and block some of the immune-suppressive effects of cortisol. The DHEA : cortisol ratio may be a good index of eustress activity (with positive effects on cell-mediated immune responses, such as moderate exercise), in contrast with distress from aversive stimuli and activities, such as maximal physical exertion in marathon running.

Growth hormone and prolactin GH is a hormone produced by cells of the anterior pituitary gland. A GH deficiency in many animals results in small, hypocellular primary and secondary lymphoid organs. The reconstitution of these deficient animals with GH restores cellularity to the lymphoid organs; restores T-cell development in the thymus; and restores antibody responses, cell-mediated responses, and NK cell activity. GH also potentiates cytotoxic T-lymphocyte activity. In animals with involution of the thymus, the administration of GH and prolactin restores thymic morphology and many T-lymphocyte functions. This reinforces the contention that GH exerts a particularly important influence on thymic function. GH also primes macrophages and neutrophils to produce superoxide anion, a functional component of phagocytosis. Surprisingly, GH is also produced by lymphocytes themselves and may act as a paracrine or autocrine signal for lymphocyte proliferation.

Prolactin is another hormone produced by cells of the anterior pituitary. The administration of prolactin contributes to the restoration of immune function in hypophysectomized animals and acts in a similar fashion with GH to help restore thymic cellularity and function in animals with involuted thymuses. Prolactin blockade decreases host resistance to some bacterial infections, such as *Listeria monocytogenes*. Mechanistic studies point toward a role for prolactin as a permissive factor or progression factor, necessary but not sufficient for IL-2-induced T-lymphocyte proliferation. A prolactin-like molecule has also been identified as a product of concanavalin A (Con A)-stimulated T lymphocytes and may be an important autocrine or paracrine lymphocyte growth factor, particularly in conjunction with a possible synergistic effect with estrogen.

Opioid peptides The opioid peptides are families of low-molecular-weight peptides, the endorphins, the enkaphalins, and the dynorphins. They are found in the CNS, the pituitary gland, and peripheral structures such as the adrenal gland. In the brain, opioid peptide interactions with their receptors can induce

analgesia, exert profound behavioral changes, and alter outflow channels to the periphery that can modulate immune responses. Some of these changes can be blocked by naloxone and other opioid blockers, whereas others cannot. The opioid peptides are cleaved from larger prohormone peptides. For example, the precursor proopiomelanocortin (POMC) is cleaved to ACTH and β-lipotropin, the latter of which gives rise to β-endorphin. β-Endorphin levels increase in the serum in parallel with ACTH levels following some stressors, suggesting that β-endorphin may be an important stress-induced neuromediator with an influence on immunocytes or immune responses. Although a review of opioid peptide actions is beyond the scope of this article, we briefly mention of some immune effects of β-endorphin.

β-Endorphin reduces antibody production in mice through μ- and κ-opioid-receptor-mediated effects. β-Endorphin inhibits lymphocyte chemotactic factor in humans and may itself act as a chemotactic factor. Some additional β-endorphin effects are thought to be nonopioid-receptor-mediated, including enhanced Con A-induced T-lymphocyte proliferation in mice, reduced phytohemagglutinin (PHA)-induced T-lymphocyte proliferation in humans and the blockade of prostaglandin E1-induced suppression of lymphocyte proliferation in rats. The opioid peptides exert very complex and varied actions on immunocytes *in vivo* and *in vitro*; sometimes exert contradictory effects *in vitro* versus *in vivo*; and can act in synergistic fashion with other neural, endocrine, and immunological mediators.

Other hormones Many other hormones, in addition to those mentioned earlier, have been shown to influence immunocytes and immune function in a variety of *in vitro* and *in vivo* models. These hormones include thyroid-stimulating hormone (TSH), thyroid hormones, gonadal steroid hormones (estrogen and androgens), posterior pituitary hormones (oxytocin and vasopressin), and melatonin (produced by the pineal gland).

Nerve Fiber Connections with Lymphoid Organs: The Hard Wiring

Peripheral nerve fibers are found in primary lymphoid organs (the bone marrow and thymus), in secondary lymphoid organs (the spleen and lymph nodes), in mucosal-associated lymphoid tissue (the gastrointestinal tract and lung), and in the skin. Tracing studies have revealed the location of some (but not all) of these connections. The two major sources of connectivity are the ANS and the primary sensory system. In the ANS, the vast majority of connections derive from the sympathetic division via a two-neuron chain, with the postganglionic component releasing NE as a major neurotransmitter. These SNS connections distribute adjacent to at least some components of all collections of lymphoid organs and tissues. Very few connections to lymphoid tissues derive from the parasympathetic division of the ANS. Classic two-neuron connections of the cholinergic parasympathetic system have not been identified in either the primary or secondary lymphoid organs; indeed, there is little evidence for cholinergic neurotransmission in these organs, despite the presence of muscarinic cholinergic receptors on some immunocytes found there. Parasympathetic connections that may influence immunocytes are found mainly in mucosal-associated lymphoid tissue and the skin.

A wide range of neuropeptides has been identified in nerve fibers in the lymphoid organs. Some of these neuropeptides (SP and CGRP) are thought to be associated mainly with sensory connections. However, very few tracing studies have demonstrated a primary sensory (afferent) origin for this neuropeptidergic innervation of lymphoid organs and tissues. Some peptides (neuropeptide Y, NPY) appear to be colocalized with other neurotransmitters in cells of the SNS. Some primary afferents, particularly the small SP fibers, have been shown to release their neurotransmitter from both proximal and distal arborizations of their axons. Thus, it is possible for a primary afferent cell to be activated and then release the neurotransmitter at the site in the periphery where the initial activating stimulus took place. It is clear that a much more thorough mapping of the cells of origin, distribution, and associations with target cells in the immune system needs to be accomplished for the nerve fiber connections that provide the innervation to cellular targets in the organs and tissues of the immune system.

Sympathetic noradrenergic nerve fibers   Postganglionic sympathetic NE nerve fibers supply primary lymphoid organs, secondary lymphoid organs, and mucosal-associated lymphoid organs with innervation. These nerve fibers distribute along the vasculature, travel with smooth muscle structures such as the trabeculae, and arborize directly into the parenchyma where they form close junctional appositions (neuroeffector junctions) with cells of the immune system. The innervation that extends into the parenchyma is associated with specific compartments of lymphoid organs and maintains that compartmentation even when involution or loss of cellularity occurs. Some neuroimmunocyte appositions are as close as 6 nm (a gap junction is 2 nm, and a classical synapse in the CNS is 20 nm). Felten and colleagues hypothesized that communication in the parenchyma of lymphoid organs occurs in both directions: (1) neurotransmitters released by sympathetic nerve endings can act on receptors on target cells of the immune system and (2) cytokines released by target cells of the immune system can modulate the extent of release of neurotransmitters such as NE. For the most part, sympathetic NE nerve terminals also colocalize NPY, although there are some terminals that contain only one and not the other. Extensive studies from the laboratory of David Felten and colleagues identified abundant innervation of lymphoid organs.

NE nerve fibers enter the bone marrow with the nutrient arteries, distribute along those arteries, and arborize extensively into the parenchyma, where they associate with stem cells and other constituents of the marrow. Most of these fibers appear to colocalize NPY. Many cells of the bone marrow possess adrenoceptors, especially β adrenoceptors. Studies using a three-dimensional bone marrow culture showed that catecholaminergic stimulation of bone marrow can augment granulocyte production. NE nerve fibers enter the thymus along the capsular surface and distribute through the septal system. Some NE fibers distribute into the thymic cortex and medulla and extend along the vasculature at the corticomedullary junction. Thymocytes possess adrenoceptors, with increasing numbers noted during thymocyte maturation. Some investigators have reported that catecholamines can suppress thymocyte proliferation through the activation of adenylate cyclase and generation of cAMP; however, this interaction may be more likely to occur during involution or during diminished cellularity, at which time the NE innervation is very dense.

NE nerve fibers enter the spleen with the splenic artery, travel along the trabecular system, and distribute extensively into the splenic white pulp. In the white pulp, NE nerve fibers follow the central artery of the white pulp, extend along the marginal sinus (where macrophages reside) and into the marginal zone, and distribute extensively into the periarteriolar lymphatic sheath. NE nerve terminals form close associations with T lymphocytes of both CD4 and CD8 subsets and with macrophages and NK cells. Very few NE fibers are found in the B-lymphocyte zones, the follicles. NE innervation appears to enhance cell-mediated immunity during the initiative phase of an immune response and has some inhibitory effect on humoral immunity in Th1-dominant animals.

NE nerve fibers enter lymph nodes with the vasculature in the hilar zone and with the capsular surface. These fibers distribute through the medullary cords, where they associate with macrophages and other cells and arborize into the cortical and paracortical zone where T lymphocytes of both CD4 and CD8 subsets reside. As in the case of the spleen, very few NE terminals distribute into the B-lymphocyte zones, the nodules. In lymph nodes, NE fibers also enhance cell-mediated immunity and, in some cases, inhibit humoral immunity, particularly in the case of auto-immune-provoking stimuli. The denervation of these NE fibers in both the spleen and lymph nodes results in diminished cell-mediated immune responses, enhanced humoral responses in Th1-dominant animals, and increased severity of autoimmune-provoking stimuli. NE also appears to exert extensive influences on cell trafficking, particularly on NK cells and T lymphocytes. Even very low concentrations of catecholamines can result in the release of marginated and organ-localized NK cells into the circulation. Interestingly, during aging, the spleen and lymph nodes progressively lose their NE innervation, according to Denise Bellinger and colleagues, due to autodestruction by oxidative metabolites of catecholamines released into the paracrine environment by NE nerve terminals in these secondary lymphoid organs. When the NE innervation is restored in old animals, with the administration of growth factor-stimulating pharmacological agents (e.g., low-dose deprenyl), IL-2 and IFN-α production is enhanced markedly, NK cell activity is elevated, and T-cell proliferation is restored.

Noradrenergic innervation is also found in mucosal-associated lymphoid organs. In the gastrointestinal tract, these fibers distribute through T-lymphocyte zones and arborize in submucosal zones.

Neuropeptide-containing nerve fibers Extensive networks of neuropeptide-containing nerve fibers distribute into both the primary and secondary lymphoid organs. A few neuropeptides, such as NPY, are colocalized with NE sympathetic nerve terminals, but most neuropeptide-containing nerve fibers are independent of the known sympathetic innervation.

Neuropeptide Y-containing terminals appear to colocalize with NE as a component of the sympathetic innervation in the bone marrow, thymus, spleen, and lymph nodes, although some non-NE NPY+ nerve terminals are present in the lymphoid organs. NPY is also found in the platelets in the spleen and is found in the circulation, apparently from release following sympathetic activation. Some immunocytes possess receptors for NPY.

SP and CGRP are found frequently as colocalized neuropeptides in non-NE nerve terminals in all lymphoid organs and tissues, as well as the skin. SP nerve fibers have been identified along the

vasculature and in the parenchyma in the bone marrow, thymus, spleen, and lymph nodes. CGRP is often colocalized with SP; however, in some sites, CGRP-containing nerve fibers distribute independently (e.g., adjacent to antigen-presenting Langerhans cells in the skin).

SP receptors have been identified on both T and B lymphocytes as well as on granulocytes and mast cells. SP is a potent regulator of inflammation and can induce extravasation and edema, attract other pro-inflammatory cells and mediators, and exacerbate inflammation in sites such as joint spaces in rheumatoid arthritis. SP can also enhance polyclonal immunoglobulin (Ig)A and IgM production by gut-associated lymphoid tissue, enhance T-cell proliferation and IL-2 production in the secondary lymphoid organs, and increase some antibody responses and lymphocyte-proliferative responses. Many of these immunoenhancing effects of SP can be counteracted by somatostatin, but an extensive understanding of somatostatin innervation of lymphoid organs is not yet available. In the skin, CGRP acts as a potent inhibitory factor on antigen presentation by Langerhans cells.

VIP-containing nerve fibers are present in Peyer's patches in the gut, thymus, and spleen. VIP receptors are present on some T lymphocytes; Cliff Ottaway showed that their expression can enhance the migration of these T cells into the gut-associated lymphoid tissue and the mesenteric lymph nodes, whereas their absence prevents such migration. VIP can also inhibit T-lymphocyte proliferation.

Many other neuropeptides have been found in the primary and secondary lymphoid organs. These neuropeptides include the opioid peptides, cholecystokinin, neurotensin, CRH, somatostatin, and galanin. Little is known about the details of the functioning of these neuropeptide-containing nerve fibers. It is particularly difficult to discern the unique role of specifically compartmentalized neuropeptides, such as the opioid peptides, that appear in neurons, pituitary cells, and immunocytes.

The origin of cell bodies for most of the neuropeptide-containing nerve fibers that distribute into the lymphoid organs and tissues is not known. Thus, we do not even know if they are components of the primary afferent system, the sympathetic or parasympathetic divisions of the ANS, or the enteric nervous system. Neuropeptide receptors are present on many specific subsets of lymphocytes, macrophages/monocytes, and other lymphoid cells. We do not yet know the details of the distribution of these receptors, the details of the second-messenger pathways in specific subsets of immunocytes, or the functional role of these receptors in immunoregulation.

Immunocyte Production of Neuropeptides

Ed Blalock, Eric Smith, and colleagues made the remarkable discovery that cells of the immune system, particularly lymphocytes and macrophages/monocytes, can synthesize neuropeptides directly. They showed that some immunocytes can synthesize the POMC gene following stimulation by a virus (Newcastle's disease) or a releasing factor (CRH). The resultant neuropeptides produced and released by the immunocytes are, for the most part, identical to their counterparts made by neurons and pituicytes. Immunocytes have been reported to produce the POMC-derived products ACTH and β-endorphin, TSH, and CRH. In some instances, the same neuropeptide can be produced by neurons, pituicytes, and immunocytes in the periphery.

Cytokine Interactions with the Nervous System

Immunologically derived mediators, the cytokines, can act directly or indirectly to influence the activity of neurons in the CNS and PNS. In addition, some supporting cells of the nervous system (microglia and astrocytes), and even a small subset of neurons in the CNS and PNS, can produce cytokines directly, particularly IL-1β. The most extensively studied cytokines with regard to effects on CNS neurons and CNS behavior are the pro-inflammatory cytokines, IL-1, IL-6, and tumor necrosis factor (TNF)-α. IL-1β can act on neurons in the CNS, particularly on hypothalamic neurons, and can induce fever, slow-wave sleep, lethargy, loss of appetite, diminished reproductive behavior, and other classic illness behaviors. Interestingly, this illness behavior can be induced by IL-1β injected by intracerebroventricular (ICV), intraperitoneal (IP), or intravenous (IV) routes; the ICV route requires lower concentrations of IL-1β to induce the illness behavior than the IP or IV routes.

Many mechanisms have been proposed by which IL-1β may exert its actions on the CNS:

1. IL-1β may cross the blood–brain barrier directly, enter into the cerebrospinal fluid, and then act directly on neurons. Banks and colleagues reported such a transport system, although the greatest extent of crossing of IL-1 into the CNS occurs in the cortex, not the hypothalamus.
2. IL-1β may act on the cells of the organum vasculosum of the lamina terminalis to release mediators such as prostaglandin E2, which, in turn, activates preoptic neurons.
3. In the circulation, IL-1β may act on endothelial cells in the brain vasculature, resulting in the release of mediators such as nitric oxide and prostaglandins that, in turn, activate neurons.
4. IL-1β may act on vagal afferents (via paraneurons) or on other afferents, according to the work of Watkins and Maier, stimulating cells in the nucleus solitarius complex, which, in turn, activate the hypothalamus.

It is likely that a combination of all of these routes operates to some extent in physiological circumstances.

IL1-β also can activate the HPA axis through its actions on the CRH neuronal system of the PVN. To a lesser extent, so can IL-6 and other cytokines. This activation of the CRH system requires the input of the A1 and A2 brain-stem NE projections to the PVN, suggesting an action of IL-1β on the central NE nerve terminals. IL-1β also activates the hypothalamic-spinal cord system, which enhances sympathetic outflow from the intermediolateral cell system of the thoracolumbar spinal cord. Thus, cytokines that activate the HPA axis and the SNS can, in and of themselves, be considered as classical stressors. In addition, viral infections and immune responses that result in the production of pro-inflammatory cytokines, such as IL-1β, also should be considered as classic stressors.

Inflammatory mediators also appear to be involved in some neurodegenerative diseases, such as Alzheimer's disease. IL-1β and many other inflammatory mediators, complement components, and acute-phase proteins can be found at the site of plaque formation and neuronal degeneration in the brains of patients with Alzheimer's disease. The long-term administration of nonsteroidal anti-inflammatory medication or specific COX-2 inhibitors appears to diminish the inflammatory response and may protect against the progression of this disease.

In the PNS, both IL-1 and IL-2 appear to act on nerve terminals of the sympathetic NE system in secondary lymphoid organs and modulate the release of NE. These findings of cytokine modulation of central and peripheral neuronal activities indicate that the immune system and nervous system are in constant communication with one another on a continuing physiological basis.

Clinical Implications of Neural-Immune Signaling

At the most basic level, neurohormones and neurotransmitters can regulate the individual cellular functions of immunocytes, such as the proliferation, differentiation, maturation, expression of cell adhesion molecules (influencing trafficking); expression of specific cell markers; synthesis of specific cell products (cytokines, immunoglobulins, and growth factors); or expression of specific portions of the genome. This can occur wherever the cell encounters an appropriate ligand, whether in an organ or in the blood.

At a more integrative level, neurohormones and neurotransmitters can also modulate immune responses, the collective interactions of multiple cell types that result in a reaction to challenge. These neural signals may either modulate aspects of innate immunity (e.g., location, number, and activity of NK cells) or modulate the acquired immune responses of both cell-mediated and humoral types. The final outcome depends on the collective impact of the specific signal molecules on antigen-presenting cells, accessory cells, lymphocytes, and any other cell types that contribute to the overall response.

The final clinical outcome is neural modulation of (1) the host response to viral, bacterial, or parasite infections, including both progression and latency; (2) wound healing; (3) inflammatory responses; (4) autoimmune reactivity; (5) immune senescence in old animals; and (6) the progression, metastatic spread, and recurrence of some specific cancers. In some instances, a single neurally derived signal may exert a predominant influence. In other instances, the collective interaction of glucocorticoids, other neurohormones, catecholamines, and neuropeptides all may contribute to the end effect. Studies demonstrate that many of these neural signals synergize with cytokines, growth factors, hormones, and other neural signals. This suggests that elucidating the integrated physiological influence of neural signaling on immune reactivity, and its potential to alter the outcome of disease processes, is a daunting but rewarding challenge.

See Also the Following Articles

Autoimmunity; Breast Cancer; Cytotoxic Lymphocytes; Immune Response; Immune Suppression; Natural Killer (NK) Cells; Opioids; Social Support.

Further Reading

Ader, R., Cohen, N. and Felten, D. L. (1995). Psychoneuroimmunology: interaction between the nervous system and the immune system. *Lancet* **345**, 99–103.

Ader, R., Felten, D. L. and Cohen, N. (1990). Interactions between the brain and the immune system. *Annual Review of Pharmacology and Toxicology* **30**, 561–5602.

Ader, R., Felten, D. L. and Cohen, N. (1991). *Psychoneuroimmunology* (2nd edn.). San Diego: Academic Press.

Bellinger, D. L., Madden, K. S., Felten, S. Y. and Felten, D. L. (1994). Neural and endocrine links between the brain and the immune system. In: Lewis, C. E., O'Sullivan, C. & Barraclough, J. (eds.) *The psychoimmunology of cancer*, pp. 55–106. New York: Oxford University Press.

Felten, D. L., Felten, S. Y., Bellinger, D. L., et al. (1993). Fundamental aspects of neural-immune signaling. *Psychotherapy and Psychosomatics* **178**, 1–10.

Kiecolt-Glaser, J. K. (1999). Stress, personal relationships, and immune function: health implications. *Brain, Behavior & Immunity* **13**, 61–72.

Madden, K. S. and Felten, D. L. (1995). Experimental basis for neural-immune interactions. *Physiological Reviews* **75**, 77–106.

Madden, K. S., Sanders, V. M. and Felten, D. L. (1995). Catecholamine influences and sympathetic neural modulation of immune responsiveness. *Annual Review of Pharmacology and Toxicology* **35**, 417–448.

McEwen, B. S. (1998). Protective and damaging effects of stress mediators. *New England Journal of Medicine* **338**, 171–179.

Reichlin, S. (1993). Neuroendocrine-immune interactions. *New England Journal of Medicine* **329**, 1246–1253.

Sheridan, J. (1998). Stress-induced modulation of anti-viral immunity. *Brain, Behavior & Immunity* **12**, 1–6.

Watkins, L., Maier, S. and Goehler, L. (1995). Cytokine-to-brain communication: a review and analysis of alternative mechanisms. *Life Sciences* **57**, 1011–1026.

Wilder, R. L. (1995). Neuroendocrine-immune system interactions and autoimmunity. *Annual Review of Immunology* **13**, 307–338.

Neuroinflammation

G Z Feuerstein, R R Ruffolo and L J Rutkowski
Wyeth Research, Collegeville, PA, USA

Inflammation and Neuroinflammation: General
  Considerations
Neuroinflammation in Stroke
Neuroinflammation in Multiple Sclerosis
Neuroinflammation in Alzheimer's Disease
Summary

Glossary

Alzheimer's disease	A neurological disorder of progressive loss of cognitive functions occurring mostly in the elderly due to the accumulation of protein deposits that damage neurons and activate glial cells.
Alzheimer's plaque	Insoluble deposits of aggregated β-amyloid protein that accumulates in the brain and cerebral blood vessels of patients with Alzheimer's disease. Amyloid plaque triggers inflammatory responses that contribute to the death of neurons and progressive dementia.
Cytokines	A family of secreted proteins originally identified as products of leukocytes that serve in innate and specific immune and inflammatory reactions. Cytokine regulate diverse functions including cell growth, differentiation, function, and disease and are regarded as pleiotropic mediators.
Inflammation	A localized protective response that follows tissue injury and aims to destroy hostile agents, resolve tissue damage, and aid in repair and rehabilitation. Inflammation involves local vascular responses, leukocyte recruitment, and tissue cell activation stimulated by both local and systemic humoral factors.
Interleukins	A family of cytokines produced by leukocytes in natural immune reactions that serve to activate or modulate the function of other leukocytes as well as nonhematopoietic cells.
Leukocytes	White blood cells that are produced in the bone marrow and lymphatic tissue and circulate in the blood. White blood cells are responsible for immune surveillance, innate immunity, and inflammation as part of host defense and tissue repair. In certain conditions, certain leukocyte subsets can mediate toxic reactions that lead to autoimmune diseases and chronic inflammatory diseases.
Lymphocytes	A subset of white blood cells that are responsible for innate and specific immune reactions. T-lymphocytes are the central arm of the acquired cellular immunity and carry receptors that largely recognize antigens of foreign origin. Following clonal expansion, T-cells acquire the ability to clear the foreign invaders. B lymphocytes are the central arm of the humoral immune response. They largely recognize soluble antigens via immunoglobulin on their surface, upon which they differentiate to memory B cells.
Magnetic resonance imaging (MRI)	A noninvasive imaging method that deploys brief magnetic pulses that polarize hydrogen atoms and then monitors energy emission. High-resolution images of soft tissue, particularly brain and spinal cord, are generated by computer algorithms. Tissue structure imaged via computerized algorithms can be deduced by differences in emission densities.
Multiple sclerosis	A neurological disease characterized by discrete white matter lesions (demyelination) and typified by intermittent, progressive, yet variable loss of motor and sensory (speech and visual) function and sometimes death.
Neurofibrillary tangles	Paired helical filaments of tau protein that accumulate inside neurons. Neurofibrillary tangles are one of the pathological hallmarks used to confirm the diagnosis of Alzheimer's disease at autopsy.
Precon-ditioning	Short and limited stress conditions that modulates tissue vulnerability to subsequent injurious events.
Prostaglandin	Lipid mediators that are produced from fatty acids and serve in local and systemic functions of diverse tissues and organs. Certain prostaglandins participate in immune and inflammatory reaction, including leukotriene B4 and thromboxane A2.
Stroke	Abrupt ischemic or hemorrhagic event in the brain that leads to loss of motor, sensory, and cognitive functions or death.

Inflammation and Neuroinflammation: General Considerations

Inflammation is a fundamental, carefully orchestrated, and highly conserved reaction of the organism meant to protect, defend, and amend diverse forms of injury. Inflammation (as well as innate immune responses) is critical for the organism's survival, yet in specific occasions, these reactions could result in a detrimental outcome. While inflammation features prominently in injuries to peripheral tissue, the situation is quite different in the central nervous system (CNS). The brain has long been considered an immunologically privileged organ. This notion is based on observations that tissue transplants into the CNS are not well rejected by the immune system, and inflammatory cells and mediators are sparse compared to peripheral tissues. The anti-inflammatory and anti-apoptosis environment in the brain and the limited access of brain-derived antigens to lymphoid organs may contribute to its immune seclusion. However, recent studies in infectious and autoimmune models have challenged this view. Injuries to the CNS activate cells within the CNS, called microglia, that like the peripheral monocyte system are capable of releasing a plethora of inflammatory mediators as well as activation of immune permissive molecules such as MHC class I. Proteins that are released from brain cells during injury can provokes acute and chronic inflammatory reactions in which both brain cells and circulating immune inflammatory cells participate.

Neuroinflammation in Stroke

Stroke Prevalence and Epidemiology

Stroke is a major medical emergency due to the resulting high rate of mortality and morbidity. In the United States alone, about 750,000 strokes, resulting in about 150,000 deaths, are estimated annually, which makes stroke the third leading cause of death in the United States. In addition, stroke management incurs a high burden of health costs due to prolonged rehabilitation, permanent (~30%) residual deficits, and loss of productive professional capabilities. The incidence of stroke has been on the decline from 1980 to 1990, primarily due to advances in aggressive management of key risk factors such as hypertension, atherosclerosis, and lipid disorders; lifestyle modifications (smoking); and in recent years, improved time to admittance to health facilities that are better equipped and organized to diagnose and treat strokes in specialized stroke care units. However, the incidence of stroke has not decreased in recent years in most of the industrialized countries while the prevalence has

actually increased due to the aging population and increased rates of comorbidities such as diabetes, heart failure, and the metabolic syndrome. In spite of the medical severity of stroke, its prevalence, and health burden, little progress has been realized in the treatment of this condition. The only specific, pharmacological treatment registered for stroke is tissue plasminogen activator (tPA), which enhances thrombolysis. This agent, however, finds limited utility (2–5% of admitted patients) due to substantial limitation of time to administration (3 h) and associated toxicity. In addition, no mortality benefits have been proven in prospective clinical trials with thrombolysis agents.

The reasons for the difficulties in discovering and developing new drugs for treatment of stroke are complex. Likely causes for failure to discover new drugs include poor understanding of the mechanism of neuronal death in stroke, which results in development of inadequate therapeutics. Also, the lack of proper experimental models for this human condition and limited insightful translational medicine may contribute. Recently, recognition of the role of inflammation in stroke has emerged, which may provide new opportunities to discover and develop effective treatment for stroke.

Cells and Mediators in Neuroinflammation in Stroke

Cerebral ischemia is marked by rapid activation of microglia, the brain cells that are part of the innate immune and inflammation cellular elements along with infiltration of inflammatory cells from the circulation into the ischemic territory (see **Figure 1**). Experimental stroke models revealed that early accumulation of blood-borne inflammatory cells in the ischemic brain persists for days to weeks after the initial insult. The early infiltration of polymorphonuclear cells (also called neutrophils) into the capillaries of the ischemic zone parallels the early activation of the glia cells (microglia and astroglia). Monocytes arrive in the injury zone much later, around 12–24 h after the ischemic injury, and are rapidly transformed into tissue macrophages displaying aggressive phagocytosis. Other immune/inflammatory cells such as lymphocytes are also observed at later time points. The significance of the exogenous leukocyte infiltration into the ischemic brain is controversial. The presence of leukocytes in the capillaries was argued to contribute to low or no flow in the capillaries due to clogging that exacerbates the ischemic insult. Furthermore, the gamut of toxic mediators released by the activated leukocytes, e.g., reactive oxygen radicals, proteases, and cytokines, has also been suspected to cause

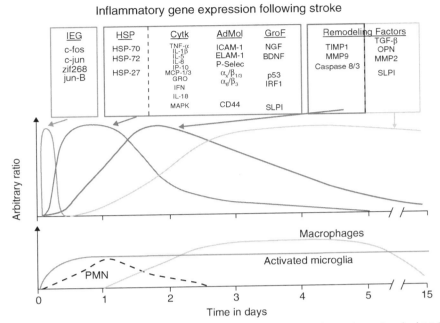

Inflammatory gene expression following stroke

Figure 1 Inflammatory cell and mediators in experimental ischemic stroke. PNM = polymorphonuclear leukocytes; SLPI = secreted leukocyte protease inhibitor; TNF = tumor necrosis factor; TIMP1 = tissue inhibitor of metalloproteinase type; MMP = matrix metalloproteinase; HSP = heat shock protein; NGF = nerve growth factor; MAPK = mitogen activated protein kinase; IL = interleukins; MCP = macrophage chemotactic protein; IFN = interferon; ICAM = intercellular adhesion molecule; ELAM = endothelium leukocyte adhesion molecule; P-sel = P- selectin; Cytk = cytokines; IEG = immediate early genes; AdMol = adhesion molecules; GroF = growth factors; OPN = osteopontin.

endothelial capillary damage in addition to neurons and other brain cells. The role of the microglia and the astroglia in the acute response to brain ischemia, while clearly evident from morphological and biochemical markers, is even more difficult to assess; they are likely to contribute to both repair and injury processes.

In addition to the evidence on the role of inflammation in stroke presented by experimental models, a role for inflammation in human stroke has also been suggested. Infectious conditions often precede stroke in humans and heighten inflammatory conditions in humans as evidenced by biomarkers such as C-reactive protein, which are associated with higher stroke risk.

Cytokine and Interleukins

Extensive research in the past decade has shed much light on inflammatory mediators that are generated following brain ischemia by either endogenous or exogenous inflammatory cells. Such mediators include eicosanoids (prostaglandins and leukotrienes), phospholipids, cytokines, chemokines, and endothelial-leukocyte adhesion molecules. Most studies in recent years focused on proinflammatory cytokines, interleukins, and cell adhesion molecules (CAMs) (see **Figure 1**), which are extremely low in normal

brain. However, in response to stroke, a large number of cytokines, interleukins, and CAMs are expressed in a typical time course (see **Figure 1**). The significance of the cytokines in mediation of brain damage in stroke is still debated, as many are pleiotropic polypeptides that have been shown to mediate numerous cellular effects such as growth, proliferation, activation, apoptosis, preconditioning, and other specific functionalities. Some of these cytokines, e.g., tumor necrosis factor-α (TNFα) and interleukin-1, have been implicated in ischemic neuronal death in some experimental models, but no clinical trial has explored the potential benefits that cytokine or interleukin modifiers might have in stroke patients. Likewise, blockade of different leukocyte adhesion molecules by genetic or pharmacological manipulations in *in vivo* experimental stroke models suggested a detrimental role of these receptors in acute ischemic brain injury. However, clinical trials with several different inhibitors of neutrophil adhesion molecules that enable leukocyte traffic across the capillary endothelium into the ischemic brain (anti-ICAM-1 antibody, enlimomab; LeukArrest, Hu23F2G, a monoclonal antibody that targets the neutrophil CD11/CD18 CAM; rNIF, recombinant neutrophil inhibitory factor, a hookworm-derived agent that reduces the inflammatory cascade by inhibiting the polymorphonuclear leukocyte adhesion to the endothelium) have failed to show efficacy.

Chemokines

Chemokines are a family of more than 50 structurally and functionally related proteins involved in inflammatory cell recruitment. These relatively small proteins are usually subdivided into four subfamilies on the basis of their structural conservation of cysteine residues. Chemokines and their receptors are constitutively expressed in normal brain cells such as microglia, astrocytes, and neurons throughout the CNS, albeit at very low levels. As shown in **Figure 1**, rapid expression of many chemokines takes place in response to acute ischemic brain injury, which corresponds with cytokine and leukocyte adhesion molecule expression. Most prominent activation has been documented for MCP-1 (monocyte attractant protein-1), interleukin-8, interferon-inducible protein-1, macrophage inflammatory protein-1, and fractalkine. While these chemokines and others seem to be expressed in the location and at the time that could lend them a role in propagation, aggravation, or repair of the ischemic injury, no agent to date has been deployed in clinical trials in stroke or other brain injury conditions. Experiments with prototypic inhibitors of certain chemokines have shown the potential for better recovery following stroke, yet proof of the concept has not been obtained in clinical studies.

Proteases and Matrix Proteins

Matrix metalloproteinases (MMPs) and serine proteases including tissue and urokinase plasminogen activators (tPA and uPA) are two large and important neutral protease gene families that are involved in the neuroinflammatory response to brain ischemia. These proteases have been the subjects of extensive research in other human diseases such as cancer and arthritis, and diverse inhibitors for many of these proteases have already been deployed to assess their role in stroke. The major pathophysiological role of MMPs has been disruption of the blood–brain barrier (BBB) and hemorrhagic transformation following ischemia. These proteases are induced, processed, and released from diverse cellular elements such as activated microglia within the ischemic zone and invading neutrophils and macrophages. However, MMPs and other proteases have many more functions that can bear on both tissue injury and repair. Angiogenesis, matrix remodeling that enables cells migration, axonal navigation, and cell–cell communication are important, understudied functions. While many MMP inhibitors have been synthesized, and some shown efficacy in

mitigation of stroke outcome in experimental models, none has been tried in human stroke. Issues regarding specificity, potency, and brain access (crossing the BBB) pose significant limitation for human trials.

Other Inflammatory Mediators

Ischemic conditions to the brain result in activation of numerous biochemical pathways including lipid degradation, neurotransmitter release, and oxygen radical generation. Most of these mediators are released in large quantities in ischemia, yet mostly in a short period of time. Lipid products such as prostaglandins (PGs), thromboxane A2 (TXA2), and leukotrienes B4 (LTB4) are potent inflammatory agents that induce strong chemotactic stimuli that facilitate inflammatory cell migration into the brain. Phospholipid products such as platelet-activating factor (PAF), a potent proinflammatory mediator, may also be important. However, while potent antagonists to PGs, TXA2, and LTB4 have been discovered, none has been tried as a potential therapeutic in stroke. Reactive oxygen radicals (RORs) have been extensively reported as a major response to brain ischemia. RORs via activation of nuclear factor-κB (NFκB) elicit diverse transcriptional events that lead to synthesis and release of many cytokines, interleukins, and other inflammatory mediators. Experimental studies with numerous antioxidant compounds have been most promising, although none has demonstrated efficacy as yet in human clinical trials.

Neuroinflammation in Multiple Sclerosis

Multiple Sclerosis: Epidemiology and Pathology

Multiple sclerosis (MS) is the most common neurological disease affecting young adults in the Western world, affecting 0.05–0.15% of Caucasians. MS prevalence varies depending on the genetic background. It is much more prevalent in Caucasians than in Africans and Asians. The disease usually begins in young adulthood, and it affects women more frequently than men. In 80–90% of cases, MS starts as a relapsing–remitting course, but over time, the number of relapses decreases, with most patients experiencing progressive neurological deficits that occur independently of relapses. In 10–20% of patients, MS begins as a primary progressive course without acute relapses. In the relapsing-remitting form of MS, acute lesions in the white matter of the brain, identified by magnetic resonance imaging (MRI), can resolve spontaneously. Disruption of the BBB, demyelination, and edema are indicative of an inflammatory process. In progressive stages, global brain atrophy and disability evolve. Contemporary concepts define MS as a chronic immune and inflammatory disease of the CNS that is focused in the myelin areas of the CNS and spinal cord resulting in axonal demyelination. The originating causes of MS are unknown, but it is widely believed to be an autoimmune and inflammatory disease process.

Inflammatory Cells and Mediators in Multiple Sclerosis

The hallmark of the brain lesion in MS is a plaque of demyelination in the white matter area of the brain where B cells, T cells, macrophages, and activated microglia are notable. The inflammatory changes are accompanied by neuronal and oligodendrocyte (myelin-producing cells) loss and astrocyte (a type of glia cell) activation. These fundamental observations were fortified by observations in an experimental model of MS, experimental allergic encephalitis (EAE), in which myelin proteins were identified as the cause of EAE. Furthermore, adoptive transfer studies suggested that CD4$^+$ T cells could transmit the disease to naive animals. Further research identified cytokines released from T helper 1 (Th1) such as interferon-γ (IFNγ), TNFβ, and IL-2 as well as the proinflammatory cytokine TNFα as the primary disease mediators. By contrast, T cells that secrete IL-4, IL-5, IL-10, and IL-13 were viewed as immune protective mechanisms. Thus, the Th1 cells have taken center stage in MS research based on information obtained in the EAE model that also shares many similarities to human MS.

However, this simplistic hypothesis has been challenged by studies that cast doubts on the distinction between Th1 and Th2 cytokines as mediators of MS and that also suggested a role for Th2-secreted cytokines as well as another subset of T cells, Th0, which secrete cytokines of both Th1 and Th2 cells. Furthermore, B cells are also likely to play a role in the mechanism of brain lesions in MS as well as the brain innate immunity and especially the microglia, which upon activation provide a proinflammatory milieu, which is permissive for T cell activation.

Immune and Inflammatory Modulators in Treatment of MS

There are currently three different immunomodulatory therapies that have been approved for the treatment of relapsing-remitting MS, as they have been shown to improve clinical or MRI symptoms and signs. These are recombinant IFN-β-1b (Betaseron and Betaferon); recombinant IFN1a (Avonex and Rebif), and glatiramer acetate (copolymer-1 or Copaxone). The discrete mechanism of action of any of these drugs is not entirely clear, but slowing disease progression toward sustained disability or annual exacerbation rate of the disease and reduction in MRI lesion burden has been demonstrated.

Neuroinflammation in Alzheimer's Disease

Alzheimer's Disease: Epidemiology and Pathology

Alzheimer's disease (AD) is the most common cause of dementia in the elderly population and the fourth leading cause of death in persons over 65 years old. AD is an incurable and progressive disease that affects millions of people worldwide. A prevalence of 10% has been cited in developed countries, with doubling in frequency every 5 years from the age of 65 to 50% at the age of 90. AD carries a substantial economic burden due to the need for intensive patient care. AD was originally described in 1906 by Dr. Alzheimer, a pathologist who noted prominent pathological features in brain of deceased patients that suffered from severe dementia. There are three pathological hallmarks in AD brain: (1) senile plaques, now known to be composed from deposits of β-amyloid protein, (2) neurofibrillary tangles, and (3) inflammation. AD etiology is heterogeneous, with about 10% of cases associated with a strong familiar background and Mendelian heritance pattern. Certain mutations in chromosome 1, 14, and 21 were identified in addition to or association with polymorphism of the ApoE gene. Metabolic and nutritional factors are often cited as confounding if not causal factors.

Neuroinflammation in Alzheimer Disease

The inflammatory condition in AD is quite different from that in stroke or MS. Most prominently, it lacks the classical T and B cell immune component so notable in MS and lacks the systemic inflammatory cell infiltration of neutrophils and macrophages seen in stroke. It is believed that the inflammation in AD is a result of microglia and astrocyte activation by the plaque material of aggregates of β-amyloid protein. In addition, advanced glycation end products (AGE) and their receptor, RAGE, have recently been implicated in the neurotoxicity of AD. Cytokines and interleukins including TNFα, IL-6, IL-1, and macrophage colony-stimulating factor (M-CSF) are the most likely mediators generated by the activated microglia and astrocytes. In addition, RORs and complement factors are often cited as players in the inflammation cascade of AD. Although the significance and contribution of inflammation to the progression of AD are a topic of debate, recent clinical (the Rotterdam Study) and epidemiological research on the use of anti-inflammatory medications in AD suggests a significant correlation between inflammation and neurodegeneration. An important set of inflammatory mediators of a potential source of therapeutics are the cyclooxygenase (COX) products of arachidonic acid metabolism, especially those generated by the COX-2 enzyme complex.

Anti-inflammatory Therapy in Alzheimer's Disease

Current treatment of AD patients is based on drugs that are supposed to increase brain levels of acetylcholine (a neurotransmitter that is associated with cognitive function). This treatment has modest and partial efficacy. Nonsteroidal anti-inflammatory drugs (NSAIDs) are presumed to have beneficial effects in AD due to reduction in microglia COX-1 or COX-2 action. However, the fact that patients who are treated with NSAIDs for reasons other than AD, such as rheumatoid arthritis, are not particularly protected from AD cast doubt on the potential efficacy of these agents. Reports on the possible efficacy of aspirin in reducing AD-associated dementia may support the COX-1/2 hypothesis since aspirin inhibits COX-1 action. Reducing platelet reactivity might be a key part of aspirin benefits. The potential of other inflammatory mediators to serve as therapeutic targets for AD remains a subject of intensive research.

Summary

Immune and inflammatory cells and mediators play an important role in health and disease. The brain is unique in its ability to secure an immune privileged environment, yet brain cells can launch inflammation when activated by an aberrant biochemical milieu (amyloid accumulation) or a physiological condition (ischemia). Brain injuries also result in the exposure to systemic immune and inflammatory processes that could contribute to damage but also provide critical repair elements. Only multiple sclerosis has gained new therapeutic opportunities in the form of immune modulators, albeit at limited efficacy. It is hoped that better understanding of the role immune and inflammatory cells play in brain diseases and injuries could lead to novel and effective treatment.

See Also the Following Articles

Alzheimer's Disease; Inflammation; Cardiovasular Disease, Stress and; Multiple Sclerosis.

Further Reading

Baecher-Allen, C., Viglietta, V. and Hafler, D. A. (2005). The potential for targeting CD4+CD25+ regulatory T-cells in the treatment of multiple sclerosis in humans. In: Taams, L. S., Akbar, A. N. & Wauben, M. H. M. (eds.) *Regulatory T-cells in inflammation*, 133–152, Basel: Birkhauser.

Bowirrat, A., Friedland, R. P. and Korcyn, A. D. (2002). Alzheimer's disease. In: Abramsky, O., Compston, A. S., Miller, A. & Said, G. (eds.) *Brain disease: therapeutics strategies and repair*. London, UK: Martin Dunitz.

de Kleer, I. M., Wedderburn, L. R., Taams, L. S., et al. (2004). CD4+CD25+ (bright) regulatory T-cells actively regulate inflammation in the joints of patients with remitting form of juvenile idiopathic arthritis. *Journal of Immunology* **172**, 6435–6443.

Feuerstein, G. (2001). In: Feuerstein, G. (ed.) *Inflammation and stroke*. Basel: Birkhauser Verlag.

Halliday, G., Robinson, S., Shepherd, C. and Kril, J. (2000). Alzheimer's disease and inflammation: a review of cellular and therapeutic mechanisms. *Clinical Experimental Pharmacology and Physiology* **27**, 1–8.

Hemmer, B., Archelos, J. and Hartung, H.-P. (2004). New concepts in the immunopathogenesis of multiple sclerosis. *Nature Reviews* **3**, 291–301.

Howard, G. and Howard, V. J. (2004). Distribution of stroke: heterogeneity of stroke by age, race and sex. In: Mohr, J. P., Choi, D. W., Grotta, J. C., Weir, B. & Wolf, P. A. (eds.) *Stroke, pathophysiology, diagnosis and management* (4th edn., pp. 3–12). Philadelphia, PA: Churchill Livingstone.

Juurlink, B. H. J. (2001). Anti-oxidant strategy to treat stroke. In: Feuerstein, G. (ed.) *Inflammation and stroke*. Basel: Birkhauser Verlag.

Lassman, H. and Ransohoff, R. M. (2004). The CD4-Th1 model for multiple sclerosis: a crucial re-appraisal. *Trends in Immunology* **25**, 132–137.

Lindsberg, P. (2001). Clinical evidence of inflammation as a risk factor in ischemic stroke. In: Feuerstein, G. (ed.) *Inflammation and stroke*. Basel: Birkhauser Verlag.

Logan-Clubb, L. and Stacy, M. (1995). An open-labeled assessment of adverse effects associated with interferon 1-beta in the treatment of multiple sclerosis. *Journal of Neuroscience Nursing* **27**, 344–347.

Minagar, A., Gonzalez Toledo, E., Alexander, J. T. and Kelley, R. E. (2004). Pathogenesis of brain and spinal cord atrophy in multiple sclerosis. *Journal of Neuroimaging* **14**, 5S–10S.

Moalem, G., Leibowitz-Amit, R., Yoles, E., et al. (1999). Autoimmune T cells protect neurons from secondary degeneration after central nervous system axotomy. *Nature Medicine* **5**, 49–55.

Rosenberg, G., Navratil, M., Barone, F. C. and Feuerstein, G. (1996). Proteolytic cascade enzymes increase in focal cerebral ischemia in rat. *Journal of Cerebral Blood Flow and Metabolism* **16**, 360–366.

Stuchbury, G. and Munch, G. (2005). Alzheimer's associated inflammation, potential drug targets and future therapies. *Journal of Neural Transmission* **112**, 429–453.

Neuron Death *See:* Glucocorticoids – Adverse Effects on the Nervous System.

Neuropeptide Y

C Carvajal, Y Dumont and R Quirion
McGill University, Montréal, Canada

The Effect of Stress on Central Neuropeptide Y Signaling
The Effect of Exogenous Neuropeptide Y on Anxiety-
    Related Behaviors
Anxiety-like Behavior in Neuropeptide Y Receptor
    Knockout and Transgenic Animals
Clinical Evidence for Neuropeptide Y in Anxiety Disorders
How Does Neuropeptide Y Regulate Emotionality?
Neuropeptide Y and Vulnerability to Disease

Glossary

Anxiety	A state of apprehension, uncertainty, or fear resulting from the anticipation of a realistic or fantasized threatening event or situation.
Depression	A mood disorder characterized by symptomatic criteria such as chronically depressed mood; low self-esteem; feelings of hopelessness, worthlessness, and guilt; and recurrent thoughts of death and suicide.
Neuropeptide Y (NPY)	A 36-amino-acid neuropeptide that is one of the most abundant within the central nervous system of all mammals, including humans.
Neuropeptide Y receptors	Receptor molecules for neuropeptide Y and the related peptides polypeptide YY (PYY) and pancreatic polypeptides (PP); they include the Y_1, Y_2, Y_4, Y_5, and Y_6 subtypes, all of which couple to G-proteins and inhibit the production of cAMP.
Sedation	A reduction of anxiety, stress, irritability, or excitement, often by using a drug.

Neuropeptide Y (NPY) was isolated from porcine brain more than 2 decades ago and is a member of a large family of peptides that also include polypeptide YY (PYY) and the pancreatic polypeptides (PP). NPY is a 36-amino-acid peptide and is one of the most abundant peptide expressed in the central nervous system (CNS) of all mammals, including humans. It is also one of the most conserved peptides in evolution, suggesting that it has an important role in the regulation of basic physiological functions. At present, five NPY receptor subtypes have been cloned and designated: Y_1, Y_2, Y_4, Y_5 and Y_6. All of them couple to G-proteins and inhibit the production of cAMP. In the rat brain, the Y_1 receptor has predominant expression in the cerebral cortex, thalamus, and brain-stem nuclei. The Y_2 receptor is abundantly expressed in the hippocampal formation and brain-stem nuclei. This subtype is considered to mostly act as presynaptic autoreceptors that provide negative feedback to NPY-ergic nerve terminals to modulate NPY release. There are only low levels of expression of the Y_4 receptor in the brain; *in situ* hybridization signals of the Y_5 receptor mRNA and its translated protein are seen in the olfactory bulb, hippocampus, and hypothalamic regions. The Y_6 receptor is not expressed in the rat and is nonfunctional in humans and primates. NPY has important modulatory functions in the immune and cardiovascular systems, circadian rhythms, food intake, and seizure activity. NPY is consistently involved in stress and anxiety-related behaviors and there is increasing support for the role of NPY in mood disorders such as depression and in various forms of addiction.

The Effect of Stress on Central Neuropeptide Y Signaling

NPY is considered an important neuromodulator in the regulation of anxiety-related behaviors. Several studies have shown that exposure to acute and chronic stress paradigms such as physical immobilization produces widespread changes in NPY expression throughout the CNS. For example, 1 h of restraint stress in Sprague–Dawley rats decreased NPY mRNA levels and NPY-like immunoreactivity (NPY-IR) by 30% in the amygdala; 2 h following restraint stress, NPY mRNA decreased by 35% in the neocortex and amygdala. However, 10 h after restraint stress, NPY-IR increased 23% in the hypothalamus. Another study

Table 1 Summary of the effects of exogenous NPY on anxiety-related behaviors[a]

Model	Treatment	Effect	Source[b]
Open field	ICV NPY	Dose-dependent anxiolytic effect	14
	NPY Y1 agonist: ICV [D-His26]NPY	Dose-dependent anxiolytic effect	14
	NPY Y2 agonist: ICV C2-NPY	No effect	14
	NPY Y5 agonist: ICV [cPP(1–7), NPY(19–23), Ala31, Aib32, Gln34]hPP	Anxiolytic-like effect	14
Elevated plus-maze	ICV NPY	↑ Time on open arms	7
		Dose-dependent anxiolytic effect	14
	ICV PYY	↑ Time on open arms	3
	ICV NPY(2–36)	↑ time on open arms	3
	NPY Y1 agonist: ICV [D-His26]NPY	Dose dependent anxiolytic effect	14
	NPY Y1 antagonist: ICV BIBP3226	Anxiogenic-like effect	9
	NPY Y1 antisense: ICV; CeA NPY Y1 antisense	Attenuated NPY-induced anxiolytic effect	4, 15
	NPY Y2 agonist: ICV C2-NPY	No effect	14
	NPY Y5 agonist: ICV [cPP(1–7), NPY(19–23), Ala31, Aib32, Gln34]hPP	Anxiolytic-like effect	14
	NPY Y1/Y4/Y5 agonist: ICV [Leu31,Pro34]NPY	↑ Time on open arms	3
	NPY Y2/Y5 agonist: ICV	↓ Time on open arms	7
	NPY(3–36)	No effect	9
Light–dark box	ICV NPY	↑ Transitions (anxiolytic-like effect)	11
Social interaction	BLA NPY	↑ Social behavior	13
	Septum NPY	↑ Social behavior	8
	NPY Y1 antagonist: BLA BIBO3304	Blocks NPY-induced ↑ in social behavior	13
	NPY Y2 agonist: BLA C2-NPY	↓ Social behavior	12
	NPY Y5 agonist: BLA [cPP(1–7), NPY(19–23), Ala31, Aib32, Gln34]hPP	Anxiolytic-like effect	12
	NPY Y2/Y5 agonist: BLA NPY(3–36)	Anxiolytic-like effect	12
	NPY Y5 antagonist: BLA Novartis 1	Blocked the anxiolytic-like effect of NPY(3–36)	12
	IP CGP71683A	No effect	10

Vogel conflict	ICV NPY	Anticonflict/anxiolytic-like effect	7
Geller–Seifter	ICV NPY	Anticonflict/anxiolytic-like effects	1, 2, 6
	NPY Y$_1$/Y$_4$/Y$_5$ agonist: ICV [Leu^{31}, Pro^{34}]NPY	Anticonflict/anxiolytic-like effects	5
Fear-potentiated startle	ICV NPY, PYY, NPY(2–36)	↓ Startle response	3
	NPY Y$_1$/Y$_4$/Y$_5$ agonist: ICV [Leu^{31}, Pro^{34}]NPY	↓ Startle response	3
	NPY Y$_2$ antagonist: ICV NPY(13–36)	No effect	3

[a] ↑, increase, ↓, decrease, BLA, injected into basolateral nucleus of the amygdala; ICV, injected intracerebroventricularly; IP, injected intraperitoneally. Adapted from Carvajal, C., Dumont, Y. and Quirion, R. (2006). Neuropeptide Y: role in emotion and alcohol dependence, CNS & Neurological Disorders – Drug Targets 5, 181–195, with permission.

[b] 1. Britton, K. T., Akwa, Y., Spina, M. G., et al. (2000). Neuropeptide Y blocks anxiogenic-like behavioral action of corticotropin-releasing factor in an operant conflict test and elevated plus maze. Peptides 21, 37–44.

2. Britton, K. T., Southerland, S., Van Uden, E., et al. (1997). Anxiolytic activity of NPY receptor agonists in the conflict test. Psychopharmacology (Berlin) 132, 6–13.

3. Broqua, P., Wettstein, J. G., Rocher, M. N., et al. (1995). Behavioral effects of neuropeptide Y receptor agonists in the elevated plus-maze and fear-potentiated startle procedures. Behavioral Pharmacology 6, 215–222.

4. Heilig, M. (1995). Antisense inhibition of neuropeptide Y (NPY)-Y1 receptor expression blocks the anxiolytic-like action of NPY in amygdala and paradoxically increases feeding. Regulatory Peptides 59, 201–205.

5. Heilig, M., McLeod, S., Brot, M., et al. (1993). Anxiolytic-like action of neuropeptide Y: mediation by Y1 receptors in amygdala, and dissociation from food intake effects. Neuropsychopharmacology 8, 357–363.

6. Heilig, M., McLeod, S., Koob, G. K., et al. (1992). Anxiolytic-like effect of neuropeptide Y (NPY), but not other peptides in an operant conflict test. Regulatory Peptides 41, 61–69.

7. Heilig, M., Soderpalm, B., Engel, J. A., et al. (1989). Centrally administered neuropeptide Y (NPY) produces anxiolytic-like effects in animal anxiety models. Psychopharmacology (Berlin) 98, 524–529.

8. Kask, A., Nguyen, H. P., Pabst, R., et al. (2001). Neuropeptide Y Y1 receptor-mediated anxiolysis in the dorsocaudal lateral septum: functional antagonism of corticotropin-releasing hormone-induced anxiety. Neuroscience 104, 799–806.

9. Kask, A., Rago, L. and Harro, J. (1996). Anxiogenic-like effect of the neuropeptide Y Y1 receptor antagonist BIBP3226: antagonism with diazepam. European Journal of Pharmacology 317, R3–R4.

10. Kask, A., Vasar, E., Heidmets, L. T., et al. (2001). Neuropeptide Y Y(5) receptor antagonist CGP71683A: the effects on food intake and anxiety-related behavior in the rat. European Journal of Pharmacology 414, 215–224.

11. Pich, E. M., Agnati, L. F., Zini, I., et al. (1993). Neuropeptide Y produces anxiolytic effects in spontaneously hypertensive rats. Peptides 14, 909–912.

12. Sajdyk, T. J., Schober, D. A. and Gehlert, D. R. (2002). Neuropeptide Y receptor subtypes in the basolateral nucleus of the amygdala modulate anxiogenic responses in rats. Neuropharmacology 43, 1165–1172.

13. Sajdyk, T. J., Vandergriff, M. G. and Gehlert, D. R. (1999). Amygdalar neuropeptide Y Y1 receptors mediate the anxiolytic-like actions of neuropeptide Y in the social interaction test. European Journal of Pharmacology 368, 143–147.

14. Sorensen, G., Lindberg, C., Wortwein, G., et al. (2004). Differential roles for neuropeptide Y Y1 and Y5 receptors in anxiety and sedation. Journal of Neuroscience Research 77, 723–729.

15. Wahlestedt, C., Pich, E. M., Koob, G. F., et al. (1993). Modulation of anxiety and neuropeptide Y-Y1 receptors by antisense oligodeoxynucleotides. Science 259, 528–531.

looked at repeated stress in Wistar–Kyoto rats. After 1 h of restraint stress, NPY mRNA increased in the arcuate nucleus of the hypothalamus by 81%, but after 3 days (1 h day^{-1}), NPY mRNA increased by 40% in the arcuate nucleus and 50% in the medial amygdala (MeA). After chronic restraint (1 h day^{-1} for 9–10 days), there was an upregulation of prepro-NPY mRNA and NPY itself in the amygdala but not in hypothalamic or cortical regions. Consequently, acute physical restraint, which promotes experimental anxiety, primarily suppressed NPY expression, but chronic physical restraint generally enhanced NPY signaling, especially in the amygdala. These results are believed to support an early hypothesis that suggests NPY may act to buffer the behavioral effects of stress-promoting signals.

The Effect of Exogenous Neuropeptide Y on Anxiety-Related Behaviors

NPY is consistently implicated in the pathogenesis of anxiety disorders, based on a significant number of findings that show NPY-induced anxiolytic activity in animal models widely used for the screening of anxiolytic compounds. NPY is reported to elicit anxiolytic-like effects in models of anxiety, including exploratory behavior-based tests such as the open field, elevated plus-maze, and light–dark compartment test, social interaction, punished responding tests, and fear-potentiated startle (see **Table 1**).

The open field test is often used to measure behavioral changes induced by anxiolytic or anxiogenic-like compounds in animal models. Anxiolytic drugs such as benzodiazepines and barbiturates increase the number of entries and time spent in the central area of the arena. Total crossings are presented as a measure of general locomotor activity in the arena. At higher doses, traditional anxiolytic drugs have significant sedative effects and suppress locomotor activity. Similarly, NPY causes dose-dependent suppression in open field activity when the intracerebroventricular (ICV) dose of NPY exceeds 5 μg. The significant effect of NPY on sedation in the open field led investigators to examine the potential anxiolytic properties of this peptide in the elevated plus-maze.

The elevated plus-maze is one of the most widely used tests for anxiety in animal models. The test is based on the conflict between the natural aversion of rodents for open spaces and the drive to explore a novel environment. Typically, the time spent on the open arms and the numbers of entries onto the open and closed arms of the maze are recorded. The percentage of open arm entries relative to the number of total arm entries is considered to be the superlative measure reflecting innate fearfulness. NPY,

administered ICV, decreased the preference for closed arm entries and increased the time spent on open arms. Higher doses of NPY (exceeding 2 nmol) suppressed entries into both closed and open arms, consistent with the sedative action of NPY observed at high doses in the open field.

A central mechanism involving the NPY Y_1 receptor subtype in the anxiolytic effect of NPY is supported by several pharmacological studies. For example, ICV administration of an antisense oligonucleotide targeted at Y_1 receptor mRNA attenuated NPY-induced anxiolytic-like effects in the elevated plus-maze and blocked the anxiolytic-like effect of NPY in the central nucleus of the amygdala (CeA) in the same test. This was confirmed in a study that demonstrated anxiolytic-like activity of the NPY, PYY, and the $Y_1/Y_4/Y_5$ agonist [Leu^{31}, Pro^{34}]NPY but not the Y_2 agonist NPY(13–36). Further support for the Y_1 receptor was revealed with the anxiogenic-like effect of the Y_1 receptor antagonist BIBP3226. The Y_2-type receptor agonist, NPY(13–36), was later shown to induce anxiogenic-like effects in this model, in mice, when administered ICV.

More recently, there was an attempt to confirm the receptor subtype(s) involved in the anxiolytic/anxiogenic action of NPY as well as to determine which receptor(s) are involved in the sedative action of NPY. This study examined ICV injection of NPY as well as the specific receptor agonists for the Y_1 receptor ([D-His^{26}]NPY), Y_2 receptor (C2-NPY), and Y_5 receptor ([cPP(1–7),NPY(19–23),Ala^{31},Aib^{32},Gln^{34}] hPP) in the elevated plus-maze and open field tests. The results revealed that NPY and the Y_1 agonists had a dose-dependent anxiolytic-like effect in both behavioral tests. However, in contrast to NPY, which caused significant sedation in the open field test, the Y_1 agonist was without sedative effect. The Y_2 agonist showed neither anxiolytic-like nor sedative effects, and the Y_5 agonist showed anxiolytic-like activity in both behavioral tests and caused sedation in the same dose range as NPY in the open field test. The authors conclude that the anxiolytic-like effects of ICV-administered NPY in rats are mediated via both Y_1 and Y_5 receptors, whereas sedation is mediated via Y_5 receptors.

Additional support for the anxiolytic-like effect of NPY has been confirmed in the light–dark compartment test in which ICV NPY increased the number of transitions between the two compartments, a validated measure of anxiolytic activity in this test. Social interaction has also been pharmacologically validated as an experimental model of anxiety. The time spent in active social behavior, as well as locomotor activity, is recorded. NPY, when microinjected into the basolateral nucleus of the amygdala (BLA) and into the caudal dorsolateral septum increases social interaction. Thus, NPY-induced anxiolysis in this paradigm of anxiety appears to be mediated by several brain regions. As in the elevated plus-maze, the involvement of the Y_1 receptor in social interaction is supported by blocking the anxiolytic-like effect of NPY with the intra-amygdalar injection of the selective Y_1 receptor antagonist BIBO3304. The role of the Y_5 receptor was also shown using [cPP(1–7),NPY (19–23),Ala^{31},Aib^{32},Gln^{34}]hPP, a selective Y_5 receptor agonist. This agonist and the mixed Y_5/Y_2 agonist NPY(3–36) caused anxiolytic-like effects when injected into the BLA. The effect of NPY(3–36) was blocked by pretreatment with a purported Y_5 antagonist, Novartis 1 (synthesized by Eli Lilly). However, the Y_5 antagonist CGP71683A did not influence anxiety in any exploratory model of anxiety.

It has also been suggested that the Y_2 NPY receptor may mediate anxiogenic-like behaviors in the amygdala in this task. One study found a dose-dependent decrease in the time spent in social interaction when the Y_2 receptor agonist C2-NPY was directly injected into the BLA. However, the authors did not attempt to reverse the anxiogenic-like effects of this molecule with a selective Y_2 receptor antagonist, such as BIIE0246. The Y_2 receptor agonists may have an anxiogenic effect because the activation of the presynaptic Y_2 receptor may lead to decreased release of NPY and a subsequent decrease in Y_1 receptor activation. Overall, in the exploratory tests of anxiety including the open field, elevated plus-maze, and social interaction, NPY produces robust anxiolytic-like activity that is mediated through the Y_1 (and possibly Y_5) receptor subtypes, whereas the anxiogenic effects of NPY are mediated through Y_2 receptors.

Several versions of operant behavioral analysis for anxiety have been developed such as the Vogel conflict test and Geller–Seifter test, which are based on conflict of motivations rather than unconditioned exploratory models. In these tests, the subject experiences opposing and concomitant tendencies of desire (e.g., to obtain a reward) and of fear (avoidance of a potentially aversive stimulus). In the Vogel conflict test, water-deprived rodents are exposed to mild and intermittent electric shock via the spout of a water bottle when attempting to drink. In this test, treatment with anxiolytic drugs increases the number of accepted shocks during the punished phase. It has been shown that ICV NPY markedly increased the number of electric shocks accepted in this test. At the doses employed, NPY was reported not to affect pain sensitivity in a shock threshold test or to affect thirst. Thus, the anticonflict effects are considered to be related to a reduction of anxiety. In the Geller–Seifter conflict test, rats are trained to respond for a food

reward and are exposed to a modest electric shock during the conflict component of the procedure. The ICV injection of NPY consistently produces dose-dependent anticonflict/anxiolytic-like effects in the Geller–Seifter test, an established animal model of anxiety especially suitable for detecting the effects of benzodiazepine-like anxiolytics. The Y_1 receptor subtype is implicated in this test as well. Intra-amygdalar injection of [Leu^{31}, Pro^{34}]NPY was shown to have anxiolytic-like effects. As in the exploratory models of anxiety, NPY can also induce anxiolysis in the conflict-based tests.

Startle is an adaptive response to acoustic stimuli that enables the individual to avoid, or reduce, the risk of an injury by a predator. In fear-potentiated startle, an acoustic stimulus is paired with an aversive intervention such as foot shock or air-puff, and after training, the stimulus alone is capable of elevating startle amplitude. As in the elevated plus-maze, ICV injections of NPY, PYY, and the Y_1/Y_4/Y_5 agonist [Leu^{31}Pro^{34}]NPY inhibited fear-potentiated startle, whereas the Y_2 agonist NPY(13–36) had no effect. The Y_1 receptor is consistently indicated across diverse animal models of anxiety to mediate the anxiolytic-like activity of NPY. However, the Y_5 receptor cannot be ignored because [Leu^{31}Pro^{34}]NPY does have some efficacy for the Y_5 receptor subtype. In addition, the Y_5–Y_2 differentiating receptor agonist NPY(2–36) has shown anxiolytic-like activity in the elevated plus-maze and fear-potentiated startle.

Anxiety-like Behavior in Neuropeptide Y Receptor Knockout and Transgenic Animals

The development of the NPY transgenic rat has provided a unique opportunity to study the effects of this peptide on anxiety-related behaviors. In this transgenic rat model, there is central overexpression of prepro-NPY mRNA and NPY peptide in the CA1 region of the hippocampus and decreased Y_1 binding sites within the hippocampus (CA1, CA2, and dentate gyrus). Recently, NPY protein levels were also shown to be significantly higher in the paraventricular, suprachiasmatic, and supraoptic nuclei of the hypothalamus and tended to be increased in the arcuate nucleus in these rats. The transgenic animals were generated using a 14.5-kb fragment of the rat NPY genomic sequence that includes the normal intronic sequence elements and is flanked by a 5-kb 5' sequence thought to contain the major regulatory elements that normally control NPY expression. Consequently, the regulation of the NPY transgene is predicted to be similar to the regulation of endogenous

NPY. These molecular and neurochemical events led to an altered anxiety profile in NPY transgenic rats that included an insensitivity to restraint stress in the elevated plus-maze and an increase in the number of punished drinking events in the Vogel conflict test. The anxiolytic-like profile of the NPY transgenic rat was replicated in a study that showed NPY transgenic animals were resistant to acute physical restraint stress measured by the elevated-plus maze and displayed anxiolytic-like activity in the open field. The behavioral profile observed in the NPY transgenic rats was not associated with any significant changes in corticosterone levels before or following a stress challenge. This suggests a mechanism other than hypothalamic-pituitary-adrenal axis modulation and supports the role of the limbic system in the modulation of anxiety-related behaviors by NPY. This may be critically important and could distinguish NPY from other substances modulating stress-responses (although there are links between NPY and corticotropin releasing hormone, CRH).

The central role of the limbic system is also supported by recent studies involving Y_2 receptor subtype knockout ($Y_2^{-/-}$) mice. Mice deficient in the Y_2 receptor subtype displayed an anxiolytic-like phenotype in the elevated plus-maze and open field test. More recently, NPY $Y_2^{-/-}$ mice displayed increase preference for the central area of the open field when compared to wild-type control ($Y_2^{+/+}$) animals without changes in locomotor activity. These findings have been confirmed by an independent laboratory using the open field, elevated plus-maze, and light–dark compartment tests. These receptors are considered to be autoreceptors that provide negative feedback to NPY-ergic nerve terminals to modulate NPY release. Consequently, $Y_2^{-/-}$ mice are predicted to have increased endogenous peptide expression, analogous to the phenotype of NPY transgenic rats, which may contribute to the underlying mechanism responsible for anxiolytic-like behaviors regulated by NPY.

There is also evidence that NPY exerts anxiolytic-like effects through Y_1 receptors within the amygdala. The predicted anxiogenic-like phenotype of NPY Y_1 knockout mice is supported by a study that found significantly higher levels of territorial aggression in Y_1 knockout mice compared to control animals using established aggression paradigms.

Interestingly, NPY knockout ($NPY^{-/-}$) mice did not show a dramatic change in anxiety-like behavior in the elevated plus-maze. $NPY^{-/-}$ mice were found to have a significant increase in the amplitude response in the acoustic startle test, and they were less active in the central part of the open field, suggesting that these animals were more anxious. Overall, the results from NPY transgenic and knockout animals provide compelling evidence for the role of NPY in the modulation of anxiety.

Clinical Evidence for Neuropeptide Y in Anxiety Disorders

In addition to the extensive preclinical data supporting NPY in the regulation of anxiety-like behaviors, a number of clinical studies have been published on the subject. In human subjects, there is a positive association between acute, uncontrollable psychological stress and robust increases in plasma levels of NPY. The increase in plasma NPY was positively correlated with increased cortisol and norepinephrine concentrations. A correlation between higher levels of stress-related NPY release and lower levels of subjective psychological distress was also found, supporting the possibility that NPY exhibits anxiolytic activity during stress in human subjects.

How Does Neuropeptide Y Regulate Emotionality?

The mechanistic action of NPY in anxiety-related behaviors is strongly associated with the amygdala. The amygdala is a key structure to the regulation of anxiety and expression of emotional responses to stress. Attention has been focused particularly on the basolateral complex (lateral, basolateral, and basomedial nuclei) and CeA. The amygdala contains NPY and significant levels of Y_1 and Y_2 receptor subtypes. These areas may be potential neural substrates to the behavioral effects of NPY on emotional regulation. NPY is also produced by neurons in the hippocampus with considerable expression of the Y_1 and Y_2 receptor subtype. In addition to the substantial evidence for the involvement of the amygdala and hippocampus, there is also evidence for the periaqueductal gray, septum, and locus coeruleus. However, the specific contribution of these anatomical regions requires further elucidation.

The interaction between CRH and NPY has been proposed as a means by which emotional behavior is regulated. In contrast to the anxiolytic-like effects of NPY, there is evidence that CRH has significant anxiogenic-like effects in animal models. For example, the ICV administration of CRH increases anxiety-like behavior in the elevated plus-maze, and CRH antagonists can block the behavioral effects of a stress challenge. The anxiogenic-like role of CRH has been confirmed in studies using CRH-overexpressing and CRH knockout mice. It has been shown that NPY can counteract the anxiogenic-like effect of CRH in the hippocampus, hypothalamus, locus coeruleus, periaqueductal gray, and septal nucleus. Moreover, deletion of Y_2 receptors causes a 60% reduction in CRH mRNA expression that might contribute to the anxiolytic-like behavior of NPY Y_2 receptor knockout mice. Thyroxine-treated adult animals displayed reduced anxiety in the motility box and elevated plus-maze, a reduction in the number of CRH-IR neurons in the CeA, and an increase in the number of NPY-IR neurons in nuclei of the basolateral complex of the amygdala.

It has also been proposed that NPY increases γ-aminobutyric acid (GABA) signaling to produce anxiolysis, analogous to many classes of anxiolytic drugs such as benzodiazepines. NPY is localized in GABAergic neurons in the amygdala, and there is evidence that NPY may directly modulate the activity of GABAergic neurons by stimulating Y_1 receptors. It has been shown that diazepam counteracts the anxiogenic effect of the Y_1 receptor antagonist BIBP3226, suggesting that the equilibrium between GABAergic and NPY-ergic neurotransmission may be important for the regulation of the emotional state in animal models. This conclusion is supported by a recent study that found chronic treatment with positive (anxiolytic) or negative (anxiogenic) regulators of $GABA_A$ receptors modulate Y_1 receptor-mediated transmission in the amygdala. The authors suggest that the NPY Y_1-mediated transmission and the GABAergic system may act together on the same postsynaptic target sites to decrease anxiety and that the Y_1 receptors might also play a role in controlling both the NPY and GABA presynaptic release.

However, it was recently shown that the anxiolytic-like effect produced by inhibiting the metabotropic glutamate receptor 5 (mGlu5) with the mGlu5 receptor antagonist MPEP is mediated by the NPY receptor and not by GABA. In order to determine the mechanism that contributes to the anxiolytic action of MPEP, the authors injected either the benzodiazepine antagonist flumazenil or the Y_1 receptor antagonist BIBO3304 into the BLA. Flumazenil antagonizes the effect of the several different classes of anxiolytic agents including the benzodiazepine diazepam, serotonergic agents, and noradrenergic ligands in animal models of anxiety through a GABA-mediated mechanism. However, the anxiolytic effects of MPEP were not changed by flumazenil; but they were abolished by BIBO3304 administration. The authors also found a decrease in NPY-IR neurons after three doses of MPEP administration, which suggests a decrease in NPY levels in the amygdala. The authors propose that the decrease in NPY levels may result from enhanced release of the peptide and that this release is responsible for the anxiolytic action of MPEP. Interestingly, the administration of metabotropic glutamate receptor antagonists into the hippocampus also produces

anxiolytic-like effects. NPY has been shown to inhibit glutamate release in the hippocampus, leading to the speculation that the anxiolytic-like effect of hippocampal NPY overexpression in NPY transgenic rats resembles the anxiolytic-like action of the metabotropic glutamate receptor antagonists. The interaction between glutamate acting via mGlu5 and NPY may represent a novel mechanism of anxiolytic action in the brain, independent of the traditional GABA-mediated benzodiazepine signaling.

Overall, these studies demonstrate that NPY and its receptor subtypes are significantly involved in the regulation of anxiety-like behaviors in both animal models and human subjects.

Neuropeptide Y and Vulnerability to Disease

Vulnerability to Depression

Depression is traditionally viewed as the manifestation of an inability to cope with various lifetime stressors that is presumably determined by genetics. Given the significance of NPY in the CNS as a modulator of anxiety, NPY may have a significant role in the etiology of depression and/or the effective reversal of symptoms. This theory is supported by preclinical data that consistently indicate a role for NPY in depression. For example, maternal deprivation is an animal model of depression/vulnerability to stress that posits that early life stress may cause changes in the CNS (e.g., hypothalamic-pituitary-adrenal dysregulation) that are associated with an increased risk of adult life depressive psychopathology. Using this model in rats for $3\,h\,day^{-1}$ during postnatal days 2–14, NPY levels were shown to be reduced in the hippocampus and striatum and increased in the hypothalamus. However, if lithium treatment was employed on days 50–83, the changes in NPY-IR induced by maternal deprivation were not observed in the hippocampus and striatum, whereas NPY levels were further increased in the hypothalamus. Consequently, early life stress has long-term effects on NPY levels in the CNS and may be a factor in the development of depression; possibly through an increased vulnerability to stress.

Additional evidence for NPY in depression is through the antidepressant-like properties of NPY. The Porsolt forced-swim test is widely used for the screening of potential antidepressant drugs. It has recently been shown that NPY displayed antidepressant-like activity in the rat forced-swim test. These results have since been confirmed in the mouse version of this test. ICV NPY administration significantly reduced immobility time in a dose-dependent manner, as did [Leu^{31}Pro^{34}]PYY. Attempts to determine the specific receptor subtype(s) involved has shown that BIBP3226 and BIBO3304 (selective Y$_1$ antagonists) and NPY(13–36) (a preferential Y$_2$ agonist) did not display any activity at the doses tested. However, pretreatment with BIBP3226 and BIBO3304 significantly blocked the anti-immobility effects of NPY. It is predicted that potentiation of NPY signaling at central postsynaptic receptors through Y$_1$ receptors is essential to reverse the behavioral characteristics of depression. The upregulation of NPY expression through Y$_1$ receptor activation may be advantageous for behavioral adaptation to stress-induced changes within the CNS. Consequently, a maladaptive response to stress may be the result of an intrinsic abnormal function of central NPY transmission that is characteristic of depressive states. Thus, NPY may be involved in the vulnerability to mood disorders through its endogenous modulation of emotional behavior.

Vulnerability to Alcoholism

Recent evidence suggests that NPY has a significant role in the neurobiological response to alcohol, including alcohol consumption, dependence, and withdrawal. NPY is beginning to emerge as an important neuromodulator in the etiology of alcoholism that is independent from the addictive and reinforcing properties of the traditional system and, instead, is strongly associated with innate emotionality. It is proposed that individuals with low innate levels of NPY and high basal levels of anxiety, or with low levels of NPY and increased anxiety caused by withdrawal, may drink increased amounts of alcohol in an attempt to reduce anxiety. There is evidence that supports this hypothesis from genetic lines of alcohol-preferring rats. For example, alcohol-preferring (P) rats have altered levels of NPY in several brain regions, including low levels of NPY in the amygdala compared to non-alcohol-preferring (NP) rats. P rats also have high basal levels of anxiety, which may predispose them to excessive alcohol drinking. The central infusion of NPY may reverse high alcohol drinking in P rats by reducing their high levels of anxiety. Studies in Wistar rats also indicate that animals with high levels of anxiety drink more alcohol than those with lower levels. Furthermore, because NPY is expressed at low levels in the amygdala following ethanol withdrawal, it is predicted that preventing this decrease in NPY expression might prevent subsequent withdrawal symptoms such as increased anxiety. Consequently, the motivational aspect of alcohol intake may be strongly tied to innate anxiety.

In summary, much evidence suggests a key role for NPY and its receptors in anxious behaviors. NPY and its congeners could also play a role in more chronic stressful situations that can possibly result in the development on depressive states or addictive behaviors.

See Also the Following Articles

Alcohol, Alcoholism and Stress: A Psychobiological Perspective; Corticotropin Releasing Factor (CRF); Depression and Manic-Depressive Illness; Depression Models.

Further Reading

Carvajal, C., Dumont, Y. and Quirion, R. (2006). Neuropeptide Y: role in emotion and alcohol dependence. *CNS & Neurological Disorders – Drug Targets* 5, 181–195.

Dumont, Y., Chabot, J. G. and Quirion, R. (2004). Receptor autoradiography as mean to explore the possible functional relevance of neuropeptides: focus on new agonists and antagonists to study natriuretic peptides, neuropeptide Y and calcitonin gene-related peptides. *Peptides* 25, 365–391.

Heilig, M. (2004). The NPY system in stress, anxiety and depression. *Neuropeptides* 38, 213–224.

Kask, A., Harro, J., von Horsten, S., et al. (2002). The neurocircuitry and receptor subtypes mediating anxiolytic-like effects of neuropeptide Y. *Neuroscience and Biobehavioral Reviews* 26, 259–283.

Lin, S., Boey, D. and Herzog, H. (2004). NPY and Y receptors: lessons from transgenic and knockout models. *Neuropeptides* 38, 189–200.

Nestler, E. J., Barrot, M., DiLeone, R. J., et al. (2002). Neurobiology of depression. *Neuron* 34, 13–25.

Pandey, S. C., Carr, L. G., Heilig, M., et al. (2003). Neuropeptide y and alcoholism: genetic, molecular, and pharmacological evidence. *Alcoholism: Clinical & Experimental Research* 27, 149–154.

Redrobe, J. P., Carvajal, C., Kask, A., et al. (2004). Neuropeptide Y and its receptor subtypes in the central nervous system: emphasis on their role in animal models of psychiatric disorders. In: Michel, M. C. (ed.) *Handbook of experimental pharmacology. Vol.162: Neuropeptide Y and related peptides*, pp. 101–136. Heidelberg: Springer.

Redrobe, J. P., Dumont, Y. and Quirion, R. (2002). Neuropeptide Y (NPY) and depression: from animal studies to the human condition. *Life Sciences* 71, 2921–2937.

Sajdyk, T. J., Shekhar, A. and Gehlert, D. R. (2004). Interactions between NPY and CRF in the amygdala to regulate emotionality. *Neuropeptides* 38, 225–234.

Thorsell, A. and Heilig, M. (2002). Diverse functions of neuropeptide Y revealed using genetically modified animals. *Neuropeptides* 36, 182–193.

Thorsell, A., Michalkiewicz, M., Dumont, Y., et al. (2000). Behavioral insensitivity to restraint stress, absent fear suppression of behavior and impaired spatial learning in transgenic rats with hippocampal neuropeptide Y overexpression. *Proceedings of the National Academy of Sciences USA* 97, 12852–12857.

Valdez, G. R. and Koob, G. F. (2004). Allostasis and dysregulation of corticotropin-releasing factor and neuropeptide Y systems: implications for the development of alcoholism. *Pharmacology Biochemistry and Behavior* 79, 671–689.

Zukowska, Z. and Feuerstein, G. (eds.) (2005). *NPY family of peptides in inflammation, immune disorders, angiogenesis, and cancer.* Basel, Switzerland: Birkhauser Verlag.

Neuropeptides, Stress-Related

A J Tilbrook
Monash University, Melbourne, Australia

Stress-Related Functions of Corticotropin Releasing Hormone and Arginine Vasopressin
Opioids
Oxytocin and Stress
Appetite-Regulating Neuropeptides and Stress

Glossary

Hypophysial portal vessel system	A highly specialized blood vessel system that plays a vital role in the rapid transport of neuropeptides produced by the hypothalamic parvicellular neurons to target cells in the anterior pituitary gland. The hypophysial portal system begins at the base of the hypothalamus with a group of capillaries (primary capillary plexus) that recombine into small portal veins, which pass down through the pituitary stalk into the anterior pituitary gland. Here they branch to form most of the anterior pituitary capillaries and sinusoids, which in turn drain into the systemic venous system. Almost all the blood supply to the anterior pituitary must first pass through the hypothalamo-hypophysial portal system, arriving via the superior hypophysial artery and leaving the anterior pituitary in the anterior hypophysial vein.
Hypothalamic-pituitary-adrenal (HPA) axis	One of the major physiological systems activated by stress; it consists of a hormonal cascade involving the hypothalamus of the brain, the anterior pituitary gland, and the cortex of the adrenal glands. The HPA axis is the humoral component of an integrated neural and endocrine system and results in the release of corticosteroid hormones from the adrenal glands. The major
	corticosteroids released during stress are the glucocorticoids, such as cortisol and corticosterone.
Median eminence	The median eminence is located at the base of the hypothalamus and is a region of confluence of neural and blood-borne messages where neuropeptides can be secreted from the terminals of neurons into the hypophysial portal vessel system.
Neuropeptides	Peptides synthesized in, stored in, and released from neural tissue.
Stress	A complex physiological state that embodies a range of integrative physiological and behavioral processes that occur when there is a real or perceived threat to homeostasis.

There are numerous neuropeptides that are involved in the regulation of stress responses and released as effector molecules as a result of stress responses. Among the most widely researched stress-related neuropeptides are corticotropin releasing hormone (CRH) and arginine vasopressin (AVP), which regulate the hypothalamic-pituitary-adrenal (HPA) axis, and the opioid peptides, which have many functions. Oxytocin is a neuropeptide now recognized as a potentially important modulator of stress responses (**Figure 1**). Other neuropeptides, such as those involved in appetite regulation, can also influence the activity of the HPA axis during stress, although there is considerable variation in the scientific literature concerning the effects of these neuropeptides.

Stress-Related Functions of Corticotropin Releasing Hormone and Arginine Vasopressin

The key stress-related action of CRH and AVP is to act as hypophysiotropic hormones to stimulate the synthesis and secretion of adrenocorticotropic hormone (ACTH) from the anterior pituitary gland (**Figure 1**).

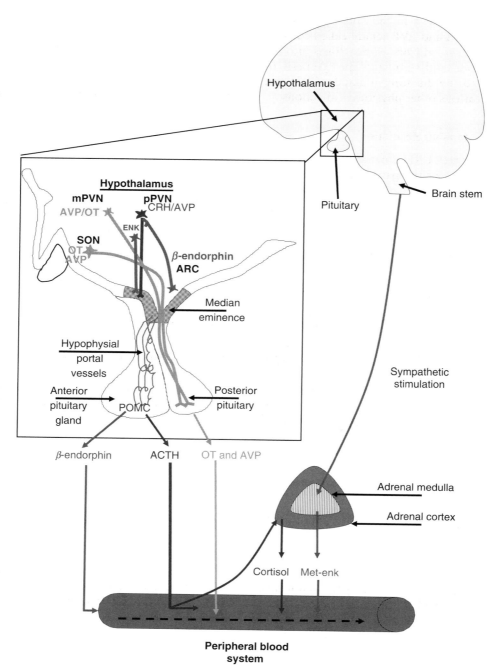

Figure 1 Diagram of some of the key neuropeptides involved in stress-related functions. Corticoptropin releasing hormone (CRH) and arginine vasopressin (AVP) are synthesized and stored in parvicellular neurons in the paraventricular nucleus of the hypothalamus (pPVN) and are released into the hypophysial portal blood to stimulate the synthesis of peptides derived from proopiomelanocortin (POMC), including adrenocorticotropic hormone (ACTH) and the opioid peptide β-endorphin, which are released into the systemic circulation. ACTH stimulates the synthesis of glucocorticoids, such as cortisol, from the adrenal cortex. Opioids such as enkephalin (ENK) and β-endorphin are synthesized in neurons in the brain and have many actions, including the modulation of stress responses. Neurons in the arcuate nucleus of the hypothalamus (ARC) that produce β-endorphin have important interactions with neurons in the pPVN that produce CRH and AVP. The opioid met-enkephalin (Met-enk) is released from the adrenal medulla due to sympathetic stimulation during stress. Oxytocin (OT) is stored in and released from neurons in the posterior pituitary as well as in the brain and acts to attenuate stress responses and reduce anxiety. Magnocellular neurons that synthesize OT and AVP have cell bodies in the magnocellular region of the PVN (mPVN) and supraoptic nucleus (SON) of the hypothalamus. There is also evidence that some neuropeptides best known for their actions in regulating appetite also influence the activity of stress systems, especially the hypothalamic-pituitary-adrenal axis.

The target endocrine cells in the anterior pituitary gland on which CRH and AVP act are called corticotropes. ACTH is released from corticotropes into the systemic circulation and stimulates the synthesis of the glucocorticoids by the adrenal glands. CRH and AVP also have various other physiological actions.

Corticotropin Releasing Hormone

The principal source of CRH is neurons located in the parvicellular division of the paraventricular nucleus of the hypothalamus, which project to the median eminence. CRH is synthesized in the cell bodies of these neurons, stored in the terminals and released into the hypophysial portal blood. It is often considered that CRH is the primary stimulator of the release of ACTH, although it is clear that AVP from parvicellular neurons located in the paraventricular nucleus also plays a role. There may be species differences in the relative importance of these neuropeptides in stimulating the release of ACTH. Various stressful stimuli (stressors) activate the HPA axis, with the consequent release of CRH and AVP into the hypophysial portal blood in a pulsatile pattern. Although the majority of CRH neurons projecting to the median eminence arise from the paraventricular nucleus, some CRH neurons from other hypothalamic nuclei project to the median eminence. CRH neurons also project to the brain stem and are found elsewhere, such as in limbic structures that are involved in processing sensory information and the regulation of the autonomic nervous system.

In addition to CRH, there are other CRH-like peptides, including urocortin I, urocortin II (or stresscopin-like peptide), and urocortin III (or stresscopin); at least two receptors (CRH-R1 and CRH-R2), and a CRH-binding protein. The CRH system is complex, and, in addition to the classic hypophysiotropic actions already described, it is important in regulating behavioral responses to stress. The activation of the HPA axis by CRH is mediated via CRH-R1, which is present in corticotropes. The binding of CRH to CRH-R1 stimulates the secretion of peptides derived from proopiomelanocortin (POMC) which, in addition to ACTH, includes β-endorphin, α-melanocyte-stimulating hormone, β-melanocyte-stimulating hormone, corticotropin-like intermediate peptide, γ-lipotropic hormone, and met-enkephalin.

Arginine Vasopressin

With the exception of the pig, all mammals studied synthesize AVP in the hypothalamus. In the pig, lysine is substituted for arginine, giving lysine vasopressin in this species. Within the hypothalamus, AVP is synthesized in parvicellular neurons that project to the median eminence and magnocellular neurons that project to the posterior pituitary (**Figure 1**). The parvicellular neurons are located in the paraventricular nucleus and synthesize AVP in the cell bodies, store it in the terminals, and release it into the hypophysial portal blood. There is an increase in AVP secretion during stress, and it travels by way of the hypophysial portal system to the anterior pituitary gland to act synergistically with CRH to stimulate the release of ACTH from corticotropes. Some parvicellular neurons synthesize and store both CRH and AVP. The cell bodies of the magnocellular neurons that produce AVP are located predominantly in the supraoptic nucleus of the hypothalamus, and AVP is stored in the terminals in the posterior pituitary from which it is released directly into the systemic circulation. AVP released from the posterior pituitary is also known as antidiuretic hormone. Although this source of AVP is generally considered to function mainly to control fluid homeostasis and, in extreme stress, effect vasoconstriction, recent studies suggest that AVP from magnocellular neurons may also stimulate ACTH secretion.

AVP acts on three different receptors (V1a, V1b, and V2), which are expressed differently in various tissues and exert different actions. The actions of AVP to stimulate the release of ACTH are mediated by the V1b receptor. Many authors consider CRH, not AVP, to be the major stimulator of ACTH synthesis and secretion. Indeed, textbooks and scientific publications often fail to recognize the role of AVP as an ACTH secretagogue. Nevertheless, it is clear that AVP plays an important role in stimulating the secretion of ACTH during stress, although its relative importance may differ between species. For example, the majority of research in rats suggests that CRH is the major ACTH secretagogue, with AVP playing more of a permissive role, perhaps potentiating the effects of CRH. In contrast, in sheep there is evidence that AVP plays a major role in stimulating ACTH secretion, although other work has suggested that CRH is more important. It also appears likely that different stressors may influence the extent to which CRH and AVP stimulate ACTH secretion.

Regulation of Corticotropin Releasing Hormone and Arginine Vasopressin Secretion

The synthesis and secretion of CRH and AVP are influenced by both excitatory and inhibitory neural inputs from various regions of the brain that process information resulting from different stressors, negative feedback by glucocorticoids, and circadian rhythms. CRH and AVP neurons in the paraventricular nucleus receive direct input from the limbic system and brain stem and indirect input from the cerebral cortex. Major excitatory input to CRH and AVP neurons arises from noradrenergic afferents of the brain stem (A_1, A_2, and A_6 noradrenergic cell groups), and there are reciprocal projections between CRH and AVP neurons in the paraventricular nucleus and neurons in the arcuate nucleus that produce POMC products, including the opioid β-endorphin. Glucocorticoids exert negative feedback by acting directly on the neurons that produce CRH and AVP and through other brain regions that have afferent inputs to the paraventricular nucleus. Glucocorticoids also act directly on pituitary corticotropes. The negative feedback actions of glucocorticoids regulating CRH and AVP synthesis are exerted via high-affinity mineralocorticoid receptors (MRs) and low-affinity glucocorticoid receptors (GRs). MRs are localized in the hippocampus and other regions of the limbic brain such as the lateral septum and amygdala, as well as hypothalamic sites. The glucocorticoids act via MRs to maintain basal activity. GRs have a more extensive distribution within the brain, being most abundant in the hypothalamus and in pituitary corticotropes, and are involved in the feedback actions of both basal and stress-induced levels of glucocorticoids. The circadian regulation of the HPA axis is illustrated by the circadian rhythms of CRH and AVP levels, which peak in the early morning and fall during the day in diurnal species. The negative feedback effects of glucocorticoids also vary in a circadian fashion.

Opioids

The opioid peptides and their receptors are distributed widely in the body. This distribution includes the central, peripheral, and autonomic nervous systems as well as several endocrine tissues and various target organs. The opioids are involved in a broad range of functions, including acting as neuropeptides to regulate stress responses. There are three classes of opioids: β-endorphin, the enkephalins (met-enkephalin and leu-enkephalin), and the dynorphins. It is often considered that the affinity of β-endorphin, the enkephalins, and dynorphins is highest for the μ-, δ-, and κ-opioid receptor subtypes, respectively. However, it is also apparent that opioids can bind to more than one receptor subtype.

Peptides Derived from Proopiomelanocortin

As previously indicated, a large number of peptides are derived from processing POMC. This includes the opioid β-endorphin. Peptides derived from POMC are found in the brain, anterior pituitary gland, gut, thyroid, thymus, adrenal medulla, pancreas, spleen, macrophages, placenta, testes, and ovaries. There is a wide distribution of β-endorphin within the brain, with the highest concentrations occurring in the medial hypothalamus and arcuate nucleus. Acting as a neuropeptide and neurotransmitter, β-endorphin is involved in a range of stress-related functions, including the modulation of CRH and AVP neurons in the paraventricular nucleus. Furthermore, during stress, the secretion of β-endorphin from the anterior pituitary gland increases in parallel with ACTH. The physiological significance of this is not known, although it is possible that this source of β-endorphin contributes to some of the known actions of β-endorphin during stress. These actions include analgesia and the regulation of blood glucose concentrations and the immune system.

Peptides Derived from Pro-Enkephalin

Pro-enkephalin (also referred to as pro-enkephalin A) is the major biological source of met-enkephalin and is a source of leu-enkephalin. Met-enkephalin-containing peptides are present in the central nervous system, adrenal medulla, gastrointestinal tract, and many other tissues. The neurons that synthesize met-enkephalin are extensively distributed throughout the central nervous system, making enkephalin the most widely distributed opioid in the brain. Pro-enkephalin neurons exist throughout the hypothalamus, including the paraventricular nucleus. The chromaffin cells of the adrenal medulla also synthesize pro-enkephalin. Met-enkephalin is often cosecreted with the catecholamines from the adrenal medulla into the peripheral circulation during stress. The biological significance of this is also unknown.

Peptides Derived from Pro-Dynorphin

Pro-dynorphin (also referred to as pro-enkephalin B) can be processed to produce dynorphin A, dynorphin B, α-neoendorphin, and β-neoendorphin. Pro-dynorphin is found in many parts of the central nervous system, including the hypothalamus, hippocampus, brain stem, amygdala, and gastrointestinal tract. The neurons that produce dynorphins in the hypothalamus are mainly located in the supraoptic nucleus and paraventricular nucleus. Dynorphins have greatest affinity for the κ-opioid receptor. Less is known about the dynorphins than the other classes of opioids, although it is apparent that they have many different physiological actions depending on their site of production. These actions include influencing the pattern of electrical activity of magnocellular neurons that produce AVP and negative feedback regulation of oxytocin secretion.

Stress-Related Functions of Opioids

Opioids exert a diverse range of stress-related actions. In particular, opioids act to attenuate or terminate stress responses. This modulatory influence on stress responses may provide a mechanism for preventing the detrimental effects of sustained or chronic stress. Specifically, opioids can inhibit the activity of the HPA axis. At least part of this mechanism involves the inhibition of the synthesis of CRH and, possibly, AVP. The reciprocal interactions between CRH and AVP neurons in the paraventricular nucleus and β-endorphin neurons in the arcuate nucleus are clearly important for this modulatory effect (**Figure 1**). Further, opioids regulate sympathetic, cardiovascular, and respiratory neural control systems and are involved in the regulation of pain, reinforcement and reward, the release of neurotransmitters, and other autonomic and neuroendocrine functions.

Opioids are involved in the control of pain and play a major role in suppressing the perception of pain (i.e., analgesia). In particular, opioids are mediators of stress-induced analgesia. The phenomenon of stress-induced analgesia is well known. There are many accounts of people being unaware of pain during a stressful experience. The origin of pain is normally at the site of intense stimulation or tissue damage, causing the discharge of impulses in a specialized set of nerve endings (nociceptors). The intensity of the excitation is regulated by local chemical signals that are released when the tissue is damaged. These include the opioids. Information about painful stimulation is carried as impulses in afferent nerve fibers that synapse in the dorsal horn of the spinal cord. Postsynaptic neurons convey the nociceptive information to the brain. Transmission at these synapses is modulated by locally released neurotransmitters, including opioids. The perception of the pain can be altered by modulation in the dorsal horn. The brain influences the processing of nociceptive input in the spinal cord, partly by activating opioid interneurons in the dorsal horn. It seems that both opioids produced in the brain and circulating opioids are involved in the induction of analgesia, with the source of the opioids that induces the analgesia varying with the type of stressor.

Oxytocin and Stress

Oxytocin is synthesized in cell bodies of magnocellular neurons located principally in the paraventricular nucleus of the hypothalamus, is stored in the terminals of these neurons in the posterior pituitary, and is released from there into the peripheral circulation (**Figure 1**). Oxytocin is also synthesized in neurons that are widely distributed within the central nervous system. The actions of oxytocin are mediated via specific high-affinity receptors that are distributed both peripherally and in many forebrain areas, including regions of the hippocampus and amygdala, bed nuclei of the stria terminalis, ventrolateral septum, and several hypothalamic nuclei. Thus, oxytocin has both peripheral and central actions, some of which concern the regulation of stress responses. The classic peripheral actions of oxytocin are to cause contraction of the myoepithelial cells of the mammary glands to stimulate milk letdown and to stimulate the myometrium of the uterus during parturition. Oxytocin also has stress-related effects, and circulating concentrations of oxytocin increase in response to some, but not all, types of stress. Oxytocin can act within the brain to reduce the responsiveness of the HPA axis to stress with reduced cortisol secretion due, at least in part, to a reduction in CRH synthesis. Oxytocin can also reduce blood pressure, increase tolerance to pain, and reduce anxiety. Oxytocin facilitates mother–infant interactions and tends to facilitate behaviors that oppose fight-or-flight behavioral responses to stress. Lactating females (in which oxytocin levels are elevated) generally display attenuated responses to stress, and although a number of different mechanisms may be involved, oxytocin is likely to play a role. Generally, oxytocin is not considered to readily cross the blood–brain barrier although this dogma has recently been challenged. It is difficult to know whether the actions of oxytocin to dampen stress responses are due to central and/or peripheral effects.

Appetite-Regulating Neuropeptides and Stress

Various neuropeptides that regulate appetite can affect the activity of the HPA axis in response to stress. These include orexin, neuropeptide Y (NPY), agouti-related protein, and cocaine and amphetamine-regulated transcript (CART).

The peptides orexin-A and orexin-B are produced in the hypothalamus and can modulate the activity of the HPA axis, both centrally and peripherally. Orexin receptors are widely distributed and are found in the paraventricular nucleus, median eminence, pituitary corticotropes, adrenal cortex, and adrenal medulla. These neuropeptides can stimulate the release of

CRH and AVP as well as having direct stimulatory effects on the adrenal cortex.

NPY may mediate the excitatory effects of orexins. Certainly NPY can influence the activity of the HPA axis, although it is not clear how because NPY has been found to both inhibit and stimulate the release of CRH. The synthesis of NPY increases in the arcuate nucleus and hilus of the dentate gyrus following restraint stress in rats.

Agouti-related protein is an appetite stimulant that is coexpressed in the arcuate nucleus with NPY, and there is differential regulation of this neuropeptide in relation to stress. For example, foot shocks in rats decreased agouti-related protein synthesis and increased NPY synthesis.

CART is synthesized in neurons in various hypothalamic structures, including the paraventricular and arcuate nuclei. Glucocorticoids can influence the synthesis of CART, and CART can act within the paraventricular nucleus to activate the HPA axis.

See Also the Following Articles

Adrenocorticotropic Hormone (ACTH); Corticotropin Releasing Factor (CRF); Glucocorticoid Negative Feedback; Hypothalamic-Pituitary-Adrenal; Anatomy of the HPA Axis; Paraventricular Nucleus; Urocortins; Vasopressin; CRH Anxiety Circuitary in Brain; Neuropeptide Y; Orexin.

Further Reading

Altemus, M. (1995). Neuropeptides in anxiety disorders: effects of lactation. *Annals of the New York Academy of Sciences* **771**, 697–707.

Charmandari, E., Tsigos, C. and Chrousos, G. (2005). Endocrinology of the stress response. *Annual Review of Physiology* **67**, 259–284.

Chrousos, G. P. (1998). Stressors, stress, and neuroendocrine integration of the adaptive response: the 1997 Hans Selye memorial lecture. *Annals of the New York Academy of Sciences* **851**, 311–335.

de Kloet, E. R. (2004). Hormones and the stressed brain. *Annals of the New York Academy of Sciences* **1018**, 1–15.

Herman, J. P., Figueiredo, H., Mueller, N. K., et al. (2003). Central mechanisms of stress integration: hierarchical circuitry controlling hypothalamo-pituitary-adrenocortical responsiveness. *Frontiers in Neuroendocrinology* **24**, 51–180.

Sapolsky, R. M. (1998). Why zebras don't get ulcers: an updated guide to stress, stress related diseases and coping. New York: W. H. Freeman.

Tilbrook, A. J., Turner, A. I. and Clarke, I. J. (2002). Stress and reproduction: central mechanisms and sex differences in non-rodent species. *Stress* **5**, 83–100.

Tilbrook, A. J. and Clarke, I. J. (2006). Neuroendocrine mechanisms of innate states of attenuated responsiveness of the hypothalamo-pituitary adrenal axis to stress. *Frontiers in Neuroendocrinology* **27**, 285–307.

Neurosis

D J Lynn
Thomas Jefferson University, Philadelphia, PA, USA

The term neurosis was used officially with confidence and authority in American psychiatry as recently as 1980, but, at least since the 1994 *Diagnostic and Statistical Manual of Mental Disorders* (4th edn.; DSM-IV), it has been officially abandoned. For official American psychiatry, it is now of primarily historical interest. To understand the evolution of the use of this term, and the related controversy, is to understand a great deal about the recent changes within American psychiatry.

The Scottish Physician William Cullen (1710–1790) introduced the term in his *First Lines of the Practice of Physic*, which first appeared in English in 1777. Cullen used the term neuroses to refer to one of four general categories of illnesses. The other three were pyrexiae (febrile diseases), cachexiae (diseases resulting from bad habits), and locales (diseases consisting of local lesions). The category Cullen named neuroses included all conditions of the central nervous system not related to fever or focal lesions.

During the nineteenth century, the term evolved into psychoneuroses, which Richard von Kraft-Ebing defined in 1872 as mental illnesses in cases in which the brain was normal.

Neuroses were at the heart of the psychoanalytic writings of Sigmund Freud (1856–1939). He was most concerned with psychoneuroses, which he distinguished from actual neuroses by their etiologies. For Freud, psychoneuroses were caused by unconscious conflicts, generally of a sexual nature, with roots in childhood. Actual neuroses were caused by current factors within the patient's awareness. In American psychiatry in the mid-twentieth century, the influence of Freud's writings and the writings of his followers was extremely strong, and in DSM-II, the term neurosis was used pervasively. In general in this era, the unconscious conflict believed to be causing the manifest neurotic symptoms attracted much more attention than the symptoms themselves. For any particular patient, the symptoms were seen as a product of, and in some sense a solution to, that patient's specific unconscious conflict. For psychoanalytically oriented psychiatrists, attention to the symptoms was important not for the purposes of arriving at a prognosis or conducting research but for delineating, and interpreting for the patient, the unconscious conflict.

DSM-III, published in 1980, was a systematic attempt to redirect attention to observable and quantifiable symptoms. Disorders were classified in a descriptive manner; the neuroses, so prominent in DSM-II, were discarded, and the term neurosis was relegated to parentheses. The authors stated that "at the present time, there is no consensus in our field as to how to define 'neurosis'" American Psychiatric Association (1980: 9). Some psychiatrists were using the term in a descriptive sense to denote a pattern of observable symptoms; others used it to designate a psychogenic etiology. DSM-III used an atheoretical approach concerning the disorders formerly termed neuroses for two stated reasons: (1) the etiology of these disorders was declared to be unknown and (2) the goal was to arrive at a system of classification that could be used by clinicians whether or not they agreed with particular theories of etiology. The editors suggested that the term neurotic disorder could be used, but only descriptively (to refer to an observable symptom pattern), and that, whenever psychiatrists wanted to convey an etiology based in unconscious conflict, the term neurotic process should be used. DSM-III-R (1987) basically continued the use of its predecessor, but DSM-IV (1994) contains no mention of the term neurosis.

For some psychoanalytic psychiatrists, these developments led to consequences that were seen as unfortunate. As Glen Gabbard put it: "although this classification accommodates the recent biological research delineating different kinds of anxiety, it also encourages clinicians to think about anxiety as an *illness* rather than as an overdetermined *symptom* of unconscious conflict".

See Also the Following Articles

Anxiety; Depression Models; Psychoanalysis.

Further Reading

American Psychiatric Association (1968). *Diagnostic and statistical manual of mental disorders* (2nd edn.). Washington, DC: APA Press.

American Psychiatric Association (1980). *Diagnostic and statistical manual of mental disorders* (3rd edn.). Washington, DC: APA Press.

American Psychiatric Association (1987). *Diagnostic and statistical manual of mental disorders* (3rd edn. rev.). Washington, DC: APA Press.

American Psychiatric Association (1994). *Diagnostic and statistical manual of mental disorders* (4th edn.). Washington, DC: APA Press.

Freud, S. (1953–1974). Anxiety, instinctual life (1933). In: Strachey, J. (ed.) *Standard edition of the complete psychological works of Sigmund Freud* (vol. 22), pp. 81–111. London: Hogarth Press.

Freud, S. (1953–1974). Sexuality in the aetiology of the neuroses (1898). In: Strachey, J. (ed.) *Standard edition of the complete psychological works of Sigmund Freud* (vol. 3), pp. 263–285. London: Hogarth Press.

Gabbard, G. O. (2000). *Psychodynamic psychiatry in clinical practice* (3rd edn.). Washington, DC: APA Press.

Person, E. S., Cooper, A. M. and Gabbard, G. O. (eds.) (2005). *The American Psychiatric Publishing textbook of psychoanalysis*. Washington, DC: APA Press.

Shorter, E. (2005). *A historical dictionary of psychiatry*. New York: Oxford University Press.

Neurotic Disorders *See:* Neurosis.

Neuroticism, Genetic Mapping of

M W Nash
King's College London, London, UK

What Is Neuroticism, and Is It Genetic?

Which Regions of the Genome Are Linked to Neuroticism?

Have Association Studies Identified Any Genes Associated with Neuroticism?

Roles of Candidate Genes in Stress

Glossary

Complex traits	Phenotypes governed by variation in many genes; often continuously and/or normally distributed. The trait does not segregate in the population following any obvious patterns. Environmental influences often account for as much as, or more than, genetic influences.
Genome	The set of all genes for a particular organism. In humans this includes both nuclear and mitochondrial DNA sequences.
5-HTTLPR	Gene polymorphism in the $5'$-promoter region of the gene encoding the serotonin (5-hydroxytryptamine; 5-HT) transporter (5-HTT) that has been implicated in susceptibility to life events/stressors.
LOD score	Logarithm of the odds score favoring linkage. The higher the score, the greater the evidence for linkage.
Mendelian or simple traits	Phenotypes governed by a single major locus or gene and hence the traits can be seen to segregate in the population following obvious additive, dominant, or recessive patterns.
Phenotype	Any observable and measurable characteristic of an organism produced by genetic and/or environmental influences.
Quantitative trait locus (QTL)	A locus implicated in genetic variation that causes a change in a continuous phenotype.

What Is Neuroticism, and Is It Genetic?

Neuroticism is a unique dimensional measure of personality thought to capture emotional stability and a temperamental sensitivity to negative stimuli. Indeed, it is a widely agreed upon higher order factor in many different personality constructs. Currently, three measures of personality are commonly used in genetic research: Eysenck's Personality Questionnaire, Cloninger's Temperament and Character Inventory, and the Neuroticism Extraversion Openness (NEO) personality inventory. For Cloninger's measure of harm avoidance (HA) and Eysenck's measure of neuroticism (EPQ-N), there is some evidence that these different personality constructs are influenced by similar genetic and environmental variables. In the case of the EPQ-N, high scorers are conceived to be overly emotional, react strongly to stimuli, and find it difficult to recover after an emotionally stimulating experience, while low scorers are conceived to be calm, even tempered, and emotionally controlled. The genetic influence on neuroticism and harm avoidance has been widely assessed, and the estimates of heritability are 40–60% of the phenotypic variance. The EPQ-N is known to overlap genetically with many internalizing disorders, such as major depression, panic disorder, and generalized anxiety disorder, and because of this, neuroticism has been used in psychiatric genetic research to identify the genetic variation causing individual differences in the susceptibility to both depression and anxiety.

Which Regions of the Genome Are Linked to Neuroticism?

Traditionally, there have been two statistical approaches to relate variation of the genome to a phenotype of interest, known as linkage mapping and association mapping. Linkage mapping has played a huge historical role in the gene mapping of Mendelian traits. In essence, the method relies on the phenomenon of allele sharing among relatives. For example, monozygotic twins share 100% of their genome, while siblings and dizygotic twins should share only 50% – on average – of their genome. To illustrate this, if two siblings are both highly neurotic, then genetic variation at a region of the genome that is truly linked to neuroticism would be expected to be shared by the siblings. If such a phenomenon is observed in more siblings than would be expected by chance, this region of the genome is declared linked to neuroticism. Linkage is a useful approach for coarse mapping, as it identifies large regions of the genome as being linked to the phenotype, but this is also a disadvantage, as large regions can contain hundreds of candidate genes. As this analysis cannot distinguish which gene or genetic variant is responsible for the linkage, it is usual after the identification of a region to perform the finer association mapping approach to localize more precisely the disease gene (see next section).

To date, there have been seven linkage studies examining a neuroticism-like phenotype. The first reported study, undertaken by Cloninger and colleagues, examined HA and observed significant linkage to the long (p) arm of chromosome 8. Additive and nonadditive interaction of the chromosome 8 peak with other loci suggested significant interaction with chromosomes 11, 18, 20, and 21. A subsequent study assessed selected regions of the genome for linkage to HA and also found linkage in an overlapping region of chromosome 8. It is not possible, however, to deduce that the same sequence variant(s) is responsible for the linkage in both these studies. Further fine mapping of the chromosome 8p region in the same sample refined the region to one around the neuregulin gene (*NRG1*), which has been implicated in schizophrenia susceptibility. The NRG1 protein is involved in signaling based on the glutamate neurotransmitter and plays a central role in neural development. Interestingly, neuroticism and HA have been reported as elevated in first-degree relatives of schizophrenics and schizotypal individuals. A re-analysis of the original data set, using a novel method, reproduced the evidence for linkage to the chromosome 8p markers. As these four studies are derived from only two samples, it is difficult to decide if a true quantitative trait locus (QTL) actually resides on chromosome 8p. The possibility that *NRG1* is a candidate for harm avoidance is intriguing, but the gene needs to be extensively examined in multiple samples before any robust conclusion can be drawn.

The first published linkage analysis of the EPQ-N was carried out by Fullerton and colleagues in a UK selected sibling sample. The main findings were QTLs on chromosomes 1, 4, 7, 12, and 13. Further evidence was presented that these loci for neuroticism might be gender specific: the QTLs on chromosomes 1, 12, and 13 appeared to be female specific, while a QTL on chromosome 8, which was not found to be genome-wide significant in the complete sample analysis, appeared to be male specific. It is interesting to note that the chromosome 8 locus is in close proximity to the chromosome 8p locus identified in HA. The second published study used a composite index of four self-report measures of anxiety and depression, including Eysenck's measure of neuroticism in a large UK-based sibship sample. As opposed to only examining Eysenck's neuroticism measure, Nash and colleagues used structural equation modeling on the four self-report measures to derive a phenotypic composite index of the shared genetic liability to both depression and anxiety. While no significant findings were obtained, linkage peaks closely approaching significance were obtained on chromosomes 1p and 6p for both the composite index and neuroticism, with a high correspondence of results between the two phenotypes. Splitting the sample by gender led to the identification of a linkage peak for females on

chromosome 12, while also indicating female specificity of the chromosome 1 peak and male specificity of the chromosome 6 peak. The most recent linkage publication on EPQ-N was performed in a New Zealand sample. While no peak reached statistical significance, a suggestive finding of linkage was obtained on chromosome 12, with nominal findings of linkages on chromosomes 1, 3, 6, 11, 15, and 17. Comparing the results from these three studies indicates a low correspondence between the results. There is possible overlap on chromosomes 1 and 12. The peak on chromosome 12 is potentially exciting, as this also overlaps with linkage peaks from both unipolar and bipolar depression. Indeed, as discussed later, variants of a gene within this peak have recently been observed to segregate with major depression and might also be associated with individual variation in neuroticism.

Similarly, comparisons between all the studies on neuroticism and harm avoidance show only slight correspondence. This is not unexpected, unless a major locus (responsible for >20% phenotypic variance) was involved. While linkage is a powerful method for simple traits with genes of major effect, its poor ability to reliably detect loci with a small phenotypic effect relegates the method to a preliminary tool providing genomic targets on which to focus fine mapping projects. Its contributions in this field at best provide suggestive evidence that chromosomes 1, 8, and 12 might harbor genetic variants that are associated with neuroticism/harm avoidance.

Have Association Studies Identified Any Genes Associated with Neuroticism?

Association mapping has historically been employed to evaluate the potential contribution of specified candidate genes, or as a follow-up, fine mapping tool to linkage analysis. Due to technological advances in speed and the reduction in expense in measuring differences in the genome, whole genome association mapping will eventually become the predominant mapping approach. The simplest version of association mapping is in case control studies of unrelated individuals and essentially examines whether or not there is a correlation between the genetic variation and the phenotype. This basic approach suffers from the fact that a much larger number of sequence variants need to be measured to capture adequately the effective genetic variation compared to linkage analysis. Nevertheless, the increased ability to detect small changes is the most attractive feature of this approach to gene mapping.

Function-Based Candidate Genes

Perhaps the biggest shift in thinking with respect to psychiatric and personality genetics has been the reduction in the expected effect size of a single genetic variant. While initial expectations were that a single genetic variant might account for around 10% of the phenotypic variance, it is now thought that 1%, or much less, is a more realistic expectation for single variants. Commonly, sample sizes are inadequate to detect such effects reliably. To tackle this problem, meta-analytic techniques can be implemented that use the results of multiple studies to estimate reliably the effect sizes and significance of genetic variants. In the only published meta-analysis of genetic polymorphisms in personality, Munafo and colleagues examined commonly researched genetic variants in the serotonin transporter (*SLC6A4*) and various dopamine genes (*DRD4, DRD2, DRD3,* and *DAT1*). Of all the results, the only significant meta-analytic association was between a polymorphism in *SLC6A4* and neurotic/avoidant traits.

Current evidence indicates that the serotonin transporter gene (*SLC6A4*), located on the long arm of chromosome 17 (17q), is probably the only gene that can be considered associated with neuroticism, albeit only weakly. The mature protein of this gene transports serotonin from the synaptic cleft back into the presynaptic neuron for reuse and is responsible for the quantity of serotonin in the synaptic cleft. A sequence variant, known as 5-HTTLPR, is present in either a short or long form in a region of the gene called the promoter, which regulates the rate at which the mRNA of the gene is made. The first study of this variant identified an association of the number of short variants with an increase in neuroticism. Subsequently, there have been many attempts at replicating this finding with varying degrees of success. To address this issue, there have been several meta-analyses of the many findings, with a general consensus supporting a small but positive association. Recently, Caspi and colleagues observed that the relationship of stressful life events and depression was mediated by 5-HTTLPR, such that individuals with two long alleles were unchanged in their risk to depression as life events increased, while the risk of depression was increased in those carrying one or more short alleles. This finding has subsequently been replicated for depression, but comprehensive studies looking only at neuroticism and 5-HTTLPR have found no mediation of the variant on the effect that life events have on neuroticism. It is highly probable that 5-HTTLPR and neuroticism are weakly associated; what is unknown, and a source of current interest, is the developmental mechanisms that 5-HTTLPR affects, which lead to its association with individual differences in neuroticism.

A more recent line of research has been driven by theories of aberrant neuronal apoptosis and neurogenesis in major depression. Based on such theories, some research has been carried out on genetic variants known to affect these mechanisms. The most studied of these is the brain-derived neurotrophic factor gene (*BDNF*), located on chromosome 11p. The BDNF protein has a well-documented role in neuronal development, survival, and plasticity, making it an attractive candidate for many psychiatric disorders. Indeed, variants in the gene have been associated with disorders such as obsessive-compulsive disorder, bipolar disorder, and major depressive disorder. Because neuroticism is genetically related to major depression and is a phenotypic marker for vulnerability to depression, genetic variants in the *BDNF* gene have been examined for their relationship with neuroticism. The original association with this gene examined a single nucleotide polymorphism that changes the 66th amino acid from a valine to a methionine and its association with neuroticism as measured by the NEO personality scale. This study found an apparently strong finding, with those individuals carrying the Met/Met genotype having substantially lower neuroticism scores than the rest of the sample. Subsequent follow-up studies using the NEO personality scale or HA have not found such strong evidence, and a recent comprehensive study examining the EPQ-N found no evidence for an association. It appears that although *BDNF* might be a plausible candidate gene for neuroticism, the data simply do not currently support this. As these studies have focused on only one variant in the gene, it is plausible that other variants in the gene are associated with neuroticism.

Position-Based Candidate Genes

Despite the promising leads from linkage studies, no positional candidates have emerged so far, but there have been some possible leads from related scientific fields. *RGS2*, or regulator of G-protein signaling 2, is a positional candidate gene from linkage studies that examined emotionality in mice. This gene is located on mouse chromosome 1 and corresponds to a region on human chromosome 1. Whether this gene is responsible for the linkage signal seen on this chromosome has not yet been established. Nevertheless, there have been reports that variants in the human version of this gene might be associated with agoraphobia. Another possible gene is *APAF1*, apoptosis protease activating factor 1, involved in the apoptosis pathway. This gene, located at 12q, was recently associated with major depression in Utah families. Functional studies indicated that only those variants that segregated with major depression had a functional effect on the apoptosis pathway. Given the genetic relationship between the EPQ-N and major depression, it is possible that *APAF1* also contributes to individual differences in neuroticism. This gene is located within the chromosome 12 linkage peak identified in two studies of neuroticism, as mentioned previously, lending weight to the suggestion that genetic variation in this gene might be associated with neuroticism.

Roles of Candidate Genes in Stress

There are a number of possible mechanisms that might explain the relationship of the aforementioned candidate genes with stress. Upon being stressed, the body enters into various response patterns, including at the molecular level an increase in firing from serotonergic neurons. As the role of the serotonin transporter is the reuptake of serotonin from the synaptic cleft, the rate at which new transporter can be made might affect the rate at which the biochemical system regains homeostasis. Because the short, low-activity 5-HTTLPR allele carriers produce less mRNA, these individuals might return to their biochemical baseline slower than long allele homozygotes. This delay might then leave these individuals more susceptible to the detrimental effects of stress. Another aspect of these detrimental effects is the neuronal toxicity of glucocorticoids, which are released as a negative feedback mechanism during response to a stressor, and it is known that glucocorticoids are capable of damaging hippocampal neurons. The rate and impact of this damage might be mediated by both BDNF and APAF1. BDNF is involved in neuronal survival, while APAF1 is involved in cell death. The functional variation that has been identified for these genes might cause some individuals to be more resilient to the toxic effects of stress, while making others more vulnerable. This model suggests that individuals who carry the S allele of 5-HTTLPR, who are homozygous for the *BDNF* Met allele, and who also have the apoptosis rate-increasing alleles of *APAF1* may be more vulnerable to the detrimental effects of stress.

See Also the Following Articles

Genetic Polymorphisms in Stress Response; Serotonin Transporter Genetic Modifications.

Further Reading

Caspi, A., Sugden, K., Moffitt, T. E., et al. (2003). Influence of life stress on depression: moderation by a polymorphism in the 5-HTT gene. *Science* 301, 386–389.

Cloninger, C. R. (1986). A unified biosocial theory of personality and its role in the development of anxiety states. *Psychiatric Developments* 4, 167–226.

Dina, C., Nemanov, L., Gritsenko, I., et al. (2005). Fine mapping of a region on chromosome 8p gives evidence for a QTL contributing to individual differences in an anxiety-related personality trait: TPQ harm avoidance. *American Journal of Medical Genetics, Part B: Neuropsychiatric Genetics* 132, 104–108.

Fullerton, J., Cubin, M., Tiwari, H., et al. (2003). Linkage analysis of extremely discordant and concordant sibling pairs identifies quantitative-trait loci that influence variation in the human personality trait neuroticism. *American Journal of Human Genetics* 72, 879–890.

Lake, R. I., Eaves, L. J., Maes, H. H., et al. (2000). Further evidence against the environmental transmission of individual differences in neuroticism from a collaborative study of 45,850 twins and relatives on two continents. *Behavior Genetics* 30, 223–233.

Lesch, K. P., Bengel, D., Heils, A., et al. (1996). Association of anxiety-related traits with a polymorphism in the serotonin transporter gene regulatory region. *Science* 274, 1527–1531.

Munafo, M. R., Clark, T. G., Moore, L. R., et al. (2003). Genetic polymorphisms and personality in healthy adults: a systematic review and meta-analysis. *Molecular Psychiatry* 8, 471–484.

Nash, M. W., Huezo-Diaz, P., Williamson, R. J., et al. (2004). Genome-wide linkage analysis of a composite index of neuroticism and mood-related scales in extreme selected sibships. *Human Molecular Genetics* 13, 2173–2182.

Neale, B. M., Sullivan, P. F. and Kendler, K. S. (2005). A genome scan of neuroticism in nicotine dependent smokers. *American Journal of Medical Genetics, Part B: Neuropsychiatric Genetics* 132, 65–69.

Sen, S., Nesse, R. M., Stoltenberg, S. F., et al. (2003). A BDNF coding variant is associated with the NEO personality inventory domain neuroticism, a risk factor for depression. *Neuropsychopharmacology* 28, 397–401.

Willis-Owen, S. A., Fullerton, J., Surtees, P. G., et al. (2005). The Val66Met coding variant of the brain-derived neurotrophic factor (BDNF) gene does not contribute toward variation in the personality trait neuroticism. *Biological Psychiatry* 58, 738–742.

Willis-Owen, S. A., Turri, M. G., Munafo, M. R., et al. (2005). The serotonin transporter length polymorphism, neuroticism, and depression: a comprehensive assessment of association. *Biological Psychiatry* 58, 451–456.

Zohar, A. H., Dina, C., Rosolio, N., et al. (2003). Tridimensional personality questionnaire trait of harm avoidance (anxiety proneness) is linked to a locus on chromosome 8p21. *American Journal of Medical Genetics, Part B: Neuropsychiatric Genetics* 117, 66–69.

Neuroticism Response to Stress, Genetic Mapping of Mice

M R Munafò
University of Bristol, Bristol, UK
J Flint
University of Oxford, Oxford, UK

Personality and Neuroticism
Animal Models of Emotionality
Genetic Mapping in Rodents
Comparisons between Rodents and Humans

Glossary

Allele	An alternative form of a genetic locus; a single allele for each locus is inherited separately from each parent.
Backcross	A cross between one animal type that is heterozygous for alleles obtained from two parental strains and a second animal type from one of those parental strains. The term is often used by itself to describe the two-generation breeding protocol of outcross followed by a backcross that is used frequently in linkage analysis.
F1	The first filial generation; the offspring resulting from the first experimental crossing of animals. The progeny produced by intercrossing F1 individuals are referred to as F2 individuals.
Heterozygous	Having two different alleles at a given locus.
Homozygous	Having two identical alleles at a given locus.
Inbred strain	Animals that result from the process of at least 20 sequential generations of brother–sister matings. This process is called inbreeding.
Intercross	A cross between two animals that have the same heterozygous genotype at designated loci, for example, between sibling F1 hybrids that were derived from an outcross between two inbred strains.
Outcross	A cross between genetically unrelated animals.
Neuroticism	A personality trait dimension that refers to emotionality, emotional instability, and stress reactivity.
Quantitative trait locus (QTL)	A locus that affects a quantitative trait.
Syntetic genes	Genes thought to reside on the same chromosome.

Personality and Neuroticism

Broad behavioral traits underlie variation in human personality, and there is general consensus that certain of these relate to individual differences in response to stress and in vulnerability to anxiety and depression in humans. Behavioral evidence of anxiety-related traits has been observed from amphibians to rodents and higher mammals. In humans, these traits have been described variously as neuroticism, trait anxiety, and harm avoidance, and there is now general agreement that any adequate trait model of personality must include a broad trait related to vulnerability to anxiety- and depression-related disorders, representing an evolutionarily conserved capacity for fear and anxiety.

The notion that a single underlying risk factor underlies vulnerability to both anxiety- and depression-related disorders is supported by evidence from twin studies in humans that these disorders share a common genetic basis. Moreover, numerous studies have arrived at similar estimates of the contribution of genetic variance to variation in trait neuroticism, with additive genetic variance estimated at approximately 30% and nonadditive variance at approximately 15%. This has led to attempts to better understand the molecular genetic architecture of trait neuroticism in humans likely to result from multiple low-magnitude genetic effects and their interactions, both with other genetic loci and environmental factors; however, this research has generally yielded disappointing and inconsistent results.

Better progress has been made in studies of animal models of emotionality, which offer several attributes useful in genetic research, including short gestation, early puberty, and large litters, as well as a greater degree of experimental control by means of directed mating and environmental control, all of which are valuable when attempting to map the genetic architecture of these traits.

Animal Models of Emotionality

Defining an animal's temperament is not easy, and operational definitions typically require the animal to show a consistent pattern of response to a behavioral task or series of tasks. For example, an animal model of emotionality might be operationally defined as the length of time it takes an animal to emerge into an aversive or threatening environment. This obviously requires relatively strong assumptions regarding the

Table 1 Animal tests of emotionality

Unconditioned responses	
Open-field arena	Activity, defecation, thigmotaxis
Elevated plus-maze	Ratio of entries to open and closed arms
Light–dark box	Emergence time
Hyponeophagia	Latency to start eating
Holeboard	Head dipping
Social interaction	Frequency of social interaction in a novel environment
Conditioned responses	
Two-way avoidance conditioning	Rate of acquisition of response
Acoustic startle	Contraction in response to loud noise
Foot shock-induced freezing	Contraction in response to conditioned stimulus
Fear-potentiated startle	Contraction in response to loud noise in conjunction with conditioned stimulus
Geller–Seifter	Frequency of conditioned response coincidental to an electrical shock
Vogel conflict	Frequency of conditioned licking coincidental to an electrical shock

extent to which this operational definition is an accurate analog of the same construct in humans. The majority of animal studies of emotionality have employed rodent models (i.e., mouse or rat). **Table 1** lists a number of tests of emotionality in animals, divided into measures that depend on unconditioned (ethological) and conditioned responses. Conditioned responses have the advantage of offering much more experimental control. These measures are founded on principles of avoidance, autonomic activation, and behavioral inhibition (i.e., the discontinuation of species-typical behaviors such as exploration).

The open-field apparatus is one widely used paradigm and consists of a circular, white, brightly lit, and fully enclosed arena that allows remote monitoring of behavior over a short period. Unfortunately, many of these tests rely on features unrelated to the trait of interest (i.e., emotionality). For example, many depend in part on the basal activity level of the animal, which may be a potential confound. A potential solution to this problem is outlined here.

Genetic Mapping in Rodents

The mouse genome is well characterized, comprising approximately 22 000 predicted genes, of which approximately 80% have an identifiable human ortholog. Inbred rodent strains exhibit substantial variability in emotionality, and these differences can be exploited for the purposes of quantitative trait mapping. Crosses between inbred strains of rodents are frequently used to map the quantitative trait loci (QTL) that give rise to the genetic component of variation in behavioral traits such as emotionality. The basic experimental design is the analysis of association between genotypic and phenotypic variation in a cross between two inbred strains of rodents (usually, but not necessarily, with contrasting emotionality

phenotypes). Several strategies exist, but in the most widely used either the offspring of the cross (the F1 generation) are mated to produce a F2 intercross or the offspring are backcrossed to either of the parental strains. Molecular genetic markers are then used to determine which chromosomal segments segregate with the trait (i.e., which chromosomal regions are shared by animals that are phenotypically similar for the trait of interest). Over the past 10 years, QTLs putatively related to emotionality have been identified on a number of chromosomes, although the molecular nature of these remains unclear.

One problem is that genetic mapping identifies a potential functional variant, rather than a gene, and functionally important variants that affect gene expression may lie some distance away from a gene or even in the location of an unrelated gene. Another problem is that this experimental design offers only a limited number of recombinants in a single generation (typically, between one and two), so that the resolution to map a specific locus is limited and may identify regions that can still contain hundreds or perhaps thousands of genes.

It is possible to remedy the problem of limited mapping resolution by mapping loci in genetically heterogeneous stocks of rodents that are generated from multiple (usually eight) inbred strains that have been successively intercrossed for maximal diversity and maintained over multiple generations through a program of pseudorandom mating. Because these animals are several generations removed from the original progenitor strains, this offers the potential of mapping a QTL to a limited number of genes, although this requires a substantial increase in marker density and the analysis is considerably more complex in this case. At present, this is most economical once broad chromosomal regions have been

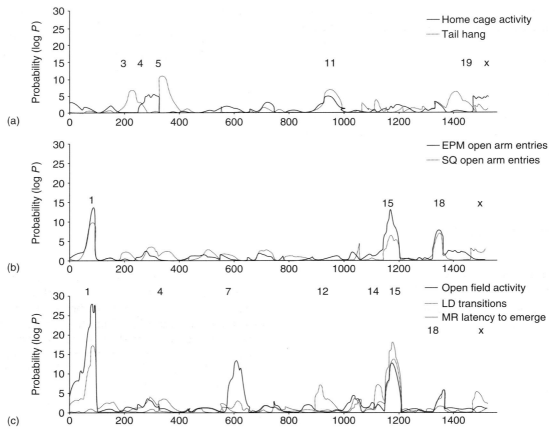

Figure 1   Quantitative trait loci that influence behavior in the De Fries strain of mice. a, Genome scan for two measures that control for putative confounds (home cage activity and tail hang); b, genome scan for two measures of emotionality (EPM open arm entries and SQ open arm entries); c, genome scan for three measures of emotionality (open field activity, LD transitions, and MR latency to emerge). Chromosomes that harbor significant genetic effects are shown as numbers on each panel. EPM, elevated plus-maze; SQ, square maze; LD, light–dark box; MR, mirror chamber. From Flint, J. (2004), The genetic basis of neuroticism, *Neuroscience Biobehavioral Review* 28, 307–316. © 2004 with permission from Elsevier.

identified, thereby limiting the number of markers required for QTL localization.

There also exists a potential solution to the problem of ensuring that the identification of loci related to emotionality in rodent models is specific to this trait. This is to attempt to identify chromosomal regions that influence multiple measures of emotionality, but not control measures, on the assumption that a single underlying trait should influence performance on multiple measures of emotionality to a comparable degree and should not influence performance on control measures.

The results of a recent attempt to do this are presented in **Figure 1**. **Figure 1a** identifies QTLs that influence control measures (i.e., potential confounds unrelated to emotionality), and **Figures 1b–c** identify QTLs that influence one or more of five tests of facets of emotionality related to emotionality (elevated plus-maze, square maze, open field arena, light–dark box, and mirror chamber).

Comparisons between Rodents and Humans

Recently, evidence for an overlap between the genetic basis for emotionality in rodent models and trait neuroticism in humans has emerged. Although a number of studies in humans have investigated individual genes, direct comparability with animal models is better achieved by a linkage analysis of human sibling pairs in which evidence of deviation from the expected value of allele sharing at a given point along the genome is evidence for the presence of a QTL at that locus. In this way, we can ask whether individuals who are behaviorally similar (i.e., have similar trait neuroticism scores) are also genetically similar (i.e., share two alleles). One locus on chromosome 1, identified in humans as potentially related to trait neuroticism, is potentially promising because it may be syntenic with loci identified in animal studies. The congruence of genetic mapping in human and animal studies may help determine whether there is a common set of genes that contribute to trait neuroticism in humans and analog models of emotionality in animals.

Further Reading

Benjamin, J., Ebstein, R. P. and Belmaker, R. H. (2002). *Molecular genetics and the human personality*. Washington, DC: APA Press.

Flint, J. (2004). The genetic basis of neuroticism. *Neuroscience Biobehavioral Reviews* **28**, 307–316.

Munafò, M. R., Clark, T. G., Moore, L. R., et al. (2004). Genetic polymorphisms in personality in healthy adults: a systematic review and meta-analysis. *Molecular Psychiatry* **9**, 471–484.

Willis-Owen, S. A. and Flint, J. (2006). The genetic basis of emotional behavior in mice. *European Journal of Human Genetics* **14**, 721–728.

Night Shiftwork

T Åkerstedt and G Lindbeck
Karolinska institutet, Stockholm, Sweden

Introduction
The Mechanism
Effects on Sleep
Alertness
Performance
Accidents
Stress Indices
Gastrointestinal Effects
Cardiovascular Effects
Mortality
Conclusion

Introduction

Shiftwork may not be the typical stressor in the classic sense, but it affects the systems of stress and restitution in a very pronounced way and causes cardiovascular disease, gastrointestinal disease, and insomnia, among other conditions. Here we review some of the connections. But before that we need to look at the phenomenon of shiftwork. This is an arrangement of work hours through which the daily duration of production/service extends to cover operation during 2–3 work days compressed into one 24-h period. Each day is called a shift. Normally, the first step of extension beyond a day shift is to introduce morning and evening shifts (6 a.m.–2 p.m. and 2 p.m.–10 p.m., respectively). When necessary, a night shift may also be used to cover the remaining 8 h. In Europe, workers often alternate among shifts, working the same shift two to four times in succession and then switching to a new shift. In transport, health care and the service sector, the shifts may be more variable in placement and duration, but the principle of alternating among different shifts remains. Even the permanent night worker alternates between a night shift and day life during his days off. Usually, the night shift is the most problematic, causing disturbed circadian rhythms, disturbed sleep, and excessive sleepiness and several diseases deriving from these disturbances.

The Mechanism

Shift work would not present a problem were it not for the biological clock that drives physiology and psychology through a 24-h cycle, with high and low periods of activity. The central oscillator is situated in the hypothalamus. It is a self-sustained oscillator and drives much of our physiology in an approximately 24-h cycle. It receives input from light and other stimuli that synchronize the pacemaker with the environmental light–dark cycle, called Zeitgebers, which entrain (influence) the biological clock to the light–dark changes of the normal environment. Essentially, light before the circadian trough (low) phase delays the biological clock (1–2 h) and light after the trough phase advances the clock.

The influence of the circadian cycle on sleep was demonstrated in monthlong isolation studies in which individuals could live according to their own preferred sleep–wake schedules. This led to the finding that some individuals developed a period of around 25 h, and that some individuals desynchronized, showing different period lengths for their sleep–wake rhythm and for their rhythm of metabolism (rectal temperature). However, the present estimate of the period length with control for light is 24.1 h.

It was later shown that whenever the sleep–wake rhythm placed sleep around the acrophase (circadian maximum) of rectal temperature, sleep was shortened, and when sleep was placed around the circadian trough phase, sleep was promoted. Thus, the biological clock interfered with sleep and wakefulness.

Effects on Sleep

The dominant health problem reported by shiftworkers is disturbed sleep and wakefulness. At least three-quarters of the shift-working population is affected. When comparing individuals with a very negative attitude to shiftwork with those with a very positive one, the strongest discriminator seems to be the ability to obtain sufficient quality of sleep during the daytime. Electroencephalograph (EEG) studies of rotating shiftworkers and similar groups showed that day sleep is 1–4 h shorter than night sleep. The shortening is due to the fact that sleep is terminated after only 4–6 h without the individual being able to return to sleep. The sleep loss is primarily taken out of stage 2 sleep (basic sleep) and stage rapid-eye movement (REM) sleep (dream sleep). Stages 3 and 4 (deep sleep) do not seem to be affected. Furthermore, the time taken to fall asleep (sleep latency) is usually shorter. Night sleep before a morning shift is also reduced, but the termination is through artificial means and the awakening is usually difficult and unpleasant. Interestingly, day sleep does not seem to improve much across series of night shifts. It appears, however, that night workers sleep slightly better (longer) than rotating workers on the night shift.

As indicated previously, shiftwork sleep duration is approximately 5.5–6 h after the night shift, and several laboratory studies have found that this amount of sleep curtailment may affect sleepiness moderately. The 2003 study by Van Dongen and colleagues indicates that the critical point for the accumulation of fatigue is approximately 7 h of sleep per night. The circadian trough and extended wakefulness (often up to 20 h) are other powerful contributors.

Alertness

Night-oriented shiftworkers complain as much about fatigue and sleepiness as they do about disturbed sleep. The sleepiness is particularly severe on the night shift, appears hardly at all on the afternoon shift, and is intermediate on the morning shift. The maximum is reached toward the early morning (5 a.m.–7 a.m.). Frequently, incidents of falling asleep occur during the night shift. At least two-thirds of the respondents report that they have experienced involuntary sleep during night work. Ambulatory EEG recordings

verify that incidents of actual sleep occur during night work in, for example, process operators. Other groups, such as train drivers or truck drivers, show clear signs of falling asleep while driving at night. This occurs toward the second half of the night and appears as repeated bursts of alpha and theta EEG activity, together with closed eyes and slow undulating eye movements. As a rule, the bursts are short (1–15 s) but frequent and seem to reflect let-downs in the effort to fend off sleep. Approximately one-quarter of the subjects recorded show the EEG/electrooculograph (EOG) patterns of fighting with sleep. This is clearly a larger proportion than is found in the subjective reports of episodes of falling asleep.

Performance

As may be expected, sleepiness on the night shift is reflected in performance. One of the classic studies in this area is by Bjerner and colleagues, who showed that errors in meter readings over a period of 20 years in a gas works had a pronounced peak on the night shift. There was also a secondary peak during the afternoon. Similar observations have been made for switchboard operators and other groups. Late-night shift performance capacity has been compared with performance following the ingestion of alcohol to a 0.08% blood alcohol level.

Accidents

If sleepiness is severe enough, interaction with the environment ceases, and if this coincides with a critical need for action, an accident may ensue. Most of the available accident data on night-shift sleepiness has been obtained from the area of transportation; the National Transportation Safety Board ranks fatigue as one of the major causes of heavy vehicle accidents.

Very little relevant data are available from conventional industrial operations, but fatal work accidents show a higher risk in shiftworkers and accidents in the automotive industry may exhibit night-shift effects. An interesting analysis has been put forward by the Association of Professional Sleep Societies Committee on Catastrophes, Sleep and Public Policy. Its consensus report notes that the nuclear plant meltdown at Chernobyl occurred at 1:35 a.m. and was due to human error (apparently related to work scheduling). Similarly, the Three Mile Island reactor accident occurred between 4 and 6 a.m. and was due not only to the stuck valve, which caused a loss of coolant water, but also, more important, to the workers' failure to recognize this event, which led to the near meltdown of the reactor. Similar incidents (although with the ultimate stage having been prevented) occurred in 1985 at the David Beese reactor in Ohio and at the Rancho Seco reactor in California. Finally, the committee also stated that the NASA Challenger space shuttle disaster stemmed from errors in judgment made in the early morning hours by people who had had insufficient sleep (because of partial night work) for days prior to the launch. Still, there is very limited support for the notion that shiftwork outside the area of transportation actually carries a higher over all accident risk.

As with sleep, the two main factors behind sleepiness and performance impairment are circadian cycle homeostatic factors. Alertness falls rapidly after awakening, but gradually levels out as wakefulness is extended. The circadian influence appears as a sine-shaped superimposition on this exponential fall in alertness. Akerstedt describes this as a three-process model of alertness regulation. Space does not permit a discussion of the derivation of these functions here.

Stress Indices

A number of studies have looked at the effect of shiftwork on endocrine and other stress-related parameters. The circadian pattern of cortisol, growth hormone, and melatonin is clearly affected by night work, but the adjustment to night work is only partial. We should also consider the increased cortisol levels and reduced insulin sensitivity following the reduction of sleep to 4 h. On the other hand, there do not seem to be any data on the long-term consequences of night work on stress indices, except perhaps for a suppression of testosterone in male nightworkers with a negative overall attitude to night shifts. Also, testosterone seems linearly related to sleep duration, as demonstrated in experimental studies of shifted sleep.

Gastrointestinal Effects

Gastrointestinal complaints are more common among night shiftworkers than among day workers. In a review of a number of reports covering 34 047 people with day or shiftwork, ulcers were found to occur in 0.3–0.7% of day workers, 5% of morning and afternoon shiftworkers, 2.5–15% of rotating shiftworkers with night shifts, and 10–30% of ex-shiftworkers. Several other studies have come to similar conclusions. Other gastrointestinal disorders, including gastritis, duodenitis, and dysfunctions of digestion are more common in shiftworkers than in day workers.

The pathophysiological mechanism underlying gastrointestinal diseases in shiftworkers is unclear, but one possible explanation is that intestinal enzymes and intestinal mobility are not synchronized with the sleep–wake pattern. Intestinal enzymes are secreted with circadian rhythmicity, and shiftworkers' intake of food is irregular compared with intestinal function. A high nightly intake of food may be related to increased lipid levels, and eating at the circadian low point may be associated with altered metabolic responses. In addition, reduced sleep affects lipid and glucose metabolism. Recently, an epidemiological study showed a large increase in ulcer risk in shiftworkers with complaints of sleep or excessive sleepiness.

Cardiovascular Effects

A number of studies have reported a higher incidence of cardiovascular disease, especially coronary heart disease, in shiftworkers than in those who work days. In a study of 504 paper-mill workers followed for 15 years a dose–response relationship was found between number of years of shiftwork and incidence of coronary heart disease in the exposure interval 1–20 years of shiftwork. A study of 79 000 female nurses in the United States gave similar results, as did studies of more than 1 million Danish men and of a cohort of Finnish workers. Again, disturbances of metabolic parameters such as lipids and glucose might contribute to this. The effects of shiftwork on metabolic changes do not seem as pronounced, however, as those of stress. Very few studies are available, but the prevalence of endocrine and metabolic diseases seems increased in shiftworkers, including increased insulin resistance.

Mortality

The mortality of shift- and day workers was studied by Taylor and Pocock, who studied 8603 male manual worker in England and Wales between 1956 and 1968. Day, shift-, and ex-shiftworkers were compared with national figures. The standardized mortality rate (SMR) can be calculated from observed and expected deaths reported in the paper. SMRs for deaths from all causes were 97, 101, and 119 for day, shift-, and ex-shiftworkers, respectively. Although the figures might indicate an increasing trend, the differences were not statistically significant. However, the reported SMR close to 100 is remarkable because the reference population was the general male population. Most mortality studies concerned with occupational cohorts reveal SMRs lower than 100, implying a healthy worker's effect. The same study showed a significantly increased incidence of neoplastic disease in shiftworkers (SMR 116).

Conclusion

Shiftwork (with night shifts) impairs sleep and alertness and increases the risk of cardiovascular and gastrointestinal disease. It also disturbs the circadian timing of the endocrine and other systems. Thus, it may serve as one form of stressor and may combine with traditional psychosocial stressors.

See Also the Following Articles

Sleep, Sleep Disorders, and Stress; Workplace Stress.

Further Reading

Åkerstedt, T. (2003). Shift work and disturbed sleep/wakefulness. *Occupational Medicine* 53, 89–94.

Bjerner, B., Holm, Å. and Swensson, Å. (1955). Diurnal variation of mental performance: a study of three-shift workers. *British Journal of Industrial Medicine* 12, 103–110.

Dijk, D.-J. and Czeisler, C. A. (1995). Contribution of the circadian pacemaker and the sleep homeostat to sleep propensity, sleep structure, electroencephalographic slow waves, and sleep spindle activity in humans. *Journal of Neuroscience* 15, 3526–3538.

Drake, C. L., Roehrs, T., Richardson, G., et al. (2004). Shift work sleep disorder: prevalence and consequences beyond that of symptomatic day workers. *Sleep* 27, 1453–1462.

Folkard, S. and Tucker, P. (2003). Shift work, safety and productivity. *Occupational and Environmental Medicine* 53, 95–101.

Harrington, J. M. (ed.) (1978). *Shift work and health: a critical review of the literature*. London: HMSO.

Hastings, M. H., Reddy, A. B. and Maywood, E. S. (2003). A clockwork web: circadian timing in brain and periphery, in health and disease. *Nature Reviews Neuroscience* 4, 649–661.

Knutsson, A. (2003). Health disorders of shift workers. *Occupational Medicine* 53, 103–108.

Mitler, M. M., Carskadon, M. A., Czeisler, C. A., et al. (1988). Catastrophes, sleep and public policy: consensus report. *Sleep* 11, 100–109.

Spiegel, K., Leproult, R. and Van Cauter, E. (1999). Impact of sleep debt on metabolic and endocrine function. *Lancet* 354, 1435–1439.

Taylor, P. J. and Pocock, S. J. (1972). Mortality of shift and day workers 1956–68. *British Journal of Industrial Medicine* 29, 201–207.

Tüchsen, F. (1993). Working hours and ischaemic heart disease in Danish men: a 4-year cohort study of hospitalization. *International Journal of Epidemiology* 22, 215–221.

Van Dongen, H. P., Maislin, G., Mullington, J. M., et al. (2003). The cumulative cost of additional wakefulness: dose-response effects on neurobehavioral functions and sleep physiology from chronic sleep restriction and total sleep deprivation. *Sleep* 26, 117–126.

Nightmares

M Hirshkowitz and A Sharafkhaneh
Baylor College of Medicine and Michael E. DeBakey
Veteran Affairs Medical Center, Houston, TX, USA

This article is a revision of the previous edition article by
M Hirshkowitz and C A Moore, volume 3, pp 49–52,
© 2000, Elsevier Inc.

Phenomenology of Frightening Awakenings
Nightmares and Posttraumatic Stress Disorder
Treatment Approaches

Glossary

Hypnagogic and hypnopompic hallucinations	Vivid sensory images occurring at the transition between sleep and wakefulness. Hypnagogic refers to hallucinations occurring as a person falls asleep while hypnopompic images occur as a person awakens. Hypnagogic imagery may be particularly vivid during rapid eye movement (REM) sleep occurring at sleep onset (as in narcolepsy). Similarly, dreamlike hypnopompic images may continue during wakefulness upon sudden or partial awakening from REM sleep. Hypnagogic and hypnopompic hallucinations may be accompanied by a complete inability to move (sleep paralysis).
Nachtmare	Nacht (night) + mare (spirit or monster). Mythologies throughout the world describe devils, demons, evil spirits, ogres, ghosts, vampires, old hags, and witches that attack individuals while they sleep. The *mare* usually sits on or crushes the sleeper's chest causing a smothering sensation and an inability to breathe. Additionally, the individual is usually unable

Night terror (also known as sleep terror) — to move. Sometimes there are sexual overtones as well with the spirit raping or assaulting the person while they lay paralyzed. This description suggests the occurrence of the parasomnia sleep paralysis accompanied by a hypnagogic or hypnopompic hallucination.

Night terror (also known as sleep terror) A sleep disorder usually arising from slow-wave sleep that involves a sudden awakening with intense fear. The afflicted individual usually emits a sharp piercing scream. Autonomic nervous system activation accompanies the awakening and the individual will often have tachycardia, tachypnea, sweating, and increased muscle tone. The individual typically acts confused, disoriented, and inconsolable during the episode; however, there may be complete amnesia about the episode upon awakening the next morning.

Parasomnia A disorder of arousal, partial arousal, or sleep stage transition. Parasomnias occur episodically during sleep and may interfere with sleep, sometimes producing insomnia or daytime sleepiness.

Rapid eye movement (REM) sleep REM sleep is one of the five sleep stages defined in humans. REM sleep was discovered by Eugene Aserinsky who noted eye movements occurring every 90–100 minutes during sleep. In initial studies, dream recall was better correlated with awakenings from REM than other sleep stages. Consequently, REM sleep came to be considered the biological substrate of dreams.

Sleep paralysis The inability to perform voluntary movements upon awakening from sleep or just before sleep onset. The individual is fully conscious, usually feels acutely anxious, typically is unable to vocalize, and may have hallucinatory activity accompanying the paralysis episode.

Nightmares, according to current terminology, are unpleasant, distressing, or frightening dreams that usually occur during rapid eye movement (REM) sleep. The International Classification of Sleep Disorders–Second Edition (ICSD-2) formally classifies the nightmare disorder as a parasomnia usually associated with REM sleep. Nightmares, as currently defined are "coherent dream sequences that seem real and become increasingly more disturbing as they unfold. Emotions usually involve anxiety, fear, or terror but frequently also anger, rage, embarrassment, disgust, and other negative feelings. Dream content most often focuses on imminent physical danger to the individual but can also involve distressing themes." The fears produced by the dream usually dissipate rapidly after awakening and clear sensorium returns.

Phenomenology of Frightening Awakenings

Although nightmares are currently conceptualized as frightening dreams that usually produce an awakening from REM sleep, the term derives from *nachtmare* which refers to a quite different phenomenon. The nachtmare (or night spirit) has taken many forms in folk lore and superstition, ranging from vampires (in Medieval Eastern Europe) to witch riders (among preAmerican Civil War slaves). Contemporary alien attacks are likely an offshoot of the same disorder. The nachtmare accompanies sleep paralysis with frightening hypnagogic or hypnopompic hallucinations and characteristically arise during the transition from wakefulness to sleep. The sleeper has difficulty breathing due to the creature sitting on his or her chest, there may also be a sense of sexual molestation, the sleeper may feel that their life force is being sucked out of them. To complicate things further, the mythical nachtmares Incubus and Succubus are commonly associated with yet as distinctly different phenomenon: the sleep terrors (*Pavor nocturnus*). Sleep terrors usually occur in slow-wave sleep, are not dreamlike, and are poorly recalled. The person may remember a frightening image; however, narrative and plot are rare.

By contrast, the nightmare in modern parlance explicitly arises from a dream, implying imagery, narrative, and plot. Individuals awakened from a dream typically recollect its content. Nightmares may afflict 10–50% of children and 50–85% of adults have at least an occasional nightmare. Overall estimates for the prevalence of nightmares range from 2–8% in the general population. Nightmares arising from either acute or posttraumatic stress disorders (PTSDs) may occur in stage 2 sleep as well as during REM sleep. However, there are other widely recognized types of awakenings associated with subjective reports of panic, dysphoria, or anxiety. These included sleep-related panic attacks, sleep terrors, and sleep paralysis with hypnagogic or hypnopompic hallucinations. These paroxysmal events arise from different stages of sleep. Like REM sleep nightmares, sleep-related panic attacks are characterized by awakening with fear. Polysomnography reveals that these episodes customarily occur during sleep stage 2, often during transition to slow-wave sleep. However, sleep-related panic attacks may occur, although rarely, at the wake-to-sleep transition.

Nightmares and Posttraumatic Stress Disorder

Nightmare frequency increases during periods of stress and after an individual experiences a distressing event (e.g., an automobile accident, burglary, rape, or death of a friend or relative). Stress and sleep deprivation are also thought to exacerbate sleep paralysis, sleep terrors, and sleep-related panic attacks. One approach to exploring the relationship between stress and these phenomena is to study the sleep in individuals with PTSD.

Silva and colleagues reported on symptoms in 131 physically or sexually abused women interviewed in a primary care setting. They found that 65% reported bad dreams, flashbacks, and/or terror attacks. These women had higher intrusion and avoidance scores. Nightmares are also reported in school age children after being involved as passengers in traffic accidents. Psychological consequences were common and persisted in 33% of children after 4–7 months. Eleven percent were thought to be severely afflicted on follow up with 17% reporting nightmares and other sleep difficulties. Nightmares related to trauma are known to persist for prolonged periods. A study of Dutch war veterans found nightmares and anxiety dreams 40 years after the traumatizing event. In a large survey of Vietnam War veterans, using a careful sampling technique, nightmare frequency strongly correlated with combat exposure. Insomnia also was associated with combat exposure but not to the same degree as nightmares. By contrast, neither chronic medical illnesses nor psychiatric disorders (panic disorder, major depression, mania, and alcohol abuse) could predict nightmare frequency.

Although recurrent distressing dreams are a key PTSD diagnostic feature according to DSM-IV, the nature of these nightmares is in question. Many clinicians assume that PTSD nightmares represent a REM sleep phenomenon; however, PTSD nightmares are poorly understood. In many respects their features conform to those present in REM sleep nightmares. They typically contain imagery, narrative, and plot. However, the repetitive, recurring nature of these nocturnal frightening phantasms makes them unusual. Another uncommon characteristic of chronic PTSD nightmares is that they narrate traumatic events, often without elaboration or symbolism. Several published descriptions of PTSD nightmares include the adrenergic concomitants tachycardia and sweating that are atypical of REM sleep. These features more commonly accompany sleep terrors. Thus, it is not surprising that some sleep experts contend that PTSD nightmares can arise from any stage of sleep. Hartmann in his extensive monograph on nightmares flatly states that PTSD nightmares "... are not typical REM nightmares; they occur sometimes in stage 2 and sometimes in all stages of sleep and even at sleep onset..." Kramer and Kinney also emphasize that PTSD nightmares can arise from both REM and stage 2 sleep.

Ross and associates argue strongly that REM sleep disturbance is closely involved in the pathogenesis of PTSD. This disturbance may be either "inappropriate recruitment of essentially normal REM sleep processes" or involvement of "inherently dysfunctional REM sleep mechanisms". They correctly contend that the vividness and recallability of PTSD nightmare content has more in common with REM than non-REM mentation. REM sleep is comprised of an array of individual features, including: low amplitude, mixed frequency electroencephalograph (EEG) activity; rapid eye movements; muscle atonia; pontine geniculate occipital (PGO) discharges; small muscle twitches; periorbital integrated potentials (PIPs); and middle ear muscle activity (MEMA). Although these activities usually occur in concert, they sometimes dissociate, as in REM sleep behavior disorder (RBD). In RBD, the atonia that characteristically accompanies REM sleep is absent. In fact, Ross and colleagues suggest RBD as a possible model for the pathophysiological mechanism underlying PTSD nightmares. In their overnight polysomnographic studies, these researchers showed that combat veterans with PTSD had elevated REM sleep percentage, longer average REM cycle duration, and increased REM density (number of eye movements per minute of REM sleep) compared to controls. These same investigators also report more phasic leg muscle activity during REM sleep in veterans with PTSD than in those without PTSD. Admittedly, the sample was small; however, these studies provide a foundation for further research.

Neuropharmacology of REM sleep clearly demonstrates involvement of cholinergic mechanisms. It is also widely accepted that acetylcholine plays an important role in the formation of memories. It has also been postulated that REM sleep mediates memory consolidation. When high adrenergic arousal accompanies a remembered experience (as occurs with acute trauma or re-experiencing a distant trauma), it appears that the memory process functions differently. Memories can be triggered by adrenergic arousal. The relationship between this arousal, flashbacks, and nightmares underlie current neuropsychiatric conceptualization of the consequences of traumatic stress. REM sleep has been characterized as a parasympathetic state with bursts of sympathetic activity (associated with phasic events). Nightmares and recurrent dreams may be considered a failure of dreamwork to handle emotionally laden, presumably adrenergically coupled experiences.

PTSD nightmares are reported in 92% of patients with flashbacks and 57% of patients without flashbacks, they seldom occur during laboratory sleep studies. This is the case even among patients who indicate having nightmares four or more times per week. Nonetheless, on several occasions during our 30 years of clinical polysomnography experience, patients had nightmares while sleeping in the laboratory. On those rare occasions, we noticed increased REM density just before awakenings associated with nightmares. Consultation with several sleep disorder medicine colleagues revealed that this is a widely held impression (e.g., Drs. Hartmann (Boston, MA), Roffwarg (Jackson, MS), Mendelson (Chicago, IL), and Mahowald (Minneapolis, MN). To the best of our collective knowledge and according to thorough search using medical databases, little systematic data exists beyond description of the phenomenon. Ross and associates mention exceedingly high REM density preceding a nightmare that fortuitously occurred during their study. We also have observed vastly increased phasic activity in combat veterans with PTSD referred to our Sleep Diagnostic Clinic for evaluation of insomnia, nightmares, or daytime sleepiness.

A phasic activity threshold likely exists that is necessary but not sufficient to produce nightmares. The level of phasic activity is elevated in patients with PTSD compared to control subjects. This conceptualization is analogous to the relationship between hypersynchronous slow-wave activity and parasomnias of arousal (confused awakening, sleepwalking, and sleep terror). Another perspective is suggested by the well-established relationship between sleep and some forms of epilepsy. Abnormal spike activity is enhanced by sleep deprivation. Interestingly, some neurophysiologically oriented researchers have posited a kindling model for flashbacks and nightmares. More research is needed to illuminate the biological substrate underlying the dysphoric mentation and paroxysmal awakenings that we call nightmares.

Treatment Approaches

Nightmares are experienced acutely (at some period during the lifetime) in many individuals. Furthermore, they typically resolve without intervention. However, persistent nightmares, particularly if the dream content is recurrent, can be a marker for significant psychopathology. In such cases, treatment is advised especially when the nightmare produces serious distress, insomnia, or interferes with daily activities. Similarly, nightmares in early childhood (preschool and early school years) are of less concern (assuming they are outgrown) than those beginning or persisting in late childhood and adolescence. In adults, the frequency of psychopathology is higher among patients suffering from chronic nightmares than in control subjects. Hartmann posits that nightmare sufferers have thin boundaries, are more vulnerable, and have weaker psychological defenses. He also suggests that these individuals are at risk for schizophrenia. In addition to this profile for patients with nightmares, traumatic events apparently can induce nightmares. The nightmares may be immediate or delayed. They may afflict the individual acutely or persist for many years. Finally, drug abuse, drug or alcohol withdrawal, and specific medications are associated with nightmares. Thus, treatment must start with a careful history emphasizing current stressors, possible traumatic experiences, psychopathology (in patient and family), alcohol and drug abuse, and medication regimen.

Several medications have been associated with increased chance of nightmares. Some of them act by potentiating REM sleep and others by producing REM sleep rebound on withdrawal. Such drugs include L-DOPA, reserpine, thiothixene, alpha methyldopa, metoprolol, propranalol, simvastatin, and atorvastatin. Interestingly, in addition to several statins appearing to induce nightmares, there is also a report by Arargun and associates (2005: 361–364) that nightmares are associated with low serum lipid levels.

Altering dose or substituting other pharmacological agents would be the first step in such cases. Alcohol or stimulant withdrawal also potentiates nightmares via presumed REM sleep mechanisms. In such cases, nightmares should be time-limited and resolve when sleep normalizes. If nightmares persist, intervention should be considered.

When psychopathology is found, it should be treated directly. Psychotherapy is thought to be beneficial. It is worth emphasizing that insomnia resulting from fear of sleep can pose a serious treatment obstacle. Sleep deprivation exacerbates nightmares, sleep terrors, and sleep paralysis attacks. Thus, the nightmare may perpetuate insomnia and thereby produce a vicious cycle. Behavioral interventions for insomnia are safe and effective in both the short and long term. Improved sleep hygiene, stimulus control therapy, sleep restriction therapy, and/or cognitive therapy are recommended. Krakow and Zadra (2006: 45–70) directly target the nightmare with imagery rehearsal therapy (IRT) with good results using four, 2-hour sessions. Another reportedly successful behavioral approach is lucid dream therapy. A lucid dream is one in which the dreamer becomes aware that he or she is dreaming. In an uncontrolled case series of five individuals that could be trained to recognize their dream state, nightmare frequency declined. Whether the decline related to increased lucidity or volitional alteration of dream content is unknown. In some cases, medications may be needed. Several medications reportedly provide some relief from nightmares when administered to patients with PTSD. Davidson and colleagues report decreased nightmare and general sleep disturbance scores in response to the atypical antidepressant nefazodone in a group of 17 patients treated with up to 600 mg day^{-1} for 12 weeks. Other antidepressants have been tried. Cavaljuga and co-workers (2003: 12–16) found fluoxetine more effective at reducing nightmares than amitriptyline; however, amitriptyline was more effective overall in acute PTSD. In another study by Gupta and co-workers, cyproheptadine (4–12 mg at bedtime) was found to be beneficial on retrospective review of nine patient charts. Response to this histamine-1 blocking, serotonin antagonist ranged from decreases in nightmare frequency (or intensity) to complete remission.

At present, the most systematic work on pharmacological treatment of nightmares is with prazosin. Peskind and colleagues (2003: 165–171) treated nine older men with posttraumatic nightmares with 2–4 mg prazosin 1 hour before bedtime. The drug substantially reduced nightmares in eight of the patients and was well tolerated. Furthermore, a 20-week, double-blind, crossover trial was conducted by Raskind and associates (2003: 371–373) in 10 Vietnam theatre combat veterans. A mean dose of 9.5 mg of prazosin was given at bedtime. Drug, compared to placebo, significantly reduced scores on recurrent distressing dreams.

In a review article concerning nightmare treatments, van Liempt (2006: 193–202) concludes that open-label reports suggest efficacy for some antidepressants, anticonvulsants, and atypical antipsychotic drugs. Placebo-controlled studies show possible efficacy with olanzapine and prazosin. We find these preliminary results are encouraging; however, more double-blind, placebo-controlled trials are needed. Finally, assorted benzodiazepines can provide relief from dream anxiety and help improve sleep. However, few randomized, placebo-controlled, clinical trials have been conducted and they had small sample sizes. Furthermore, the withdrawal effects from pharmacotherapeutic interventions have not been systematically studied.

Further Reading

Arargun, M. Y., Gulec, M., Cilli, A. S., et al. (2005). Nightmares and serum cholesterol level: a preliminary report. *Canadian Journal of Psychiatry* 50, 361–364.

Bell, C. C., Shakoor, B., Thompson, B., et al. (1984). Prevalence of isolated sleep paralysis in black subjects. *Journal National Medical Association* 76, 501–508.

Boriani, G., Biffi, M., Strocchi, E., et al. (2001). Nightmares and sleep disturbances with simvastatin and metoprolol. *Annals of Pharmacotherapy* 35, 1292.

Cavaljuga, S., Licanin, I., Mulabegovic, N., et al. (2003). Therapeutic effects of two antidepressant agents in the treatment of posttraumatic stress disorder (PTSD). *Bosnian Journal of Basic Medical Sciences* 3, 12–16.

Davidson, J. R., Weisler, R. H., Malik, M. L., et al. Treatment of posttraumatic stress disorder with nefazodone. *International Clinical Psychopharmacology* 13, 111–113.

Diagnostic Classification Steering Committee. (1990). *International classification of sleep disorders – 2nd edition: diagnostic and coding manual*. Westchester, IL, USA: American Academy of Sleep Medicine.

Ermin, M. K. (1987). Dream anxiety attacks (nightmares). *Psychiatric Clinics of North America* 10, 667–674.

Firestone, M. (1985). The "old hag" sleep paralysis in Newfoundland. *Journal of Psychoanalytic Anthropology* 8, 47–66.

Gupta, S., Popli, A., Bathurst, E., et al. (1998). Efficacy of cyproheptadine for nightmares associated with posttraumatic stress disorder. *Comprehensive Psychiatry* 39, 160–164.

Hartmann, E. (1984). *The nightmare: the psychology and biology of terrifying dreams*. New York: Basic Books.

Hauri, P. J., Friedman, M. and Ravaris, C. L. (1989). Sleep in patients with spontaneous panic attack. *Sleep* 12, 323–337.

Kales, A., Soldatos, C., Caldwell, A., et al. (1980). Nightmares: clinical characteristics and personality patterns. *American Journal of Psychiatry* 137, 1197–1201.

Krakow, B. and Zadra, A. (2006). Clinical management of chronic nightmares: imagery rehearsal therapy. *Behavioral Sleep Medicine* 4, 45–70.

Kramer, M. and Kinney, L. (1988). Sleep patterns in trauma victims with disturbed dreaming. *Psychiatric Journal of the University of Ottawa* 13, 12–16.

Morin, C. M., Colecchi, C., Stone, J., et al. (1999). Behavioral and pharmacological therapies for late-life insomnia: a randomized controlled trial. *JAMA* 17, 991–999.

Neylan, T. C., Marmar, C. R., Metzler, T. J., et al. (1998). Sleep disturbance in the Vietnam generation: findings from a nationally representative sample of male Vietnam veterans. *American Journal of Psychiatry* 155, 929–933.

Peskind, E. R., Bonner, L. T., Hoff, D. J., et al. (2003). Prazosin reduces trauma-related nightmares in older men with chronic posttraumatic stress disorder. *Journal of Geriatric Psychiatry and Neurology* 16, 165–171.

Raskind, M. A., Peskind, E. R., Kanter, E. D., et al. (2003). Reduction of nightmares and other PTSD symptoms in combat veterans by prazosin: a placebo-controlled study. *American Journal of Psychiatry* 160, 371–373.

Ross, R. J., Ball, W. A., Sullivan, K. A., et al. (1989). Sleep disturbance as the hallmark of PTSD. *American Journal of Psychiatry* 146, 697–707.

Silva, C., McFarlane, J., Soeken, K., et al. (1997). Symptoms of post-traumatic stress disorder in abused women in a primary care setting. *Journal of Womens Health* 6, 543–552.

van Liempt, S., Vermetten, E., Geuze, E., et al. (2006). Pharmacotherapy for disordered sleep in post-traumatic stress disorder: a systematic review. *International Clinical Psychopharmacology* 21, 193–202.

Woodward, S. H., Arsenault, N. J., Murray, C., et al. (2000). Laboratory sleep correlates of nightmare complaint in PTSD inpatients. *Biological Psychiatry* 48, 1081–1087.

Nitric Oxide

S M McCann
Louisiana State University, Baton Rouge, LA, USA

Role of Nitric Oxide in Physiological Release of Hypothalamic Neuropeptides and Transmitters

Role of Nitric Oxide in Stress-Induced Alterations in Hypothalamic-Pituitary Function

Effect of Infection on Cytokine and Nitric Oxide Formation in the Pineal Gland and in Other Organ Systems

The Role of Nitric Oxide in Reproduction

The Nitric Oxide Hypothesis of Aging

Conclusion

Glossary

Adrenocorticotropic hormone (ACTH)	A polypeptide hormone secreted from the corticotropes of the anterior pituitary that stimulates the secretion of glucocorticoids (cortisol in human, corticosterone in rat) from the adrenal cortex.
Cytokine	A polypeptide or small protein secreted classically by cells of the immune system, such as lymphocytes, monocytes, and macrophages, and now known to be secreted by other cells, such as endothelial cells and adipocytes. In many instances, cytokines have autocrine, paracrine, and endocrine effects to alter growth and function of their target cells.
Follicle-stimulating hormone (FSH)	A heterodimeric glycoprotein secreted by gonadotropes of the anterior pituitary that promotes follicular growth in the ovaries and spermatogenesis in the testes and interacts with the luteinizing hormone to produce estrogen secretion by the ovarian follicles.
Growth hormone (GH)	A protein hormone secreted by the somatotropes of the anterior pituitary that is responsible for growth by anabolic effects in many tissues often mediated by insulin-like growth factor I, secreted principally by the liver.
Interferon γ	One of several interferons that particularly has antiviral activity in contrast to the antibacterial activity of many of the interleukins.
Interleukin (IL)	A group of cytokines. IL-1 is a pro-inflammatory cytokine and was the first cytokine to be characterized; two closely related proteins, IL-1α and β, have similar actions on closely related receptors in many tissues. Subsequently characterized cytokines were named in the order of their discovery. IL-2 is a pro-inflammatory cytokine. IL-10, IL-13, and IL-1 receptor antagonist are anti-inflammatory cytokines.
Luteinizing hormone (LH)	A heterodimeric glycoprotein secreted by gonadotropes of the anterior pituitary that induces ovulation and corpus luteum formation, estradiol secretion from the follicle, and progesterone secretion from the corpus luteum of female mammals and stimulates the interstitial tissue of the testis to secrete testosterone in males.
Prolactin (PRL)	A protein hormone, related to growth hormone, secreted by the lactotropes of the anterior pituitary. Its best known function is to stimulate the growth and secretion of milk from the mammary gland. In males, it affects male sex accessories. It also has actions on the cells of the immune system that enhance immune responses.
Thymosin α_1	A polypeptide cytokine secreted by the thymus that has paracrine and hormonal actions.
Thyroid-stimulating hormone (TSH)	A heterodimeric glycoprotein secreted by the thyrotrope of the anterior pituitary that stimulates the secretion of thyroid hormones.

Tumor necrosis factor α	A pro-inflammatory cytokine mediating local inflammatory and systemic responses to infection. It was named according to its originally described action; also known as cachectin.

Stress may be defined as any stimulus that distorts homeostasis in the organism. Therefore, stress can be physical, as in the case of excessive heat or cold, trauma, surgical operations, or infection, or it can be emotional and psychological. Selye, who coined the term, even talked about the stress of life itself. It is the stresses of life that contribute to degenerative disease and old age.

Stress can affect every organ system in the body, but the principal mediators of the response to stress are the sympathetic nervous system and the hypothalamic-pituitary-adrenal axis. Various hypothalamic-releasing and -inhibiting hormones are released from their axon terminals in the median eminence (ME) into the capillaries of the hypophysial portal veins that transport them to the anterior lobe of the pituitary gland. There they stimulate or inhibit the release of the various pituitary hormones that act either directly on body tissues or on their target glands, which in turn release hormones that act on various tissues of the body. Examples of the latter are adrenocorticotropic hormone (ACTH), follicle-stimulating hormone (FSH), luteinizing hormone (LH), and thyroid-stimulating hormone (TSH); examples of the former are prolactin (PRL) and growth hormone (GH).

In the dozen years since the discovery of nitric oxide (NO) in the body and the enzymes forming it, it has become evident that NO plays a pivotal role in the function of every organ system of the body. This article first examines the role of NO under physiological conditions and then indicates how this role is affected by stress. In this connection, most attention has focused on the role of NO in the induction of the responses to infection. Little attention has been given so far to its role in psychological and other types of stress.

Role of Nitric Oxide in Physiological Release of Hypothalamic Neuropeptides and Transmitters

Corticotropin Releasing Hormone

The release of corticotropin releasing hormone (CRH) from hypothalami incubated *in vitro* is controlled by muscarinic cholinergic receptors because it can be blocked by atropine. The acetylcholine-producing interneurons in the hypothalamus release

acetylcholine, which stimulates a muscarinic-type receptor, which in turn stimulates CRH release from the CRH neurons. Neural NO synthase (nNOS) has been located in neurons in the paraventricular nucleus (PVN) of the hypothalamus. Stimulated CRH release can be blocked by N^G-monomethyl-L-arginine (NMMA), a competitive inhibitor of all forms of NOS. Consequently, CRH release from the neurons in the PVN is stimulated by cholinergic neurons that synapse on these NOergic neurons to activate NOS. NOS synthesizes NO, which diffuses into the CRH neurons and activates CRH release by activating cyclooxygenase I (COX I), leading to the generation of prostaglandin E_2 (PGE_2) from arachidonate (AA). PGE_2 activates CRH via the activation of adenylyl cyclase and the generation of cyclic adenosine monophosphate (cAMP). cAMP activates protein kinase A, which induces the exocytosis of CRH secretory granules into the hypophysial portal vessels that then activate ACTH release from the corticotrophs of the anterior pituitary gland. NO activates not only COX, but also lipoxygenase (LOX), which also plays a role in the activation of CRH release. NO also activates guanylyl cyclase (GC), which converts guanosine triphosphate into cyclic guanosine monophosphate (cGMP). cGMP is postulated to increase intracellular $[Ca^{2+}]$, which is required to activate phospholipase A_2, which converts membrane phospholipids into AA, the substrate for COX and LOX, permitting the generation of prostaglandins (PGs) and leukotrienes, respectively. The activation of CRH release can be blocked by the synthetic glucocorticoid dexamethasone and also by blockers of the three pathways of AA metabolism (e.g., clotrimazol, which blocks epoxygenase, which converts AA into epoxides, and indomethacin, which inhibits COX) and by 5′ 8′ 11-eicisotrinoic acid, which blocks LOX. Thus, CRH release is activated by the AA cascade. α-Melanotropic-stimulating hormone (α-MSH) also inhibits CRH release. Cyclosporin inhibits CRH release as well, probably by inhibiting calcineurin. Calcineurin dephosphorylates NOS, rendering it active.

Luteinizing Hormone-Releasing Hormone

The role of NO in luteinizing hormone-releasing hormone (LHRH) release has been elucidated. Norepinephrine (NE), glutamic acid (GA), and oxytocin stimulate LHRH release by activation of nNOS. The pathway is as follows. Oxytocin and/or GA activate NE neurons in the medial basal hypothalamus (MBH), which activate NOergic neurons by $α_1$-adrenergic receptors. The NO released diffuses into LHRH terminals and induces LHRH release by the activation of GC and COX. NO controls not only the release of

LHRH bound for the pituitary, but also that which induces mating activity by actions in the brain stem. The adipocyte hormone, leptin, also increases the release of LHRH from medial basal hypothalamic explants by stimulating the release of NO. However, β-endorphin and γ-aminobutyric acid (GABA) block the activation of LHRH release by NO. In contrast to the clear evidence for the stimulation of LHRH release by NO, it apparently has no effect on FSH release mediated by the FSH releasing factor.

Other Hypothalamic Peptides

Evidence from *in vivo* experiments suggests that NO also stimulates the release of GH releasing hormone (GHRH), and *in vitro* experiments clearly show that it also stimulates the release and synthesis of somatostatin. The release of oxytocin and vasopressin from the hypothalamus is suppressed by NO. NO stimulates the release of the PRL-inhibiting hormone, dopamine.

Effects of Nitric Oxide on the Release of Pituitary Hormones

nNOS is present in folliculostellate (FS) cells, a cell type of the anterior pituitary not previously thought to produce hormones but that is now known to produce several cytokines. nNOS has also been found in LH gonadotrophs. NO produced by this nNOS in the pituitary has important functions in altering pituitary hormone secretion. Intravenous injection of nitro-arginine methyl ester (NAME) augments vasopressin-induced ACTH release, so NO probably blocks ACTH secretion induced by vasopressin or CRH, but this has not been studied directly. NO inhibits PRL secretion. Apparently, NO from FS cells diffuses to adjacent lactotrophs where it induces the production of cGMP by activating GC. cGMP then inhibits PRL release by blocking the exocytosis of PRL secretory granules.

The principal PRL-inhibiting hormone, dopamine, apparently acts on cell surface D2 receptors on FS cells to activate NOS followed by NO production. However, the action of FSH-releasing factor (FSHRF), LHRH, and leptin to stimulate not only FSH but also LH is brought about by their action on specific receptors on gonadotrophs to activate nNOS, thereby generating cGMP, which, instead of inhibiting, as in the case of lactotropes, promotes hormone secretion. Specificity of action of these compounds on gonadotropin release is accomplished by specific receptors for each of these ligands that increase intracellular $[Ca^{2+}]$, thereby activating nNOS. Both LHRH and leptin preferentially stimulate LH with a lesser potency to release FSH, whereas FSHRF selectively releases FSH and has a lower potency to release

LH. In this way, it is possible to have differential effects of various stimuli on FSH and LH secretion. This mechanism accounts for the pulses of FSH alone generated by FSHRF and of LH alone generated by LHRH.

Role of Nitric Oxide in Stress-Induced Alterations in Hypothalamic-Pituitary Function

Nearly all types of stress elicit a stereotyped pattern of pituitary hormone secretion in humans that consists of a rapid increase in ACTH, PRL, and GH secretion (in rats, GH secretion is inhibited) and inhibition of the secretion of LH, TSH, and, to a lesser extent, FSH. The pattern is caused primarily by alterations in the secretion of hypothalamic-releasing and -inhibiting hormones.

Immediate Response to Infection

The role of NO has been studied extensively in a model of the stress from infections that consists of injecting bacterial lipopolysaccharide (LPS) intravenously (IV) or intraperitoneally (IP). This induces an identical pattern of pituitary hormone secretion as that seen in infection. There is a very rapid increase in plasma ACTH and PRL within a few minutes following the IV injection of LPS. The response is dose-related and is accompanied by a rapid inhibition of LH and TSH (but not FSH) secretion. GH secretion is stimulated in humans but suppressed in rats. This initial response to LPS is mediated by the constitutive nNOS present in the brain. There is no participation of the NO synthesized by inducible NOS (iNOS) in this initial response. Indeed, the initial response must be due to action on receptors for LPS on the endings of vagal afferents and also in areas where the blood–brain barrier is not present, such as the choroid plexus, ME, organum vasculosum lamina terminalis (OVLT), area postrema, and other circumventricular organs. LPS alters the release of the various hypophysiotropic hormones, increasing the release of CRH and vasopressin, GHRH, and somatostatin, particularly in the rat, which overpowers the effect on the release of GHRH. LPS decreases the release of dopamine, the PRL-inhibiting hormone; LHRH; and TRH (but not FSHRF). All of these pathways involve the participation of nNOS as described earlier. Input to the hypothalamus from LPS by vagal afferents occurs, at least in part, by activation of the locus ceruleus, which sends noradrenergic axons to the hypothalamus to activate CRH release.

In the authors' studies, LPS itself had no acute effect on ACTH release from hemianterior pituitaries *in vitro*. However, LPS induces cytokine production in the pituitary. Cytokine production would be increased in a few hours and undoubtedly would modify the responses of the pituitary to the continued altered secretion of releasing and inhibiting hormones.

Delayed Response

Central nervous system (CNS) infection is a powerful inducer of cytokine production in glia and neurons of the brain, which causes the induction of iNOS and the production of potentially toxic quantities of NO. Following IV injection of an intermediate dose of LPS, there was an induction of IL-1α immunoreactive neurons in the preoptic-hypothalamic region. These cells were shown to be neurons by the fact that double staining revealed the presence of neuron-specific enolase. The neurons were found in saline-injected control animals, suggesting that they are normally present, but they increased in number by a factor of two within 2 h following injection of LPS. They are located in a region that also contains thermosensitive neurons. They may be the neurons that are stimulated to induce fever following the injection of LPS. They have short axons that did not project clearly to the areas containing the various hypothalamic-releasing and -inhibiting hormones, but they could also be involved in the stimulation or inhibition of their release, which occurs following infection.

This study led to further research that demonstrated that the IP injection of a moderate dose of LPS induced IL-1β and iNOS mRNA in the brain, anterior pituitary, and pineal glands. The results were very exciting because an induction of IL-1β and iNOS mRNA occurred with the same time course as found in the periphery following the injection of LPS, namely, clear induction of IL-Iβ followed by iNOS mRNA within 2 h, reaching a peak in 4–6 h, followed by a decline to near basal levels at the next measurement by 24 h after the injection. The induction of both mRNAs occurred in the meninges; choroid plexus; circumventricular organs, such as the subfornical organ and ME; ependymal cells lining the ventricular system; and, very surprisingly, parvocellular neurons of the PVN and arcuate nucleus (AN), areas of particular interest because they contain hypothalamic-releasing and -inhibiting hormone-producing neurons and also other neurotransmitters controlled by NO. The greatest induction occurred in the anterior lobe of the pituitary, where the iNOS mRNA was increased at 2 h by a factor of 45 and in the pineal where the activity was increased at 6 h by a factor of 7, whereas the increase in the PVN was fivefold. At 6 h, the medial basal hypothalamus was found to have an increased content of NOS measured *in vitro* and the collected cerebrospinal fluid (CSF) had

increased concentrations of the NO metabolite nitrate. These results indicate that the increase in iNOS mRNA was followed by the *de novo* synthesis of iNOS that liberated NO into the tissue and also into the CSF. Presumably, LPS was bound to its receptors in the circumventricular organs and in the choroid plexus. These receptors, as in macrophages, activated DNA-directed IL-1β mRNA synthesis, which, in turn, caused the synthesis of IL-1β. IL-1β then activated iNOS mRNA and synthesis.

How can neurons in the AN and PVN be activated inside the blood–brain barrier? In the case of the AN, the neurons may have axons that project to the ME. These neurons may have LPS receptors on their cell surface, which then induce IL-β mRNA and IL-1β synthesis. IL-1β then induces iNOS mRNA followed by NO synthesis. Alternatively, LPS, acting on its receptors, may induce IL-β mRNA and iNOS mRNA simultaneously.

Active transport mechanisms for IL-1 and other cytokines, and perhaps LPS, are present in the choroid plexus. On the basis of the authors' results, cells of the choroid plexus must have LPS receptors on them. LPS then stimulates IL-1β and iNOS mRNA, followed by the synthesis of IL-1β and iNOS in the choroid plexus. LPS and IL-1β are then transported into the CSF. LPS is carried by CSF flow to the third ventricle, where it either crosses the ependyma or acts on terminals of PVN neurons in the ependyma to induce IL-1β and iNOS mRNA. This massive delayed increased NO production should further increase the effects of NO to maintain the pattern of hypothalamic hormone secretion already induced by LPS. Unfortunately, the effect of inhibitors of NOS on these later stages in the response to LPS or infection has not yet been studied. Interestingly enough, in studies on LHRH release induced by NO, it has been shown that increasing concentrations of NO provided by the release from sodium nitroprusside (NP) produce a bell-shaped dose–response curve in terms of LHRH release, with values reaching a peak and then declining as the concentration of NO increases. Therefore, the massive increase in NO produced by iNOS, several hours after injection of LPS, might actually reduce the effects of NO on releasing hormone discharge below the peaks achieved earlier.

In addition to inducing the production of pro-inflammatory cytokines such as IL-1, IL-2, IL-6, and TNF-α, LPS also induces the production of anti-inflammatory cytokines such as IL-10 and L-13 and the IL-1 receptor antagonist in the brain, pituitary, and pineal gland. In the periphery, these inhibit the inflammatory response induced by the pro-inflammatory cytokines. Limited studies indicate that these anti-inflammatory cytokines antagonize the actions of the pro-inflammatory cytokines in the brain as well as the hypothalamic-pituitary response to infection.

Direct Actions of Lipopolysaccharide, Cytokines, and Nitric Oxide on the Anterior Pituitary Gland during Infection

As indicated earlier, LPS had no acute direct effect to alter ACTH release from incubated pituitaries. Thus, the initial LPS-induced changes in pituitary hormone secretion are mediated by the altered release of hypophysiotropic hormones; however, LPS induces a massive induction of cytokine and, consequently, iNOS production in the anterior pituitary. Therefore, after the first few hours these cytokines and the massive release of NO will certainly modify the response of the gland to the hypothalamic factors. Unfortunately, these later times after LPS have not been studied experimentally.

Interleukin 1   The effects of IL-1β and several other cytokines released by LPS have been studied extensively *in vitro*. It was reported that IL-1 releases ACTH and other pituitary hormones from perifused pieces of pituitary glands. In the case of the other cytokines, the authors have found actions on the pituitary gland; however, it required a period of 1–2 h for these actions to become manifest.

Tumor necrosis factor α   After at least 1 h of incubation, TNF-α stimulated the release of ACTH, GH, TSH, and minimally PRL from either overnight-cultured dispersed pituitary cells or hemipituitaries; however, the minimal effective dose (MED) for these actions of TNF-α was 100-fold greater with dispersed cells than with hemipituitaries. We speculate that this decreased sensitivity in the dispersed cell preparation is due either to the loss of receptors or to paracrine actions of various pituitary cells to augment the effects on other pituitary cells in the hemipituitary preparation. There was a bell-shaped dose–response curve of response of the pituitaries, and the MED of 10^{-12} M for the hemipituitaries is within the concentrations that might be encountered *in vivo* in infection. Consequently, the authors concluded that cachectin may play an important role in altering pituitary hormone release by direct actions on the gland in infection; however, because of the relatively slow onset of these actions, it is likely that the acute response to infection is brought about by alterations in the release of hypothalamic-releasing and -inhibiting hormones, which then affect the gland. During more chronic infection, the actions at the pituitary

modulate the effects on the release of the hypothalamic peptides.

Interleukin 6   The incubation of IL-6 with hemipituitaries *in vitro* for at least 2 h increased the release of ACTH and GH only into the culture medium at the single concentration of 10^{-13} M. Concentrations of 10^{-14} or $^{-12}$M were ineffective. Again, there was a bell-shaped dose–response curve with the abolition of the actions with higher doses. Using 4-day monolayer-cultured cells, Spangelo and co-workers found not only an IL-6-induced increase in GH release but also an increase in PRL release. These differences may be accounted for by the different preparations of IL-6 used or, perhaps more likely, by their use of the dispersed cell system. This system may result in up- or downregulation of receptors for IL-6 in the relative absence of endogenous ligand and loss of paracrine actions because of separation of the cells. Because IL-6 is clearly produced by the pituitary gland itself and the production is increased by LPS (see earlier discussion), it is quite likely that IL-6 has important direct actions on the pituitary to modify pituitary hormone release. These actions probably modulate the effects of the cytokine on the release of hypothalamic hormones mentioned previously.

Therefore, the effect of IL-6 released from the hypothalamus and pituitary and also reaching the gland after release in the periphery during infection is the result of its actions at both the hypothalamic and pituitary levels, which induces a stimulation of ACTH and GH, and a decrease in TSH release in acute situations *in vivo*.

The authors have not investigated chronic exposure to IL-6. It is quite likely that there might be other effects, perhaps similar to those that occur in infection, with chronic exposure to this IL. Indeed, the acute effects of most of the cytokines at hypothalamic and pituitary sites can be characterized over a short period of an hour or two; however, much more research should be done to characterize the effects of more prolonged exposure of both the hypothalamus and the pituitary gland to these substances.

Interleukin 2   IL-2 is the most potent agent known to act directly on the pituitary to alter pituitary hormone release. At a concentration of 10^{-15} M, it elevated PRL and TSH release and inhibited the release of FSH, LH, and GH from hemipituitaries *in vitro*. ACTH release was induced with a higher concentration (10^{-12}–10^{-10} M). After reaching the minimal effective stimulatory or inhibitory concentration, the dose–response curve was flat, but at much higher concentrations (10^{-9} or 10^{-8} M), responses tended to diminish to insignificant values. Again, a bell-shaped dose–response curve was obtained similar to those observed with other cytokines.

Interferon-γ The incubation of INF-γ with hemipituitaries *in vitro* revealed no effect on the release of PRL, TSH, and GH, and it revealed a stimulation of ACTH release only at the relatively high concentration of 10^{-8} M. Later studies revealed that, at a concentration of 10^{-12} M, INF-γ also decreased the release of GH from pituitaries incubated *in vitro*. At a much higher concentration ($10^{-8}M$), it potentiated GH release induced by growth releasing hormone (GRH) but had no direct effect by itself. Because this is a 10,000-fold increase in dose over that which produced the inhibition of release, the authors question whether it is of pathophysiological significance. This inhibitory action on GH release vanished with higher doses, again giving the bell-shaped dose–response curve indicated earlier.

Thymosin α₁ Thymosin α_1 evoked a dose-dependent release of TSH and ACTH, although there was no effect on the release of PRL and GH from hemipituitaries incubated *in vitro*. There was a remarkable ability of the peptide to stimulate LH in a dose-related manner at a dose as low as 10^{-12} M, whereas FSH release was unaltered. Because thymosin α_1 has been localized to both the hypothalamus and the pituitary, it may have physiological significance in neuroendocrine immunology. As in the case of the other cytokines, both hypothalamic and pituitary sites of action may be of importance for the induction of changes in pituitary hormone release.

Therefore, although LPS does not alter pituitary hormone secretion directly, it induces cytokine release that in turn stimulates iNOS synthesis. The NO generated, together with the direct actions of the cytokines, produces modifications in the pituitary response to the altered pattern of hypothalamic peptides reaching the gland. Unfortunately, again, there have been no studies of these later events in terms of pituitary hormone release. From what is known, the general pattern that occurs immediately after the injection of LPS is maintained. Further studies of these later times are essential.

Role of Nitric Oxide in the Pattern of Pituitary Hormone Secretion in Other Physical and Psychological Stresses

In contrast to the extensive research carried out on the effects of LPS to mimic the effects of infection, little attention has been paid to the role of NO in mediating the effects of psychological stresses on the hypothalamic-pituitary axis. It has been shown that restraint stress increases the expression of nNOS, but not iNOS, with the same time course and in the same regions in which LPS induces iNOS. Furthermore, the injection of nitroarginine methyl ester (L-NAME), an inhibitor of NOS, blocked ACTH release induced by foot shock and other physical-emotional stresses.

Effect of Infection on Cytokine and Nitric Oxide Formation in the Pineal Gland and in Other Organ Systems

Space limitations limit this article mostly to the effect of NO on the hypothalamic-pituitary axis; however, as described earlier, LPS causes the induction of IL-1β mRNA followed by iNOS mRNA in the pineal as well, and experiments indicate that a similar response occurs in the heart and kidney. It is probably a uniform response throughout all organ systems of the body. Under normal conditions, NO exercises an important role in practically every, if not every, organ system of the body. The massive increase in NO production following infection is already known to be responsible for the production of toxic shock, and its toxicity probably contributes to the malaise that occurs during infections.

The Role of Nitric Oxide in Reproduction

Because LHRH induces ovulation by releasing LH and because animals go into heat around the time of ovulation, it occurred to me that LHRH could induce mating behaviour. Indeed, this turns out to be the case. Mating behaviour in female rats is brought about by LHRH neural axons that extend to the brain stem and release NO, which activates descending pathways and induces the lordosis reflex. Efferents from the pelvic spinal cord activate the pelvic ganglia, which send axons that extend to the corpora cavernosa of the penis and release Ach, which, in turn, acts on the muscle that releases NO, which activates GC to generate cGMP, which dilates the corpora leading to erection. In the presence of stress or infection, these pathways are inactive because stress blocks LHRH release. Viagra (sildenafil) promotes penile erection by inhibiting the phosphodiesterase 5 in the corpora cavernosa, thus slowing the inactivation of cGMP and prolonging the erection. The role of NO in mating behaviour is established, but its action in the external genitalia of women is not certain, although we predict that it would induce clitoral erection to facilitate orgasm.

The Nitric Oxide Hypothesis of Aging

As indicated earlier, NO generated by endothelial NOS (eNOS) and nNOS plays a ubiquitous role in the body in controlling the function of almost every, if not every, organ system. Bacterial and viral products, such as bacterial LPS, induce iNOS synthesis, which produces massive amounts of NO toxic to the invading viruses and bacteria but also to host cells by the inactivation of enzymes leading to cell death. The actions of all forms of NOS are mediated not only by the free-radical oxidant properties of this soluble gas but also by its activation of GC, leading to the production of cGMP, which mediates many of its physiological actions. In addition, NO activates COX and LOX, leading to the production of physiologically relevant quantities of PGE_2 and leukotrienes.

The authors' hypothesis is that recurrent infections over the life span play a significant role in producing aging changes in all systems of the body via the release of toxic quantities of NO. NO may be a major factor in the development of coronary heart disease (CHD). Considerable evidence has accrued indicating

a role for infections in the induction of CHD and, indeed, patients treated with a tetracycline derivative had 10 times less complications of CHD than their controls. Stress, inflammation, and infection have all been shown to cause the induction of NOS in rats, and it is likely that this triad of events is very important in the progression of coronary arteriosclerosis leading to coronary occlusion. The aging of the anterior pituitary and pineal, with the resultant decreased secretion of pituitary hormones and the pineal hormone melatonin, respectively, may be caused by NO.

Inside the blood–brain barrier, the induction of iNOS in the temperature-regulating centers by infections may cause the decreased febrile response in the aged by loss of thermosensitive neurons. iNOS induction in the PVN may cause the decreased nocturnal secretion of GH and PRL that occurs with age, and its induction in the AN may destroy LHRH neurons, thereby leading to a decreased release of gonadotropins. Recurrent infections may play a role in the aging

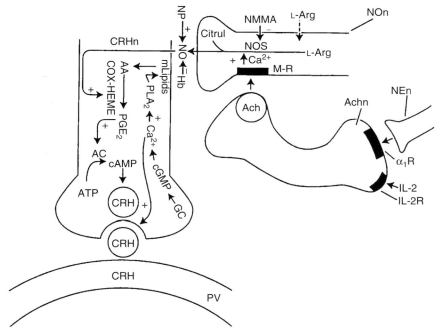

Figure 1 Diagram of the mechanism of action of cytokines such as IL-2 to release CRH by nitric oxide. In the case of systemic administration of inflammatory cytokines such as IL-2 or pain stimuli, afferent input occurs by vagal afferents that project to the locus ceruleus, a small brain-stem nucleus that contains many norepinephrinergic neurons (NEn) that project axons to the PVN, where they are visualized to act on α_1 receptors (α_1R) on acetylcholine interneurons (Achn) there. When IL-2 is in the circulation, it can also reach these neurons and act on its receptors there (IL-2R) to activate the Achn. This releases acetylcholine (Ach) from synaptic vesicle Ach from the cholinergic neuron, which acts on muscarinic receptors (M-R) on the nitric oxidergic neuron (NOn), increasing intracellular free calcium, which combines with calmodulin to activate nitric oxide synthase (NOS). This converts L-arginine within the neuron, which is also pumped into the neuron by an active transport mechanism in the presence of oxygen and various cofactors into citrulline (Citrul) and nitric oxide (NO) that diffuses over to the CRH neuron to activate guanylyl cyclase (GC), which causes the production of cGMP, which increases intracellular free calcium. The increased intracellular calcium not only plays a role in exocytosis of CRH granules, but also activates phospholipase A_2, which converts membrane phospholipids to arachidonic acid (AA). NO activates cyclooxygenase by interacting with the heme group on the molecule, leading to the conversion of AA to prostaglandin E_2 (PGE_2), which activates adenylyl cyclase (AC), which generates cAMP from ATP, which also leads to the extrusion of CRH synaptic vesicles into the hypophysial portal veins (PV), which carry it to the anterior pituitary to release ACTH. CRHn, corticosterone releasing hormone (CRH) neuron; mLipids, membrane lipids; NMDA, N-methyl-D-aspartic acid; PLA2, phospholipase A2.

of other parts of the brain because there are increased numbers of astrocytes expressing IL-1β throughout the brain in aged patients. IL-1 and products of NO activity accumulate around the plaques of Alzheimer's disease and may play a role in the progression of the disease. Flu encephalitis during World War I possibly induced iNOS in cells adjacent to substantia nigra dopaminergic neurons, leading to the death of these cells, which, coupled with ordinary aging fallout, led to early-onset Parkinsonism. The CNS pathology in acquired immunodeficiency syndrome (AIDS) patients bears a striking resemblance to aging changes and may also be largely caused by the action of iNOS. Antioxidants, such as melatonin, vitamin C, and vitamin E, probably play an important acute and chronic role in reducing or eliminating the oxidant damage produced by NO.

Conclusion

NO clearly plays a very important role in mediating the response to stress of every organ system in the body. This article concentrates on its actions mediating the response to stress and infection of the hypothalamic-pituitary axis. Afferent input (e.g., by LPS acting on receptors on vagal afferents) reaches the brain stem, where it activates the locus ceruleus, an important nucleus containing neuroadrenergic neurons that project to the hypothalamus (**Figure 1**). In the case of the CRH-ACTH-adrenocortical axis, the NE released in the vicinity of the PVN activates CRH release by stimulating cholinergic interneurons that release Ach, which in turn activates NOergic neurons by muscarinic receptors. The NO released then triggers CRH release. LPS also acts on receptors in circumventricular neurons, such as the ME and organum vasculosum lamina terminalis, to activate the NOergic control of CRH release. CRH passes down the hypophysial portal vessels and activates ACTH release. CRH releases ACTH from the corticotropes of the anterior pituitary gland, which circulates to the adrenal cortex to stimulate the release of cortisol. Cortisol exerts negative feedback to suppress CRH release and decrease the pituitary response to the CRH released. Continued stimulation by stress, such as LPS, maintains the stimulatory drive, maintaining the elevated ACTH and cortisol concentrations.

Acknowledgments

This work was supported by NIH Grants DK 43900 and MH51853. We thank Judy Scott and Jill Lucius for their excellent secretarial assistance.

See Also the Following Articles

Adrenocorticotropic Hormone (ACTH); Aging and Stress, Biology of; Cytokines; Neuroimmunomodulation.

Further Reading

Banks, W. A., Kastin, A. J., Huang, W., et al. (1996). Leptin enters the brain by a saturable system independent of insulin. *Peptides* **17**, 305–311.

McCann, S. M., Karanth, S., Kamat, A., et al. (1994). Induction by cytokines of the pattern of pituitary hormone secretion in infection. *Neuroimmunomodulation* **1**, 2–13.

McCann, S. M., Licinio, J., Wong, M.-L., et al. (1998). The nitric oxide hypothesis of aging. *Experimental Gerontology* **33**, 813–826.

McCann, S. M., Mastronardi, C., Walczewska, A., et al. (2003). The role of nitric oxide in control of LHRH release that mediates gonadotropin release and sexual behavior. *Current Pharmaceutical Design* **9**, 381–390.

Rettori, V., Dees, W. L., Hiney, J. K., et al. (1994). An interleukin-1-alpha-like neuronal system in the preoptic-hypothalamic region and its induction by bacterial lipopolysaccharide in concentrations which alter pituitary hormone release. *Neuroimmunomodulation* **1**, 251–258.

Rivier, C. (1998). Role of NO and carbon monoxide in modulating the ACTH response to immune and nonimmune signals. *Neuroimmunomodulation* **5**, 203–213.

Wong, M.-L., Bongiorno, P. B., Rettori, V., et al. (1997). Interleukin (IL) 1β, IL-1 receptor antagonist, IL-10, and IL-13 gene expression in the central nervous system and anterior pituitary during systemic inflammation: pathophysiological implications. *Proceedings of the National Academy of Sciences USA* **94**, 227–232.

Wong, M.-L., Rettori, V., Al-Shekhlee, A., et al. (1996). Inducible nitric oxide synthase gene expression in the brain during systemic inflammation. *Nature Medicine* **2**, 581–584.

Norepinephrine *See:* Adrenaline.

Northern Ireland, Post Traumatic Stress Disorder in

P Bell
South and East Belfast Health and Social Services
Trust, Belfast, UK

This article is a revision of the previous edition article by
P Bell, volume 3, pp 62–65, © 2000, Elsevier Inc.

Early Survey of Survivors of Violence
The Enniskillen Bombing
The Kegworth Air Disaster
Theoretical Model Used in Debriefing

Glossary

Posttraumatic stress disorder (PTSD)	A psychological injury after violence, characterized by reexperiencing trauma, hyperarousal, and withdrawal.

Psychiatrists in Northern Ireland had been treating the survivors of violence for more than 10 years, since PTSD was defined in the *Diagnostic and Statistical Manual of Mental Disorders* (DSM-III; 3rd edn.). In general psychiatry, most of the patients encountered are suffering from a psychiatric illness. This results when an individual who is vulnerable is subjected to a stressor. In the 1970s, the concept of psychological injury was not well developed, and so people who suffered from psychological problems after exposure to violence were viewed according to the psychiatric illness model. Either these patients were assumed to have some constitutional vulnerability to anxiety or depression and that a neurotic illness had been precipitated by an adverse life event or else the psychological injuries were dismissed as a normal reaction. Previous attempts to define psychological injuries, such as shell shock and combat neurosis, had been discredited because these diagnoses carried with them some secondary gain. In the early 1980s, a group of psychiatrists based at the Mater Hospital decided to examine the diagnosis of PTSD in order to see whether it applied to the victims of violence in Northern Ireland. The diagnosis had considerable appeal because of the clear operational definition involving a pattern of symptoms. However, local psychiatrists were skeptical about the diagnosis for three main reasons. First, community surveys in Northern Ireland had indicated that the number of cases of psychiatric morbidity in the province was no higher than in England or Scotland. Second, experience with survivors of violence indicated that they were a very different population from the archetypal Vietnam veteran. In particular, there seemed little evidence of impulsive violence or substance abuse. And the final reason for skepticism about the diagnosis of PTSD was the fact that this diagnosis had already begun to fall into disrepute in the United States, where veterans of the Vietnam War were able to obtain a higher pension if they were given this diagnosis.

Early Survey of Survivors of Violence

This first study conducted in Northern Ireland had a simple methodology. The case notes of almost 700 patients were examined retrospectively, and for each case a total of 80 items of information were recorded. These 80 items of information included the symptoms of PTSD, social and environmental factors, and a number of other items that might be expected to predispose to psychological problems. The results of the survey were valuable because of the large number of patients involved and because the retrospective nature of this study (normally a disadvantage) meant that both the patients and interviewers were naïve to the diagnosis of PTSD and, thus, that the symptoms could not have been feigned. Eighty items of information were analyzed by the computer department of Queen's University, Belfast, where a mainframe computer applied the diagnostic criteria defined in DSM-III to the symptom checklists. The research team was surprised by the results.

Despite the skepticism of psychiatrists, when the diagnosis of PTSD was applied to this group of patients, 23% fulfilled the diagnostic criteria. This percentage is very high, especially considering that the symptoms of PTSD were not specifically being looked for at the time when the patients were interviewed. A number of factors were found to be significantly associated with the diagnosis. These findings were very much in keeping with literature on PTSD from other parts of the world, in that female, elderly, and unmarried individuals were more likely to develop PTSD. However, the negative findings were perhaps more striking than the positive findings. Despite the large numbers involved, there was no significant association of PTSD with a past history of psychiatric illness, family history of psychiatric illness, or any of the other putative vulnerability factors that were examined in this study.

It was also striking that 75% of the population had recovered from the psychological difficulties within 18 months. This indicated that most people had recovered before litigation issues had been settled. At that time, the conventional wisdom was the view of Millar, that psychological injuries do not resolve until compensation issues have been resolved.

The results of this study forced psychiatrists in Northern Ireland to reappraise their views on the psychological effects of violence. For the first time, PTSD began to be seen as a true psychological injury. Until then, it was not uncommon for victims of violence to be told by their doctors, "Of course, you're upset. It is normal to be upset when you have been involved in an explosion." Psychiatrists began to realize that saying this to patients was rather like saying to the victim of a road-traffic accident, "Of course, you've got a broken leg. It is normal to have a broken leg when you have been run down by a bus."

It was becoming clear that PTSD is an injury analogous to a grief reaction, in that it is a psychological reaction that happens to normal people when placed under extreme stress, and that there is a natural course of healing after such an injury which takes about 1.5 years. The analogy with grief reaction goes further in that certain circumstances at the time of the trauma might produce a delayed injury and that, if the natural course of the healing process is disrupted, a chronic injury may result. People in Northern Ireland were well aware that a grief reaction is normal and that allowances have to be made for normal people who suffer psychological problems for a year or so after a bereavement. Through a process of education, the public has become aware that psychological injuries after trauma do not imply any psychological weakness and that people with these injuries usually recover with the passage of time.

This study contained a large number of individuals with a wide spectrum of traumatic experiences, ranging from being a casual witness to a bombing to surviving a specific assassination attempt (e.g., one individual had survived an attempted sectarian murder; a gun was put to his head but jammed when the trigger was pulled). In addition, there were a number of individuals who experienced traumatic events unrelated to the Troubles, including common assault and sexual assault. When these different types of traumatic experience were grouped together, the researchers were surprised to find that there was no significant difference in the rate of PTSD among these different groups. It seemed that the seriousness of the traumatic event and the objective level of danger were less important in producing PTSD than the individual's subjective experience of the event.

The study raised a number of questions, which were addressed in a later study. A number of speculative suggestions have been put forward to explain the paradox that individuals affected by violence are psychologically ill and yet no increase in morbidity is seen in the community as a whole. The nature of violence in Northern Ireland changed during the 1970s from widespread civil unrest to attacks on specific targets. A much smaller number of individuals were involved in these violent incidents, and so community surveys might not be sensitive enough to pick up the small numbers involved. Anecdotally, psychiatrists noticed that the level of functioning of certain marginal individuals improved in an atmosphere of violence. It was believed that this might be because sectarian polarization had produced tightly knit ghettos with increased community spirit and support. Durkheim pointed out the importance of these social factors in determining the mental health of a community, and it might be that the detrimental psychological effects of violence for the individuals directly involved might be partly compensated for by the increased community spirit in tightly knit sectarian ghettos. The hypothesis was proposed that a blitz spirit in these communities might be masking the psychological ill effects on those directly effected by violence. If this is the case, it was proposed that, if the Troubles were to end and Northern Ireland returned to more normal social functioning, we might see an upsurge in psychological morbidity.

During the 1980s, a number of scientific papers were published describing survivors of various civilian disasters from all parts of the world. These papers emphasized the validity of the concept of PTSD. It was striking that the psychological sequelae seen after trauma were remarkably similar in different cultures and with different types of trauma. It became clear from the growing literature and from clinical experience that there is a core group of symptoms, involving hyperarousal, emotional constriction, and reliving the event, that are experienced after all types of trauma and that, in addition, to these symptoms there are a variety of other symptoms that depend on the type of trauma experienced. For example, passive victims of violence in Northern Ireland had low rates of substance abuse, survivor guilt, and acting as if the incident were reoccurring compared to active participants in violence such as Vietnam veterans. The survivors of hostage situations seemed to develop symptoms of learned helplessness in addition to the core syndrome of PTSD, and victims of sexual violence often suffered the additional symptoms of post-rape syndrome, including obsessional cleanliness, mistrust of members of the opposite sex, and an aversion to sexual stimuli. The definition of PTSD became more focused in subsequent revisions of DSM-III, and the difference between the symptoms experienced by adults and children were more clearly delineated.

The Enniskillen Bombing

A terrorist bomb exploded in the town square at Enniskillen on Remembrance Sunday 1987 as the town gathered to remember the dead in two world wars. A group of survivors were followed up at 6 months and 12 months in order to determine the relationship between their physical and psychological injuries. Millar had said that there is an inverse relationship between physical injuries and psychological injuries after a traumatic event. This was found to be true when the survivors were followed up at 6 months, but at 12 months it seemed that those individuals who suffered more severe physical injuries tended to develop delayed PTSD after 6 months. This group of survivors were particularly unfortunate because their psychological injuries were only beginning to emerge at a time when other victims of the trauma were beginning to put the incident behind them. In working with survivors of the Enniskillen bombing, researchers emphasized the importance of local supports, debriefing, and education. Many survivors and their families were relieved to be told that the psychological reactions that they were seeing were, in fact, normal under the circumstances and were likely to improve within 18 months or so. Families were also relieved to hear that the withdrawal and irritability, which they were finding so hard to live with, were in fact predictable parts of a recognized psychological injury that tended to improve with time. In this way, education was able to prevent one of the main complications of PTSD, namely marital disharmony.

The Kegworth Air Disaster

A passenger jet carrying over 90 people traveling between London and Belfast in 1989 crashed on to a stretch of motorway as it was diverted to East Midlands Airport. Research teams followed up the survivors on both sides of the Irish Sea. The relationship between physical and psychological injuries was once more explored in some detail. One of the most striking findings from this piece of research, which was not reported in the original paper, was that individuals from England and Scotland (68%) were significantly more likely to develop PTSD than residents of Northern Ireland (43%) (**Table 1**). A number of possible reasons have been put forward to explain this result. It may be that even when applying the research criteria psychiatrists in Northern Ireland

Table 1 Rates of PTSD according to home address (%)[a]

	England/Scotland	Northern Ireland
No PTSD	7	24
PTSD	15	19

[a]PTSD, posttraumatic stress disorder.

tend to be more reluctant to make the diagnosis of PTSD, perhaps applying the research criteria more strictly than our colleagues in mainland United Kingdom. Another possible reason is that individuals living in Northern Ireland have been in some way inured to violence and were, therefore, less traumatized than individuals from mainland United Kingdom, who had less direct experience of traumatic situations. Anecdotal experience indicates that individuals may suffer a series of traumatic events without any psychological ill effects, only to break down very severely after a relatively minor trauma. This suggests that repeated exposure to trauma can strengthen defense mechanisms up to a certain point, but once these defense mechanisms have been overwhelmed the psychological injury seems more severe than otherwise would be the case.

Theoretical Model Used in Debriefing

Successful debriefing seems to depend on making PTSD understandable to the individual involved. Models that are too technical or difficult to believe are of little value. The following model has been developed from various sources, as well as from direct experience of PTSD in Northern Ireland.

Three groups of symptoms are involved in PTSD: hyperarousal, reliving the incident, and emotional constriction. The hyperarousal is best explained as part of the fight-or-flight response to stress. This is one of the survival mechanisms by which nature has equipped us to deal with dangerous or threatening situations. Symptoms such as increased aggression, increased startle reaction, sleep disturbance, and hypervigilance are seen. These symptoms may improve an individual's chances of survival in a dangerous situation and arguably improve the functioning of a combat soldier.

The symptoms of reexperiencing the incident in the form of flashbacks and nightmares is best understood according to Janet's model of traumatic memory. Under normal circumstances, long-term memories are laid down in a process of digesting experience. Long-term memory is not a factual record of events but a story that we tell ourselves to explain the past. It seems that traumatic memories are portions of experience so threatening to the individual that they cannot be digested by this process. In this way, the traumatic event remains recorded as a factual record, almost like a videotape. Individuals can remember what they had for breakfast on the day of a traumatic event 15 years after the incident. Perhaps this is why listening to the accounts of survivors is so distressing – the events are recorded so literally and usually accurately. These traumatic memories are so distressing that they are phobically avoided. They are suppressed, and the conscious mind attempts to keep them in the subconscious. However, they reemerge when the individual is off-guard (e.g., when asleep). It may be that it is this phobic element that is improved when individuals undergo eye movement desensitization.

Emotional constriction and estrangement from others can be viewed as a loss of innocence. This assumes a state of normal denial, in which most people believe that the world is a safe place and that death and mutilation are things that happen to other people. However, traumatic events force us to confront our own mortality and destroy this normal denial. Thus, people with PTSD are living in a different – more dangerous – world than those individuals around them, who continue to convince themselves that the world is a safe place. In order to be normal again, individuals with PTSD must convince themselves once more that the world is a safe place, and they attempt to do this by suppressing the memory, thus leading to the development of traumatic memories that reemerge in the form of nightmares and flashbacks.

This model has been found to be very useful in talking to survivors of violence. People with PTSD often think of themselves as members of an elite club who are able to see the truth when those around them remain naïve. It is perhaps for this reason that group therapy can be successful in PTSD, although there is a strong danger of scapegoating in groups because of the high levels of free-floating anger that survivors suffer as part of PTSD.

The Clinical Resource and Efficacy Support Team for Northern Ireland reviewed the Northern Ireland literature and produced guidelines for management of PTSD in June 2003. This found strong evidence that a single-session individual debriefing was not helpful and may well be harmful. The team also found evidence that brief programs of cognitive-behavior therapy were effective, as well as pharmacological treatment with selective serotonin reuptake inhibitors (SSRIs), monoamine oxidase inhibitors (MAOIs), and tricyclic antidepressants (TCAs). Eye movement desensitization and supportive group therapy were also found to be effective, and there was evidence that nonprofessional and practical assistance reduced the frequency of avoidance and intrusion symptoms.

Because individuals with PTSD are normal, they often do not respond well to mental health professionals. Normal supports are more useful in supporting these individuals (e.g., family, friends, employment, and church), but debriefing and education are useful in reducing the suffering for survivors and their families. Symptomatic relief can be offered, but, if PTSD persists beyond 1.5 years, the prognosis becomes less positive and the response to treatment is usually incomplete, leaving lasting emotional scars.

Further Reading

Bell, P., Kee, M., Loughrey, G. L., et al. (1988). Post traumatic stress disorder in N. Ireland. *Acta Psychiatricia Scandinavian* 77, 166–170.

Cairns, E. and Wilson, R. (1985). Psychiatric aspects of stress in N. Ireland. *Stress Medicine* 1, 193–196.

Loughrey, G. L., Curran, P. S. and Bell, P. (1993). Post traumatic stress disorder and civil violence in N. Ireland. In: Wilson, J. P. & Raphael, B. (eds.) *The international handbook of traumatic stress syndromes*, pp. 377–380. New York: Plenum.

Lyons, H. A. (1979). Civil violence – the psychological aspects. *Journal of Psychosomatic Research* 23, 373–376.

Nuclear Warfare, Threat of

J Thompson
University College London, London, UK

This article is a revision of the previous edition article by
J Thompson, volume 3, pp 66–70, © 2000, Elsevier Inc.

Threat of Nuclear Warfare

Evaluating the Threat

Questionnaires: The Chief Method of Studying
   Nuclear Anxiety

Individual Studies

Summary

Glossary

Anxiety	The fearful anticipation of potential harm.
Denial	A concept of psychoanalytic origin implying an unwillingness to face unpleasant facts.
Questionnaire	A French word, meaning a list of questions, usually on a particular subject of psychological interest, with a common restricted format for answers. If properly standardised and validated on relevant populations they can be useful in estimating psychological characteristics and states of mind.

Threat of Nuclear Warfare

One thing can be said for certain about nuclear anxiety – it is not an innate fear. On the contrary, no other anxiety depends so much on an appreciation of a wide range of political, cultural, and military threats. Anxiety about the threat of nuclear warfare is caused by the belief that a nuclear war may happen and that it will bring widespread destruction to civilization. This anxiety is linked to powerful images of the explosive power of nuclear weapons and to the dreadful consequences for individuals, society, and the environment if they should come to be used. If all anxiety is based on an assessment of threat, even though the assessment may be faulty, then anxiety about nuclear war is threat assessment at its most difficult.

Evaluating the Threat

A balanced, rational assessment of the threat of nuclear war includes assessing the following issues: the destructive power of the weapons, the reliability of the weapons-delivery systems, the protection afforded by buildings and shelters, the viability of countermeasures, the extent of the damage caused by the weapons to national infrastructure, the effects of radiation, the effects of major fires on the climate, the possibilities of reconstruction, the nature of enemies, the international political scene, the personalities of the nuclear weapons operators and political leaders, the mood of people in countries that have nuclear weapons, the reliability of warning systems, the possibilities of false alarms, the likelihood of terrorist actions, and the spread of nuclear weapons capability to other nations and to armed groups. By the very nature of the threat, such a list can never be exhaustive. To complicate matters, nuclear weapons are now often categorized as weapons of mass destruction, so the risks are conflated with chemical and biological warfare risks. A less rational assessment of the likelihood of nuclear war is subject to the distorting effects of personal depression, selective monitoring of news, paranoid ideas about other nations, and generalized sociopolitical anxiety.

As a consequence, any proper evaluation of the topic must contrast the objective threat with the perceived threat and then explain any identified differences. In fact, it has been extremely hard for the average citizen to evaluate this threat, which has been with us in various forms for over 50 years. Much of this uncertainty relates to the secrecy that has surrounded nuclear warfare and to the difficulty of determining the intentions of opposed nations.

One approach to getting a more objective assessment is to look at the Doomsday Clock, which was established by the *Bulletin of the Atomic Scientists* in 1947 as a way of showing the consensus view of scientists of the likelihood of nuclear war. Assuming for the moment that these scientists know more about the risks than the average person, the highest danger point, at 2 min to midnight, came in 1953 with the hydrogen bomb tests. The next closest, at 3 min to midnight, came in 1949 when the Soviet Union exploded its first atomic bomb and in 1984 when the arms race accelerated. By 1991 the clock had achieved a safety high point, with a leisurely 17 min to midnight, as arms reductions took place and the Soviet Union contracted. It currently stands at 7 min to midnight, unchanged since February 2002 as a consequence of political extremism and the proliferation of weapons.

There is little doubt that the destructive power of nuclear weapons is very great and has increased greatly over successive decades. However, many citizens find it difficult to comprehend the destructive power of these weapons, which is so far outside normal human experience, and at the same time may incorrectly believe that everything will be destroyed during a nuclear war. Although it is very hard to be sure about the consequences, there are a range of possibilities.

A full-scale nuclear war might destroy some nations immediately by so damaging their cities and infrastructures that is renders them incapable of providing basic services to their citizens, in the same way that conventional wars have damaged many parts of the world and left the local population destitute, without shelter and food, and dependent on outside help for survival. Such a general world war with nuclear weapons could well leave the survivors incapable of maintaining themselves at their former level of living, in the way that the Black Death disrupted the medieval world. Strategists argue as to whether it would be possible to have a limited nuclear war, many feeling that a nuclear war would quickly spread out of control.

However, from the perspective of the beginning of a new century, the threat of the immediate destruction of civilization may seem remote. The end of the cold war has brought about a change of mood as well as a change in the real level of threat of war between superpowers. Nuclear weapons have come to be seen as an ancient terror, last year's music. Yet the number of nuclear nations has grown, and the threat of regional nuclear conflicts has increased. It would indeed be a cruel fate for our global society to perish from an unfashionable cause.

Questionnaires: The Chief Method of Studying Nuclear Anxiety

Where would the study of anxiety be without the questionnaire? No other method in the social sciences has borne so heavy a load and has been pressed into service in so many campaigns and in so many different theatres of research. The procedure is as follows. The authors make a list of questions to which they would like answers, sometimes drawn from their own interests and imaginations, sometimes drawn from matters of public debate, and even sometimes drawn from opposed points of view. The answers given by willing subjects are often reported in raw form by giving the percentages of respondents who agree with a particular proposition. Sometimes the question list is subjected to item analysis to detect faulty questions and to factor analysis in order to search for an underlying structure to the answers. This generally

leads to revisions of the question list and the methods for scoring the answers to produce subscores with greater explanatory power. The questionnaire is now judged fit for wider use, and comparative studies follow with different populations. Done well, this can be a considerable help in understanding the answers to the questions and can produce interesting comparisons between different groups. Done badly, it can produce many ineffective lists of questions leading to a confusing mass of contradictory findings.

A more profound problem with questionnaires is trying to understand what questionnaire responses really mean. Do they tap real opinions that may lead to real actions, or are they little more than party chatter, the surface moods and immediate responses of the disengaged? In plain terms, is a person who says he or she is anxious about nuclear war really anxious about nuclear war, and what does the person's anxiety amount to? Does it restrict the person in the way that a phobia might? Does the person experience the agony of someone who fears flying but must travel by air for some urgent reason?

To answer those questions, the questionnaire approach must be supplemented with appropriate observations and suitable cross-checks. So, if someone is anxious that there will be a nuclear war, how will he or she behave? If the person believes that war is imminent, some of his or her behaviors ought to be obvious, but if the person cannot be sure how soon the war will start, then it is harder to make predictions. We might surmise that the person would be less likely to make long-term investments and preparations, that he or she would have some sort of emergency nuclear war plan, and that he or she would frequently refer to possible nuclear wars when contemplating all other plans. Such behavioral indicators of nuclear anxiety have been studied infrequently.

The typical subjects of questionnaire studies are captive student populations, although occasionally a proper epidemiological sample is obtained. The ages of the subjects are generally 11 and above, and usually the subjects are tested on one occasion, without much reference to other measures such as intelligence, personality, medical history, school records, spare-time activities, and other interests. Although some questionnaires are used in comparative studies, question lists tend to proliferate and to tap different domains, and often they advertise their purpose in a way that may influence the answers that respondents give. For example, people may be moderately optimistic until faced with a list of dangers and then they become more fearful as they contemplate all the threats that face them. The demand characteristics of the questionnaire may lead to self-serving distortions.

Individual Studies

Nuclear Warfare Anxiety

The category of nuclear warfare anxiety may contain a number of related fears. These include fears about death, from whatever cause; worries about the dangers of technology and the pace of change in industrial societies; despair at not being able to bring about political change on the nuclear weapons issue; and a general sense of foreboding about the future. Nonetheless, when questionnaires are appropriately refined, nuclear weapons can be shown to be a cause of anxiety in their own right.

How Common Is Nuclear Anxiety?

In the 1980s and early 1990s, nuclear anxiety was common. It was generally cited as being in the top three worries of most young people, although the rate declined as the cold war diminished. The death of parents, doing very badly at school, getting cancer, and being unemployed were the other most common worries. The mid-1980s seem to have been the peak, with as high as 54% of U.S. and 93% of USSR adolescents responding that they were worried about nuclear war. A few years later, the rates had diminished by approximately 10%. Large-scale epidemiological studies show big variations in the rates, with as high as 80% of Finnish adolescents and as (relatively) low as 30% of English and Austrian adolescents reporting such fears. Interestingly, most of the literature on this subject dates from before 1993; after that year, there are far fewer published findings.

Who Is Affected by Nuclear Anxiety?

Most people are affected by nuclear anxiety to some extent. Despite some early anxieties about biased questionnaire samples, nuclear anxiety is not restricted to wealthy, politicized families but is found in all social strata, including profoundly disadvantaged teenagers living in violent inner-city neighborhoods (who might be thought to be too much at present risk to worry about future dangers). In this last group, despite not having activist parents and despite personally despairing about being able to do anything about the nuclear threat, teenagers ranked nuclear war (in 1991) as their second worry – after fear of being murdered – and this fear was higher in those who had actually experienced violence.

Those with nuclear anxiety tend to be more aware of global issues; have good self-esteem; believe that they, and not outside forces, are responsible for their success in life; be not unusually anxious in general; be not religious; have a healthy optimism about the future; and have a tendency toward political activism. Women generally are more likely than men to experience nuclear anxiety.

Does Nuclear Anxiety Run in Families?

The few studies that matched children with their parents found an understandable similarity of attitudes. Nuclear concern is higher in higher-income families; scholastically able children are more knowledgeable and more fearful about nuclear war; and children's hopelessness about the arms race increases as parents' worry about nuclear war increases. Girls express more worry than boys. Interestingly, children with a high degree of general anxiety do not indicate a high degree of nuclear fears. However, parents are often poor at predicting nuclear anxiety in their children and are more likely to deny their own anxiety than are their children.

How Do People Cope with Nuclear Anxiety?

One coping mechanism is to downplay a real anxiety. Keilin sought to go beyond questionnaire studies by subjecting those who reported themselves to be high or low on nuclear anxiety to a laboratory investigation of their emotional responses to nuclear images. People with low nuclear anxiety, although reporting lower levels of emotionality, were more emotional when shown nuclear war stimuli, as reflected by several physiological and behavioral measures. People with high nuclear anxiety were also anxious about relevant social issues, but did not have a greater disposition to be anxious. Keilin interpreted these findings as supporting the existence of nuclear war-related denial processes on the part of the low-anxiety-reported group but only when faced with highly salient and dramatic nuclear stimuli. So, some people repress their nuclear anxieties and others sensitize themselves to the emotional threat, and questionnaires may pick up their preferred coping styles rather than their real emotions.

Another approach is to become an activist. Peace activists sometimes find that their initial anxiety about nuclear war subsides after they have been active for a period of time. They see activism as intrinsically valuable, something they turned to at periods of flux in their lives, believing that they should act to prevent current problems caused by the arms race and not just the anticipated damage from a nuclear war.

How Do the Nuclear Anxious Differ from Others?

Anti-nuclear activists tend to be cooperation-oriented individuals who express spontaneous nuclear concern, have high nuclear anxiety, and also have feelings of empowerment on personal and nuclear issues. They possess feminine traits and are generally tolerant of ambiguity, are open-minded, and have low manipulative tendencies in interpersonal relationships. They are likely to believe that chance does not determine nuclear outcomes and that nuclear war cannot be survived. The most common contrasting group has been those who are pro-defense, that is to say, those who believe that the best protection against nuclear war is to hold nuclear weapons as a deterrent. Pro-defense activists tend to be strength-oriented individuals who express low nuclear anxiety and tend to be masculine, dogmatic, persuasive, and intolerant of ambiguity. They are likely to believe that nuclear issues are controlled by powerful others and chance. This is a very clear differentiation between attitudes and suggests a profoundly different worldview, leading to widely differing rates of nuclear anxiety.

Does Nuclear Anxiety Cause Psychological Disorders?

Specific anxiety about nuclear war does not appear to lead to psychological disorders, although despair about the future (which may show up as nuclear anxiety on general questionnaires) may be linked with adolescent depression. Those with nuclear anxiety followed up 8 years later were very slightly more likely to have psychosomatic health complaints and emotional distress but not drug, relationship, or work problems.

Summary

Nuclear anxiety appears to be somewhat different from more trait-based stress conditions in that it is a reaction to real-world events and it seems to have subsided with the passing of the cold war. In terms of the usual imperfect measures, it appears that children survived their upbringing in the nuclear age. Although it is hard to prove identifiable major effects of nuclear anxiety, it would be surprising if so widespread a perceived danger had no effect at all. Perhaps the main effect has been to frighten many, to reduce their confidence in the future, and to goad some into activism, leading to considerable relief for all when the arms race ended in a truce.

See Also the Following Article

Hiroshima Bombing, Stress Effects of.

Further Reading

Keilin, W. J. (1987). Reactions to the threat of nuclear war: An investigation of emotional and defensive processes. PhD thesis, Colorado State University.

National Academy of Sciences (1986). *The medical implications of nuclear war.* Washington, DC: Institute of Medicine.

Schatz, R. and Fiske, S. T. (1992). International reactions to the threat of nuclear war: the rise and fall of concern in the eighties. *Political Psychology* 13, 1–30.

Nutrition

J E Morley
Saint Louis University Medical School, St. Louis, MO, USA

This article is reproduced from the previous edition, volume 3, pp 71–74, © 2000, Elsevier Inc.

Introduction
Stress-Induced Eating: the Tail-Pinch Model
Stress-Induced Anorexia
Anorexia of Aging: a Response to a Physiological Stressor
Stress, Chewing, and Feeding in Humans
Conclusion

Glossary

Corticotropin-releasing hormone (CRH)	A neurotransmitter that plays a role in co-ordinating the response to stress. Administration of CRH causes anorexia, and it appears to be the major neurotransmitter responsible for stress-induced anorexia.
Stress-induced anorexia	Decreased food ingestion secondary to a severe stressor that can be either exteroceptive or interoceptive.
Stress-induced eating	Eating induced in response to an external stressor.
Tail-pinch eating	Eating induced in rodents or cats by gently pinching their tail. It is mainly due to activation of an endogenous opioid, dynorphin.

Introduction

There are numerous interactions between stress and nutrition. Nutrition insecurity is one of the most important stressors of the human race. The need to maintain nutritional intake is the primal driving force of human beings. Simple organisms, such as the *Pleurobranchea,* spend the majority of their life eating and only when adequately nourished (their state of eustress) do they release a satiety hormone that stops eating and then results in egg laying. Severely malnourished women lose the ability to produce luteinizing hormone surges and become amenorrheic. Malnutrition leads to immune dysfunction, including a marked decline in CD4+ T lymphocytes producing a similar picture of immune function to that seen in patients with AIDS. Malnutrition increases the propensity of organisms to develop a variety of infections, which, with associated cytokine release, lead to activation of the stress response. Thus, deficient nutritional intake can be associated with both psychological and physical stressors.

Much of the long-term injury produced by repetitive stress is due to damage produced by free radicals.

A number of nutrients such as vitamins C and E and the trace mineral selenium play an important role as free radical scavengers and as such may limit stress-induced damage.

In addition to the effects of nutrition as a stressor and stress alleviator, an important component of the stress response is alterations in food ingestion. Dependent on the kind and duration, stress can either increase or decrease food intake. A number of psychiatric diseases, such as depression and anorexia nervosa, produce alterations in food intake secondary to activation of the classic stress response. Obesity, which has become a national epidemic in the United States, has been associated with a variety of psychological stressors in relationship to the alteration in body image. Release of stress hormones, such as cortisol, can alter fat deposition, resulting in an increase in visceral obesity. Visceral obesity is associated with an increase in diabetes mellitus, hypertension, myocardial infarction, stroke, and mortality. Aging is a physiological stressor that is associated with anorexia.

Figure 1 summarizes the potential interactions between nutrition and stress.

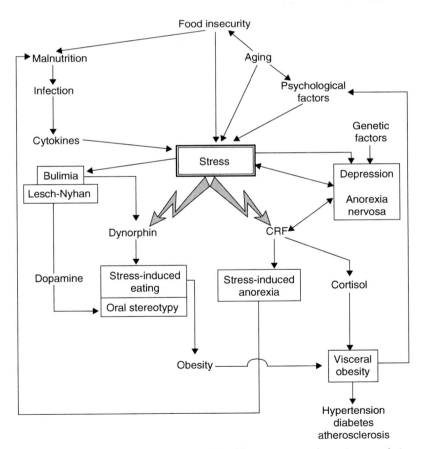

Figure 1 Nutrition and stress interrelate at multiple levels. Nutritional factors can produce stress and stress can lead to under- or overnutrition. Eventually a vicious cycle develops. CRF, corticotropin releasing factor, synonymous with CRH, corticotropin-releasing hormone.

Stress-Induced Eating: the Tail-Pinch Model

Stress-induced ingestion has been classically described in the ethology literature. Eating is commonly observed during boundary disputes in a variety of birds. Pecking at the ground is common, and the frequency can be increased experimentally by replacing the substratum with grain. Ciclid fish bite at the substratum during intervals between fighting. Electric shocks given to sticklebacks result in feeding similar to that seen with food deprivation. Handling rats may increase food intake. Electric shocks induce chewing in monkeys and rabbits. These findings led researchers to develop a stress-induced eating model, namely mild tail pinch in cats, rats, and mice. The stressor appears to be the pinch as a mild pinch to other parts of the body also induced feeding.

The tail-pinch model represents a stimulus-bound behavior in that the rodent stops eating as soon as the pinch is removed. The phenomenon generalizes to sweetened milk but not to water ingestion. Tail pinch appears to drive chewing to a greater degree than it drives ingestive behaviors. Tail pinch may also induce other behaviors such as copulation and maternal behaviors. Tail pinch demonstrates a number of similarities to the behavior seen following electrical stimulation of the lateral hypothalamus.

The neurochemistry involved in tail pinch-induced eating has been explored in some detail with pharmacological approaches. Both dopamine and endogenous opioids appear to play a central role in the modulation of tail-pinch eating. Dopamine appears to be involved predominantly in the production of chewing behaviors, whereas opioids appear to be more involved in ingestive behaviors.

A number of neurotransmitters and peptide hormones have been shown to decrease tail pinch-induced ingestive behaviors. Centrally, these include serotonin, prostaglandin E2, and thyrotropin-releasing hormone. Peripherally, both cholecystokinin and bombesin decrease food intake in the tail-pinch model.

Prolonged chronic tail pinch eventually results in weight loss and naloxone-perceptible withdrawal symptoms. These animals show similar changes to those seen in morphine-addicted animals.

In summary, tail pinch-induced eating appears to be an excellent model of stress-induced eating, which is predominantly dependent on the activation of dopaminergic and opioid neurotransmitters.

Stress-Induced Anorexia

Severe stressors, such as restraint stress, in rodents result in anorexia and weight loss. Corticotropin-releasing hormone (CRH) has been demonstrated to be a potent anorectic agent when administered intracerebroventricularly to rodents. CRH levels increase in the hypothalamus during restraint stress. Inhibition of CRH with antibodies or antagonists reverses the anorexia associated with restraint stress.

Anorexia produced by CRH can be attenuated by tail pinch, suggesting a delicate balance between stress-induced eating and stress-induced anorexia.

Overall, considerable evidence shows that stress-induced anorexia is due to the activation of CRH. CRH also appears to play an important role in stress-induced anorexia in humans (*vide infra*).

Anorexia of Aging: a Response to a Physiological Stressor

The aging process can be conceived to be a physiological stressor that produces its effects over the life span. Over the life span there is approximately a 30% decrease in food intake. This is predominantly due to a decrease in the central opioid-feeding drive. There does not appear to be an alteration in the effects of CRH with aging. In addition to the central neurotransmitter changes with aging, there are also peripheral alterations in adaptive relaxation of the fundus of the stomach due to decreased nitric oxide synthase activity. This leads to early antral filling and a greater degree of satiation for a given amount of food ingested.

The anorexia of aging makes the older individual at greater risk for developing severe anorexia and weight loss when exposed to stressors. The release of cytokines from varying sources has a potent anorectic effect in older persons secondarily to activation of the CRH stress cascade.

Stress, Chewing, and Feeding in Humans

Stress has long been recognized as a cause of masticatory muscle contraction. As pointed out by St. Matthew, "and there shall be a weeping and gnashing of teeth." Biting into a hard object was used by early surgeons to decrease the pain of surgery in the days antedating anesthesia. Anxiety increases bruxism (tooth grinding). In Lesch–Nyhan syndrome (hypoxanthine–guanine phosphoribosyltransferase deficiency), oral stereotypy is increased markedly during periods of emotional distress.

In humans, approximately two-thirds become anorectic when stressed, whereas one-third overeat. In stressed overeaters the act of chewing appears to be as important as the actual ingestion of food. When the stressor is boredom, overeating is the most common associated behavior. Bulimia (binge eating, which may be associated with subsequent vomiting) is often precipitated by a traumatic event.

Anorexia nervosa represents a classic pathological example of intrapsychic stress resulting in anorexia and severe weight loss. Patients with anorexia nervosa have been demonstrated to have elevated CRH levels in the cerebrospinal fluid.

Depression represents a major intrapsychic stressor. Two-thirds of depressed persons tend to be anorectic, and in these individuals, CRH levels in the cerebrospinal fluid are increased.

Conclusion

There is now ample evidence that not only does nutritional insufficiency result in stress, but stressors can lead to either over- or undereating in human beings. Both the endogenous opioid system (dynorphin) and CRH have been demonstrated to be neurotransmitters playing a role in the alterations in ingestive behavior produced by stress. A number of diseases that have a predominant component of altered food ingestion, such as anorexia nervosa and bulimia, appear to be precipitated by stress. Nutrient intake remains the most important behavior for the survival of all organisms. It is not surprising, therefore, that nutrition and stress are intertwined so intimately.

See Also the Following Articles

Diet and Stress, Non-Psychiatric; Eating Disorders and Stress; Obesity, Stress and; Diet and Stress, Psychiatric.

Further Reading

Greeno, C. G. and Wing, R. R. (1994). Stress-induced eating. *Psychological Bulletin* **115**, 444–464.

Grunberg, N. E. and Straub, R. O. (1992). The role of gender and taste class in the effects of stress on eating. *Health Psychology* **11**, 97–100.

Morley, J. E. and Levine, A. S. (1980). Stress-induced eating is mediated through endogenous opiates. *Science* **209**, 1259–1261.

Morley, J. E., Levine, A. S. and Rowland, N. E. (1983). Stress induced eating. *Life Sciences* **32**, 2169–2182.

Nemeroff, C. B. (1988). The role of corticotropin-releasing factor in the pathogenesis of major depression. *Pharmacopsychiatry* **21**, 76–82.

Troop, N. A., Holbrey, A., Trowler, R., et al. (1994). Ways of coping in women with eating disorders. *Journal of Nervous and Mental Disease* **182**, 535–540.

Weinstein, S. E., Shide, D. J. and Rolls, B. J. (1997). Changes in food intake in response to stress in men and women: psychological factors. *Appetite* **28**, 7–18.